D1602192

The American Cancer Society's Principles of Oncology
Prevention to Survivorship

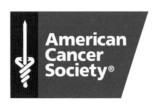

The American Cancer Society is a global grassroots force of nearly 2 million volunteers dedicated to saving lives, celebrating lives, and leading the fight for a world without cancer. From breakthrough research, to free lodging near treatment, a 24/7/365 live helpline, free rides to treatment, and convening powerful activists to create awareness and impact, the Society is the only organization attacking cancer from every angle. For more information go to www.cancer.org.

The American Cancer Society's

Principles of Oncology

Prevention to Survivorship

Edited by The American Cancer Society

Atlanta, Georgia, USA

WILEY Blackwell

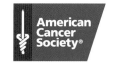

Registered Office(s)
John Wiley & Sons, Inc., 111 River Street, Hoboken, NJ 07030, USA
John Wiley & Sons Ltd, The Atrium, Southern Gate, Chichester, West Sussex, PO19 8SQ, UK

Editorial Office
9600 Garsington Road, Oxford, OX4 2DQ, UK

For details of our global editorial offices, customer services, and more information about Wiley products visit us at www.wiley.com.

Wiley also publishes its books in a variety of electronic formats and by print-on-demand. Some content that appears in standard print versions of this book may not be available in other formats.

Library of Congress Cataloging-in-Publication Data

Names: American Cancer Society, editor.
Title: The American Cancer Society's principles of oncology : prevention to survivorship /
   edited by the American Cancer Society.
Other titles: Principles of oncology
Description: Hoboken, NJ : Wiley, 2018. | Includes bibliographical references and index. |
Identifiers: LCCN 2017040597 (print) | LCCN 2017041494 (ebook) | ISBN 9781119468875 (pdf) |
   ISBN 9781119468882 (epub) | ISBN 9781119468844 (cloth)
Subjects: | MESH: Neoplasms–prevention & control | Neoplasms–therapy | Survivors |
   Early Medical Intervention–standards | United States | Practice Guideline
Classification: LCC RC268 (ebook) | LCC RC268 (print) | NLM QZ 250 | DDC 616.99/4052–dc23
LC record available at https://lccn.loc.gov/2017040597

Cover design by Wiley
Cover image: © Tendo/Shutterstock

Set in 9.5/11.5 pt Warnock by SPi Global, Pondicherry, India
Printed and bound in Singapore by Markono Print Media Pte Ltd

10 9 8 7 6 5 4 3 2 1

Contents

List of Contributors

Catherine M. Alfano, PhD
Vice President
Survivorship
Cancer Control
American Cancer Society
Atlanta, Georgia, USA

Joseph E. Bauer, PhD
Strategic Director
Statistics and Evaluation Center
American Cancer Society
Atlanta, Georgia, USA

Shrujal S. Baxi, MD, MPH
Medical Oncologist
Department of Medicine
Memorial Sloan Kettering Cancer Center
New York, New York, USA

Victoria Blinder, MD, MSc
Medical Oncologist
Department of Medicine
Memorial Sloan Kettering Cancer Center
New York, New York, USA

Otis W. Brawley, MD
Chief Medical Officer
American Cancer Society
Atlanta, Georgia, USA

Paul Brittain, MD
Second Year Fellow
University of Colorado Anschutz Medical Campus
Aurora, Colorado, USA

Eduardo Bruera, MD
Department Chair
Department of Palliative Care and Rehabilitation Medicine
University of Texas MD Anderson Cancer Center
Houston, Texas, USA

Jeanne Carter, PhD
Head, Female Sexual Medicine and Women's Health Program
Gynecology Service
Department of Surgery
Memorial Sloan Kettering Cancer Center
New York, New York, USA

Bradley C. Carthon, MD, PhD
Assistant Professor, Hematology and Medical Oncology
Medical Director, Inpatient Medical Oncology
Winship Cancer Institute
Emory University School of Medicine
Atlanta, Georgia, USA

Alejandro Chaoul, PhD
Assistant Professor
Palliative, Rehabilitation and Integrative Medicine
University of Texas MD Anderson Cancer Center
Houston, Texas, USA

Lorenzo Cohen, PhD
Professor
Palliative, Rehabilitation, and Integrative Medicine
University of Texas MD Anderson Cancer Center
Houston, Texas, USA

Dexter L. Cooper, MPH
Research Assistant II
Morehouse School of Medicine
Atlanta, Georgia, USA

Kerry S. Courneya, PhD
Professor
Faculty of Physical Education and Recreation
University of Alberta
Edmonton, Alberta, Canada

Diwakar Davar, MD
Assistant Professor of Medicine
Division of Hematology-Oncology
University of Pittsburgh Medical Center
Pittsburgh, Pennsylvania, USA

S. Lindsey Davis, MD
Assistant Professor of Medical Oncology
University of Colorado Anschutz Medical Campus
Aurora, Colorado, USA

Wendy Demark-Wahnefried, PhD, RD
Professor of Nutrition Sciences
Associate Director for Cancer Prevention and Control
University of Alabama at Birmingham
Birmingham, Alabama, USA

Rony Dev, DO
Associate Professor
Department of Palliative Care and Rehabilitation Medicine
University of Texas MD Anderson Cancer Center
Houston, Texas, USA

Curtiland Deville, Jr., MD
Assistant Professor of Radiation Oncology and Molecular
Radiation Sciences
Department of Radiation Oncology and Molecular Radiation
Sciences
Johns Hopkins University School of Medicine
Baltimore, Maryland, USA

Maura N. Dickler, MD
Medical Oncologist
Gynecology Service, Department of Surgery
Memorial Sloan Kettering Cancer Center
New York, New York, USA

Colleen Doyle, MS, RD
Managing Director
Nutrition and Physical Activity
Cancer Control
American Cancer Society
Atlanta, Georgia, USA

Deborah L. Driscoll, BA
Program Manager
Statistics and Evaluation Center
American Cancer Society
Atlanta, Georgia, USA

S. Gail Eckhardt, MD
Professor and Co-Division Head of Medical Oncology
University of Colorado Anschutz Medical Campus
Aurora, Colorado, USA

Stacey Fedewa, PhD, MPH
Strategic Director
Risk Factors and Screening Surveillance
Intramural Research
American Cancer Society
Atlanta, Georgia, USA

Darren R. Feldman, MD
Medical Oncologist
Department of Medicine
Memorial Sloan Kettering Cancer Center
New York, New York, USA

Ted Gansler, MD, MPH, MBA
Strategic Director
Pathology Research
American Cancer Society
Atlanta, Georgia, USA

Heidi Ganzer, MS, RD, CSO, LD
Nutrition Therapy Director
Minnesota Oncology
St. Paul, Minnesota, USA

Susan M. Gapstur, PhD, MPH
Vice President
Epidemiology Research Program
American Cancer Society
Atlanta, Georgia, USA

M. Kay Garcia, DrPH, MSN, RN, LAc
Associate Professor
Oncology/Integrative Medicine Program
University of Texas MD Anderson Cancer Center
Houston, Texas, USA

Emily Glogowski, MS, MSc, LCGC
Genomics Consultant
GeneDx
Gaithersburg, Massachusetts, USA

Thomas J. Glynn, PhD
Consulting Professor
School of Medicine
Stanford University
Palo Alto, California, USA

Shari B. Goldfarb, MD
Medical Oncologist
Department of Surgery
Memorial Sloan Kettering Cancer Center
New York, New York, USA

Frederick L. Greene, MD, FACS
Clinical Professor of Surgery
UNC School of Medicine
Chapel Hill, North Carolina, USA

Olwen M. Hahn, MD
Associate Professor of Hematology-Oncology
The University of Chicago
Chicago, Illinois, USA

R. Donald Harvey, PharmD, BCOP, FCCP, FHOPA
Associate Professor
Hematology, Medical Oncology, and Pharmacology
Winship Cancer Institute
Emory University School of Medicine
Atlanta, Georgia, USA

William J. Hogan, MB, BCh
Internist
Division of Hematology
Mayo Clinic
Rochester, Minnesota, USA

Andreas M. Hötker, MD
Clinical Research Fellow
Department of Radiology
Memorial Sloan-Kettering Cancer Center
New York, New York, USA

Hedvig Hricak, MD, PhD
Professor of Radiology
Department of Radiology
Memorial Sloan-Kettering Cancer Center
New York, New York, USA

Arti Hurria, MD
Professor
Department of Medical Oncology and Therapeutics Research
City of Hope Comprehensive Cancer Center
Duarte, California, USA

Richard D. Hurt, MD
Emeritus Medical Director
Nicotine Dependence Center
Primary Care Internal Medicine
Rochester, Minnesota, USA

Eric J. Jacobs, PhD, MS
Strategic Director
Pharmacoepidemiology
Epidemiology Research Program
American Cancer Society
Atlanta, Georgia, USA

Adrienne Jaeger, BA, RN
Advanced Nursing Program
Yale School of Nursing
Yale University
New Haven, Connecticut, USA

Ahmedin Jemal, DVM, PhD
Vice President
Surveillance and Health Services Research
American Cancer Society
Atlanta, Georgia, USA

Christopher G. Kanakry, MD
Assistant Clinical Investigator
National Cancer Institute
Experimental Transplantation and Immunology Branch
Bethesda, Maryland, USA

Elizabeth Kessler, MD
Assistant Professor of Medical Oncology
University of Colorado Anschutz Medical Campus
Aurora, Colorado, USA

Fadlo R. Khuri, MD
Professor, Hematology and Medical Oncology
Adjunct Professor of Medicine, Pharmacology and Otolaryngology
Winship Cancer Institute
Emory University School of Medicine
Atlanta, Georgia, USA

John M. Kirkwood, MD
Usher Professor of Medicine Dermatology and Translational Science Division of Hematology-Oncology
University of Pittsburgh Medical Center
Pittsburgh, Pennsylvania, USA

Lauren A. Kosinski, MD
Managing Partner
The Seed House
Chestertown, Maryland, USA

Elizabeth Kvale, MD
Associate Professor of Medicine
Department of Medicine
University of Alabama at Birmingham
Birmingham, Alabama, USA

Richard Lee, MD
Associate Professor of Medicine
Case Western Reserve University
Cleveland, Ohio, USA

Stephen Leong, MD
Associate Professor of Medical Oncology
University of Colorado Anschutz Medical Campus
Aurora, Colorado, USA

Mark A. Lewis, MD
Hematology/Oncology
Intermountain Healthcare,
Salt Lake City, Utah, USA

Benjamin D. Li, MD, FACS
Cancer Center Director
MetroHealth System
Cleveland, Ohio, USA

Christopher H. Lieu, MD
Assistant Professor, Division of Medical Oncology
Director, Colorectal Medical Oncology
University of Colorado Anschutz Medical Campus
Aurora, Colarado, USA

Jennifer A. Ligibel, MD
Director
Leonard P. Zakim Center for Integrative Therapies Senior Physician
Associate Professor of Medicine
Dana-Farber Cancer Institute,
Boston, Massachusetts, USA

Gabriel Lopez, MD
Medical Director, Integrative Medicine Program
Assistant Professor, Palliative, Rehabilitation and Integrative Medicine
University of Texas MD Anderson Cancer Center
Houston, Texas, USA

Leo Luznik, MD
Associate Professor of Oncology
Johns Hopkins Hospital
Sidney Kimmel Comprehensive Cancer Center
Bethesda, Maryland, USA

Matthew Matasar, MD, MS
Hematologic Oncologist
Department of Medicine
Memorial Sloan Kettering Cancer Center
New York, New York, USA

Marji L. McCullough, ScD, RD
Strategic Director
Nutritional Epidemiology
Intramural Research
American Cancer Society
Atlanta, Georgia, USA

Jeffrey A. Meyerhardt, MD, MPH
Clinical Director
Gastrointestinal Cancer Center
Associate Professor of Medicine
Dana-Farber Cancer Institute
Boston, Massachusetts, USA

Maura Miccò, MD
Clinical Research Fellow
Department of Radiology
Memorial Sloan-Kettering Cancer Center
New York, New York, USA

Kimberly D. Miller, MPH
Epidemiologist
Surveillance and Health Services Research
American Cancer Society
Atlanta, Georgia, USA

Timothy J. Moynihan, MD
Oncologist
Department of Medical Oncology
Mayo Clinic
Rochester, Minnesota, USA

John P. Mulhall, MD
Director
Male Sexual and Reproductive Medicine Program
Memorial Sloan Kettering Cancer Center
New York, New York, USA

Christian J. Nelson, PhD
Psychologist
Gynecology Service, Department of Surgery
Memorial Sloan Kettering Cancer Center
New York, New York, USA

Danielle Novetsky Friedman, MD
Pediatrician
Department of Pediatrics
Memorial Sloan Kettering Cancer Center;
Weill Cornell Medical College
New York, New York, USA

Kevin C. Oeffinger
Professor
Division of Medical Oncology
Department of Medicine
Memorial Sloan Kettering Cancer Center
New York, New York, USA

Kenneth Offit, MD, MPH
Chief
Clinical Genetics Service
Department of Medicine
Memorial Sloan Kettering Cancer Center
New York, New York, USA

Sumanta K. Pal, MD
Assistant Clinical Professor
Department of Medical Oncology and Therapeutics Research
City of Hope Comprehensive Cancer Center
Duarte, California, USA

David M. Panicek, MD, FACR
Vice Chair for Clinical Affairs
Department of Radiology
Memorial Sloan-Kettering Cancer Center
New York, New York, USA

Alpa V. Patel, PhD
Strategic Director
CPS-3
Intramural Research
American Cancer Society
Atlanta, Georgia, USA

John D. Pfeifer, MD, PhD
Professor of Pathology and Immunology
Department of Pathology and Immunology
Washington University Medical Center
St. Louis, Missouri, USA

William C. Phelps, PhD
Vice President
Extramural Research
American Cancer Society
Atlanta, Georgia, USA

Ramesh Rengan, MD, PhD
Medical Director
SCCA Proton Therapy Center
Department of Radiation Oncology
University of Washington
Seattle, Washington, USA

Laura Q. Rogers, MD, MPH, FACP, FACSM
Professor of Nutrition Sciences
University of Alabama at Birmingham
Birmingham, Alabama, USA

Andrew J. Roth, MD
Psychiatrist
Department of Psychiatry and Behavioral Sciences
Memorial Sloan-Kettering Cancer Center;
Weill Cornell Medical Center
New York, New York, USA

Talya Salz, PhD
Assistant Attending Outcomes Research Scientist
Department of Epidemiology and Biostatistics
Memorial Sloan Kettering Cancer Center
New York, New York, USA

Charles Saxe, PhD
Director
Extramural Grants
American Cancer Society
Atlanta, Georgia, USA

Richard L. Schilsky, MD, FACP, FASCO
Senior Vice President and Chief Medical Officer
American Society of Clinical Oncology
Alexandria, Virginia, USA

Arvind M. Shinde, MD, MBA, MPH
Attending Physician
Hematology and Oncology
Samuel Oschin Comprehensive Cancer Institute
Cedars-Sinai
Los Angeles, California, USA

Kasmintan A. Schrader, MBBS, FRCPC, PhD
Assistant Professor
Department of Medical Genetics
University of British Columbia
Vancouver, British Columbia, Canada

Armin Shahrokni
Internist and Hematologic Oncologist
Department of Medicine
Memorial Sloan Kettering Cancer Center
New York, New York, USA

Gaurav Shukla, MD, PhD
Resident Physician
Department of Radiation Oncology
Thomas Jefferson University
Philadelphia, Pennsylvania, USA

M. Andrew Sicard, MD
Surgeon
Department of Surgery
Surgical Associates of Opelousas
Opelousas, Louisiana, USA

Rebecca L. Siegel, MPH
Strategic Director
Surveillance Information Services
Intramural Research
American Cancer Society
Atlanta, Georgia, USA

Edgar P. Simard, PhD, MPH
Adjunct Assistant Professor
Epidemiology Department
Rollins School of Public Health
Emory University
Atlanta, Georgia, USA

Gopal K. Singh, PhD, MS, MSc
Senior Health Equity Advisor
Office of Health Equity
US Department of Health and Human Services
Health Resources and Services Administration
Office of Health Equity
Rockville, Maryland, USA

Robert A. Smith, PhD
Vice President
Cancer Screening
Cancer Control
American Cancer Society
Atlanta, Georgia, USA

Tenbroeck Smith, MA
Strategic Director
Behavioral Research Center
American Cancer Society
Atlanta, Georgia, USA

Yukio Sonoda, MD
Surgeon
Ovarian Cancer Surgery
Gynecology Service
Department of Surgery
Memorial Sloan Kettering Cancer Center
New York, New York, USA

Kevin D. Stein, PhD
Adjunct Associate Professor
Department of Behavioral Sciences and Health Education,
Emory University Rollins School of Public Health
Atlanta, Georgia, USA

Nicole L. Stout, DPT, CLT-LANA
Cancer Rehabilitation Project Lead
Office of Strategic Research
Department of Rehabilitation Medicine
National Institutes of Health Clinical Center
Bethesda, Maryland, USA

Kelly L. Stratton, MD
Assistant Professor
Department of Urology
Stephenson Cancer Center
Oklahoma City, Oklahoma, USA

Ahmad A. Tarhini, MD, PhD
Associate Professor of Medicine
Division of Hematology-Oncology
University of Pittsburgh Medical Center
Pittsburgh, Pennsylvania, USA

Charles R. Thomas, Jr., MD
Professor and Chair
Department of Radiation Medicine
Oregon Health and Science University
Portland, Oregon, USA

Cynthia A. Thomson, PhD, RD
Professor, Mel and Enid Zuckerman College
of Public Health
Director, Canyon Ranch Center for Prevention
and Health Promotion
University of Arizona Cancer Center
Tucson, Arizona, USA

Emily Tonorezos, MD, MPH
Internist
Department of Medicine
Memorial Sloan Kettering Cancer Center
New York, New York, USA

Lindsey A. Torre, MSPH
Senior Epidemiologist
Surveillance and Health Services Research
American Cancer Society
Atlanta, Georgia, USA

Andrew C. Walls, MD
Instructor in Dermatology
Brigham and Women's Hospital
Harvard Medical School
Boston, Massachusetts, USA

Elizabeth Ward, PhD
Senior Vice President
Intramural Research
American Cancer Society
Atlanta, Georgia, USA

Martin A. Weinstock, MD, PhD
Professor of Dermatology
Brown University School of Public Health
Providence, Rhode Island, USA

Richard C. Wender, MD
Chief Cancer Control Officer
American Cancer Society
Atlanta, Georgia, USA

J. Lee Westmaas, PhD
Strategic Director
Tobacco Control Research
American Cancer Society
Atlanta, Georgia, USA

Andreas G. Wibmer, MD
Clinical Research Fellow
Department of Medical Physics
Memorial Sloan-Kettering Cancer Center
New York, New York, USA

Mark R. Wick, MD
Professor of Pathology
Associate Director of Surgical Pathology
Department of Pathology
University of Virginia Health System
Charlottesville, Virginia, USA

Joshua F. Zeidner, MD
Assistant Professor of Medicine
Division of Hematology/Oncology
University of North Carolina
Lineberger Comprehensive Cancer Center
Chapel Hill, North Carolina, USA

Amelia B. Zelnak, MD, MSc
Medical Oncologist
Atlanta Cancer Care
Northside Hospital Cancer Institute
Atlanta, Georgia, USA

Introduction

The American Cancer Society (ACS) published its first textbook in 1963 with the objective of introducing students and practicing clinicians to the rapidly emerging field of oncology. Since then, eleven editions of this book have been published under a variety of titles. These books have steadily grown in size, reflecting the accumulation of cancer-related knowledge. Due to the growing body of cancer information available, we have divided the content into two books to cover the information we considered most essential.

In this first book, *The American Cancer Society's Principles of Oncology: Prevention to Survivorship,* we review the epidemiological and biological principles relevant to cancer prevention and cancer screening; introduce the principles and methods of cancer diagnosis and modalities of cancer treatment; and review follow-up and survivorship concepts and recommendations, symptom management, and other quality-of-life-related topics.

The last edition of the ACS textbook was published in 2001, and our hiatus was based in part on uncertainty regarding the value of textbooks in the era of ubiquitous access to online information. Our return to this project was motivated by a constant stream of requests from physicians, nurses, public health professionals, cancer registrars, and others, as well as a decisive survey of academic oncologists involved in teaching medical students and residents. Recognizing the distinction between chunks of reference material available online and textbooks that present a coherent and coordinated body of knowledge, this textbook and its companion (*The American Cancer Society's Oncology in Practice: Clinical Management*) are written for those who are new to this field or to a particular aspect of multidisciplinary cancer control, and for experienced practitioners who have not recently updated their general knowledge of cancer or some aspect thereof.

These books are comprised of the contributions of the distinguished chapter authors who took time from their busy clinical and/or research schedules to organize and summarize their knowledge on a particular aspect of cancer control. We sincerely thank them for their time and expertise.

In addition to the authors, I would like to thank our editorial board of prominent experts who selected chapter authors and reviewed/edited chapter manuscripts; the additional reviewers (listed in the frontmatter) who added their expertise to the editorial process; our dedicated colleagues at Wiley Blackwell who patiently navigated us through production; and the American Cancer Society staff who helped organize and coordinate this project. And of course, this book and everything else done by the American Cancer Society depends on the support of our volunteers and donors, and is inspired by our constituents.

Ted Gansler, MD, MBA, MPH

Section 1

Cancer Causes, Prevention, and Early Detection

1

Descriptive Epidemiology

Rebecca L. Siegel, Kimberly D. Miller, and Ahmedin Jemal

Surveillance and Health Services Research, American Cancer Society, Atlanta, Georgia, USA

Introduction

Cancer was the eighth leading cause of death in the United States (US) in 1900 [1], but has been the second leading cause of death, after heart disease, during the last half of the twentieth century, accounting for approximately one in every four deaths [2]. Despite its prevalence throughout history, the recording of cancer incidence at the population level has only been available in the US since the mid-1970s.

Cancer Surveillance in the US

Cancer surveillance is the systematic collection and analysis of data about cancer diagnoses, including information about the patient (e.g., date of birth, sex, race), the tumor (e.g., site of origin, stage, histology), and the initial course of treatment. Cancer registration is useful to the public health in many important ways. These data are used to measure cancer occurrence in the population, including incidence, mortality, survival, and patterns of care; to plan and evaluate cancer control programs; to prioritize the allocation of healthcare resources; and to advance population-based epidemiologic and health services research. Population-based cancer statistics can also be used to corroborate medical hypotheses. For example, the rapid rise and fall of endometrial cancer incidence rates that mirrored the rise and fall in the use of unopposed estrogen as menopausal hormone therapy affirmed the association between estrogen and endometrial cancer risk [3,4]. Likewise, the dramatic 7% decline in breast cancer incidence from 2002 to 2003 reflects the abrupt decrease in menopausal hormone use after the Women's Health Initiative study reported its association with increased breast cancer risk [5,6].

The coverage and quality of cancer surveillance data have improved greatly over time. The current system of cancer registration in the US involves hospital registries, which furnish data for the evaluation of care within the hospital, and population-based registries, which are usually associated with state health departments or related institutions. Hospital registries also serve as the primary data source for central state registries. The cancer registrar carries the major responsibility for data collection and other day-to-day registry operations [7]. As patients are increasingly being diagnosed and treated in outpatient settings, case finding by cancer registrars at central registries has expanded to other medical facilities, including physician offices, pathology laboratories, and freestanding treatment centers.

Registry operations and the quality of the data collected by the registrar are guided by standards established by the Commission on Cancer (CoC) of the American College of Surgeons, the Surveillance, Epidemiology, and End Results (SEER) Program of the National Cancer Institute (NCI), the National Program of Cancer Registries (NPCR) of the Centers for Disease Control and Prevention (CDC), the American Joint Committee on Cancer (AJCC), and the North American Association of Central Cancer Registries (NAACCR).

Surveillance, Epidemiology, and End Results Program

The NCI's SEER Program was established as a result of the National Cancer Act of 1971, which mandated the collection, analysis, and dissemination of data to aid in the prevention, treatment, and diagnosis of cancer in the US [8]. Case ascertainment began on January 1, 1973. The original catchment area, known as SEER 9, covered 9% of the US population and included registries in five states (Connecticut, Iowa, New Mexico, Utah, and Hawaii) and four metropolitan areas (Detroit, Michigan; San Francisco–Oakland, California; Atlanta, Georgia; and Seattle–Puget Sound, Washington). The SEER 9 data are the only source for long-term, population-based cancer incidence and survival trends in the US. The SEER program expanded over time to include 18 registries covering 28% of the population, including 26% of African Americans, 38% of Hispanics, 44% of American Indians and Alaska Natives, 50% of Asians, and 67% of Hawaiian/Pacific Islanders [9]. Since its inception, quality control has been an integral component of the SEER program, which is considered the gold standard for cancer registration around the world. Cancer incidence and survival data from SEER and cancer mortality data from the National Center for Health Statistics are published annually in the *SEER Cancer Statistics Review*.

National Program of Cancer Registries

In 1992, Congress enacted the Cancer Registries Amendment Act to establish the NPCR at the CDC [10]. At the time this legislation was passed, 10 states had no cancer registry and most states with registries lacked the resources necessary to achieve minimum reporting standards. Today, NPCR supports central cancer registries in 45 states, the District of Columbia, Puerto Rico, and the US Pacific Island Jurisdictions [11]. Together, the SEER Program and NPCR collect and disseminate data that approaches 100% coverage of the US population.

North American Association of Central Cancer Registries

The NAACCR was established in 1987 as an umbrella organization to provide support to cancer registries and tumor registrars in the US and Canada. The organization works collaboratively with government agencies, professional associations, and private and nonprofit organizations toward the compatibility of cancer registry data. The NAACCR sets reporting standards, certifies central registries based on data quality criteria, and aggregates and distributes surveillance data for epidemiologic research. Registry-specific and combined national cancer incidence rates for the US have been published annually in *Cancer Incidence in North America* (*CINA*) for the past 26 years.

National Cancer Data Base

In contrast to population-based SEER and NPCR registries, the National Cancer Data Base (NCDB) is a hospital-based registry jointly sponsored by the American Cancer Society and the American College of Surgeons. The NCDB includes approximately 70% of all cancer diagnoses in the US from more than 1,400 hospitals accredited by the American College of Surgeons' CoC [12]. The database was established in 1989 and now contains more than 26 million records. One of the primary purposes of the NCDB is to provide information back to CoC treatment facilities about their quality of care. Additionally, the NCDB is a rich data source for cancer epidemiologists who study outcomes because it contains standardized data on patient demographics and insurance status; cancer type, histology, and staging; and first course of treatment. However, these data are somewhat limited for research purposes because they are not representative of the general population and because cancer cases that tend to be diagnosed and treated in nonhospital settings (e.g., melanoma and prostate cancer) are less likely to be captured.

National Center for Health Statistics

The National Center for Health Statistics (NCHS) is an agency within the CDC that serves as the principal repository for vital and health statistics in the US. State legislation requires that death certificates be completed for all deaths, and federal legislation requires national collection and reporting of deaths. Causes of death and other patient information are reported by certifying physicians on standard death certificates filed in the states and then processed and consolidated by the NCHS. For cancer mortality statistics, the underlying cause of death is classified according to the procedures specified by the World Health Organization's International Classification of Diseases (ICD) codes, which are periodically updated and currently in the 10th revision.

Measuring the Cancer Burden

The key measures for describing the occurrence of cancer are prevalence, incidence, mortality, and survival. Incidence and mortality data are also used by American Cancer Society researchers to estimate the number of new cancer cases and cancer deaths that will occur in the US in the current year [13,14]. These estimates are useful because cancer incidence and death data lag 2–4 years behind the current year due to the time required for collection, compilation, quality control, and dissemination. While these model-based projections are not informative for tracking temporal trends, they provide an estimate of the contemporary cancer burden and are widely cited by researchers, cancer control advocates, and public health planners.

Prevalence

Cancer prevalence refers to the number of individuals living in a population with a previous cancer diagnosis. It is a mixture of new and pre-existing cases, and thus is a function of incidence and survival. Population prevalence may be estimated for diagnoses within a specified time period (limited-duration) or for all diagnoses (complete). The complete prevalence estimate is often referred to as the number of cancer survivors.

Incidence

Cancer incidence is the number of newly diagnosed cases during a specified time period in a defined population. It is usually expressed as an annual rate per 100,000 population such that the numerator is the number of new cancer cases and the denominator is the size of the population at risk. For example, the denominator for cancers that only occur in one sex is the sex-specific population. Sometimes the appropriate denominator is not straightforward. For example, the population at risk for uterine cancer is not the entire female population, but the fraction of women (approximately 80%) who have not had a hysterectomy (surgical removal of the uterus). Routine reporting of uterine cancer incidence rates typically fail to account for hysterectomy and thus substantially underestimate the burden of this disease [15].

Cancer registry data are corrected and updated over time due to delays or errors in case reporting. To account for the effect of reporting delays on registry data, NCI and NAACCR provide delay-adjusted rates. Delay-adjustment has the largest effect on data in the most recent time period for cancers that are frequently diagnosed in outpatient settings, such as melanoma, leukemia, and prostate cancer [16]. For example, leukemia incidence rates in the most recent reporting year are 14% higher after delay-adjustment [8]. Cancer incidence rates presented in this chapter were adjusted for delays in reporting whenever possible.

Mortality

Cancer mortality refers to the number of individuals who die from cancer during a specified time period in a defined population. Like incidence, it is typically expressed as an annual rate per 100,000 population such that the numerator is the number of cancer deaths in a given year and the denominator is the population size. The cancer death rate represents the risk of death among the entire population as opposed to the risk specifically among cancer patients. Therefore, it is a function of both incidence and survival.

Cancer death rates are calculated based on information obtained from death certificates, including age at death, sex, place of residence, and underlying cause of death. On the US Standard Certificate of Death, the underlying cause of death is the disease or injury that initiated the chain of events leading to death, as opposed to the final disease condition. For example, the death of a patient who died from sepsis as a result of lung cancer would be coded as lung cancer. The accuracy of death certificate data depends on the cause of death (e.g., rapidly fatal diseases are recorded more accurately) and the physician who records the death (e.g., attending physician versus the coroner).

Age Standardization

The risk of cancer diagnosis or death increases exponentially with age. For this reason, cancer-related vital statistics are conventionally reported as either age-specific or age-standardized rates. Age-standardized rates have been weighted to a common population age distribution to eliminate the effect of age on cancer rates and allow valid comparison between populations with different age structures. For example, without age-standardization, the risk of cancer appears much higher in Florida (572 per 100,000) than in Alaska (370 per 100,000) because Florida has a much older population. However, after age adjustment, the incidence rates in these states are quite similar (438 versus 432 per 100,000, respectively). Current cancer incidence and death rates for the US are generally weighted to the 2000 US standard population [17] unless they are being compared to international rates, when the world standard population is used.

Survival

The cancer survival rate is the percentage of patients who are alive at a specified time following cancer diagnosis, usually 5 years. There are several different methods of calculating survival. Observed survival represents overall survival and includes death from cancer as well as other causes. Relative survival is the ratio of the proportion of survivors in a cohort of cancer patients to the proportion of expected survivors in a comparable group of cancer-free individuals [18]. For example, a relative survival rate of 100% indicates that the likelihood of survival after a cancer diagnosis is the same as survival in the general population. Cancer-specific survival is the probability of surviving cancer in the absence of other causes of death [19]. Relative and cancer-specific survival are measures of net survival because they estimate cancer survival in the absence of death from other causes.

Relative survival is the measure most often presented in cancer surveillance reports because it is useful for tracking trends and comparing survival between populations. It is typically expressed as a 5-year rate, although it may be presented for 10 or even 15 years postdiagnosis for less fatal cancers.

Although survival rates are useful for monitoring progress in the early detection and treatment of cancer, they have several limitations and should be interpreted with caution. First, they do not reflect the most recent advances in treatment because they are based on the experiences of patients who were diagnosed several years ago due to both the lag time in data reporting (typically 2–4 years) and the necessity for sufficient follow-up time. Second, survival statistics are not useful for predicting individual prognosis because factors that strongly influence survival, such as treatment protocols, comorbidities, and biological and behavioral differences in tumor and patient characteristics, cannot be controlled. Third, survival rates for cancers with early detection practices (e.g., prostate, breast) are subject to lead time bias, as discussed in Chapter 11 [20]. This bias, for example, is reflected in the 5-year relative survival rate for prostate cancer in the US, which increased from 68% in the mid-1970s to nearly 100% since around 2000 [8,21].

Lifetime, Relative, and Attributable Risk

Epidemiologists use the word *risk* in several ways. Lifetime risk refers to the probability that an individual will be diagnosed with or die from cancer over the course of a lifetime. For example, in the US, the lifetime risk of developing lung cancer is approximately one in 14 for men and one in 17 for women [8]. Risk can also be assessed for particular age groups; for instance, one in 29 women who are cancer-free at age 59 will develop breast cancer by age 69 [2].

Relative risk in cancer studies measures the strength of the relationship between a specific risk factor and cancer by comparing risk among persons with a specific trait or exposure to risk among persons without the trait or exposure. For example, the relative risk of lung cancer death among smokers is 26 for women and 25 for men [22]; in other words, smoking increases the risk of dying from lung cancer about 25-fold. Most relative risks are not this large, however.

Attributable risk, or attributable fraction, refers to the contribution of a particular exposure or trait to the cancer burden. In other words, it is the difference in the disease burden between exposed and unexposed populations who are similar in other respects. For example, an analysis of smoking-attributable mortality (SAM) found that 83% of lung cancer deaths in men in 2011 were attributable to smoking [23].

Cancer Occurrence Patterns in the US

Prevalence

The NCI estimates that there were 15.5 million Americans with a history of cancer alive on January 1, 2016, a number that will grow to about 20 million by 2026 [24]. The number of survivors is growing rapidly because of advances in the early detection and treatment of cancer, which have lengthened survival times, as well as the growth and aging of the population. Almost half of cancer survivors are 70 years of age or older. The most common diagnoses among male survivors are prostate or colorectal cancer, while among women they are breast or uterine corpus cancers.

Incidence

In the US, the lifetime risk of developing cancer is slightly less than one in two for men and a little more than one in three for women [8]. An estimated 1,688,780 persons received a new cancer diagnosis in 2017 [2]. Historically, the occurrence of cancer has increased over time; however, from about 2000 to 2013, incidence rates decreased in men and were stable in women (Figure 1.1). The four most common cancer types – prostate, female breast, lung and bronchus, and colorectal – account for about half of all new cancer cases and thus strongly influence overall trends (Figure 1.2).

Cancer incidence trends reflect changes in behavior and medical practice. For example, much of the rise in male cancer incidence rates between 1975 and 1992 was due to increased detection of clinically asymptomatic prostate cancer, first via transurethral resection of the prostate (TURP) [25] and later

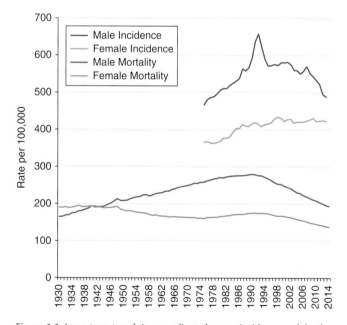

Figure 1.1 Long-term trends in age-adjusted cancer incidence and death rates, 1930–2014. *Source:* Incidence – Surveillance, Epidemiology, and End Results Program (SEER) 9 registries (San Francisco, Connecticut, Detroit, Hawaii, Iowa, New Mexico, Seattle, Utah, and Atlanta), November 2015 submission, National Cancer Institute. Rates were adjusted for delays in reporting. Mortality – US Mortality Volumes 1930–1959; US Mortality Data 1960–2014, National Center for Health Statistics, Centers for Disease Control and Prevention.

via prostate-specific antigen (PSA) testing [26]. In less than two decades, prostate cancer incidence rates more than doubled, from 94 cases per 100,000 men in 1975 to 237 cases per 100,000 men in 1992 [8]; rates subsequently fell rapidly as the proportion of men undergoing a first PSA test diminished [27] (Figure 1.3).

Cancer incidence trends have also been strongly influenced by tobacco use. Most (80%) lung cancers in the US are due to smoking [23]. As a result of the smoking epidemic, lung cancer among men catapulted from a rare disease to the most commonly diagnosed cancer during the first half of the twentieth century [28,29]. Lung cancer rates and trends vary by sex because of historic differences in smoking patterns between men and women; smoking prevalence peaked at 65% around 1950 among men and at 38% around 1960 among women [30]. The lag period between peak population smoking prevalence and peak lung cancer rates is 30–40 years. Circa 1930, lung cancer rates began a long period of increase that peaked in the 1980s in men and around 2005 in women (Figures 1.3 and 1.4) [8]. During the most recent 5 years of data (2009–2013), lung cancer incidence rates declined annually by 2.9% in men and 1.4% in women.

Breast cancer is the most commonly diagnosed cancer among women (Figure 1.2). Breast cancer incidence rates increased rapidly from 1980 to 1987 because of increased diagnosis of asymptomatic tumors due to the widespread dissemination of mammography screening (Figure 1.4) [31]. Breast cancer rates have also been influenced over time by changes in reproductive patterns (e.g., later age at first birth, fewer births) that often accompany economic growth and are associated with an increased risk of breast cancer. Incidence rates gradually increased by 0.4% per year from 2004 to 2013, driven by trends in non-White women [8].

Cancers located in the colon or rectum are the third most commonly diagnosed cancers in both men and women (Figure 1.2). Colorectal cancer is one of only two cancer types (cervical cancer is the other) that can be prevented with screening. Screening prevents colorectal cancer by detecting and allowing for the removal of adenomatous polyps, from which most malignancies in the colorectum develop [32,33]. Colorectal cancer incidence rates have been decreasing since the mid-1980s, with similar patterns for men and women [8]. It has been estimated that half of this decline is due to changes in risk factors and half is due to colorectal cancer screening [34]. However, the recent acceleration in the pace of decline has been attributed primarily to increased colonoscopy uptake [34,35].

Survival and Mortality

Advances in cancer screening strategies and targeted therapies have greatly improved cancer outcomes. Over the past 70 years, the 5-year relative survival rate for cancer has more than doubled, from 24% in men and 33% in women for diagnoses between 1935 and 1940 [28] to 67% in both sexes for diagnoses between 2006 and 2012 [8]. Still, one in four men and one in five women will die from cancer [36], the equivalent of approximately 600,920 people in 2017 [2]. The median age of death from cancer is 72 years [8].

Estimated New Cases*

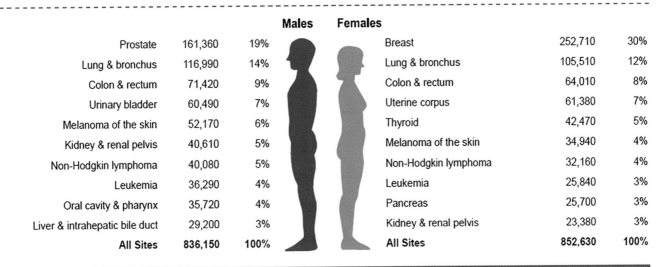

Males			Females		
Prostate	161,360	19%	Breast	252,710	30%
Lung & bronchus	116,990	14%	Lung & bronchus	105,510	12%
Colon & rectum	71,420	9%	Colon & rectum	64,010	8%
Urinary bladder	60,490	7%	Uterine corpus	61,380	7%
Melanoma of the skin	52,170	6%	Thyroid	42,470	5%
Kidney & renal pelvis	40,610	5%	Melanoma of the skin	34,940	4%
Non-Hodgkin lymphoma	40,080	5%	Non-Hodgkin lymphoma	32,160	4%
Leukemia	36,290	4%	Leukemia	25,840	3%
Oral cavity & pharynx	35,720	4%	Pancreas	25,700	3%
Liver & intrahepatic bile duct	29,200	3%	Kidney & renal pelvis	23,380	3%
All Sites	**836,150**	**100%**	**All Sites**	**852,630**	**100%**

Estimated Deaths

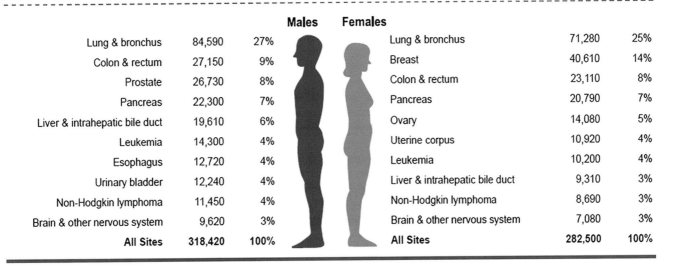

Males			Females		
Lung & bronchus	84,590	27%	Lung & bronchus	71,280	25%
Colon & rectum	27,150	9%	Breast	40,610	14%
Prostate	26,730	8%	Colon & rectum	23,110	8%
Pancreas	22,300	7%	Pancreas	20,790	7%
Liver & intrahepatic bile duct	19,610	6%	Ovary	14,080	5%
Leukemia	14,300	4%	Uterine corpus	10,920	4%
Esophagus	12,720	4%	Leukemia	10,200	4%
Urinary bladder	12,240	4%	Liver & intrahepatic bile duct	9,310	3%
Non-Hodgkin lymphoma	11,450	4%	Non-Hodgkin lymphoma	8,690	3%
Brain & other nervous system	9,620	3%	Brain & other nervous system	7,080	3%
All Sites	**318,420**	**100%**	**All Sites**	**282,500**	**100%**

Figure 1.2 Leading new cancer cases and deaths in the US in 2017. Ranking is based on modeled projections and may differ from the most recent observed data. *Estimates are rounded to the nearest 10 and cases exclude basal cell and squamous cell skin cancers and *in situ* carcinoma except urinary bladder. *Source:* Siegel *et al.*[2]. Reproduced with permission of John Wiley & Sons.

Notable improvements in 5-year relative survival rates over the past three decades have occurred among both Whites and Blacks (Table 1.1). Advances in treatment have resulted in particularly dramatic improvement in survival for most types of leukemia. For example, in large part due to the discovery of the targeted drug imatinib, the 5-year relative survival rate for chronic myeloid leukemia increased from 31% for cases diagnosed between 1990 and 1992 to 66% for diagnoses between 2006 and 2012 [8,37]. Survival rates for some cancers, such as lung and pancreas, have been slow to improve.

Currently cancer death rates among men are about 40% higher than those among women, although historically rates were higher among women (Figure 1.1). Cancer death rates among men increased 70% from 1930 to 1990, but have since declined by 31%. Cancer death rates among women have been less variable, declining by 21% since 1991.

Lung cancer is the leading cause of cancer death among both men and women, accounting for more than one-quarter of all cancer deaths in the US (Figure 1.2). Lung cancer death rates among men increased 21-fold from 1930 to 1990 as a result of the smoking epidemic, although they have since decreased by 43% (Figure 1.5). Similarly, lung cancer death rates among women increased 16-fold before beginning to drop in 2003 (Figure 1.6) [8]. Due to few early symptoms, the majority (57%) of lung cancer cases are diagnosed at a distant stage, for which the 5-year relative survival rate is 4%. For the 16% of cases diagnosed at a localized stage, survival increases to 55%.

Breast cancer is the second leading cause of cancer death among women, accounting for 14% of all female cancer deaths (Figure 1.2). Breast cancer death rates fluctuated little from 1930 to 1989, but have since decreased by 38% [8] (Figure 1.6). Approximately half of this decline has been attributed to

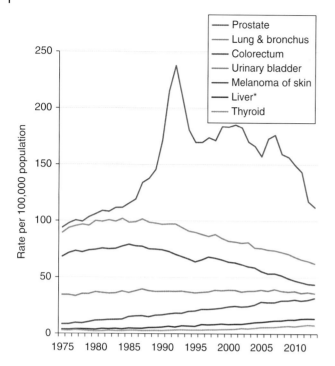

Figure 1.3 Long-term trends in age-adjusted cancer incidence rates among men, 1975–2013. *Source:* Surveillance, Epidemiology, and End Results Program (SEER) 9 registries (San Francisco, Connecticut, Detroit, Hawaii, Iowa, New Mexico, Seattle, Utah, and Atlanta), November 2015 submission. Rates were adjusted for delays in reporting. *Includes intrahepatic bile duct.

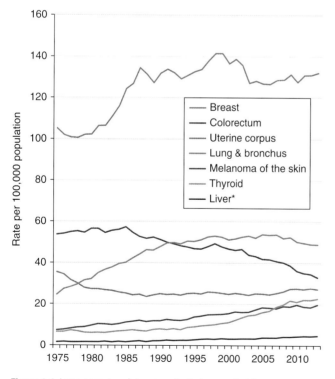

Figure 1.4 Long-term trends in age-adjusted cancer incidence rates among women, 1975–2013. *Source:* Surveillance, Epidemiology, and End Results Program (SEER) 9 registries (San Francisco, Connecticut, Detroit, Hawaii, Iowa, New Mexico, Seattle, Utah, and Atlanta), November 2015 submission. Rates were adjusted for delays in reporting. *Includes intrahepatic bile duct.

mammography screening and half to improvements in adjuvant treatment [38]. Most breast cancers (61%) are diagnosed at a localized stage, for which the 5-year relative survival rate is 99%; survival drops to 85% or 26% for women whose cancer has reached a regional or distant stage, respectively, by the time of diagnosis [8].

Prostate cancer accounts for about 8% of male cancer deaths (Figure 1.2). Prostate cancer death rates increased during the first half of the twentieth century, were relatively stable for several decades, then rose and fell concurrently with the distinct peak in incidence rates associated with widespread uptake of PSA testing (Figure 1.5). This rapid rise and fall in mortality rates is thought to be a result of attribution bias: deaths due to other causes mistakenly attributed to prostate cancer on death certificates because of a prevalent prostate cancer diagnosis [39]. However, the continued decrease since the mid-1990s is likely to be real and due to advances in both primary and salvage treatments, as well as early detection, although results from randomized clinical trials evaluating the efficacy of PSA testing have been equivocal [40,41]. Prostate cancer death rates decreased by 3.4% per year from 2010 to 2014 [8]. Ninety-two percent of prostate cancer patients are diagnosed at a localized or regional stage, for which the 5-year relative survival rate approaches 100%.

Colorectal cancer accounts for 8–9% of all cancer deaths in men and women (Figure 1.2). Colorectal cancer death rates have been declining since around 1950 among women and since the mid-1980s among men (Figures 1.5 and 1.6). Mortality declines from 1975 to 2000 have been attributed to screening (53%), changes in risk factors (35%), and improvements in treatment (12%) [34]. From 2010 to 2014, death rates declined by 2.5% per year among men and 2.8% per year among women [8]. Although several different screening tests effectively diagnose colorectal cancer early, less than half (39%) of patients are diagnosed with local stage disease, for which 5-year relative survival is 90% [8]. One in five colorectal cancer patients is still diagnosed with distant stage disease, for which the 5-year survival rate is just 14%; for those diagnosed with regional stage disease, 5-year survival is 71%.

Demographic and Geographic Patterns

The occurrence of cancer is strongly influenced by demographic characteristics, including age, sex, race, socioeconomic status, and place of residence. One of the strongest risk factors for cancer is increasing age. This is primarily because 10 or more years usually pass between exposure to external factors and detectable cancer. Between 2009 and 2013, slightly more than half (53%) of new cancer cases and 69% of cancer deaths occurred among individuals who were age 65 years or older [8]. Sex also influences cancer risk; the lifetime probability of developing cancer is slightly higher for men than for women – 41% versus 38% between 2011 and 2013. Reasons for this disparity are not completely understood, but are likely related to differences in risk factor behaviors, hormone exposure, and healthcare utilization [42].

Race and ethnicity substantially modify cancer risk (Table 1.2 and Table 1.3). Of the five major racial and ethnic groups in the US (non-Hispanic White, non-Hispanic Black, Asian/Pacific Islander, American Indian/Alaska Native, and Hispanic), Black

Table 1.1 Trends in 5-year relative survival rates[1] (%) by race, US, 1975–2012.

	All races			White			Black		
	1975–77	1987–89	2006–12	1975–77	1987–89	2006–2012	1975–77	1987–89	2006–12
All sites	49	55	69	50	57	70	39	43	63
Brain and other nervous system	22	29	35	22	28	33	25	32	44
Breast (female)	75	84	91	76	85	92	62	71	82
Colon and rectum	50	60	66	50	60	67	45	52	59
Esophagus	5	9	21	6	11	22	4	7	13
Hodgkin lymphoma	72	79	89	72	80	89	70	72	86
Kidney and renal pelvis	50	57	75	50	57	75	49	55	75
Larynx	66	66	62	67	67	64	58	56	52
Leukemia	34	43	63	35	44	64	33	35	58
Liver and intrahepatic bile duct	3	5	18	3	6	18	2	3	13
Lung and bronchus	12	13	19	12	13	19	11	11	16
Melanoma of the skin	82	88	93	82	88	93	57[2]	79[2]	69
Myeloma	25	27	50	24	27	50	29	30	52
Non-Hodgkin lymphoma	47	51	73	47	51	74	49	46	65
Oral cavity and pharynx	53	54	67	54	56	69	36	34	47
Ovary	36	38	46	35	38	46	42	34	38
Pancreas	3	4	9	3	3	9	2	6	8
Prostate	68	83	99	69	84	>99	61	71	97
Stomach	15	20	31	14	18	30	16	19	30
Testis	83	95	97	83	95	97	73[2,3]	88	90
Thyroid	92	94	98	92	94	99	90	92	97
Urinary bladder	72	79	79	73	80	79	50	63	66
Uterine cervix	69	70	69	70	73	71	65	57	58
Uterine corpus	87	82	83	88	84	86	60	57	66

Source: Howlader *et al.* [8].
[1] Rates are adjusted for normal life expectancy and are based on cases diagnosed in the SEER 9 areas from 1975 to 1977, 1987 to 1989, and 2006 to 2012, all followed through 2013.
[2] The standard error is between 5 and 10 percentage points.
[3] Survival rate is for cases diagnosed from 1978 to 1980.

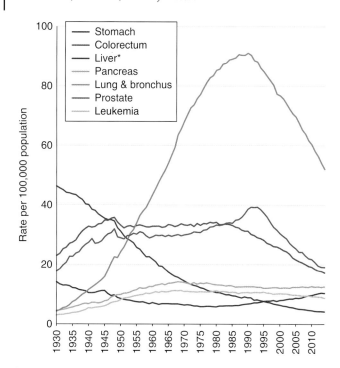

Figure 1.5 Long-term trends in age-adjusted male cancer death rates by site, 1930–2014. *Source:* US Mortality Volumes 1930–1959; US Mortality Data 1960–2014, National Center for Health Statistics, Centers for Disease Control and Prevention. *Includes intrahepatic bile duct.

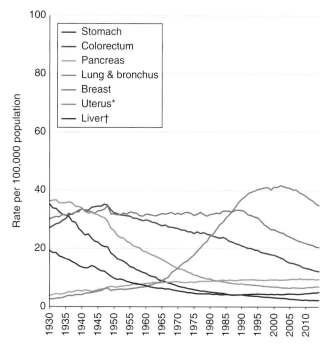

Figure 1.6 Long-term trends in age-adjusted female cancer death rates by site, 1930–2014. *Source:* US Mortality Volumes 1930–1959; US Mortality Data 1960–2014, National Center for Health Statistics, Centers for Disease Control and Prevention. *Uterus refers to uterine corpus and uterine cervix combined. †Includes intrahepatic bile duct.

men have the highest overall rates of cancer incidence and death and Black females have the lowest survival rates [8]. Racial inequalities in the cancer burden primarily reflect obstacles to receiving healthcare services related to cancer prevention, early detection, and high-quality treatment, as opposed to biological differences [43].

While Americans of Asian, Hispanic, or American Indian descent generally have lower rates than non-Hispanic Whites or Blacks for the most common cancers, they have a higher burden of cancers related to infectious agents, such as cancers of the liver (hepatitis B and C viruses), stomach (*Helicobacter pylori*), and cervix (human papillomavirus) [2]. Factors that contribute to this disparity include a higher prevalence of cancer-related infections in immigrant countries of origin for Hispanics and Asian/Pacific Islanders [44] and lower rates of screening for cervical cancer [41]. In addition, some groups of American Indians and Alaska Natives have substantially higher rates of lung and kidney cancers, which is thought to reflect the higher prevalence of risk factors for these cancers, such as smoking, obesity, hypertension, and end-stage renal disease [45]. It is important to note that because cancer surveillance data in the US are reported for very broadly defined racial and ethnic categories, important differences in the cancer burden within groups is masked. For example, the age-adjusted cancer death rate among Cuban men is approximately 15% higher than that among Mexican men [46]. In addition, race misclassification among American Indians and Alaska Natives continues to be a challenge in accurately measuring the cancer burden in this population.

Poverty is the driving factor for the majority of health inequalities in the US. Members of minority populations are substantially more likely than Whites to be economically disadvantaged; in 2015, 24% of Blacks and 21% of Hispanics lived in poverty compared to 9% of non-Hispanic Whites [47]. Importantly, however, persons of lower socioeconomic status have disproportionately higher cancer death rates than those who are more affluent, regardless of race or ethnicity. One study estimated that eliminating socioeconomic disparities would prevent twice as many premature cancer deaths as eliminating racial disparities [48].

Cancer rates also vary geographically. For example, male lung cancer incidence rates from 2009 to 2013 ranged from 34 (cases per 100,000 men) in Utah to 118 in Kentucky [2]. Lung cancer shows the largest geographic variation of any cancer type because it is driven by historical smoking prevalence, which varies dramatically by state [49]. In 2015, smoking prevalence ranged from 9% in Utah to 26% in Kentucky and West Virginia [50]. State smoking prevalence is influenced by differences in state and local tobacco control activities, tobacco industry marketing, and social norms about tobacco use.

Conclusion

Cancer is a major public health problem in the US, as well as many other parts of the world. Cancer surveillance is essential for monitoring the cancer burden; identifying high-risk populations; quantifying progress in prevention, early detection, and

Table 1.2 Incidence rates by site, race, and ethnicity, US, 2009–2013.[1]

	All races combined	Non-Hispanic White	Non-Hispanic Black	Asian/Pacific Islander	American Indian/ Alaska Native[2]	Hispanic
All sites						
Male	512.1	519.3	577.3	310.2	426.7	398.1
Female	418.5	436.0	408.5	287.1	387.3	329.6
Breast (female)	123.3	128.3	125.1	89.3	98.1	91.7
Colorectum						
Male	46.9	46.1	58.3	37.8	51.4	42.8
Female	35.6	35.2	42.7	27.8	41.2	29.8
Kidney and renal pelvis						
Male	21.7	21.9	24.4	10.8	29.9	20.7
Female	11.3	11.3	13.0	4.8	17.6	11.9
Liver and intrahepatic bile duct						
Male	11.8	9.7	16.9	20.4	18.5	19.4
Female	4.0	3.3	5.0	7.6	8.9	7.5
Lung and bronchus						
Male	75.0	77.7	90.8	46.6	71.3	42.2
Female	53.5	58.2	51.0	28.3	56.2	25.6
Prostate	123.2	114.8	198.4	63.5	85.1	104.9
Stomach						
Male	9.2	7.8	14.7	14.4	11.2	13.1
Female	4.6	3.5	7.9	8.4	6.5	7.8
Uterine cervix	7.6	7.0	9.8	6.1	9.7	9.9

Source: Siegel *et al.* [2]. Reproduced with permission of John Wiley & Sons.

Hispanic origin is not mutually exclusive from Asian/Pacific Islander or American Indian/Alaska Native.

[1] Rates are per 100,000 population and age adjusted to the 2000 US standard population.

[2] Data based on Indian Health Service Contract Health Service Delivery Areas and exclude data from Kansas.

Table 1.3 Death rates by site, race, and ethnicity, US, 2010–2014.[1]

	All races combined	Non-Hispanic White	Non-Hispanic Black	Asian/Pacific Islander	American Indian/ Alaska Native[2]	Hispanic
All sites						
Male	200.4	204.0	253.4	122.7	183.6	142.5
Female	141.5	145.5	165.9	88.8	129.1	97.7
Breast (female)	21.2	21.1	30.0	11.3	14.1	14.4
Colorectum						
Male	17.7	17.3	25.9	12.4	19.5	15.0
Female	12.4	12.3	16.9	8.8	14.0	9.2
Kidney and renal pelvis						
Male	5.6	5.8	5.7	2.7	8.9	4.9
Female	2.4	2.5	2.5	1.1	4.2	2.3
Liver and intrahepatic bile duct						
Male	9.2	8.0	13.3	14.3	14.9	13.1
Female	3.7	3.3	4.6	6.1	6.8	5.8
Lung and bronchus						
Male	55.9	58.3	69.8	31.7	46.2	27.3
Female	36.3	39.8	35.5	18.0	30.8	13.4
Prostate	20.0	18.7	42.8	8.8	19.4	16.5
Stomach						
Male	4.4	3.4	8.7	7.1	7.5	6.9
Female	2.3	1.7	4.2	4.3	3.8	4.1
Uterine cervix	2.3	2.1	3.9	1.7	2.8	2.6

Source: Siegel *et al.* [2]. Reproduced with permission of John Wiley & Sons.

Hispanic origin is not mutually exclusive from Asian/Pacific Islander or American Indian/Alaska Native.

[1] Rates are per 100,000 population and age adjusted to the 2000 US standard population.

[2] Data based on Indian Health Service Contract Health Service Delivery Areas.

treatment strategies; and informing cancer control programs. Descriptive cancer epidemiology research has also greatly contributed to the current understanding of cancer. The foundation of cancer surveillance is population-based cancer registration. The expansion in population coverage of high-quality cancer

data collection in the US, from 9% in the mid-1970s to almost 100% today, is a major public health milestone. This achievement has the potential to further reduce the cancer burden by facilitating widespread, targeted interventions at the community level, where health inequalities arise.

References

1 Linder FE, Grove RD. *Vital Statistics Rates in the United States 1900–1940*. Washington: United States Government Printing Office, 1947.

2 Siegel R, Miller KD, Jemal A. Cancer Statistics, 2017. *CA Cancer J Clin* 2017;67:7–30.

3 Weiss NS, Szekely DR, Austin DF. Increasing incidence of endometrial cancer in the United States. *N Engl J Med* 1976;294:1259–62.

4 Ziel HK, Finkle WD. Increased risk of endometrial carcinoma among users of conjugated estrogens. *N Engl J Med* 1975;293:1167–70.

5 Coombs NJ, Cronin KA, Taylor RJ, Freedman AN, Boyages J. The impact of changes in hormone therapy on breast cancer incidence in the US population. *Cancer Causes Control* 2010;21:83–90.

6 Ravdin PM, Cronin KA, Howlader N, et al. The decrease in breast-cancer incidence in 2003 in the United States. *N Engl J Med* 2007;356:1670–74.

7 Hutchison C, Menck H, Burch M, Gottschalk R. *Cancer Registry Management: Principals and Practice, 2nd edn.* National Cancer Registrar's Association, Inc., 2004.

8 Howlader N, Noone AM, Krapcho M, et al. *SEER Cancer Statistics Review, 1975–2013*. Bethesda: National Cancer Institute, 2016.

9 National Cancer Institute. Surveillance, Epidemiology, and End Results Program. Available from: seer.cancer.gov (accessed 11 May 2017).

10 Centers for Disease Control and Prevention. State cancer registries: status of authorizing legislation and enabling regulations–United States, October 1993. MMWR 1994;43:71,74–5.

11 Centers for Disease Control and Prevention. National Program of Cancer Registries. Available from: cdc.gov/cancer/npcr/about.htm (accessed 11 May 2017).

12 Bilimoria KY, Stewart AK, Winchester DP, Ko CY. The National Cancer Data Base: a powerful initiative to improve cancer care in the United States. *Ann Surg Oncol* 2008;15:683–90.

13 Chen HS, Portier K, Ghosh K, et al. Predicting US- and state-level cancer counts for the current calendar year: Part I: evaluation of temporal projection methods for mortality. *Cancer* 2012;118:1091–9.

14 Zhu L, Pickle LW, Ghosh K, et al. Predicting US- and state-level cancer counts for the current calendar year: Part II: evaluation of spatiotemporal projection methods for incidence. *Cancer* 2012;118:1100–9.

15 Siegel RL, Devesa SS, Cokkinides V, Ma J, Jemal A. State-level uterine corpus cancer incidence rates corrected for hysterectomy prevalence, 2004 to 2008. *Cancer Epidemiol Biomarkers Prev* 2013;22:25–31.

16 Clegg LX, Feuer EJ, Midthune DN, Fay MP, Hankey BF. Impact of reporting delay and reporting error on cancer incidence rates and trends. *J Natl Cancer Inst* 2002;94:1537–45.

17 Day JG. *Population Projections of the United States by Age, Sex, Race, and Hispanic Origin: 1995 to 2050*. US Government Printing Office, Washington, DC: US Bureau of the Census, 1996.

18 Ederer F, Axtell LM, Cutler SJ. The Relative Survival Rate: A Statistical Methodology. *National Cancer Institute Monograph* 6; 101–21, 1961.

19 Marubini E, Valsecchi MG. *Analysing Survival Data from Clinical Trials and Observational Studies*. New York: John Wiley & Sons, Inc., 1995.

20 Hutchison GB, Shapiro S. Lead time gained by diagnostic screening for breast cancer. *J Natl Cancer Inst* 1968;41:665–81.

21 Brawley OW. Trends in prostate cancer in the United States. *J Natl Cancer Inst Monogr* 2012;2012:152–6.

22 Thun MJ, Carter BD, Feskanich D, et al. 50-year trends in smoking-related mortality in the United States. *N Engl J Med* 2013;368:351–64.

23 Siegel RL, Jacobs EJ, Newton CC, et al. Deaths due to cigarette smoking for 12 smoking-related cancers in the United States. *JAMA Intern Med* 2015;175(9):1574–6.

24 Miller KD, Siegel RL, Lin CC, et al. Cancer treatment and survivorship statistics, 2016. *CA Cancer J Clin* 2016;66:271–89.

25 Potosky AL, Kessler L, Gridley G, Brown CC, Horm JW. Rise in prostatic cancer incidence associated with increased use of transurethral resection. *J Natl Cancer Inst* 1990;82:1624–8.

26 Potosky AL, Miller BA, Albertsen PC, Kramer BS. The role of increasing detection in the rising incidence of prostate cancer. *JAMA* 1995;273:548–52.

27 Legler JM, Feuer EJ, Potosky AL, Merrill RM, Kramer BS. The role of prostate-specific antigen (PSA) testing patterns in the recent prostate cancer incidence decline in the United States. *Cancer Causes Control* 1998;9:519–27.

28 Griswold MH, Wilder CS, Cutler SJ, Pollack ES. *Cancer in Connecticut 1935–1951*. Hartford, Connecticut: Connecticut State Department of Health, 1955.

29 Proctor RN. Tobacco and the global lung cancer epidemic. *Nat Rev Cancer* 2001;1:82–6.

30 Weiss W. Cigarette smoking and lung cancer trends. A light at the end of the tunnel? *Chest* 1997;111:1414–6.

31 DeSantis CE, Fedewa SA, Goding Sauer A, et al. Breast Cancer Statistics, 2015. *CA Cancer J Clin* 2015;66:31–42.

32 Stryker SJ, Wolff BG, Culp CE, et al. Natural history of untreated colonic polyps. *Gastroenterology* 1987;93:1009–13.

33 Winawer SJ, Zauber AG, Ho MN, et al. Prevention of colorectal cancer by colonoscopic polypectomy. *The National Polyp Study Workgroup. N Engl J Med* 1993;329:1977–81.

34 Edwards BK, Ward E, Kohler BA, *et al.* Annual report to the nation on the status of cancer, 1975–2006, featuring colorectal cancer trends and impact of interventions (risk factors, screening, and treatment) to reduce future rates. *Cancer* 2010;116:544–73.

35 Cress RD, Morris C, Ellison GL, Goodman MT. Secular changes in colorectal cancer incidence by subsite, stage at diagnosis, and race/ethnicity, 1992–2001. *Cancer* 2006;107:1142–52.

36 DevCan: Probability of Developing or Dying of Cancer, Version 6.7.4 Statistical Methodology and Applications Branch, Surveillance Research Program, National Cancer Insititute, 2015.

37 O'Brien S, Berman E, Borghaei H, *et al.* NCCN clinical practice guidelines in oncology: chronic myelogenous leukemia. *J Natl Compr Canc Netw* 2009;7:984–1023.

38 Berry DA, Cronin KA, Plevritis SK, *et al.* Effect of screening and adjuvant therapy on mortality from breast cancer. *N Engl J Med* 2005;353:1784–92.

39 Feuer EJ, Merrill RM, Hankey BF. Cancer surveillance series: interpreting trends in prostate cancer--part II: cause of death misclassification and the recent rise and fall in prostate cancer mortality. *J Natl Cancer Inst* 1999;91:1025–32.

40 Etzioni R, Gulati R, Tsodikov A, *et al.* The prostate cancer conundrum revisited: treatment changes and prostate cancer mortality declines. *Cancer* 2012;118:5955–63.

41 Fedewa SA, Sauer AG, Siegel RL, Jemal A. Prevalence of major risk factors and use of screening tests for cancer in the United States. *Cancer Epidemiol Biomarkers Prev* 2015;24:637–52.

42 Cook MB, Dawsey SM, Freedman ND, *et al.* Sex disparities in cancer incidence by period and age. *Cancer Epidemiol Biomarkers Prev* 2009;18:1174–82.

43 Bach PB, Schrag D, Brawley OW, *et al.* Survival of blacks and whites after a cancer diagnosis. *JAMA* 2002;287:2106–13.

44 Torre LA, Bray F, Siegel RL, *et al.* Global cancer statistics, 2012. *CA Cancer J Clin* 2015;65:87–108.

45 Espey DK, Wu XC, Swan J, *et al.* Annual report to the nation on the status of cancer, 1975–2004, featuring cancer in American Indians and Alaska Natives. *Cancer* 2007;110:2119–52.

46 Siegel RL, Fedewa SA, Miller KD, *et al.* Cancer statistics for Hispanics/Latinos, 2015. *CA Cancer J Clin* 2015;65:457–80.

47 Proctor BD, Semega JL, Kollar MA. US Census Bureau Current Population Reports, P60-252. Income and Poverty in the United States: 2015. Washington, D.C.: U.S. Census Bureau, 2016.

48 Siegel R, Ward E, Brawley O, Jemal A. Cancer statistics, 2011: the impact of eliminating socioeconomic and racial disparities on premature cancer deaths. *CA Cancer J Clin* 2011;61:212–36.

49 Jemal A, Thun MJ, Ries LA, *et al.* Annual report to the nation on the status of cancer, 1975–2005, featuring trends in lung cancer, tobacco use, and tobacco control. *J Natl Cancer Inst* 2008;100:1672–94.

50 Behavioral Risk Factor Surveillance System (BRFSS), Centers for Disease Control and Prevention, 2015. Public Use Data File, 2016.

2

Fundamentals of Cancer Epidemiology

Susan M. Gapstur and Eric J. Jacobs

Epidemiology Research Program, American Cancer Society, Atlanta, Georgia, USA

"An ounce of prevention is worth a pound of cure"

Benjamin Franklin

Introduction

Epidemiology (from Greek "epi" = upon and "demos" = people) is the study of the factors that influence health and disease occurrence and distribution in populations, and is the scientific foundation of public health and preventive medicine.

Several early observations were critical in launching the field of cancer epidemiology. For example, in 1713, Bernardino Ramazzini, an Italian physician, reported the virtual absence of cervical cancer and relatively high incidence of breast cancer in nuns, and hypothesized that these findings were related to their celibate lifestyle. These observations were an important first step towards understanding the role of sexually transmitted infections and hormones in cancer etiology. In 1761, John Hill, a London physician, wrote the book *Cautions Against the Immoderate Use of Snuff* in which he linked tobacco (snuff) to cancer risk. These observations led to epidemiologic research in the 1950s and early 1960s that established smoking as a cause of lung cancer, which was recognized in the 1964 United States (US) Surgeon General's report on *Smoking and Health*. In 1775, Percivall Pott, an English surgeon, described cancer of the scrotum in chimney sweeps, establishing a link between an occupational exposure and cancer. This research led to many studies identifying other carcinogenic occupational exposures that informed the development of policies to establish limits on those exposures [1].

Critically important methodological developments subsequently contributed to advancements in cancer epidemiology. William Farr and Marc d'Espine created a nomenclature system for grouping diseases in the mid-nineteenth century. This nomenclature formed the basis for the International Classification of Disease, which is used to code cause of death. In the early part of the twentieth century, the first population-based cancer registries were established for the collection of information on newly diagnosed cancer cases. In the US, cancer registries now exist in all 50 states and Puerto Rico, and play a critical role in identifying cancer cases for epidemiologic studies. Over the past century, new laboratory and computer technologies, study designs and statistical methods for data analyses have enhanced the contribution of cancer epidemiology to cancer surveillance and to the identification of host, lifestyle, and environmental factors that increase or reduce risk of cancer.

A comprehensive review of epidemiologic methods is beyond the scope of this chapter, and can be found in many epidemiology textbooks. Instead, this chapter is intended to provide the reader with a fundamental understanding of key terminology, different types of study design, measures of associations, threats to validity, approaches to combining results from several studies, and criteria for judging causal relationships. Understanding these concepts is important because evidence from well-designed epidemiologic research guides clinical and public health practice, regulations, policies, and guidelines.

Exposures and Disease Occurrence

In epidemiologic investigations, the term "exposure" is used broadly to describe a factor that may be associated with higher or lower risk of disease. Exposures may relate to an agent (sometimes broadly referred to as "environmental" factor), person, place, or time. More specifically, exposures can include sociodemographic factors (e.g., age, sex, race, ethnicity, education, income), behavioral or lifestyle factors (e.g., tobacco smoking, alcohol consumption, poor diet or nutrition, physical inactivity, sun exposure), medical factors (e.g., high body mass index, diabetes mellitus status, reproductive characteristics), biomarkers (e.g., circulating markers, urinary markers), genetic and epigenetic factors (e.g., white blood cell telomere length, germline genetic variants), and classical environmental factors including aspects of the chemical, physical, and biological

Table 2.1 Basic measures of cancer occurrence or burden used in epidemiology.

Measure	Definition
Case counts	Number of cancer cases or deaths (usually new cases or deaths in a year)
Prevalence	Proportion of the population with cancer at one point in time
Incidence rate	Number of new cancer cases per 100,000 persons per year
Mortality rate	Number of new cancer deaths per 100,000 persons per year
Survival rate	Proportion of cancer patients surviving for a given period of time (usually 5 years in cancer)

environment such as exposure to ozone or infectious organisms. Detailed information on cancer-specific risk factors, including genetic and medical factors, reproductive factors, infectious agents, occupational and environmental contaminants, and lifestyle factors such as tobacco, nutrition, physical activity, and sun exposure are described in other chapters of this textbook.

Several different measures describe the burden of cancer as defined in Table 2.1. Understanding the differences between these measures is essential for medical and public health professionals.

Case counts are the number of individuals with a specific type of cancer (e.g., invasive breast cancer or multiple myeloma) at one point in time, or who develop or die of cancer over a given period. They are used in the numerator for computing prevalence, incidence, mortality, and survival statistics. Case counts are generally identified through hospital, state and national registries, or death certificates. The prevalence of a cancer (also called point prevalence) is the number of people with that cancer (regardless of when it was diagnosed) divided by the total number of people in the population at a particular point in time. While prevalence is sometimes referred to as a prevalence rate, this is incorrect because, by definition, it does not specify any unit of time over which the cases occurred. By themselves, case counts and prevalence estimates are most useful for planning and allocation of resources and less useful for epidemiologic investigations of disease causation.

Measures frequently used in cancer surveillance and etiology research include incidence rates, mortality rates, and survival rates. An incidence rate is the number of new cases of a disease (e.g., cancer) in a population during a specified time period, divided by the total number of person-years in that population. Similarly, the mortality rate is the number of deaths from a disease (e.g., cancer) in a population during a specified time period, divided by the total number of person-years in that population. These measures can provide quite different information. For example, among women aged 55 and older in the US, the incidence rate and prevalence of breast cancer is higher than the incidence rate and prevalence of lung cancer. However, because of the low survival rate among women with lung cancer, the lung cancer mortality rate is considerably higher than that for breast cancer.

Study Designs

Epidemiologic studies are often classified as either descriptive or analytic. Descriptive epidemiologic studies typically report patterns of disease occurrence or health-related factors (e.g., the prevalence of smoking) by demographic characteristics, place, and/or time. Such studies can provide early clues about etiology and generate hypotheses, but are not designed to test specific hypotheses about exposure–disease associations.

Descriptive studies often use routinely collected data including cancer registry or surveillance data, national surveys, census information, employment records, or clinical records. Cancer surveillance data, often gathered by cancer registries, are used to compute annual cancer incidence rates, mortality rates, prevalence, and survival. Such surveillance data are useful for describing cancer occurrence for specific geographic regions, over time and among demographic groups such as those based on age, race/ethnicity, and gender. In addition, cross-sectional surveys are used to describe the prevalence of a health condition or risk factor in a population at specific points in time. For example, using data from the National Health and Nutrition Examination Survey, researchers described the prevalence of obesity in the US for different categories of sex, age, and race/ethnicity, and over time [2]. Case reports or case series can be considered descriptive studies, as they may include detailed information about a specific patient or group of patients with suggestive patterns of exposure. However, because case reports or case series lack a comparison group of people without the condition of interest, they are not suitable for making sound inferences about disease causation. Overall, the information generated from descriptive studies is important for identifying high-risk populations, for monitoring progress in cancer prevention, early detection and treatment, and for informing analytic studies of exposure–disease relationships.

Analytic epidemiologic studies, unlike descriptive studies, are specifically designed to test hypotheses about exposure–disease associations. There are two broad groups of epidemiologic study designs – experimental and observational. In an experimental study (discussed in more detail later in this section) the investigator increases or decreases exposure to the factor(s) of interest, usually based on random assignment, though not always. In contrast, in an observational analytic epidemiologic study, the investigator does not control the exposure of research study participants, but rather observes, records, and analyzes information as it exists.

There are several different types of observational study designs, including *ecologic studies, cross-sectional studies, case-control studies*, and *cohort studies*. Because these study designs have different strengths and limitations, it is useful to be able to distinguish them. The type of study design used will depend on factors including the characteristics of the cancer to be studied, the nature of the exposure (e.g., occupational, diet, medical) or intervention (e.g., screening tool), and the type and availability of pre-existing data.

Ecologic studies compare a group level measure of an exposure with a group level measure of an outcome. For example, an early ecologic study of diet and breast cancer showed a strong positive correlation between per capita fat intake and breast cancer mortality rates across 39 countries [3]. However, countries with high fat intake may differ substantially in many ways from countries with low fat intake. It is possible that other breast cancer risk factors correlated with per capita fat intake, such as body mass index, explained the observed correlation with breast cancer mortality. Because only country level information on fat intake was available, it was difficult to determine if this association also existed at the level of the individual. This potential difference in detecting an association at the group vs the individual level is known as the "ecologic fallacy". Ecologic studies are typically less able to statistically adjust for correlated risk factors than studies with detailed information collected from individuals. Therefore, studies that rely on individual level data are often preferable to ecological studies.

Cross-sectional studies can be used to examine exposure–disease relationships at one point in time based on individual level data, and often rely on data that already exist or data that can be collected relatively quickly and cost-effectively. Cross-sectional studies can be informative about exposure–disease relationships when the exposure does not change as a result of the disease and the disease is unlikely to be fatal. For example, a cross-sectional study would be reasonable for examining an association between germ-line genetic mutations, which do not change as a result of the outcome, and the prevalence of colorectal polyps, which for most people does not lead to premature death. However, if the exposure changes as a result of the disease or if the disease has a poor survival, then the estimate of association between an exposure and a disease might not be valid. For example, in a cross-sectional study examining the association between heavy alcohol drinking and the prevalence of pancreatic cancer, individuals with pancreatic cancer might have reduced their alcohol consumption because they were not feeling well, potentially underestimating the true association between alcohol consumption and risk of pancreatic cancer. Moreover, as pancreatic cancer is usually rapidly fatal, individuals alive with pancreatic cancer at any point in time will tend to be those with less rapidly fatal forms of the disease, and therefore are unlikely to be representative of pancreatic cancer cases in general.

Case-control studies and *cohort* studies are the two most commonly used study designs in analytic epidemiology. In a case-control study of cancer, newly diagnosed cancer cases in a defined population and time period are identified and enrolled, and their exposure history is compared to that of a random sample of "control" individuals from the same source population as the cases, without the cancer of interest. In a case-control study, exposure information collected from cases and controls must refer to the time period prior to disease so that temporal relationships between an exposure and a disease can be reasonably inferred. An example of a case-control study is the Western Australia Bowel Health Study [4]. In that study, colorectal cancer cases diagnosed between 2005 and 2007 were identified through the Western Australia state cancer registry, and randomly selected controls were identified from the Western Australia state voter registration rolls from the same time period (voter registration is compulsory in Australia). Both cases and controls then completed a questionnaire asking about colorectal cancer risk factors, such as physical activity.

Case-control studies are a valuable research design, and are particularly well-suited for studying rare diseases, including many cancers, which can be difficult to study in cohort studies. Compared to cohort studies, they require fewer participants and can often provide results more quickly. However, they generally examine only a single type of cancer outcome. Several different biases can arise in case-control studies and should be kept in mind. For example, recall bias can occur in a case-control study if cases report their prior exposure differently than controls. Evidence of recall bias is well-illustrated in studies of induced abortion and breast cancer. Early case-control studies were suggestive of a positive association between induced abortion and risk of breast cancer. However, the stigma of induced abortion can create the appearance of associations between abortion and breast cancer risk where there is none. That is, cases (women with breast cancer) are more likely to report their reproductive history accurately, including that they had an induced abortion, than controls (women without breast cancer). This "recall bias" in case-control studies led to a positive estimate of the association between induced abortion and breast cancer risk that was not subsequently replicated in prospective cohort studies, leading a number of groups with expertise on this topic, including the American College of Obstetricians and Gynecologists, to determine that induced abortion is not associated with an increased risk [5].

In *cohort* studies, information about exposures is collected from a group of generally healthy individuals, or individuals without the disease of interest, and then this group is followed over time to determine who develops disease. Cohort studies can be either prospective or retrospective. In *a prospective cohort study*, exposure information is collected at the start of the study and then cases of disease are identified as they occur over time, usually over many years or even decades. Prospective cohort study populations can be defined and selected on the basis of different factors. For example, some prospective cohorts are defined by geographic area (e.g., the Iowa Women's Health Study, a population-based cohort of postmenopausal women [6]), or by occupation (e.g., the Nurses' Health Study) [7]. The study population for other cohorts can be more broadly defined, such as the American Cancer Society's (ACS) Cancer Prevention Study-II, which includes men and women recruited by ACS volunteers nationwide [8]. In a *retrospective cohort study*, previously recorded information on exposure and disease occurrence over time in a defined group of people is assembled and analyzed. Retrospective cohort study designs are commonly used to investigate occupational exposure–disease relationships.

Cohort studies have both notable advantages and disadvantages. Compared to case-control studies, there is little potential for bias from "differential" recall of exposure, because recall is unlikely to differ systematically between those who go on to develop cancer and those who do not. In addition, unlike in case-control studies, absolute incidence and mortality rates can be calculated within the cohort, and many different disease outcomes can be studied. However, prospective cohort studies can be costly due to the high cost of following a large number of participants over time, and many years may be needed to obtain results, particularly for rare cancers. Despite these disadvantages, a well-conducted prospective cohort study – particularly one in which follow-up exposure information is updated and loss of study participants is minimized – can provide strong evidence for or against causal associations between risk factors and disease outcomes, including cancer.

Participants in cohort studies are usually not representative of the general population. Although this does not threaten the internal validity of associations observed within a cohort, the generalizability of associations observed in cohorts to other populations should be considered. However, experience has shown that biologic associations between exposure and disease are usually generalizable. For example, while participants in the British Doctors Study from the 1950s were in no way representative of the British general population, the association between cigarette smoking and risk of lung cancer observed in the British Doctors Study has subsequently been observed in a wide variety of other study populations [9].

Experimental (or intervention) studies are conducted among individuals or among groups to evaluate the efficacy or effectiveness of treatments, procedures, behavioral or lifestyle changes, programs, or services on a specific outcome or outcomes. Unlike an observational study in which the investigator does not intervene to change the participants' exposure, in an experimental study participants are assigned to different groups in an attempt to modify exposure to a specific factor. In a "single-blinded" experimental study, study subjects do not know which exposure groups (i.e., treatment vs placebo or standard of care) they have been assigned to whereas in a "double-blinded" study neither the study subject nor the investigator knows who is assigned to which exposure group. Therefore, in a single-blinded study, potential bias introduced by the perceptions of study subjects is minimized, whereas in a double-blinded study potential bias from both the perceptions of the study subjects and the investigators is minimized.

In most experimental studies (though not all) assignment of individuals or groups to the exposure is done randomly. Studies in which the exposure is randomly assigned are usually referred to as randomized trials or randomized clinical trials. Random assignment assures that the exposure groups are, on average, comparable on all other factors – both known and unknown – except the exposure (often a treatment or intervention), making it unlikely that differences in outcomes between exposure groups can be explained by other factors. When feasible, randomized trials are considered to provide the most reliable evidence that an exposure causes or prevents a disease.

Despite the important advantages of randomized trials, they cannot be used to answer all research questions. Randomized trials are usually costly and, particularly for cancer outcomes, can take many years. In addition, it is unethical to assign participants to a potentially hazardous exposure from which they would be unlikely to benefit, such as a potent pesticide.

Measures of Association

Data collected in epidemiologic studies are used to quantitatively estimate associations between an exposure and a disease outcome. In cancer epidemiology, a common measure of association is the *rate ratio* (RR), sometimes referred to as the *risk ratio*. The rate ratio is the incidence rate of disease in individuals

Table 2.2 Hypothetical data from 1 year of follow-up in a cohort study of 400,000 men.

	Developed bladder cancer?		Total number of men
	Yes	No	
Current smokers (exposed)	400	99,600	100,000
Never smokers (not exposed)	300	299,700	300,000

with a particular exposure divided by the incidence rate in individuals without this exposure. For example, consider a hypothetical cohort study of men aged 55 years and older. If the observed incidence rate of bladder cancer among current cigarette smokers in this study was 400 per 100,000 person-years, and the observed incidence rate of bladder cancer among never smokers was 100 per 100,000 person-years, then the rate ratio for current smoking would be 4.0.

A closely related measure is the *relative risk*, which is the proportion of study participants in the exposed group who develop the disease during a defined time period divided by the same proportion among study participants in the unexposed group. For example, consider the hypothetical data shown in Table 2.2 from a cohort study that included only men aged 55 years and older who were current cigarette smokers or never smokers, and followed them for 1 year. The relative risk is 400/100,000 divided by 300/300,000, or 4.0. The relative risk is technically a different measure than the rate ratio because it is based on counts while the rate ratio is based on rates that include person-years in the denominator. However, the relative risk will be virtually identical to the rate ratio when the disease outcome is relatively uncommon (as is true in most studies of cancer) and/or when the time period under observation is relatively short.

Odds ratios from case-control studies of incident cancer outcomes can nearly always be interpreted the same way as a relative risk. For example, it would be accurate to say that in this study current smoking compared to never smoking was associated with fourfold higher risk of developing bladder cancer. More comprehensive explanations of the derivation and use of these and other measures of associations can be found in standard epidemiology textbooks.

As described later in this section, the size of rate ratios, relative risks and odds ratios is one of several criteria used when assessing whether an association is causal. Once an association is established as causal, however, measures of *absolute risk* are more relevant than measures of relative risk, both clinically and for public health.

Absolute risk due to an exposure is often measured by the *attributable risk*, sometimes referred to as the *risk difference*, or *rate difference*. Attributable risk is defined as the difference in incidence or mortality rates between the exposed and unexposed, and represents the excess rate of disease in the exposed group that can be attributed to the exposure.

Table 2.3 illustrates relative risks and attributable risks using results from a large ACS study comparing men who were

Table 2.3 Relative risk and attributable risk of cancer mortality by pipe smoking.

	Rate per 100,000 person-years in pipe smokers	Rate per 100,000 person-years in never smokers	Relative risk	Attributable risk per 100,000 person years
Pancreatic cancer	45.9	29.1	1.6	16.8
Esophageal cancer	14.4	6.0	2.5	8.4

exclusive pipe smokers with those who had never smoked [10]. The relative risk associated with pipe smoking was greater for esophageal cancer mortality (2.5) than for pancreatic cancer mortality (1.6). However, because deaths from esophageal cancer were less common than deaths from pancreatic cancer, the attributable risk was greater for pancreatic cancer mortality than for esophageal cancer mortality. These results therefore suggested that a man's pipe smoking is more likely to cause him to die from pancreatic cancer than from esophageal cancer.

Another measure of absolute risk is the *population attributable risk*, which provides an estimate of the health impact of an exposure on a population taking into account how common the exposure is. The population attributable risk is defined as the difference between the incidence or mortality rate in the overall population (both exposed and unexposed) and that in just the exposed portion of the population. For example, if the incidence rate of pancreatic cancer in the entire population of women in the US aged 55 years and older was 50 per 100,000 person-years, and the incidence rate among women of this age in the US who had never smoked was 40 per 100,000 person-years, then the population attributable risk for smoking would be 10 per 100,000 person-years. The population attributable risk depends on both the strength of the exposure–disease association (i.e., the relative risk) and how common the exposure is. A common exposure with a relatively low relative risk may have a larger population attributable risk than a rare exposure with a high relative risk.

Threats to Validity

Before an association can be considered potentially causal it is important to consider the possibility that it is a chance finding (random error), or a result of systematic error caused by information bias, selection bias, and/or confounding. These systematic errors can result from limitations in the study design, data collection, or statistical analysis.

The role of chance, or random error, needs to be considered in the interpretation of epidemiologic results. Most epidemiologic investigations test hypotheses about whether an exposure increases or decreases the risk of disease based on data collected from a sample of a larger underlying population. Statistical hypothesis testing begins with stating the null hypothesis, which, for example, is that the risk of disease in the exposed group is the same as that in the unexposed group. Then statistical techniques are used to ask, if the null hypothesis is true, what is the probability of detecting an association as large as or larger than the one observed? This probability is known as the *P*-value. In biomedical research, an association with a *P*-value of 0.05 or smaller is often described as "statistically

significant", and interpreted as being less likely to be due to chance. For any given true association, the size of the *P*-value is closely related to the sample size (a.k.a., power) of the study. The larger the sample size, the lower the *P*-value is likely to be, and the more likely the association will be found to be statistically significant. Conversely, studies with small sample sizes are less likely to find an association to be statistically significant.

Even very low *P*-values cannot be used to infer causality because other information also is necessary to draw such conclusions. Indeed, an observed association that is "statistically significant" may still be due purely to chance. The plausibility of an association needs to be taken into account when assessing how likely it is to be due to chance. For example, a statistically significant association between astrological sign and cancer risk may be more likely to be a chance finding than a similar association between cigarette smoking and cancer risk.

As mentioned previously, when interpreting results of a study it is important to rule out systematic errors. Information bias is a type of systematic error that occurs when the exposure and/or outcome data are assessed inaccurately. Information bias is a particular concern when exposure assessment differs between those with disease (or who go on to develop disease) and those without disease. One type of information bias is recall bias, which was described above for the association between induced abortion and risk of breast cancer in the section on case-control studies. In that scenario, cases recalled and reported their history of induced abortion more accurately than controls resulting in an increased risk that was not replicated in cohort studies where all participants report their history before breast cancer occurs.

Selection bias is a second type of systematic error, which can occur when the participation rates of potential study subjects differ based on both exposure and disease status. Using the same example of induced abortion and breast cancer risk, selection bias would occur if cases that agreed to participate represented all cases in the population but women with a history of induced abortion were less likely to agree to participate as controls. Information and selection bias can be minimized by using a carefully developed study protocol, properly training data collection staff, and maintaining high study response rates and data quality.

Confounding is a third type of systematic error which can occur when another exposure (i.e., the confounder) is related to both the main exposure of interest and the disease outcome. Confounding is well-illustrated by a study of the relationship between coffee drinking and risk of oral/pharyngeal cancer. In many populations, heavy coffee drinkers are more likely to smoke cigarettes and drink alcohol than people who do not drink coffee. In addition, cigarette smoking and alcohol consumption increase risk of oral/pharyngeal cancer. Without proper consideration of smoking and drinking, heavy coffee consumption will be associated with increased risk of oral/pharyngeal cancer even if coffee has no effect on oral/pharyngeal cancer (or possibly even if it was beneficial). Therefore, examination of the relationship between coffee consumption and risk of oral/pharyngeal cancer requires approaches to deal with confounding by cigarette smoking and alcohol drinking.

Several approaches can be used to deal with confounding in observational epidemiologic studies. One approach is to adjust for smoking and drinking history using commonly available statistical methods during the study analysis. Indeed, in a recent analysis of data from a large prospective cohort study of men and women, before adjustment for smoking history, the relative risk for consumption of more than four cups/day of coffee compared to no coffee consumption in relation to fatal oral/pharyngeal cancer was 1.52; however, after statistical adjustment for smoking history, alcohol consumption and other potential confounding factors, the relative risk was 0.58 [11]. An alternative approach for minimizing or eliminating the effects of known confounding factors is to exclude participants who have been or are exposed to the known confounding factors, effectively eliminating the confounding factor. In addition, in case-control studies, the investigator may consider selecting cases and controls who are matched on one or more known confounders, although such matching must be accounted for in the statistical analysis and will make it impossible to examine the association of the matching factor with risk of the disease outcome. Although these approaches can be quite effective, particularly when confounders are known and well-measured, no observational study can entirely rule out confounding, as not all confounding factors may be known.

Summarizing or Combining Data from Multiple Studies

Summarizing evidence from epidemiologic studies on specific exposure–disease relationships can be useful when findings from different studies are inconsistent, or when individual studies are limited in size, particularly if the strength of association is weak. Approaches for summarizing epidemiologic evidence include traditional narrative reviews, meta-analyses, and pooled analyses. Traditional narrative reviews provide a qualitative assessment of the state of the evidence from multiple individual observational and/or experimental studies. Epidemiologic meta-analyses typically combine published relative risks or odds ratios from multiple individual studies to calculate a summary estimate of the relative risk. The contribution of each study to the summary risk estimate is weighted according to its size, so that larger studies have more influence. In contrast, in pooled analyses, data on individual study participants from several studies are combined into a single data set, which is then used to calculate an overall risk. If well-conducted, all of these approaches can be useful for better understanding the association between an exposure and risk of cancer.

Narrative reviews, meta-analyses, and pooled analyses have all become increasingly available and it is important to understand their strengths and limitations. A strength of narrative reviews and meta-analyses is that they can be done quickly as they make use of already published results. However, published studies often vary widely in study design and quality. It is critical that narrative reviews, meta-analyses and pooled analyses consider and discuss differences between studies as well as the potential limitations of the individual studies they include. Both meta-analyses and pooled analyses provide more precise measures of exposure–disease relationships by combining results from individual studies. However, different studies are likely to have used different questions or other methods to assess exposure. Therefore, one concern in both meta-analyses and pooled analyses is that the level of detail included in a summary estimate for given exposure may sometimes be reduced to that of the study with the minimum amount of information.

Both reviews and meta-analyses can be affected by publication bias, which occurs when studies with null findings are less likely to be published than those with statistically significant results. Therefore, reviews or meta-analyses may overestimate the true strength of an association. Methods for detecting publication bias have been developed and can be incorporated into meta-analyses and reviews [12, 13]. Publication bias, however, may be less likely to occur in pooled analyses, because even when a study has not been published due to imprecise or null findings, investigators are often willing to contribute data to a pooled analysis. Through efforts such as the National Cancer Institute's Cohort Consortium [14], there is a growing body of research using pooled analyses to examine uncommon exposures (for example low frequency genetic variants) and/or rare cancers (e.g., male breast cancer).

"Proof" of Causality

The strongest evidence for a causal association between an exposure and a disease comes from randomized trials that compare incidence or mortality rates between individuals who were randomized to receive an exposure and those who were not. However, as noted above, it is unethical to conduct experiments exposing humans to agents that cause or are suspected to cause diseases such as cancer. Therefore, it is often necessary to assess evidence carefully for causality from the body of observational epidemiologic studies.

Guiding principles about the total body of epidemiologic evidence that constitutes "proof" of a causal relationship have been proposed to help inform public health and clinical policies, guidelines and recommendations. In the 1964 Surgeon General's Report on Smoking and Health, the Advisory Committee of the US Public Health Service described five principles that were considered in determining that the associations between smoking and several diseases found in observational epidemiologic studies were causal [15]. These principles were subsequently expanded by Sir Austin Bradford Hill and are described in Table 2.4 [16]. Importantly, no single principle is sufficient to infer that an exposure is causally related to a disease.

Organizations such as the World Health Organization's International Agency for Research on Cancer (IARC) apply

Table 2.4 Criteria for assessing causality between an exposure and cancer incidence and/or mortality.

(1)	Strength	A large (strong) relative risk or odds ratio is more likely to support a causal relationship than a small (weak) one. However, a small relative risk or odds ratio does not exclude the possibility of a causal relationship.
(2)	Consistency	The association is replicated in several studies of the same or different design, conducted by different investigators, under different circumstances and in different populations.
(3)	Specificity	The exposure is specific in causing tumors at one site or of one morphological/histological type. However, evidence of causality can be supported if the exposure causes cancer at multiple sites that share common carcinogenic pathways.
(4)	Temporality	There is evidence that the exposure preceded the onset of disease.
(5)	Gradient	The strength of association increases as dose or intensity of the exposure increases, or the association decreases as exposure decreases or is removed. However, the absence of a biologic gradient does not preclude a causal relationship.
(6)	Plausibility	A causal relationship is supported if there is evidence that the association is biologically plausible.
(7)	Coherence	The epidemiologic evidence is consistent with evidence from other types of research, and does not conflict with other types of research evidence or what is known about the exposure and the disease.
(8)	Experiment	Experimental evidence that removal of the exposure (e.g., in an occupational setting) reduces risk, or evidence from a clinical trial showing that administration of a treatment or preventive agent (e.g., selective estrogen receptor modulator prevention of breast cancer in high-risk women). This type of evidence is not always available.
(9)	Analogy	A similar exposure (e.g., chemical classes, hormonal factors) to the one of interest shows evidence of a causal relationship.

Source: adapted from Hill (1965) [16].

these and other criteria to support inferences about causal relationships between an exposure and cancer risk. Indeed, since the 1970s IARC has convened expert working groups to review the strength of scientific evidence on the carcinogenic effects of chemical, occupational, physical, biological, and lifestyle factors in order to identify the causes of human cancer. The information reviewed by the working groups and their conclusions are published in the *IARC Monographs on the Evaluation of Carcinogenic Risks to Humans* [17]. There are four primary areas of scientific evidence that are summarized and evaluated by the working groups: (1) exposure data based on production, use, occurrence and exposure levels in the environment, workplace and human body tissue/fluids; (2) human evidence based on epidemiological studies, including dose-response and other quantitative data if available; (3) evidence-based research in experimental animals; and (4) mechanistic and other relevant data including toxicokinetics and other mechanism(s) of carcinogenesis. The overall evaluation of the carcinogenicity of an agent to humans is based on the strength of the evidence derived from the entire body of research, and ultimately, the working group classifies an agent into one of five groups: Group 1, The agent is carcinogenic to humans; Group 2A, The agent is probably carcinogenic to humans; Group 2B, The agent is possibly carcinogenic to humans; Group 3, The agent is not classifiable as to its

carcinogenicity to humans; and Group 4, The agent is probably not carcinogenic to humans. A more detailed description of these classifications can be found in Chapter 8 of this textbook. Overall, these IARC reviews contributes to the scientific evidence on which international and national health agencies set policies to reduce human exposure to occupational and environmental carcinogens, and to promote healthy lifestyles.

Summary

Epidemiology has evolved considerably over the past century and has made critical contributions to what we know about the role of occupational, environmental, lifestyle, medical and host factors in cancer etiology. New advancements in molecular and genetic technologies continue to emerge, and epidemiologists are working in transdisciplinary teams with laboratory and clinical scientists to apply these methods to identify individuals at high risk of developing cancer. These results will be helpful for informing who might benefit from enhanced screening or chemoprevention recommendations (such as anti-estrogen use for prevention of breast cancer). Regardless, rigorous epidemiologic methodology and careful assessment of causality remain the foundation on which public health policies and guidelines are established.

References

1 Greenwald P, Dunn BK. Landmarks in the history of cancer epidemiology. *Cancer Res* 2009;69(6):2151–62.

2 Flegal KM, Carroll MD, Kit BK, Ogden CL. Prevalence of obesity and trends in the distribution of body mass index among US adults, 1999–2010. *JAMA* 2012;307(5):491–7.

3 Carroll KK. Experimental evidence of dietary factors and hormone-dependent cancers. *Cancer Res* 1975;35(11):3374–83.

4 Boyle T, Fritschi L, Heyworth J, Bull F. Long-term sedentary work and the risk of subsite-specific colorectal cancer. *Am J Epidemiol* 2011;173(10):1183–91.

5 Committee on Gynecologic Practice. ACOG Committee Opinion No. 434: induced abortion and breast cancer risk. *Obstet Gynecol* 2009;113(6):1417–8.

6 Folsom AR, Kushi LH, Anderson KE, *et al.* Associations of general and abdominal obesity with multiple health outcomes in older women: the Iowa Women's Health Study. *Arch Intern Med* 2000;160(14):2117–28.

7 Belanger CF, Hennekens CH, Rosner B, Speizer FE. The nurses' health study. *Am J Nurs* 1978;78(6):1039–40.

8 Calle EE, Rodriguez C, Jacobs EJ, *et al.* The American Cancer Society Cancer Prevention Study II Nutrition Cohort: rationale, study design, and baseline characteristics. *Cancer* 2002;94(2):500–11.

9 Doll R, Hill AB. The mortality of doctors in relation to their smoking habits; a preliminary report. *Br Med J* 1954;1(4877):1451–5.

10 Henley SJ, Thun MJ, Chao A, Calle EE. Association between exclusive pipe smoking and mortality from cancer and other diseases. *J Natl Cancer Inst* 2004;96(11):853–61.

11 Hildebrand JS, Patel AV, McCullough ML, *et al.* Coffee, tea, and fatal oral/pharyngeal cancer in a large prospective US cohort. *Am J Epidemiol* 2013;177(1):50–8.

12 Ioannidis JP, Trikalinos TA. The appropriateness of asymmetry tests for publication bias in meta-analyses: a large survey. *CMAJ* 2007;176(8):1091–6.

13 Ferguson CJ, Brannick MT. Publication bias in psychological science: prevalence, methods for identifying and controlling, and implications for the use of meta-analyses. *Psychol Methods* 2012;17(1):120–8.

14 National Cancer Institute Cohort Consortium. Available from: http://epi.grants.cancer.gov/Consortia/cohort.html (accessed 11 May 2017).

15 US Department of Health EaW, Public Health Service. *Smoking and Health: Report of the Advisory Comittee to the Surgeon General of the Publc Health Service.* United States Public Health Service, Office of the Surgeon General, Washington, D.C., 1964.

16 Hill AB. The environment and disease: association or causation? *Proc Roy Soc Med* 1965;58:295–300.

17 IARC Monographs on the Evaluation of Carcinogenic Risks to Humans. Available from: http://monographs.iarc.fr (accessed May 11 2017).

3

Socioeconomic Inequalities in Cancer Incidence and Mortality

Gopal K. Singh[1] and Ahmedin Jemal[2]

[1] *US Department of Health and Human Services, Health Resources and Services Administration, Office of Health Equity, Rockville, Maryland, USA*
[2] *Surveillance and Health Services Research, American Cancer Society, Atlanta, Georgia, USA*

Introduction

Monitoring health inequalities according to socioeconomic status (SES) and other key demographic factors such as race/ethnicity and rural/urban residence has long been an important focus of epidemiologic and public health research in the United States (US) [1–3]. Reduction of health inequalities by these characteristics has been an integral part of the national health policy initiative in the US for the past four decades [1, 2]. Previous research has shown the dynamic nature of socioeconomic disparities in cancer rates as the association between SES and incidence and mortality from major cancers has changed markedly during the past five decades [4–6]. Temporal patterns have changed largely as a result of differential rates of decline or increase in mortality among those in various SES or deprivation groups and changing socioeconomic patterns in major cancer risk factors such as smoking, diet, obesity, and physical inactivity [3–6].

Association between cancer mortality or incidence and SES, whether measured at the individual- or area-level, varies for specific cancers [3–15]. Area-based association is determined using cancer and socioeconomic data aggregated to a community or geographic area of residence such as counties or census tracts. Contemporary data indicate that higher SES is associated with lower rates of lung, stomach, liver, cervical, esophageal, and oropharyngeal cancer and higher rates of breast cancer and melanoma [3–17]. The major behavioral determinants of cancer, such as smoking, diet, alcohol use, obesity, physical inactivity, reproductive behavior, occupational and environmental exposures, and cancer screening are themselves substantially influenced by individual- and area-level socioeconomic factors [2, 3, 6, 14, 17–19].

Analyzing socioeconomic patterns in cancer mortality and incidence is important because it allows us to quantify cancer-related health disparities between the least and most advantaged socioeconomic groups and to identify areas or population groups that are at greatest risk of cancer diagnosis and mortality and who may therefore benefit from focused social and medical interventions [3, 6]. Such an analysis is also useful for tracking progress toward reducing health disparities in cancer as recent estimates of cancer disparities can be compared with those that prevailed in the previous decades [3, 6]. Comparison of cancer rates and trends across population groups or areas may provide important insights into the impact of cancer control interventions, such as smoking cessation, cancer screening, physical activity campaigns, and cancer treatment [3–6, 9].

Reliable individual-level SES data for all ages, particularly for ages 65 and older, are lacking on US death certificates, which provide the basis for computing cancer mortality rates for various demographic groups and geographic areas [3–6, 9, 20]. Individual-level data on education, income, and occupation are not available for cancer patients in the SEER database, which has been the primary source of data on cancer incidence, stage at diagnosis, treatment, and survival patterns in the US for the past four decades [6, 9, 15, 21]. Given such data limitations, population-based studies of socioeconomic disparities in cancer rates in the US have generally utilized area-based socioeconomic data linked to both individual- and aggregate-level cancer data [3–6, 9, 13, 16, 17]. Recent linkages of the census and Current Population Survey records with the National Death Index and cancer patient medical records have led to the development of the National Longitudinal Mortality Study (NLMS) and the SEER-NLMS Record Linkage Study [10, 15, 22, 23]. These longitudinal, cohort databases allow the estimation and analysis of cancer incidence, mortality, disease stage, and survival patterns according to individual-level socioeconomic characteristics [10, 15, 22, 23].

In this chapter, we examine temporal area–socioeconomic disparities in US all-cancer, lung, colorectal, prostate, breast, and cervical cancer mortality, and present area–socioeconomic patterns in cancer incidence using the SEER database. Using the linked NLMS data, we also present socioeconomic inequalities in mortality and incidence from all cancers combined and lung, colorectal, prostate, breast, cervical, stomach, liver, and esophageal cancers. Lung cancer is the leading cause of cancer mortality, and colorectal, prostate, and breast cancers are among the most commonly diagnosed cancers; these sites, along with stomach, liver, esophageal, and cervical cancer, contribute greatly to the overall cancer burden in the US [3, 20, 21, 24, 25].

Taken together, these cancers account for more than half of all cancer deaths and new cancer cases in the US [21, 24, 25]. Additionally, breast, cervical, colorectal, and prostate cancers are the cancer sites for which established screening tests have been introduced into the general population [3, 6, 25].

Data Sources and Methodology

Socioeconomic disparities in cancer mortality and incidence are examined by using three national data sources: the national mortality database, the NLMS, and the SEER cancer registry database [2, 3, 10, 20–22]. Since the vital-statistics-based national mortality database lacks reliable socioeconomic data for all ages, socioeconomic patterns in mortality were derived by linking census-based county-level socioeconomic data with the national mortality statistics [3–6, 9, 16]. A composite socio-economic deprivation index, developed for various census time periods, was used to define the socioeconomic standing of all 3,141 counties in the US and census tracts in the 11 SEER cancer registries. Indicators of education, occupation, wealth, income distribution, unemployment rate, poverty rate, and housing quality were used to construct the deprivation index [3–5, 26]. Higher index scores denote higher levels of SES and lower levels of deprivation. Index scores were categorized into five area groups, ranging from being the most deprived (first quintile) to the least disadvantaged (fifth quintile) county or neighborhood groups [3–6, 26]. Details of the US deprivation index are provided elsewhere [3–5, 26].

Cancer mortality and incidence rates for each county, area deprivation, or individual-level socioeconomic group were age-adjusted by the direct method using the age-composition of the 2000 US population as the standard [6, 15, 20, 21]. Log-linear models were used to estimate annual rates of change in SES-specific mortality trends from 1950 to 2013 [16, 17]. Socioeconomic disparities in mortality and incidence, estimated separately for men and women, were described by rate ratios (relative risks) and rate differences (absolute inequalities), which were tested for statistical significance at the 0.05 level. When using the NLMS data, cohort-based incidence and mortality rates were computed using the person-years approach [15, 22].

Socioeconomic Disparities in Cancer Mortality Based on Aggregate County-Level Data

Figure 3.1 shows changing socioeconomic patterns in US all-cancer mortality rates over time. Between 1950 and 2007, there was a gradual change from higher cancer mortality in high-SES areas to higher mortality in low-SES areas. The correlation between area-level SES and all-cancer mortality rates changed

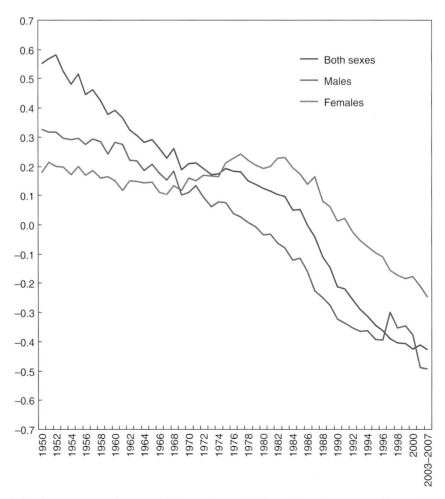

Figure 3.1 Weighted correlations between area socioeconomic index and county-level age-adjusted cancer mortality rates, US, 1950–2007.

from +0.55 in 1950 to −0.43 in 2007. The relationship between SES and all-cancer mortality rates reversed earlier for males than females. Between 1950 and 2007, the correlation changed from +0.33 to −0.50 for males and from +0.18 to −0.25 for females. Currently, there is a consistent, inverse SES gradient in all-cancer mortality rates. From 2009 to 2013, those in the most-deprived groups had a 19% higher mortality rate than those in the least-deprived group. Socioeconomic gradients and absolute inequalities are steeper for men than for women.

Compared to their counterparts in the least-deprived group, men had 25% higher mortality and women 11% higher mortality in the most-deprived group (data not shown).

Socioeconomic trends in lung cancer mortality differed for men and women. From 1950 to 1974, men in more affluent areas had higher lung cancer mortality than those in more deprived areas. Socioeconomic differentials reversed and started to widen by the early 1980s for men and by 2002 for women (Figure 3.2). From 2009 to 2013, socioeconomic

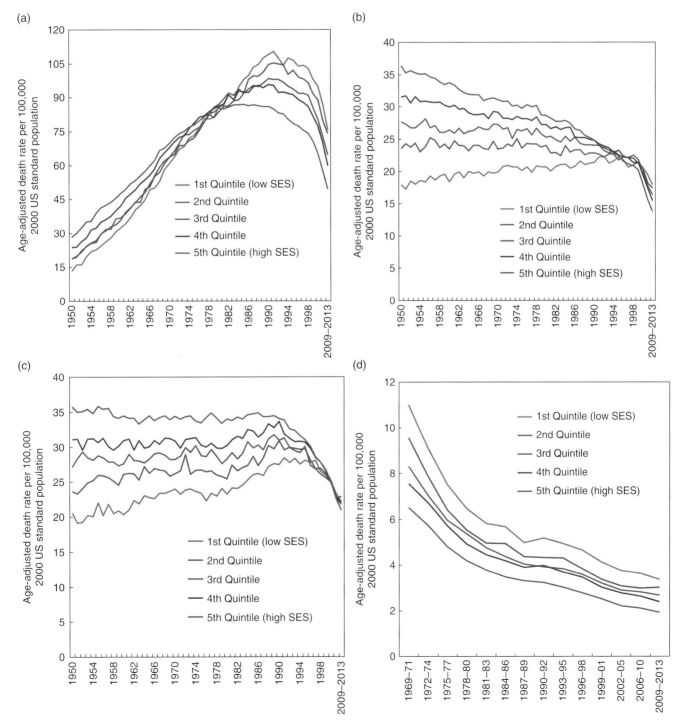

Figure 3.2 Trends in (a) lung, (b) colorectal, (c) female breast, and (d) cervical cancer mortality rates by area socioeconomic deprivation index, US, 1950–2013.

inequalities in lung cancer mortality were larger and more consistent for men than for women. Men and women in the most-deprived group had 54% and 16% higher lung cancer mortality rates than their most affluent counterparts, respectively.

From 1950 to 1990, lung cancer mortality among men increased at 5.1% per year in the most-deprived group, significantly faster than the annual rate of increase of 2.8% for men in the most-affluent group. Moreover, from 1991 to 2013, lung cancer mortality fell at a more rapid pace for men in the more affluent groups (2.53% annually in the most-affluent group vs 1.61% in the most-deprived group). From 1950 to 2013, there were marked increases in lung cancer mortality among women in all deprivation groups, although the annual rate of increase in mortality was somewhat higher in the more deprived groups.

Socioeconomic trends in US colorectal cancer mortality changed dramatically between 1950 and 2013, with the positive SES gradients in mortality narrowing over time and then reversing at the turn of the twenty-first century (Figure 3.2). From 2009 to 2013, there was an inverse SES gradient, with those in the two most-deprived groups having 30% and 27% higher rates of colorectal cancer mortality than their most-affluent counterparts, respectively. From 1950 to 2013, colorectal cancer mortality increased at 0.25% per year in the most-deprived group, whereas it fell consistently in the higher SES groups; the annual rates of decline in mortality in the two most-affluent groups were 1.24% and 0.87%, respectively. Socioeconomic trends in colorectal cancer mortality were generally similar for men and women.

Prostate cancer mortality did not vary appreciably over time by area deprivation. However, during the past two decades, an inverse socioeconomic gradient in prostate cancer mortality was found, with mortality rates falling similarly in all deprivation groups between 1995 and 2013. From 2009 to 2013, men in the most-deprived group had 19% higher prostate cancer mortality than men in the most-affluent group.

Socioeconomic differences in breast cancer mortality have narrowed over time and appear to have reversed during the past decade, as higher deprivation levels are now associated with higher breast cancer mortality rates. The reversal of the trend has occurred as breast cancer mortality rates have declined over time for more affluent women and have increased or remained stable for women in more deprived groups. From 1950 to 2013, the breast cancer mortality rate increased by 0.54% annually for women in the most-deprived group, while it decreased by 0.48% per year for women in the most-affluent group. From 2009 to 2013, women in the most-deprived group had 6% higher mortality than their most-affluent counterparts. In 1950, women in the most-deprived group had 42% lower mortality than women in the most-affluent group (Figure 3.2).

Cervical cancer mortality rates in the US have declined consistently for the past six decades, and rates of mortality decline among women in all deprivation groups have been similar. However, despite the decline, substantial inverse socioeconomic gradients in cervical cancer mortality have persisted. From 2009 to 2013, women in the two most-deprived groups had 76% and 58% higher cervical cancer mortality rates, respectively, than their most-advantaged counterparts, a pattern of inequality that also characterized the trends from 1969 to 2010 (Figure 3.2).

Socioeconomic Disparities in Cancer Mortality Based on Individual-level Data

All-cancer mortality rates among men varied consistently by individual-level education and income levels. Men with less than a high school education had 70% higher cancer mortality than those with a college degree, whereas men below the poverty level had 43% higher cancer mortality than men with incomes ≥600% of the poverty level (Table 3.1). Although higher cancer mortality was associated with lower education and income levels in women, the gradients were less marked in women than in men. Socioeconomic inequalities in lung cancer mortality, especially among men, were very marked, with men with less than a high school education having 2.4 times higher lung cancer mortality, and those below the poverty level having 1.8 times higher mortality than their more educated and affluent counterparts. Education and income were also inversely related to female lung cancer mortality, with education having a stronger impact than income.

Both education and income were significantly associated with colorectal cancer mortality; men with less than a high school education had 53% higher mortality risk than those with a college degree. Both prostate and breast cancer mortality rates did not vary by education and income levels. There were steep education and income gradients in cervical cancer mortality, with women with less than a high school education and below the poverty level having 2.5 and 4.4 times higher cervical cancer mortality than women with the highest education and income levels, respectively. Rates of stomach, liver, and esophageal cancer mortality also varied substantially and inversely by education and income levels (Table 3.1). More recent follow-up data from the NLMS need to be analyzed to determine if the magnitude of SES disparities in major cancers has increased.

Socioeconomic Disparities in Site-Specific Cancer Incidence

The patterns of socioeconomic disparities in cancer incidence are generally similar to those in cancer mortality [6, 9]. According to the analysis of the 1988–1992 SEER data, higher neighborhood SES was associated with higher cancer incidence rates for the total population and for women in particular (data not shown) [6]. The male lung cancer incidence rate was 61% higher in the most-deprived than the least-deprived neighborhoods. Lung cancer incidence in women did not vary by neighborhood deprivation. Prostate cancer incidence rates increased with increasing neighborhood SES; men in the most-affluent neighborhoods had a 36% higher prostate cancer incidence rate than men in the most-deprived neighborhoods. Higher neighborhood SES levels were associated with higher breast cancer incidence rates. Women in the most-affluent neighborhoods had 47% higher breast cancer incidence rates than their most-disadvantaged counterparts. Cervical cancer incidence increased consistently with increasing deprivation levels. Women in the most-deprived neighborhoods had a 2.7 higher risk of cervical cancer than women in the most-affluent neighborhoods. Higher

Table 3.1 Age-adjusted all-cancer and site-specific cancer mortality rates per 100,000 population and relative risk (RR) of mortality among those aged ≥25 years by educational attainment and poverty status.

	Age-adjusted mortality			Age-adjusted mortality			Age-adjusted mortality		
	Rate	SE	RR	Rate	SE	RR	Rate	SE	RR
	All cancers combined, male			**All cancers combined, female**			**Lung cancer, male**		
Educational attainment (years)									
<12	418.15	4.14	1.57*	251.18	3.05	1.23*	153.05	2.53	2.36*
12	351.49	4.44	1.32*	228.32	2.59	1.12*	111.67	2.38	1.72*
13–15	334.57	6.92	1.26*	218.20	4.30	1.07	95.40	3.53	1.47*
16+	265.88	5.34	1.00	204.40	4.66	1.00	64.94	2.56	1.00*
Poverty status (ratio of family income to poverty threshold)									
<100%	425.92	8.01	1.43*	264.01	4.60	1.26*	151.81	4.82	1.83*
100–150%	418.24	7.99	1.40*	245.02	5.06	1.17*	146.93	4.83	1.77*
150–200%	396.53	7.47	1.33*	235.06	4.93	1.12*	138.87	4.44	1.67*
200–400%	360.04	3.99	1.21*	225.60	2.74	1.08*	115.51	2.20	1.39*
400–600%	320.14	5.35	1.07	216.11	3.90	1.03	99.99	2.86	1.20*
Above 600%	298.19	6.15	1.00	208.97	4.60	1.00	83.04	3.06	1.00
	Lung cancer, female			**Colorectal cancer, male**			**Colorectal cancer, female**		
Educational attainment (years)									
<12	58.82	1.51	1.83*	40.81	1.25	1.53*	29.21	0.95	1.16
12	52.84	1.22	1.65*	40.11	1.52	1.51*	25.91	0.89	1.03
13–15	46.06	1.98	1.44*	37.27	2.33	1.40*	24.45	1.46	0.97
16+	32.08	1.87	1.00	26.65	1.70	1.00	25.12	1.67	1.00
Poverty status (ratio of family income to poverty threshold)									
<100%	58.97	2.24	1.28*	39.54	2.41	1.24*	29.59	1.44	1.29*
100–150%	54.19	2.43	1.17*	41.59	2.47	1.31*	29.30	1.62	1.28*
150–200%	49.28	2.26	1.07	41.12	2.39	1.29*	28.20	1.63	1.23
200–400%	48.83	1.27	1.06	39.08	1.33	1.23*	25.75	0.93	1.12
400–600%	48.70	1.80	1.05	37.16	1.88	1.17	26.05	1.39	1.13
Above 600%	46.18	2.13	1.00	31.77	2.05	1.00	22.96	1.56	1.00
	Prostate cancer			**Breast cancer, female**			**Cervical cancer**		
Educational attainment (years)									
<12	49.50	1.29	1.03	39.76	1.30	0.89	6.76	0.58	2.49*
12	43.49	1.74	0.91	41.58	1.11	0.93	3.87	0.34	1.42
13–15	48.18	2.92	1.00	42.24	1.86	0.94	2.76	0.46	1.01
>16	47.97	2.49	1.00	44.88	2.12	1.00	2.72	0.53	1.00
Poverty status (ratio of family income to poverty threshold)									
<100%	45.36	2.51	0.95	44.84	1.98	1.13	8.34	0.90	4.39*
100–150%	49.93	2.52	1.04	41.39	2.22	1.04	6.29	0.88	3.31*
150–200%	47.62	2.53	0.99	42.70	2.17	1.08	4.99	0.79	2.63*
200–400%	49.60	1.58	1.03	41.78	1.19	1.05	3.88	0.36	2.04*
400–600%	43.90	2.22	0.92	38.86	1.64	0.98	2.61	0.42	1.37
Above 600%	47.95	2.78	1.00	39.69	1.98	1.00	1.90	0.45	1.00

(Continued)

Table 3.1 (Continued)

	Age-adjusted mortality			Age-adjusted mortality			Age-adjusted mortality		
	Rate	SE	RR	Rate	SE	RR	Rate	SE	RR
	Stomach cancer, male			**Stomach cancer, female**			**Liver and IBD cancer, male**		
Educational attainment (years)									
<12	14.50	0.76	1.92*	7.38	0.51	1.74*	8.47	0.60	1.34*
12	9.15	0.70	1.21	4.85	0.38	1.14	6.60	0.61	1.05
13–15	8.98	1.12	1.19	3.80	0.57	0.89	7.98	1.04	1.27
16+	7.56	0.92	1.00	4.25	0.68	1.00	6.30	0.76	1.00
Poverty status (ratio of family income to poverty threshold)									
<100%	14.00	1.44	1.65*	6.47	0.69	1.20*	10.47	1.27	1.43*
100–150%	13.89	1.41	1.64*	6.64	0.81	1.24*	8.43	1.16	1.15
150–200%	11.94	1.30	1.41*	6.03	0.79	1.12*	7.46	1.05	1.02
200–400%	11.61	0.71	1.37*	5.39	0.42	1.00*	6.74	0.53	0.92
400–600%	7.69	0.82	0.91	4.18	0.57	0.78	6.29	0.72	0.86
Above 600%	8.46	1.03	1.00	5.37	0.75	1.00	7.34	0.90	1.00
	Liver and IBD cancer, female			**Esophageal cancer, male**			**Esophageal cancer, female**		
Educational attainment (years)									
<12	4.20	0.40	1.84*	10.22	0.67	1.89*	3.02	0.34	1.24
12	3.13	0.30	1.37	10.13	0.71	1.88*	2.25	0.26	0.93
13–15	3.08	0.52	1.35	8.01	0.98	1.48*	2.76	0.49	1.14
16+	2.28	0.50	1.00	5.40	0.67	1.00	2.43	0.52	1.00
Poverty status (ratio of family income to poverty threshold)									
<100%	4.52	0.59	1.91*	13.77	1.48	1.90*	3.39	0.55	1.22
100–150%	5.25	0.74	2.22*	9.59	1.27	1.32	2.67	0.50	0.96
150–200%	3.44	0.58	1.45	10.72	1.24	1.48	3.32	0.60	1.19
200–400%	2.77	0.31	1.17	8.85	0.61	1.22	2.12	0.26	0.76
400–600%	2.83	0.45	1.19	7.42	0.75	1.02	2.19	0.40	0.78
Above 600%	2.37	0.49	1.00	7.24	0.87	1.00	2.79	0.54	1.00

Source: 1979–1998 National Longitudinal Mortality Study.
Mortality rates are age-adjusted to the 2000 US standard population.
* $P < 0.05$.

deprivation levels were associated with higher rates of stomach, liver, and esophageal cancer incidence. Compared to their most-affluent counterparts, those in the most-deprived neighborhoods had 64%, 90%, and 93% higher rates of stomach, liver, and esophageal cancer incidence, respectively.

The linked SEER-NLMS data show slightly different individual-level SES patterns in cancer incidence than the area-level patterns [15]. This is partly due to the different time periods covered in the two databases. Overall cancer incidence rates were 12–13% higher among the poor and those with less than a high school education compared to their most-educated or affluent counterpart [15]. Men and women with less than a high school education had 3.0 and 2.0 times higher lung cancer incidence rates, respectively than those with a college degree [15]. Those below the poverty level had 52–72% higher lung cancer incidence rates than their counterparts with incomes at ≥600% of the poverty level [15]. Individuals with the lowest education and income levels had higher colorectal cancer incidence rates

than their most-advantaged counterpart [15]. Higher education and income levels were associated with higher prostate and breast cancer incidence rates; men and women with less than a high school education had 21% and 26% lower prostate and breast cancer incidence rates, respectively, than their counterparts with a college degree [15]. Consistent with the neighborhood pattern, women with less than a high education had 3.2 times higher cervical cancer incidence than those with a college degree [15].

Summary and Conclusions

In this chapter, we have examined socioeconomic disparities in mortality and incidence from all cancers combined and from major cancers using both aggregate community- and individual-level data. Analysis of long-term trends and contemporary SES inequalities in cancer adds to the voluminous literature on

Table 3.2 Prevalence (%) of current smoking, obesity, and cancer screening by education and income/poverty level in the United States.

	Current smoking (male)	Current smoking (female)	Obesity (male)	Obesity (female)	Mammogram within the past 2 years[1]	Pap test within the past 3 years[1]	Ever had a Colonoscopy[1]
Educational attainment (years)							
Total	17.9	14.4	31.6	30.8	73.2	82.7	65.3
<High school	27.2	20.1	31.7	37.1	63.1	74.1	50.6
High school graduate	25.7	20.1	36.0	34.8	68.7	76.2	62.6
Some college/associate degree	19.7	17.0	37.0	35.2	73.7	82.4	66.4
College graduate +	7.2	5.7	23.8	21.8	80.2	89.0	73.4
Poverty status (ratio of family income to poverty threshold)							
<100%	34.1	26.4	31.7	40.4	64.1	76.8	48.0
100–200%	26.2	19.5	31.5	38.2	64.3	77.9	55.4
200–300%	19.8	15.9	33.9	33.1	69.1	80.5	64.4
300–400%	18.9	12.3	33.8	32.3	74.3	83.3	69.8
400–500%	13.3	9.4	31.7	26.7	78.0	87.4	70.7
Above 500%	9.7	7.8	30.0	21.6	81.0	88.2	73.7

Source: The 2014–2015 National Health Interview Survey.

Note: ages were ≥ 40 years for mammography, 25–64 years for Pap test, ≥50 years for colonoscopy, and ≥25 years for obesity and smoking.

[1] 2015 National Health Interview Survey, Cancer Control Supplement.

SES and cancer disparities. Socioeconomic patterns in US cancer mortality have reversed over time, and the continued widening of the inverse socioeconomic gradients in all-cancer, lung, and colorectal cancer mortality appears to be consistent with those observed for all-cause and cardiovascular disease mortality in the US [2, 3, 26].

Socioeconomic inequalities in cancer incidence and mortality in the US are particularly marked in lung, cervical, stomach, and liver cancer [3–6, 9, 10, 15]. Substantial socioeconomic disparities exist not only in cancer incidence and mortality but also in stage at cancer diagnosis and survival [3, 6, 9, 15, 23]. Such inequalities have been shown to exist for Whites, Blacks, and other major racial/ethnic groups such as Hispanics, Asians/Pacific Islanders, and American Indians/Alaska Natives [3, 6, 9].

Socioeconomic disparities in incidence and mortality from various cancers may reflect differences in smoking prevalence, dietary fat intake, obesity, physical inactivity, reproductive factors (e.g., delayed childbearing, childlessness, and breastfeeding), alcohol use, human papillomavirus (HPV) infection, cancer screening, and healthcare factors [3, 5, 6, 11, 14, 19, 27]. Higher smoking rates are more prevalent among men and women in lower SES groups and in more deprived areas (Table 3.2) [2, 5, 16, 19, 28]. Smoking rates have fallen more rapidly for those in higher SES groups, which largely explains temporal SES trends in all-cancer and lung cancer mortality rates [2, 4–6]. Dietary factors such as fat intake, red meat consumption, and high calorie intake have been mentioned as risk factors for colorectal, prostate, and breast cancer and inequalities in both incidence and mortality may in part reflect differences in these factors [3, 5, 6, 14]. Studies have found higher consumption of lower-quality diets and energy-dense foods and lower intakes of fruits and vegetables among lower SES groups but higher total calorie and fat intake among higher SES groups [2, 3, 18]. The higher prostate and breast cancer incidence rates in the more advantaged groups may partly reflect their higher utilization of screening.

Disparities in healthcare factors play a prominent role in producing socioeconomic disparities in mortality from colorectal, prostate, breast, and cervical cancer. Low-SES individuals and residents of more deprived neighborhoods have substantially higher rates of late-stage diagnoses of lung, colorectal, prostate, breast, and cervical cancer and significantly lower rates of cancer survival than their counterparts from more affluent neighborhoods or SES backgrounds [6, 9, 15, 23, 29–35]. Lack of health insurance, limited access to care, and lower rates of regular pap smear, mammography, and colorectal cancer screening among lower SES individuals (as shown in Table 3.2) and among residents of more disadvantaged areas may account for their higher rates of late-stage cancer diagnoses [2, 3, 6, 31–33]. However, lower cancer survival rates among the disadvantaged may not only reflect their higher rates of late-stage cancer diagnoses, but also less favorable cancer treatment or medical care [3, 6, 33].

Research suggests that SES and area deprivation levels do not fully account for racial/ethnic disparities in cancer incidence, mortality, and outcomes in the US [3, 6, 9, 10, 13]. For example, within each deprivation group, Blacks have higher all-cancer mortality rates than Whites. Indeed, the overall cancer mortality and incidence rates for Blacks in the most-affluent group are similar to or exceed those for Whites in the most-deprived group [3, 6]. Within each SES or deprivation group, black women have approximately two times higher cervical cancer mortality and 50% higher breast cancer mortality than white women [3, 6]. Black men in each deprivation group have at least two times higher prostate cancer mortality rates than their white counterparts [3, 6]. Such marked racial inequalities may exist partly because Blacks are socially and materially worse off than Whites across different socioeconomic strata [2, 3]. Moreover, they are more likely to be disadvantaged than Whites in health-risk behaviors, healthcare access and use, and cancer treatment and survival within each deprivation group [2, 3, 6].

Detection of cancer at an early, localized stage may be considered a marker for access to healthcare and preventive health services, including cancer screening [6, 25]. Studies have shown significant black–white and socioeconomic disparities in stage at cancer diagnosis [6, 9]. Within each SES or deprivation group, Blacks have a higher likelihood than Whites of being diagnosed with advanced-stage colorectal, prostate, breast, and cervical cancers [6, 9]. Additionally, even after controlling for stage at diagnosis, Blacks, in each deprivation group, have significantly lower survival rates from colorectal, prostate, breast, and cervical cancer than Whites [6, 9, 36–38].

Comparison with International Patterns

Although studies of cancer inequalities vary widely in their use of socioeconomic measures and coverage of time periods, socioeconomic disparities in US cancer mortality and incidence are generally consistent with patterns observed for the other industrialized countries [3, 11, 14]. Consistent with the US pattern, all-cancer mortality rates in England from 2004 to 2006 increased consistently by area deprivation levels [39]. In several European populations, cancer mortality rates are significantly higher among both males and females in lower education groups [11]. Consistent with the US pattern, lung cancer mortality rates for both men and women in Canada increased in relation to deprivation levels [40]. Higher lung cancer mortality rates are found among men in lower SES groups in many European countries [11, 41]. Inverse socioeconomic gradients in US colorectal cancer mortality rates are compatible with occupational and educational patterns in mortality observed among several European countries [11, 42]. Marked socioeconomic disparities in US cervical cancer mortality reported here are generally consistent with those shown for other industrialized countries. An approximately twofold higher cervical cancer mortality was found among women in low- rather than high-SES groups in a study that compared inequalities in various low/middle income countries, North America, and Europe, although the magnitude of socioeconomic inequalities was greater in North America than in Europe [39, 43, 44].

Caution should be exercised when comparing area-based SES effects with individual-level effects. Area socioeconomic measures are qualitatively different from individual-level SES and should be viewed as community, neighborhood, or social structural influences. Although area-based socioeconomic patterns in cancer mortality and incidence reported here are generally consistent with those at the individual level, the area-level effects are smaller in magnitude than individual-level SES effects [3, 6–10, 15]. This may partly be due to the compositional heterogeneity of the counties examined, which are socioeconomically more heterogeneous than census tracts [3–6]. Unfortunately, the national mortality database does not include census-tract geocodes because of confidentiality concerns [3, 20].

Cancer is the leading cause of mortality in the US for those aged <85 years and is the most prominent cause of death in terms of years of potential life lost [2, 3, 20]. The extent of socioeconomic disparities in cancer mortality and incidence reported here contributes greatly to overall health inequalities in the US. With large socioeconomic inequalities in smoking, obesity, and physical inactivity among young people continuing to persist, inequalities in US cancer mortality and incidence are not expected to diminish in the foreseeable future [2, 3]. Efforts to reduce cancer disparities, especially those in lung cancer, therefore might include tobacco control policies at the national and local levels that place greater smoking restrictions or legislate against smoking in public places, ban tobacco marketing, reduce tobacco availability, increase financial and other barriers to smoking, and provide targeted smoking cessation programs for those with low SES or in disadvantaged areas [3, 6]. Healthcare inequalities in the US have also risen in both absolute and relative terms and socioeconomic disparities in stage at diagnosis and survival from major cancers have persisted [3, 6]. These trends would also imply continuation of socioeconomic inequalities in cancer mortality and incidence. Health policies therefore should also enhance access to cancer screening programs among socioeconomically disadvantaged populations or those in rural and medically underserved areas. Lastly, social policy measures aimed at improving the broader social determinants, such as general living conditions and the social and physical environments, are needed to tackle health inequalities, including those in cancer mortality and incidence [3, 6].

The views expressed are the authors' and not necessarily those of the Health Resources and Services Administration or the US Department of Health and Human Services.

References

1 US Department of Health and Human Services. Healthy People 2020. Available from: http://www.healthypeople.gov/2020/default.aspx (accessed 11 May 2017).

2 National Center for Health Statistics. *Health, United States, 2011 with Special Feature on Socioeconomic Status and Health.* Hyattsville, MD: US Department of Health and Human Services, 2012.

3 Singh GK, Williams SD, Siahpush M, Mulhollen A. Socioeconomic, rural-urban, and racial inequalities in US cancer mortality: part I – all cancers and lung cancer and Part II–colorectal, prostate, breast, and cervical cancers. *J Cancer Epidemiol* 2012:1–27.

4 Singh GK, Miller BA, Hankey BF, Feuer EJ, Pickle LW. Changing area socioeconomic patterns in U.S. cancer mortality, 1950–1998: part I - all cancers among men. *J Natl Cancer Ins* 2002; 94(12):904–15.

5 Singh GK, Miller BA, Hankey BF. Changing area socioeconomic patterns in U.S. cancer mortality, 1950–1998: part II - lung and colorectal cancers. *J Natl Cancer Inst* 2002;94(12):916–25.

6 Singh GK, Miller BA, Hankey BF, Edwards BK. Area Socioeconomic Variations in U.S. Cancer Incidence, Mortality, Stage, Treatment, and Survival, 1975–1999. NCI Cancer Surveillance Monograph Series, No.4. Bethesda, MD: National Cancer Institute, 2003. NIH Publication No. 03-5417. Available from: http://seer.cancer.gov/publications/ses/index. html (accessed 11 May 2017).

7 Faggiano F, Partanen T, Kogevinas M, Boffetta P. Socioeconomic differentials in cancer incidence and mortality. *IARC Sci Publ* 1997;138:65–176.

8 Davey Smith G, Leon D, Shipley M, Rose G. Socioeconomic differentials in cancer among men. *Int J Epidemiol* 1991;20:339–45.

9 Singh GK, Miller BA, Hankey BF, Edwards BK. Persistent area socioeconomic disparities in U.S. incidence of cervical cancer, mortality, stage, and survival, 1975–2000. *Cancer* 2004;101(5):1051–7.

10 Singh GK, Siahpush M. All-cause and cause-specific mortality of immigrants and native born in the United States. *Am J Public Health* 2001;91(3):392–9.

11 Menvielle G, Kunst AE, Stirbu I, *et al.* Educational differences in cancer mortality among women and men: a gender pattern that differs across Europe. *Br J Cancer* 2008;98(5):1012–19.

12 Steenland K, Henley J, Thun M. All-cause and cause-specific death rates by educational status for two million people in two American Cancer Society cohorts, 1959–1996. *Am J Epidemiol* 2002;156(1):11–21.

13 Chu KC, Miller BA, Springfield SA. Measures of racial/ethnic health disparities in cancer mortality rates and the influence of socioeconomic status. *J Natl Med Assoc* 2007;99(10): 1092–104.

14 Kogevinas M, Pearce N, Susser M, Boffetta P. Social inequalities and cancer. *IARC Sci Publ* 1997;138:1–15.

15 Clegg LX, Reichman ME, Miller BA, *et al.* Impact of socioeconomic status on cancer incidence and stage at diagnosis: selected findings from the surveillance, epidemiology, and end results: National Longitudinal Mortality Study. *Cancer Causes Control* 2009; 20(4):417–35.

16 Singh GK, Siahpush M, Williams SD. Changing urbanization patterns in US lung cancer mortality, 1950–2007. *J Community Health* 2012;37(2):412–20.

17 Singh GK, Siahpush M, Altekruse SF. Time trends in liver cancer mortality, incidence, and risk factors by unemployment level and race/ethnicity, United States, 1969–2011. *J Community Health* 2013;38(5):926–40.

18 Singh GK, Siahpush M, Hiatt RA, Timsina LR. Dramatic increases in obesity and overweight prevalence and body mass index among ethnic-immigrant and social class groups in the United States, 1976–2008. *J Community Health* 2011;36(1):94–110.

19 Blackwell DL, Lucas JW, Clarke TC. Summary health statistics for U.S. adults: National Health Interview Survey, 2012. *Vital Health Stat* 2012;10(260):1–161.

20 Xu JQ, Murphy, SL, Kochanek KD, Bastian BA. Deaths: final data for 2013. *Nat Vital Stat Rep* 2016;64(2):1–118.

21 Howlader N, Noone AM, Krapcho M, *et al.* (eds) *SEER Cancer Statistics Review, 1975–2013.* Bethesda, MD: National Cancer Institute, 2016. Available from: http://seer.cancer.gov/ csr/1975_2013/ (accessed 11 May 2017).

22 US Census Bureau. National Longitudinal Mortality Study, Reference Manual. US Census Bureau, 2012. Available from: http://www.census.gov/did/www/nlms Washington, DC: /publications/reference.html (accessed 11 May 2017).

23 Du XL, Lin CC, Johnson NJ, Altekruse S. Effects of individual-level socioeconomic factors on racial disparities in cancer treatment and survival: findings from the National Longitudinal Mortality Study, 1979–2003. *Cancer* 2011;117(14):3242–51.

24 Jemal A, Simard EP, Dorell C, *et al.* Annual report to the nation on the status of cancer, 1975–2009, featuring the burden and trends in human papillomavirus (HPV)-associated cancers and HPV vaccination coverage levels. *J Natl Cancer Inst* 2013;105(3):175–201.

25 American Cancer Society. *Cancer Facts & Figures 2016.* Atlanta: American Cancer Society, 2016.

26 Singh GK. Area deprivation and widening inequalities in US mortality, 1969–1998. *Am J Public Health* 2003;93(7):1137–43.

27 Rim SH, Joseph DA, Steele, Thompson TD, Seeff LC. Colorectal cancer screening – United States, 2002, 2004, 2006, and 2008. *MMWR* 2011;60(Suppl):42–6.

28 National Center for Health Statistics. *The National Health Interview Survey, Questionnaires, Datasets, and Related Documentation: 2014–2015 Public Use Data Files.* Hyattsville, MD: US Department of Health and Human Services; 2015. Available from: http://www.cdc.gov/nchs/nhis/nhis_ questionnaires.htm (accessed 11 May 2017).

29 Mandelblatt J, Andrews H, Kerner J, Zauber A, Burnett W. Determinants of late stage diagnosis of breast and cervical cancer: the impact of age, race, social class, and hospital type. *Am J Public Health* 1991;81(5):646–9.

30 Parikh-Patel A, Bates JH, Campleman S. Colorectal cancer stage at diagnosis by socioeconomic and urban/rural status in California, 1988–2000. *Cancer* 2006;107(5 Supplement): 1189–95.

31 Baade PD, Turrell G, Aitken J. Geographic remoteness, area-level socio-economic disadvantage, and advanced breast cancer: a cross-sectional, multilevel study. *J Epidemiol Community Health* 2011;65(11):1037–43.

32 Kogevinas M, Porta M. Socioeconomic differences in cancer survival: a review of the evidence. *IARC Sci Publ* 1997;138:177–206.

33 Auvinen A, Karjalainen S. Possible explanations for social class differences in cancer patient survival. *IARC Sci Publ* 1997;138:65–176.

34 Coleman MP, Babb P, Sloggett A, *et al.* Socioeconomic inequalities in cancer survival in England after the NHS cancer plan. *Br J Cancer* 2010;103(4):446–53.

35 Bradley CJ, Given CW, Roberts C. Race, socioeconomic status, and breast cancer treatment and survival. *J Natl Cancer Inst* 2002;94(7):490–6.

36 McCarthy AM, Dumanovsky T, Visvanathan, *et al.* Racial/ethnic and socioeconomic disparities in mortality among women diagnosed with cervical cancer in New York City, 1995–2006. *Cancer Causes Control* 2010; 21(10)1645–55.

37 Robbins AS, Whittemore AS, Thom DH. Differences in socioeconomic status and survival among white and black men with prostate cancer. *Am J Epidemiol* 2000;151(4):409–16.

38 Marcella S, Miller JE. Racial differences in colorectal cancer mortality: the importance of stage and socioeconomic status. *J Clin Epidemiol* 2001;54(4):359–66.

39 Department of Health. Tackling Health Inequalities: 2007 *Status Report on the Programme for Action.* London: Health Inequalities Unit, Department of Health, 2007.

40 Wilkins R, Berthelot J, Ng E. Trends in mortality by neighbourhood income in urban Canada from 1971 to 1996. *Health Rep* 2002;13(Suppl):1–27.

41 Van der Heyden JHA, Schapp MM, Kunst AE, *et al.* Socioeconomic inequalities in lung cancer mortality in 16 European populations. *Lung Cancer* 2009;63(3):322–30.

42 Aarts MJ, Lemmens VEPP, Louwman MWJ, *et al.* Socioeconomic status and changing inequalities in colorectal cancer? A review of the associations with risk, treatment and outcome. *Eur J Cancer* 2010;46:2681–95.

43 Ng E, Wilkins R, Fung MFK, Berthelot J. Cervical cancer mortality by neighbourhood income in urban Canada from 1971 to 1996. *CMAJ* 2004;170(10):1545–9.

44 Parikh S, Brennan P, Boffetta P. Meta-analysis of social inequality and the risk of cervical cancer. *In J Cancer* 2003;105:687–91.

4

The Global Burden of Cancer

Ahmedin Jemal and Lindsey A. Torre

Surveillance and Health Services Research, American Cancer Society, Atlanta, Georgia, USA

Introduction

Global variations in cancer rates largely reflect differences in environmental risk factors rather than biologic differences [1, 2]. Early evidence of this came from studies documenting that cancer rates in successive generations of migrants shifted toward those of the host country. For example, colorectal cancer rates in 1950 in the third generation of Japanese immigrants to California approached those of white Californians [1, 2]. In general, cancers related to smoking, dietary patterns, and reproductive behaviors are the most common cancers in economically developed countries, whereas cancers related to infections predominate in economically developing countries (Figure 4.1). However, the cancer pattern in economically developing countries is changing; cancers associated with smoking, unhealthy diet, and overweight and obesity, such as lung, breast, and colorectal cancers, are becoming more common due in part to increasingly sedentary lifestyles associated with urbanization, as well as targeted advertisements by the tobacco and the food/beverage industries. The cancer burden in developing countries also is increasing because of the aging and growth of the population. This chapter provides an overview of the global descriptive epidemiology of commonly diagnosed cancers.

International Cancer Data Sources

Major sources of data for research on global cancer include national or regional cancer registries for incidence and national or regional vital registration for mortality. The World Health Organization's IARC (International Agency for Research on Cancer) compiles global cancer incidence and mortality data which is publicly available on its website (http://www-dep.iarc.fr/). IARC also estimates incidence, mortality, and prevalence for every country in the world using the best available data; these estimates are also publicly available at the GLOBOCAN website (globocan.iarc.fr). Issues affecting global cancer information include lack of cancer registries and/or vital registration in many countries, incomplete coverage of the population, or inadequate quality of registration.

Incidence and death rates in the IARC database and given in this chapter are age standardized to the 1960 world standard population (see Chapter 1 for description of age standardization). Therefore, these rates cannot be compared with rates age-standardized to a different standard population, for example, the 2000 US population as given in Chapter 1 of this book, or elsewhere.

All Cancer Sites

A total of 14.1 million new cancer cases and 8.2 million cancer deaths were estimated to have occurred in 2012 worldwide, with over 55% of the cases and 65% of the cancer deaths occurring in economically developing countries (Table 4.1). Although the overall cancer incidence rate in economically developed countries in both males and females is nearly twice as high as the rate in economically developing countries, overall cancer mortality rates are generally similar between economically developed and developing countries. Reasons for this pattern include differences in awareness, detection practice, completeness of case reporting, and survival. Overall, survival after a diagnosis of cancer is poorer in economically developing countries due to later stage at diagnosis and limited access to standard treatment (Figure 4.2). Further, the most commonly diagnosed cancers in economically developing countries are more likely to be fatal. For example, while the most common cancers among men in developed countries are prostate, lung, and colon and rectum, the most common cancers in developing countries are lung, liver, and stomach (Figure 4.1).

The American Cancer Society's Principles of Oncology: Prevention to Survivorship, First Edition. Edited by The American Cancer Society.
© 2018 The American Cancer Society. Published 2018 by John Wiley & Sons, Inc.

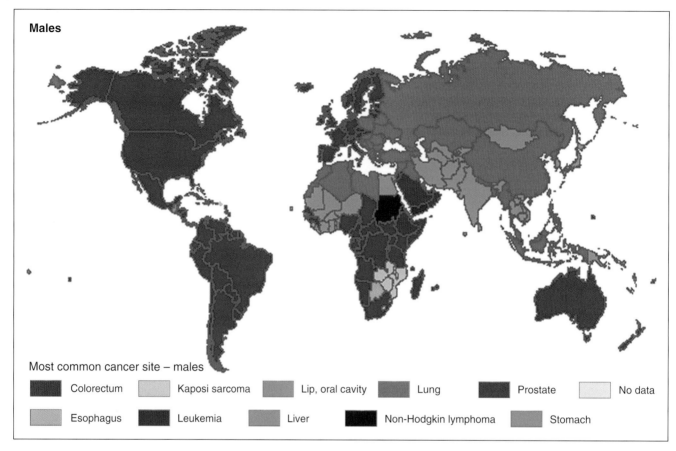

Most common cancer site – males

Colorectum	Kaposi sarcoma	Lip, oral cavity	Lung	Prostate	No data
Esophagus	Leukemia	Liver	Non-Hodgkin lymphoma	Stomach	

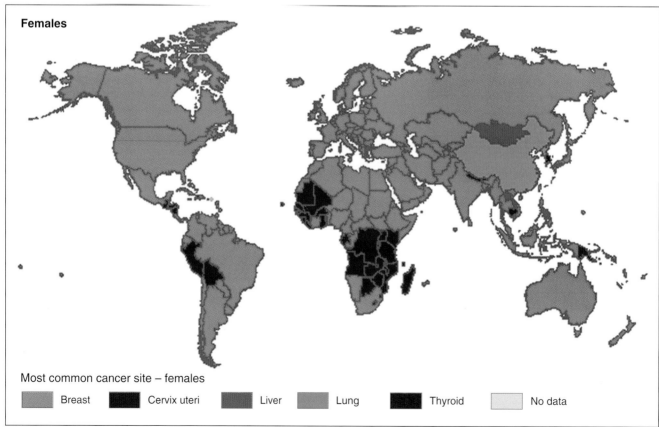

Most common cancer site – females

Breast	Cervix uteri	Liver	Lung	Thyroid	No data

Figure 4.1 Most commonly diagnosed cancers worldwide by sex, 2012. *Source:* Ferlay *et al.* [5]. Reproduced with permission of IARC.

Table 4.1 Incidence and mortality rates and number of cases and deaths by sex and cancer site for more and less developed areas, 2012.

	World				More developed areas				Less developed areas			
	Incidence		Mortality		Incidence		Mortality		Incidence		Mortality	
	ASR	Cases	ASR	Deaths	ASR	Cases	ASR	Deaths	ASR	Cases	ASR	Deaths
Males												
All cancers[1] (C00-97, but C44)	204.9	7,410,000	126.3	4,653,000	307.1	3,227,000	138.0	1,592,000	163.0	4,184,000	120.1	3,062,000
Bladder (C67)	9.0	330,000	3.2	123,000	16.9	196,000	4.5	59,000	5.3	134,000	2.6	64,000
Brain, nervous system (C70–72)	3.9	140,000	3.0	106,000	5.9	48,000	4.0	37,000	3.3	91,000	2.6	70,000
Colorectum (C18–21)	20.6	746,000	10.0	374,000	36.3	399,000	14.7	175,000	13.7	347,000	7.8	198,000
Esophagus (C15)	9.0	323,000	7.7	281,000	6.4	68,000	5.2	56,000	10.1	255,000	9.0	225,000
Gallbladder (C23–24)	2.1	77,000	1.6	60,000	2.3	28,000	1.5	19,000	2.0	49,000	1.6	41,000
Hodgkin lymphoma (C81)	1.1	39,000	0.4	15,000	2.3	16,000	0.4	4,000	0.8	23,000	0.4	12,000
Kidney (C64–66)	6.0	214,000	2.5	91,000	12.6	125,000	4.2	48,000	3.4	89,000	1.7	43,000
Larynx (C32)	3.9	138,000	2.0	73,000	5.1	51,000	2.2	23,000	3.5	87,000	2.0	51,000
Leukemia (C91–95)	5.6	201,000	4.1	151,000	8.8	80,000	4.6	51,000	4.4	120,000	3.7	100,000
Lip, oral cavity (C00–08)	5.5	199,000	2.7	98,000	7.0	68,000	2.3	23,000	5.0	131,000	2.8	75,000
Liver (C22)	15.3	554,000	14.3	521,000	8.6	92,000	7.1	80,000	17.8	462,000	17.0	441,000
Lung (C33–34)	34.2	1,242,000	30.0	1,099,000	44.7	490,000	36.8	417,000	30.0	751,000	27.2	682,000
Melanoma of skin (C43)	3.3	121,000	0.9	31,000	10.2	99,000	2.0	21,000	0.8	21,000	0.4	10,000
Multiple myeloma (C88 + C90)	1.7	62,000	1.2	43,000	3.3	36,000	1.8	22,000	1.0	26,000	0.8	21,000
Nasopharynx (C11)	1.7	61,000	1.0	36,000	0.6	5,000	0.2	2,000	2.0	56,000	1.3	33,000
Non-Hodgkin lymphoma (C82–85, C96)	6.0	218,000	3.2	115,000	10.3	102,000	3.5	41,000	4.3	116,000	2.8	75,000
Other pharynx (C09–10, C12–14)	3.2	115,000	2.2	78,000	4.7	44,000	2.2	21,000	2.8	71,000	2.2	56,000
Pancreas (C25)	4.9	178,000	4.7	174,000	8.6	95,000	8.3	93,000	3.3	83,000	3.2	81,000
Prostate (C61)	30.6	1,095,000	7.8	307,000	68.0	742,000	10.0	142,000	14.5	353,000	6.6	165,000
Stomach (C16)	17.4	631,000	12.7	469,000	15.6	175,000	9.2	107,000	18.1	456,000	14.4	362,000
Testis (C62)	1.5	55,000	0.3	10,000	5.2	33,000	0.3	2,000	0.7	23,000	0.3	8,000
Thyroid (C73)	1.9	68,000	0.3	13,000	3.6	30,000	0.3	4,000	1.4	39,000	0.4	9,000

(Continued)

Table 4.1 (Continued)

	World				More developed areas				Less developed areas			
	Incidence		Mortality		Incidence		Mortality		Incidence		Mortality	
	ASR	Cases	ASR	Deaths	ASR	Cases	ASR	Deaths	ASR	Cases	ASR	Deaths
Females												
All cancers[1] (C00–97, but C44)	165.2	6,658,000	82.9	3,548,000	239.9	2,827,000	86.2	1,287,000	135.8	3,831,000	79.8	2,261,000
Bladder (C67)	2.2	99,000	0.9	42,000	3.7	58,000	1.1	21,000	1.5	42,000	0.7	21,000
Brain, nervous system (C70–72)	3.0	117,000	2.1	83,000	4.4	41,000	2.7	30,000	2.7	76,000	1.9	53,000
Breast (C50)	43.1	1,671,000	12.9	522,000	73.4	788,000	14.9	198,000	31.3	883,000	11.5	324,000
Cervix uteri (C53)	14.0	528,000	6.8	266,000	9.9	83,000	3.3	36,000	15.7	445,000	8.3	230,000
Colorectum (C18–21)	14.3	614,000	6.9	320,000	23.6	338,000	9.3	158,000	9.8	276,000	5.6	163,000
Corpus uteri (C54)	8.2	320,000	1.8	76,000	14.7	168,000	2.3	35,000	5.5	152,000	1.5	41,000
Esophagus (C15)	3.1	133,000	2.7	119,000	1.2	18,000	0.9	15,000	4.1	114,000	3.6	104,000
Gallbladder (C23–24)	2.3	101,000	1.8	82,000	2.0	35,000	1.4	26,000	2.4	66,000	2.0	57,000
Hodgkin lymphoma (C81)	0.7	27,000	0.3	10,000	1.9	13,000	0.3	3,000	0.5	14,000	0.3	7,000
Kidney (C64–66)	3.0	124,000	1.2	53,000	6.2	75,000	1.7	27,000	1.8	49,000	0.9	26,000
Larynx (C32)	0.5	19,000	0.2	10,000	0.6	7,000	0.2	3,000	0.4	12,000	0.3	7,000
Leukemia (C91–95)	3.9	151,000	2.8	114,000	5.8	61,000	2.8	40,000	3.2	90,000	2.6	74,000
Lip, oral cavity (C00–08)	2.5	101,000	1.2	47,000	2.6	33,000	0.6	10,000	2.5	69,000	1.4	38,000
Liver (C22)	5.4	228,000	5.1	224,000	2.7	42,000	2.5	43,000	6.6	186,000	6.4	182,000
Lung (C33–34)	13.6	583,000	11.1	491,000	19.6	268,000	14.3	210,000	11.1	315,000	9.8	281,000
Melanoma of skin (C43)	2.8	111,000	0.6	24,000	9.3	92,000	1.2	15,000	0.7	20,000	0.3	9,000
Multiple myeloma (C88+C90)	1.2	52,000	0.8	37,000	2.2	31,000	1.2	21,000	0.7	20,000	0.6	16,000
Nasopharynx (C11)	0.7	26,000	0.4	15,000	0.2	2,000	0.1	1,000	0.8	24,000	0.5	14,000
Non-Hodgkin lymphoma (C82–85, C96)	4.1	168,000	2.0	84,000	7.1	89,000	2.0	34,000	2.8	80,000	1.8	50,000
Other pharynx (C09–10, C12–14)	0.7	27,000	0.5	19,000	0.8	9,000	0.3	4,000	0.7	18,000	0.5	14,000
Ovary (C56)	6.1	239,000	3.7	152,000	9.1	100,000	5.0	66,000	5.0	139,000	3.1	86,000
Pancreas (C25)	3.6	160,000	3.4	157,000	5.9	93,000	5.5	91,000	2.4	67,000	2.3	65,000
Stomach (C16)	7.5	320,000	5.7	254,000	6.7	99,000	4.2	68,000	7.8	221,000	6.5	186,000
Thyroid (C73)	6.1	230,000	0.6	27,000	11.1	93,000	0.4	7,000	4.7	137,000	0.7	20,000

Source: GLOBOCAN 2012.

ASR indicates age-standardized rate per 100,000. Rates are standardized to the World Standard Population.

[1] Excluding nonmelanoma skin cancer

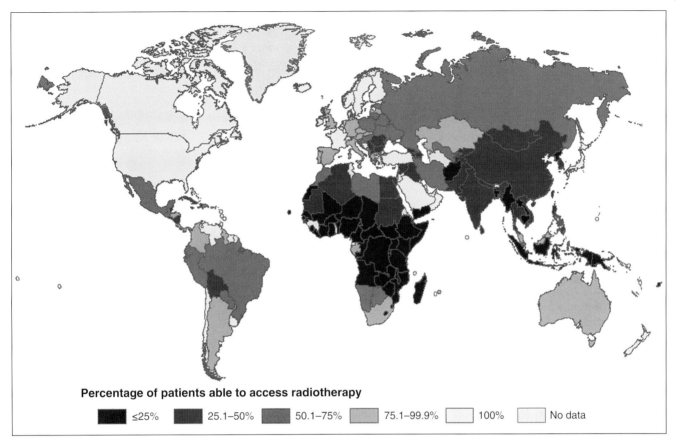

Percentage of patients able to access radiotherapy

| ≤25% | 25.1–50% | 50.1–75% | 75.1–99.9% | 100% | No data |

Figure 4.2 Estimated radiotherapy availability worldwide, 2013. *Countries with 100% of patients able to access radiotherapy may also include countries where radiotherapy supply is greater than demand, although disparities in access may still exist within these countries. *Source:* Jemal *et al.* The Cancer Atlas, 2nd edn. Atlanta, GA: American Cancer Society, 2015.

Lung Cancer

Lung cancer is the leading cause of cancer death in men and the second leading cause of cancer death in women, with an estimated 1,099,000 deaths in men and 491,000 deaths in women in 2012 (Table 4.1). Smoking is the predominant cause of lung cancer, accounting for 80% of lung cancer deaths in men and 50% in women [3]. Global variations in lung cancer rates and trends reflect differences in the stage and degree of the tobacco epidemic; lung cancer rates peak 30–40 years after peak smoking prevalence [4]. In men, the highest lung cancer mortality rates (per 100,000) are found in Eastern Europe and the lowest in Sub-Saharan Africa, ranging from 0.4 in Niger to 66.6 in Hungary [5]. In females, rates are highest in Eastern and Northern Europe and North America and lowest in Sub-Saharan Africa, ranging from fewer than three in most countries of Africa to 28.4 in the United States (US). The relatively high lung cancer rates in Chinese and North Korean women (30.7 and 18.0 per 100,000 females) despite their low smoking prevalence (<2% current smokers) are thought to reflect indoor air pollution from unventilated coal-fueled stoves and cooking fumes [6]. In addition to smoking and air pollution, other factors that increase lung cancer risk include environmental and occupational exposures to radon, asbestos, arsenic, certain metals (e.g., nickel, chromium, cadmium), and radiation [7, 8].

In those countries where the tobacco epidemic was established first such as the United Kingdom (UK), the US, Australia, and Canada, lung cancer rates have been decreasing over the past two decades in men and began to plateau or decrease in the past 10 years in women [9–12]. In these countries, the tobacco epidemic was established before or around the middle of the twentieth century, with women generally taking up smoking in large numbers later than men. In those countries where the tobacco epidemic was established later, such as Eastern European, Asian, and South American countries, lung cancer mortality rates among men are continuing to increase or have only peaked recently; rates continue to increase among women in many of these countries [12].

Lung cancer is the most preventable cause of cancer death. Quitting smoking at any age substantially decreases lung cancer risk, although the benefit decreases with quitting at older ages [13–15]. Public health policies and interventions that promote smoking cessation among adults and deter smoking initiation among adolescents include increased cigarette excise taxes, restricting smoking in public places, restriction of advertising tobacco products, and education and counter advertising on the health hazards of smoking. The implementation of these interventions in countries such as the US and the UK, though at a suboptimal level, has led to decreases in lung cancer rates and other smoking-related diseases [16–18]. In 2005, the World

Health Organization Framework Convention on Tobacco Control (FCTC) came into force to coordinate governments around the world to combat the global tobacco epidemic through implementation of proven tobacco policies. Measurable progress in implementation of these policies has been noted, although at a slower pace.

Lung cancer is one of the most fatal cancers with little variation in survival rates across countries by economic development; 5-year relative survival worldwide ranges from about 10 to 20% (Table 4.2). Survival is greatly reduced if lung cancer is diagnosed at later stages [7]. A recent randomized screening trial for lung cancer using computed tomography (CT) scans showed a

Table 4.2 Five-year net survival[1](%) for selected cancers among adults aged 15 and older in select countries, 2005–2009.

	Stomach	Colon	Rectum	Liver	Lung	Female breast	Cervix	Ovary	Prostate	Leukemia
Africa										
Algerian registries	10[2]	57[2]	46[2]	18[2]	15[2]	60[2]	55[2]	42[2]	59[2]	14[2]
South Africa (Eastern Cape)	–	–	–	10[2]	19[2]	53	55	91[2]	100[2]	
Asia										
Chinese registries	31	55	53	13	18	81	60	39	64	21
Indian registries	19	37	29	4	10	60	46	14[2]	58	6[2]
Indonesia (Jakarta)	18	28	58	20	12[2]	78	65	40[†]	44	40
Israel	29	69	67	14[2]	24	87	66	42	94	50
South Korea	58	66	66	20	19	83	77	44	82	23
Mongolia	15	31	16	9	7	57	60	52	40	36
Thai registries	12	50	40	8	8	71	56	41	58	14
Turkey (Izmir)	17	53	45	14	10	79	61	39	81	33
Northern America										
Canada	25	63	63	18	17	86	67	38	92	55
US registries	29	65	64	15	19	89	63	41	97	52
Central and Southern America										
Brazilian registries	25	58	56	12[2]	18	87	61	32	96	20[2]
Chilean registries	18	43	38	8[2]	6	77	51	32	89	16
Colombian registries	17	43	–	5	9	76	59	31	79	20
Ecuadorian registries	32[2]	68	53	18[2]	29[2]	83	62	47	92	34
Europe										
Austria	33	63	62	13	18	83	66	42	91	46
Belgium	33	65	65	20	17	85	65	43	93	59
Czech Republic	23	55	50	7[2]	12	80	65	37	83	46
Denmark	18	56	58	6	11	82	65	37	77	57
Finland	25	63	63	8	12	87	65	45	93	51
German registries	32	65	62	14	16	85	65	40	91	54
Italian registries	32	63	60	18	15	86	68	39	90	47
Poland	19	50	47	10[2]	13	74	53	34	74	49
Slovenia	27	56	55	5	11	80	69	38	78	38
Spanish registries	27	59	58	16	13	84	65	38	87	52
United Kingdom	19	54	57	9	10	81	60	36	83	47
Oceania										
Australian registries	28	64	64	15	15	86	67	38	89	51
New Zealand	27	62	61	17	12	84	64	34	89	58

Source: Allemani *et al.* [47]. Reproduced with permission of Elsevier.
[1] Survival percentages are age-standardized.
[2] Data are subject to limitations. Please see source.

20% decreased lung cancer mortality among individuals aged 55–74 years with a 30 pack-year smoking history [19]. However, the high cost, as well as the infrastructure and technical expertise required, precludes adoption of CT lung cancer screening in developing countries in the immediate future.

Colon and Rectum Cancer

Colon and rectum cancer is the second most common cancer in females and the third in males, with an estimated 614,000 cases in females and 746,000 cases in males in 2012 (Table 4.1, Figure 4.1). The incidence rates per 100,000 vary substantially, ranging from 1 in Mozambique and The Gambia to 35.8 in Norway among females and from 1.5 in Mozambique to 61.6 in Slovakia among males [5]. In general, the highest rates are found in North America, Australia, Europe, and Japan and the lowest rates in Africa and South-Central Asia. Reasons for these regional variations include differences in risk factors such as obesity, smoking, and consumption of red and processed meat [20].

Colorectal cancer incidence rates are rapidly increasing in both males and females in many parts of the world, including Eastern Europe, Asia, and select countries in South America and Africa. Between 1983–1987 and 1998–2002, incidence rates among men increased by 90% in select regions in Japan, by 87% in Spain, and by ≥45% in the Czech Republic, Slovakia, and Slovenia [21]. In fact, the rates among males in the Czech Republic and Slovakia have already exceeded the peak rates observed in long-standing developed countries such as the US. The incidence trends in these countries reflect their obesity and tobacco epidemics. In contrast, incidence rates in most Western and Northern European countries are increasing slightly or leveling off. The US is one of few countries with decreasing incidence rates in both males and females. This favorable trend in the US is thought to be largely due to wider dissemination of colorectal cancer screening, specifically endoscopy, which can detect precancerous lesions for removal [21]. In other countries with decreasing incidence and more recent introduction of screening, risk factor changes probably play a large role [22]. Mortality rates are decreasing in many countries, likely due to improved treatment as well as screening. While these declines are occurring in both developed and developing countries, some lower-resource countries in South America and Eastern Europe continue to experience increasing mortality rates [20].

Colorectal cancer can be prevented by addressing its primary risk factors, such as unhealthy body weight and diet as well as smoking, and by removing precancerous lesions detected by screening. Japan and a number of countries in Europe have screening programs; most of these countries use the fecal occult blood test [20]. The introduction of colorectal cancer screening using endoscopy in most parts of Asia, South America, and Africa may not be feasible or recommended because of high cost and infrastructure requirements as well as the relatively low burden of the disease in these areas [23]. Survival rates substantially vary internationally according to the availability of early detection and treatment services (Table 4.2) [24, 25]. Five-year survival in the US increases to 90% if the disease is at the local stage [26].

Breast Cancer

Breast cancer is the most commonly diagnosed cancer in both developed and developing countries, with 1.7 million newly diagnosed cases in 2012. It is the leading cause of cancer death in women in developing countries and the second leading cause of cancer death in developed countries, with a total of 522,000 deaths (Table 4.1, Figure 4.1). Generally, the highest incidence rates are found in North America, Europe, and Australia and New Zealand and the lowest in Africa and Asia (except Israel), with rates (per 100,000 females) ranging from fewer than 10 to over 100. These variations are thought to reflect differences in disease awareness and detection practice, as well as reproductive factors such as age at menarche and full-term pregnancy, number of pregnancies, breastfeeding, and use of menopausal hormone therapy.

Incidence rates are decreasing or stabilizing in many areas with the highest rates, including the US, the UK, and Australia, likely due to declining use of menopausal hormone therapy after publication of a major study in 2002 that linked use of menopausal therapy to breast cancer and other conditions [27]. Rates may also be declining or stable in Western countries because of longstanding screening programs, which reduce the number of prevalent cases to be detected in the population, or a leveling-off of participation in screening [28]. In contrast, incidence rates are rapidly increasing in areas with lower rates or in economically developing countries. Between the 1970s and early 2000s, incidence rates more than doubled in Miyagi (Japan) and increased by about 40% in Chennai (India). These increases are thought to reflect changes in reproductive factors, obesity, and physical inactivity, as well as increased awareness and screening.

Breast cancer mortality rates are decreasing in many high income countries due to early detection and improved treatment [29]. In contrast, rates are increasing in low income countries because of increasing prevalence of risk factors (obesity, alcohol consumption, and physical inactivity), as well as lack of early detection services and standard treatment (Figure 4.2).

Mammography screening at the population level may not be feasible for many low-resource countries; however, in these countries, awareness of signs and symptoms and clinical breast examination are recommended for early intervention [30]. When detected early (local stage), breast cancer survival is about 90% or more in developed countries, compared to about 75% in select developing countries [31]. Survival for late (distant)-stage breast cancer ranges from about 15% in developing countries to 25% in developed countries [31].

Prostate Cancer

Prostate cancer is the second most frequently diagnosed cancer and the fifth leading cause of cancer deaths worldwide among men, with an estimated 1.1 million new cases and 307,000 deaths in 2012 (Table 4.1). The highest incidence rates are found in North America, Northern and Western Europe, and parts of Oceania (Australia and New Zealand), while the lowest rates are found in Asia and North Africa. Incidence rates vary by over

100-fold across countries (0.7 per 100,000 in India to 178.6 in US Blacks). Although the highest incidence rates are found in high-income countries, the highest death rates are mainly found in low-income areas, including Sub-Saharan Africa and the Caribbean.

Advanced age, black race, and family history are the only well-established risk factors for prostate cancer [32]. About 10% or fewer of prostate cancer cases are estimated to be due to genetics [32]. Other suspected risk factors include diets high in processed meats, calcium, or dairy foods. It has been suggested that much of the contemporary international variation in prostate cancer incidence rates is due to differences in detection practices through the PSA test [33], although substantial variations were also noted before the dissemination of this test.

Incidence trends in select high-income countries such as the US, Canada, and Australia have closely followed trends in the use of PSA testing to screen for prostate cancer [33]. Incidence rates rapidly increased from the late 1980s through the early 1990s due to the introduction and wide utilization of PSA testing. In subsequent years, rates sharply decreased and then leveled off due to fewer prevalent cases as well as reduced screening. In contrast, incidence rates in Southern and Western European countries increased at a slower rate, because of gradual adoption of PSA testing. Rates are also increasing in several low- and middle-income countries where PSA utilization is not common, such as Thailand, which may be due to increasing prevalence of suspected risk factors, such as obesity and consumption of a diet rich in animal fat.

Mortality rates are decreasing in most high-income countries due in part to improved treatment (surgery and radiation therapy for early stage disease and hormone therapy for advanced disease); the contribution of screening to the decreasing mortality rates is unclear [34]. In contrast, mortality rates are increasing in most low- and middle-income countries, paralleling the incidence trends in these countries.

Although the modifiable causes of prostate cancer have not been well defined, it is possible that risk can be reduced through healthy body weight, adequate physical activity, and a healthy diet low in processed meats and fats and high in fruits and vegetables. Uncertainty regarding benefits and harms of PSA testing is discussed in Chapter 11.

Comparisons of international prostate cancer survival rates can be difficult to interpret, as "lead time bias" associated with PSA testing can affect the amount of time that a person is observed to be alive following diagnosis. Five-year survival in the US, where PSA testing is common, is 99%. In the UK, where PSA testing is less common, 5-year survival is 83% (Table 4.2).

Liver Cancer

Liver cancer is the sixth most commonly diagnosed cancer and the second leading cause of cancer death worldwide, with an estimated 782,000 new cases and 746,000 deaths in 2012 (Table 4.1, Figure 4.1). Nearly 85% of these cancers occur in the developing world, with China alone accounting for 50% of the total. The highest rates are found in Eastern Asia (China, North and South Korea) and in West and Central Africa; rates are lowest in Europe, Oceania, North America and parts of South-Central Asia (e.g., India). Hepatocellular carcinoma (HCC), a cancer of the parenchymal cells of the liver, accounts for 75–90% of liver cancers worldwide. Cholangiocarcinoma, a cancer of cells lining the bile duct, is a less common form of liver cancer worldwide, but the dominant form in Thailand due to the high prevalence of liver fluke infection.

The most important risk factor for HCC is chronic infection with hepatitis B (HBV) or hepatitis C (HCV) virus [35, 36]. HBV and HCV, which are bloodborne infections that can be transmitted through childbirth, unprotected sexual contact (HBV), or contaminated injections or blood transfusions, account for 59% and 33% respectively of HCC in economically developing countries. The corresponding percentages in economically developed countries are 23% and 20% [36]. Other known risk factors for HCC include dietary aflatoxin exposure, type 2 diabetes mellitus, smoking, and cirrhosis related to alcohol or non-alcoholic fatty liver disease (associated with obesity), with each of these accounting for variable proportions of the disease across regions [37, 38].

Liver cancer (HCC) incidence rates are increasing in areas with lower rates such as the US, the UK, and Australia. This may be in part due to the high prevalence of chronic HCV infection due to use of contaminated needles and blood products and intravenous drug use, which was common in the 1960s and 1970s. It is also possible that the obesity epidemic and the associated rise in diabetes mellitus contributed to this pattern. Incidence rates also have increased in some developing countries such as Egypt. The increase in Egypt has been attributed in part to HCV infection from contaminated needles used for antischistosomal therapy between the 1950s and 1980s [39].

Incidence rates have been decreasing in areas with historically higher rates, especially in Asia, including China and Japan. The decrease in China may reflect improved sanitary conditions and reduced contamination of food with aflatoxin B1 through improved food storage.

Liver cancer survival is extremely poor; 5-year survival is 20% or less in all countries. However, the primary causes of HCC can be prevented through public health measures. HBV vaccine has been available since 1982; as of 2011, 179 countries had introduced the vaccination into their routine immunization schedules [40], and the vaccine has also been made affordable for developing countries. Universal HBV childhood vaccination in Taiwan since the 1980s has led to a dramatic decrease in liver cancer incidence rates in children and adolescents [41], although these programs are too recent to have contributed to the overall decrease in liver cancer rates. While no vaccine for HCV exists, HCV incidence can be reduced through public health measures to curb HCV transmission in medical settings involving injection and blood transfusions, as well as interventions with injecting drug users [35]. A reduction in HCC risk has been shown with the use of antiviral treatments for individuals who are already infected with HBV or HCV, but these treatments can be costly and difficult for patient adherence and are unlikely to be feasible in resource-constrained settings [38]. Limited studies on mortality reduction through screening of high-risk individuals have had mixed results [37, 38].

Cervical Cancer

Cervical cancer is the fourth most commonly diagnosed cancer and the fourth leading cause of cancer death among women worldwide, with an estimated 528,000 new cases and 266,000 deaths in 2012 (Table 4.1, Figure 4.1). About 85% of cervical cancer cases and deaths occur in economically developing countries, with India accounting for 25% of deaths. The highest incidence rates are found in Sub-Saharan Africa, South-Central Asia, and parts of South America, while the lowest are found in Europe, North America, Australia and New Zealand. Cervical cancer is primarily caused by the human papillomavirus (HPV; see Chapter 7). International variations in the burden of cervical cancer are largely due to differences in screening, which can not only detect cervical cancer early but also prevent cervical cancer through the detection of treatable precancerous lesions [25].

Cervical cancer incidence rates have decreased by as much as 70% over the past five decades in Western countries due to cervical cytology screening (the Papanicolaou [Pap] smear and, more recently, liquid-based cytology), which can detect precancerous lesions and cancer. Incidence rates in India and in some parts of Sub-Saharan Africa and South America have decreased little, and cervical cancer remains the leading cause of cancer deaths in these countries largely because of lack of early detection services.

When cervical cancer is detected early (local stage), 5-year survival is about 70% [31]. However, when it is detected at the distant stage, survival decreases to 19% in developed countries and 7% in developing countries [31]. The healthcare infrastructures in most developing countries cannot support the introduction of cytology screening due to technical and infrastructure requirements. However, alternative cost-effective early detection methods, such as visual inspection using Lugol's iodine or acetic acid, and testing for HPV DNA in cervical cell samples, can also detect precancerous cells or cancer in its earlier stages. Vaccination against HPV is the most promising preventive measure for substantially reducing the future burden of cervical cancer in economically developing countries. Vaccines which protect against the two types of HPV that cause the majority (70%) of cervical cancer cases have been available since 2006, and a new vaccine which protects against nine types of HPV and can prevent about 90% of cervical cancer cases was licensed by the US Food and Drug Administration in 2014 [42]. However, broad vaccination in developing countries depends on the cost of the vaccine. Recent negotiations have resulted in the manufacturers lowering the price for developing countries, although it may still be prohibitively high for most of the countries where the vaccines are needed the most.

Stomach Cancer

Stomach cancer is the fifth most commonly diagnosed cancer and the third leading cause of cancer death worldwide, with an estimated 952,000 new cancer cases and 723,000 deaths in 2012 (Table 4.1, Figure 4.1). Generally, rates are twice as high in males as in females. The highest incidence rates are found in Eastern Asia and lowest rates in Africa and North America, with rates (per 100,000 population) varying from 1.3 in men and 0.5 in women in Mozambique to 62.3 in men and 24.7 in women in Korea. These variations are thought to reflect differences in prevalence of *Helicobacter pylori* (*H. pylori*) infection, which accounts for about 90% of noncardia gastric cancers worldwide [43]. Other known risk factors include smoking, obesity, and diets rich in smoked foods, salted meat or fish, and pickled vegetables [44].

Stomach cancer incidence and mortality rates have been steadily decreasing in most parts of the world, although the decrease began much earlier in Western countries. In the US, rates have decreased by about 80% since 1950. Reasons for this decrease are unclear but are thought to reflect the increased use of refrigerators, which made salting and curing for preservation of food obsolete and increased the availability of fresh fruit and vegetables, as well as reduced prevalence of *H. pylori* infection due to improved hygiene and use of antibiotics. It is also possible that increased screening activity in Japan [45, 46] and reductions in smoking prevalence in the US, the UK, Australia, and Canada may have contributed to the decreasing stomach cancer mortality rates [45].

Five-year survival ranges from about 15 to 30% in Western countries (Table 4.2). In Japan and Korea, survival is over 50% [47], likely due to early detection through stomach cancer screening programs. Primary prevention of stomach cancer through reduction in risk factors includes not smoking, decreasing consumption of smoked foods, salted meat or fish, and pickled vegetables, and increasing consumption of fresh fruits and vegetables. Treatment of *H. pylori* for the prevention of stomach cancer is currently being evaluated. In recent randomized trials in Asia, screening for and eradication of *H. pylori* using antibiotics was shown to reduce the risk of stomach cancer [48]. While this approach requires further research, it may represent a promising new way to decrease stomach cancer rates further in countries where chronic *H. pylori* infection is common; however, there are concerns about antibiotic resistance or increases in gastroesophageal reflux from this type of treatment [49]. Some countries with a very high burden of gastric cancer, such as Japan and South Korea, have introduced national screening, but its role in reducing mortality at the population level is debated [46]. Screening programs are not recommended for countries with a lower burden of stomach cancer.

Esophageal Cancer

Esophageal cancer is the eighth most commonly diagnosed cancer and the sixth leading cause of cancer death worldwide, with 456,000 new cases and 400,000 deaths estimated in 2012 (Table 4.1, Figure 4.1). The highest incidence rates are found in Asia, including China, and Eastern and Southern Africa, and the lowest rates are in North and Central Africa, parts of Europe, and South America, with rates varying by 100-fold among these regions (<1 per 100,000 in several countries of Oceania and North and Central Africa to >20 in Turkmenistan and Malawi). Generally, rates are three to four times higher in males than in females.

There are two major histologic forms of esophageal cancer, squamous cell carcinoma and adenocarcinoma, each with distinct anatomic and geographic patterns. Squamous cell carcinoma occurs mostly in the middle or upper third of the esophagus, whereas most adenocarcinomas occur in the lower one third or the gastroesophageal junction. Major risk factors for squamous cell carcinoma are smoking and alcohol consumption; for adenocarcinoma they are smoking, overweight and obesity, gastroesophageal reflux disease, and Barrett's esophagus [50]. Squamous cell carcinoma represents over 90% of the cases in high risk areas, particularly in Iran and North Central China. Reasons for these high rates are unknown, but are thought to reflect poor nutrition and drinking of hot beverages [51]. In contrast, smoking and alcohol consumption account for 90% of squamous cell carcinoma in the US and other Western countries. While incidence rates for squamous cell carcinoma of the esophagus have been decreasing in many Western countries because of reductions in smoking and alcohol consumption [52], rates of adenocarcinoma of the esophagus have been increasing in these same countries in part because of the obesity epidemic and possibly decreases in *H. pylori* infection due to improved hygiene [53].

Risk of both types of esophageal cancer can be lowered by consumption of a diet high in fruits and vegetables [54]. Squamous cell carcinoma in Western countries can be prevented through decreasing smoking and alcohol consumption [54], although further research is needed to identify preventive strategies for squamous cell carcinoma in high-risk areas of Iran, China, and Eastern and Southern Africa where the risk factors are not well understood [25]. No preventive strategies for esophageal adenocarcinoma have yet been completely validated, but it is possible that weight reduction, treatment of gastroesophageal reflux disease, management of Barrett's esophagus, or use of nonsteroidal anti-inflammatory drugs or statins may decrease the risk of esophageal adenocarcinoma [53, 54]. Early detection of esophageal cancer or precursor lesions using endoscopic screening among high-risk populations has the potential to lower mortality at the population level, although this too has not yet been demonstrated [53, 54]. As endoscopy is costly and requires significant infrastructure, it is unlikely to be feasible in low-resource settings. As no effective early detection strategies for esophageal cancer have yet been developed, esophageal cancer is often diagnosed at a later stage and thus has low survival. Five-year survival is about 20% or less in both developed and developing countries [55].

Oral Cavity and Pharyngeal Cancers

Oral cavity and pharyngeal cancers account for 3% of cancer cases (443,000) and deaths (241,000) worldwide (Table 4.1), with 65% of cases occurring in developing countries. The incidence rates of oral cavity and pharyngeal cancer vary more than 20-fold across countries, ranging from <1 in Cape Verde and The Gambia to 27.2 in Papua New Guinea. Generally, the highest rates are found in South-Eastern and South-Central Asia and Eastern Europe and the lowest rates in Africa, Eastern Asia, and parts of South America. In high-incidence areas such as

India, oral cavity cancer is the most commonly diagnosed cancer in men (Figure 4.1). Cigarette smoking, chewing tobacco or betel quid, and alcohol consumption are known risk factors for oral cavity and pharyngeal cancers. Certain subsites of the oral cavity and pharynx (the oropharynx, including base of tongue and tonsil) are strongly associated with HPV [56]. The proportional contribution of risk factors to the burden of oral cavity and pharyngeal cancers varies across regions.

International variations in temporal trends in oral cavity and pharyngeal cancer rates as a whole reflect the stage and the degree of the tobacco epidemic. In places such as Hungary, Slovakia, and Taiwan, where the tobacco epidemic was established recently, oral cavity cancer incidence and mortality rates are increasing. In contrast, rates are decreasing in countries such as the US, the UK, and Australia, where the tobacco epidemic was established at the beginning of the last century. However, incidence rates for oropharyngeal cancer have been increasing rapidly in the US and other Western countries, which is thought to reflect increases in HPV infection due to changes in sexual behavior, specifically oral sex [57].

As tobacco and excessive alcohol consumption are the major causes of cancers of the oral cavity and pharynx, reduction of these risk factors is the best prevention method [58]. It is likely that avoiding HPV infection through safer sex practices or HPV vaccination can reduce the risk of HPV-associated cancers of the oral cavity and pharynx, although this has not yet been demonstrated [57]. Studies have not shown that screening for cancers of the oral cavity and pharynx in the general population is effective in reducing mortality [59–61]. A study in a high-prevalence area of India found that screening reduced mortality among high-risk tobacco and alcohol users, but these results need to be confirmed before recommendations can be made [59, 61–63]. Limited studies of screening for oral HPV infection have not shown reduced risk of oral cavity and pharyngeal cancers [64, 65]. Five-year survival for oral cavity cancer ranges from about 40 to 60% in Western countries and 20 to 45% in developing countries [55, 66]. Survival for oropharyngeal cancer is lower at about 20–45% [55].

Conclusion

The global burden of cancer is increasing due to the aging and growth of the population, as well as increased prevalence of known risk factors (e.g., physical inactivity, obesity, and smoking) associated with urbanization, and tobacco and food and beverage industry marketing. In addition to increases in risk of cancers associated with these risk factors, developing countries continue to bear a disproportionate burden of infection-related cancers. The global burden of cancer could be substantially reduced by implementing existing cancer control measures in all countries according to each country's economic resources. The establishment and/or strengthening of population-based cancer registries should be an integral part of any cancer control program for evaluating the effectiveness of the program and monitoring progress. Further research is also needed across the cancer continuum for many cancers from risk factors (causation) to prevention, early detection, and treatment.

References

1 Buell P, Dunn JE, Jr. Cancer mortality among Japanese Issei and Nisei of California. *Cancer* 1965;18:656–64.

2 Kolonel L, Wilkens L. Migrant studies. In: D Schottenfeld, JF Fraumeni Jr (eds) *Cancer Epidemiology and Prevention*, 3rd edn. New York: Oxford University Press, 2006:189–201.

3 Ott JJ, Ullrich A, Mascarenhas M, Stevens GA. Global cancer incidence and mortality caused by behavior and infection. *J Pub Health* 2011;33(2):223–33.

4 Lopez AD, Collishaw N, Piha T. A descriptive model of the cigarette epidemic in developed countries. *Tob Control* 1994;3(3):242–7.

5 Ferlay J, Soerjomataram I, Ervik M, *et al.* GLOBOCAN 2012 v1.0, Cancer Incidence and Mortality Worldwide: IARC CancerBase No. 11 [Internet]. Lyon, France: International Agency for Research on Cancer. Available from: http://globocan.iarc.fr (accessed 11 May 2017).

6 Mu L, Liu L, Niu R, *et al.* Indoor air pollution and risk of lung cancer among Chinese female non-smokers. *Cancer Causes Control* 2013;24(3):439–50.

7 Spitz MR, Wu X, Wilkinson A, Wei Q. Cancer of the lung. In: D Schottenfeld, JF Fraumeni Jr (eds) *Cancer Epidemiology and Prevention*, 3rd edn. New York: Oxford University Press, 2006:638–58.

8 Cogliano VJ, Baan R, Straif K, *et al.* Preventable exposures associated with human cancers. *J Natl Cancer Inst* 2011;103(24):1827–39.

9 Bosetti C, Levi F, Lucchini F, Negri E, La Vecchia C. Lung cancer mortality in European women: recent trends and perspectives. *Ann Oncol* 2005;16(10):1597–604.

10 Jemal A, Simard EP, Dorell C, *et al.* Annual report to the nation on the status of cancer, 1975–2009, featuring the burden and trends in human papillomavirus (HPV)-associated cancers and HPV vaccination coverage levels. *J Natl Cancer Inst* 2013;105(3):175–201.

11 Malvezzi M, Bosetti C, Rosso T, *et al.* Lung cancer mortality in European men: trends and predictions. *Lung Cancer* 2013;80(2):138–45.

12 Youlden DR, Cramb SM, Baade PD. The International Epidemiology of Lung Cancer: geographical distribution and secular trends. *J Thorac Oncol* 2008;3(8):819–31.

13 Peto R, Darby S, Deo H, *et al.* Smoking, smoking cessation, and lung cancer in the UK since 1950: combination of national statistics with two case-control studies. *Br Med J* 2000;321(7257):323–9.

14 Pirie K, Peto R, Reeves GK, Green J, Beral V. The 21st century hazards of smoking and benefits of stopping: a prospective study of one million women in the UK. *Lancet* 2013;381(9861):133–41.

15 Thun MJ, Carter BD, Feskanich D, *et al.* 50-year trends in smoking-related mortality in the United States. *N Engl J Med* 2013;368(4):351–64.

16 Warner KE, Mendez D. Tobacco control policy in developed countries: yesterday, today, and tomorrow. *Nicotine Tob Res* 2010;12(9):876–87.

17 Britton J, Bogdanovica I. Tobacco control efforts in Europe. *Lancet* 2013;381(9877):1588–95.

18 Jemal A, Thun MJ, Ries LA, *et al.* Annual report to the nation on the status of cancer, 1975–2005, featuring trends in lung cancer, tobacco use, and tobacco control. *J Natl Cancer Inst* 2008;100(23):1672–94.

19 Smith RA, Brooks D, Cokkinides V, Saslow D, Brawley OW. Cancer screening in the United States, 2013: a review of current american cancer society guidelines, current issues in cancer screening, and new guidance on cervical cancer screening and lung cancer screening. *CA Cancer J Clin* 2013;63(2):88–105.

20 Center MM, Jemal A, Smith RA, Ward E. Worldwide variations in colorectal cancer. *CA Cancer J Clin* 2009;59(6):366–78.

21 Center MM, Jemal A, Ward E. International trends in colorectal cancer incidence rates. *Cancer Epidemiol Biomarkers Prev* 2009;18(6):1688–94.

22 Arnold M, Sierra MS, Laversanne M, *et al.* Global patterns and trends in colorectal cancer incidence and mortality. *Gut* 2017;66(4):683–91.

23 Potter MB. Strategies and resources to address colorectal cancer screening rates and disparities in the United States and globally. *Annu Rev Public Health* 2013;34:413–29.

24 Coleman MP, Forman D, Bryant H, *et al.* Cancer survival in Australia, Canada, Denmark, Norway, Sweden, and the UK, 1995–2007 (the International Cancer Benchmarking Partnership): an analysis of population-based cancer registry data. *Lancet* 2011;377(9760):127–38.

25 Torre LA, Bray F, Siegel RL, *et al.* Global cancer statistics, 2012. *CA Cancer J Clin* 2015;65(2):87–108.

26 Siegel RL, Miller KD, Jemal A. Cancer statistics, 2015. *CA Cancer J Clin* 2015;65(1):5–29.

27 Rossouw JE, Anderson GL, Prentice RL, *et al.* Risks and benefits of estrogen plus progestin in healthy postmenopausal women: principal results from the Women's Health Initiative randomized controlled trial. *JAMA* 2002;288(3):321–33.

28 Youlden DR, Cramb SM, Dunn NA, *et al.* The descriptive epidemiology of female breast cancer: an international comparison of screening, incidence, survival and mortality. *Cancer Epidemiol* 2012;36(3):237–48.

29 Berry DA, Cronin KA, Plevritis SK, *et al.* Effect of screening and adjuvant therapy on mortality from breast cancer. *New Engl J Med* 2005;353(17):1784–92.

30 Anderson BO, Cazap E, El Saghir NS, *et al.* Optimisation of breast cancer management in low-resource and middle-resource countries: executive summary of the Breast Health Global Initiative consensus, 2010. *Lancet Oncol* 2011;12(4):387–98.

31 Sankaranarayanan R, Swaminathan R, Brenner H, *et al.* Cancer survival in Africa, Asia, and Central America: a population-based study. *Lancet Oncol* 2010;11:165–73.

32 Platz EA, Giovannucci E. Prostate Cancer. In: D Schottenfeld, J Fraumeni Jr (eds) *Cancer Epidemiology and Prevention*, 3rd edn. New York: Oxford University Press, 2006.

33 Center MM, Jemal A, Lortet-Tieulent J, *et al.* International variation in prostate cancer incidence and mortality rates. *Eur Urol* 2012;61(6):1079–92.

34 Baade PD, Youlden DR, Krnjacki LJ. International epidemiology of prostate cancer: geographical distribution and secular trends. *Mol Nutr Food Res* 2009;53(2):171–84.

35 London WT, McGlynn KA. Liver Cancer. In: D Schottenfeld, JF Fraumeni Jr (eds) *Cancer Epidemiology and Prevention*, 3rd edn. New York: Oxford University Press, 2006:763–86.

36 Parkin DM. The global health burden of infection-associated cancers in the year 2002. *Int J Cancer* 2006;118(12):3030–44.

37 El-Serag HB. Hepatocellular carcinoma. *New Engl J Med* 2011;365(12):1118–27.

38 Mittal S, El-Serag HB. Epidemiology of hepatocellular carcinoma: consider the population. *J Clin Gastroenterol* 2013;47(Suppl):S2–S6.

39 Frank C, Mohamed MK, Strickland GT, *et al*. The role of parenteral antischistosomal therapy in the spread of hepatitis C virus in Egypt. *Lancet* 2000;355(9207):887–91.

40 World Health Organization. Hepatitis B 2012. Available from: http://www.who.int/immunization/topics/hepatitis_b/en/index.html (accessed 11 May 2017).

41 Chiang CJ, Yang YW, You SL, Lai MS, Chen CJ. Thirty-year outcomes of the national hepatitis B immunization program in Taiwan. *JAMA* 2013;310(9):974–6.

42 Herrero R, Gonzalez P, Markowitz LE. Present status of human papillomavirus vaccine development and implementation. *Lancet Oncol* 2015;16(5):e206–16.

43 Plummer M, Franceschi S, Vignat J, Forman D, de Martel C. Global burden of gastric cancer attributable to pylori. *Int J Cancer* 2015;136(2):487–90.

44 Shibata A, Parsonnet J. Stomach cancer. In: D Schottenfeld, JF Fraumeni Jr (eds) *Cancer Epidemiology and Prevention*, 3rd edn. New York: Oxford University Press, 2006:707–20.

45 Bertuccio P, Chatenoud L, Levi F, *et al*. Recent patterns in gastric cancer: a global overview. *Int J Cancer* 2009;125(3):666–73.

46 Leung WK, Wu MS, Kakugawa Y, *et al*. Screening for gastric cancer in Asia: current evidence and practice. *Lancet Oncol* 2008;9(3):279–87.

47 Allemani C, Weir HK, Carreira H, *et al*. Global surveillance of cancer survival 1995–2009: analysis of individual data for 25,676,887 patients from 279 population-based registries in 67 countries (CONCORD-2). *Lancet* 2015;385(9972):977–1010.

48 Herrero R, Parsonnet J, Greenberg ER. Prevention of gastric cancer. *JAMA* 2014;312(12):1197–8.

49 Mazzoleni LE, Francesconi CF, Sander GB. Mass eradication of Helicobacter pylori: feasible and advisable? *Lancet* 2011; 378(9790):462–4.

50 Kamangar F, Chow WH, Abnet CC, Dawsey SM. Environmental causes of esophageal cancer. *Gastroenterol Clin North Am* 2009;38(1):27–57, vii.

51 Islami F, Boffetta P, Ren JS, *et al*. High-temperature beverages and foods and esophageal cancer risk–a systematic review. *Int J Cancer* 2009;125(3):491–524.

52 Bosetti C, Levi F, Ferlay J, *et al*. Trends in oesophageal cancer incidence and mortality in Europe. *Int J Cancer* 2008;122(5): 1118–29.

53 Lagergren J, Lagergren P. Recent developments in esophageal adenocarcinoma. *CA Cancer J Clin* 2013;63(4):232–48.

54 Blot WJ, McLaughlin JK, Fraumeni Jr JF. Esophageal Cancer. In: D Schottenfeld, JF Fraumeni Jr (eds) *Cancer Epidemiology and Prevention*, 3rd edn. New York: Oxford University Press, 2006:697–706.

55 World Health Organization International Agency for Research on Cancer. Cancer survival in Africa, Asia, and the Caribbean and Central America. Lyon, 2011.

56 Forman D, de Martel C, Lacey CJ, *et al*. Global burden of human papillomavirus and related diseases. *Vaccine* 2012;30(Suppl 5):F12–23.

57 Gillison ML, Alemany L, Snijders PJ, *et al*. Human papillomavirus and diseases of the upper airway: head and neck cancer and respiratory papillomatosis. *Vaccine* 2012;30 (Suppl 5):F34–54.

58 Mayne ST, Morse DE, Winn DM. Cancers of the Oral Cavity and Pharynx. In: D Schottenfeld, JF Fraumeni Jr (eds) *Cancer Epidemiology and Prevention*, 3rd edn. New York: Oxford University Press, 2006:674–96.

59 Brocklehurst P, Kujan O, Glenny AM, *et al*. Screening programmes for the early detection and prevention of oral cancer. *UOF – Cochrane Database Syst Rev* 2006;(3):CD004150. PMID: 16856035. Cochrane database of systematic reviews (Online). 2010(11):CD004150.

60 Mitka M. Evidence lacking for benefit from oral cancer screening. *JAMA* 2013;309(18):1884.

61 Olson CM, Burda BU, Beil T, Whitlock EP. *Screening for Oral Cancer A. Targeted Evidence Update for the U.S. Preventive Services Task Force. Evidence Synthesis No. 102. AHRQ Publication No. 13-05186-EF-1*. Rockville, MD: Agency for Healthcare Research and Quality, 2013.

62 Sankaranarayanan R, Ramadas K, Thara S, *et al*. Long term effect of visual screening on oral cancer incidence and mortality in a randomized trial in Kerala, India. *Oral Oncol* 2013;49(4):314–21.

63 Sankaranarayanan R, Ramadas K, Thomas G, *et al*. Effect of screening on oral cancer mortality in Kerala, India: a cluster-randomised controlled trial. *Lancet* 2005;365(9475): 1927–33.

64 Fakhry C, Rosenthal BT, Clark DP, Gillison ML. Associations between oral HPV16 infection and cytopathology: evaluation of an oropharyngeal "pap-test equivalent" in high-risk populations. *Cancer Prev Res (Phila)* 2011;4(9):1378–84.

65 Kreimer AR, Chaturvedi AK. HPV-associated oropharyngeal cancers–are they preventable? *Cancer Prev Res (Phila)* 2011;4(9):1346–9.

66 Sant M, Allemani C, Santaquilani M, *et al*. EUROCARE-4. Survival of cancer patients diagnosed in 1995–1999. Results and commentary. *Eur J Cancer* 2009;45(6):931–91.

5

Counseling and Testing for Inherited Predisposition to Cancer

Emily Glogowski[1], Kasmintan A. Schrader[2], Kelly L. Stratton[3], and Kenneth Offit[4]

[1] *GeneDx, Gaithersburg, Massachusetts, USA*
[2] *University of British Columbia, Vancouver, British Columbia, Canada*
[3] *Stephenson Cancer Center, Oklahoma City, Oklahoma, USA*
[4] *Memorial Sloan Kettering Cancer Center, New York, New York, USA*

Introduction

Predispositions to cancers of the breast, colon, ovary, uterus, and other organs affect tens of thousands of Americans each year, and increase risks for additional neoplasms in cancer survivors. Inherited cancer risk falls on a spectrum [1], arising from single or combined low-, moderate-, or high-risk germline (heritable) gene mutations (more recently termed pathogenic variants). Most cancer diagnoses in the population are considered "sporadic"; these are diagnosed at later ages, without a relevant family history, and are traditionally believed to have little or no relation to the patient's genetic inheritance. Less often, the same cancer type may be diagnosed in multiple family members, at typical ages for that cancer type. Possible explanations for these "familial clusters" include chance, moderate-risk genetic factors, and/or shared environmental factors.

Only 5–10% of most common cancer types are caused by inherited pathogenic variants in single high-risk (high-penetrance) genes [2]. Features of these so-called "hereditary cancer syndromes" include multiple affected relatives, bilateral and/or multifocal disease, and/or early ages of diagnosis. Most hereditary syndromes increase cancer risk to several organs, often with specific histological features, although significant clinical variability exists. Sometimes characteristic skin lesions and other benign features can present diagnostic clues to an underlying syndrome (Table 5.1).

Most cancer syndromes display autosomal dominant inheritance, with 50% risk for each sibling and child to inherit the predisposition. Some adult syndromes can also have pediatric manifestations, in light of the early and variable ages of disease-onset. Age at presentation is likely modified by the particular cellular pathway of the mutated gene, interactions with environmental factors or other cellular pathways ("modifier" genes). In some circumstances, biallelic (two) pathogenic variants in common syndromes can predispose to childhood tumors, such as Fanconi anemia and constitutional (biallelic) mismatch repair

deficiency (Table 5.1). For these, screening of carriers' partners may be worthwhile due to the population carrier frequency. Additionally, a host of individually rare pediatric cancer syndromes exist that warrant genetic counseling for children and their families [3]. Noteworthy examples are retinoblastoma, Wilm's tumor, and the bone marrow failure syndromes [4].

This chapter aims to describe the common adult "hereditary cancer syndromes" (as defined above), as detailed in Table 5.1 and elsewhere [1, 3, 5]. "Familial cancer" is addressed in the last section, although the distinction between these two categories is becoming blurred with advances in understanding of underlying molecular causes. The proportion of hereditary and familial cancers (combined) that is explained by known genetic factors is outlined in Figure 5.1, and further discussed below.

Genetic Counseling and Testing

For the past two decades, clinical testing for pathogenic variants in cancer predisposition genes has increasingly influenced clinical oncology practice [2]. Identification of "high-risk individuals" provides opportunities for tailored management, including intensive surveillance from an early age, risk-reducing surgeries, and pharmacoprevention (or "chemoprevention"). Subspecialty societies have published guidelines for the responsible clinical translation of genetic information [6–8], recommending that genetic testing be offered in the context of counseling regarding possible medical and psychosocial consequences. Informed consent is required, and even legally mandated in some states. Counseling includes a discussion of the benefits, accuracy, and limitations of genetic testing; implications of positive, negative, and uncertain results; and possible psychosocial consequences including emotional upset and genetic discrimination (Figure 5.2). Mathematical models that incorporate an individual's personal and/or family history (Figure 5.3) can be used to estimate a patient's risk of testing positive or developing

Table 5.1 Major adult cancer predisposition syndromes, with associated features and genes. Associated malignancies are listed first, followed by less common tumors and benign features. Modified from Weitzel *et al.* [1]. The incidences of these syndromes are listed elsewhere [138]. Human Genome Organisation (HUGO)-approved gene abbreviations can be found at http://www.genenames.org/. This list is not exhaustive. Syndromes and familial clusters that are poorly characterized genetically are not included (see text).

Syndrome	Primary cancer types and other manifestations	Inheritance	Gene(s)
Hereditary breast cancer syndromes			
Cowden (includes *PTEN*-hamartomatous tumor, Bannayan-Riley- Ruvalcaba, Proteus syndromes)	Breast, thyroid (follicular type), endometrial, renal; hamartomatous polyps, oral mucosal papillomas, skin trichilemmomas, macrocephaly, benign breast, thyroid, vascular, genitourinary disease	Dominant	*PTEN, KILLIN*
BRCA-associated breast and ovarian cancer	Breast (female and male), ovarian, fallopian tube, peritoneal, prostate, pancreas, skin	Dominant	*BRCA1, BRCA2*
(includes *Fanconi anemia* FANCD1)	*Fanconi:* Leukemia, solid tumors of head, neck, skin, GI, genital; bone marrow failure, developmental delay, congenital malformations	Recessive	Biallelic *BRCA2*
Li-Fraumeni	Breast, brain, sarcomas, adrenocortical, childhood, many other cancer types	Dominant	*TP53*
Hereditary endocrine tumor syndromes			
Carney complex (=Carney-Stratakis syndrome)	Thyroid; schwannoma, myxoid subcutaneous tumors, primary adrenocortical nodular hyperplasia, testicular Sertoli cell tumor, atrial myxoma, pituitary adenoma, fibroadenoma, blue nevus	Dominant	*PRKAR1A*
Multiple endocrine neoplasia, Type 1	Pancreatic islet cell, pituitary (prolactinoma), parathyroid and adrenocortical tumors, endocrine tumors of the gastro-entero-pancreatic tract (Zollinger-Ellison syndrome), carcinoids	Dominant	*MEN1, CDKN1B/*p27, *CDKN2B/*p15
Multiple endocrine neoplasia, Type 2	Thyroid (medullary type); pheochromocytoma, parathyroid hyperplasia	Dominant	*RET*
Hereditary paraganglioma and pheochromocytoma	Paraganglioma, renal (clear cell, chromophobe, papillary, oncocytoma), breast, thyroid; pheochromocytoma	Dominant	*SDHB, SDHD, SDHC, SDHA SDHAF2, MAX, TMEM127 (*also *VHL, RET, NF1)*
Hereditary gastroenterologic syndromes			
Familial adenomatous polyposis (FAP) (includes *attenuated FAP* phenotype, *Turcot variant* and *APC-deletion syndrome*)	Colon, duodenal and upper GI carcinomas and adenomas, thyroid, infant hepatoblastoma; desmoid tumors, jaw osteomas, dental anomalies, congenital hypertrophy of the retinal pigment epithelium, lipomas, fibromas, epidermoid cysts, nasopharyngeal angiofibromas; *Turcot:* medulloblastoma; *Deletion syndrome:* developmental delay	Dominant	*APC*
Familial gastrointestinal stromal tumor (GIST)	GIST, cutaneous hyperpigmentation, esophageal stenosis (dysphagia)	Dominant	*KIT, PDGFRA (*also *NF1, PRKAR1A)*
Hereditary diffuse gastric cancer	Gastric (diffuse type), breast (lobular type)	Dominant	*CDH1*
Hereditary pancreatitis	Pancreatic; pancreatitis	Dominant	*PRSS1, SPINK1, CFTR, CASR, CTRC*
Juvenile polyposis syndrome (occasional overlap with *hereditary hemorrhagic telangiectasia (HHT)*	Stomach, small intestine and colorectal polyps (of hamartomatous or "juvenile" type) and cancers, pancreatic; *HHT:* arteriovenous malformations and mucocutaneous telangiectases	Dominant	*SMAD4, BMPR1 (ENG, ALK1* in HHT*)*
Lynch syndrome (=hereditary nonpolyposis colorectal cancer) (includes *Turcot* and *Muir-Torre* variants)	Colon, endometrial, ovarian upper GI (including pancreas), ovarian, renal pelvis, ureter, bladder, possible breast; *Turcot:* glioblastoma *Muir-Torre:* sebaceous neoplasia, keratoacanthomas	Dominant	*MLH1, MSH2, MSH6, PMS2, EPCAM/ TACSTD1* (MMR genes)
(Includes *constitutional mismatch repair [CMMR] deficiency*)	*CMMR:* childhood hematologic, brain, colon; café-au-lait skin macules	Recessive	Biallelic MMR carriers
MYH-associated polyposis	Colon and upper GI carcinomas and adenomas, possible Lynch- and FAP-associated tumors	Recessive	*MYH (=MUTYH)*
Peutz-Jeghers syndrome	Colorectal, stomach, pancreatic, breast, adenoma malignum of cervix; small intestine, stomach, colon and nasal polyps (of hamartomatous or "Peutz-Jeghers" type), sex cord (SCTAT) and Sertoli tumors, mucocutaneous hyperpigmentation	Dominant	*STK11*

Table 5.1 (Continued)

Syndrome	Primary cancer types and other manifestations	Inheritance	Gene(s)
Hereditary genitourinary cancer syndromes			
Birt-Hogg-Dube syndrome	Renal cell carcinoma (RCC) (mixed chromophobe, oncocytic, clear cell); fibrofolliculomas, trichodiscoma, acrochordon, lung blebs, pneumothorax	Dominant	*FLCN*
Hereditary leiomyomatosis and renal cell carcinoma	Papillary RCC type II (*FH*-associated); skin and uterine leiomyomata	Dominant	*FH*
Hereditary papillary renal cancer	Papillary RCC (type I)	Dominant	*MET*
Tuberous sclerosis	RCC (and cysts), angiomyolipomas, giant cell astrocytoma; ependymoma, cardiac rhabdomyoma, characteristic CNS and skin anomalies	Dominant	*TSC1, TSC2*
Von Hippel-Lindau syndrome	RCC (and cysts); pheochromocytomas, hemangioblastomas (CNS), angiomas (retina), endolymphatic sac tumors, pancreatic cysts, epididymal cystadenoma	Dominant	*VHL*
Hereditary genodermatoses			
Familial atypical multiple mole melanoma (includes hereditary melanoma pancreatic syndrome)	Melanoma, pancreatic; nevi	Dominant	*CDKN2A* (p16), *CDK4, CMM*
Gorlin syndrome (=nevoid basal cell carcinoma syndrome)	Basal cell, medulloblastoma (childhood); palmar/plantar pits, cardiac/ovarian fibromas, jaw keratocysts, macrocephaly, facial and skeletal features	Dominant	*PTCH1*
Neurofibromatosis 1	Neurofibrosarcomas (nerve sheath tumors); neurofibromas, pheochromocytomas, optic/CNS gliomas, meningiomas, Lisch nodules, axillary/inguinal freckling, café-au-lait spots, skeletal/learning disabilities	Dominant	*NF1*

cancer [1, 6, 9, 10]. Post-test counseling includes: results communication and interpretation; consideration of additional genetic tests; recommendations for surveillance, risk-reducing surgeries, and pharmacoprevention; and referrals for ongoing care. In some settings, such as familial adenomatous polyposis (FAP) and von Hippel-Lindau disease (VHL), genotype-phenotype correlations allow for loose predictions of clinical manifestations based on the region of the gene affected. With any germline test, a proportion of results are variants of uncertain clinical significance. These require careful interpretation and follow-up. Counseling also includes a discussion of risks to offspring and other relatives. Identification of a family's pathogenic variant allows for cost-effective risk-stratification of relatives, by tailoring screening recommendations for those with or without the variant. A discussion of modern reproductive options, such as preimplantation genetic diagnosis, has become integrated into routine counseling.

Any person with personal and/or family features suspicious for a hereditary cancer syndrome should be considered for genetic counseling and testing. Common indications include (but are not limited to) any patient with the following cancer types: early-onset breast, triple negative breast, male breast, epithelial ovarian, metastatic prostate, early colon, mismatch repair deficient colon, early-onset endometrial [6, 11], more than 10 colon adenomas, or a known germline pathogenic variant in the family. Certain rare tumors can also provide an indication for referral, regardless of family history (Table 5.2) [12]. Publicly-available consensus criteria for referral, syndrome reviews and recommendations for management, can be found on the National Comprehensive Cancer Network® (NCCN®) (www.

nccn.org) and GeneReviews (www.genereviews.org) websites [11, 13]. Providers should be familiar with local clinical genetics services; searchable listings can be found online at GeneTests™ (www.geneclinics.org), National Society of Genetic Counselors (www.nsgc.org), and the National Cancer Institute (http://www.cancer.gov/cancertopics/genetics/directory).

Hereditary Breast and Gynecologic Cancer Syndromes

Hereditary breast and ovarian cancer susceptibility is commonly caused by dominantly-inherited germline pathogenic variants in the *BRCA1* and *BRCA2* genes. Women from high-risk families who carry *BRCA1* or *BRCA2* gene pathogenic variants have an estimated 45–84% lifetime risk of developing breast cancer [14], compared to a general population risk of 12% (1 in 8) [15]. Female *BRCA1* and *BRCA2* pathogenic variant carriers have an estimated 11–62% lifetime risk of ovarian cancer, as well as fallopian tube and peritoneal cancers [14], compared to about 1.4% (1 in 73) for the general population [16]. *BRCA1*-related risks are generally higher than *BRCA2*. These wide ranges reflect the differences between the original highest-risk versus later population-based studies. As these ranges are confusing to patients, a large meta-analysis is helpful for counseling [14]. Knowledge that *BRCA1*-driven breast tumors are often, but not exclusively, histologically "triple negative" (negative for estrogen receptors, progesterone receptors, and Her2) can guide genetic testing [17]. Evidence to date has not demonstrated altered prognosis, outside of standard prognostic

(a)

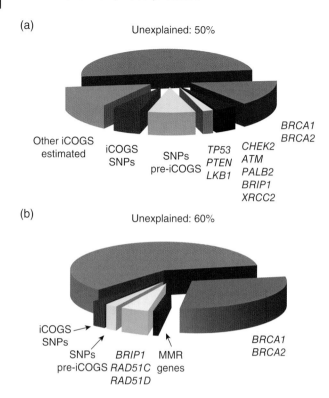

Unexplained: 50%

Other iCOGS estimated   iCOGS SNPs   SNPs pre-iCOGS   *TP53 PTEN LKB1*   *CHEK2 ATM PALB2 BRIP1 XRCC2*   *BRCA1 BRCA2*

(b)

Unexplained: 60%

iCOGS SNPs   SNPs pre-iCOGS   *BRIP1 RAD51C RAD51D*   MMR genes   *BRCA1 BRCA2*

Figure 5.1 Estimated proportions of familial (a) breast, (b) ovarian cancer. Most cancer is sporadic, although familial aggregation is also observed for most cancer types. Most familial cancer remains unexplained. The proportion attributable to known, high-risk syndromes (*BRCA1/2*, MMR genes, *TP53*) is not large. Past genome-wide association studies (GWAS) have identified numerous low-penetrance loci (pre-iCOGS), and recent international consortia, such as the Illumina Collaborative Oncological Gene-environment Study (iCOGS), are uncovering additional loci. In the figure, "pre-iCOGS" and "iCOGS" refer to susceptibility loci (SNPs) identified before and after use of the iCOGS array, respectively. "Other iCOGS estimated" refers to loci anticipated to be discovered as studies with the array progress [140]. SNP, single nucleotide polymorphism. *Source:* Bahcall 2013 [140]. Reproduced with permission of Nature Publishing Group.

factors, for *BRCA*-associated breast cancers [18]. Affected carriers have a 25–30% risk of developing a second breast cancer in the 10 years after their first diagnosis [18]. By contrast, a survival advantage has been demonstrated in *BRCA*-associated *ovarian* cancers, linked to platinum-based chemotherapy response. Male *BRCA1*, and predominantly, *BRCA2* pathogenic variant carriers have increased risks for male breast and aggressive prostate cancers [19]. So-called "founder mutations" occur in genetically-isolated populations, such as in one out of 40 individuals of Ashkenazi Jewish origin [20], and other groups.[6]

Women with *BRCA* pathogenic variants should be referred for high-risk breast cancer surveillance including annual magnetic resonance imaging (MRI), starting at age 25–30 [21], and offered risk-reducing mastectomies [22]. Pharmacopreventive options include tamoxifen and raloxifene for breast protection [23, 24] and oral contraceptives for ovarian [25] protection. The efficacy of ovarian cancer surveillance is limited [26] so

prophylactic removal of the ovaries and fallopian tubes is recommended after childbearing [27, 28]. This surgery may additionally reduce breast cancer risk, presumably due to induction of premature menopause. Unfortunately, occult or peritoneal carcinomas can occur during or following ovarian removal [29]. Male carriers should monitor their breast tissue, seek medical evaluation for any anomalies, and screen for prostate cancer at age 40 [30]. Breast imaging techniques have not been studied in men, but can be performed if anatomically feasible. Poly(ADP-ribose) polymerase (PARPi) inhibitors, such as FDA-approved olaparib, have been developed to target ovarian, metastatic breast [31], and prostate [32] cancers, and hold promise for others such as pancreatic [33] cancer in *BRCA1/2* pathogenic variant carriers [34].

Less common breast cancer syndromes should be considered in *BRCA1/2*-negative breast cancer families (Table 5.1). Macrocephaly and oral papules can raise suspicion for Cowden syndrome, which would imply additional thyroid, endometrial, and other cancer risks [35, 36]. In Li-Fraumeni syndrome, germline *TP53* pathogenic variants cause increased and early-onset risks for many cancer types, including breast [37]. International screening trials using frequent biochemical testing with rapid total body, breast and brain MRI, have been encouraging and consensus guidelines have been proposed [38]. Lynch syndrome (LS) [39] and Peutz-Jeghers syndrome (PJS) [40], described below, are also contributors to gynecologic malignancies.

Hereditary Colorectal Cancer Syndromes

A large proportion of high-risk colorectal cancer (CRC) predisposition stems from LS and the polyposis syndromes. LS is caused by dominantly-inherited pathogenic variants in the mismatch repair (MMR) genes (*MLH1, MSH2, MSH6,* or *PMS2*). Through a different mechanism, deletions in the 3' region of *TACSTD1/EPCAM* can cause downstream epigenetic silencing of *MSH2*. Dysfunctional MMR genes allow for buildup of DNA replication errors in tumors. This phenomenon, known as microsatellite instability (MSI), can be used to identify LS-related tumors [41]. Likewise, immunohistochemical (IHC) stains of tumor tissue can demonstrate loss of MMR protein expression, and guide germline testing in a patient [42]. IHC and MSI results correlate, and signify an underlying somatic or germline MMR deficiency [43]. This MMR phenotype is also present in about 15% of nonhereditary colon cancer, explained by somatic hypermethylation of the *MLH1* promoter [44] or other somatic MMR pathogenic variants [45]. Clinical criteria, known as the revised Bethesda guidelines [46] and revised Amsterdam criteria [47], have traditionally been used to identify individuals who would benefit from genetic evaluation for LS. Many institutions now evaluate many or all newly-diagnosed CRC and endometrial tumors for MMR deficiency, using MSI and/or IHC [33, 48].

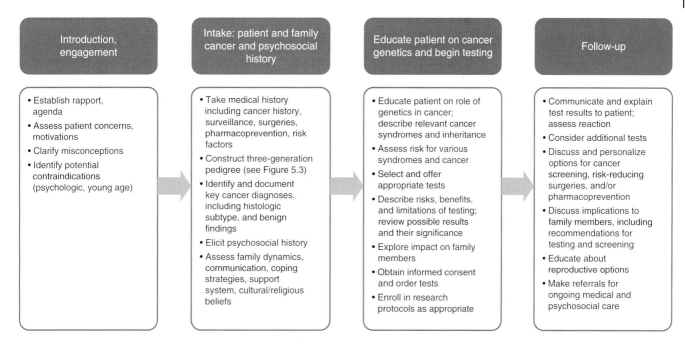

Figure 5.2 Elements of hereditary/familial cancer genetic counseling.

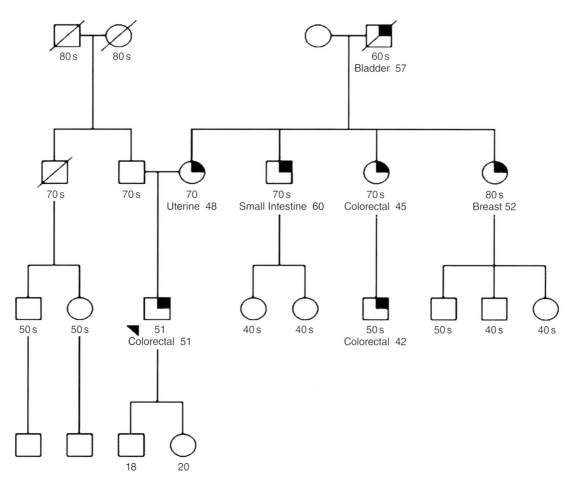

Figure 5.3 Sample pedigree, suggestive of Lynch syndrome. Typical pedigree taken during genetic counseling, used for risk assessment. Arrow indicates the proband (consultant); circles represent women; squares men. Horizontal alignment indicates a generation; vertical lines show offspring/parents. Shading indicates a cancer diagnosis. Diagonal line indicates individual is deceased. Here, the proband was diagnosed with colorectal cancer at age 51 and his maternal family history meets Amsterdam criteria [47] for Lynch syndrome.

Table 5.2 Tumors/cancers that are strongly associated with a germline cancer predisposition. Each of the tumors/cancers listed here (organized by organ system) should trigger a referral for genetic counseling [139], regardless of other medical/family history. This list is not meant to be comprehensive, and does not include combinations of different tumor types.

Organ/system affected	Cancer/tumor subtype
Brain/nervous system	Atypical teratoid/malignant rhabdoid tumor
	Choroid plexus carcinoma
	Hemangioblastomas (brain, spine)
	Lhermitte-Duclos disease (adult, cerebellar)
	Malignant peripheral nerve sheath tumor
	Meningioma (< age 25)
Circulatory	Juvenile myelomonocytic leukemia
Eye	Retinal angiomas
	Optic glioma
	Retinoblastoma
Ear	Endolymphatic sac
	Vestibular schwannomas (bilateral)
Thyroid	Medullary
	Papillary cribriform-morular variant
Abdomen	Desmoids
Stomach	Diffuse (< age 40)
Liver	Hepatoblastoma (< age 15)
Adrenal/neuroendocrine	Adrenocortical carcinoma
	Paraganglioma
	Pheochromocytoma
	Primary pigmented nodular adrenocortical dysplasia
Kidney/urinary tract	Chromophobe (multiple/bilateral)
	Hybrid oncocytic
	Papillary renal cell type 2 (or FH-associated)
Reproductive	Adenoma malignum of cervix
	Ovarian, fallopian tube, or primary peritoneal
	Papillary cystadenomas of the epididymis or broad ligament
	Male breast
	Sex cord tumors with annular tubules
Skin	Trichilemmomas
	Leiomyomas
	Sebaceous adenoma/carcinoma

The highest cancer risks in LS are CRC (25–75%), with an accelerated adenoma-to-carcinoma progression, and endometrial carcinoma (30–45%) in women [49]. In comparison, the average risks are 5% for colorectal [50] and 2.6% (of women) for endometrial cancers [51]. Other cancer risks, including upper gastrointestinal, urologic and ovarian, are present to a lesser degree (Table 5.1) [12]. Genotype–phenotype correlations are emerging. A child who inherits two MMR pathogenic variants can manifest childhood and hematologic malignancies (Table 5.1) [52]. Surveillance colonoscopy every 1–2 years from age 20 to 25 halves CRC incidence and mortality [53, 54]. Screening for extracolonic tumors, such as with upper endoscopies, urinalysis, and for females, transvaginal ultrasounds, endometrial biopsies, and/or CA-125 blood tests, may be considered by age 35, although their efficacy is unproven [12, 55]. Evidence suggests protective effects of long-term aspirin use [56]. Identification of LS at the time of, or prior to, CRC diagnosis can impact clinical management. Risk-reducing subtotal colectomy, instead of segmental resection, should be offered to address the risk of metachronous CRC [28, 57]. Risk-reducing hysterectomy with bilateral salpingo-oophorectomy should be offered to women during colectomy and/or after childbearing [28, 55, 58]. The demonstration of tumor mismatch-repair status in predicting clinical benefit of immune checkpoint blockade has opened the door to new lines of therapy in this patient group [59].

Classic familial adenomatous polyposis (FAP) displays hundreds to thousands of adenomatous colon polyps in the teenage years, with a 90% CRC risk by age 45, and other benign and malignant findings (Table 5.1) [14, 60]. In 25% of cases, family history is absent due to *de novo* (new) pathogenic variants that are sometimes mosaic [61]. Genetic testing is offered in childhood. Consensus guidelines recommend management with annual sigmoidoscopy or colonoscopy starting age 10–15, until surgery is performed. Risk-reducing colectomy is the treatment of choice once adenomas appear, usually in the late teens, with continued surveillance of the ileal pouch [28]. Extracolonic monitoring includes upper endoscopy and physical examination with thyroid and abdominal palpation [14, 62]. Pharmacopreventive considerations include COX II inhibitors [63]. In attenuated FAP (AFAP), with under 100 adenomas and CRC onset 10–20 years later [64], surgical intervention is guided by polyp number/size/histology, genotype associations, patient preference, and screening compliance.

One quarter of polyposis patients who test negative for *APC* pathogenic variants carry biallelic *MUTYH* pathogenic variants [65, 66], with a high lifetime CRC risk [67]. Benign and malignant extracolonic manifestations may resemble attenuated or classic FAP [68], although the full spectrum of disease is still under study. *MUTYH*-associated polyposis (MAP) is managed according to the clinical phenotype, with frequent colonoscopies and upper endoscopies, and possibly risk-reducing colectomy and/or [14] pharmacoprevention. *MUTYH* carriers comprise 1–2% of populations of European descent [65], and may have a marginally increased colon cancer risk [67].

Uncommon polyposis syndromes include PJS, juvenile polyposis syndrome (JPS), Cowden syndrome (Table 5.1) [11, 14, 69], and others. PJS displays polyps and cancer risks throughout the upper and lower GI tract and other organs, with characteristic brown or blue buccal markings [40]. Pathogenic variants in *STK11* are responsible in most cases [70]. JPS presents clinically with multiple polyps with "juvenile" histology and cancer risks throughout the gastrointestinal (GI) tract. Around 50–60% of JPS cases are caused by pathogenic variants in *SMAD4* or *BMPR1A* [71]. The syndrome can co-occur with hereditary hemorrhagic telangiectasia (HHT) [72], causing potentially lethal arteriovenous malformations when undetected. Cowden syndrome, mentioned previously, involves GI dysplastic polyps of varied histologies [73].

A significant fraction of polyposis is unexplained by the known syndromes. Historically, the terms "mixed" or "hyperplastic" polyposis referred to the presence of varied or nonadenomatous polyp types, respectively. Polyp classifications are not yet standardized, and the nomenclature is confusing. Criteria for a combined "serrated polyposis syndrome" have been proposed, based on the number, location, and size of hyperplastic or serrated colon polyps [14]. Heterozygous *GREM1* pathogenic variants are implicated in a fraction [74].

Hereditary Upper Gastrointestinal Cancer Syndromes

Importantly, upper GI manifestations occur in most of the hereditary cancer syndromes described above [14]. Particularly in PJS, risks to the small intestine include obstruction, bleeding due to polyps, and cancer [40]. Risks for pancreatic adenocarcinoma (PAC) are seen in PJS, LS [75] and possibly JPS [71]. PAC may be caused by hereditary breast–ovarian cancer syndrome in 12–17% of familial cases [76, 77]; hereditary pancreatitis explains a few [78]. PAC is seen with multiple nevi and melanomas in familial atypical multiple-mole melanoma (Table 5.1) [79]. Genes causing Fanconi anemia, including *PALB2/FANCN*, also predispose to PAC [80, 81]. In all of these categories, PAC is usually seen in conjunction with other component tumors of the syndrome. There is no proven method of screening for PAC. However, patients may join ongoing trials investigating MRI cholangiopancreatography, endoscopic ultrasound, tumor marker measurement, and other techniques [82].

Hereditary diffuse gastric cancer (HDGC) syndrome is characterized by susceptibility to gastric cancer of the diffuse type (DGC) and breast cancer of the lobular type (LBC). Germline pathogenic variants in *CDH1* are found in 30–50% of HDGC families, with geographic variability [83]. The International Gastric Linkage Consortium's genetic testing criteria [84] are: DGC under age 40; two DGC cases at any age (one confirmed DGC), and families with both DGC and LBC (one diagnosed before age 50). Testing may also be considered in patients with bilateral or familial LBC under age 50, DGC and cleft lip/palate, and those with precursor lesions for signet ring cell carcinoma. HDGC shows virtually complete penetrance for small foci of *in situ* or invasive cancer, with 70% chance of gastric cancer for males and 56% for females by age 80 [85]. Since endoscopic surveillance is ineffective, carriers require prophylactic total gastrectomies. Unfortunately, this surgery has a significant effect on quality of life. Such families should be managed by a multidisciplinary expert team. Female carriers need intensive breast cancer surveillance with breast MRI [85], due to the 42% LBC risk. Additional genes have been linked.

Mesenchymal stromal tumors of the GI tract (GIST) occur in the small bowel due to constitutively-activated pathogenic variants in *KIT* and *PDGFRA* [86]. Specific dermatologic and ocular features can assist in distinguishing these from neurofibromatosis type 1-associated GIST [87] and Carney–Stratakis-associated

GIST. Use of the selective tyrosine kinase inhibitor, imatinib, can stabilize esophageal GIST in patients harboring *c-KIT* pathogenic variants [88].

Hereditary Endocrine Syndromes

Multiple endocrine neoplasia type 1 (MEN1) syndrome predisposes to at least 20 endocrine and nonendocrine tumors, especially parathyroid adenomas causing hyperparathyroidism and hypercalcemia; pituitary tumors such as prolactinoma; and well-differentiated endocrine tumors of the gastro-enteropancreatic tract. Tumors present with growth effects or hormone overproduction. Thymic carcinoids can be aggressive in males and smokers. In multiple endocrine neoplasia type 2 (MEN2), prophylactic thyroidectomy is performed in childhood or earlier, due to the near certainty of aggressive medullary thyroid carcinoma [89]. Pheochromocytomas and parathyroid disease also occur. In both MEN1 [90] and MEN2 [89], screening involves targeted imaging and biochemical studies from an early age. Cowden and Carney–Stratakis syndromes also have endocrine manifestations, including nonmedullary thyroid cancers (Table 5.1).

The hereditary paraganglioma and pheochromocytoma syndromes mainly result from pathogenic variants in the succinate dehydrogenase (*SDH*) complex genes, named by their subunit (Table 5.1) [91]. They predispose to neuroendocrine tumors, specifically, hormone-producing adrenal pheochromocytomas, and nonfunctioning extra-adrenal paragangliomas with malignant potential [92]. Symptoms of catecholamine excess include hypertension, profuse sweating, or palpitations. Kidney cancers occur, especially with *SDHB* pathogenic variants [93], and display a breadth of histologies [94]. Lifelong imaging and biochemical measurement in these families can reduce risk of malignancy and hypertensive crises [95]. Pheochromocytomas occur elsewhere, as a lesser feature of von Hippel-Lindau disease (VHL), neurofibromatosis type 1, and MEN2 [91]. Together, hereditary syndromes account for at least one quarter of these tumors [96].

Hereditary Kidney Cancer Syndromes

Hereditary syndromes involving renal cancer [97–99] garner increasing attention, due to their recent elucidation and potential amelioration with targeted therapies. VHL patients, with central nervous system or ocular hemangioblastomas (angiomas), have a 70% risk of renal cell carcinoma (RCC) from early to late adulthood [100]. Screening for early manifestations, starting in infancy, has shifted the primary cause of mortality from cerebellar hemangioblastomas to RCC later in life [101]. Hereditary papillary renal cell carcinoma (HPRCC) displays variable penetrance, causing the development of multiple type 1 papillary RCCs. Identification can be challenging, secondary to small hypovascular lesions with poor enhancement and reduced penetrance at late ages [102]. Targeted therapy with *MET* inhibitors has been proposed [103]. Birt-Hogg-Dubé syndrome (BHD) is characterized by mixed renal cell cancer histologies and cysts [104], with skin fibrofolliculomas, pulmonary cysts, and spontaneous pneumothorax [105]. For VHL, HPRCC, and BHD, renal management involves surveillance of kidney lesions under 3 cm, with conservative surgical management of larger tumors, to attempt to preserve renal function [106, 107].

Hereditary leiomyomatosis and renal cell cancer (HLRCC) syndrome, caused by fumarate hydratase gene (*FH*) pathogenic variants, can cause unilateral type II papillary RCC or collecting duct RCC [108]. Red or brown skin leiomyomas develop and may be confused with acne, precluding diagnosis. Affected women develop symptomatic uterine fibroids at an early age, commonly requiring hysterectomy [109]. Unlike other syndromes, HLRCC is associated with solitary lesions that carry metastatic potential even when small. Their aggressive nature precludes observation and warrants removal of all identifiable lesions [110].

Cowden syndrome and the hereditary paraganglioma syndromes include RCC as a minor feature. Tuberous sclerosis syndrome associates with clear cell RCC (Table 5.1). RCC families rarely have constitutional translocations involving chromosome 3 [98], or other known and unknown genes [98]. Lynch syndrome causes urothelial carcinomas of the renal pelvis and ureter, and possibly bladder cancer, but not RCC.

New Directions and Research

Historically, candidate genes for hereditary cancer syndromes were uncovered by examining specific regions of the genome, in large cancer families, for cosegregation with disease. Thereafter, large-scale genome association studies found common single nucleotide polymorphisms (SNPs) that only marginally alter risk [111]. Now, "next-generation" sequencing (NGS) technologies are being used for partial or entire genome sequencing, and are setting the stage for novel disease-susceptibility gene discovery. A recent example is a dominant predisposition to pre-B cell acute lymphoblastic leukemia, which we have termed *PAX5-*associated neoplasia (PABN) [112]. Other genes identified with this approach include *BAP1, GREM1*[74], *MAX, PALB2, POLE,* and *POLD1* [113]. Large consortia, such as the Breast and Ovarian Cancer Association Consortia (BCAC and OCAC), and the Illumina Collaborative Oncological Gene-environment Study (iCOGS), are pursuing SNP-based association studies of breast, ovarian and prostate cancers [114]. COMPLEXO unites researchers who use next generation sequencing to study breast and ovarian cancer heritability [115]. The Consortium of Investigators of Modifiers of *BRCA1/2* (CIMBA) highlights the potential for certain alleles to modulate cancer risk in individuals with known hereditary syndromes [116, 117]. Meanwhile, NGS technologies are being applied to the *somatic* analysis of human malignancies, through international collaborations such as The Cancer Genome Atlas (TCGA, http://cancergenome.nih.gov) and the International Cancer Genome Consortium (ICGC, https://www.icgc.org). Altogether, this exciting wave of research is beginning to uncover additional rare, highly-penetrant, susceptibility variants, as well as moderate-penetrance alleles (Figure 5.4). Through them, we may ultimately learn the genetic causes behind most familial cancer risk.

Combinations of newly-discovered moderate-penetrance genes almost certainly play a role in sporadic as well as familial

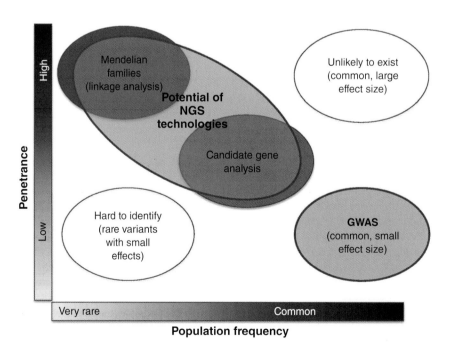

Figure 5.4 The utility of different methods of genetic and genomic analyses used to define cancer susceptibility factors plotted as a function of penetrance and population frequency. Traditional approaches such as linkage analysis in large affected families have successfully defined the established rare and highly penetrant cancer syndromes, discussed in this chapter (shown at the top left). GWAS (genome-wide association studies) of large numbers of individuals affected and unaffected with common sporadic cancers have identified common variants with small effects (bottom right). The anticipated utility of NGS (next-generation sequencing) stems from its potential to identify additional moderate-to-high risk cancer susceptibility genes in smaller cancer families. *Source:* adapted from Stadler *et al.* 2014 [137]. Reproduced with permission of American Society of Clinical Oncology.

cancers. For example, breast cancer susceptibility is heterogeneous and implicates *ATM, BRCA1, BRCA2* [118], *CDH1, CHEK2, NBN, NF1, PALB2* [119], *TP53, PTEN, STK11*, and a host of other genes, in familial and/or sporadic cases [120–122]. Similarly, next generation sequencing has implicated *BRIP1*, mismatch repair genes (*MSH1, MLH1, MSH6, PMS2, EPCAM*), *RAD51C, RAD51D, STK11* (non-epithelial), in addition to *BRCA1* and *BRCA2*, in ovarian cancer. These gene lists are constantly evolving and updates can be found on www.nccn.org. Familial, nonsyndromic, colorectal cancer comprises at least 15% of all CRC [123], and high-risk families with microsatellite stable tumors are termed "familial CRC type X" to acknowledge their unknown etiology [124, 125]. Similarly, familial cancers of the pancreas, stomach (intestinal type), esophagus, thyroid (nonmedullary), prostate [126], testicular, brain [127], lung, lymphoproliferative diseases, sarcomas [128], melanoma, and other cancer types are observed. Multiple contributing genes have been implicated, yet much remains unexplained. Most likely, their etiology is complex and/or heterogeneous; these families remain excellent candidates for large-scale genomic studies. Finally, advances in genetics understanding should not draw attention from the study of environmental contributions. For example, cigarette smoking and high body mass index have been shown to magnify cancer risk in Lynch syndrome [129]. Moving forward, studies of the interplay between genetic variations and endogenous or exogenous exposures will be critical for cancer prevention and control.

"Multiplex" cancer panels that simultaneously analyze multiple genes are now commercially available for clinical use [130]. Patients may increasingly present to their primary care, gynecology, oncology, and other physicians with a "personalized medicine" report, requesting interpretation and possibly follow-up tests. Such patients may be referred for formal genetic counseling, as their results will reflect a mixture of clinically major, minor, and uncertain contributions to disease-risk, each of which may or may not be medically-actionable [131].

The Prospective Registry of MultiPlex Testing, or PROMPT (www.promptstudy.org) has been formed to study variants in these genes. ClinVar (www.clinvar.com; part of ClinGen) is a public archive of relationships among human genetic variants and phenotypes. Clinically, large-scale somatic analysis of tumor genomes, accompanied by germline analysis for a control comparison, may become the standard of care at large academic centers. Through these processes, "incidental" discoveries of patients' risks for other cancers, as well as noncancerous diseases, needs to be addressed [132, 133, 134, 135]. The development of methods to convey, or not convey, such incidental findings is ongoing (for example, see the publically-available decision aid www.genomicsadviser.com). These changes are defining new challenges in cancer genetic and genomic counseling [130, 136, 137].

Special thanks to Marina Corines, Amy Plofker, Michael Newman, Rohini Rau-Murthy, and Anne Lincoln for their tireless efforts and expert assistance with editing, figures, and other aspects of this text.

References

1 Weitzel JN, Blazer KR, Macdonald DJ, Culver JO, Offit K. Genetics, genomics, and cancer risk assessment: state of the art and future directions in the era of personalized medicine. *CA Cancer J Clin* 2011;61(5):327–59. doi:10.3322/caac.20128.

2 Offit K. *Clinical Cancer Genetics: Risk Counseling and Management.* New York: Wiley-Liss, 1998.

3 Lindor NM, McMaster ML, Lindor CJ, Greene MH. Concise Handbook of Familial Cancer Susceptibility Syndromes, 2nd edn. *J Nat Cancer Inst Monogr* 2008;(38):3–93. Epub 2008 June 1. doi:10.1093/jncimonographs/lgn001.

4 Alter BP. Diagnosis, genetics, and management of inherited bone marrow failure syndromes. Hematology Am Soc Hematol Educ Program 2007:29–39.

5 Garber JE, Offit K. Hereditary cancer predisposition syndromes. *J Clin Oncol* 2005;23(2):276–92.

6 Berliner JL, Fay AM, Cummings SA, Burnett B, Tillmanns T. NSGC practice guideline: risk assessment and genetic counseling for hereditary breast and ovarian cancer. *J Genet Couns* 2013;22(2):155–63.

7 American Society of Clinical Oncology. American Society of Clinical Oncology policy statement update: genetic testing for cancer susceptibility. *J Clin Oncol* 2003;21(12):2397–406.

8 Robson ME, Storm CD, Weitzel J, Wollins DS, Offit K. American Society of Clinical Oncology policy statement update: genetic and genomic testing for cancer susceptibility. *J Clin Oncol* 2010;28(5):893–901.

9 Balmana J, Balaguer F, Castellvi-Bel S, *et al.* Comparison of predictive models, clinical criteria and molecular tumour screening for the identification of patients with Lynch syndrome in a population-based cohort of colorectal cancer patients. *J Med Genet* 2008;45(9):557–63.

10 Fischer C, Kuchenbacker K, Engel C, *et al.* Evaluating the performance of the breast cancer genetic risk models BOADICEA, IBIS, BRCAPRO and Claus for predicting BRCA1/2 mutation carrier probabilities: a study based on 7352 families from the German Hereditary Breast and Ovarian Cancer Consortium. *J Med Genet* 2013;50(6):360–7.

11 Kohlmann W, Gruber SB. Lynch Syndrome. February 5 2004 [updated 22 May 2014]. In: RA Pagon, MP Adam, HH Ardinger, *et al.* (eds) GeneReviews® [Internet]. Seattle: University of Washington, Seattle, 1993–2017. Available from: https://www.ncbi.nlm.nih.gov/books/NBK1211/

12 Banks KC, Moline JJ, Marvin ML, Newlin AC, Vogel KJ. 10 rare tumors that warrant a genetics referral. *Fam Cancer* 2013;12(1):1–18.

13 Jasperson KW, Patel SG, Ahnen DJ. APC-Associated Polyposis Conditions. December 18 1998 [updated 2 February 2017]. In: RA Pagon, MP Adam, HH Ardinger, *et al.* (eds) GeneReviews® [Internet]. Seattle: University of Washington, Seattle, 1993–2017. Available from: https://www.ncbi.nlm.nih.gov/books/NBK1345/

14 Chen S, Parmigiani G. Meta-analysis of *BRCA1* and *BRCA2* penetrance. *J Clin Oncol* 2007;25(11):1329–33.

15 American Cancer Society Cancer Statistics Center. Probability of developing cancer, 2011–2013. https://cancerstatisticscenter.cancer.org/#/ (accessed 7 June 7 2017).

16 National Cancer Institute; Surveillance, Epidemiology, and End Results. SEER stat fact sheets: ovary. http://seer.cancer.gov/statfacts/html/ovary.html (accessed 15 May 2017).

17 Hartman AR, Kaldate RR, Sailer LM, *et al.* Prevalence of BRCA mutations in an unselected population of triple-negative breast cancer. *Cancer* 2012;118(11):2787–95.

18 Robson ME. Treatment of hereditary breast cancer. *Semin Oncol* 2007;34(5):384–91.

19 Lecarpentier J, Silvestri V, Kuchenbaecker KB, *et al.* Prediction of breast and prostate cancer risks in male BRCA1 and BRCA2 mutation carriers using polygenic risk scores. *J Clin Oncol* 2017; April 27.

20 Roa BB, Boyd AA, Volcik K, Richards CS. Ashkenazi Jewish population frequencies for common mutations in BRCA1 and BRCA2. *Nature Genet* 1996;14(2):185–7.

21 Robson ME, Offit K. Breast MRI for women with hereditary cancer risk. *JAMA* 2004;292(11):1368–70.

22 Kurian AW, Sigal BM, Plevritis SK. Survival analysis of cancer risk reduction strategies for BRCA1/2 mutation carriers. *J Clin Oncol* 2010;28(2):222–31.

23 King MC, Wieand S, Hale K, *et al.* Tamoxifen and breast cancer incidence among women with inherited mutations in BRCA1 and BRCA2: National Surgical Adjuvant Breast and Bowel Project (NSABP-P1) Breast Cancer Prevention Trial. *JAMA* 2001;286(18):2251–6.

24 Gronwald J, Tung N, Foulkes WD, *et al.* Tamoxifen and contralateral breast cancer in BRCA1 and BRCA2 carriers: an update. *Int J Cancer* 2006;118(9):2281–4.

25 Cibula D, Zikan M, Dusek L, Majek O. Oral contraceptives and risk of ovarian and breast cancers in BRCA mutation carriers: a meta-analysis. *Expert Rev Anticancer Ther* 2011;11(8):1197–207.

26 Long KC, Kauff ND. Screening for familial ovarian cancer: a ray of hope and a light to steer by. *J Clin Oncol* 2013;31(1):8–10.

27 Kauff ND, Domchek SM, Friebel TM, *et al.* Risk-reducing salpingo-oophorectomy for the prevention of BRCA1- and BRCA2-associated breast and gynecologic cancer: a multicenter, prospective study. *J Clin Oncol* 2008;26(8):1331–7.

28 Guillem JG, Wood WC, Moley JF, *et al.* ASCO/SSO review of current role of risk-reducing surgery in common hereditary cancer syndromes. *J Clin Oncol* 2006;24(28):4642–60.

29 Reitsma W, de Bock GH, Oosterwijk JC, *et al.* Support of the 'fallopian tube hypothesis' in a prospective series of risk-reducing salpingo-oophorectomy specimens. *Eur J Cancer* 2013;49(1):132–41.

30 Bancroft EK, Page EC, Castro E, *et al.* Targeted prostate cancer screening in BRCA1 and BRCA2 mutation carriers: results from the initial screening round of the IMPACT study. *Eur Urol* 2014;66(3):489–99.

31 Robson M, Im SA, Senkus, *et al.* Olaparib for Metastatic Breast Cancer in Patients with a Germline BRCA Mutation. *N Engl J Med* 2017;377(6): 523–533.

32 Ramakrishnan Geethakumari P, Schiewer MJ, Knudsen KE, Kelly WK. PARP Inhibitors in Prostate Cancer. *Curr Treat Options Oncol* 2017;18(6):37.

33 Luo G, Lu Y, Jin K, Cheng H, *et al.* Pancreatic cancer: BRCA mutation and personalized treatment. *Expert Rev Anticancer Ther* 2015;15(10):1223–31.

34 Fong PC, Boss DS, Yap TA, *et al.* Inhibition of poly(ADP-ribose) polymerase in tumors from BRCA mutation carriers. *N Engl J Med* 2009;361(2):123–34.

35 Pilarski R. Cowden syndrome: a critical review of the clinical literature. *J Genet Couns* 2009;18(1):13–27.

36 Tan MH, Mester JL, Ngeow J, *et al.* Lifetime cancer risks in individuals with germline PTEN mutations. *Clin Cancer Res* 2012;18(2):400–7.

37 Gonzalez KD, Noltner KA, Buzin CH, *et al.* Beyond Li Fraumeni Syndrome: clinical characteristics of families with p53 germline mutations. *J Clin Oncol* 2009;27(8): 1250–6.

38 Kratz CP, Achatz MI, Brugières L, *et al.* Cancer screening recommendations for individuals with Li-Fraumeni Syndrome. *Clin Cancer Res* 2017;23(11):e38–e45.

39 Lu KH, Dinh M, Kohlmann W, *et al.* Gynecologic cancer as a "sentinel cancer" for women with hereditary nonpolyposis colorectal cancer syndrome. *Obstet Gynecol* 2005;105(3):569–74.

40 Beggs AD, Latchford AR, Vasen HFA, *et al.* Peutz–Jeghers syndrome: a systematic review and recommendations for management. *Gut* 2010;59(7):975–86.

41 Zhang L. Immunohistochemistry versus microsatellite instability testing for screening colorectal cancer patients at risk for hereditary nonpolyposis colorectal cancer syndrome. Part II. The utility of microsatellite instability testing. *J Mol Diagn* 2008;10(4):301–7.

42 Shia J. Immunohistochemistry versus microsatellite instability testing for screening colorectal cancer patients at risk for hereditary nonpolyposis colorectal cancer syndrome. Part I. The utility of immunohistochemistry. *J Mol Diagn* 2008;10(4):293–300.

43 Hampel H, Frankel WL, Martin E, *et al.* Feasibility of screening for Lynch syndrome among patients with colorectal cancer. *J Clin Oncol* 2008;26(35):5783–8.

44 Cunningham JM, Kim CY, Christensen ER, *et al.* The frequency of hereditary defective mismatch repair in a prospective series of unselected colorectal carcinomas. *Am J Hum Genet* 2001;69(4):780–90.

45 Haraldsdottir S, Hampel H, Tomsic J, *et al.* Colon and endometrial cancers with mismatch repair deficiency can arise from somatic, rather than germline, mutations. *Gastroenterology* 2014;147(6):1308–16.e1.

46 Umar A, Boland CR, Terdiman JP, *et al.* Revised Bethesda Guidelines for hereditary nonpolyposis colorectal cancer (Lynch syndrome) and microsatellite instability. *J Natl Cancer Inst* 2004;96(4):261–8.

47 Vasen HF, Watson P, Mecklin JP, Lynch HT. New clinical criteria for hereditary nonpolyposis colorectal cancer (HNPCC, Lynch syndrome) proposed by the International Collaborative group on HNPCC. *Gastroenterology* 1999;116(6):1453–6.

48 Recommendations from the EGAPP Working Group: genetic testing strategies in newly diagnosed individuals with colorectal cancer aimed at reducing morbidity and mortality from Lynch syndrome in relatives. *Genet Med* 2009;11(1):35–41.

49 Barrow E, Hill J, Evans DG. Cancer risk in Lynch Syndrome. *Fam Cancer* 2013;12(2):229–40.

50 American Cancer Society. Key statistics about colorectal cancer. http://www.cancer.org/cancer/colonandrectumcancer/ detailedguide/colorectal-cancer-key-statistics (accessed 15 May 2017).

51 American Cancer Society. Key statistics for endometrial cancer? http://www.cancer.org/cancer/endometrialcancer/ detailedguide/endometrial-uterine-cancer-key-statistics (accessed 15 May 2017).

52 Wimmer K, Etzler J. Constitutional mismatch repair-deficiency syndrome: have we so far seen only the tip of an iceberg? *Hum Genet* 2008;124(2):105–22.

53 Jarvinen HJ, Aarnio M, Mustonen H, *et al*. Controlled 15-year trial on screening for colorectal cancer in families with hereditary nonpolyposis colorectal cancer. *Gastroenterology* 2000;118(5):829–34.

54 de Vos Tot Nederveen Cappel WH, Jarvinen HJ, Lynch PM, *et al*. Colorectal surveillance in Lynch syndrome families. *Fam Cancer* 2013;12(2):261–5.

55 Vasen HF, Blanco I, Aktan-Collan K, *et al*. Revised guidelines for the clinical management of Lynch syndrome (HNPCC): recommendations by a group of European experts. *Gut* 2013;62(6):812–23.

56 Burn J, Gerdes AM, Macrae F, Mecklin JP, *et al*. Long-term effect of aspirin on cancer risk in carriers of hereditary colorectal cancer: an analysis from the CAPP2 randomised controlled trial. *Lancet* 2011;378(9809):2081–7.

57 Parry S, Win AK, Parry B, *et al*. Metachronous colorectal cancer risk for mismatch repair gene mutation carriers: the advantage of more extensive colon surgery. *Gut* 2011;60(7):950–7.

58 Schmeler KM, Lynch HT, Chen L-M, *et al*. Prophylactic surgery to reduce the risk of gynecologic cancers in the Lynch syndrome. *N Engl J Med* 2006;354(3):261–9.

59 Le DT, Uram JN, Wang H, *et al*. PD-1 Blockade in tumors with mismatch-repair deficiency. *N Engl J Med* 2015;372(26):2509–20.

60 Galiatsatos P, Foulkes WD. Familial adenomatous polyposis. *Am J Gastroenterol* 2006;101(2):385–98.

61 Aretz S, Stienen D, Friedrichs N, *et al*. Somatic APC mosaicism: a frequent cause of familial adenomatous polyposis (FAP). *Hum Mutat* 2007;28(10):985–92.

62 Vasen HF, Moslein G, Alonso A, *et al*. Guidelines for the clinical management of familial adenomatous polyposis (FAP). *Gut* 2008;57(5):704–13.

63 Steinbach G, Lynch PM, Phillips RK, *et al*. The effect of celecoxib, a cyclooxygenase-2 inhibitor, in familial adenomatous polyposis. *N Engl J Med* 2000;342(26): 1946–52.

64 Knudsen AL, Bisgaard ML, Bulow S. Attenuated familial adenomatous polyposis (AFAP). A review of the literature. *Fam Cancer* 2003;2(1):43–55.

65 Sieber OM, Lipton L, Crabtree M, *et al*. Multiple colorectal adenomas, classic adenomatous polyposis, and germ-line mutations in MUTYH. *N Engl J Med* 2003;348(9):791–9.

66 Al-Tassan N, Chmiel NH, Maynard J, *et al*. Inherited variants of MUTYH associated with somatic G:C-- > T:A mutations in colorectal tumors. *Nat Genet* 2002;30(2):227–32.

67 Theodoratou E, Campbell H, Tenesa A, *et al*. A large-scale meta-analysis to refine colorectal cancer risk estimates associated with MUTYH variants. *Br J Cancer* 2010;103(12):1875–84.

68 Vogt S, Jones N, Christian D, *et al*. Expanded extracolonic tumor spectrum in MUTYH-associated polyposis. *Gastroenterology* 2009;137(6):1976–85.

69 Ngeow J, Heald B, Rybicki LA, *et al*. Prevalence of germline PTEN, BMPR1A, SMAD4, STK11, and ENG mutations in patients with moderate-load colorectal polyps. *Gastroenterology* 2013;144(7):1402–9.e5.

70 Aretz S, Stienen D, Uhlhaas S, *et al*. High proportion of large genomic STK11 deletions in Peutz-Jeghers syndrome. *Hum Mutat* 2005;26(6):513–9.

71 Brosens LA, Langeveld D, van Hattem WA, Giardiello FM, Offerhaus GJ. Juvenile polyposis syndrome. *World J Gastroenterol* 2011;17(44):4839–44.

72 Faughnan ME, Palda VA, Garcia-Tsao G, *et al*. International guidelines for the diagnosis and management of hereditary haemorrhagic telangiectasia. *J Med Genet* 2011;48(2): 73–87.

73 Levi Z, Baris HN, Kedar I, *et al*. Upper and lower gastrointestinal findings in PTEN mutation-positive Cowden syndrome patients participating in an active surveillance program. *Clin Transl Gastroenterol* 2011;2:e5. doi:10.1038/ctg.2011.4.

74 Jaeger E, Leedham S, Lewis A, *et al*. Hereditary mixed polyposis syndrome is caused by a 40-kb upstream duplication that leads to increased and ectopic expression of the BMP antagonist GREM1. *Nat Genet* 2012;44(6):699–703.

75 Kastrinos F, Mukherjee B, Tayob N, *et al*. Risk of pancreatic cancer in families with Lynch syndrome. *JAMA* 2009;302(16): 1790–5.

76 Hahn SA, Greenhalf B, Ellis I, *et al*. BRCA2 germline mutations in familial pancreatic carcinoma. *J Natl Cancer Inst* 2003;95(3):214–21.

77 Murphy KM, Brune KA, Griffin C, *et al*. Evaluation of candidate genes MAP2K4, MADH4, ACVR1B, and BRCA2 in familial pancreatic cancer: deleterious BRCA2 mutations in 17%. *Cancer Res* 2002;62(13):3789–93.

78 Rebours V, Boutron-Ruault M-C, Schnee M, *et al*. Risk of pancreatic adenocarcinoma in patients with hereditary pancreatitis: a national exhaustive series. *Am J Gastroenterol* 2008;103(1):111–9.

79 Lynch HT, Fusaro RM, Lynch JF, Brand R. Pancreatic cancer and the FAMMM syndrome. *Fam Cancer* 2008;7(1):103–12.

80 Klein AP. Genetic susceptibility to pancreatic cancer. *Mol Carcinog* 2012;51(1):14–24.

81 Tischkowitz MD, Sabbaghian N, Hamel N, *et al*. Analysis of the gene coding for the BRCA2-interacting protein PALB2 in familial and sporadic pancreatic cancer. *Gastroenterology* 2009;137(3):1183–6.

82 Ludwig E, Olson SH, Bayuga S, *et al*. Feasibility and yield of screening in relatives from familial pancreatic cancer families. *Am J Gastroenterol* 2011;106(5):946–54.

83 Kaurah P, MacMillan A, Boyd N, *et al*. Founder and recurrent CDH1 mutations in families with hereditary diffuse gastric cancer. *JAMA* 2007;297(21):2360–72.

84 Van der Post RS, Carneiro F, Guilford P, *et al*. Hereditary diffuse gastric cancer: updated clinical guidelines with an emphasis on germline CDH1 mutation carriers. *J Med Genet* 2015;52(6):361–74.

85 Hansford S, Kaurah P, Li-Chang H, *et al*. Hereditary diffuse gastric cancer syndrome: CDH1 mutations and beyond. *JAMA Oncol* 2015;1(1):23–32.

86 Agarwal R, Robson M. Inherited predisposition to gastrointestinal stromal tumor. *Hematol Oncol Clin North Am* 2009;23(1):1–13, vii.

87 Pasmant E, Vidaud M, Vidaud D, Wolkenstein P. Neurofibromatosis type 1: from genotype to phenotype. *J Med Genet* 2012;49(8):483–9.

88 Graham J, Debiec-Rychter M, Corless CL, *et al*. Imatinib in the management of multiple gastrointestinal stromal tumors associated with a germline KIT K642E mutation. *Arch Pathol Lab Med* 2007;131(9):1393–6.

89 Kloos RT, Eng C, Evans DB, *et al*. Medullary thyroid cancer: management guidelines of the American Thyroid Association. *Thyroid* 2009;19(6):565–612.

90 Thakker RV, Newey PJ, Walls GV, *et al*. Clinical practice guidelines for multiple endocrine neoplasia type 1 (MEN1). *J Clin Endocrinol Metab* 2012;97(9):2990–3011.

91 Fishbein L, Nathanson KL. Pheochromocytoma and paraganglioma: understanding the complexities of the genetic background. *Cancer Genet* 2012;205(1–2):1–11.

92 Pacak K, Eisenhofer G, Ahlman H, *et al*. Pheochromocytoma: recommendations for clinical practice from the First International Symposium. *Nat Clin Pract End Met* 2007;3(2):92–102.

93 Ricketts CJ, Forman JR, Rattenberry E, *et al*. Tumor risks and genotype-phenotype-proteotype analysis in 358 patients with germline mutations in SDHB and SDHD. *Hum Mutat* 2010;31(1):41–51.

94 Henderson A, Douglas F, Perros P, Morgan C, Maher ER. SDHB-associated renal oncocytoma suggests a broadening of the renal phenotype in hereditary paragangliomatosis. *Fam Cancer* 2009;8(3):257–60.

95 Lenders J, Duh Q, Eisenhofer G, *et al*. Pheochromocytoma and paraganglioma: an endocrine society clinical practice guideline. *J Clin Endocrinol Metab* 2014;99(6):1915–42.

96 Neumann HP, Bausch B, McWhinney SR, *et al*. Germ-line mutations in nonsyndromic pheochromocytoma. *N Engl J Med* 2002;346(19):1459–66.

97 Coleman JA, Russo P. Hereditary and familial kidney cancer. *Curr Opin Urol* 2009;19(5):478–85.

98 Verine J, Pluvinage A, Bousquet G, *et al*. Hereditary renal cancer syndromes: an update of a systematic review. *Eur Urol* 2010;58(5):701–10.

99 Stratton KL, Alanee S, Glogowski EA, *et al*. Outcome of genetic evaluation of patients with kidney cancer referred for suspected hereditary cancer syndromes. *Urol Oncol* 2016;34(5):238.e1–7.

100 Maher ER, Neumann HP, Richard S. von Hippel-Lindau disease: a clinical and scientific review. *Eur J Hum Genet* 2011;19(6):617–23.

101 Lonser RR, Glenn GM, Walther M, *et al*. von Hippel-Lindau disease. *Lancet* 2003;361(9374):2059–67.

102 Zbar B, Glenn G, Lubensky I, *et al*. Hereditary papillary renal cell carcinoma: clinical studies in 10 families. *J Urol* 1995;153(3 Pt 2):907–12.

103 Schmidt LS, Nickerson ML, Angeloni D, *et al*. Early onset hereditary papillary renal carcinoma: germline

104 Pavlovich CP, Walther MM, Eyler RA, *et al*. Renal tumors in the Birt-Hogg-Dube syndrome. *Am J Surg Pathol* 2002;26(12):1542–52.

105 Houweling AC, Gijezen LM, Jonker MA, *et al*. Renal cancer and pneumothorax risk in Birt-Hogg-Dube syndrome; an analysis of 115 FLCN mutation carriers from 35 BHD families. *Br J Cancer* 2011;105(12):1912–9.

106 Shuch B, Singer EA, Bratslavsky G. The surgical approach to multifocal renal cancers: hereditary syndromes, ipsilateral multifocality, and bilateral tumors. *Urol Clin North Am* 2012;39(2):133–48, v.

107 Pavlovich CP, Grubb RL, 3rd, Hurley K, *et al*. Evaluation and management of renal tumors in the Birt-Hogg-Dube syndrome. *J Urol* 2005;173(5):1482–6.

108 Merino MJ, Torres-Cabala C, Pinto P, Linehan WM. The morphologic spectrum of kidney tumors in hereditary leiomyomatosis and renal cell carcinoma (HLRCC) syndrome. *Am J Surg Pathol* 2007;31(10):1578–85.

109 Menko F, Maher E, Schmidt L, *et al*. Hereditary leiomyomatosis and renal cell cancer (HLRCC). Renal cancer risk, surveillance and treatment. *Fam Cancer* 2014;13(4):637–44.

110 Grubb RL, 3rd, Franks ME, Toro J, *et al*. Hereditary leiomyomatosis and renal cell cancer: a syndrome associated with an aggressive form of inherited renal cancer. *J Urol* 2007;177(6):2074–9; discussion 9–80.

111 Stadler ZK, Thom P, Robson ME, *et al*. Genome-wide association studies of cancer. *J Clin Oncol* 2010;28(27):4255–67.

112 Shah S, Schrader KA, Waanders E, *et al*. A recurrent germline PAX5 mutation confers susceptibility to pre-B cell acute lymphoblastic leukemia. *Nat Genet* 2013;45(10):1226–31.

113 Palles C, Cazier JB, Howarth KM, *et al*. Germline mutations affecting the proofreading domains of POLE and POLD1 predispose to colorectal adenomas and carcinomas. *Nat Genet* 2013;45(2):136–44.

114 Focus on cancer risk (iCOGS Focus). *Nat Genet* 2013;45(4): 339–465.

115 Southey MC, Park DJ, Nguyen-Dumont T, *et al*. COMPLEXO: identifying the missing heritability of breast cancer via next generation collaboration. *Breast Cancer Res* 2013;15(3):402.

116 Bojesen SE, Pooley KA, Johnatty SE, *et al*. Multiple independent variants at the TERT locus are associated with telomere length and risks of breast and ovarian cancer. *Nat Genet* 2013;45(4):371–84, 84e1–2.

117 Mulligan AM, Couch FJ, Barrowdale D, *et al*. Common breast cancer susceptibility alleles are associated with tumour subtypes in BRCA1 and BRCA2 mutation carriers: results from the Consortium of Investigators of Modifiers of BRCA1/2. *Breast Cancer Res* 2011;13(6):R110. doi:10.1186/bcr3052.

118 Seal S, Thompson D, Renwick A, *et al*. Truncating mutations in the Fanconi anemia J gene BRIP1 are low-penetrance breast cancer susceptibility alleles. *Nat Genet* 2006;38(11):1239–41.

119 Rahman N, Seal S, Thompson D, *et al*. PALB2, which encodes a BRCA2-interacting protein, is a breast cancer susceptibility gene. *Nat Genet* 2007;39(2):165–7.

missense mutations in the tyrosine kinase domain of the met proto-oncogene. *J Urol* 2004;172(4 Pt 1):1256–61.

120 Easton DF, Pooley KA, Dunning AM, *et al*. Genome-wide association study identifies novel breast cancer susceptibility loci. *Nature* 2007;447(7148):1087–93.

121 Foulkes WD. Inherited susceptibility to common cancers. *N Engl J Med* 2008;359(20):2143–53.

122 Comprehensive molecular portraits of human breast tumours. *Nature* 2012;490(7418):61–70.

123 Cannon-Albright LA, Skolnick MH, Bishop DT, Lee RG, Burt RW. Common inheritance of susceptibility to colonic adenomatous polyps and associated colorectal cancers. *N Engl J Med* 1988;319(9):533–7.

124 Lindor NM, Rabe K, Petersen GM, *et al*. Lower cancer incidence in Amsterdam-I criteria families without mismatch repair deficiency: familial colorectal cancer type X. *JAMA* 2005;293(16):1979–85.

125 Ku CS, Cooper DN, Wu M, *et al*. Gene discovery in familial cancer syndromes by exome sequencing: prospects for the elucidation of familial colorectal cancer type X. *Mod Pathol* 2012;25(8):1055–68.

126 Pritchard CC, Mateo J, Walsh MF, *et al*. Inherited DNA-repair gene mutations in men with metastatic prostate cancer. *N Engl J Med* 2016;375(5):443–53.

127 Vijapura C, Saad Aldin E, Capizzano AA, *et al*. Genetic Syndromes Associated with Central Nervous System Tumors. *Radiographics* 2017;37(1):258–280.

128 Chan SH, Lim WK, Ishak NDB, *et al*. Germline Mutations in Cancer Predisposition Genes are Frequent in Sporadic Sarcomas. *Sci Rep* 2017;7(1):10660.

129 van Duijnhoven FJ, Botma A, Winkels R, *et al*. Do lifestyle factors influence colorectal cancer risk in Lynch syndrome? *Fam Cancer* 2013; epub 2013 May 9.

130 Domchek SM, Bradbury A, Garber JE, Offit K, Robson ME. Multiplex genetic testing for cancer susceptibility: out on the high wire without a net? *J Clin Oncol* 2013;31(10): 1267–70.

131 Tung N, Domchek SM, Stadler Z, *et al*. Counselling framework for moderate-penetrance cancer-susceptibility mutations. *Nature reviews. Clin Oncol* 2016;13(9):581–8.

132 Lohn Z, Adam S, Birch PH, Friedman JM. Incidental findings from clinical genome-wide sequencing: a *review. J Genet Couns* 2013; epub May 26, 2013.

133 Green RC, Berg JS, Grody WW, *et al*. ACMG recommendations for reporting of incidental findings in clinical exome and genome sequencing. *Genet Med* 2013;15(7):565–74.

134 Schrader KA, Cheng DT, Joseph V, *et al*. Germline Variants in Targeted Tumor Sequencing Using Matched Normal DNA. *JAMA Oncol* 2016;2(1):104–11.

135 Mandelker D, Zhang L, Kemel Y, *et al*. Mutation Detection in Patients With Advanced Cancer by Universal Sequencing of Cancer-Related Genes in Tumor and Normal DNA vs Guideline-Based Germline Testing. *JAMA* 2017;318(9): 825–83.

136 Bombard Y, Robson M, Offit K. Revealing the incidentalome when targeting the tumor genome. *JAMA* 2013;310(8):795–6.

137 Stadler ZK, Schrader KA, Vijai J, Robson M, Offit K. Cancer genomics and inherited risk. *J Clin Oncol* 2014;32(7):687–98.

138 Abeloff MD, Armitage JO, Niederhuber JE, Kastan MB, McKenna WG. *Abeloff's Clinical Oncology*, 4th edn. Philadelphia: Churchill Livingstone/Elsevier, 2008.

139 Hampel H, Bennett RL, Buchanan A, Pearlman R. A practice guideline from the American College of Medical Genetics and Genomics and the National Society of Genetic Counselors: referral indications for cancer predisposition assessment. 2015;17(1):70–87.

140 Bahcall OG. Common variation and heritability estimates for breast, ovarian and prostate cancers [primer #1]. https://doi.org/10.1038/ngicogs.1 (accessed 15 May 2017). Online-only hypertext essay on: Focus on cancer risk. *Nat Genet* 2013; 45(4):339–465.

6

Tobacco

Thomas J. Glynn[1], Richard D. Hurt[2], and J. Lee Westmaas[3]

[1] *School of Medicine, Stanford University, Palo Alto, California, USA*
[2] *Nicotine Dependence Center, Primary Care Internal Medicine, Rochester, Minnesota, USA*
[3] *Tobacco Control Research, American Cancer Society, Atlanta, Georgia, USA*

Introduction

Cigarette smoking and other forms of tobacco use are the primary preventable causes of disease and premature death in the United States (US). The use of tobacco, particularly through cigarettes, causes more than 30% of all cancers and contributes significantly to the incidence of cardiovascular and pulmonary diseases, reproductive abnormalities, and childhood illnesses, and exacerbates such conditions as chronic renal disease, diabetes, and asthma [1].

Despite the terrible toll from tobacco use, on both health and the economy – there are more than 480,000 tobacco-related deaths in the US alone each year and the cost to the US economy exceeds $289 billion annually [1] – significant progress has been made over the past 50 years in addressing this most stubborn of public health challenges. When the first US Surgeon General's Report on Smoking and Health was published in 1964 [2], more than 42% of the US population smoked cigarettes but, in 2015, the Centers for Disease Control and Prevention (CDC) reported that the prevalence of smoking in the US had dropped to 15.1%, the lowest level in nearly a century, since the period just after World War I [3].

This chapter will examine, in a relatively abbreviated format, the full range of reasons and circumstances that have led to the relative success of the tobacco control movement up to the present time and what still needs to be done if this success is to be made permanent and expanded upon.

Epidemiology

Tobacco use in the Americas predates the time of Columbus, but does not appear to have been used anywhere else in the world prior to this. After Columbus brought tobacco leaf and plants with him upon returning from his first voyage, however, tobacco cultivation and use spread rapidly from Europe eastward. By the 1600s, tobacco use, in a variety of forms, predominantly chewing tobacco, snuff, pipes and cigars but not cigarettes, had become a worldwide phenomenon [4, 5].

Native Americans introduced early colonists to tobacco cultivation, curing, and consumption practices. By the mid-1600s, tobacco exports had become an important source of revenue for the colonies, as well as a pastime at home, social gatherings, and in commerce [4, 5].

Tobacco was subjected to considerable scrutiny from the 1600s on and developed a wide range of both proponents and opponents. French diplomat Jean Nicot treated Queen Catherine de Medici's migraines with tobacco and European physicians recommended tobacco as a cure for all manner of ailments, whereas English King James I described smoking as "loathsome" and a death penalty for smoking tobacco was imposed in Turkey and in the Qing Dynasty of China [4, 6].

And now, 500 years after tobacco began its circumnavigation of the globe, it has at least 1.3 billion users, predominantly cigarettes, is killing more than 14,500 people *every day*, and is debilitating and sickening many times that number [6]. Yet it is only in the past 50 years that tobacco science has begun, in painstaking, evidence-based fashion, to detail its chemical composition, the psychology and physiology of its use, its dependence-producing properties, and the appalling human and economic costs it has rendered in the past and continues to incur in the present.

US Epidemiology of Tobacco Use

Tobacco use in the form of cigarettes in the US was relatively low until the twin events of US entry into World War I and the advent of automated cigarette manufacturing ushered in an era of accelerated use of tobacco. The decline in tobacco use finally began after the publication of the first US Surgeon General's Report on Tobacco and Health in 1964, which built on previous studies and provided new evidence that helped to conclusively link cigarette smoking to lung cancer and heart disease. At the time of the publication of that report, over 40% of the adult population were regular smokers, including more than 50% of all men and about 28% of all women [2]. Per capita consumption of cigarettes rose to nearly 4300 by 1965 [7].

By 2015, the prevalence rate of cigarette smoking had dropped to 15%, more specifically 17% of all men and 14% of all women. Per capita consumption of cigarettes in 2011 was 1232 [8], reflecting not only the lower prevalence, but also a substantial reduction in the number of cigarettes smoked per day among those who remained smokers and the increase in the population.

The reduction in the number of cigarettes smoked per day, which by 2011 was only 28% the number that was being smoked daily in 1965 [7, 8], is particularly striking. This reduction represents a dual trend – a reduction in the number of cigarettes smoked each day by daily smokers and an increase in the number of smokers who smoke only occasionally, for example only on weekends. Both trends represent public health advances; since the damage from cigarette smoking is dose and time related, damage to health is multiplied by the number of cigarettes smoked and the number of years one has smoked [9]. Nevertheless, since health risks are increased even among occasional users and when as few as one to five cigarettes are smoked daily [10], the public health message must remain focused on convincing smokers, and those who have not begun to smoke, to refrain from any use of cigarettes.

Other notable trends in the epidemiology of tobacco use in the US, which will require careful monitoring in the future, include: the narrowing of the gap between male and female cigarette smokers, from more than 25% in 1965 and to just 3% in 2015; the increase in the use of small cigars among youth; the relative stability of smokeless tobacco use prevalence; the introduction of forms of tobacco use from abroad, such as kreteks and hookah; the introduction of new tobacco products such as dissolvable tobacco and electronic cigarettes; the increasing concentration of cigarette smoking among low-income, low-education, LGBT, and psychiatric groups in the US; and the slow decline of youth tobacco use between 2000 and 2011, after a sharp rise in such use in the 1990s [1].

Health Risks from Tobacco Use

Although it is difficult to identify a specific point at which knowledge of the disease consequences of tobacco use was accepted by the global health community, many believe that it was the series of studies conducted in Germany during the 1930s and early 1940s [11], culminating in the 1950 publications by Wynder and Graham, and Doll and Hill [12, 13]. These studies marked the beginning of the documentation in a clear, scientifically indisputable way that tobacco use was a cause of death and disease in humans.

This scientific documentation linking tobacco use to a wide range of debilitating illnesses and disease continued and accelerated through the 1950s and early 1960s (including the key Joint Report of the Study Group on Smoking and Health, based on the 1957 US panel assembled by the National Cancer Institute, the American Heart Association, the National Heart Institute, and the American Cancer Society to examine the scientific evidence concerning the effects of tobacco smoking on health) [14–17]. Then, in 1962 and 1964, respectively, two landmark documents, the Report of the Royal College of Physicians in the United Kingdom, and the Report of the Advisory Committee to the Surgeon General of the Public Health Service in the US [2, 18], firmly established in all but the most jaundiced eyes, as well as those of the tobacco industry, the causal relation between tobacco use and disease.

Cigarette smoke is now known to contain more than 7,000 chemicals and chemical compounds, including cyanide, benzene, formaldehyde, ammonia, arsenic, vinyl chloride, polonium-210, and heavy metals such as cadmium, nickel, and lead. More than 60 of these ingredients have been identified as carcinogens [9]. Many of these substances occur naturally in the tobacco leaf, some are added during the manufacturing process, and still others are formed from the combustion caused when cigarettes are lit.

Additionally, smokeless tobacco, which comes in a number of forms (e.g., moist and dry snuff, snus, dissolvable lozenges and tablets) contains many of the same chemicals and carcinogens found in cigarette smoke. Smokeless tobacco is used by about 3% of American adults, a rate which has remained steady for more than a decade. These products – although they differ considerably in ingredients and harm potential – should not be considered safe. Most can cause oral, esophageal, and pancreatic cancers among their users and are also implicated in the development of cardiovascular disease [19, 20]. While there is general agreement that smokeless tobacco products are less lethal than combusted cigarettes, the evidence remains sparse about their effectiveness as aids to quitting cigarettes. While some researchers cite the experience of snus use in Sweden – which has the lowest lung cancer rates in Western Europe – as evidence that snus, with its lower nitrosamine levels, can be a safe alternative to combusted cigarettes, the Swedish experience is not necessarily comparable to what might transpire in the US and awaits sound, objective data before serious discussion of such use can be undertaken in the US [21].

The most serious health consequences from tobacco occur, however, when any tobacco product is burned and inhaled, particularly from cigarettes, pipes, or cigars. Consider that tobacco use and, especially cigarette smoking [1, 9, 22]:

- Accounts for more than 480,000 premature deaths, or nearly one in five of all deaths, each year in the US
- Reduces life expectancy, on average, by at least 10 years
- Causes more than 8 million Americans to be sick with a tobacco-caused illness or disease at any given time
- Causes more premature deaths in the US each year than HIV, illegal drug use, alcohol use, motor vehicle injuries, suicides, and murders *combined*
- Causes or contributes to the development of the following cancers: acute myeloid leukemia, bladder cancer, cancer of the cervix, cancer of the esophagus, kidney cancer, cancer of the larynx, lung cancer, cancer of the oral cavity, pancreatic cancer, cancer of the pharynx, colon polyps and colon cancer and stomach cancer
- Causes nearly one of every three cancer deaths in the US
- Causes approximately 85% of all lung cancer deaths in the US
- Increases men's risk of dying from lung cancer by 22 times and women's risk by 12 times
- Causes approximately 90% of all premature deaths from chronic obstructive lung disease

- Increases the risk of dying prematurely from coronary heart disease or stroke by two to four times
- Triples middle-aged men's and women's risk of dying from heart disease
- Increases men's and women's risk of dying from bronchitis or emphysema by 10 times
- Increases the risk of many adverse reproductive and early childhood effects, including infertility, preterm delivery, stillbirth, low birth weight, lower respiratory illnesses, middle ear disease, reduced lung function, asthma, and sudden infant death syndrome (SIDS)
- Causes more than 1000 annual deaths and many thousands of injuries due to smoking-caused fires
- Is associated with lower bone density and hip fractures among women.

In addition to these direct health effects of smoke inhalation and use of smokeless tobacco by the tobacco user him or herself, there are also numerous health effects that *nonsmokers* suffer through the inhalation of secondhand smoke emanating either from the cigarette itself or the exhalation of smoke by the smoker. These effects, caused by the more than 250 chemicals in secondhand smoke that are known to be toxic or carcinogenic, and in addition to the reproductive and early childhood effects noted above, are responsible for more than 49,000 premature deaths per year in the US, primarily from coronary heart disease, but also including more than 3,000 lung cancer deaths [23].

In summary, several Surgeons General of the US, and the reports on tobacco and health that they have issued, are very clear in stating that there is no risk-free level of exposure to tobacco and that use of tobacco in any form, and especially cigarette smoking, carries with it a highly significant risk of premature disease and death.

Economic Effects of Tobacco Use

While the effects of tobacco use in the US are correctly focused on its human toll – the death and disease it causes – there are also substantial economic costs associated with tobacco use. These costs, which have a debilitating effect on individuals, families, and local, state, and national economies, include [1]:

- More than $133 billion in public and private healthcare expenditures, including at least $31 billion in Medicaid payments, $27 billion in Medicare payments, and $10 billion in other Federal government healthcare-related costs due to tobacco use (e.g., through the Veterans Administration healthcare system)
- More than $151 billion in work productivity losses, which includes only productivity losses due to work lives shortened by tobacco-caused death, and *not* productivity lost due to smoking-caused disability and sick days, or to reductions in productivity while working, such as for smoking breaks
- More than $500 million in residential and commercial property damages from cigarette-caused fires
- Approximately $3 billion tobacco-related cleaning and maintenance costs in residential and commercial property
- Approximately $70 billion in taxpayer burden – or $611 per household – from smoking-caused government spending

- Nearly $3 billion in annual expenditures through Social Security Survivors Insurance for the more than 300,000 children who have lost at least one parent due to a smoking-caused premature death
- Individual expenditures of an average of $2,201 for cigarettes per year for a pack-a-day smoker, meaning that, in a US household at the median income level with two smokers, each smoking one pack per day, nearly 8% of pre-tax income is spent on cigarettes
- A cost of $10.47 to the US economy for every pack of cigarettes sold.

As important as it is to collect epidemiologic data regarding tobacco use and the morbidity and mortality associated with it, the World Health Organization (WHO) also emphasizes the importance of collecting and analyzing economic data related to tobacco use and its effects, such as those examples noted above [24].

Among the important reasons cited by the WHO for collecting these economic data are: the need to measure the impact of smoking and tobacco use on healthcare delivery and financing, in order to best plan for providing an effective infrastructure (e.g., sufficient trained healthcare providers, lung and heart disease treatment facilities, etc.) for the future treatment of tobacco-caused disease in the population; to inform the adoption of economic interventions, such as increases in cigarette taxes and financial incentives for not smoking or using tobacco; to determine damages in smoking-related litigation, which is an increasingly common tool used in tobacco control; to guide in the development and financing of health policy and health planning for tobacco control initiatives; to inform national and local legislators and policymakers not only about the health burden from tobacco use on their constituents, but also the economic burden; and to provide an economic framework for tobacco control program evaluation.

Current Approaches to the Control of Tobacco Use

Tobacco control is, in the broadest sense, any effort to reduce or eliminate the devastating health and economic effects of tobacco use on individuals and populations.

In the US, the modern era of tobacco control began informally in the 1950s when newspaper and magazine articles began to publish information about studies linking cigarette smoking to lung cancer and questioning whether some form of warning or awareness campaigns for the public were justified or needed. The US tobacco industry, with its exceptional political access, influence, and economic power, recognized the danger of broad public awareness of the health dangers of cigarettes to their business and began a counter-campaign to alleviate and distract public and official concerns about the dangers of cigarette smoking. The industry itself had been aware of these dangers for many years, but had conspired among themselves to keep this information from the public and the medical community.

After spending considerable resources on shoring up their political support, the tobacco industry – including manufacturers' and growers' associations – published on January 4, 1954, what they called "A Frank Statement to Cigarette Smokers" in more than 400 US newspapers [25]. This statement questioned the science suggesting that cigarette smoking was a major cause of lung cancer and established what was called the "Tobacco Industry Research Committee" which would, the Frank Statement claimed, conduct objective investigations of health claims against cigarette smoking. This openly defiant, anti-science stance by the tobacco industry in 1954 galvanized its critics and the science community and can be reasonably called the beginning of the tobacco control movement in the US

Due to the great power of the industry, however, efforts to inform the public about the accumulating scientific evidence regarding the health dangers from cigarette smoking and the need to control tobacco use moved slowly. In 1957, newly appointed US Surgeon General Leroy Burney, after commissioning a study of the evidence to date, declared that it was the official position of the US Public Health Service (USPHS) that the evidence pointed to a causal relationship between cigarette smoking and lung cancer [26]. This declaration spurred further research and public debate.

Outside the US, other countries were also taking notice of the growing scientific evidence connecting cigarette smoking to a variety of diseases, with cancer most prominent among them. The British Medical Research Council, and similar panels in Denmark, the Netherlands, Norway, Sweden, Finland, and Canada all studied the issue and came to conclusions similar to those of Dr Burney [27]. Building on this momentum, in 1959, Dr Burney published a "special article" in *The Journal of the American Medical Association (JAMA)* in which he, and the USPHS, were even more explicit than in the 1957 report, declaring that "…the weight of evidence at present implicates smoking as the principal factor in the increased incidence of lung cancer" [28]. More than 50 years later, this conclusion seems simple, straightforward, and obvious, but the uncertainty created by the tobacco industry's campaign of misinformation and questions regarding the validity of the science surrounding smoking and disease caused even the American Medical Association, the publisher of *JAMA*, to write an editorial questioning the accuracy of Dr Burney's statement, noting that "…A number of authorities who have examined the same evidence cited by Dr Burney do not agree with his conclusions" [29].

Nevertheless, the scientific data continued to accumulate and two vital events in the early 1960s built on Dr Burney's official concerns and statements. The first was a letter written in June 1961 to newly-elected President John F. Kennedy from the American Cancer Society, the American Heart Association, the National Tuberculosis Association, and the American Public Health Association [30]. This letter called on the President to establish a Presidential Commission on Smoking and stated that:

"On the basis of the weight of scientific evidence on the relationship of cigarette smoking to cancer, especially cancer of the lung, to cardiovascular diseases and to other debilitating and fatal diseases, we believe that such a Commission should examine the social responsibilities of business, of voluntary agencies, and of government in the education of the youth of America; and should recommend various ways to protect the public, weighing the costs against the benefits to be achieved and seeking a

solution of this health problem that would interfere least with the freedom of industry or the happiness of individuals."

The President took this request seriously and asked his newly-appointed Surgeon General, Dr Luther L. Terry to establish an advisory committee to "look into the matter of smoking and health". Dr Terry undertook this assignment in early 1962, and just months later, as he and his staff were in the process of assembling their advisory committee, in March 1962, *"A Report of the Royal College of Physicians on Smoking in Relation to Cancer of the Lung and Other Diseases"* was published in Britain [18]. The Royal College report was considered to be the first truly definitive review of the smoking and health issue and received wide media coverage, not only in Britain, but globally. The aim of the report was to inform the public, the health provider community, and the British government about the strong epidemiological case that could now be made connecting cigarette smoking to a wide variety of health issues. It called upon the government to implement a wide range of public health measures to reduce smoking and on physicians to advise patients about illnesses caused and exacerbated by smoking and to help patients to stop smoking.

Finally, on January 11, 1964, the advisory committee assembled by Dr Terry at the behest of President Kennedy held a press conference to issue its final report, *"Smoking and Health: A Report of the Advisory Committee to the Surgeon General of the Public Health Services"* [2]. This 387-page report – even more comprehensive than the 1962 Royal College report – was the culmination of more than 14 months of work by an expert committee of 10 physicians and scientists, a technical staff of more than 20 people, and more than 150 consultants. The press conference was held on Saturday, both to minimize the expected negative effect on the stock market and to obtain as much coverage as possible in the Sunday newspapers. As Dr Terry recalled some time afterwards, the contents of the report "…hit the country like a bombshell. It was front page news and a lead story on every radio and television station in the US and many abroad" [30].

Although the tobacco industry would continue to dispute and distort the scientific basis of the Royal College and Terry reports for many years, the foundation had been laid for a 50-year campaign to control tobacco use and the death and disease that it causes. The very next year after the Terry report was delivered the US Congress passed the Cigarette Labeling and Advertising Act, requiring that health warning labels (e.g., "Cigarettes may be hazardous to your health") be placed on cigarette packages sold in the US – the modern era of organized tobacco control began.

What "Works" in Tobacco Control?

While cigarette smoking is still the major cause of preventable premature death and disability in the US, and much more needs to be done to eliminate its unconscionable health and economic effects, it has nevertheless been estimated that the success of public health efforts to control tobacco use in the 50 years after the Terry report was issued has averted more than 8 million premature deaths and hundreds of millions of illnesses in the US alone [1, 31].

Before attempting to describe what interventions have been perhaps most successful in reducing the toll of tobacco-caused disease in the US, it is essential to point out that none of this progress could have been made without the strong scientific research – including basic and applied research and surveillance – which is the foundation on which all public health interventions in tobacco control have been built. Without this research – which must continue into the future – we would not know, for example, how and why nicotine, when delivered rapidly and in high doses, creates such a strong dependence on tobacco smoking, how even the secondhand smoke from cigarettes can be deadly, how cigarette prices affect youth and adult smoking rates, or how to develop medications and treatment protocols to help smokers quit.

What "Works"

There have been concerted efforts over the past several decades to apply good science to tobacco control efforts, perhaps nowhere more energetically and systematically than in Australia [32] and, in the US, in California [33]. In both cases, a tax on cigarettes was used to fund a broad array of tobacco control efforts, including countermarketing advertising, public education, sharply decreasing the number of public spaces where smoking was allowed, and increasing the availability of tobacco dependence treatment options, all with the aim of "denormalizing" tobacco use, thereby demonstrating to both children and adults that the tobacco industry is not a "normal" business but is, instead, one that has lied to the American public for decades, and that tobacco use, and especially cigarette smoking, is an unhealthy, socially unacceptable, non-normative behavior in which most people do not engage.

The successes in Australia and California led to attempts to summarize the most effective interventions that have been developed for the prevention and control of tobacco use. Three of these efforts stand out due to the painstaking, science-based process in which they were developed, and their broad adoption throughout the world. They are the World Health Organization's MPOWER protocol [34], the Centers for Disease Control and Prevention's Best Practices for Comprehensive Tobacco Control Programs [35], and the United Nation's treaty, the Framework Convention on Tobacco Control (FCTC) [36].

A common theme among each of these approaches is that no single intervention applied at one point in time has been shown to be more than marginally effective. Instead, each provides clear data demonstrating that a comprehensive approach to tobacco control – multiple interventions applied simultaneously over an extended period – is the most effective means of preventing and reducing tobacco use.

The three approaches cited above provide insights into many interventions that have been shown to be effective when applied comprehensively. The FCTC [36], for example, recommends the widest array of approaches, including:

- Raising prices/taxes on tobacco
- Reducing illicit trade in tobacco
- Increasing secondhand smoke bans
- Banning tobacco advertising, sponsorship, and promotion
- Increasing litigation aimed at the tobacco industry
- Conducting tobacco control media campaigns

- Regulating all tobacco products
- Conducting surveillance of tobacco use practices
- Placing large, graphic health warning on all tobacco products
- Conducting public education campaigns
- Reducing youth access to tobacco
- Banning misleading tobacco product claims/descriptors
- Isolating tobacco in international trade agreements, and
- Providing easily accessible tobacco dependence treatment of all tobacco users.

Do all these approaches "work"? Data suggest that they do, although some "work" better than others and all work best when applied simultaneously over an extended period. Since applying all the interventions suggested above by the FCTC can be a daunting challenge, the WHO undertook in 2008 an effort to distill the FCTC interventions, and the CDC's, into a more manageable package, which they have called "MPOWER" [34] and consists of:

- Monitor tobacco use and prevention policies
- Protect people from tobacco smoke
- Offer help to quit tobacco use
- Warn about the dangers of tobacco
- Enforce bans on tobacco advertising, sponsorship, and promotion
- Raise taxes on tobacco.

The WHO MPOWER package of interventions have now been shown to "work". In countries and regions where they have been implemented simultaneously and over time, they have begun to affect behaviors and attitudes toward tobacco use, that is the "denormalization" effects seen in the long-term Australia and California campaigns.

In the US recently, there has been an effort to even further streamline the MPOWER package and many public health groups, while continuing their efforts to educate, keep tobacco out of trade agreements, reduce advertising, etc., now focus many of their tobacco control intervention efforts on these three interventions which we know to "work":

- Raise taxes on tobacco products
- Promote smoke-free environments
- Increase availability of easily accessible, affordable tobacco dependence treatment for those who wish to quit.

Special Emphasis Section: Treatment of Tobacco Dependence

In 1999, Jha and Chaloupka estimated that approximately 180 million premature deaths could be averted in the first half of the twenty-first century if adult cigarette smoking were halved by 2020 [37]. While acknowledging that prevention of youth smoking uptake is an essential element in tobacco control, Jha and Chaloupka's data clearly showed that a distinct focus of resources on tobacco dependence treatment would bring adult smoking rates down sharply, and be the best "investment" in public health that could be made in the early twenty-first century.

There is sufficient evidence that treating tobacco dependence "works"; the combination of face-to-face, group, telephone, and more recently, social media, approaches, in concert with pharmacotherapies, enables many smokers to quit and stay quit [38]. Reducing the number of adult smokers also has a salutary effect on youth uptake by providing fewer smoking role models for them to emulate.

In 2008, the USPHS released a comprehensive update of its 2000 Guideline for Treating Tobacco Use and Dependence [39]. This evidence-based Guideline was updated by a panel of experts who distilled a literature of more than 8,700 peer-reviewed articles and performed comprehensive meta-analyses of the available data. The Guideline emphasizes that tobacco dependence is a chronic medical condition that often requires repeated intervention and multiple attempts to stop. In the US, approximately 70% of smokers want to stop smoking and approximately half make a serious attempt to stop smoking every year (i.e. quitting for 24 hours or more). Unfortunately, these efforts are usually unaided and unsuccessful; only approximately 4–7% of smokers who attempt to stop smoking are able to do so on their own [40].

The authors of the 2008 Guideline note that substantial progress has been made since the first Guideline was published in 1996. The Guideline points to the increased coverage of tobacco dependence treatments by health plans, Medicare, and Medicaid. The subsequent passage and implementation of the Affordable Care Act in the US is also enabling millions more smokers to obtain treatment for their dependence [41]. Additionally, the Joint Commission now requires tobacco dependence interventions for hospitalized smokers with a diagnosis of acute myocardial infarction, congestive heart failure, or pneumonia [42]. The Guideline also notes that progress has been made in disseminating treatment options on the population level. Telephone quitlines have been particularly effective in providing wide access to counseling, and many quitlines provide nicotine replacement therapy (NRT) at no cost to the smoker, which can significantly improve a quitline caller's chances of successfully quitting [43].

Each Guideline recommendation is supported by a meta-analysis of scientific studies to provide a strong base of evidence designed to encourage clinicians to advise their tobacco-using patients about effective tobacco dependence counseling and medications. The Guideline also recommends that health systems, insurers, and purchasers assist clinicians in making such effective treatments available. For this to occur, clinicians and healthcare delivery systems need consistently to identify and document tobacco use status and treat every tobacco user seen in a healthcare setting. The Guideline recommends that an office-wide system be implemented to ensure that every patient at every clinic visit is queried regarding their tobacco use status and that this status is then documented. One easy way to accomplish this is to expand the collection and monitoring of vital signs to include tobacco use [44], as many clinical practices and hospitals now do.

The Guideline also recommends that clinicians should encourage every patient who is willing to attempt to stop using tobacco and direct them toward effective counseling and medications. For the patient who is unwilling to set a quit date, the Guideline recommends using the technique of motivational interviewing [45] to maintain patient engagement in the treatment process. Even brief tobacco counseling interventions are effective for improving tobacco abstinence outcomes compared with no intervention or self-help materials. Because there is a dose response for counseling interventions, longer or more intensive treatments result in better smoking abstinence outcomes compared with brief behavioral therapy. This is true regardless of the format used for the counseling intervention (i.e., individual, group, or telephone counseling).

Two components of counseling are especially effective and the Guideline recommends that clinicians use these when counseling patients to stop tobacco use. The first is *Practical Counseling*, a problem-solving and skills-training approach used to help the patient recognize thoughts, behaviors, and situations that may lead to increased smoking or relapse, and that helps the patient identify and practice coping or problem-solving skills to deal with them. Practical counseling also includes providing basic information concerning the neurobiology of tobacco dependence and withdrawal symptoms that might be experienced. The second is *Intra-treatment Support*, in which the clinician can provide support to the smoking patient in a variety of ways and begins with encouraging the patient to make an attempt to stop. The clinician should communicate in a caring, nonjudgmental manner and also encourage the patient to openly discuss perceived barriers to stopping smoking. Telephone counseling and return visits are a clear demonstration of intratreatment support [38].

The Guideline also recommends seven first-line, FDA-approved, medications that may be used either individually or in combinations. These medications include five nicotine replacement medications (nicotine gum, a nicotine vapor inhaler, nicotine lozenges, nicotine nasal spray, and nicotine patches) and two non-nicotine medications (bupropion, an antidepressant, and varenicline, a partial nicotine agonist).

The Guideline states that all smokers trying to quit should be offered medication, except where contraindicated or among specific populations for which there is, as yet, insufficient evidence of effectiveness (e.g.,pregnant women, smokeless tobacco users, light smokers, and adolescents). The Guideline also points out that while counseling and medication are effective when used by themselves, the combination of counseling and medication(s) is more effective than either used alone. Detailed guidance for use of the seven first-line, FDA-approved medications are in Table 6.1.

In addition to the consensus-driven advice about medication use in the USPHS Guideline, the FDA has considered updating its guidance on pharmacotherapy use for tobacco dependence treatment to include modifications in package labeling which permit, among other changes, longer duration of use for nicotine replacement medications, after consultation with the patient's healthcare provider [46]. Other recent guidance for the most effective use of pharmacotherapy in the treatment of tobacco dependence include the 2014 US Surgeon General's Report on Smoking and Health [1] and a JAMA Clinical Evidence Synopsis [47].

The Guideline also emphasizes that telephone quitline counseling is effective with diverse populations and has a broad reach. In the US, telephone quitlines are available in every state; therefore, both clinicians and healthcare delivery systems should ensure patient access to quitlines and promote quitline use. The national quitline number is 1-800-QUITNOW, which connects smokers to a routing system that redirects them to their free state quitline service.

Table 6.1 Guidance for use of the seven first-line, FDA-approved medications.

Medication	Cautions/warnings	Side effects	Dosage	Use	Availability (check insurance)
Bupropion SR 150	Not for use if you: • Currently use monoamine oxidase (MAO) inhibitor • Use bupropion in any other form • Have a history of seizures • Have a history of eating disorders • See FDA package insert warning regarding suicidality and antidepressant drugs when used in children, adolescents, and young adults	• Insomnia • Dry mouth	• Days 1–3: 150 mg each morning • Days 4–end: twice daily	Start 1–2 weeks before quit date; use 2–6 months	Prescription only: • Generic • Zyban • Wellbutrin SR
Nicotine gum (2 mg or 4 mg)	• Caution with dentures • Do not eat or drink 15 min before or during use	• Mouth soreness • Stomach ache	• 1 piece every 1–2 h • 6–15 pieces per day • If <24 cigs: 2 mg • If >25 cigs per day or chewing tobacco: 4 mg	Up to 12 weeks or as needed	OTC only: • Generic • Nicorette
Nicotine inhaler	• May irritate mouth/throat at first (but improves with use)	• Local irritation of mouth and throat	• 6–16 cartridges per day • Inhale 80 times per cartridge • May save partially used cartridge for next day	Up to 6 months; taper at end	Prescription only: • Nicotrol inhaler
Nicotine lozenge (2 mg or 4 mg)	• Do not eat or drink 15 min before or during use • One lozenge at a time • Limit 20 in 24 h	• Hiccups • Cough • Heartburn	• If you smoke/chew <30 min after waking: 2 mg • If you smoke/chew >30 min after waking: 4 mg • Weeks 1–6: 1 every 1–2 h • Weeks 7–9: 1 every 2–4 h • Weeks 10–12: 1 every 4–8 h	3–6 months	OTC only: • Generic • Commit
Nicotine nasal spray	• Not for patients with asthma • May irritate nose (improves over time) • May cause dependence	• Nasal irritation	• 1 "dose" = 1 squirt per nostril 1–2 doses per h • 8–40 doses per day • Do NOT inhale	3–6 months; taper at end	Prescription only: • Nicotrol NS
Nicotine patch	• Do not use if you have severe eczema	• Local skin reaction • Insomnia	• One patch per day • If >10 cigs per day: 21 mg 4 weeks, 7 mg 2–4 weeks • If <10 per day: 14 mg 4 weeks, then 7 mg 4 weeks	8–12 weeks	OTC or prescription: • Generic • Nicoderm CQ • Nicotrol
Varenicline	Use with caution in patients: • With significant renal impairment • With serious psychiatric illness • Undergoing dialysis • FDA Warning: Varenicline patients have reported depressed mood, agitation, changes in behavior, suicidal ideation, and suicide. • See www.fda.gov for further updates regarding recommended safe use of Varenicline	• Nausea • Insomnia • Abnormal, vivid, or strange dreams	• Days 1–3: 0.5 mg every morning • Days 4–7: 0.5 mg twice daily • Day 8–end: 1 mg twice daily	Start 1 week before quit date; use 3–6 months	Prescription only: • Chantix
Combinations: 1) Patch + bupropion 2) Patch + gum 3) Patch + lozenge + inhaler	• Only patch + bupropion is currently FDA approved • Follow instructions for individual medications	See individual medications above	See individual medications above	See above	See above

Based on the 2008 Clinical Practice Guideline: Treating Tobacco Use and Dependence, US Public Health Service, May 2008. See the FDA website for additional dosing and safety information, including safety protocols.

Finally, as highlighted in the Guideline, counseling and pharmacotherapy are proven effective strategies to help smokers stop smoking. Higher taxes for cigarettes and smoke-free workplace policies are two effective public health policies that may prompt a smoker to make an attempt to stop and often help them stop.

New Technologies for Treating Tobacco Dependence

Since the 2008 Guideline update, new approaches and technologies have been developed to reach more smokers who would like to quit. Interventions have recently included websites, computer or web-based programs, email programs, texting programs for mobile phones, and smartphone "apps" (applications) that attempt to provide the advice and support of in-person clinical treatments.

These are potentially valuable public health tools because of their availability to anyone with a computer or smartphone, and the ability to provide cost-free, clinically-relevant information to smokers. Earlier versions of web-based or computer programs provided mainly static information designed to help the smoker quit, for example, information on pharmacotherapy, or strategies for dealing with cravings. Subsequent iterations have added algorithms that use information provided by the smoker, such as his or her habits, triggers, urges, etc. to provide individually-tailored support and information.

Moreover, with the now-widespread availability and use of social media platforms such as Facebook and Twitter, web-based programs have recently incorporated features to allow users to reach out to members of their social network for support for quitting (e.g., becomeanex.org and smokefree.gov). In one such program, QuitNet, the social aspect is particularly emphasized, as it is designed primarily for smokers and former smokers to provide mutual emotional and informational support for quitting. These programs have been generally effective, with several reviews demonstrating they can help smokers quit at a higher rate compared to quitting on one's own [48, 49].

One review found that internet-based programs using a theoretical framework (e.g., theory of planned behavior) were associated with greater efficacy, as was delivery of more behavior change techniques, and the addition of other ways of maintaining contact with participants such as through email or, preferably, text messaging [50]. Some programs, however, fail to provide evidence-based assistance recommended by the Guideline, or do not take full advantage of the interactive and tailoring capabilities of the internet [51]. It may be difficult, therefore, for some smokers to determine which web-based program should be selected to provide maximal assistance.

With the advent of smartphones, many of the functions of computer-delivered programs became available to mobile phone users through computer applications ("apps") that can be downloaded. Given that more than 70% of smokers say they would like to quit, demand for apps to help do so is strong, with hundreds of thousands of such apps of being downloaded monthly [52]. As with computer programs for cessation, however, there is a wide range of quality among these apps. A report that evaluated the most popular apps on the iPhone and Android platforms for content found that the majority were missing several basic evidence-based practices such as referrals to a quitline and recommending approved medications and counseling. In addition, many apps did not take advantage of texting and tailoring capabilities, which have been found in prior research to facilitate smoking cessation [53].

A more positive aspect of recent apps, however, is the inclusion of features that allow a user to access social support through social media platforms such as Facebook and Twitter. Other features of smartphones, for example their GPS (global positioning system) function could potentially be exploited in the future (e.g., by recognizing venues where smoking occurs, such as at a bar, and sending messages to help the user resist temptation). Individual tailoring of messages, which has been found to be effective in computer interventions for smoking cessation [54] is another feature that could conceivably be incorporated into apps. Although some apps (e.g., NCI's QuitPal) include several evidence-based practices, these often do not top the list of app searches. Thus, apps that do show efficacy in ongoing randomized control trials will need to be marketed appropriately and sufficiently to facilitate their use among smokers who wish to quit.

While these new technologies offer a host of opportunities for clinicians to recommend a new or different approach to quitting and for smokers to try, it is also difficult for both clinicians and patients to determine which of these new technologies, especially smartphone apps, will offer the most help in quitting. Since these technologies are new, as noted above, there are few scientifically-proven criteria in place to help guide the clinician or patient to the most useful of these technologies.

Nevertheless, until such criteria become available, it is reasonable to consider using technologies and apps developed by health-based organizations with an established reputation for scientific accuracy, such as the Legacy Foundation (now called the Truth Initiative, www.truthinitiative.org) and the American Cancer Society (www.cancer.org), or by government organizations such as the National Cancer Institute (www.cancer.gov). Also, clinicians and patients can explore whether a given technology or app has used an established, scientifically-derived approach in developing their quit-smoking plan, such as a reference to the USPHS Guideline, or if consultants from leading medical institutions have helped develop the technology. While this guidance is certainly not foolproof – with so many new technologies and apps on the market now and without regulation, the user must be cautious – it should help both clinicians and patients choose another approach to the vital, and continuing, effort to quit smoking.

Current Issues and Controversies in Tobacco Control

There is remarkable agreement in the public health community regarding the most effective approaches to addressing the tobacco epidemic: increasing smoke-free environments, raising and indexing tobacco taxes, making access to tobacco dependence treatment as widely available as possible, conducting hard-hitting counter-advertising campaigns, eliminating tobacco advertising and promotions to children and youth, etc. Yet, there remain some issues around which uncertainty or controversy remains.

E-Cigarettes/Harm Reduction

Among the newer, additional approaches to tobacco control which the 2014 Surgeon General's Report on Smoking and Health suggests for consideration is whether ending the use of the most harmful tobacco product, combusted tobacco, while decreasing the potential harm from newer, innovative products such as e-cigarettes, may be a reasonable goal [1].

This concept of "harm reduction" – an approach to risky behavior that prioritizes minimizing the damage from a given behavior, rather than eliminating the behavior itself – has, of course, been used in other areas of public health, for example providing clean needles to IV drug users, rather than attempting the more herculean task of ending drug abuse altogether. In tobacco control, however, "harm reduction" has traditionally been viewed as a controversial ideology, with one side arguing that the only path to eliminating the scourge of cigarette smoking is abstinence from all forms of tobacco, while another side argues that "…it is nonsensical to dismiss a (less harmful) alternative by demanding absolute safety". In practice, of course, the path to reducing and eliminating the dangers of cigarette smoking will weave between these two positions. It is in this context that a relatively new product – the electronic cigarette, or e-cigarette – has brought the concept of harm reduction to the forefront of tobacco control discussions [e.g., 55–58].

What are E-Cigarettes and Why are they Controversial?

E-cigarettes have been described by many of their proponents as a possible game-changing product which can end the use of combustible cigarettes once and for all, and by their detractors as the first step down a slippery slope to an expansion of the combusted cigarette-caused epidemic [59].

Proponents of e-cigarettes – both in the public health community and among e-cigarette manufacturers – emphasize their potential for expanding the tools available for smokers who want to quit: their comforting similarity to regular cigarettes for smokers; the likelihood that they are considerably safer than combusted cigarettes; and their absence of harmful secondhand smoke. Many of these proponents urge the public health community, the federal government (especially the Food and Drug Administration [FDA]), and state and local governments, to drop any objections to e-cigarettes, and take actions to promote rather than reduce their use and move them further towards mainstream social and scientific acceptance. Doing so, they argue, could enable e-cigarettes to largely or wholly replace the use of combusted cigarettes, which are known to be harmful, killing nearly half their users. E-cigarettes, their proponents argue, while not harmless, certainly do not approach the harm levels of combusted cigarettes and, therefore, will result in net benefit to public health – less combusted smoking-caused disease and premature death [55–59].

Opponents of e-cigarettes, and of harm reduction approaches more broadly, however, urge more caution concerning their widespread use and: emphasize the considerable lack of accumulated scientific knowledge about their safety for long-term inhalation; their effectiveness as smoking cessation aids; their appeal to youth; the effects of the e-cigarette industry's marketing strategies; the potential for dual-use of both e-cigarettes and combusted cigarettes; the effects of the mainstream tobacco industry's entry into the e-cigarette marketplace; and the potential for "renormalization" of combusted cigarette use. They urge the public to remain wary of e-cigarette use, the FDA to take the necessary actions to bring e-cigarettes under their full regulatory authority, and e-cigarette manufacturers to open their doors to independent testing, disclosure, and regulatory standards for their products, as well as to provide evidence for any product claims [55–60].

We can expect the harm reduction controversy to continue as the tobacco industry and others continue to expand the range of nicotine delivery products, such as e-cigarettes, that are less harmful than combusted cigarettes, but whose ultimate contribution to reducing the health and economic burden of tobacco use will remain uncertain while awaiting results from independent, longitudinal research.

FDA Regulation of Tobacco

In 2009, the US Congress passed the Family Smoking Prevention and Tobacco Control Act [61, 62]. This legislation completed a decades-long effort to give the US FDA the authority to regulate tobacco products. In doing so, Congress enabled the FDA to establish the Center for Tobacco Products (CTP), which is charged with regulating the manufacture, marketing, and distribution of tobacco products in order to reduce tobacco use by children under 18 and protect public health.

More specifically, the Tobacco Control Act authorizes the FDA to act in a number of ways, including:

- Restricting tobacco sales, distribution, and marketing
- Requiring stronger health warnings on packaging and in advertisements
- Requiring disclosure of tobacco product ingredients
- Reducing (but not eliminating) the amount of nicotine in tobacco products
- Creating standards for tobacco products
- Regulating "modified risk" (i.e. potentially harm reducing) tobacco products, such as e-cigarettes, snus, dissolvables, heat-not-burn, etc.

Brief History of the Tobacco Control Act

There had been discussions about the potential for bringing tobacco under the regulatory powers of the FDA ever since the 1964 Surgeon General's Report established that tobacco smoke causes cancer and heart disease. However, serious discussion of this issue only began during Dr David Kessler's tenure as FDA Commissioner in the early 1990s. To use this power, the FDA needed to determine if there was evidence that the nicotine in cigarettes and smokeless tobacco was a drug under federal law. Therefore, beginning in 1992, Dr Kessler and his staff conducted a thorough review of the science, drawing from the tobacco industry's research, published studies, and any precedents set from other laws and regulations.

Congressional hearings were then conducted in 1994, which included the now iconic scene of the CEOs of the seven major US tobacco companies swearing that they did not believe that nicotine was addictive. After these hearings, and after the formal scientific and legal investigation was completed, the FDA determined in 1995 that nicotine could, indeed, be considered a drug under the terms of the Food, Drugs, and Cosmetics Act of 1938.

Dr Kessler and the FDA then proposed regulations regarding tobacco. US tobacco companies immediately sued to stop the FDA from enforcing the proposed regulations. In 2000, the US Supreme Court declared that the proposed FDA regulations were not within the FDA's existing powers and said that to make it legal, Congress would have to pass a law establishing the FDA's authority to regulate tobacco. Passing such a law did not get much traction in the ensuing years until the Obama administration renewed interest in the issue. With bipartisan support, Congress passed the Family Smoking Prevention and Tobacco Control Act in the spring of 2009 and, as noted above, President Obama signed it into law on June 22, 2009.

Accomplishments to Date

The Tobacco Control Act is a work in progress. Under any circumstances, it is challenging to be charged with the fast-track creation of an enormously wide-ranging, staff-intensive enterprise within an existing Federal agency, all the more so given the intense scrutiny of the Tobacco Control Act and the FDA from the tobacco industry, the public health community, Congress, and others. To date, a range of specific actions have been taken, including:

- Requiring tobacco companies to disclose to the FDA harmful/potentially harmful chemicals in their products
- Enforcing the existing prohibition on misleading tobacco product claims (e.g., "light", "low-tar")
- Requiring, for the first time, graphic health warnings on tobacco packages and ads (this is currently suspended due to the tobacco companies' lawsuit to block this requirement)
- Issuing regulations to stop sales of tobacco to minors
- Commissioning a first-ever study of tobacco use and behavior, which will follow a group of tobacco users over an extended period, so that we can better understand how to help people not start, or stop, using tobacco
- Prohibiting tobacco companies' brand-name sponsorship of sporting events and concerts in order to keep them from advertising to minors
- Releasing a detailed description of research priorities, which will help establish a science-based store of information which the FDA can use to make the most effective use of its regulatory powers to reduce tobacco use
- Providing support to states to keep children and youth from using tobacco products
- Issuing guidance for new tobacco product applications
- Banning flavored cigarettes, which appeal to children and youth.

These actions, and the many others taken to date by the FDA under the authority of the Tobacco Control Act, are a significant step forward in addressing tobacco control in the US and, while the FDA and the CTP have acted to put the Tobacco Control Act into action, there is considerably more action needed, including:

- Addressing whether the FDA will continue to allow cigarettes with menthol flavoring to be marketed
- Addressing whether gradually reducing nicotine in cigarettes would keep people from starting smoking and/or help them quit

- Determining standards for allowable levels of naturally-occurring ingredients and additives in tobacco products and tobacco smoke
- Developing a comprehensive strategy across the FDA to regulate nicotine, which would recognize that there is a range, or continuum, of risk for different tobacco products
- Determining how the tobacco industry will be able to make claims about tobacco products that may be less harmful than traditional smokeable products in order to protect consumers
- How to appropriately regulate the growing range of alternative tobacco products (e.g., e-cigarettes, dissolvables, snus, etc.).

Further, the FDA and the CTP regulatory actions, while essential to ongoing efforts to reduce tobacco-caused death and disease, are not being conducted in a vacuum. Local and state governments, and other parts of the FDA and the Federal government as a whole, are also involved in tobacco policy change, and their actions interact with and expand the effectiveness of the CTP's actions. The public health community also continues to play a role in supporting and, where appropriate, constructively criticizing, the actions of the FDA and CTP. Each of these entities must, however, continue to cooperate and work together if the full effect of the Act – to make a healthier, more tobacco-free country – is to be felt by tobacco users and non-users alike.

On May 8, 2016, the FDA took a significant step forward in establishing a more comprehensive approach to tobacco product regulation by issuing its so-called "deeming rule", through which it extended its authority over *all* tobacco products. As the roll-out of this authority continues over the next several years, the tobacco industry, alternative nicotine product industry, and the public health and tobacco control communities will be carefully monitoring the effect of this rule on tobacco use prevalence and its effects on public health.

Vaccines

There has been considerable interest in recent years in the development of vaccines to aid in smoking cessation, relapse prevention, and even in the prevention of smoking uptake. The basic premise behind these vaccines is to reduce, or even eliminate, the amount of nicotine that reaches the brain after it is inhaled by a smoker.

While the development of a safe and effective vaccine has the potential to be a major advance in the effort to end tobacco use, candidate vaccines developed to date have been shown to be safe but not yet sufficiently effective in enhancing long-term smoking cessation or preventing relapse. Research is continuing on this potentially breakthrough technology [63].

Tobacco and International Trade

While, at first glance, the connection between tobacco control efforts in the US and international trade issues may not be obvious, there is growing evidence that, by increasing the primacy of health over commerce in trade agreements, tobacco control and public health are enhanced.

Due to the ubiquity and lucrative nature of tobacco growth and sales, tobacco products are often included in negotiations surrounding global, regional, or country-to-country trade agreements. For many years, tobacco products were treated no differently than fruits, textiles, or metals. The appalling health effects of tobacco products were not considered as negotiators made arguments about the size of tariffs, the types of tobacco products, and the amount of unprocessed leaf, etc. that would be included in a given agreement. In recent years, however, due to the resistance some countries, such as Thailand, have offered in demanding that tobacco imports not always be a natural part of any trade agreement, there has been a growing recognition that excluding tobacco from free-trade agreements would protect health.

Successful arguments have been made that excluding tobacco from trade agreements is compatible with international law, which provides for other harmful products, such as certain poisons, to be exempted. In addition, the World Trade Organization (WTO) has declared that human health is an important consideration and that, if necessary, governments may "put aside WTO commitments" to protect human life. Allowing and encouraging trade negotiators to permit health to "trump" trade would directly protect the health of citizens affected by trade agreements, which are expected to increase as the world continues to recover from the global recession that occurred between 2008 and 2009. It also would provide a clear message to policymakers and all citizens that tobacco needs to be treated differently, similar to any inherently dangerous product such as weapons or landmines [64–66].

The Tobacco "Endgame"

A recent concept that has attracted wide attention in the US and global tobacco control and public health communities is the tobacco "endgame" – the elimination or virtual elimination of tobacco use as a public health concern. This has emerged as a somewhat controversial concept, with some feeling that it is premature and distracting to focus on eliminating tobacco use when it is still on the rise in many countries and regions, while others feel that it is a necessary consideration and goal in order to maintain and expand energy, resources, and actions devoted to further controlling, and eventually eliminating, tobacco use.

The degree of interest surrounding the endgame concept is evident in the convening of a recent global conference [67] and special journal issue [68] devoted to the idea. While there is no universal agreement on just what constitutes an "endgame" – for example, tobacco use prevalence rates of 10% or less? 5% or less? no tobacco use at all? – a number of countries where tobacco use has been in decline for some time, such as New Zealand, Scotland, and Finland [69], have now set deadlines for their countries to become, in essence, tobacco-free.

In the US, with an adult smoking prevalence rate of 15% in 2015 [3], discussion of a tobacco endgame may seem premature, but many consider it a goal worth pursuing. The 2014 US Surgeon General's Report recognizes the desirability of developing, over time, an endgame strategy in the US and devotes an entire chapter to a discussion of a variety of endgame strategies which the US might consider as we continue to move toward a smoke- and tobacco-free society [1].

There are, of course, many other issues and controversies surrounding tobacco control in the US, for example, the usefulness of mandating the reduction of nicotine in cigarettes to nonaddicting levels, the reduction/elimination of menthol flavoring in cigarettes, the role of litigation in reducing the influence of the tobacco industry, etc. The existence of these issues and controversies demonstrate, rather than weakness, the strength of the tobacco control movement as it further matures and continues to be guided by science and public health principles.

Global Tobacco Control Issues and Considerations

While this chapter focuses primarily on tobacco use and control from a US perspective, it is becoming increasingly difficult for any country or region to address tobacco solely from their own perspective. As noted above, issues such as global trade and the increasing availability and use of social media platforms are acting to make tobacco use and control a global, rather than country- or region-specific concern.

As tobacco use declines in the high-income countries, for example in Western Europe, the US and Canada, Australia, and New Zealand, the data are very clearly indicating that the tobacco epidemic has now expanded to, and become more focused on, the world's low- and middle-income countries (LMIC), due largely to the expansion of the multinational tobacco industry's marketing efforts in Eastern Europe, Asia, Africa, and Latin America [70–72]. Tobacco use kills more than 6 million people annually worldwide. If current trends continue, tobacco use will kill 8 million people annually by 2030, 83% of whom reside in low- and middle-income countries [73].

Fortunately, although the sharply increasing tobacco use prevalence rates in these regions is cause for considerable alarm and need for action, the deadly experience of the high-income nations over the past century need not be wholly repeated in the LMICs. Resources not available in the mid-1960s at the height of the tobacco epidemic in the high-income nations are now widely available to the LMICs, such as the WHO's FCTC and its MPOWER report, and funding sources both large (such as the Michael R. Bloomberg Foundation, the Bill and Melinda Gates Foundation, the US NIH's Fogarty International Center, and the Pfizer Foundation) and more modest (such as Canada's International Development Research Corporation, the Norwegian Cancer Society, the American Cancer Society, and Cancer Research UK). In addition, there is a significant body of tobacco-focused public health research and intervention experience, as well as experience in addressing both communicable and noncommunicable diseases (NCDs), on which the LMICs may now draw as they address the tobacco epidemic in their regions [24, 74–76]. A specific global focus on NCDs – cancer, heart disease, lung disease, and diabetes, each of which is partially caused and exacerbated by tobacco use, especially cigarette smoking – has been accelerated by the convening of a High-Level UN Meeting on this issue in 2011 [77].

The FCTC in particular has been a global galvanizing force for the past decade, serving, as its name implies, as a framework and road map for global tobacco control efforts. Now, in the early part of the twenty-first century, with the FCTC in force in more than 175 countries, covering approximately 90% of the world's population [78], governments and civil society are looking anew at, and taking stock of, the challenges facing tobacco control.

While the primary focus in global tobacco control efforts remain on promoting those interventions that, as discussed above, are known to have significant impact on the reduction of the incidence and prevalence of tobacco use (e.g., increasing tobacco taxes; promoting smoke-free environments; banning tobacco advertising, sponsorships, and promotions, making tobacco dependence treatment widely available), parties to the FCTC treaty are also now beginning to deploy the full range of tobacco control interventions and tools that the FCTC provides to them, including efforts, as discussed above, to carve tobacco out of international trade agreements, to reduce cigarette smuggling (which keeps prices low and encourages uptake and maintenance of smoking), to engage in litigation against domestic and multinational tobacco companies, to require larger and more graphic health warnings on cigarette packages, and to reduce tobacco industry targeting of children and women.

If these global efforts to address the full range of tobacco challenges can be applied widely, consistently, and over an extended period, the possibility then exists to reduce, and perhaps significantly reduce, the expected one billion tobacco-caused deaths anticipated during this twenty-first century.

Conclusion

Enormous progress has been made in reducing the health and economic impact of tobacco use in the US over the past half-century. Millions of premature deaths have been averted and smoking prevalence rates among adults have plummeted from 42% and more than 4000 cigarettes smoked annually per capita in 1964, to 15% and just over 1200 cigarettes smoked annually per capita currently. For the first time in 50 years, the number of smokers in the US has dropped below 40 million since modern recording started in 1965 [3]. Sophisticated, science-based tools, interventions, and treatments are now available to medical professionals, public health practitioners, and policymakers in order to help them address individual and population-wide use of tobacco. A Federal agency now has the authority to regulate tobacco, and the tobacco industry itself has been convicted [79], on the basis of millions of previously secret documents, of mail and wire fraud and racketeering due to its long, and now recognized as felonious, attempts to keep the truth about the dangers of tobacco use from the American public.

Yet, 36.5 million American adults and 3 million youth continue to smoke. The tobacco companies, despite their status as convicted felons, continue to sell, and fight every attempt to protect Americans from their deadly products. Further, the tobacco industry, seeing that its sales in the high-income nations are finally falling, as in the US, are now re-focusing their efforts on new markets in the low- and middle-income nations, which the WHO predicts will now cause one *billion* premature deaths globally this century.

The counterbalancing effects of the progress of the past 50 years, and the ongoing threats to that progress, make it clear that efforts to reduce tobacco use, both in the US and abroad, must continue and be expanded, and that research and surveillance to support those efforts must, as well, continue and be expanded.

References

1 U.S. Department of Health and Human Services. The Health Consequences of Smoking – 50 Years of Progress: A Report of the Surgeon General. Atlanta, GA: U.S. Department of Health and Human Services, Centers for Disease Control and Prevention, National Center for Chronic Disease Prevention and Health Promotion, Office on Smoking and Health, 2014.

2 U.S. Department of Health, Education, and Welfare. *Smoking and Health: Report of the Advisory Committee to the Surgeon General of the Public Health Service*. Washington: U.S. Department of Health, Education, and Welfare, Public Health Service, Center for Disease Control, 1964. PHS Publication No. 1103.

3 Current Cigarette Smoking Among Adults – United States, 2005–2015. *Morbidity and Mortality Weekly Report*, November 11, 2016;65(44):1205–11.

4 Burns E. *The Smoke of the Gods: A Social History of Tobacco*. Philadelphia: Temple University Press, 2007.

5 Borio G. Tobacco Timeline. Available at: http://archive.tobacco.org/History/Tobacco_History.html (accessed 8 June 2017).

6 Shafey O, Eriksen M, Ross H, Mackay J. *The Tobacco Atlas*, 3rd edn. Atlanta: American Cancer Society, 2009.

7 *Tobacco Situation and Outlook Report Yearbook*. U.S. Department of Agriculture. Washington, DC, October 2007.

8 Consumption of Cigarettes and Combustible Tobacco – United States, 2000–2011. *Morbidity and Mortality Weekly*, August 3, 2012;61(30):565–9.

9 Centers for Disease Control and Prevention, Office on Smoking and Health. How Tobacco Smoke Causes Disease: The Biology and Behavioral Basis for Smoking-Attributable Disease: A Report of the Surgeon General. Atlanta, GA, 2010.

10 Bjartveit K, Tverdal A. Health consequences of smoking 1–4 cigarettes per day. *Tobacco Control* 2005;14;315–20.

11 Muller FH. Tabakmissbrauch und Lungencarcinom. *Z Krebsforsch* 1939;49:57–85.

12 Wynder EL, Graham EA. Tobacco smoking as a possible etiologic factor in bronchiogenic carcinoma; a study of 684 proved cases. *JAMA* 1950;143:329–36.

13 Doll R, Hill AB. Smoking and carcinoma of the lung; preliminary report. *Br Med J* 1950;2:739–48.

14 Doll R, Hill AB. The mortality of doctors in relation to their smoking habits; a preliminary report. *Br Med J* 1954;1:1451–5.

15 Hammond EC, Horn D. The relationship between human smoking habits and death rates: a follow-up study of 187,766 men. *JAMA* 1954;155:1316–28.

16 Hammond EC, Horn D. Smoking and death rates; report on forty-four months of follow-up of 187,783 men. *I. Total mortality. JAMA* 1958;166:1159–72.

17 Smoking and Health: joint report of the Study Group on Smoking and Health. *Science* 1957;125(3258):1129–33.

18 Royal College of Physicians of London. *Smoking and Health. A Report of the Royal College of Physicians of London on Smoking in Relation to Cancer of the Lung and Other Diseases*. London, UK: Royal College of Physicians, London, 1962.

19 International Agency for Research on Cancer. Smokeless Tobacco and Some Tobacco-Specific N-Nitrosamines. Lyon, France: World Health Organization International Agency for Research on Cancer, 2007. IARC Monographs on the Evaluation of Carcinogenic Risks to Humans Volume 89.

20 Tobacco Product Use Among Adults – United States, 2012–2013. *Morbidity and Mortality Weekly Report*, June 27, 2014;63(25):542–7.

21 Rutqvist, LE. Report on the Swedish Snus Experience, submitted to the FDA Tobacco Product Scientific Advisory Committee. http://www.fda.gov/downloads/ advisorycommittees/committeesmeetingmaterials/ tobaccoproductsscientificadvisorycommittee/ ucm293256.pdf (accessed 16 May 2017).

22 Fiore, MC. Schroeder, SA. Baker, TB. Smoke, the chief killer – strategies for targeting combustible tobacco use. *NEJM* 2014;370(4):297–9.

23 Centers for Disease Control and Prevention, Office on Smoking and Health. The Health Consequences of Involuntary Exposure to Tobacco Smoke: A Report of the Surgeon General. Atlanta, GA, 2006.

24 WHO Report on the Global Tobacco Epidemic, 2008: *The MPOWER package*. Geneva: World Health Organization, 2008.

25 Tobacco.org. http://archive.tobacco.org/History/540104frank. html (accessed 16 May 2017).

26 American Bar Association. http://www.abajournal.com/ magazine/article/july_12_1957_surgeon_general_links_ smoking_and_lung_cancer/ (accessed 16 May 2017).

27 Proctor, RN. *Golden Holocaust: Origins of the Cigarette Catastrophe and the Case for Abolition*. Berkeley: University of California Press, 2011.

28 Burney LE. Special article: smoking and lung cancer: Statement by the Public Health Service. *JAMA* 1959;171:1829–37.

29 Talbot J. Smoking and lung cancer. *JAMA* 1959;171:2104.

30 The Pump Handle. http://scienceblogs.com/ thepumphandle/2012/10/02/public-health-classic-surgeon-generals-1964-report-on-smoking-and-health/ (accessed 16 May 2017).

31 Holford TR, Meza R, Warner KE, *et al*. Tobacco control and the reduction in smoking-related premature deaths in the United States, 1964–2012. *JAMA* 2014;311(2):164–71.

32 Commonwealth of Australia. National Tobacco Control Strategy 2012–2018. Canberra, Australia, 2012.

33 California Tobacco Control Program. https://archive.cdph.ca.gov/ programs/Tobacco/Pages/default.aspx (accessed 8 June 2017).

34 World Health Organization – MPOWER Protocol. http:// www.who.int/tobacco/mpower/en/ (accessed 16 May 2017).

35 Centers for Disease Control and Prevention. Best Practices for Comprehensive Tobacco Control Programs. Atlanta, GA: U.S. Department of Health and Human Services, Centers for Disease Control and Prevention, National Center for Chronic Disease Prevention and Health Promotion, Office on Smoking and Health, 2014.

36 World Health Organization – framework Convention on Tobacco Control. http://www.who.int/fctc/text_download/en/ (accessed 16 May 2017).

37 Jha P, Chaloupka FJ. *Curbing the Epidemic: Governments and the Economics of Tobacco Control*. Washington, DC: World Bank, 1999.

38 Hurt, RD, Ebbert, JO, Hays, JT, McFadden, DD. Treating tobacco dependence in a medical setting. *CA Cancer J Clin* 2009;59(5):314–26.

39 Fiore M, Baker T, Jaen C, *et al*. Treating Tobacco Use and Dependence: 2008 Update. Clinical Practice Guideline. Rockville: US Department of Health & Human Services, Public Health Service, 2008.

40 Quitting Smoking Among Adults – United States, 2001–2010. *Morbidity and Mortality Weekly Report*, November 11, 2011;60(44):1513–19.

41 American Lung Association. http://www.lung.org/ our-initiatives/tobacco/cessation-and-prevention/ tobacco-cessation-and-affordable-care-act. html?referrer=https://www.google.com/ (accessed 8 June 2017).

42 Fiore MC, Goplerud E, Schroeder SA. The Joint Commission's new tobacco-cessation measures – will hospitals do the right thing? *N Engl J Med* 2012;366:1172–4.

43 Centers for Disease Prevention and Control – The Guide to Community Preventive Services. http://www. thecommunityguide.org/tobacco/RRquitlines.html (accessed May 16 2017).

44 Ahluwalia, JS, Gibson, CA, Kenney, RE, Wallace, DD, Resnicow, K. Smoking status as a vital sign. *J Gen Intern Med* 1999;14(7):402–8.

45 Lai DTC, Cahill K, Qin Y, Tang JL. Motivational interviewing for smoking cessation. Cochrane Database of Systematic Reviews 2010, Issue 1.

46 Fucito, LM, Bars, MP, Forray, A, *et al*. Addressing the evidence for FDA nicotine replacement therapy label changes: a policy statement of the Association for the Treatment of Tobacco Use and Dependence and the Society for Research on Nicotine and Tobacco. *Nicotine Tob Res* 2014;16(7):909–14.

47 Cahill, K, Stevens, S, Lancaster, T. Pharmacological treatments for smoking cessation. *JAMA* 2014;311(2):193–4.

48 Myung SK, McDonnell DD, Kazinets G, Seo HG, Moskowitz JM. Effects of web- and computer-based smoking cessation programs: meta-analysis of randomized controlled trials. *Arch Intern Med* 2009;169(10):929–37.

49 Walters ST, Wright JA, Shegog R. A review of computer and internet-based interventions for smoking behavior. *Addict Behav* 2006;31(2):264–77.

50 Webb TL, Joseph J, Yardley L, Michie S. Using the internet to promote health behavior change: a systematic review and meta-analysis of the impact of theoretical basis, use of behavior change techniques, and mode of delivery on efficacy. *J Med Internet Res* 2010; 12(1):e4.

51 Bock B, Graham A, Sciamanna C, *et al*. Smoking cessation treatment on the internet: content, quality, and usability. *Nicotine Tob Res* 2004;6(2):207–19.

52 Abroms L, Westmaas JL, Bontemps-Jones J, Ramani R, Mellerson J. A content analysis of popular smartphone apps for smoking cessation. *Am J Prev Med* 2013;45(6):732–6.

53 Free C, Whittaker R, Knight R, *et al*. Txt2stop: a pilot randomised controlled trial of mobile phone-based smoking cessation support. *Tob Control* 2009;18(2):88–91.

54 Strecher VJ, Shiffman S, West R. Randomized controlled trial of a web-based computer-tailored smoking cessation program as a supplement to nicotine patch therapy. *Addiction* 2005;100(5):682–8.

55 Fairchild A, Colgrove J. Out of the Ashes: The Life, Death, and Rebirth of the "Safer" Cigarette in the United States. *Am J Public Health* 2004;94(2):192–204.

56 Rooke, C. Harm reduction and the medicalization of tobacco use. *Sociol Health Illn* 2013;35(3):361–76.

57 Martin, EG, Warner, KE, Lantz, PM. Tobacco harm reduction: what do the experts think? *Tob Control* 2004;13:123–8.

58 Fairchild, AL, Bayer, R, Colgrove, J. The renormalization of smoking? E-Cigarettes and the tobacco endgame. *N Eng J Med* 2014;370:293–5.

59 Glynn, TJ. E-Cigarettes and the future of tobacco control. *CA Cancer J Clin* 2014;64(3): 164–8.

60 U.S. Food and Drug Administration. E-Cigarettes: impact on individual and population health. Tob Control 2014;23:Supplement 2.

61 Family Smoking Prevention and Tobacco Control Act. http://www.fda.gov/TobaccoProducts/Guidance ComplianceRegulatoryInformation/ucm237092.htm (accessed 16 May 2017).

62 Overview of the Family Smoking Prevention and Tobacco Control Act: Consumer Fact Sheet. http://www.fda.gov/ tobaccoproducts/guidancecomplianceregulatoryinformation/ ucm246129.htm (accessed 16 May 2017).

63 Hartmann-Boyce J, Cahill K, Hatsukami D, Cornuz J. Nicotine Vaccines for Smoking Cessation, 2012, Cochrane Database of Systematic Reviews, *Issue* 8.

64 Shaffer RE, Brenner JE, Houston T. International trade agreements: a threat to tobacco control policy. *Tob Control* 2005;14:19–25.

65 World Health Organization, Tobacco-Free Initiative. *Confronting the Tobacco Epidemic in a New Era of Trade and Investment Liberalization*. Geneva: World Health Organization, 2012.

66 McGrady, B. *Trade and Public Health: The WTO, Tobacco, Alcohol, and Diet*. London: Cambridge University Press, 2014.

67 International Conference on Public Health Priorities in the 21st Century. http://www.world-heart-federation.org/ publications/heart-beat-e-newsletter/heart-beat-december-2013/advocacy-news/endgame-conference/ (accessed 8 June 2017).

68 The Tobacco Endgame. Tob Control 2013;22:Supplement 1.

69 Cobiac LJ, Ikeda T, Nghiem N, Blakely T, Wilson N. Modeling the implications of regular increases in tobacco taxation in the tobacco endgame. *Tob Control* 2015;24(e2):154–60.

70 McKay J. Implementing tobacco control policies. *Br Med Bull* 2012;102(1):5–16.

71 Stoklosa M, Ross H. Tobacco control funding for low-income and middle-income countries in a time of economic hardship. *Tob Control* 2014;23(e2):e122–6

72 Yach D, Pratt A, Glynn TJ, Reddy KS. Research to stop tobacco deaths. *Global Health*, 2014;10:39–45.

73 Global Tobacco Control. http://www.cancer.org/aboutus/ globalhealth/tobacco-control (accessed 16 May 2017).

74 Norwegian Knowledge Center for the Health Services. *Interventions for Tobacco Control in Low- and Middle-income Countries: Evidence from Randomised and Quasi-Randomised Studies*. Oslo, Norway: Norwegian Knowledge Center for the Health Services, 2012.

75 CDC Grand Rounds: Global Tobacco Control. *Morbidity and Mortality Weekly Report*, 2014;63(13):277–80.

76 Glynn T, Seffrin JR, Brawley OW, Grey N, Ross H. The globalization of tobacco use: 21 challenges for the 21st century. *CA Cancer J Clin* 2010;60(1):51–60.

77 Non-Communicable Disease Alliance. http://www.ncdalliance. org/sites/default/files/rfiles/Key%20Points%20of%20 Political%20Declaration.pdf (accessed 16 May 2017).

78 World Health Organization. Parties to the WHO Framework Convention on Tobacco Control. http://www.who.int/fctc/ signatories_parties/en/ (accessed 16 May 2017).

79 The Daily Washington Law Reporter. RICO Convictions of Major Tobacco Companies Affirmed. http://www.dwlr.com/ blog/2011-05-12/rico-convictions-major-tobacco-companies-affirmed (accessed 16 May 2017).

7

Microbial Carcinogens

Edgar P. Simard[1] and Ahmedin Jemal[2]

[1] Rollins School of Public Health, Emory University, Atlanta, Georgia, USA
[2] Surveillance and Health Services Research, American Cancer Society, Atlanta, Georgia, USA

Introduction

Human microbial carcinogens include a diverse grouping of viruses, bacteria, and parasitic worms. This chapter focuses on those classified as "Group 1" agents with sufficient evidence to conclude they are carcinogenic to humans based on a rigorous review of evidence by the International Agency for Research on Cancer [1]. This chapter provides a historical background, a discussion of carcinogenic mechanisms, and for each carcinogen, an overview of their biologic and epidemiologic features.

The hypothesis of a causal role for infectious agents and cancer has been explored for centuries, largely informed by animal studies that revealed numerous carcinogenic viruses, although none caused disease in humans [2]. In the early twentieth century, flukes (*Schistosoma* infections) were noted to be associated with bladder cancer, but it was not until 50 years later with the development of new laboratory methods, that other microbial carcinogens were discovered [2–4]. In the late 1950s, Dennis Burkitt observed that childhood lymphomas were clustered in equatorial Africa, which fueled speculation of an infectious cause of the disease and spurred laboratory studies that led to the discovery of Epstein–Barr virus, which is now known to be related to a number of human cancers [2, 5, 6]. Advances in molecular and genetic techniques have led to an expanded understanding of relationships between established microbial carcinogens and additional cancer sites, as well as the discovery of new carcinogens.

Microbial carcinogens are somewhat unique in that unlike most chemical and other carcinogens, they exhibit tissue tropism causing specific cancer types (e.g., human papillomavirus [HPV] type 16 infection is associated with squamous cell carcinomas). Their mechanisms can be conceptualized into three broad groups: direct carcinogens that integrate their genetic material into host cells disrupting normal cellular functions; indirect carcinogens that act via chronic inflammation; and indirect carcinogens that act via immune suppression (Table 7.1) [1].

Epstein–Barr Virus

Epstein–Barr virus (EBV) is a DNA gamma *Herpesvirus* and infection among humans is ubiquitous [7]. The natural history of infection involves an initial primary and subsequent latent infection that remains largely undetected and asymptomatic for a lifetime. Lymphocytes are the major cellular target of EBV and the virus is predominantly B-lymphotropic, although T-lymphocytes and epithelial cells may also be infected [1]. EBV is transmitted through premastication of food and other salivary routes associated with low socioeconomic status, including crowding, in resource-limited countries where infection is acquired during childhood. In contrast, in developed countries, infection is often acquired during young adulthood with transmission occurring via intimate oral contact; infectious mononucleosis can manifest as a result [8]. There is no vaccine to prevent infection.

Epstein–Barr nuclear antigens code for viral transcription programs that result in the expression of gene products associated with reactivation, directly influencing malignant outcomes (Table 7.1 provides a classification of each microbial carcinogen as direct or indirect) [9, 10]. This process occurs in the presence of understudied cofactors, including immunosuppression [11]. There are several EBV-related cancers, including: nasopharyngeal carcinoma (NPC), non-Hodgkin lymphomas (NHLs) including Burkitt lymphoma (BL), as well as other subtypes, Hodgkin lymphoma, and natural killer (NK)/T-cell lymphomas (Table 7.2) [12]. Risk of EBV-related malignancies is elevated among people with immune suppression related to human immunodeficiency virus (HIV) infection and with iatrogenic immunosuppression following solid organ or hematopoietic stem cell transplantation. Malarial infection is a cofactor in endemic African BL although

Table 7.1 Microbial carcinogens: summary of biologic mechanisms.

Classification/carcinogen	Biologic mechanisms
Direct carcinogen, infection results in direct transformation of normal to malignant cells	
EBV	Viral genome can usually be detected in each cancer cell
HPV	Virus can immortalize after growth of target cells *in vitro*
HTLV-1	Virus expresses oncogenes that interact with cellular proteins
KSHV	leading to the disruption of cell-cycle checkpoints, inhibition of apoptosis, and cell immortalization
Indirect carcinogen, infection results in chronic inflammation	
HBV	Chronic infections results in persistent inflammation that produces
HCV	inflammatory cytokines, chemokines, and prostaglandins, secreted
Helicobacter pylori	by infected and/or inflammatory cells
Schistosoma haematobium	This process also leads to the production of reactive oxygen
Opistorchis viverrini	species which have direct mutagenic effects resulting in the
Clonorchis sinensis	deregulation of the immune system and the promotion of angiogenesis, processes essential for tumour survival
Indirect carcinogen, infection results in immune suppression	
HIV-1	Immune suppression as a result of infection with HIV leads to decreased immune surveillance increasing cancer risk

Source: adapted from IARC Monograph Volume 100B: Biologic Agents, A Review of Human Carcinogens (2012) [1].
Note: restricted to those microbial carcinogens that are known to have a known causal association with human cancer as assessed by the International Agency for Research on Cancer.
Abbreviations: EBV, Epstein-Barr virus; HBV, hepatitis B virus; HCV, hepatitis C virus; HIV-1, human immunodeficiency virus type-1; HPV, human papillomavirus; HTLV-1, human T-cell lymphotropic virus type-1. KSHV, Kaposi sarcoma-associated herpesvirus.

Table 7.2 Microbial carcinogens and their associated cancer sites.

Microbial carcinogen	Associated cancer
EBV	Burkitt lymphoma, immune-suppression-related non-Hodgkin lymphoma, NK/T-cell lymphoma, Hodgkin lymphoma
HBV	Hepatocellular carcinoma
HCV	Hepatocellular carcinoma, non-Hodgkin lymphoma
KSHV	Kaposi sarcoma, primary effusion lymphoma
HIV-1	Kaposi sarcoma, non-Hodgkin lymphoma, Hodgkin lymphoma, cancer of the cervix, anus, conjunctiva
HPV 16	Cancer of the cervix, vulva, vagina, penis, anus, oral cavity and oropharynx
HTLV-1	Adult T-cell leukaemia and lymphoma (ATLL)
Helicobacter pylori	Non-cardia gastric carcinoma, low-grade B-cell mucosa-associated lymphoid tissue (MALT) gastric lymphoma
Clonorchis sinensis	Cholangiocarcinoma
Opisthorchis viverini	Cholangiocarcinoma
Schistosoma haematobium	Urinary bladder cancer

Source: adapted from IARC Monograph Volume 100B: Biologic Agents, A Review of Human Carcinogens (2012) [1].
Note: associated cancers are restricted to those with sufficient evidence to conclude causality as assessed by the International Agency for Research on Cancer. Abbreviations: EBV, Epstein-Barr virus; HBV, hepatitis B virus; HCV, hepatitis C virus; HIV-1, human immunodeficiency virus type-1; HPV, human papillomavirus; HTLV-1, human T-cell lymphotropic virus type-1; KSHV, Kaposi sarcoma-associated herpesvirus.

the mechanisms by which malaria and EBV interact to increase cancer risk are unclear [13]. The majority of endemic BL cases are attributable to EBV (>95%) whereas the role of EBV is usually less significant in other NHLs and Hodgkin lymphomas, with variation by geography and subtype [14]. EBV infection is generally associated with a two- to fourfold increased cancer risk relative to EBV negative individuals (although relative risk is greater for some subtypes, like BL) [1].

For all EBV-related NHLs, immunosuppression resulting in decreased T-cell surveillance that promotes unchecked EBV replication in B-lymphocytes is important in carcinogenesis [15]. Similar mechanisms play a role in the transformation of the pathognomonic Reed–Sternberg cell (of B-cell lineage) in Hodgkin lymphomas. For EBV-related NPC, salted fish consumption is an important cofactor in Asian countries where NPC is common [16].

Hepatitis B Virus

Hepatitis B virus (HBV) is a hepatotrophic DNA *Hepadnaviridae* virus. HBV is transmitted via percutaneous or permucosal exposure to infected blood or other fluids such as semen and vaginal secretions [17]. Transmission risk factors include intravenous drug use, unprotected sex with an HBV-infected partner, sharing of blood-contaminated household items (e.g., razors), unsafe injections, transfusion of unscreened blood, and birth of an infant to an HBV-infected mother. Perinatal transmission is common in endemic areas without infant postexposure prophylaxis and routine vaccination. Young age at exposure increases risk of chronic (lifelong) infection associated with risk of hepatocellular carcinoma (HCC) [18]. Globally, approximately 53% of all HCC cases are attributable to HBV, although the proportion is higher in many Asian and sub-Saharan African countries reflecting geographic differences in HBV endemicity levels (Figure 7.1) [19].

Cofactors in the natural history of HBV infection include viral genotype, tobacco and alcohol use, aflatoxin exposure, and coinfection with other oncogenic viruses (e.g., hepatitis C virus and HIV) [1]. As an indirect carcinogen (Table 7.1), chronic infection initiates a decades-long progression of host immune response promoting intermittent hepatocytic necrosis, regeneration, and proliferation. This process results in fibrosis and cirrhosis, increasing HCC risk (Table 7.2). Risk of HCC among

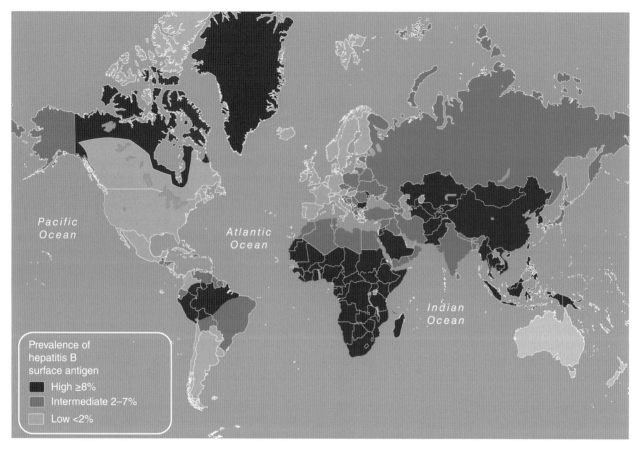

Figure 7.1 Global prevalence of chronic hepatitis B virus infection. *Source:* Centers for Disease Control and Prevention. CDC Health Information for International Travel 2012. New York: Oxford University Press, 2012.

chronic HBV-infected persons is elevated approximately 20-fold [20].

Primary infection and related sequelae (including HCC) may be prevented through prophylactic vaccination, which has been available in the United States (US) since 1981 [17]. Routine vaccination is recommended in the US for all children and high-risk adults [21, 22]. Childhood vaccination is widespread in developed countries [23] but progress is needed to scale-up vaccination in low-resource areas where HBV infection remains endemic [24]. Infection may also be prevented through safer sexual practices (e.g., condom use), sterile injection practices, and other means. Successful antiviral therapy of chronic HBV infection also reduces HCC risk.

Hepatitis C Virus

Hepatitis C virus (HCV) is a hepatotrophic RNA *Flavivirus*. Percutaneous blood exposure is the primary route of transmission occurring mainly through injection drug use, unsafe therapeutic injections, and unscreened transfusions. Mother-to-child (vertical) transmission and sexual transmission are less common [25]. As a result, transmission predominantly occurs in adulthood and approximately 70% of those acutely infected will develop chronic infection that increases risk of HCC [1]. Approximately 25% of all cases of cirrhosis and HCC occur among individuals with chronic HCV infection [19]. There is substantial geographic heterogeneity in prevalence of infections (Figure 7.2) which mirrors patterns in HCV-related outcomes. Cofactors in HCV natural history include viral genotype (genotype 1 is worse than others), coinfection with HBV and/or HIV, alcohol and tobacco use, and obesity and diabetes [1, 25, 26].

The virus acts indirectly (Table 7.1) by stimulating inflammation resulting in hepatocyte damage and leading to fibrosis and cirrhosis. HCC risk is elevated approximately 20-fold among HCV-infected individuals [20]. HCV proteins also act directly with the host, changing signalling pathways regulating cell metabolism and division [1]. Chronic infection is also associated with extrahepatic manifestations (including nonmalignant mixed cryoglobulinemia) and an increased risk of NHL (NHL risk is approximately 2.5-fold higher for HCV-positive individuals) [1, 20]. This may occur as a result of chronic B lymphocyte proliferation through persistent antigenic stimulation and/or chromosomal translocations.

There is no vaccine to prevent HCV infection. However, avoiding exposure to HCV-infected blood and other infectious body fluid reduces infection risk. One time HCV screening of all persons born between 1945 and 1965 is recommended by the Centers for Disease Control and Prevention to identify those with chronic infection in the US [27]. Identifying and successfully treating this population would reduce the risk of HCV-related sequelae, including HCC.

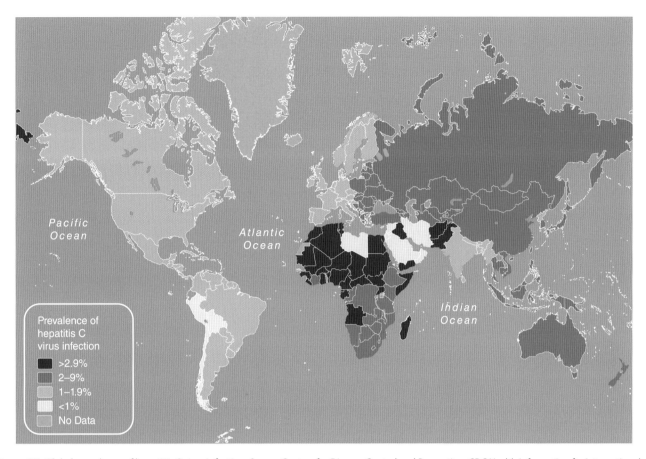

Figure 7.2 Global prevalence of hepatitis C virus infection. *Source:* Centers for Disease Control and Prevention. CDC Health Information for International Travel 2012. New York: Oxford University Press, 2012.

Kaposi Sarcoma Herpesvirus

Kaposi sarcoma herpesvirus (KSHV) or human herpesvirus type-8 (HHV-8) is a DNA *Herpesvirus*. Infection prevalence varies by global region, country, and sociodemographic groups within countries. These patterns are evident in the spectrum of malignant outcomes associated with infection. KSHV is thought to be transmitted primarily by saliva [1, 28]. In resource-limited settings, transmission (believed to be from salivary exposure) occurs during childhood whereas in more developed areas transmission occurs during adulthood concurrent with sexual activity. In the US, KSHV infection is rare among the general population (seroprevalence is approximately 7%) but common among men who have sex with men (MSM, 20–60%), especially those co-infected with HIV [29–32]. Oral sexual practices appear important for transmission among MSM [33].

Primary infection establishes a lifelong latent infection, during which viral proteins reactivate, resulting in lytic (productive) virus replication. The virus has been isolated in a number of cell types, including endothelial cells of KS lesions [1, 34]. Several latent and lytic viral proteins are involved in carcinogenesis and protein expression can result in genomic instability, DNA damage, and other events directly involved in cellular transformation (Table 7.1) [1, 33].

Kaposi sarcoma (KS) is a tumour of vascular or lymphatic endothelial cells and the most common KSHV-related malignancy. KHSV is associated with all clinical variants of the disease (endemic, sporadic, AIDS-related) and a large proportion of rare primary effusion lymphomas (Table 7.2) [1]. Both malignancies occur at great excess among HIV-infected persons and transplant recipients, underscoring immunosuppression as a cofactor. KSHV is also associated with about 50% of multicentric Castleman disease cases, a lymphoproliferative disorder. While there is no primary prevention, among immunosuppressed populations, cancer risk may be decreased by immune restoration (e.g., through effective HIV therapies) [35–37].

Human Immunodeficiency Virus Type-1

Human immunodeficiency virus type-1 (HIV-1) is an RNA *Retrovirus*. Humans are the natural host and the virus targets CD4+ T-lymphocytes, macrophages expressing specific protein receptors, and dendritic cells [1, 38]. The virus can be detected in a variety of tissues, as infected target cells are found throughout the body. Global infection prevalence ranges from less than 0.5% in developed regions to more than 30% in parts of sub-Saharan Africa [1]. Similar to other bloodborne oncogenic viruses, HIV is transmitted via permucosal and percutaneous exposures and vertically from mother to child. Primary infection results in a lifelong chronic infection characterized by the progressive depletion of CD4+ T-lymphocytes. Due to their shared risk factors and transmission routes, co-infection with one or more additional oncogenic viruses is common.

Many cancers associated with HIV are themselves caused by oncogenic viruses. Cancer risk in the HIV-1-infected individual is elevated indirectly by immunosuppression and the increased expression of the effects of other oncogenic viruses (Table 7.1). HIV-1 infection alone does not lead to cell transformation or immortalization. In the presence of their necessary primary cause, HIV-1 causes KS, NHL, Hodgkin lymphoma, cervical and anal cancers, and conjunctival cancer (Table 7.2) [1]. For example, risk of KS is elevated in people with HIV because it likely induces lytic replication of KSHV [39]. For the three main NHL subtypes associated with HIV (primary brain lymphoma, large-cell immunoblastic lymphoma, and BL) hyperactivation of B cells and unchecked EBV replication are important [15]. For cervical and anal cancers, HIV-1 may promote replication of HPV-infected cells [1]. Immunosuppression also increases risk for squamous cell conjunctival cancer due to ultraviolet radiation exposure [40, 41]. These cancers also occur in HIV-negative persons making it difficult to qualify the fraction of cases attributable to HIV.

There is no HIV vaccine although exposure may be prevented in similar ways to those for other bloodborne viruses. Effective HIV treatment resulting in partial immune reconstitution dramatically decreases risk for some, but not all, HIV-associated cancers [37, 42].

Human Papillomavirus

There are more than 100 HPV types belonging to the DNA *Papillomaviridae* family that can be divided based on tissue tropism: skin-trophic (associated with benign warts) and mucosal-trophic (some of which are associated with malignancy). The mucosal-trophic types can be further divided into high or low risk based on their cancer associations, and target squamous epithelial cells. HPV 16 and HPV 18 are considered to be the most common carcinogenic HPV types (other carcinogenic types are HPV 31, HPV 33, HPV 35, HPV 39, HPV 45, HPV 51, HPV 52, HPV 56, HPV 58, HPV 59, HPV 66, and HPV 68) [1, 43]. Infection with mucosal tropic HPVs is commonly acquired soon after sexual debut, and HPV is transmitted through genital contact, including vaginal, anal, and oral sex. Because HPV infection incidence and clearance rates are high, a single prevalence estimate is difficult to assess and most people will have at least one infection during their lifetime. Host immune response usually clears the infection although some people develop a persistent infection, especially those infected with HPV 16 [44].

HPV infection is a necessary cause of all cervical cancers, approximately 90% of anal cancers, and more than 60% of specific subsites of oropharyngeal cancer (e.g., tonsil, oral cavity, Waldeyer's ring) and vaginal, vulvar, and penile cancers (Tables 7.1 and 7.2) [45]. Specifically, two HPV-encoded oncoproteins (E6 and E7) are involved in the regulation of cell growth and overcoming apoptosis to promote HPV DNA replication leading to genomic instability [1, 43]. The natural history of cervical carcinogenesis includes the development of precursor *in-situ* lesions and subsequent tumour invasion, although many infections and lesions spontaneously regress [46]. Cofactors in cervical neoplasia include smoking and hormonal (e.g., oral contraceptive use) and reproductive characteristics (e.g., early

age at sexual debut) [46, 47]. Immunosuppression is also important and HPV-related cancers occur in excess among HIV-infected people [37, 42, 48]. The mechanistic pathways for other HPV-related cancers are thought to be similar to that of cervical cancer but are less clear [1, 43, 49]. HPV 6 and 11 are associated with anogenital warts and respiratory papillomatosis.

Primary prevention of HPV infection and type-related outcomes may be achieved through prophylactic vaccination. The currently approved HPV vaccines (bivalent – HPV 16/18; quadrivalent – HPV 6/11/16/18; and 9-valent – HPV 6/11/16/18/31/33/45/52/58) protect against high-risk HPV 16 and 18 which account for approximately 70% of all cervical cancers worldwide and most noncervical HPV-related cancers [50–54]. Proper and consistent use of condoms may also provide some protection against infection [55].

Human T-cell Lymphotropic Virus

Human T-cell lymphotropic virus type-1 (HTLV-1) is an RNA *Retrovirus* [56, 57]. Similar to other bloodborne viruses it may be transmitted vertically, sexually, and through blood-to-blood contact [58]. Transmission via breast feeding is high in some endemic areas like Japan [1]. Infection prevalence is varied and endemic in only specific regions (i.e., parts of Japan, sub-Saharan Africa, South America and the Caribbean) [58]; these patterns also manifest in the spectrum of diseases associated with HTLV-1.

Infection is a necessary cause of adult T-cell leukaemia/lymphoma (ATLL), which occurs among approximately 2–4% of HTLV-1 carriers [1] (Table 7.2). Male gender is an important factor in risk of this cancer and the latency period ranges from 10 to 60 years, based on geographic region [1]. The virus targets $CD4^+$ T-lymphocytes and is monoclonally integrated into their genome, directly influencing cancer risk of the host (Table 7.1). The Tax protein (considered an oncoprotein) can directly immortalize and transform T-cells [3, 10].

There is no vaccine to prevent HTLV-1 infection. Prevention methods are similar to other bloodborne pathogens. Counselling infected mothers about the risk of transmission via breast feeding can reduce mother-to-child transmission [58].

Helicobacter Pylori

Infection with the bacterium *Helicobacter pylori* (*H. pylori*) is common throughout the world (50% prevalence) with significant variation in prevalence between countries [1]. *H. pylori* is transmitted through close person-to-person contact and transmission is common among members of the same households and within families. Low socioeconomic status is a risk factor, perhaps as a proxy for hygienic conditions and crowding. In resource-limited settings infection is commonly acquired during childhood and persists for life unless treated with antibiotics [1]. *H. pylori* colonizes the gastric epithelial mucosa and frequent genetic mutations of the bacteria contribute to infection persistence [1].

Cancer risk is increased indirectly in ways that involve characteristics of the bacterium (e.g., genetic) and the host (e.g., inflammatory response) (Table 7.1). For example, strains with the Cag-A gene appear to have increased carcinogenicity. Gastritis as a result of *H. pylori* infection results in epithelial cell hypermethylation and altered cell turnover rates [1, 59]. *H. pylori* infection confers an approximately twofold increase in cancer gastric cancer risk and is associated with approximately 75% of cases of non-cardia gastric adenocarcinomas (Table 7.2) [20, 60]. Cofactors such as dietary practices (e.g., diets low in fruits and vegetables and high in salted and/or smoked foods) as well as smoking and alcohol intake also appear to increase gastric cancer risk [61]. Genetic polymorphisms involved with lymphomagenesis provide a link for *H. pylori* and gastric low-grade B-cell mucosa-associated lymphoid tissue lymphoma (MALT lymphoma), and infection is responsible for more than 75% of gastric MALT lymphoma cases [1, 60].

There is no vaccine to prevent *H. pylori* infection. However, a screen and treat paradigm using proton pump inhibitors coupled with antibiotics has been shown to be effective in the prevention of both gastric cancer and MALT lymphoma and as therapy for early-stage gastric MALT lymphoma [62–64].

Schistosoma Haematobium

Schistosoma haematobium (*S. haematobium*) is a trematode worm with a complex life cycle involving both humans and water-dwelling snail hosts. Infection is endemic in parts of sub-Saharan Africa and Egypt [1]. The parasite enters the human host through exposure with contaminated fresh water. Infection may be common among fishermen and agricultural workers and women and children with water exposure. Most people in these regions have multiple infections throughout their lifetime that are asymptomatic and do not result in any disease.

The parasites' eggs are deposited in the urinary bladder and invoke a series of host responses that indirectly influence urinary bladder cancer risk (Tables 7.1 and 7.2) [1]. Regional dietary patterns may also act synergistically with infections [65]. The inflammatory response results in increased oxidative stress and DNA damage promoting malignant transformation [1]. Approximately 40% of urinary bladder cancer cases in endemic regions have evidence of *S. haematobium* infection [60]. Prevention of infection in endemic areas is difficult as it is acquired during activities necessary for daily living, although eradication of the snail host has been achieved in limited areas. Treatment of *S. haematobium* may reduce cancer risk, but reinfection is likely unless individuals migrate from endemic areas [66].

Opisthorchis Viverrini and Clonorchis Sinesis

Liver flukes *Opisthorchis viverrini* (*O. viverrini*) *and Clonorchis sinesis* (*C. sinesis*) have a complicated life cycle requiring multiple hosts and environmental factors. When the feces of humans with live fluke infection contaminate water sources, snails can ingest their eggs, which then develop into cercariae that migrate to the skin of freshwater fish. When raw or undercooked fish are consumed by humans the flukes are transmitted. Human infection is endemic in many Asian countries including China

and Thailand, and approximately 75% of infections are from *C. sinensis* [1]. Similar to other infection-related cancers, the geographic patterns of cholangiocarcinoma (bile duct cancer) associated with liver flukes are striking and rates are dramatically high in parts of Thailand (mainly due to *O. viverrini*). *C. sinensis* infection can persist for decades and *O. viverrini* infection persists for about 10 years [1].

Mature flukes reside in the bile duct where eggs are deposited. Infection promotes cell proliferation and oxidative stress that can lead to DNA damage and adduct formation, indirectly increasing cholangiocarcinoma risk (Tables 7.1 and 7.2). Other factors, for example, genetic characteristics, also play a role in carcinogenesis. In endemic regions, infection is responsible for most cases of bile duct cancer. While liver fluke infections are treatable, reinfection is also common due to frequent fish consumption [67].

Conclusions

Both the burden of microbial carcinogens and their associated malignant outcomes disproportionately affect individuals in low resource settings. Incidence rates of such cancers are elevated several fold in less developed regions of the world, where infection-related cancers are leading causes of morbidity and mortality. In 2008, 22.9% of incident cancers were attributable to infectious causes in less developed countries versus 7.4% in more developed countries [60]. Specifically, HCC, cervical cancer, and gastric adenocarcinoma account for the majority of infection-related cancers in less developed countries (Table 7.3) [60]. The causes of these disparities are multifactorial and include societal, environmental, and individual characteristics. Furthermore, cancer-related outcomes are typically poor in these settings because treatment options are scarce and cost-prohibitive. However, scaling-up access to low-cost cancer prevention activities, including HBV and HPV vaccination programs may help reduce the burden of cancer in the future [24]. Clinicians who care for patients in or from countries where microbial infections are prevalent should be aware of these associated cancer risks and follow established screening and treatment guidelines to reduce cancer risk.

This chapter focused on known human microbial carcinogens. Some of the carcinogens discussed are associated with additional cancers but the strength of epidemiologic and mechanistic data preclude decisions regarding causality [1]. In addition, with advances in molecular detection techniques, the discovery of new microbial carcinogens is likely. For example, Merkel cell polyomavirus is considered to have oncogenic potential and is associated with a rare neuroendocrine tumour, Merkel cell carcinoma [68]. However, it is not known if infection is necessary for cancer development. Continued research into the mechanistic pathways for these cancers is also warranted along with prevention research. For many of the microbial carcinogens discussed, vaccine research is on-going and would likely prevent both the primary infections and their related cancer outcomes. Additional research is also warranted to develop low-cost and low-technology prevention measures for use in resource-limited settings where the burden of infection-related cancers is the highest.

Table 7.3 Number of new cancer cases in 2008 attributable to infection, by infectious agent and development status.

Infectious agent	Less-developed regions	More developed regions	World
Hepatitis B and C viruses	520,000 (32.0%)	80,000 (19.4%)	600,000 (29.5%)
Human papillomavirus	490,000 (30.2%)	120,000 (29.2%)	610,000 (30.0)
Helicobacter pylori	470,000 (28.9%)	190,000 (46.2%)	660,000 (32.5%)
Epstein–Barr virus	96,000 (5.9%)	16,000 (3.9%)	110,000 (5.4%)
Kaposi sarcoma herpes virus	39,000 (2.4%)	4,100 (1.0%)	43,000 (2.1%)
Human T-cell lymphotropic virus type-1	660 (0.0%)	1,500 (0.4%)	2,100 (0.1%)
Opisthorchis viverrini and *Clonorchis sinensis*	2,000 (0.1%)	0 (0.0%)	2,000 (0.1%)
Schistosoma haematobium	6,000 (0.4%)	0 (0.0%)	6,000 (0.3%)
Total	1,600,000 (100.0%)	410,000 (100.0%)	2,000,000 (100.0%)

Source: adapted from de Martel C *et al.* [60].

Data are number of new cancer cases attributable to a particular infectious agent (proportion of the total number of new cases attributed to infection that is attributable to a specific agent).

References

1 Biological agents. Volume 100 B. A review of human carcinogens. IARC monographs on the evaluation of carcinogenic risks to humans/World Health Organization, *International Agency for Research on Cancer* 2012;100B (Pt B):1–441.

2 Epstein MA. Historical background. *Philos Trans R Soc Lond B, Biol Sci* 2001;356(1408):413–20.

3 zur Hausen H. *Infections Causing Human Cancer.* Weinheim, Germany: Wiley-Blackwell, 2011.

4 Parsonnet J (ed.) *Microbes and Malignancy: Infection as a Cause of Human Cancers.* New York: Oxford University Press, 1999.

5 Burkitt D. A children's cancer dependent on climatic factors. *Nature* 1962;194:232–4.

6 Epstein MA, Achong BG, Barr YM. Virus Particles in Cultured Lymphoblasts from Burkitt's Lymphoma. *Lancet* 1964;1 (7335):702–3.

7 de-The G, Day NE, Geser A, *et al.* Sero-epidemiology of the Epstein–Barr virus: preliminary analysis of an international study – a review. *IARC Sci Publ* 1975;11(2):3–16.

8 Papesch M, Watkins R. Epstein-Barr virus infectious mononucleosis. *Clin Otolaryngol Allied Sci* 2001;26(1):3–8.

9 Thorley-Lawson DA. EBV the prototypical human tumor virus – just how bad is it? *J Allergy Clin Immunol* 2005;116(2):251–61; quiz 62.

10 Carrillo-Infante C, Abbadessa G, Bagella L, Giordano A. Viral infections as a cause of cancer (review). *Int J Oncol* 2007;30(6):1521–8.

11 Young L. Epstein-Barr virus: general features. In: B Mahy, M van Regenmortel (eds) *Encyclopedia of Virology.* New York: Oxford University Press, 2008:148–57.

12 Carbone A, Gloghini A, Dotti G. EBV-associated lymphoproliferative disorders: classification and treatment. *Oncologist* 2008;13(5):577–85.

13 Thorley-Lawson DA, Allday MJ. The curious case of the tumour virus: 50 years of Burkitt's lymphoma. *Nat Rev Microbiol* 2008;6(12):913–24.

14 Thompson MP, Kurzrock R. Epstein-Barr virus and cancer. *Clin Cancer Res* 2004;10(3):803–21.

15 Engels EA. Infectious agents as causes of non-Hodgkin lymphoma. *Cancer Epidemiol Biomarkers Prev* 2007;16(3):401–4.

16 Yuan JM, Wang XL, Xiang YB, *et al.* Preserved foods in relation to risk of nasopharyngeal carcinoma in Shanghai, China. *Int J Cancer* 2000;85(3):358–63.

17 Shepard CW, Simard EP, Finelli L, Fiore AE, Bell BP. Hepatitis B virus infection: epidemiology and vaccination. *Epidemiol Rev* 2006;28:112–25.

18 McMahon BJ, Alward WL, Hall DB, *et al.* Acute hepatitis B virus infection: relation of age to the clinical expression of disease and subsequent development of the carrier state. *J Infect Dis* 1985;151(4):599–603.

19 Perz JF, Armstrong GL, Farrington LA, Hutin YJ, Bell BP. The contributions of hepatitis B virus and hepatitis C virus infections to cirrhosis and primary liver cancer worldwide. *J Hepatol* 2006;45(4):529–38.

20 Parkin DM. 11. Cancers attributable to infection in the UK in 2010. *Br J Cancer* 2011;105 Suppl 2:S49–56.

21 Mast EE, Margolis HS, Fiore AE, *et al.* A comprehensive immunization strategy to eliminate transmission of hepatitis B virus infection in the United States: recommendations of the Advisory Committee on Immunization Practices (ACIP) part 1: immunization of infants, children, and adolescents. *MMWR Recomm Rep* 2005;54(RR-16):1–31.

22 Mast EE, Weinbaum CM, Fiore AE, *et al.* A comprehensive immunization strategy to eliminate transmission of hepatitis B virus infection in the United States: recommendations of the Advisory Committee on Immunization Practices (ACIP) Part II: immunization of adults. *MMWR Recomm Rep* 2006;55(RR-16):1–33; quiz CE1-4.

23 Global routine vaccination coverage, 2011. *MMWR Morb Mortal Wkly Rep* 2012;61(43):883–5.

24 Simard EP, Jemal A. Commentary: infection-related cancers in low- and middle-income countries: challenges and opportunities. *Int J Epidemiol* 2013;42(1):228–9.

25 Alter MJ. Epidemiology of hepatitis C virus infection. *World J Gastroenterol* 2007;13(17):2436–41.

26 Nainan OV, Alter MJ, Kruszon-Moran D, *et al.* Hepatitis C virus genotypes and viral concentrations in participants of a general population survey in the United States. *Gastroenterology* 2006;131(2):478–84.

27 Smith BD, Morgan RL, Beckett GA, *et al.* Recommendations for the identification of chronic hepatitis C virus infection among persons born during 1945–1965. *MMWR Recomm Rep* 2012;61(RR-4):1–32.

28 Pauk J, Huang ML, Brodie SJ, *et al.* Mucosal shedding of human herpesvirus 8 in men. *N Engl J Med* 2000;343(19):1369–77.

29 Engels EA, Atkinson JO, Graubard BI, *et al.* Risk factors for human herpesvirus 8 infection among adults in the United States and evidence for sexual transmission. *J Infect Dis* 2007;196(2):199–207.

30 Martin JN, Ganem DE, Osmond DH, *et al.* Sexual transmission and the natural history of human herpesvirus 8 infection. *N Engl J Med* 1998;338(14):948–54.

31 Melbye M, Cook PM, Hjalgrim H, *et al.* Risk factors for Kaposi's-sarcoma-associated herpesvirus (KSHV/HHV-8) seropositivity in a cohort of homosexual men, 1981–1996. *Int J Cancer* 1998;77(4):543–8.

32 O'Brien TR, Kedes D, Ganem D, *et al.* Evidence for concurrent epidemics of human herpesvirus 8 and human immunodeficiency virus type 1 in US homosexual men: rates, risk factors, and relationship to Kaposi's sarcoma. *J Infect Dis* 1999;180(4):1010–7.

33 Dourmishev LA, Dourmishev AL, Palmeri D, Schwartz RA, Lukac DM. Molecular genetics of Kaposi's sarcoma-associated herpesvirus (human herpesvirus-8) epidemiology and pathogenesis. *Microbiol Mol Biol Rev* 2003;67(2):175–212.

34 Chang Y, Cesarman E, Pessin MS, *et al.* Identification of herpesvirus-like DNA sequences in AIDS-associated Kaposi's sarcoma. *Science* 1994;266(5192):1865–9.

35 Biggar RJ, Chaturvedi AK, Goedert JJ, Engels EA. AIDS-related cancer and severity of immunosuppression in persons with AIDS. *J Natl Cancer Inst* 2007;99(12):962–72.

36 Engels EA, Pfeiffer RM, Fraumeni JF, Jr, *et al.* Spectrum of cancer risk among US solid organ transplant recipients. *JAMA* 2011;306(17):1891–901.

37 Simard EP, Pfeiffer RM, Engels EA. Spectrum of cancer risk late after AIDS onset in the United States. *Arch Intern Med* 2010;170(15):1337–45.

38 Barre-Sinoussi F, Chermann JC, Rey F, *et al.* Isolation of a T-lymphotropic retrovirus from a patient at risk for acquired immune deficiency syndrome (AIDS). *Science* 1983;220(4599):868–71.

39 Varthakavi V, Smith RM, Deng H, Sun R, Spearman P. Human immunodeficiency virus type-1 activates lytic cycle replication of Kaposi's sarcoma-associated herpesvirus through induction of KSHV Rta. *Virology* 2002;297(2):270–80.

40 de Koning MN, Waddell K, Magyezi J, *et al.* Genital and cutaneous human papillomavirus (HPV) types in relation to conjunctival squamous cell neoplasia: a case-control study in Uganda. *Infect Agents Cancer* 2008;3:12.

41 Sun EC, Fears TR, Goedert JJ. Epidemiology of squamous cell conjunctival cancer. *Cancer Epidemiol Biomarkers Prev* 1997;6(2):73–7.

42 Engels EA, Pfeiffer RM, Goedert JJ, *et al.* Trends in cancer risk among people with AIDS in the United States 1980–2002. *AIDS* 2006;20(12):1645–54.

43 Human Papillomaviruses. IARC monographs on the evaluation of carcinogenic risks to humans/World Health Organization, *International Agency for Research on Cancer* 2007;90:1–636.

44 Munoz N, Hernandez-Suarez G, Mendez F, *et al.* Persistence of HPV infection and risk of high-grade cervical intraepithelial neoplasia in a cohort of Colombian women. *Br J Cancer* 2009;100(7):1184–90.

45 Gillison ML, Chaturvedi AK, Lowy DR. HPV prophylactic vaccines and the potential prevention of noncervical cancers in both men and women. *Cancer* 2008;113(10 Suppl):3036–46.

46 Schiffman M, Wentzensen N. Human papillomavirus infection and the multistage carcinogenesis of cervical cancer. *Cancer Epidemiol Biomarkers Prev* 2013;22(4):553–60.

47 Luhn P, Walker J, Schiffman M, *et al.* The role of co-factors in the progression from human papillomavirus infection to cervical cancer. *Gynecol Oncol* 2013;128(2):265–70.

48 Goedert JJ, Cote TR, Virgo P, *et al.* Spectrum of AIDS-associated malignant disorders. *Lancet* 1998;351(9119):1833–9.

49 Zandberg DP, Bhargava R, Badin S, Cullen KJ. The role of human papillomavirus in nongenital cancers. *CA Cancer J Clin* 2013;63(1):57–81.

50 FDA licensure of bivalent human papillomavirus vaccine (HPV2, Cervarix) for use in females and updated HPV vaccination recommendations from the Advisory Committee on Immunization Practices (ACIP). *MMWR Morb Mortal Wkly Rep* 2010;59(20):626–9.

51 Recommendations on the use of quadrivalent human papillomavirus vaccine in males. Advisory Committee on Immunization Practices (ACIP), 2011. *MMWR Morb Mortal Wkly Rep* 2011;60(50):1705–8.

52 Markowitz LE, Dunne EF, Saraiya M, *et al.* Quadrivalent Human Papillomavirus Vaccine: Recommendations of the Advisory Committee on Immunization Practices (ACIP). *MMWR Recomm Rep* 2007;56(RR-2):1–24.

53 Petrosky E, Bocchini Jr J, Hariri S, *et al.* Use of 9-Valent Human Papillomavirus (HPV) Vaccine: Updated HPV Vaccination Recommendations of the Advisory Committee on Immunization Practices. *MMWR Morb Mortal Wkly Rep* 2015;64(11):300–4.

54 Saslow D, Andrews KS, Manassaram-Baptiste D, *et al.* Human papillomavirus vaccination guideline update: American Cancer Society guideline endorsement. *CA Cancer J Clin* 2016;66(5):375–85.

55 Manhart LE, Koutsky LA. Do condoms prevent genital HPV infection, external genital warts, or cervical neoplasia? A meta-analysis. *Sex Transm Dis* 2002;29(11):725–35.

56 Hinuma Y, Nagata K, Hanaoka M, *et al.* Adult T-cell leukemia: antigen in an ATL cell line and detection of antibodies to the antigen in human sera. *Proc Natl Acad Sci USA* 1981;78(10):6476–80.

57 Poiesz BJ, Ruscetti FW, Gazdar AF, *et al.* Detection and isolation of type C retrovirus particles from fresh and cultured lymphocytes of a patient with cutaneous T-cell lymphoma. *Proc Natl Acad Sci USA* 1980;77(12):7415–19.

58 Proietti FA, Carneiro-Proietti AB, Catalan-Soares BC, Murphy EL. Global epidemiology of HTLV-I infection and associated diseases. *Oncogene* 2005;24(39):6058–68.

59 Peek RM, Jr, Blaser MJ. Helicobacter pylori and gastrointestinal tract adenocarcinomas. *Nat Rev Cancer* 2002;2(1):28–37.

60 de Martel C, Ferlay J, Franceschi S, *et al.* Global burden of cancers attributable to infections in 2008: a review and synthetic analysis. *Lancet Oncol* 2012;13(6):607–15.

61 Bonequi P, Meneses-Gonzalez F, Correa P, Rabkin CS, Camargo MC. Risk factors for gastric cancer in Latin America: a meta-analysis. *Cancer Causes Control* 2013;24(2):217–31.

62 Fuccio L, Minardi ME, Zagari RM, *et al.* Meta-analysis: duration of first-line proton-pump inhibitor based triple therapy for Helicobacter pylori eradication. *Ann Intern Med* 2007;147(8):553–62.

63 Malfertheiner P, Megraud F, O'Morain CA, *et al.* Management of Helicobacter pylori infection – the Maastricht IV/ Florence Consensus Report. *Gut* 2012;61(5):646–64.

64 Stolte M, Bayerdorffer E, Morgner A, *et al.* Helicobacter and gastric MALT lymphoma. *Gut* 2002;50(Suppl 3):III19–24.

65 Mayer DA, Fried B. The role of helminth infections in carcinogenesis. *Adv Parasitol* 2007;65:239–96.

66 Mostafa MH, Sheweita SA, O'Connor PJ. Relationship between schistosomiasis and bladder cancer. *Clin Microbiol Rev* 1999;12(1):97–111.

67 Parkin DM, Ohshima H, Srivatanakul P, Vatanasapt V. Cholangiocarcinoma: epidemiology, mechanisms of carcinogenesis and prevention. *Cancer Epidemiol Biomarkers Prev* 1993;2(6):537–44.

68 Spurgeon ME, Lambert PF. Merkel cell polyomavirus: a newly discovered human virus with oncogenic potential. *Virology* 2013;435(1):118–30.

8

Environmental and Occupational Carcinogens

Elizabeth Ward

Intramural Research, American Cancer Society, Atlanta, Georgia, USA

Introduction

The term carcinogen usually refers to an exogenous exposure that increases the probability of developing a malignancy. The term can apply to a single chemical such as benzene, to physical agents such as X-rays or ultraviolet light, to infectious agents such as hepatitis C or to specific occupations or industries (e.g., nickel refining). Furthermore, a carcinogenic exposure can act at any point on a continuum of tumor initiation, promotion, and/or progression. It may directly affect the structure or function of a cell's DNA, by causing mutations or inactivating genes that control cell differentiation and survival. Alternatively, it may act by increasing the rate of cell turnover, which favors the survival and proliferation of genetically damaged cells [1]. The broadest definition of environmental carcinogen includes all factors other than heritable genetic characteristics that increase the risk of cancer. By this definition, it is estimated that about two thirds of cancers are environmental in origin. Important environmental risk factors for cancer in the general population include tobacco use, poor nutrition and physical inactivity, and certain medications and medical treatments [2]. This chapter will focus on a narrower group of environmental carcinogens to which individuals may be involuntarily exposed, including contaminants in indoor and outdoor air, water and food, consumer products and workplaces.

Environmental causes of cancer have always been present in the human environment. Prior to the development of modern industry, humans were exposed to combustion products in indoor heating and cooking, nitrates and nitrites in food preservation, polycyclic aromatic hydrocarbons in charred meats, ultraviolet radiation from the sun, mycotoxins in grains, and arsenic in drinking water. Environmental causes of cancer in preindustrial environments also included infectious agents such as *Helicobacter pylori* and Epstein–Barr virus, discussed in other chapters of this book. Even today, natural contaminants in soil and water, prevalence of certain infectious diseases, and dietary and lifestyle practices are important causes of variation in human cancer rates throughout the world.

Industrial development and growth of the chemical industry brought new hazards into the human environment. Some carcinogenic materials that were always present in the environment, such as uranium, asbestos, and certain metals, began to be mined, extracted and used in large scale industrial processes, bringing humans in contact with airborne contaminants [2]. The petrochemical industry developed methods to extract and concentrate chemicals such as benzene from crude oil, and to develop and synthesize new chemical compounds. Use of radioactive materials in medical, commercial, and military applications resulted in new carcinogenic hazards in the workplace and general environment. As these hazards were identified, methods were developed to study the occurrence of cancer related to occupational and environmental exposures in human populations and use animal models and toxicological testing systems to predict the potential carcinogenicity of substances before widespread human exposure. By the end of the twentieth century, exposure to toxic substances in the general environment and workplaces had been markedly reduced in the US and Europe. Nonetheless, exposure continues for many substances that are recognized to be carcinogenic based on laboratory studies but are not regulated as such in consumer products and/or occupational and environmental settings [3]. This chapter will introduce the reader to criteria for evaluating toxicologic and epidemiologic evidence for carcinogenicity, provide information about occupational and environmental exposures that are recognized to be carcinogenic to humans and highlight the importance of research to resolve the carcinogenicity of common exposures that have been documented to cause cancer in animals but for which human evidence is limited or unavailable. Finally, the chapter will provide perspectives that may be helpful for clinicians in discussing occupational and environmental carcinogens with patients and the public.

Criteria for Classifying Agents as Carcinogenic to Humans

The conclusion that an agent is carcinogenic to humans, and the impetus for public health and regulatory actions to reduce exposure, most often relies on a combination of data from epidemiologic and experimental studies. In some instances, an exposure may be classified as carcinogenic based on epidemiologic studies alone. In other instances, an agent may be classified as a human carcinogen based on evidence of carcinogenicity in animals and data that supports a similar mechanism for causing cancer in humans. High-quality epidemiologic studies can provide strong evidence that a specific exposure causes cancer. Occupational cohorts often provide the best opportunity for such studies because of relatively high level and well-documented exposures, but opportunities to conduct such studies are limited. It often takes 20 years or more from the time a carcinogenic exposure begins until a carcinogenic hazard can be detected in an occupational cohort. Thus, epidemiologic studies must either identify a population that began exposure a long time ago, or identify a population now and study their cancer incidence or mortality for a long period in the future. Unfortunately, for some occupational carcinogens, including asbestos, millions of people had been exposed before epidemiologic studies documented the hazard. Thus, the prevention of occupational and environmental cancer hazards being introduced into the human environment must rely on extrapolation of toxicological studies to humans.

The type of toxicological study considered to be most definitive in the evaluation of potential carcinogens is the 2-year rodent bioassay. This assay involves test groups of 50 rats and 50 mice of both sexes and at two or three doses of the test agent. In the US, the B6C3F1 mouse and the F344 rat are commonly used. At about 8 weeks of age, test animals are placed on the test agent (or placebo) for the remaining 96 weeks of their lifespan. The test agent may be administered in feed, by gavage (forced feeding), or by inhalation. The maximum dose level used in a 2-year bioassay is determined by the estimated maximally tolerated dose (MTD), usually derived from a 90-day study. The MTD is defined by the Environmental Protection Agency (EPA) as "the highest dose that causes no more than a 10% weight decrement, as compared to appropriate control groups; and does not produce mortality, clinical signs of toxicity, or pathological lesions (other than those that may be related to a neoplastic response) that would be predicted to shorten the animal's natural lifespan". These tests often, but not always, involve exposure of animals to much higher doses than occur in humans. High exposure levels are used to allow carcinogenic effects to be seen even in relatively small groups of animals, and the assumption is made that an exposure that causes cancer at higher doses will also do so at lower doses [4]. This type of study is extremely expensive, and a variety of shorter term tests are used, in combination with data on extent of human exposure, to prioritize substances for testing.

To better identify environmental chemicals that may pose human health risks, the EPA, the National Institute of Environmental Health Sciences National Toxicology Program, the National Center for Advancing Translational Sciences, and the FDA formed the Toxicology Testing in the 21st Century

(Tox21) consortium in 2008 to use quantitative high-throughput screening methods to test thousands of chemicals across dozens of *in vitro* assays representing known toxicity pathways. A subset of high-throughput screening assays have been mapped to the 10 key characteristics of carcinogens developed by the International Agency for Research on Cancer to support chemical hazard assessment [5]. As part of the Cancer Moonshot Initiative, the Tox21 consortium will work to develop an expanded suite of high-throughput *in vitro* assays that fill current assay gaps and more comprehensively cover the 10 key characteristics. Using robotic technology, the consortium will screen the entire Tox21 chemical library of approximately 10,000 environmental and industrial chemicals, pesticides, and food additives across the expanded assay set to identify chemicals that may possess previously unknown carcinogenic characteristics or that may be acting through multiple characteristics to produce synergies in environmental carcinogenesis [6].

There are several organizations which systematically review evidence for potential human carcinogens [7]. Two of the most widely cited are the International Agency for Research on Cancer Monographs Program (IARC Monographs) which is part of the World Health Organization (WHO)[1] and the National Toxicology Programs Review of Carcinogens (NTP ROC), which is an Interagency Program administered by the National Institute of Environmental Health Sciences (NIEHS) [8].

The IARC Monograph Program was initiated in 1969 to evaluate the carcinogenic risk of chemicals to humans and to produce monographs on individual chemicals (information on the program can be obtained at http://monographs.iarc.fr/). The program assembles international groups of experts to critically review and evaluate evidence on the carcinogenicity of a wide range of human exposures. Published data regarding an agent, mixture, or exposure circumstance are reviewed to determine the level of evidence for carcinogenicity in humans and experimental animals.

The IARC monograph program criteria for sufficient evidence of carcinogenicity are stringent. For humans, sufficient evidence for carcinogenicity requires that "… a positive relationship has been observed between the exposure and cancer in studies in which chance, bias and confounding could be ruled out with reasonable confidence". For animals, sufficient evidence for carcinogenicity generally requires "…an increased incidence of malignant neoplasms in (a) two or more species of animals or (b) in two or more independent studies in one species carried out at different times or in different laboratories or under different protocols. Based on separate evaluations of carcinogenicity in humans and experimental animals, the agent, mixture, or exposure circumstance is classified into one of five groups. The category Group 1, *carcinogenic to humans*, is used when there is sufficient evidence of carcinogenicity in humans, or exceptionally, when the evidence in humans is less than sufficient but there is sufficient evidence of carcinogenicity in animals and strong evidence in exposed humans that the agent acts through a relevant mechanism of carcinogenicity. The category Group 2A, *probably carcinogenic to humans*, is used when there is limited evidence of carcinogenicity in humans and sufficient evidence for carcinogenicity in animals. In some cases, an agent may be placed in this category when there is inadequate evidence of carcinogenicity in humans and strong evidence of both carcinogenicity in animals and a common mechanism of action in humans and animals [1]. Most of the environmental carcinogens discussed in this chapter are in IARC Group 1 and 2A. As of 21 October, 2016 the IARC Monographs Program lists 118 substances in Group 1 and 79 in Group 2A. An additional 291 agents are listed in Group 2B, *possibly carcinogenic to humans*. This category is used for agents when there is limited evidence of carcinogenicity in humans and less than sufficient evidence of carcinogenicity in experimental animals, when there is inadequate evidence of carcinogenicity in humans but sufficient evidence of carcinogenicity in experimental animals and in some instances, when there is inadequate evidence of carcinogenicity in humans and less than sufficient evidence of carcinogenicity in experimental animals together with supporting evidence from mechanistic and other relevant data. An agent may also be classified in this category solely on the basis of strong evidence from mechanistic and other relevant data [1].

The NTP also has a systematic process for evaluating human carcinogens, which classifies agents, mixtures of substances, and exposure circumstances as "Known To Be Human Carcinogens" or "Reasonably Anticipated To Be Human Carcinogens". The 13th Report on Carcinogens, issued by NTP in 2011, listed 56 substances as "Known To Be Human Carcinogens", and 187 as "Reasonably Anticipated To Be Human Carcinogens" [9].

Selected Occupational and Environmental Exposures

This chapter will focus on agents and exposure circumstances for which there is the strongest evidence for carcinogenicity in humans; those which the IARC has classified as having sufficient evidence for cancer in one or more cancer sites in humans. This data stems from a comprehensive update of data on carcinogenicity by the IARC of all carcinogens which had previously been designated in Group 1 as known human carcinogens, published in the IARC Monographs 100A through F, and subsequent Monographs. In Monograph 100 and subsequent Monographs, in addition to the classification of animal, human, and overall evidence for carcinogenicity, IARC working groups voted on which cancer sites had *sufficient* or *limited* evidence for carcinogenicity in humans.

Occupational and Environmental Agents and Exposure Circumstances with *Sufficient* Evidence for Causing Lung Cancer in Humans

Table 8.1 lists agents that have been classified by the IARC as having *sufficient* evidence for lung cancer based on exposures in occupational and environmental settings [10]. The lung is the most common target organ for occupational and environmental carcinogens; an estimated 20% of lung cancers in the US are attributable to occupational exposures [11]. The lung is an important route of entry for airborne carcinogens because of its large surface area and the volume of air that is inhaled and exhaled daily. Although many substances are absorbed rapidly from the lung into the bloodstream, other materials, including metals, fibers, and dusts may reside in the lung for long periods

of time. Radioactive materials, such as radon progeny, that remain trapped in the lung, emit radiation as they continue their radioactive decay. Many carcinogenic particulates and fibers induce inflammation in the lung, resulting in free radicals and/or fibrosis that can lead to pulmonary diseases such as silicosis and asbestosis. Selected occupational and environmental lung carcinogens to which there is widespread human exposure are discussed below.

Asbestos is a particularly important cause of occupationally-related lung cancer. The term "asbestos" refers to a group of naturally-occurring minerals containing fibrous silicates that are highly resistant to heat and chemical degradation. Asbestos was widely used for insulation and fire protection in the US before health effects were recognized and use was curtailed in the 1970s and 80s. In addition to lung cancer, asbestos causes asbestosis and malignant mesothelioma, a rare and highly fatal cancer arising in the pleura, peritoneum, or pericardium. An estimated 27.5 million workers were occupationally exposed to asbestos from 1940 to 1979; thus many older Americans had significant occupational asbestos exposure early in their working careers and continue to be at risk for asbestos-related cancer and lung disease. It was projected in 1982 that annual mortality from asbestos-related cancer in the US would peak in the year 2000 at about 9,700 deaths (including approximately 3,000 from mesothelioma and 4,700 from lung cancer) and then decline, but remain substantial, for another three decades [12]. The projections turned out to be fairly accurate for mesothelioma death rates, which fell from 11.3 per million in 2001, representing 2,509 deaths, to 10.7 per million in 2010, representing 2,745 deaths [13]. Although exposure to asbestos has been markedly reduced in the US and many other countries, it is estimated that 125 million people globally are occupationally exposed to asbestos each year [14]. In addition to causing lung cancer and mesothelioma, the most recent IARC review of asbestos found sufficient evidence for associations of laryngeal and ovarian cancer and limited evidence for colorectal, pharyngeal and stomach cancer associated with asbestos exposure.

Exposure to *radon decay products* is a particularly important cause of environmentally-related lung cancer, estimated to contribute to 8–15% of lung cancer deaths in Europe and North America [15]. Radon-222 (radon) is a naturally occurring radioactive decay product of uranium 238 and radium 226, existing as a gas that is produced in most soils and rocks in widely varying concentrations. People can be exposed to significant levels of radon in indoor air because it diffuses through walls and accumulates in basements and unventilated underground spaces. Radon was found to cause lung cancer in studies of uranium miners who were exposed to very high concentrations in underground mines [16]. Although average radon concentrations in the indoor air of most homes are about an order of magnitude (10-fold) lower than those in uranium mines, epidemiologic studies have documented increased risks of lung cancer associated with residential radon exposures in the same range as those predicted based on extrapolating results from higher dose occupational studies to lower doses [17, 18]. Although radon cannot be completely eliminated from homes and workplaces, the EPA sets action levels for concentration of radon in homes, and provides information about how it is measured and how levels can be reduced.

Table 8.1 Agents that the IARC has classified as having sufficient evidence of causing lung cancer in humans based on IARC Monograph 100 and subsequent monographs. Highlighted agents or exposure circumstances are discussed in the text.

Carcinogenic agent or exposure circumstance	Year first designated as Group 1 carcinogen	Cancer sites with *sufficient evidence* in humans	Cancer sites with *limited evidence* in humans
Aluminum production	1987	Lung Urinary bladder	
Arsenic and inorganic arsenic compounds	1987	Lung Skin Urinary bladder	Kidney Liver Prostate
Asbestos (all forms)	1987	Larynx Lung Mesothelioma Ovary	Colorectum Pharynx Stomach
Beryllium and beryllium compounds	1993	Lung	
Bis(chloromethyl) ether	1987	Lung	
Cadmium and cadmium compounds	1993	Lung	Kidney Prostate
Chromium(VI) compounds	1990	Lung	Nasal cavity and paranasal sinus
Coal gasification	1984	Lung	
Coal, indoor emissions from household combustion	2006	Lung	
Coal-tar pitch	1973	Lung Skin	Urinary bladder
Coke production	1984	Lung	
Engine exhaust, diesel		Lung	Urinary bladder
Hematite mining (underground)	1972	Lung	
Iron and steel founding	1987	Lung	
Nickel compounds	1973	Lung Nasal cavity and paranasal sinus	
Outdoor air pollution	2016	Lung	
Painting	1989	Lung Urinary bladder	Childhood leukemia (maternal exposure)
Particulate matter in outdoor air pollution	2016	Lung	
Radon-222 and its decay products	1988	Lung	Leukemia
Rubber production industry		Lung	
Silica dust, crystalline (in the form of quartz or crystobalite)	1997	Lung	
Soot	1985	Lung Skin	Urinary bladder
Sulfur mustard	1975	Lung	
Tobacco smoke, secondhand		Lung	Larynx Pharynx
X-radiation, gamma radiation	1999	Lung, salivary gland, esophagus, stomach, colon, bone, basal cell of the skin, female breast, kidney, urinary bladder, brain and CNS, thyroid and leukemia (excluding chronic lymphocytic leukemia)	Rectum, liver, pancreas, ovary, prostate, non-Hodgkin lymphoma, multiple myeloma

In general, smokers exposed to occupational and environmental lung carcinogens have a much greater risk of developing lung cancer than individuals with either exposure alone. A recent study compared lung cancer mortality among 2,377 insulators with long-term high levels of asbestos exposure to a referent group of blue collar workers from the American Cancer Society Cancer Prevention Study (CPS) II cohort [19]. This study found that asbestos workers who smoked had a 28-fold increased risk of lung cancer compared to nonsmoking men in the CPS II cohort, while nonsmoking workers had a fivefold increased risk. Importantly, lung cancer risks declined substantially among former insulators who stopped smoking. Similar patterns of combined risks for smoking and radon exposure were found among radon-exposed uranium miners [20].

Unlike asbestos and radon, whose carcinogenicity has been recognized for decades, strong evidence documenting that exposure to crystalline silica and diesel exhaust causes lung cancer has only recently become available.

Crystalline silica is an important industrial compound found abundantly in the earth's crust; it is estimated that 2.2 million US workers are exposed to silica. Hazardous occupational exposures to silica dust have long been known to occur in a variety of industrial operations, including mining, quarrying, sandblasting, rock drilling, road construction, pottery making, stone masonry, and tunneling operations. Recently, hazardous silica exposures have been newly documented during hydraulic fracturing of gas and oil wells and during fabrication and installation of engineered stone countertops [21]. It has long been known that inhalation of crystalline silica dust causes silicosis, a progressive disabling and incurable disease of the lung. There has been increasing evidence that silica exposure also increases lung cancer risk, but it was unclear whether this increased risk occurred only among workers with silicosis or could result from silica exposure even in the absence of lung disease. Several recent studies have provided evidence that silica exposure causes lung cancer. One such study, of 34,000 tungsten miners, iron miners, and pottery workers found a statistically significant positive exposure-response trend for cumulative silica exposure and lung cancer both among individuals who had been diagnosed with silicosis and those who had not. An increased relative risk for lung cancer was also observed in silica-exposed never smokers [22, 23]. Based on evidence that silica exposure causes cancer, the US Occupational Health and Safety Administration (OSHA) recently reduced the occupational exposure limit, providing greater protection for workers exposed to silica dust [24].

Diesel exhaust is a common exposure in occupational and environmental settings. Sources of exposure include motor vehicle exhausts, exhausts from other diesel engines (such as diesel trains and ships), and from power generators. It is estimated that 1.4 million workers in the US and 3 million workers in Europe are occupationally exposed to diesel engine exhaust [25]. For decades there has been evidence from epidemiologic studies of increased lung cancer risks in occupational groups such as truck drivers with high levels of diesel exhaust exposure. However, few of these studies were able to measure diesel exposure levels and/or account for potential differences in smoking between study and comparison populations. In 2012, definitive epidemiologic studies confirming strong associations between diesel exhaust exposure and lung cancer were published [26, 27]. These studies included workers employed in nonmetal mining facilities which had high air levels of diesel exhaust underground but low levels of potential occupational confounders (i.e., radon, silica, asbestos). Quantitative estimates of exposure were developed for each individual and a strong and consistent relationship between exposure to diesel exhaust and increased risk of dying from lung cancer was demonstrated. Among heavily exposed workers, the risk of dying from lung cancer was approximately three times greater than among the least exposed workers. A similar exposure-response trend was observed for workers who had never smoked tobacco. The results of these studies led the IARC to classify diesel exhaust as a known human carcinogen in 2012.

Diesel exhaust contributes to *outdoor air pollution* in urban areas, which has also been associated with lung cancer. The component of outdoor air pollution most strongly associated with lung cancer is particulate matter (PM), a general term for a mixture of solid particles and liquid droplets found in the air and, in particular, $PM_{2.5}$ which are fine particulates less than 2.5 μm in diameter. Sources of particulate matter in air include forest fires, road dust, electrical power plants, industrial processes, and cars and trucks are primary sources. Secondary sources give off gases that react with sunlight and water in the air to form particles. Coal-fired power plants and exhaust from cars and trucks are common secondary sources [28]. Epidemiologic studies in the US and Europe have examined associations between outdoor air pollution levels and death rates from all causes, nonmalignant heart and lung disease, and lung cancer. In one series of studies, ACS epidemiologists collaborated with outside researchers who study air pollution to assess the health effects of exposure to outdoor air pollution in the ACS CPS II population [29]. This study used information about air pollution levels in 151 US metropolitan areas in which cohort members were residing, along with information about their individual risk factors, such as cigarette smoking. The study found that people living in the most polluted areas had higher death rates from all causes, non-malignant heart and lung disease, and lung cancer than those in the least polluted areas. Results of this study contributed to the decision by the US EPA to issue more stringent standards in 1997 limiting exposure to air pollutants, including the first standard for $PM_{2.5}$. An updated and expanded analysis of the ACS study was published in 2002 [30]. This study estimated that each $10 \, \mu g/m^3$ elevation in fine particulate air pollution ($PM_{2.5}$) was associated with a 4%, 6% and 8% increased risk of all-cause, heart and lung disease, and lung cancer mortality, respectively. A re-analysis of the updated data file by independent investigators estimated a 14% increase in lung cancer mortality associated with a $10 \, \mu g/m^3$ elevation in $PM_{2.5}$ [31]. More recently, analyses in the ACS cohort indicated that a $10 \, \mu g/m^3$ increase in $PM_{2.5}$ concentration was associated with a statistically significant 15–27% increase in lung-cancer mortality in never smokers [32]. Additional evidence for an association between $PM_{2.5}$ levels in outdoor air and lung cancer comes from the Harvard Six Cities Study; the most recent update of which found a statistically significant 37% increase in lung cancer mortality (for each $10 \, \mu g/m^3$ increase in $PM_{2.5}$ [33]. Levels of air pollution vary markedly throughout the world, and are particularly high in densely populated urban areas in middle income countries. In October 2013, the IARC classified "outdoor air pollution" and "particulate matter" as

Group 1 carcinogens, noting that the most recent estimates suggest that in 2010, 223,000 deaths from lung cancer worldwide resulted from outdoor air pollution.

Indoor air pollution from combustion of solid fuels is an important cause of lung cancer globally. This association was brought to light by the very high lung cancer rates observed among nonsmoking women in regions of China where unventilated indoor coal stoves have traditionally been used for cooking and heating [34]. Combustion products of coal include fine particulates, sulfur dioxide, arsenic, and polycyclic aromatic hydrocarbons. Burning of crude biomass fuels – such as crop residues, animal dung, and wood – for cooking and heating in developing countries has been less strongly associated with lung cancer, but also results in high levels of indoor air pollution, resulting in increased risk for acute respiratory infections and chronic obstructive pulmonary disease [35]. In 2006, the IARC concluded that there is sufficient evidence in humans for the carcinogenicity of household combustion of coal, and limited evidence for the carcinogenicity of household combustion of biomass fuel (primarily wood). The WHO estimates that over 4 million people a year die prematurely from illness attributable to indoor air pollution due to solid fuel use, 12% due to pneumonia, 34% from stroke, 26% from ischemic heart disease, 22% from chronic obstructive pulmonary disease (COPD), and 2% from lung cancer [36]. WHO is a leading partner in a new Global Alliance for Clean Cookstoves that is promoting improved biomass cookstove designs that can substantially reduce indoor air pollution. as well as use of alternative cleaner fuel sources for household heating and cooking.

Occupational and Environmental Agents and Exposure Circumstances with *Sufficient* Evidence for Causing Cancers of the Blood and Lymph System in Humans

An estimated 0.8–2.8 of leukemias in the US are attributable to occupational exposures [11]. Table 8.2 lists occupational and environmental carcinogens primarily associated with cancers of the blood and lymph system.

Benzene was one of the first recognized human leukemogens. Historically, numerous case reports documented that high levels of benzene exposure in occupational settings caused pancytopenia and aplastic anemia; at lower levels chronic benzene exposure causes hematologic suppression [37, 38]. Case reports of leukemia, often with short latency from onset of exposure, were observed in the same industrial settings. Two epidemiologic studies, published in 1977 and 1978, demonstrated statistically significant excess leukemia mortality in workers exposed to benzene, but did not have sufficient data on benzene exposure to permit examination of quantitative dose–response relationships [39, 40]. A study published in 1977, which provided such information, was the basis for a proposed OSHA standard for benzene of 1-ppm [41]. During the following decade, the dose–response relationship in the single study with available information was extensively re-examined, and debate about the exposure–response relationship between low levels of benzene exposure and leukemia continued, largely in response to attempts to regulate the allowable concentrations of benzene in air and water in the general environment and in the occupational setting [42]. Subsequently, a very large epidemiologic study, conducted by the Chinese Academy of Preventive Medicine and the National Cancer Institute in the US among benzene-exposed workers in China and an unexposed referent group, demonstrated increased risks of leukemia at cumulative exposure levels lower than 10 ppm years, as well as associations between benzene exposure, myelodysplastic syndrome and non-Hodgkin lymphoma. Benzene was first evaluated by the IARC and found to have sufficient evidence for carcinogenicity in humans in 1982. In its most recent review of benzene, the IARC concluded that there is strong evidence that occupational exposure to benzene causes acute nonlymphocytic leukemia and limited evidence that it causes acute and chronic lymphocytic leukemia, multiple myeloma, and non-Hodgkin lymphoma.

Benzene is a gaseous pollutant that is ubiquitous in the environment. Cigarette smoke is the major source of benzene exposure for smokers and for those who live or work with smokers [43]. Elevated benzene exposures occur in the homes

Table 8.2 Agents that the IARC has classified as having sufficient evidence of causing leukemia or lymphoma in humans based on IARC Monograph 100 and subsequent monographs. Highlighted agents or exposure circumstances are discussed in the text.

Carcinogenic agent	Year first designated as Group 1 carcinogen	Cancer sites with *sufficient evidence* in humans	Cancer sites with *limited evidence* in humans
Benzene	1982	Leukemia (acute nonlymphocytic)	Leukemia (acute lymphocytic, chronic lymphocytic, multiple myeloma, non-Hodgkin lymphoma)
1,3-Butadiene	2008	Hematolymphatic organs	
Formaldehyde	2006	Leukemia, nasopharynx	Nasal cavity and paranasal sinus
Lindane	2015	Non-Hodgkin lymphoma	
Rubber production industry	1982	Leukemia, lymphoma, urinary bladder, lung, stomach	Prostate, esophagus, larynx
X-radiation, gamma radiation	1999	Leukemia (excluding chronic lymphocytic leukemia), lung, salivary gland, esophagus, stomach, colon, bone, basal cell of the skin, female breast, kidney, urinary bladder, brain and CNS, and thyroid	Non-Hodgkin lymphoma, multiple myeloma, rectum, liver, pancreas, ovary, prostate

of smokers, the interiors of automobiles and buses, and in the vicinity of gasoline stations and heavily traveled highways [44]. Epidemiologic studies do not provide direct evidence that exposure to benzene at levels present in urban air, motor vehicles or gasoline stations increase the risk of leukemia in the general population. Low level, common exposures like air pollution by benzene are difficult to study because it is difficult to characterize individual exposure accurately and because very large study sizes are necessary to detect small risks. A number of studies have investigated potential associations of benzene exposure with childhood leukemia, with increasing evidence of a positive association with parental, *in utero* and early life benzene exposure [45, 46]. Recent studies have substantiated concerns about health effects of low levels of benzene exposure in occupational settings. A study of petroleum distribution workers with low levels of benzene exposure in the range of current occupational exposure limits found evidence for an increased risk of myelodysplasia among workers with higher cumulative exposures [47]. Another study found cumulative exposure related increased risks for acute myeloid leukaemia and multiple myeloma among 25,000 offshore drilling workers exposed to low levels of benzene [48].

Formaldehyde is also a common contaminant in outdoor and indoor air. It is produced in combustion processes and present in emissions from motor vehicles, power plants, incinerators, refineries, wood stoves and kerosene heaters. It may be released from particle boards and similar building materials, carpets, paints and varnishes, during cooking of some foods, and during its use as a disinfectant. It is also present in tobacco smoke. Automobile exhaust is a major source of formaldehyde in ambient air. Occupational exposure to formaldehyde can occur in a wide variety of occupations and industries. Formaldehyde also occurs as a natural product in most living systems and in the environment [49].

Formaldehyde is highly reactive and most formaldehyde that is inhaled is absorbed in the upper respiratory tract; formaldehyde exposure also causes irritation in the eyes, nose, and throat of exposed humans. Administration of formaldehyde by inhalation in rats showed an excess of squamous cell carcinomas of the nasal cavities and a number of epidemiologic studies have demonstrated excess risks of nasopharyngeal cancer mortality, consistent with the target site that might be predicted from toxicological data. However, an unexpected excess of leukemia mortality has been observed in a number of studies of occupational groups exposed to formaldehyde, including medical and other professionals exposed to formaldehyde in embalming fluid and several groups of industrial workers. Despite conflicting evidence of no increased risk of leukemia mortality in one well-done epidemiologic study, the IARC concluded that there is *sufficient* evidence that formaldehyde causes leukemia in humans in 2012.

X-radiation and gamma-radiation is known to cause cancer of many sites and types based on studies of populations exposed at high levels, including atomic bomb survivors, and patients treated with therapeutic radiation for benign and malignant conditions.

Exposure to X-radiation and gamma-radiation at lower levels in occupational settings has been associated with leukemia. A meta-analysis of epidemiologic studies of workers in several industries with protracted exposure to low-dose gamma radiation found an increased risk of leukemia (excluding chronic lymphocytic leukemia) per 100 mGy of radiation consistent with that expected from the Life Span Study cohort of Japanese atomic bomb survivors [50]. A study of long-term mortality in nearly 44,000 US radiologists compared to nearly 65,000 psychiatrists found increased death rates for acute myeloid leukemia and/or myelodysplastic syndrome that was driven by high rates among radiologists who graduated before 1940, likely due to their higher radiation exposure [51]. Several cytostatic drugs cause an increased risk of leukemias and/or lymphomas in patients who receive high doses; although such risks have not been documented in healthcare workers, potential routes of exposure in healthcare environments have been documented and precautions to minimize exposure are warranted [52].

Occupational and Environmental Agents and Exposure Circumstances with Sufficient Evidence for Causing Transitional Cell Carcinoma of the Bladder

Arsenic contamination in water is a major cause of environmentally related bladder cancer throughout the world. Arsenic is a naturally occurring element widely distributed in the earth's crust. Exposure to high levels of arsenic in drinking water has been recognized for many decades in some regions of the world, notably in the People's Republic of China, Taiwan (China), and some countries in Central and South America. More recently, several other regions have reported drinking water that is highly contaminated with arsenic [53]. Very high (greater than 20-fold) elevated risks of bladder cancer mortality have been observed among populations whose water supplies are highly contaminated with arsenic compared to regions in the same country with lower level contamination. Consumption of arsenic contaminated water also causes excess risks of cancer of the lung and skin cancer. In addition to areas where arsenic-contaminated drinking water sources have been used for decades, water supplies in some areas of the world were more recently contaminated. For example, most of the water supply in Bangladesh is drawn from tube wells that were installed in the 1970s to reduce ingestion of pathogen-contaminated surface waters; water from many of these relatively shallow wells has been found to contain high concentrations of arsenic. Extensive contamination of drinking water in Bangladesh with arsenic is predicted to cause excess cancer deaths as well as other chronic diseases, and reproductive and developmental defects. Mitigation of these hazards would require installing deeper wells and/or developing other safe sources of drinking water. Despite the potential benefits to public health and feasibility of these interventions, they have not been widely applied.

An estimated 7–19% of bladder cancers in men and 3–19% in women in the US are attributable to occupational exposures [11]. *Aromatic amine* exposure is an important cause of occupational bladder cancer. Aromatic amines are also present in mainstream and sidestream smoke and may contribute to the elevated risk of bladder cancer observed in smokers.

The potential for exposure to certain aromatic amines to cause large excesses in bladder cancer was recognized in the

Table 8.3 Agents that the IARC has classified as having sufficient evidence of causing cancer of the urinary bladder in humans based on IARC Monograph 100 and subsequent monographs. Highlighted agents or exposure circumstances are discussed the in text.

	Year first designated as Group 1 carcinogen	Cancer sites with *sufficient evidence* in humans	Cancer sites with *limited evidence* in humans
Aluminum production	1987	Lung Urinary bladder	
4-Aminobiphenyl	1972	Urinary bladder	
Arsenic and inorganic arsenic compounds	1973	Lung, skin, urinary bladder	Kidney, liver, prostate
Auramine production	1972	Urinary bladder	
Benzidine	1999	Urinary bladder	
Magenta production	1987		
2-Naphthylamine	1974	Bladder	
Ortho-Toluidine	2010	Urinary bladder	
Painting	1989	Urinary bladder, lung, mesothelioma,	Maternal exposure, childhood leukemia
X-radiation, gamma radiation	1999	Urinary bladder, lung, salivary gland, esophagus, stomach, colon, bone, basal cell of the skin, female breast, kidney, brain and CNS, thyroid and leukemia (excluding chronic lymphocytic leukemia)	Rectum, liver, pancreas, ovary, prostate, non-Hodgkin lymphoma, multiple myeloma

first half of the twentieth century when reports began to accumulate about excess numbers of bladder cancers occurring in dye manufacturing industries. In 1954, a study was published linking the high incidence of bladder cancer among workers in the British dye manufacturing industry to 4-aminobiphenyl and *B*-naphthylamine [54]. Recent studies have linked exposure to *ortho*-toluidine, another aromatic amine used in the manufacture of rubber chemicals, to high risks of bladder cancer [55].

Other occupational exposures have been associated with bladder cancer. Workers in the aluminum industry and painters have excess risks of bladder cancer, although specific agents have not been identified (Table 8.3). Numerous studies have associated occupations with exposure to metal working fluids with bladder cancer [56]. More recently studies have been able to associate bladder cancer risks with specific types of metal working fluid exposure [57].

Disinfection by-products in drinking water are an emerging concern with respect to risk of bladder cancer in the general population. Drinking water disinfectants can react with organic matter to form disinfection by-products including trihalomethanes which can be absorbed through the skin when showering, bathing and swimming in pools as well as taken into the body by ingestion [58]. There are a large variety of disinfection by-products which vary in toxicity and some have been shown to be mutagenic or genotoxic. Epidemiologic studies have suggested that disinfection by-products may be related to bladder cancer risk. Studies of the potential association are complicated by the difficulty in assessing individual exposure and the variability in level and nature of contaminants [59].

Occupational and Environmental Agents and Exposure Circumstances with Sufficient Evidence of Causing Cancers of Target Organs other than Lung, Leukemia/Lymphoma and Transitional Cell Carcinoma of the Bladder

Most human carcinogens cause cancer in a relatively small number of target organs, which are often target organs for other types of acute and chronic toxicity associated with the exposure (Table 8.4). Only a few carcinogens are associated with cancers of many or all sites, the most important of which is 2,3,7,8-TCDD (TCDD), which causes cancer and other health effects through binding to the aryl hydrocarbon hydroxylase receptor (AhR) which is expressed in almost all mammalian tissues. TCDD has a very long half-life in the body. The binding of TCDD to the AhR triggers adaptive cellular responses that alter the cell's ability to proliferate, migrate, apoptose, senesce and terminally differentiate. TCDD binding may also up-regulate drug metabolizing enzymes, thus increasing the presence of highly reactive intermediates that form during metabolic activation of exogenous and endogenous substances. TCDD has been most strongly associated with increased risks for cancer of all sites in epidemiologic studies. It also causes tumors in a wide variety of sites in experimental animals. TCDD has never been intentionally manufactured for large-scale commercial use, but was a contaminant in chlorophenoxy herbicides, including 2,4,5-trichlorophenoxyacetic acid (2,4,5-T), which were widely used in the 1960s and 1970s to control weeds and as a defoliant during the Vietnam war. TCDD may also be produced in thermal processes such as incineration, in metal processing, and in the bleaching of paper pulp with free chlorine. Most human

Table 8.4 Agents that the IARC has classified as having sufficient evidence of causing cancer sites other than lung, leukemia/lymphoma or urinary bladder in humans based on IARC Monograph 100 and subsequent monographs. Highlighted agents or exposure circumstances are discussed in the text.

Carcinogenic agent or exposure circumstance	Year first designated as Group 1 carcinogen	Cancer sites with *sufficient evidence* in humans	Cancer sites with *limited evidence* in humans
Isopropyl alcohol production	1977	Larynx	
Leather dust	1981	Nasal cavity and paranasal sinus	
Mineral oils, treated or mildly treated	1973	Skin (non-melanoma)	
Polychlorinated biphenyls		Skin (melanoma)	
Solar radiation	1992	Skin (basal cell carcinoma, squamous cell carcinoma, melanoma)	Eye (squamous cell carcinoma, melanoma), lip
2,3,7,8-TCDD	1997	All sites combined	Lung Non-Hodgkin lymphoma Soft tissue sarcoma
Vinyl chloride	1974	Liver angiosarcoma Hepatocellular cancer	
Wood dust	1995	Nasopharynx, nasal cavity and paranasal sinus	
X-radiation, gamma radiation	1999	Lung, salivary gland, esophagus, stomach, colon, bone, basal cell of the skin, female breast, kidney, urinary bladder, brain and CNS, thyroid and leukemia (excluding chronic lymphocytic leukemia)	Rectum, liver, pancreas, ovary, prostate, non-Hodgkin lymphoma, multiple myeloma

exposure to TCDD occurs as a result of eating meat, milk, eggs, fish and related products, as TCDD is persistent in the environment and accumulates in animal fat. Since the mid-1980s, mean tissue concentrations of TCDD in the general population have decreased by two- to threefold [49].

Importance of Continued Research

In contrast to the carcinogenic exposures described in this chapter for which human cancer risks have been adequately studied and documented, there are many agents that have not been adequately studied in either experimental systems or humans. From the public health and cancer prevention perspective, it is particularly important to resolve the carcinogenicity of substances for which there is widespread human exposure and sufficient evidence for carcinogenicity in animals. As we have gained more knowledge about how exogenous agents interact with the body to increase risk of cancer, it has become apparent that carcinogens often act through multiple mechanisms.

Perspectives That May Be Helpful for Clinicians in Discussing Occupational and Environmental Carcinogens with Their Patients and the General Public

- Environmental and occupational carcinogens are a serious concern. Although the most important steps that individuals can take to reduce their chances of developing and dying from cancer are to avoid tobacco smoking, maintain a healthy weight, and have recommended cancer screening tests, some of the most important things societies and governments can

do to prevent cancer are to support research on the causes of cancer and to regulate carcinogens and other health hazards in workplaces and the general environment.

- Most cancers related to occupational and environmental exposures are clinically indistinguishable from other cancers. Only a few occupational and environmental carcinogens been identified as causing rare histologic types of cancer; these include angiosarcoma of the liver associated with exposure to vinyl chloride monomer, small cell lung cancer associated with bis chloromethyl ether exposure, and mesothelioma associated with asbestos exposure. However, for the most part, cancers that arise from occupational and environmental carcinogens are of the common histologic types for the organs where they develop, and large scale and carefully designed epidemiologic studies are needed to determine whether a particular exposure increases cancer risks.
- In the absence of data from well-designed and large-scale epidemiologic studies in humans, which may not be feasible for many potential environmental and occupational carcinogens, substances that cause cancer in animal studies should be treated as if they have potential to cause cancer in humans.
- It is important to review each patient's occupational history to determine if they have been exposed to occupational or environmental carcinogens. Occupational exposures associated with high risks of lung cancer, such as asbestos, should be considered in determining whether individuals should be offered low dose CT screening. Although randomized trials have not been performed to estimate the potential mortality benefit of bladder cancer screening for individuals exposed to aromatic amines associated with high risks of bladder cancer, bladder cancer screening programs have been offered to occupational cohorts with known high risks in the hope that detecting and treating early lesions will reduce the morbidity and mortality associated with muscle-invasive disease.

References

1 *Preamble: IARC Monographs on the Evaluation of Carcinogenic Risks to Humans*. Lyon, France: International Agency for Research on Cancer, World Health Organization, 2006.

2 Fontham ET, Thun MJ, Ward E, *et al*. American Cancer Society perspectives on environmental factors and cancer. *CA Cancer J Clin* 2009;59(6):343–51.

3 Ward EM, Schulte PA, Straif K, *et al*. Research recommendations for selected IARC-classified agents. *Environ Health Perspect* 2010;118(10):1355–62.

4 Bucher JR. The National Toxicology Program rodent bioassay: designs, interpretations, and scientific contributions. *Ann N Y Acad Sci* 2002;982:198–207.

5 Smith MT, Guyton KZ, Gibbons CF, *et al*. Key characteristics of carcinogens as a basis for organizing data on mechanisms of carcinogenesis. *Environ Health Perspect* 2016;124(6):713–21.

6 Cancer Moonshot: Report of the Cancer Moonshot Task Force, https://www.whitehouse.gov/sites/default/files/docs/final-whcmtf-report-1012161.pdf, 2016.

7 Cogliano VJ, Baan RA, Straif K, *et al*. The science and practice of carcinogen identification and evaluation. *Environ Health Perspect* 2004;112(13):1269–74.

8 National Toxicology Program. Report on Carcinogens, 12th edn. Research Triangle Park, NC: U.S. Department of Health and Human Services, Public Health Service, 2011.

9 National Toxicology Program. Report on Carcinogens, 13th edn. Research Triangle Park, NC: U.S. Department of Health and Human Services, Public Health Service, 2014.

10 Field RW, Withers BL. Occupational and environmental causes of lung cancer. *Clin Chest Med* 2012;33(4):681–703.

11 Steenland K, Burnett C, Lalich N, Ward E, Hurrell J. Dying for work: the magnitude of US mortality from selected causes of death associated with occupation. *Am J Ind Med* 2003;43(5):461–82.

12 Nicholson WJ, Perkel G, Selikoff IJ. Occupational exposure to asbestos: population at risk and projected mortality – 1980–2030. *Am J Ind Med* 1982;3(3):259–311.

13 Mortality Data: Malignant Mesothelioma, National Organization for Occupational Safety and Health, Centers for Disease Control. https://wwwn.cdc.gov/eworld/Grouping/Malignant_mesothelioma/100 (accessed 18 May 2017).

14 Elimination of asbestos-related diseases, 2006. http://whqlibdoc.who.int/hq/2006/WHO_SDE_OEH_06.03_eng.pdf (accessed 18 May 2017).

15 Krewski D, Lubin JH, Zielinski JM, *et al*. Residential radon and risk of lung cancer: a combined analysis of 7 North American case-control studies. *Epidemiology* 2005;16(2):137–45.

16 *Anomymous. Health effects of exposure to radon BEIR VI*. Washington, DC: National Academy Press, 1999.

17 Lubin JH. Studies of radon and lung cancer in North America and China. *Radiat Prot Dosimetry* 2003;104(4):315–19.

18 Darby S, Hill D, Deo H, *et al*. Residential radon and lung cancer--detailed results of a collaborative analysis of individual data on 7148 persons with lung cancer and 14,208 persons without lung cancer from 13 epidemiologic studies in Europe. *Scand J Work Environ Health* 2006;32 Suppl 1:1–83.

19 Markowitz SB, Levin SM, Miller A, Morabia A. Asbestos, asbestosis, smoking, and lung cancer. New findings from the North American insulator cohort. *Am J Resp Crit Care Med* 2013;188(1):90–6.

20 Schubauer-Berigan MK, Daniels RD, Pinkerton LE. Radon exposure and mortality among white and American Indian uranium miners: an update of the Colorado Plateau cohort. *Am J Epidemiol* 2009;169(6):718–30.

21 Bang KM, Mazurek JM, Wood JM, *et al*. Silicosis mortality trends and new exposures to respirable crystalline silica - United States, 2001–2010. *MMWR Morb Mortal Wkly Rep* 2015;64(5):117–20.

22 Steenland K, Ward E. Silica: a lung carcinogen. *CA Cancer J Clin* 2014;64(1):63–9.

23 Liu Y, Steenland K, Rong Y, *et al*. Exposure-response analysis and risk assessment for lung cancer in relationship to silica exposure: a 44-year cohort study of 34,018 workers. *Am J Epidemiol* 2013;178(9):1424–33.

24 Occupational Exposure to Respirable Crystalline Silica: A Rule by the Occupational Safety and Health Administration. https://www.federalregister.gov/documents/2016/03/25/2016-04800/occupational-exposure-to-respirable-crystalline-silica (accessed 18 May 2017).

25 IARC Working Group on the Evaluation of Carcinogenic Risks to Humans. Diesel and Gasoline Engine Exhausts and Some Nitroarenes. *IARC Monogr Eval Carcinog Risks Hum* 2014;105:9–699.

26 Attfield MD, Schleiff PL, Lubin JH, *et al*. The Diesel Exhaust in Miners study: a cohort mortality study with emphasis on lung cancer. *J Natl Cancer Inst* 2012;104(11):869–83.

27 Silverman DT, Samanic CM, Lubin JH, *et al*. The Diesel Exhaust in Miners study: a nested case-control study of lung cancer and diesel exhaust. *J Natl Cancer Inst* 2012;104(11):855–68.

28 Health Impacts of Fine Particles in Air, Centers for Disease Control and Prevention. http://ephtracking.cdc.gov/showAirHIA.action (accessed 18 May 2017).

29 Pope CA, 3rd, Thun MJ, Namboodiri MM, *et al*. Particulate air pollution as a predictor of mortality in a prospective study of U.S. adults. *Am J Respir Crit Care Med* 1995;151(3 Pt 1):669–74.

30 Pope CA, 3rd, Burnett RT, Thun MJ, *et al*. Lung cancer, cardiopulmonary mortality, and long-term exposure to fine particulate air pollution. *JAMA* 2002;287(9):1132–41.

31 Krewski D, Burnett R, Jerrett M, *et al*. Mortality and long-term exposure to ambient air pollution: ongoing analyses based on the American Cancer Society cohort. *J Toxicol Environ Health A* 2005;68(13–14):1093–109.

32 Turner MC, Krewski D, Pope CA, 3rd, *et al*. Long-term ambient fine particulate matter air pollution and lung cancer in a large cohort of never-smokers. *Am J Resp Crit Care Med* 2011;184(12):1374–81.

33 Lepeule J, Laden F, Dockery D, Schwartz J. Chronic exposure to fine particles and mortality: an extended follow-up of the Harvard Six Cities study from 1974 to 2009. *Environ Health Perspect* 2012;120(7):965–70.

34 Boffetta P, Nyberg F. Contribution of environmental factors to cancer risk. *Br Med Bull* 2003;68:71–94.

35 Zhang J, Smith KR. Indoor air pollution: a global health concern. *Br Med Bull* 2003;68:209–25.

36 WHO. Household Air Pollution and Health Factsheet No. 292, 2014.

37 Ward E, Hornung R, Morris J, *et al.* Risk of low red or white blood cell count related to estimated benzene exposure in a rubberworker cohort (1940–1975). *Am J Ind Med* 1996;29(3):247–57.

38 Lan Q, Zhang L, Li G, *et al.* Hematotoxicity in workers exposed to low levels of benzene. *Science* 2004;306 (5702):1774–6.

39 Infante PF, Rinsky RA, Wagoner JK, Young RJ. Leukaemia in benzene workers. *Lancet* 1977;2(8028):76–8.

40 Ott GM, Townsend JC, Fishbeck WA, Langner RA. Mortality among individuals occupationally exposed to benzene. *Arch Environ Health* 1978;33:3–10.

41 Rinsky RA, Smith AB, Hornung R, *et al.* Benzene and leukemia. An epidemiologic risk assessment. *N Engl J Med* 1987;316(17):1044–50.

42 Paustenbach DJ, Bass RD, Price P. Benzene toxicity and risk assessment, 1972–1992: implications for future regulation. *Environ Health Perspect* 1993;101 Suppl 6:177–200.

43 Goldstein BD, Liu Y, Wu F, Lioy P. Comparison of the effects of the US Clean Air Act and of smoking prevention and cessation efforts on the risk of acute myelogenous leukemia. *Am J Public Health* 2011;101(12):2357–61.

44 Wallace L. Environmental exposure to benzene: an update. *Environ Health Perspect* 1996;104 Suppl 6:1129–36.

45 Buffler PA, Kwan ML, Reynolds P, Urayama KY. Environmental and genetic risk factors for childhood leukemia: appraising the evidence. *Cancer Invest* 2005;23(1):60–75.

46 Carlos-Wallace FM, Zhang L, Smith MT, Rader G, Steinmaus C. Parental, in utero, and early-life exposure to benzene and the risk of childhood leukemia: a meta-analysis. *Am J Epidemiol* 2016;183(1):1–14.

47 Schnatter AR, Glass DC, Tang G, Irons RD, Rushton L. Myelodysplastic syndrome and benzene exposure among petroleum workers: an international pooled analysis. *J Natl Cancer Inst* 2012;104(22):1724–37.

48 Stenehjem JS, Kjaerheim K, Bratveit M, *et al.* Benzene exposure and risk of lymphohaematopoietic cancers in 25,000 offshore oil industry workers. *Br J Cancer* 2015;113(11):1641.

49 IARC. *IARC Monographs on the Evaluation of Carcinogenic Risks to Humans. Vol 100 F, Chemical agents and related occupations.* Lyon, France: International Agency for Research on Cancer, 2012.

50 Daniels RD, Schubauer-Berigan MK. A meta-analysis of leukaemia risk from protracted exposure to low-dose gamma radiation. *Occup Environ Med* 2011;68(6):457–64.

51 Berrington de Gonzalez A, Ntowe E, Kitahara CM, *et al.* Long-term mortality in 43 763 U.S. radiologists compared with 64 990 U.S. *psychiatrists. Radiology* 2016;281(3):847–57.

52 Connor TH, McDiarmid MA. Preventing occupational exposures to antineoplastic drugs in health care settings. *CA Cancer J Clin* 2006;56(6):354–65.

53 IARC. *IARC Monographs on the Evauation of Carcinogenic Risks to Humans. Vol 100C, Arsenic, metals, fibres and dusts.* Lyon, France: International Agency for Research on Cancer, 2012.

54 Case RA, Hosker ME, McDonald DB, Pearson JT. Tumours of the urinary bladder in workmen engaged in the manufacture and use of certain dyestuff intermediates in the British chemical industry. I. The role of aniline, benzidine, alpha-naphthylamine, and beta-naphthylamine. *Br J Ind Med* 1954;11(2):75–104.

55 Carreon T, Hein MJ, Hanley KW, Viet SM, Ruder AM. Bladder cancer incidence among workers exposed to o-toluidine, aniline and nitrobenzene at a rubber chemical manufacturing plant. *Occup Environ Med* 2014;71(3):175–82.

56 Colt JS, Karagas MR, Schwenn M, *et al.* Occupation and bladder cancer in a population-based case-control study in Northern New England. *Occup Environ Med* 2011;68(4):239–49.

57 Friesen MC, Costello S, Eisen EA. Quantitative exposure to metalworking fluids and bladder cancer incidence in a cohort of autoworkers. *Am J Epidemiol* 2009;169(12):1471–8.

58 Villanueva CM, Cantor KP, Grimalt JO, *et al.* Bladder cancer and exposure to water disinfection by-products through ingestion, bathing, showering, and swimming in pools. *Am J Epidemiol* 2007;165(2):148–56.

59 Villanueva CM, Kogevinas M, Cordier S, *et al.* Assessing exposure and health consequences of chemicals in drinking water: current state of knowledge and research needs. *Environ Health Perspect* 2014;122(3):213–21.

9

Nutrition and Physical Activity for Cancer Prevention

Stacey Fedewa[1], Rebecca L. Siegel[1], Colleen Doyle[2], Marji L. McCullough[1], and Alpa V. Patel[1]

[1] *Intramural Research, American Cancer Society, Atlanta, Georgia, USA*
[2] *Cancer Control, American Cancer Society, Atlanta, Georgia, USA*

Introduction

Approximately 20% of all cancers diagnosed in the United States (US) are attributable to unhealthy diet, excess alcohol consumption, physical inactivity, and body fatness [1–7]. In addition, excess weight, poor diet, and physical inactivity are related to several chronic diseases including cardiovascular disease, type 2 diabetes, hypertension, and sleep disorders. Several public health and governmental organizations provide general recommendations for physical activity, nutrition, and maintaining a healthy body weight aimed at improving the overall health in the US. The guidelines issued by the American Cancer Society (ACS), which were last updated in 2012 and also provide recommendations for individual choices as well as community action regarding physical and social environments that influence individual food and activity behavior, will be used as the basis for this chapter [1]. These recommendations are important for reducing cancer incidence and mortality. Adults who most closely adhere to the ACS recommendations for individual choices are 10% to 20% less likely to be diagnosed with any cancer and 20–30% less likely to die from the disease than those who are least adherent [8–10]

The four main recommendations of the ACS guideline for nutrition and physical activity are summarized in Table 9.1 and each component of these guidelines is discussed in further detail below.

Overweight and Obesity

Weight recommendations for individuals of differing height are usually described by ranges of body mass index (BMI). BMI can be calculated as a person's weight in kilograms/(height in meters)^2 or by (weight in pounds $\times$ 703)/(height in inches)^2. Adults with a BMI from 18.5 to 24.9 kg/m^2 are considered to have a healthy weight; those with a BMI of 25.0 to 29.9 kg/m^2 or 30.0 kg/m^2 or higher are classified as overweight or obese,

respectively. Criteria for overweight and obesity among children are also based on BMI, but consider percentile BMI rankings by age and gender [11, 12].

Achieving and maintaining a healthy body weight requires an appropriate balance between energy intake (from food and beverages) and energy expenditures (from physical activity) [13, 14]. Effective strategies for achieving this balance include a diet with an emphasis on plant foods and wholegrains, limited consumption of high-calorie foods and beverages, and smaller portion sizes; limiting between-meal snacks; tracking food intake; increasing intentional physical activity; and limiting time spent in sedentary behaviors [1, 15, 16].

Unhealthy dietary patterns, physical inactivity, and excessive weight gain often begin during childhood and persist into adulthood. Consequently, 70% of those who are overweight by adolescence will remain overweight as adults [17, 18] with elevated risk of several forms of cancer and other chronic health problems. Therefore, establishing healthful lifestyle behaviors that prevent overweight and obesity in children and adolescents is important for reducing the risk of several chronic diseases that typically occur decades later [19, 20].

Body Weight and Cancer Risk

Overweight and obesity are clearly associated with increased risk for developing cancers of the breast (in postmenopausal women), colon and rectum, endometrium, kidney, pancreas, and esophagus (adenocarcinoma), and are probably associated with increased risk of cancers of the liver, cervix, and ovary; multiple myeloma; non-Hodgkin lymphoma; and aggressive prostate cancer [1]. These associations are thought to be mediated by several mechanisms, some of which are specific to certain cancers. In general, the association between obesity and cancer is mediated by effects on fat and sugar metabolism, immune function, and levels of peptide and steroid hormones (including insulin, insulin-like growth factors, leptin, and estrogens) [1, 21–24]. Specifically, the association between excess weight and endometrial and breast cancer is mediated by

Table 9.1 ACS Guidelines on Nutrition and Physical Activity for Cancer Prevention.

Recommendations for Individual Choices

Achieve and maintain a healthy weight throughout life.

- Be as lean as possible throughout life without being underweight.
- Avoid excess weight gain at all ages. For those who are currently overweight or obese, losing even a small amount of weight has health benefits and is a good place to start.
- Engage in regular physical activity and limit consumption of high-calorie foods and beverages as key strategies for maintaining a healthy weight.

Adopt a physically active lifestyle.

- Adults should engage in at least 150 min of moderate-intensity or 75 min of vigorous-intensity physical activity each week, or an equivalent combination, preferably spread throughout the week.
- Children and adolescents should engage in at least 1 h of moderate- or vigorous-intensity physical activity each day, with vigorous-intensity activity at least 3 days each week.
- Limit sedentary behavior such as sitting, lying down, and watching television and other forms of screen-based entertainment.
- Doing any intentional physical activity above usual activities, no matter what the level of activity, can have many health benefits.

Consume a healthy diet, with an emphasis on plant sources.

- Choose foods and beverages in amounts that help achieve and maintain a healthy weight.
- Limit consumption of processed meat and red meats.
- Eat at least two-and-a-half cups of vegetables and fruits each day.
- Choose wholegrain instead of refined-grain products.

Limit alcohol consumption, if you drink at all.

- Drink no more than one drink per day for women or two per day for men.

Recommendations for Community Action

Public, private, and community organizations should work collaboratively at national, state, and local levels to implement environmental policy changes that:

- Increase access to affordable, healthy foods in communities, worksites, and schools, and decrease access to and marketing of foods and beverages of low nutritional value, particularly to youth.
- Provide safe, enjoyable, and accessible environments for physical activity in schools and worksites, and for transportation and recreation in communities.

---

increases in estrogen levels. Inflammation due to fatty liver is thought to be the mechanism by which excess weight increases the risk for liver cancer. Excess weight may lead to acid reflux and gallstones, increase inflammation in these areas, and positively influence the risk of esophageal and gallbladder cancer, respectively [22]. Additionally, results from studies of weight loss interventions (including lifestyle and behavioral interventions, pharmacologic interventions, and bariatric surgery) have shown that even modest weight loss (5% of body weight) improves biomarkers of metabolic and inflammatory processes that are thought to contribute to the relationship between BMI and certain cancers [22, 25].

Prevalence of Overweight and Obesity in the US

Among adults aged 20–74 years, the prevalence of obesity doubled between 1976 and 1980 (15%) and 1999 and 2000 (31%), but has remained stable since 2003 at 32–34% [11, 26]. From 2011 to 2012, more than two-thirds of American adults were overweight or obese [26]. Individual characteristics such as race, ethnicity, gender, state of residence, and sexual orientation are significantly associated with prevalence of obesity. Hispanic men (41%) and women (45%) and non-Hispanic black women (57%) were most likely to be obese, whereas prevalence is lowest among Asian American men and women (11%); one-third of non-Hispanic white men and women were obese [27]. Across all race/ethnicities, prevalence is higher among those who were US-born compared to foreign born, with duration of residence conferring greater risk of obesity [28–30]. Prevalence is also more common among women with lower incomes compared to women with higher incomes; however, this pattern is not observed in men. While non-Hispanic white lesbians are more likely to be overweight (55%) than heterosexual women (51%), gay men are substantially less likely to be overweight (56%) than heterosexual men (69%) [31]. Regionally, obesity prevalence is generally highest in the South and lowest in the West.

Physical Activity and Cancer Prevention

The ACS physical activity recommendation for adults is to engage in at least 150 min of moderate-intensity activity or 75 min of vigorous-intensity activity per week, or an equivalent combination, preferably spread throughout the week (Table 9.1). In addition, individuals should decrease sedentary behaviors, replacing and/or disrupting them, when possible, with light to moderate activity (such as incidental walking and "moving about").

Usual physical activity is generally of low intensity in short bouts during a person's daily routine. Intentional physical activities are moderate or vigorous in intensity, associated with exercise or transportation (bike riding or brisk walking), and utilize large muscle groups, causing a noticeable increase in heart rate, breathing depth and frequency, and perspiration (see Table 9.2 for examples). Walking is accessible and inexpensive, confers health benefits with few adverse effects, and is the most frequently reported physical activity among US adults [7, 32]. The optimal intensity, duration, and frequency of physical activity needed to reduce cancer risk is not fully known, and may vary for different cancer types. However, studies suggest that amounts of physical activity that exceed the minimum ACS recommendations are likely to provide even greater reductions in cancer risk [1, 13, 14]. Despite this evidence, most US adults do not meet the minimum ACS recommendations for aerobic activity, which are discussed in further detail below [27].

For people who are mostly inactive or just beginning to increase their activity level, engaging in any amount and intensity of intentional physical activity is likely to be beneficial. In fact, the greatest reduction in mortality risk is seen when going from no intentional activity to any activity [33]. Men older than 40, women older than 50, and other people with chronic illnesses and/or known cardiovascular risk factors should seek medical clearance before beginning a physical activity program.

The ACS recommends that children and adolescents should be physically active at moderate- to vigorous-intensity for at least 60 min daily [1, 34]. Daily high-quality physical education programs and other opportunities for physical activity should

Table 9.2 Examples of moderate and vigorous physical activity.

	Moderate-intensity Activities	Vigorous-intensity Activities
Exercise and leisure	Walking, dancing, leisurely bicycling, ice and roller skating, horseback riding, canoeing, power yoga	Jogging or running, fast bicycling, circuit weight training, aerobic dance, martial arts, jumping rope, swimming
Sports	Volleyball, golfing (without a cart), softball, baseball, badminton, doubles tennis, downhill skiing	Soccer, field or ice hockey, lacrosse, singles tennis, racquetball, basketball, cross-country skiing
Home activities	Mowing the lawn, general yard and garden maintenance	Digging, carrying, and hauling, masonry, carpentry
Occupational activity	Walking and lifting as part of the job (custodial work, farming, auto or machine repair)	Heavy manual labor (forestry, construction, fire-fighting)

be provided for children at school, while sedentary recreation, such as watching television and playing video games, should be minimized at home [35, 36].

Physical Activity and Cancer Risk

In addition to its role in maintaining a healthy body weight, physical activity is associated with improved regulation of sex hormones, insulin, prostaglandins, and immune function [1]. Physical activity, independent of obesity, is inversely associated with the risk of several types of cancer, including those of the breast, colon, and endometrium [3]. Further, regular physical activity reduces the risk of overall mortality and several chronic diseases including cardiovascular disease, type 2 diabetes, osteoporosis, and hypertension [1, 37, 38]. Long periods of sedentary behavior, defined as ≤1.5 metabolic equivalents increase the likelihood of becoming obese, of developing type-2 diabetes, cardiovascular disease, and various types of cancers, and increase overall mortality independent of physical activity. [39, 40]

Prevalence of Physical Activity and Sedentary Behavior

In 2013, 31% of adults reported no leisure-time physical activity during an average week. Approximately half of adults (50% overall, 54% of men and 46% of women) reported meeting ACS recommended levels of aerobic activity [27]. Physical activity levels vary substantially by sociodemographic factors. For example, 62% of those aged 18–24 years met recommended levels of aerobic activity levels compared to 35% of adults 65 years and older. Compliance ranged from 42% in non-Hispanic blacks to 54% in non-Hispanic whites among race and ethnic groups, and from 31% in adults without a high school diploma to 62% in college graduates by level of education.

From 2009 to 2010, the self-reported average time spent sitting daily among adults aged 20 years and older was 285 min for men and 281 min for women. Mexican Americans reported lower average amounts of sitting in an average day compared to non-Hispanic whites and blacks, a pattern that was consistent across sex [41].

In 2013, only 27% of US high school students met or exceeded minimum levels of physical activity recommended by the ACS, and only 29% attended physical education classes daily. Notably, larger percentages reported three or more hours daily of television

viewing (33%) or video gaming or non-school related computer screen time (41%) [27]. The proportion of high school students who met recommended physical activity ranged widely by state, from 16% in the District of Columbia to 39% in Oklahoma.

Nutrition, Dietary Factors, and Alcohol Consumption and Cancer Prevention

Unhealthy dietary patterns may increase cancer risk either directly, independent of BMI, or indirectly through excessive caloric consumption that lead to overweight and obesity. The largest percentage of calories in the American diet comes from foods and beverages that are high in fat, added sugar, and refined carbohydrates, and add little nutritional value [42]. Limiting portion sizes, especially of calorie-dense foods and beverages, will reduce caloric intake. Several other aspects of diet associated with increased cancer risk are described below.

Processed and Red Meats

High intake of processed meat (e.g., lunch meats, bacon, hot dogs) or red meat (e.g., beef, lamb, pork) has been convincingly associated with increased risk of colorectal cancer [43] and limited evidence suggests an association with pancreatic cancer [44]. The International Agency for Research on Cancer (IARC) recently reviewed the evidence and classified processed meat as a Class I carcinogen, and concluded that red meat is a probable carcinogen [45]. Higher consumption of meat is also associated with modest but statistically significant increases in overall cancer incidence and mortality, as well as death from other causes [3, 46]. Nitrates or nitrites used to preserve processed meats can contribute to the formation of nitrosamines, which are mutagens involved in carcinogenesis [46]. Additionally, cooking meats at high temperatures produces heterocyclic amines, which is thought to damage human DNA, increasing cancer risk [47, 48]. In addition, heme iron present in red meat damages colon surface epithelium [47]. The ACS recommends limiting consumption of processed and red meats by choosing smaller portions (e.g., served as a side dish rather than the focus of a meal) and by substituting fish, poultry, or legumes, which are rich in nutrients that may protect against cancer and can serve as a healthier source of protein than meat.

Vegetables and Fruits

Vegetables (including legumes) and fruits contain numerous bioactive substances (including vitamins, minerals, fiber, and carotenoids) that may help prevent cancer. There is evidence suggesting that greater consumption of nonstarchy vegetables (such as broccoli, green beans, lettuce, and squash) and fruits is associated with lower risk of oral, pharyngeal, laryngeal, esophageal, gastric, and estrogen-receptor negative breast cancers [49, 50]. Higher prediagnostic blood concentrations of carotenoids, such as beta-carotene and lycopene, are associated with a lower risk of breast cancer [51]. Foods rich in these compounds include sweet potatoes, green leafy vegetables, carrots, and tomato products. Randomized controlled trials of individual vitamin supplements, such as beta-carotene, vitamin C, vitamin E, selenium, and folic acid generally do not lower cancer risk and may even cause harm [52, 53]. Individual supplements may provide too high a dose, potentially not "in balance" with other nutrients in the diet. Therefore, it is recommended that individuals obtain nutrients from foods, rather than individual supplements. The potential benefits of vegetable and fruit consumption on cancer risk may also be in part mediated by their replacement of more calorie-dense foods and associated maintenance of a healthy weight [15].

Consumption of vegetables and fruits remains lower than is recommended among US adults and children [15], due to lack of affordable produce, preparation time and taste preferences, and the abundance of relatively inexpensive options (e.g., processed snacks, sugared sodas, and fast food) that compete with healthier choices [54].

The ACS recommendation for consuming at least two-and-a-half cups of vegetables and fruits each day is based on evidence regarding cancer risk. However, for overall health, the ACS supports the recommendation in the 2015–2020 Dietary Guidelines for Americans for consuming higher levels and encourages consumers to fill half of their plate with vegetables and fruits for meals and snacks [14].

In 2013, only 15.1% of US adults consumed three or more servings of vegetables per day and 29.8% reported eating two or more servings of fruits daily. Among US high school students surveyed during 2013, only 15.7% reported consuming vegetables three or more times per day and 33.2% consumed 100% fruit juice or fruit two or more times a day [27].

Wholegrain

Compared to refined flour products, wholegrain foods (made from the entire grain seed) are lower in caloric density and higher in fiber, certain vitamins, and minerals [14]. Studies support an inverse association of intake of wholegrain foods and dietary fiber with the risk of colorectal cancer [43]. In addition, wholegrains are part of an overall diet pattern rich in fruits, vegetables and low in red meat and processed meat, which has been consistently associated with lower risk of death from cancer [55]

Alcohol consumption

ACS recommends that people who drink alcohol should limit their intake to no more than two drinks per day for men and one drink (defined as 12 ounces of beer, five ounces of wine, or 1.5 ounces of 80-proof distilled spirits) per day for women [14]. Lower limits are recommended for women because of their smaller body size and slower metabolism of alcohol.

Alcohol consumption is an established risk factor for oral, pharyngeal, laryngeal, esophageal, liver, colorectal, and female breast cancers, and evidence also suggests an association with pancreatic cancer [1, 3, 56, 57]. The combination of tobacco use and alcohol consumption increases the risk for oral, pharyngeal, laryngeal, esophageal cancers far more than the independent effect of either exposure alone [3]. Even a few drinks per week result in a modest but consistent increase in breast cancer risk, which continues to increase with alcohol consumption at progressively higher levels [58]. Alcohol consumption is one of the few modifiable risk factors associated with incidence of breast cancer. Alcohol may influence cancer risk through a variety of mechanisms, which vary by cancer site. There is strong evidence that acetaldehyde, a component of alcohol, induces DNA damage and is involved in head and neck, esophageal, and liver carcinogenesis. Alcohol intake may also increase estrogen concentration, thereby increasing the risk of breast cancer. There is moderate evidence that alcohol acts as a solvent for other carcinogens, increases oxidative stress, and interferes with folate metabolism, increasing the risk of several cancers.

Although low to moderate intake of alcoholic beverages has been associated with decreased risk of coronary heart disease, this is not a compelling reason for nondrinkers to start consuming alcohol. Risk of cardiovascular disease can be reduced by medications, as well as by lifestyle changes (not smoking, consuming a diet low in saturated and trans fats and high in a variety of plant foods, maintaining a healthy weight, and staying physically active) that also reduce risk of cancer and other health problems [59, 60].

The prevalence of consuming one or more drinks per day for women and two or more drinks per day for men during 2012 was around 5% for US adults aged 18 years and older [61]. Annual US per capita alcohol consumption decreased from 2.8 gallons in 1980 to less than 2.1 gallons in 1998, and then slightly increased to 2.3 gallons in 2011 [62].

Community Action

Experience in tobacco control and other public health initiatives has shown that public policies and environmental strategies can be powerful tools to alter structural socioenvironmental factors to influence population-level behavior. Measures such as smoke-free laws and increases in cigarette excise taxes have been highly effective in deterring tobacco use. To avert an epidemic of obesity-related cancer and other chronic disease, similar purposeful changes in public policy and in the community environment that support healthy behaviors throughout a person's life cycle are needed to address the prevailing socioenvironmental factors contributing to increased obesity [1, 38]. These factors include logistical and economic barriers to obtaining healthful food (in contrast to the ubiquitous presence and marketing of unhealthful foods), and limited access to safe, convenient and affordable opportunities for recreational physical activity [63]. Other social, economic, and environmental factors that adversely influence patterns of nutrition and physical activity include a decrease in walking as a mode of transportation and increased reliance on automobiles, increased sedentary work, more meals eaten away from home, increased availability of cheap but calorie-dense processed foods, price structures that promote purchasing and consumption of larger portions, and increased consumption of sugar-sweetened beverages [1, 15, 54, 63].

Many experts as well as governmental and nongovernmental organizations recognize that obesity is a complex problem that requires implementation of a broad range of effective approaches at the level of individuals and populations [1, 38]. The ACS believes that a multilevel public health strategy that includes public education as well as policies that promote environments in which it is easier for individuals to make healthy choices will be most effective [1, 38, 64].

Community Action Strategies

Public and private organizations at the local, state, and national levels can develop policies and allocate or expand resources to facilitate positive changes in nutrition and physical activity patterns [19, 20]. For example:

- States, school districts, and schools can set and implement science-based standards for physical education programs and for all foods and beverages sold and served in schools.
- Employers can implement worksite health promotion programs [19, 20] but should not tie health insurance premiums to health behaviors or health status.
- Healthcare professionals can take an "assess, advise, and assist" approach to helping their patients to achieve and maintain a healthful BMI [65, 66]. The US Preventive Services Task Force recommends behavioral counseling to promote a healthy lifestyle among people at high risk for cardiovascular disease [67] and behavioral counseling for weight loss among youth and adults who are obese [68, 69].
- At the state and local level, community leaders can promote policies such as regulation of the school food environment, zoning changes and tax incentives to attract food stores that carry fresh vegetables and fruits into poor neighborhoods, and the creation of safe spaces that promote physical activity [17].

References

1 Kushi LH, Doyle C, McCullough M, *et al.* American Cancer Society Guidelines on nutrition and physical activity for cancer prevention: reducing the risk of cancer with healthy food choices and physical activity. *CA Cancer J Clin* 2012;62(1):30–67.

2 World Cancer Research Fund International. *Continuous Update Project: Cancer Preventability Estimates for Diet, Nutrition, Body Fatness, and Physical Activity.* London: World Cancer Research Fund International, 2015.

3 World Cancer Research Fund and American Institute for Cancer Research. *Food, Nutrition, Physical Activity and the Prevention of Cancer: A Global Perspective.* Washington DC, 2007.

4 World Cancer Research Fund and American Institute for Cancer Research, *Policy and Action for Cancer Prevention.* Washington DC, 2009.

5 Eheman, C, Henley SJ, Ballard-Barbash R, *et al.* Annual Report to the Nation on the status of cancer, 1975–2008, featuring cancers associated with excess weight and lack of sufficient physical activity. *Cancer* 2012;118(9):2338–66.

6 Doll R, Peto R. *The Causes of Cancer: Quantitative Estimates of Avoidable Risks of Cancer in the United States Today.* Oxford: Oxford University Press, 1981: 1197–312.

7 Centers for Disease Control and Prevention. Vital signs: walking among adults – United States, 2005 and 2010. *MMWR Morb Mortal Wkly Rep* 2012; 61:595–601.

8 Kabat GC, Matthews CE, Kamensky V, Hollenbeck AR, Rohan TE. Adherence to cancer prevention guidelines and cancer incidence, cancer mortality, and total mortality: a prospective cohort study. *Am J Clin Nutr* 2015;101(3):558–69.

9 Thomson CA, McCullough ML, Wertheim BC, *et al.* Nutrition and physical activity cancer prevention guidelines, cancer risk, and mortality in the women's health initiative. *Cancer Prev Res (Phila)*;2014;7(1):42–53.

10 McCullough ML, Patel AV, Kushi LH, *et al.* Following cancer prevention guidelines reduces risk of cancer, cardiovascular disease, and all-cause mortality. *Cancer Epidemiol Biomarkers Prev* 2011;20(6):1089–97.

11 Fryar C, Carroll M, Ogden CL. Prevalence of Overweight, Obesity, and Extreme Obesity Among Adults: United States, Trends 1960–1962 through 2009–2010. National Center for Health Statistics. September 2012. Available from: http://www.cdc.gov/nchs/data/hestat/obesity_adult_09_10/obesity_adult_09_10.pdf (accessed 19 May 2017).

12 Centers for Disease Control and Prevention. About Child & Teen BMI. 2015 Available from: http://www.cdc.gov/healthyweight/assessing/bmi/childrens_bmi/about_childrens_bmi.html (accessed 19 May 2017).

13 International Agency for Research on Cancer, IARC Handbooks of Cancer Prevention. Volume 6: *Weight Control and Physical Activity.* Lyon, France: IARC Press, 2002.

14 US Department of Health and Human Services and US Department of Agriculture. Dietary Guidelines for Americans 2015–2020, 8th edn. Available from: http://health.gov/dietaryguidelines/2015/guidelines (accessed 19 May 2017).

15 Krebs-Smith SM, Guenther PM, Subar AF, Kirkpatrick SI, Dodd KW. Americans do not meet federal dietary recommendations. *J Nutr* 2010;140(10):1832–8.

16 Mitchell, JA, Bottai M, Park Y, Marshall SJ, Moore SC, Matthews CE. A prospective study of sedentary behavior and changes in the body mass index distribution. *Med Sci Sports Exerc* 2014;46(12):2244–52.

17 US Department of Health and Human Services. *The Surgeon General's Call to Action to Prevent and Decrease Overweight and Obesity.* Washington, DC: US Department of Health and Human Services, 2001.

18 Patton, GC, Coffey C, Carlin JB, *et al.* Overweight and obesity between adolescence and young adulthood:

a 10-year prospective cohort study. *J Adolesc Health* 2011;48(3):275–80.

19 Institute of Medicine and National Research Council, *Local Government Actions to Prevent Childhood Obesity*. Washington, DC: The National Academies Press, 2009.

20 White House Task Force on Childhood Obesity Report to the President. Solving the Problem of Childhood Obesity within a Generation, 2010.

21 Calle EE, Kaaks R. Overweight, obesity and cancer: epidemiological evidence and proposed mechanisms. *Nat Rev Cancer* 2004;4(8):579–91.

22 Byers T, Sedjo RL. Body fatness as a cause of cancer: epidemiologic clues to biologic mechanisms. *Endocr Relat Cancer* 2015;22(3):R125–34.

23 Giovannucci, E., Ascherio A, Rimm EB, Colditz GA, Stampfer MJ, Willett WC. Physical activity, obesity, and risk for colon cancer and adenoma in men. *Ann Intern Med* 1995;122(5):327–34.

24 Patel AV, Rodriguez C, Bernstein L, *et al.* Obesity, recreational physical activity, and risk of pancreatic cancer in a large U.S. Cohort. *Cancer Epidemiol Biomarkers Prev* 2005;14(2): 459–66.

25 Byers T, Sedjo RL. Does intentional weight loss reduce cancer risk? *Diabetes Obes Metab* 2011;13(12):1063–72.

26 Ogden CL, Carroll MD, Kit BK, Flegal KM. Prevalence of childhood and adult obesity in the United States, 2011–2012. *JAMA* 2014;311(8):806–14.

27 American Cancer Society. *Cancer Prevention & Early Detection Facts & Figures 2015–2016*. Atlanta: American Cancer Society, 2015.

28 Akresh IR. Overweight and obesity among foreign-born and U.S.-born Hispanics. *Biodemography Soc Biol* 2008;54(2): 183–99.

29 Mehta NK, Elo IT, Ford ND, Siegel KR. Obesity Among U.S.- and Foreign-Born Blacks by Region of Birth. *Am J Prev Med*, 2015. 49(2):269–73.

30 Goel, M.S., McCarthy EP, Phillips RS, Wee CC. Obesity among US immigrant subgroups by duration of residence. *JAMA* 2004;292(23):2860–7.

31 Deputy NP, Boehmer U. Weight status and sexual orientation: differences by age and within racial and ethnic subgroups. *Am J Public Health* 2014;104(1):103–9.

32 Ogilvie D, Foster CE, Rothnie H *et al.* Scottish Physical Activity Research Collaboration. *Interventions to promote walking: systematic review. BMJ* 2007;334:1204.

33 Moore SC, Patel AV, Matthews CE, *et al.* Leisure time physical activity of moderate to vigorous intensity and mortality: a large pooled cohort analysis. *PLoS Med* 2012; 9(11):e1001335.

34 US Department of Health and Human Services. Physical Activity Guidelines for Americans, 2008. *Washington*, DC: US Department of Health and Human Services.

35 Strong W, Malina RM, Blimkie CJ, *et al.* Evidence based physical activity for school-age youth. *J Pediatr* 2005;146(6):732–7.

36 Community Preventive Services Task Force. Obesity Prevention and Control: Behavioral Interventions that Aim to Reduce Recreational Sedentary Screen Time Among Children. Available from: http://www.thecommunityguide.org/obesity/behavioral.html (accessed 19 May 2017).

37 Samitz G, Egger M, Zwahlen M. Domains of physical activity and all-cause mortality: systematic review and dose-response meta-analysis of cohort studies. *Int J Epidemiol* 2011:40(5):1382–400.

38 Kumanyika SK, Obarzanek E, Stettler N, *et al.* Population-based prevention of obesity: the need for comprehensive promotion of healthful eating, physical activity, and energy balance: a scientific statement from American Heart Association Council on Epidemiology and Prevention, Interdisciplinary Committee for Prevention (formerly the expert panel on population and prevention science). *Circulation* 2008;118(4):428–64.

39 Patel AV, Bernstein L, Deka A, *et al.* Leisure time spent sitting in relation to total mortality in a prospective cohort of US adults. *Am J Epidemiol* 2010;172(4):419–29.

40 Proper KI, Singh AS, van Mechelen W, Chinapaw MJ. Sedentary behaviors and health outcomes among adults: a systematic review of prospective studies. *Am J Prev Med* 2011;40(2):174–82.

41 Harrington DM, Barreira TV, Staiano AE, Katzmarzyk PT. The descriptive epidemiology of sitting among US adults, NHANES 2009/2010. *J Sci Med Sport*, 2014;17(4):371–5.

42 Marriott BP, Olsho L, Hadden L, Connor P. Intake of added sugars and selected nutrients in the United States, National Health and Nutrition Examination Survey (NHANES) 2003–2006. *Crit Rev Food Sci Nutr* 2010;50(3):228–58.

43 World Cancer Research Fund and American Institute for Cancer Research. Continuous Update Project Report. *Food, Nutrition, Physical Activity, and the Prevention of Colorectal Cancer*. London: Imperial College, 2011.

44 World Cancer Research Fund and American Institute for Cancer Research. Continuous Update Project Report. *Food, Nutrition, Physical Activity, and the Prevention of Pancreatic Cancer*. London, UK: Imperial College, 2012.

45 Bouvard V, Loomis D, Guyton KZ, *et al.* International Agency for Research on Cancer Monograph Working Group. Carcinogenicity of consumption of red and processed meat. *Lancet Oncol* 2015;16(16):1599–600.

46 Sinha R, Cross AJ, Graubard BI, Leitzmann MF, Schatzkin A. Meat intake and mortality: a prospective study of over half a million people. *Arch Intern Med* 2009;169:562–71.

47 Kim E, Coelho D, Blachier F. Review of the association between meat consumption and risk of colorectal cancer. *Nutr Res* 2013;33(12):983–94.

48 Butler LM, Sinha R, Millikan RC, *et al.* Heterocyclic amines, meat intake, and association with colon cancer in a population-based study. *Am J Epidemiol* 2003; 157(5):434–45.

49 Jung S, Spiegelman D, Baglietto L, *et al.* Fruit and vegetable intake and risk of breast cancer by hormone receptor status. *J Natl Cancer Inst* 2013;105(3):219–36.

50 World Cancer Research Fund and American Institute for Cancer Research. *Food, Nurition, Physical Acitivity and the Prevention of Cancer: A Global Perspective*, Washington DC, 2007.

51 Eliassen AH, Hendrickson SJ, Brinton LA, *et al.* Circulating carotenoids and risk of breast cancer: pooled analysis of eight prospective studies. *J Natl Cancer Inst* 2012; 104(24):1905–16.

52 Omenn GS, Goodman GE, Thornquist MD, *et al.* Effects of a combination of beta carotene and vitamin A on lung cancer

and cardiovascular disease. *N Engl J Med* 1996; 334(18):1150–5.

53 Klein EA, Thompson IM Jr, Tangen CM, *et al*. Vitamin E and the risk of prostate cancer: the Selenium and Vitamin E Cancer Prevention Trial (SELECT). *JAMA* 2011;306(14):1549–56.

54 Darmon N, Drewnowski A. Does social class predict diet quality? *Am J Clin Nutr* 2008; 87:1107–17.

55 Liese AD, Krebs-Smith SM, Subar AF, *et al*. The Dietary Patterns Methods Project: synthesis of findings across cohorts and relevance to dietary guidance. *J Nutr* 2015; 145(3):393–402.

56 Secretan B, Straif K, Baan R, *et al*. WHO International Agency for Research on Cancer Monograph Working Group. A review of human carcinogens—Part E: tobacco, areca nut, alcohol, coal smoke, and salted fish. *Lancet Oncol* 2009;10(11):1033–4.

57 International Agency for Research on Cancer. *IARC Monographs on the Evaluation of Carcinogenic Risks to Humans*. Volume 83: Alcohol Drinking. Lyon: IARC Press, 1988.

58 Narod SA. Alcohol and risk of breast cancer. *JAMA* 2011;306(17):1920–1.

59 Waxman A and World Health Assembly. WHO global strategy on diet, physical activity and health. *Food Nutr Bull* 2004;25(3):292–302.

60 Estruch R, Ros E, Salas-Salvadó J, *et al*. PREDIMED Study Investigators. Primary prevention of cardiovascular disease with a Mediterranean diet. *N Engl J Med* 2013;368(14): 1279–90.

61 National Center for Health Statistics. *Health, United States, 2013: With a Special Feature on Prescription Drugs*. Hyattsville, MD, 2014,

62 LaVallee RA, Trinh K, Yi H. Apparent Per Capita Alcohol Consumption: National, State and Regional Trends, 1977–2012. Available from: http://pubs.niaaa.nih.gov/publications/surveillance98/CONS12.htm, 2014 (accessed 19 May 2017).

63 Fakhouri TH, Hughes JP, Burt VL, *et al*. Physical activity in U.S. youth aged 12–15 years, 2012. *NCHS Data Brief* 2014;141:1–8.

64 Khan LK, Sobush K, Keener D, *et al*. Centers for Disease Control and Prevention. Recommended community strategies and measurements to prevent obesity in the United States. *MMWR Recomm Rep* 2009;58(RR-7):1–26.

65 Brawer R, Brisbon N, Plumb J. Obesity and cancer. *Prim Care* 2009;36(3):509–31.

66 Orzano AJ, Scott JG. Diagnosis and treatment of obesity in adults: an applied evidence-based review. *J Am Board Fam Pract* 2004;17(5):359–69.

67 LeFevre ML and U. S. Preventive Services Task Force. Behavioral counseling to promote a healthful diet and physical activity for cardiovascular disease prevention in adults with cardiovascular risk factors: U.S. Preventive Services Task Force Recommendation Statement. *Ann Intern Med* 2014;161(8):587–93.

68 U. S. Preventive Services Task Force, Screening for obesity in children and adolescents: US Preventive Services Task Force recommendation statement. *Pediatrics* 2010; 125(2):361–7.

69 Moyer VA and U.S.P.S.T. Force. Screening for and management of obesity in adults: U.S. Preventive Services Task Force recommendation statement. *Ann Intern Med* 2012; 157(5):373–8.

10

Sun Protection

Andrew C. Walls[1] and Martin A. Weinstock[2]

[1] *Brigham and Women's Hospital; Harvard Medical School, Boston, Massachusetts, USA*
[2] *Brown University School of Public Health, Providence, Rhode Island, USA*

Introduction

Skin cancer is the most common type of cancer in the United States (US) and each year there are more new cases of skin cancer diagnosed than all other forms of cancer combined [1]. This chapter will highlight the epidemiology, causes, risk factors, and methods of prevention for the three major types of cutaneous cancer: melanoma, basal cell carcinoma (BCC) and squamous cell carcinoma (SCC).

The cancers are named after the skin cells they histologically resemble. The main cellular component of the epidermis, also known as keratinocytes, are comprised of cells in different stages of maturation; squamous keratinocytes comprise the superficial layers of the skin while their progenitor cells, basal cells, are found along the base of the epidermis, attached to the basement membrane. Melanocytes are found at the interface between basal and squamous keratinocytes and produce melanin pigment. Melanocytes are also the primary cell type that comprises benign and atypical nevi. As both basal and squamous cell carcinomas are comprised of cells that resemble those of keratinocyte origin, the term keratinocyte carcinoma is used to describe them collectively, whereas melanoma is a malignant neoplasm of melanocytes.

For all three of these skin cancers, exposure to ultraviolet radiation (UVR), through sunlight or artificial sources (such as tanning beds) is the primary avoidable cause. Prevention of these cancers is predicated upon proper sun exposure behaviors, identification of individuals most at risk of developing these tumors and early identification of suspicious skin lesions.

Epidemiology

The incidence of BCC, SCC and melanoma has been steadily increasing. Whites comprise the majority of BCC, SCC and melanoma diagnoses and deaths and both incidence and mortality are highest in the elderly, particularly males. However, recently increased incidence of all three cancers has been noted in young adults as well, particularly melanoma in women aged 15–39.

Mortality

Basal and squamous cell carcinomas are the most common skin cancers, while melanoma is the deadliest and accounts for more deaths than any other skin disease; it is estimated melanoma will result in approximately 9,730 deaths during 2017 alone [2]. While overall melanoma mortality has remained relatively stable in the US it has been decreasing in people younger than 50 and increasing in people older than 50 [1, 3].

Melanoma does not affect all ages and populations equally. Men are approximately 60% more likely to be diagnosed with melanoma, and their mortality is more than double that of women. Men are more likely to be diagnosed with more advanced disease, but even in men and women with the same stage of melanoma, risk of death is still higher in men. Elderly (≥65 years) non-Hispanic white men have the highest death rate of any population in the US, approximately three times that of elderly white women (24.4/100,000 and 8.6/100,000, respectively) [4]. Moreover, mortality is increasing more in this age group than in younger groups (6.6 annual percent change in men, 0.6 in women) [2].

Mortality data for BCC and SCC is less well-known as these cancers are not followed by major cancer registries. SCC is responsible for the majority of deaths due to keratinocyte carcinomas; BCC is a locally destructive tumor, but metastasis and subsequent death is a rare event (<1%), while SCC metastasizes to lymph nodes or distant sites in approximately 3–4% of those diagnosed, resulting in death in an estimated 2–4% of SCC diagnosed [5, 6].

Incidence and Burden of Healthcare

Melanoma incidence rates have steadily increased for the past 30 years and the American Cancer Society predicts 87,110 new cases of melanoma during 2017. This increase has been in both sexes, in all age groups and for all tumor thicknesses [1–3, 7]. Similar trends have been seen in other continents, namely Europe and Australia, and worldwide incidence has increased by approximately 30% between 1990 and 2008 [8, 9].

Incidence of BCC is higher than that of SCC, occurring at an approximate 4:1 ratio [10]. Collectively, BCC and SCC represent the majority of skin cancer diagnoses in the US and by all accounts, their incidence is also rising. The most recent data estimates that there were 3.5 million new cases of keratinocyte carcinoma in the US, doubling since the early 1990s, and resulting in billions of dollars of healthcare-related costs [11, 12]. As with melanoma, this trend has been observed internationally [13]. Of note, the incidence of keratinocyte carcinoma appears to be increasing not just in the elderly populations, but in younger individuals [14].

Risk Factors

The overall trend of increasing skin cancer in the US and worldwide is multifactorial but has largely been attributed to an increase in recreational sun exposure, the recent increased use of tanning beds, and a lack of effective practices to prevent skin cancer. Exposure to UVR is the primary risk factor for all three main types of skin cancers. Most other significant risk factors, such as fair skin, red hair, sunburns and the strength of one's immune system relate to the host's susceptibility to the molecular damage induced by UVR. Geographic distributions of skin cancer, studies of the timing and patterns of sun exposure as well as the molecular consequences of DNA damage induced by UVR all support the role of UVR in skin cancer pathogenesis.

Sun Exposure and Skin Cancers

Geography
Skin cancer does not occur equally in all geographic regions. The incidence of BCC and SCC is significantly higher in areas of lower latitude. For example, the incidence of SCC in Arizona is three times higher than that in New Hampshire and 25–45 times higher than in Finland [15–17]. Similarly, incidence rates of BCC in Hawaii are the highest in the US and triple the rate seen in Minnesota [18]. Australia, a population of primarily UK origin, has the highest rates of BCC, SCC, and melanoma in the world, much higher than current estimates for those still living in the UK [13, 19].

Timing and Pattern of Sun Exposure
While sun exposure is a common etiologic agent for BCC, SCC and melanoma, the timing and pattern of exposures varies slightly for each cancer. Chronic, continuous UVR exposure appears to play a predominant role in the etiology of keratinocyte carcinomas, whereas evidence suggests that intermittent exposure, such as sunburns is more closely related to development of melanoma. This is supported by the fact that the majority of SCC and BCC occur on the most photoexposed areas of the body: the head, neck, dorsal hands and arms. SCC is thought to be linked to total cumulative hours exposed to UVR, usually at an intensity less than that which causes sunburns in the individual [20]. For BCC, it appears that a complex combination of

cumulative radiation plus intense intermittent exposure may be most important [21]. Finally, for melanoma, sunburns, the product of bursts of intense sun exposure, appears to preferentially lead to melanocyte proliferation; melanoma often appears in areas of the body that receive intermittent sun exposure, such as the trunk in men and the lower extremities in women [22].

There has been much study into the timing of sun exposure in an individual's life. Sunburns sustained during childhood or adolescence elevate lifetime risk of melanoma (and likely BCC as well), even many years later [22]. This notion is supported by migrant studies showing that for individuals who immigrate from areas of low sun exposure to high sun exposure (e.g., the UK to Australia), an elevated risk of melanoma is seen only in those who move at young age [23]. Furthermore, the rising incidence of all skin cancer types in young adults, particularly women, has been primarily attributed to the use of tanning beds [24, 25]. However, sun exposure later in life is also important to the pathogenesis of skin cancer and recent meta-analyses have shown a persistent increased risk for melanoma with sunburns at all ages [26]. Moreover, individuals with melanoma can reduce their risk of developing a second primary lesion through sun avoidance practices [27] and the number of keratinocyte carcinomas are reduced in transplant patients that use sunscreen following their first diagnosis of skin cancer [28].

Tanning Beds

The use of indoor tanning beds as a source of UVR contributes to the pathogenesis of all three major forms of skin cancer and has been classified by the World Health Organization as a Group 1 Carcinogen ("known to cause cancer in humans"), placing artificial sources of UVR in the same category as tobacco, asbestos, and nuclear fission products [29].

Melanoma
The systematic review and meta-analysis by the International Agency for Research on Cancer (IARC) led to classification of tanning bed exposure as a group 1 agent (carcinogenic to humans) [30]. The results demonstrated a statistically significant association between first tanning bed exposure before the age of 35 and a 75% increase in melanoma risk. Subsequent studies from the US and Australia have confirmed this finding and demonstrate, after controlling for confounding, a dose–response relationship for the number of hours spent in tanning booths, the number of tanning sessions, and the number of years spent using tanning beds [31, 32]. The Australian study, which focused on melanomas occurring at a younger age, estimated that tanning bed use was responsible for 76% of all melanoma diagnosed in 18–29 year olds. Further compelling evidence has been seen in Iceland [33] where from 1992 to 2001 melanoma incidence in young women increased rapidly, increasing at a rate greater than 15% per year. The sharp increase was attributed to the use of tanning beds; subsequent public health campaigns and the closure of half of available tanning beds brought about a decline in melanoma incidence.

Basal and Squamous Cell Carcinoma
As early as 2002 it was demonstrated that those using tanning beds had 2.5 times the risk for developing SCC and 1.5 times the

risk for BCC [34]. More recently, a large study of 73,000 White nurses in the US demonstrated a dose–response relationship for tanning bed use and the development of both SCC and BCC [35]. Use during high school/college was associated with the greatest risk of developing BCC. A third study of individuals with young-onset BCC (<40 years) found tanning bed use increased risk of young-onset BCC by 69% [24]. Risk was higher for females and an estimated 43% of the young-onset BCC was thought to be preventable by having never been exposed to a tanning bed.

Mechanisms of UVR-induced Carcinogenesis

UVR is nonvisible light radiation that falls between X-rays and visible light on the electromagnetic spectrum. It has a shorter wavelength, and therefore higher energy than visible light. UVR is divided into three subsets according to wavelength: UVA (400–320 nm), UVB (320–280 nm), and UVC (280–200 nm). The ozone layer blocks the majority of the higher energy UVC and UVB light emitted from the sun. Approximately 95% of the UVR reaching the earth's surface is comprised of UVA, and the remainder is UVB.

UVA and UVB have differential effects on the skin although both are individually capable of inducing skin cancer. UVB, with its short wavelength and higher energy, only superficially penetrates the skin, with subsequent damage predominantly in the epidermis. Direct DNA damage occurs, resulting in cyclobutane pyrimidine dimers that affect proper cell replication and induce carcinogenesis [36]. UVA radiation indirectly damages DNA through the generation of reactive oxygen species [37]. When either form of UVR-induced DNA damage occurs in key cell cycle and tumor suppressor genes, oncogenic transformation may occur. There are many mutations described and each skin cancer is induced through disruption of a different signaling pathway, although mutations in *TP53* – a stress-response, oncosuppressive gene crucial to cell cycle regulation – can be found in melanoma, BCC and SCC [38].

UV-induced skin erythema (sunburn) is the result of cellular injury, leading to vasodilation and therefore erythema and edema of the skin [39]. Concomitantly, damaged keratinocytes undergo apoptosis and melanocytes are stimulated to upregulate melanin production, thus increasing visible skin pigmentation ("a tan") [36, 38]. However, even without preceding erythema, this upregulation of pigment can only result from DNA damage. Therefore, skin tanning is typically due to radiation-induced DNA damage even in the absence of overt burning.

As UVB is principally responsible for the skin burning response, UVA was previously thought to be responsible for photoaging but incapable of carcinogenesis, a conclusion that inspired the development of "safe" UVA-only tanning beds. This misconception has been disproven by the previously mentioned discoveries in UVA-induced molecular damage, cancer induction in laboratory animals by UVA, the cancers attributed to these tanning beds, as well as studies of psoriasis patients receiving long-term UVA light therapy. Follow-up of patients receiving therapeutic psoralen (a photosensitizing agent) and UVA light treatment has been demonstrated to result in the increased incidence of BCC, SCC, and melanoma [40, 41].

Host Phenotype

The amount of damage caused to the skin by UVR is the product of host pigmentary characteristics. Sunburn sensitivity, as characterized by light skin tones that burn easily and tan poorly, is a strongly documented independent factor for all three cancers, as are associated pigmentary characteristics: freckling, red or blonde hair, and light eye color [42–45]. However, melanoma and keratinocyte cancers also diverge in risk factors. In addition to sunburns and pigmentary characteristics, family history of melanoma and the number of melanocytic nevi (moles) are important risk factors for melanoma, whereas markers of actinic damage and a personal history of keratinocyte carcinoma strongly predict risk for SCC and BCC.

Age

Despite recent increases in younger populations, skin cancers are primarily a disease of the elderly; onset for all three is common in the fifth and sixth decades and incidence continues to rise thereafter. The reasons for this are likely multifactorial and a result of the accumulation of sun exposure, latency between sun exposure and the emergence of skin cancers, and an age-related decrease in immunosurveillance in the skin. The incidence of SCC increases with age. Individuals aged 75 and older have greater than 50 times the incidence rates of those under 45 [16, 46]. Similarly, incidence of BCC increases dramatically with age, with those aged 55–75 having an incidence rate a 100 times greater than those under 20 [47]. As noted previously, both melanoma incidence and mortality are rising disproportionately in those over 65 years of age.

Nevi

Acquired melanocytic nevi, both benign and atypical, are closely associated with risk for melanoma. While it is possible for a melanoma to arise within a nevus, most melanomas arise *de novo* and nevi serve as a phenotypic marker of increased melanoma risk [48]. Nevi are acquired as the result of early-life sun exposure in genetically predisposed individuals [49]. They typically increase in number until the third and fourth decade of life. Benign, or typical nevi are the most common form of nevi and are ≤5 mm with regular borders and pigment patterns. Risk for melanoma is associated with total-body nevus counts and increases with increasing nevus burden; those with over 100 total nevi have an estimated ninefold risk, even after adjusting for skin tone [50, 51].

Atypical nevi, which tend to be larger and more variable in color, are more strongly associated with melanoma risk. Elevated risk for melanoma has been seen in individuals with a single atypical nevus and risk again increases with higher numbers of atypical nevi [50, 52].

Family History

Family history is an important risk factor in melanoma. There is some evidence that nonsyndromic family history may play a role in the development of BCC or SCC although this has yet to be fully elucidated, and familial occurrence of melanoma is more prominent than in BCC or SCC.

Melanoma

A family history of melanoma in one or more first-degree relatives elevates risk [53, 54]. Concomitant family history of other cancers, especially pancreatic cancer, should further the index of suspicion. Many associated familial mutations have been described in melanoma; the best described are mutations in the *CDKN2A* tumor suppressor gene which encodes the important p16 cell cycle regulator and its effectors [55]. However, even in families with multiple melanomas, a *CDKN2A* mutation is only found in 20–40% of individuals and a causative mutation is most often not identified [56]. Regardless, these patients are still considered to be a high-risk population and are at risk for the development of single as well as multiple primary melanomas [57].

Basal and Squamous Cell Carcinoma

The contribution of a family history of a first-degree relative with keratinocyte carcinoma is undefined and the topic has not been studied in detail. One large study in Sweden found that a first-degree relative with SCC was associated with a two- to threefold increase in risk, although it is impossible to ascertain if there is a genetic basis or if it is the product of similar sun exposure and skin pigmentation within a family [58]. In BCC, recent genome-wide association studies (GWAS) have found genetic polymorphisms in a variety of cell-signaling and skin pigmentation molecular pathways [59, 60] although the clinical value of these findings has yet to be elucidated.

Previous Skin Cancer

Individuals with previous skin cancers are at significant risk to develop more. This is true for both melanoma and keratinocyte carcinomas. For individuals with a history of keratinocyte carcinoma, the risk of developing a subsequent keratinocyte carcinoma may be as high as 50% [61]. Further studies have elucidated this risk specifically in individuals with previous BCC and have found risk of a second BCC to be between 40 and 55% at 5 years [62, 63]. These risks have been found to be increased in males, older individuals, those who sunburn easily, and have markers of actinic damage.

Risk for melanoma is higher in those with a preceding melanoma and increases further for those with atypical nevi and family history of melanoma [57, 64]. Notably, risk is highest within 1 year of diagnosis of the first melanoma but remains elevated for at least 20 years thereafter [65]. For patients with two primary melanomas, risk for a third may be 30% at 5 years [64]. There is also evidence that a history of keratinocyte carcinoma can elevate risk of later developing melanoma. Therefore, clinicians should remain vigilant for all forms of skin cancer in these individuals [66, 67].

Immunosuppression

Chronic immunosuppression is a major risk factor for skin cancer; it is predominantly seen in organ transplant recipients (OTR), although it has been seen in patients using anti-TNF biologic therapies or long-term glucocorticoids, and in those with HIV infection. UVR is still the primary etiologic agent in immunosuppressed individuals, as their cancers still occur in typical sun-exposed locations and incidence rates are increased in sunnier climates [68]. The increased incidence of skin cancers in immunosuppressed populations underscores the human immune system's role in recognizing and eradicating UVR-damaged cells from the skin.

Skin cancer, 95% of which are keratinocyte carcincomas, is the single most common malignancy in OTRs [68]. Contrary to the general population, SCC is the most common keratinocyte carcinoma in this population with a higher incidence of aggressive subtypes and metastasis [69]. Risk increases with the duration of immunosuppression and varies by the dosing and type of immunosuppressive regimens used but overall risk of SCC is thought to be 65-fold, BCC 10-fold, and melanoma three- to fivefold in the OTR population [68]. The use of sunscreen has been shown to reduce the number of subsequent keratinocyte carcinomas in OTRs [28].

Skin Cancer and Disease

A wide variety of diseases predispose individuals to the development of skin cancer (often SCC) in areas of chronic inflammation and injury. Diseases of pigment loss or dysfunction, faulty DNA repair or germline genetic mutations may also predispose to keratinocyte cancers and melanoma.

Chronic Inflammation

Occurrence of SCC is well-documented in areas of chronic inflammation including wounds, burns, scars, and osteomyelitis drainage tracts; these factors account for most incident SCC in dark-skinned populations [70]. Skin diseases resulting in chronic inflammation, such as lichen sclerosus et atrophicus and epidermolysis bullosa, predispose to SCC; death from cutaneous SCC is common in certain variants of epidermolysis bullosa [71].

Xeroderma Pigmentosum

Xeroderma pigmentosum is a rare genetic disorder but confers extremely high risk for SCC, BCC, and melanoma. These individuals have decreased functionality in proteins required for repair of UVR-induced DNA damage and develop all forms of skin cancer in early childhood; risk before age 20 is elevated 10,000-fold [72].

Oculocutaneous Albinism

Individuals affected by oculocutaneous albinism have deficiencies in melanin synthesis and are therefore much more vulnerable to UVR. An elevated risk of skin cancers, predominantly SCC, is seen, again with the potential for childhood onset, especially in sunny climates [73, 74].

Voriconazole

The systemic antifungal medication voriconazole has been associated with both SCC and melanoma development. It is proposed to occur through photosensitization, although the mechanism is not currently well understood. Moreover, described cases are in concomitantly immunosuppressed patients [75, 76].

Prevention of Skin Cancers

Sun Protection

As UVR is the most significant etiologic agent in skin carcinogenesis, prevention of all three cancers should be possible with minimization of this exposure. Recent review of data from national surveys has demonstrated alarming rates of sun exposure and low rates of proper sun protection practices [77,78]. Overall, at least 38% of all US adults and 69% of adolescents had a sunburn within the past year (78). According to a survey from 2010: 32.1% of adults reported always or often using sunscreen when outside for an hour or more on a warm, sunny day; 37.1% reported seeking shade; 12.8% reported wearing hats; and 11.5% wore long-sleeved shirts. A survey of high school students reported that during 2013 only 10.1% reported using sunscreen routinely [77].

As of 2013, 4.4% of American adults (1.8% of men and 6.9% of women) and 12.8% of high school students (5.3% of boys and 20.2% of girls) reported using a tanning bed within the last year. The highest prevalence was 30.7, among female non-Hispanic White high school students [77]. As of December 2016, 12 states (CA, DE, HI, IL, LA, MN, NC, NH, NV, OR, TX, VT) and the District of Columbia have now banned use of tanning beds for those under 18 years of age with most others requiring parental permission [79].

Minimizing UVR exposure, through sun protection and tanning bed avoidance, should be an individual's primary preventative practice. Proper sun protection with UV-safe clothing and appropriate sunscreen use on exposed body sites is key when outdoors and the sun is high in the sky. The National Council on Skin Cancer Prevention, comprised of more than 45 skin cancer organizations, including the American Cancer Society and the American Academy of Dermatology (AAD), has published the following recommendations [80]:

- Do Not Burn or Tan: avoid intentional tanning. Avoid tanning beds. Ultraviolet light from the sun and tanning beds causes skin cancer and wrinkling.
- Seek Shade: when the sun's rays are the strongest between 10 a.m. and 4 p.m.
- Wear Protective Clothing: long-sleeved shirt and pants. A wide-brimmed hat and sunglasses.
- Generously Apply Sunscreen: use a broad spectrum sunscreen with sun protection factor (SPF) 30 or higher for protection from UVA and UVB radiation. and reapply every 2 hours.
- Use Extra Caution Near Water, Snow and Sand: these surfaces reflect the damaging rays of the sun, which can increase your chance of sunburn.
- Get Vitamin D Safely: through a healthy diet or vitamin supplements.
- Carefully Examine All of Your Skin Once a Month: a new or changing spot should be evaluated.

Clothing

In 1996, the Australian Radiation Protection and Nuclear Safety Agency (ARPANSA) developed a set of testing criteria to assess the ultraviolet protection factor (UPF) for fabrics to allow for proper labeling of sun protective clothing. This is currently used by American clothing manufacturers. Clothing is rated on a scale of 15–50+. Those fabrics with a UPF score of 40 or higher effectively block 97.5% or more of UVR, while those with the minimal score of 15 block an estimated 93.3%. The following factors contribute to the UPF rating of fabric [81]:

- Tightness of the weave or knit (tighter improves the rating)
- Composition of the yarns (cotton, polyester, etc.)
- Color (darker colors are generally better)
- Stretch (more stretch lowers the rating)
- Moisture (many fabrics have lower ratings when wet)
- Condition (worn and faded garments may have reduced ratings)
- Finishing (some fabrics are treated with UV-absorbing chemicals).

Sunscreen

Sunscreen use has been shown to prevent SCC, actinic keratoses, nevi, and melanoma, but not yet BCC [82–85]. The strongest evidence in support of the use of sunscreen derives from a randomized trial in Queensland, Australia. In this trial, 1,621 individuals were randomized to daily use of SPF 16 sunscreen, versus discretionary use for a 4-year period. Ten years after the conclusion of the trial, invasive melanoma risk was decreased by 73% and SCC risk was reduced by 40% [84, 85]. BCC rates were reduced, but not significantly. It is important to note that the youngest enrollees in the study were 25 years old and the authors hypothesize that an even more dramatic effect could be seen had the daily sunscreen use begun in childhood or adolescence and had used a SPF higher than 16. Sunscreen use in school children leads to lower nevus counts, especially in freckled children [86]. As nevus counts may serve as a marker of melanocyte-stimulating sun exposure, this finding provides indirect evidence that sunscreen use may reduce risk of invasive melanoma. Similar results have been seen in children using clothing to prevent sun exposure [87, 88].

The AAD currently recommends an SPF of 30 or greater [89]. SPF is calculated experimentally as a multiplier of the dose of UVB needed to induce erythema on human skin under experimental conditions (2 mg of sunscreen is applied per cm^2). Studies have shown that only 25–50% of this amount is applied during normal usage conditions, reducing the SPF to an unsatisfactory level [90]. The current AAD guidelines for sunscreen application are:

- Reapply at least every 2 h, sooner if exposed to sweat, water, or mechanical friction
- Use broad spectrum, water-resistant sunscreen providing UVA and UVB protection.

Vitamin D

As sun avoidance and sunscreen use may put individuals at risk for vitamin D deficiency, the AAD currently recommends a vitamin D-rich diet with oral supplementation of 600–800 IU daily in adults [91].

Chemoprevention

A number of agents have been investigated as chemopreventative agents as a means to delay, reverse, suppress, or prevent skin cancer. Overall, there is very little evidence to date that chemopreventative medications have efficacy in preventing skin cancers. Moreover, any potential risk reduction must be weighed against the inherent adverse effects and complications of these medications.

Keratinocyte Carcinoma

Retinoids/Vitamin A

Evidence for chemoprevention of SCC with oral retinoids exists in high-risk patient populations. Use of retinol (vitamin A) 25,000 IU has demonstrated 26% risk reduction for SCC in those with two or more previous SCCs [92]. In psoriasis patients receiving PUVA therapy, oral retinoids were associated with a reduced risk of SCC but not BCC [93]. Additionally, oral isotretinoin has been shown to be effective in preventing keratinocyte carcinomas in patients with xeroderma pigmentosum [94], while acitretin in renal transplant patients has shown benefit is some studies [95, 96], but not others [97]. Topical tretinoin has not been shown to be effective in preventing skin cancer [98] and currently no treatment recommendations for use of vitamin A or retinoids exist.

Nonsteroidal Anti-inflammatory Drugs (NSAIDs)

The use of NSAIDs for the prevention of SCC has been suggested by animal models; human studies have shown reduced SCC with NSAID use [99, 100], while others have not [101, 102].

ACE (angiotensin-converting enzyme) Inhibitors/
Angiotensin Receptor Blockers

Data are limited but a recent cohort study of individuals at high risk observed a significant risk reduction for both SCC and BCC [103]. This finding has also been observed in a smaller group of renal transplant recipients [104].

Melanoma

Fibrates or Statins

The findings of three large systematic reviews of randomized controlled trials have not found evidence of a protective effect of statins or fibrates in reducing risk for melanoma. Risk is often reduced, but has never been found to be significant in meta-analyses [105–107].

NSAIDs

NSAIDs have been an ongoing source of investigation and controversy in melanoma risk. Some studies have suggested that NSAIDs, particularly aspirin, may have a protective effect [100, 108, 109], but multiple other studies have found no reduction of risk [110–112].

Vitamin D

Similar to NSAIDs, a theoretical role for a vitamin-D-mediated reduction of melanoma has been demonstrated in animal models, but in humans results are conflicting [113–115]. A randomized controlled trial in women showed a melanoma risk reduction only for a subset analysis of women with previous keratinocyte carcinoma taking vitamin D and calcium. However, there was no protective effect for the total population [116].

Screening for Skin Cancer

In addition to primary prevention of skin cancers, early detection of these lesions is important. In melanoma, the depth of invasion of the tumor is the single most important prognostic feature and therefore early detection of melanoma lesions may translate to a decrease in mortality. However, as it has been estimated that in order to achieve sufficient power to assess this reduction in melanoma mortality in the US, a randomized control trial would require 800,000 people [117]. The scale and cost of such an undertaking is prohibitive. Currently, there are no formal recommendations or guidelines for routine skin cancer screening for average-risk populations. The American Cancer Society recommends that, "… the best way to detect skin cancer early is to be aware of new or changing skin growths, particularly those that look unusual. Any new lesions, or a progressive change in a lesion's appearance (size, shape, color, etc.) should be evaluated promptly by a physician" [1].

The current recommendation of the US Services Preventative Task Force is that, "… the current evidence is insufficient to assess the balance of benefits and harms of visual skin examination by a clinician to screen for skin cancer in adults" but also notes that, "This recommendation applies to asymptomatic adults who do not have a history of premalignant or malignant skin lesions. Patients who present with a suspicious skin lesion or who are already under surveillance because of a high risk of skin cancer, such as those with a familial syndrome (eg, familial atypical mole and melanoma syndrome), are outside the scope of this recommendation statement." [118].

There is, however, emerging evidence that screening for melanoma may reduce mortality. In Northern Germany, screening was offered to all residents in the state of Schleswig-Holstein at the hands of dermatologists and specially trained primary care physicians [119, 120]. These screening exams were offered for 1 year and with only 19% of the population participating, at 5 years, melanoma mortality rates were decreased by nearly 50%; 90% of melanomas detected were <1 mm. There was no change in melanoma mortality to the nearby unscreened populations to the north, south, east, or west. Based on these findings, Germany has initiated a national screening program for all adults ages 35 and older although results are not yet available. A melanoma screening effort in the US at the Lawrence Livermore National Laboratory from 1984 to 1996 demonstrated an increase in *in situ* lesions and decrease in thick lesions (>0.75 mm). Most importantly, mortality was reduced [121].

Further studies have shown that melanoma, when found by a physician (as opposed to the patient or family member) is thinner [122–124] and that having had a recent clinical exam reduces risk of thick melanoma [125]. Moreover, patients who conduct skin self-examination are likely to have thinner melanoma than those who do not [126]. Technique for proper skin self-examination can be found on the ACS website [127]. While the skin exam itself is fast and well-tolerated by the patient, there is potential cost and morbidity associated with increased skin biopsies, overdiagnosis, and skin surgeries.

Higher Risk Populations

The US Preventive Services Taskforce (USPSTF) notes that it "did not examine the outcomes related to surveillance of patients at extremely high risk, such as those with familial syndromes" and that clinicians should be aware that those with fair skin, men and women older than 65, patients with atypical moles, more than 50 moles, family history, or considerable past sun exposure are "groups at substantially increased risk for melanoma". [118]. While there are no USPSTF recommendations for these individuals, the AAD recommends self-examination and regular checkups for any individuals who have [128]:

- A close blood relative who has/had melanoma, several more distant relatives who have a history of melanoma, or a family history of other skin cancers
- A personal history of skin cancer
- A history of exposure to ultraviolet (UV) rays from the sun, tanning beds, or sun lamps – whether intermittent or year round, even if the exposure was years ago
- Experienced severe, especially blistering, sunburns
- Fair skin, especially when the person has blond or red hair and blue, green, or gray eyes
- Skin that is sun sensitive, or tends to burn and freckle rather than tan
- Large, asymmetrical, or unusual-looking mole(s)

- Fifty-plus moles
- A history of X-ray treatments for acne
- A history of taking immunosuppressive medications for severe arthritis or to prevent organ rejection.

Furthermore, as it has become evident that those older than 65, especially men, and those of lower socioeconomic class and lower healthcare access are bearing a disproportionate share of advanced melanoma disease in the US, there has been a recent call for focused education and targeted outreach for these groups [129].

Conclusion

Collectively, skin cancer diagnoses exceed those of all other cancers combined. The three predominant subtypes are BCC, SCC, and melanoma. For all three skin cancers, exposure to UVR, through sunlight or artificial sources (i.e. tanning beds) is the avoidable cause and prevention of these cancers is predicated upon proper sun exposure behaviors. Individuals with fair skin, a history of sunburns or tanning bed use, numerous nevi, prolonged immunosuppression or a family history of melanoma appear at greatest risk for skin cancers and therefore would likely benefit from screening as early identification of suspicious skin lesions may be life-saving.

References

1 ACS. Cancer Facts and Figures. Atlanta: American Cancer Society, 2017. Available from: https://www.cancer.org/content/dam/cancer-org/research/cancer-facts-and-statistics/annual-cancer-facts-and-figures/2017/cancer-facts-and-figures-2017.pdf (accessed 23 May 2017).

2 Siegel RL, Miller KD, Jemal A. Cancer statistics, 2017. *CA Cancer J Clin* 2017;67(1):7–30.

3 Jemal A, Saraiya M, Patel P, *et al*. Recent trends in cutaneous melanoma incidence and death rates in the United States, 1992–2006. *J Am Acad Dermatol* 2011;65(5 Suppl 1):S17–25 e1–3.

4 Howlader N, Noone AM, Krapcho M, *et al*. (eds). SEER Cancer Statistics Review, 1975–2013, National Cancer Institute. Bethesda, MD. http://seer.cancer.gov/csr/1975_2013/, based on November 2015 SEER data submission, posted to the SEER website, April 2016. Accessed 23 May 2016.

5 Karia PS, Han J, Schmults CD. Cutaneous squamous cell carcinoma: estimated incidence of disease, nodal metastasis, and deaths from disease in the United States, 2012. *J Am Acad Dermatol* 2013;68(6):957–66.

6 Osterlind A, Hjalgrim H, Kulinsky B, Frentz G. Skin cancer as a cause of death in Denmark. *Br J Dermatol* 1991;125(6):580–2.

7 Linos E, Swetter SM, Cockburn MG, Colditz GA, Clarke CA. Increasing burden of melanoma in the United States. *J Invest Dermatol* 2009;129(7):1666–74.

8 Parkin DM, Pisani P, Ferlay J. Estimates of the worldwide incidence of 25 major cancers in 1990. *Int J Cancer* 1999;80(6):827–41.

9 Ferlay J, Shin HR, Bray F, *et al*. Estimates of worldwide burden of cancer in 2008: GLOBOCAN 2008. *Int J Cancer* 2010;127(12):2893–917.

10 Alam M, Ratner D. Cutaneous squamous-cell carcinoma. *N Engl J Med* 2001;344(13):975–83.

11 Rogers HW, Weinstock MA, Harris AR, *et al*. Incidence estimate of nonmelanoma skin cancer in the United States, 2006. *Arch Dermatol* 2010;146(3):283–7.

12 Bickers DR, Lim HW, Margolis D, *et al*. The burden of skin diseases: 2004 a joint project of the American Academy of Dermatology Association and the Society for Investigative Dermatology. *J Am Acad Dermatol* 2006;55(3):490–500.

13 Lomas A, Leonardi-Bee J, Bath-Hextall F. A systematic review of worldwide incidence of nonmelanoma skin cancer. *Br J Dermatol* 2012;166(5):1069–80.

14 Christenson LJ, Borrowman TA, Vachon CM, *et al*. Incidence of basal cell and squamous cell carcinomas in a population younger than 40 years. *JAMA* 2005;294(6):681–90.

15 Harris RB, Griffith K, Moon TE. Trends in the incidence of nonmelanoma skin cancers in southeastern Arizona, 1985–1996. *J Am Acad Dermatol* 2001;45(4):528–36.

16 Karagas MR, Greenberg ER, Spencer SK, Stukel TA, Mott LA. Increase in incidence rates of basal cell and squamous cell skin cancer in New Hampshire, USA. New Hampshire Skin Cancer Study Group. *Int J Cancer* 1999;81(4):555–9.

17 Hannuksela-Svahn A, Pukkala E, Karvonen J. Basal cell skin carcinoma and other nonmelanoma skin cancers in Finland from 1956 through 1995. *Arch Dermatol* 1999;135(7):781–6.

18 Chuang TY, Popescu A, Su WP, Chute CG. Basal cell carcinoma. A population-based incidence study in Rochester, Minnesota. *J Am Acad Dermatol* 1990;22(3):413–17.

19 Erdmann F, Lortet-Tieulent J, Schuz J, *et al*. International trends in the incidence of malignant melanoma

1953–2008 – are recent generations at higher or lower risk? *Int J Cancer* 2013;132(2):385–400.

20 Gallagher RP, Hill GB, Bajdik CD, *et al.* Sunlight exposure, pigmentation factors, and risk of nonmelanocytic skin cancer. II. Squamous cell carcinoma. *Arch Dermatol* 1995;131(2): 164–9.

21 Rubin AI, Chen EH, Ratner D. Basal-cell carcinoma. *N Engl J Med* 2005;353(21):2262–9.

22 Elwood JM, Jopson J. Melanoma and sun exposure: an overview of published studies. *Int J Cancer* 1997;73(2):198–203.

23 Oliveria SA, Saraiya M, Geller AC, Heneghan MK, Jorgensen C. Sun exposure and risk of melanoma. *Arch Dis Child* 2006;91(2):131–8.

24 Ferrucci LM, Cartmel B, Molinaro AM, *et al.* Indoor tanning and risk of early-onset basal cell carcinoma. *J Am Acad Dermatol* 2012;67(4):552–62.

25 Cust AE, Jenkins MA, Goumas C, *et al.* Early-life sun exposure and risk of melanoma before age 40 years. *Cancer Causes Control* 2011;22(6):885–97.

26 Macbeth AE, Grindlay DJ, Williams HC. What's new in skin cancer? An analysis of guidelines and systematic reviews published in 2008–2009. *Clin Exp Dermatol* 2011;36(5):453–8.

27 Kricker A, Armstrong BK, Goumas C, *et al.* Ambient UV, personal sun exposure and risk of multiple primary melanomas. *Cancer Causes Control* 2007;18(3):295–304.

28 Ulrich C, Jurgensen JS, Degen A, *et al.* Prevention of non-melanoma skin cancer in organ transplant patients by regular use of a sunscreen: a 24 months, prospective, case-control study. *Br J Dermatol* 2009;161 Suppl 3:78–84.

29 El Ghissassi F, Baan R, Straif K, *et al.* A review of human carcinogens – part D: radiation. *Lancet Oncol* 2009;10(8):751–2.

30 IARC Working Group on Artificial Ultraviolet Light and Skin Cancer. The association of use of sunbeds with cutaneous malignant melanoma and other skin cancers: a systematic review. *Int J Cancer* 2007;120(5):1116–22.

31 Lazovich D, Vogel RI, Berwick M, *et al.* Indoor tanning and risk of melanoma: a case-control study in a highly exposed population. *Cancer Epidemiol Biomarkers Prev* 2010; 19(6):1557–68.

32 Cust AE, Armstrong BK, Goumas C, *et al.* Sunbed use during adolescence and early adulthood is associated with increased risk of early-onset melanoma. *Int J Cancer* 2011;128(10): 2425–35.

33 Hery C, Tryggvadottir L, Sigurdsson T, *et al.* A melanoma epidemic in Iceland: possible influence of sunbed use. *Am J Epidemiol* 2010;172(7):762–7.

34 Karagas MR, Stannard VA, Mott LA, *et al.* Use of tanning devices and risk of basal cell and squamous cell skin cancers. *J Natl Cancer Inst* 2002;94(3):224–6.

35 Zhang M, Qureshi AA, Geller AC, *et al.* Use of tanning beds and incidence of skin cancer. *J Clin Oncol* 2012;30(14):1588–93.

36 Lim HW, James WD, Rigel DS, *et al.* Adverse effects of ultraviolet radiation from the use of indoor tanning equipment: time to ban the tan. *J Am Acad Dermatol* 2011;64(5):893–902.

37 Agar NS, Halliday GM, Barnetson RS, *et al.* The basal layer in human squamous tumors harbors more UVA than UVB fingerprint mutations: a role for UVA in human skin carcinogenesis. *Proc Natl Acad Sci USA* 2004;101(14):4954–9.

38 Hussein MR. Ultraviolet radiation and skin cancer: molecular mechanisms. *J Cutan Pathol* 2005;32(3):191–205.

39 Buckman SY, Gresham A, Hale P, *et al.* COX-2 expression is induced by UVB exposure in human skin: implications for the development of skin cancer. *Carcinogenesis* 1998;19(5):723–9.

40 Stern RS. The risk of melanoma in association with long-term exposure to PUVA. *J Am Acad Dermatol* 2001;44(5):755–61.

41 Stern RS, Liebman EJ, Vakeva L. Oral psoralen and ultraviolet-A light (PUVA) treatment of psoriasis and persistent risk of nonmelanoma skin cancer. PUVA Follow-up Study. *J Natl Cancer Inst* 1998;90(17):1278–84.

42 Cho E, Rosner BA, Feskanich D, Colditz GA. Risk factors and individual probabilities of melanoma for whites. *J Clin Oncol* 2005;23(12):2669–75.

43 Zanetti R, Rosso S, Martinez C, *et al.* The multicentre south European study 'Helios'. I: Skin characteristics and sunburns in basal cell and squamous cell carcinomas of the skin. *Br J Cancer* 1996;73(11):1440–6.

44 Grodstein F, Speizer FE, Hunter DJ. A prospective study of incident squamous cell carcinoma of the skin in the nurses' health study. *J Natl Cancer Inst* 1995;87(14):1061–6.

45 Olsen CM, Carroll HJ, Whiteman DC. Estimating the attributable fraction for melanoma: a meta-analysis of pigmentary characteristics and freckling. *Int J Cancer* 2010;127(10):2430–45.

46 Gray DT, Suman VJ, Su WP, *et al.* Trends in the population-based incidence of squamous cell carcinoma of the skin first diagnosed between 1984 and 1992. *Arch Dermatol* 1997;133(6):735–40.

47 Scotto J, Fears, TR, Fraumeni Jr, JF, *et al.* Incidence of nonmelanoma skin cancer in the United States in collaboration with Fred Hutchinson Cancer Research Center. NIH publication No 83–2433, US Department of Health and Human Services, Public Health Service, National Institutes of Health, National Cancer Institute, Besthesda, MD, 1983; xv:113.

48 Purdue MP, From L, Armstrong BK, *et al.* Etiologic and other factors predicting nevus-associated cutaneous malignant melanoma. *Cancer Epidemiol Biomarkers Prev* 2005;14(8):2015–22.

49 Harrison SL, MacLennan R, Speare R, Wronski I. Sun exposure and melanocytic naevi in young Australian children. *Lancet* 1994;344(8936):1529–32.

50 Olsen CM, Carroll HJ, Whiteman DC. Estimating the attributable fraction for cancer: a meta-analysis of nevi and melanoma. *Cancer Prev Res (Phila)* 2010;3(2):233–45.

51 Bataille V, Bishop JA, Sasieni P, *et al.* Risk of cutaneous melanoma in relation to the numbers, types and sites of naevi: a case-control study. *Br J Cancer* 1996;73(12):1605–11.

52 Gandini S, Sera F, Cattaruzza MS, *et al.* Meta-analysis of risk factors for cutaneous melanoma: I. Common and atypical naevi. *Eur J Cancer* 2005;41(1):28–44.

53 Gandini S, Sera F, Cattaruzza MS, *et al.* Meta-analysis of risk factors for cutaneous melanoma: III. Family history, actinic damage and phenotypic factors. *Eur J Cancer* 2005;41(14):2040–59.

54 Olsen CM, Carroll HJ, Whiteman DC. Familial melanoma: a meta-analysis and estimates of attributable fraction. *Cancer Epidemiol Biomarkers Prev* 2010;19(1):65–73.

55 Chatzinasiou F, Lill CM, Kypreou K, *et al*. Comprehensive field synopsis and systematic meta-analyses of genetic association studies in cutaneous melanoma. *J Natl Cancer Inst* 2011;103(16):1227–35.

56 Goldstein AM, Chan M, Harland M, *et al*. Features associated with germline CDKN2A mutations: a GenoMEL study of melanoma-prone families from three continents. *J Med Genet* 2007;44(2):99–106.

57 Siskind V, Hughes MC, Palmer JM, *et al*. Nevi, family history, and fair skin increase the risk of second primary melanoma. *J Invest Dermatol* 2011;131(2):461–7.

58 Hussain SK, Sundquist J, Hemminki K. The effect of having an affected parent or sibling on invasive and in situ skin cancer risk in Sweden. *J Invest Dermatol* 2009;129(9):2142–7.

59 Stacey SN, Sulem P, Jonasdottir A, *et al*. A germline variant in the TP53 polyadenylation signal confers cancer susceptibility. *Nat Genet* 2011;43(11):1098–103.

60 Zhang M, Liang L, Morar N, *et al*. Integrating pathway analysis and genetics of gene expression for genome-wide association study of basal cell carcinoma. *Hum Genet* 2012;131(4):615–23.

61 Karagas MR, Stukel TA, Greenberg ER, *et al*. Risk of subsequent basal cell carcinoma and squamous cell carcinoma of the skin among patients with prior skin cancer. *Skin Cancer Prevention Study Group. JAMA* 1992;267(24):3305–10.

62 Robinson JK. Risk of developing another basal cell carcinoma. A 5-year prospective study. *Cancer* 1987;60(1):118–20.

63 Dyer R, Weinstock M, Cohen T, Rizzo A, Bingham S. Predictors of basal cell carcinoma in high risk patients in the VATTC (VA Topical Tretinoin Chemoprevention) Trial. *J Invest Dermatol* 2012;132(11):2544–51.

64 Ferrone CR, Ben Porat L, Panageas KS, *et al*. Clinicopathological features of and risk factors for multiple primary melanomas. *JAMA* 2005;294(13):1647–54.

65 Goggins WB, Tsao H. A population-based analysis of risk factors for a second primary cutaneous melanoma among melanoma survivors. *Cancer* 2003;97(3):639–43.

66 Marghoob AA, Slade J, Salopek TG, *et al*. Basal cell and squamous cell carcinomas are important risk factors for cutaneous malignant melanoma. *Screening implications. Cancer* 1995;75(2 Suppl):707–14.

67 Kahn HS, Tatham LM, Patel AV, Thun MJ, Heath CW, Jr. Increased cancer mortality following a history of nonmelanoma skin cancer. *JAMA* 1998;280(10):910–2.

68 Zwald FO, Brown M. Skin cancer in solid organ transplant recipients: advances in therapy and management: part I. Epidemiology of skin cancer in solid organ transplant recipients. *J Am Acad Dermatol* 2011;65(2):253–61.

69 Berg D, Otley CC. Skin cancer in organ transplant recipients: epidemiology, pathogenesis, and management. *J Am Acad Dermatol* 2002;47(1):1–17.

70 Gloster HM, Jr, Neal K. Skin cancer in skin of color. *J Am Acad Dermatol* 2006;55(5):741–60.

71 Fine JD, Johnson LB, Weiner M, Li KP, Suchindran C. Epidermolysis bullosa and the risk of life-threatening cancers: the National EB Registry experience, 1986–2006. *J Am Acad Dermatol* 2009;60(2):203–11.

72 DiGiovanna JJ, Kraemer KH. Shining a light on xeroderma pigmentosum. *J Invest Dermatol* 2012;132(3 Pt 2):785–96.

73 Schulze KE, Rapini RP, Duvic M. Malignant melanoma in oculocutaneous albinism. *Arch Dermatol* 1989;125(11): 1583–6.

74 Cruz-Inigo AE, Ladizinski B, Sethi A. Albinism in Africa: stigma, slaughter and awareness campaigns. *Dermatol Clin* 2011;29(1):79–87.

75 Cowen EW, Nguyen JC, Miller DD, *et al*. Chronic phototoxicity and aggressive squamous cell carcinoma of the skin in children and adults during treatment with voriconazole. *J Am Acad Dermatol* 2010;62(1):31–7.

76 Miller DD, Cowen EW, Nguyen JC, McCalmont TH, Fox LP. Melanoma associated with long-term voriconazole therapy: a new manifestation of chronic photosensitivity. *Arch Dermatol* 2010;146(3):300–4.

77 American Cancer Society. *Cancer Prevention & Early Detection Facts & Figures 2015–2016*. Atlanta: American Cancer Society, 2015. http://www.cancer.org/acs/groups/content/@research/documents/webcontent/acspc-045101.pdf (accessed 23 May 2017).

78 Tripp MK, Watson M, Balk SJ, Swetter SM, Gershenwald JE. State of the science on prevention and screening to reduce melanoma incidence and mortality: the time is now. *CA Cancer J Clin* 2016;66(6):460–80.

79 NCSL. *Indoor Tanning Restrictions for Minors: A State-by-State Comparison*. Washington, DC: National Conference of State Legislation; 2012. Available from: http://www.ncsl.org/research/health/indoor-tanning-restrictions.aspx (accessed 23 May 2107).

80 NFSCP. Skin Cancer Prevention. National Council on Skin Cancer Prevention 2012. Available from: http://www.skincancerprevention.org/skin-cancer/prevention-tips (accessed 23 May 2017).

81 ARPANSA. About Ultraviolet Protection Factor Testing. Australian Radiation Protection and Nuclear Safety Agency 2012. Available from: www.arpansa.gov.au/services/upf/index.cfm (accessed 23 May 2017).

82 Lee TK, Rivers JK, Gallagher RP. Site-specific protective effect of broad-spectrum sunscreen on nevus development among white schoolchildren in a randomized trial. *J Am Acad Dermatol* 2005;52(5):786–92.

83 Thompson SC, Jolley D, Marks R. Reduction of solar keratoses by regular sunscreen use. *N Engl J Med* 1993;329(16):1147–51.

84 Green AC, Williams GM, Logan V, Strutton GM. Reduced melanoma after regular sunscreen use: randomized trial follow-up. *J Clin Oncol* 2011;29(3):257–63.

85 van der Pols JC, Williams GM, Pandeya N, Logan V, Green AC. Prolonged prevention of squamous cell carcinoma of the skin by regular sunscreen use. *Cancer Epidemiol Biomarkers Prev* 2006;15(12):2546–8.

86 Gallagher RP, Rivers JK, Lee TK, *et al*. Broad-spectrum sunscreen use and the development of new nevi in white children: a randomized controlled trial. *JAMA* 2000;283(22):2955–60.

87 English DR, Milne E, Jacoby P, *et al*. The effect of a school-based sun protection intervention on the development of melanocytic nevi in children: 6-year follow-up. *Cancer Epidemiol Biomarkers Prev* 2005;14(4):977–80.

88 Bauer J, Buttner P, Wiecker TS, Luther H, Garbe C. Effect of sunscreen and clothing on the number of melanocytic nevi in 1,812 German children attending day care. *Am J Epidemiol* 2005;161(7):620–7.

89 AAD. Sunscreens. American Academy of Dermatology, 2012. Available from: https://www.aad.org/media/stats/prevention-and-care/sunscreen-faqs (accessed 21 August 2017).

90 Neale R, Williams G, Green A. Application patterns among participants randomized to daily sunscreen use in a skin cancer prevention trial. *Arch Dermatol* 2002;138(10): 1319–25.

91 AAD. Vitamin D Position Statement. American Academy of Dermatology, 2012. Available from: https://www.aad.org/media/stats/prevention-and-care/vitamin-d-and-uv-exposure (accessed 21 August 2017).

92 Moon TE, Levine N, Cartmel B, *et al*. Effect of retinol in preventing squamous cell skin cancer in moderate-risk subjects: a randomized, double-blind, controlled trial. Southwest Skin Cancer Prevention Study Group. *Cancer Epidemiol Biomarkers Prev* 1997;6(11):949–56.

93 Nijsten TE, Stern RS. Oral retinoid use reduces cutaneous squamous cell carcinoma risk in patients with psoriasis treated with psoralen-UVA: a nested cohort study. *J Am Acad Dermatol* 2003;49(4):644–50.

94 Kraemer KH, DiGiovanna JJ, Moshell AN, Tarone RE, Peck GL. Prevention of skin cancer in xeroderma pigmentosum with the use of oral isotretinoin. *N Engl J Med* 1988;318 (25):1633–7.

95 George R, Weightman W, Russ GR, Bannister KM, Mathew TH. Acitretin for chemoprevention of non-melanoma skin cancers in renal transplant recipients. *Australas J Dermatol* 2002;43(4):269–73.

96 Bavinck JN, Tieben LM, Van der Woude FJ, *et al*. Prevention of skin cancer and reduction of keratotic skin lesions during acitretin therapy in renal transplant recipients: a double-blind, placebo-controlled study. *J Clin Oncol* 1995;13(8):1933–8.

97 de Sevaux RG, Smit JV, de Jong EM, van de Kerkhof PC, Hoitsma AJ. Acitretin treatment of premalignant and malignant skin disorders in renal transplant recipients: clinical effects of a randomized trial comparing two doses of acitretin. *J Am Acad Dermatol* 2003;49(3):407–12.

98 Weinstock MA, Bingham SF, Digiovanna JJ, *et al*. Tretinoin and the prevention of keratinocyte carcinoma (Basal and squamous cell carcinoma of the skin): a veterans affairs randomized chemoprevention trial. *J Invest Dermatol* 2012;132(6):1583–90.

99 Elmets CA, Viner JL, Pentland AP, *et al*. Chemoprevention of nonmelanoma skin cancer with celecoxib: a randomized, double-blind, placebo-controlled trial. *J Natl Cancer Inst* 2010;102(24):1835–44.

100 Johannesdottir SA, Chang ET, Mehnert F, *et al*. Nonsteroidal anti-inflammatory drugs and the risk of skin cancer: a population-based case-control study. *Cancer* 2012;118 (19):4768–76.

101 Asgari MM, Chren MM, Warton EM, Friedman GD, White E. Association between nonsteroidal anti-inflammatory drug use and cutaneous squamous cell carcinoma. *Arch Dermatol* 2010;146(4):388–95.

102 Butler GJ, Neale R, Green AC, Pandeya N, Whiteman DC. Nonsteroidal anti-inflammatory drugs and the risk of actinic keratoses and squamous cell cancers of the skin. *J Am Acad Dermatol* 2005;53(6):966–72.

103 Christian JB, Lapane KL, Hume AL, Eaton CB, Weinstock MA. Association of ACE inhibitors and angiotensin receptor blockers with keratinocyte cancer prevention in the randomized VATTC trial. *J Natl Cancer Inst* 2008;100 (17):1223–32.

104 Moscarelli L, Zanazzi M, Mancini G, *et al*. Keratinocyte cancer prevention with ACE inhibitors, angiotensin receptor blockers or their combination in renal transplant recipients. *Clin Nephrol* 2010;73(6):439–45.

105 Dellavalle R, Drake A, Graber M, *et al*. Statins and fibrates for preventing melanoma. Cochrane Database of Systematic Reviews 2005(4):Art. No.: CD003697.

106 Freeman SR, Drake AL, Heilig LF, *et al*. Statins, fibrates, and melanoma risk: a systematic review and meta-analysis. *J Natl Cancer Inst* 2006;98(21):1538–46.

107 Bonovas S, Nikolopoulos G, Filioussi K, *et al*. Can statin therapy reduce the risk of melanoma? A meta-analysis of randomized controlled trials. *Eur J Epidemiol* 2010;25(1):29–35.

108 Curiel-Lewandrowski C, Nijsten T, Gomez ML, *et al*. Long-term use of nonsteroidal anti-inflammatory drugs decreases the risk of cutaneous melanoma: results of a United States case-control study. *J Invest Dermatol* 2011;131(7):1460–8.

109 Joosse A, Koomen ER, Casparie MK, *et al*. Non-steroidal anti-inflammatory drugs and melanoma risk: large Dutch population-based case-control study. *J Invest Dermatol* 2009;129(11):2620–7.

110 Asgari MM, Maruti SS, White E. A large cohort study of nonsteroidal anti-inflammatory drug use and melanoma incidence. *J Natl Cancer Inst* 2008;100(13):967–71.

111 Cook NR, Lee IM, Gaziano JM, *et al*. Low-dose aspirin in the primary prevention of cancer: the Women's Health Study: a randomized controlled trial. *JAMA* 2005;294(1):47–55.

112 Jacobs EJ, Thun MJ, Bain EB, *et al*. A large cohort study of long-term daily use of adult-strength aspirin and cancer incidence. *J Natl Cancer Inst* 2007;99(8):608–15.

113 Reichrath J, Rech M, Moeini M, *et al*. In vitro comparison of the vitamin D endocrine system in 1,25(OH)2D3-responsive and -resistant melanoma cells. *Cancer Biol Ther* 2007; 6(1):48–55.

114 Asgari MM, Maruti SS, Kushi LH, White E. A cohort study of vitamin D intake and melanoma risk. *J Invest Dermatol* 2009;129(7):1675–80.

115 Millen AE, Tucker MA, Hartge P, *et al*. Diet and melanoma in a case-control study. *Cancer Epidemiol Biomarkers Prev* 2004;13(6):1042–51.

116 Tang JY, Fu T, Leblanc E, *et al*. Calcium plus vitamin D supplementation and the risk of nonmelanoma and melanoma skin cancer: post hoc analyses of the women's health initiative randomized controlled trial. *J Clin Oncol* 2011;29(22):3078–84.

117 Wolff T, Tai E, Miller T. Screening for skin cancer: an update of the evidence for the U.S. Preventive Services Task Force. *Ann Intern Med* 2009;150(3):194–8.

118 USPSTF. Screening for Skin Cancer. U.S. Preventive Services Task Force, 2016. Available from: https://www.uspreventiveservicestaskforce.org/Page/Document/RecommendationStatementFinal/skin-cancer-screening2 (accessed 21 August 2017).

119 Breitbart EW, Waldmann A, Nolte S, *et al*. Systematic skin cancer screening in Northern Germany. *J Am Acad Dermatol* 2012;66(2):201–11.

120 Katalinic A, Waldmann A, Weinstock MA, *et al*. Does skin cancer screening save lives?: an observational study comparing trends in melanoma mortality in regions with and without screening. *Cancer* 2012;118(21): 5395–402.

121 Schneider JS, Moore DH, 2nd, Mendelsohn ML. Screening program reduced melanoma mortality at the Lawrence Livermore National Laboratory, 1984 to 1996. *J Am Acad Dermatol* 2008;58(5):741–9.

122 Terushkin V, Halpern AC. Melanoma early detection. *Hematol Oncol Clin North Am* 2009;23(3):481–500.

123 Geller AC, Johnson TM, Miller DR, *et al*. Factors associated with physician discovery of early melanoma in middle-aged and older men. *Arch Dermatol* 2009;145(4):409–14.

124 Schwartz JL, Wang TS, Hamilton TA, *et al*. Thin primary cutaneous melanomas: associated detection patterns, lesion characteristics, and patient characteristics. *Cancer* 2002;95(7):1562–8.

125 Aitken JF, Elwood M, Baade PD, Youl P, English D. Clinical whole-body skin examination reduces the incidence of thick melanomas. *Int J Cancer* 2010;126(2):450–8.

126 Carli P, De Giorgi V, Palli D, *et al*. Dermatologist detection and skin self-examination are associated with thinner melanomas: results from a survey of the Italian Multidisciplinary Group on Melanoma. *Arch Dermatol* 2003;139(5):607–12.

127 ACS. Skin Cancer Prevention and Early Detection: Skin Exams, 2012. Available from: http://www.cancer.org/Cancer/CancerCauses/SunandUVExposure/SkinCancerPreventionandEarlyDetection/skin-cancer-prevention-and-early-detection-skin-exams (accessed 23 May 2017).

128 AAD. When to see a dermatologist. American Academy of Dermatology: Skin CancerNet, 2012 Available from: http://www.skincarephysicians.com/skincancernet/whentosee.html.

129 Geller AC, Swetter SM, Oliveria S, Dusza S, Halpern AC. Reducing mortality in individuals at high risk for advanced melanoma through education and screening. *J Am Acad Dermatol* 2011;65(5 Suppl 1):S87–94.

11

Screening and Early Detection

Robert A. Smith, Otis W. Brawley, and Richard C. Wender

American Cancer Society, Atlanta, Georgia, USA

Introduction

A common feature of many cancers is that outcomes generally are more favorable when treatment is initiated early in the disease's natural history. This observation has motivated researchers and clinicians to develop screening technologies to detect occult disease, and organizations to issue guidelines and recommendations related to screening. Today, the health systems of most developed nations and many developing nations support screening the population for one or more of the common cancers. Cancer screening is defined as testing to detect presymptomatic disease in a population to reduce the incidence rate of advanced disease and initiate treatment earlier. For some cancers, detecting and treating precursor lesions also is a goal, thus also contributing to reduced morbidity and mortality through reductions in the incidence of invasive disease.

The Decision to Screen – Key Criteria

The observation that treatment of early stage disease is associated with improved survival is not sufficient evidence of the benefit of screening. Although such observations are commonly the first evidence that screening could reduce the risk of cancer death, aside from being an untrustworthy proxy for reduced disease-specific mortality, other factors must be considered, including the burden of disease, understanding the natural history of the disease, the characteristics of the screening test, the balance of benefits and harms experienced by adults undergoing screening, the cost and acceptability of screening, and the values of the target population [1, 2]. These criteria were outlined in 1968 (Table 11.1) [3]. Although each criterion is important, there are no consensus thresholds alone or in combination that policy makers can look to when making decisions about whether to invite the population to screening. Thus, not only does a health system's decision to offer screening require considering these criteria collectively and making a judgment,

but national systems and organizations examining the same data may differ in their judgment about the value of screening overall, or how it is applied in the population [1, 2, 4].

Disease Burden

Cancers that are associated with significant mortality, morbidity, or both, are potentially suitable for screening. Cancers with lower overall disease burden may become candidates for screening if a subgroup of the population at higher risk can be identified. Because the incidence of cancer increases as adults gets older, examination of the age-incidence curve can reveal an age-specific incidence rate of invasive disease or precursor lesions in average or high risk individuals that be judged to be sufficiently high to begin screening. Consideration should also be given to an age or overall health status when screening is no longer likely to be beneficial.

Characteristics of the Disease

If a disease is judged to be sufficiently important to be considered for screening, it also is necessary to understand its age–incidence curve, disease latency period, the period within the latency period when it is detectable, and the period within which treatment before the onset of clinically apparent disease has a prognostic advantage compared with treatment after the disease is symptomatic.

The Detectable Preclinical Phase and Lead Time

The screening interval must be set to ensure that most cancers will be detected at an early stage in a population undergoing screening. While most cancers have a long preclinical phase, generally it is late in the preclinical phase, but before the onset of symptoms, that an invasive cancer may become detectable by a screening test. This detectable preclinical phase, also referred to as the tumor *sojourn time*, is the estimated duration of time during which an occult tumor can be detected by a screening test before the onset of symptoms [5]. The duration of time

The American Cancer Society's Principles of Oncology: Prevention to Survivorship, First Edition. Edited by The American Cancer Society.
© 2018 The American Cancer Society. Published 2018 by John Wiley & Sons, Inc.

Table 11.1 Key factors in the decision to introduce screening.

Disease burden: the disease should be an important health problem, as measured by morbidity, mortality, and other measures of disease burden.

The natural history of the disease: the disease should have a detectable preclinical phase, and the length of this phase should be known in order to set the screening intervals.

Effectiveness of treatment: treatment of disease detected before the onset of symptoms should offer benefits compared with treatment after the onset of symptoms.

Effectiveness of the screening test: the screening test should meet acceptable levels of accuracy and cost.

Acceptability: the screening test and follow-up requirements should be acceptable to individuals at risk and to their healthcare providers.

Benefits versus harms: there should be clear evidence that the potential benefits of screening outweigh the potential harms.

within the sojourn time that detection by screening advances the time of diagnosis is known as the *lead time*. For screening to be successful, the screening interval should be shorter than the mean sojourn time to ensure that the schedule of periodic screening provides the opportunity to detect most disease in the target population *before* the onset of symptoms. When the screening interval equals or exceeds the mean sojourn time, too many cancers will be detected clinically after symptoms develop. Tailoring the screening interval to the sojourn time also discourages screening too frequently, which is wasteful of resources and will increase the rate of false positive findings. The interrelationship between the sojourn time and the lead time is shown in Figure 11.1.

For some cancers the age to begin screening and the screening interval also may be influenced by the prevalence of precursor lesions, which if identified and treated may prevent progression to invasive disease. For example, the most likely abnormal finding resulting from screening for cervix cancer and colon cancer are precancerous lesions; these lesions have long preclinical phases before some of these abnormalities develop into invasive and eventually symptomatic cancers.

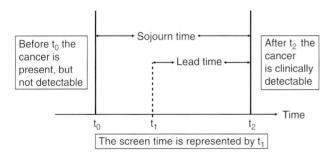

Figure 11.1 The relationship between sojourn time and lead time in cancer screening. The cancer is asymptomatic, but detectable by screening, i.e., the *sojourn time* ($t_0 – t_2$). Lead time gained = ($t_2 – t_1$).

The Benefit of Early Treatment

Treatment of screen-detected cancers or precursor lesions should offer clear advantages compared with treatment of symptomatic disease. These advantages principally are measured by a lower disease-specific mortality rate, but also may be

measured by other outcomes or combinations of outcomes, including reduced incidence, reduced morbidity associated with therapy, and improved quality of life.

Efficacy and Effectiveness

Although reports of better outcomes when cancer is detected in asymptomatic individuals suggest the potential benefit for screening, the validation of the efficacy of a screening test must be established with an experimental study, that is, a prospective randomized controlled trial (RCT). Evaluations of screening tests using nonexperimental designs prior to the establishment of efficacy with an RCT generally are not acceptable as a basis for policy since nonexperimental study designs are subject to biases that may invalidate the appearance of benefit, such as lead-time and length biases, overdiagnosis, and self-selection bias.

Threats to Validity in the Evaluation of Screening

Lead time Bias

The point within the sojourn time when the cancer is detected by screening is known as the lead time, and gaining lead time by advancing the time of diagnosis before symptoms develop is the purpose of screening. However, comparisons of survival rates in screened and unscreened populations may be misleading because lead time advances the point at which survival begins to be measured. Thus, it is possible that screening only moves forward the timing of the patient's diagnosis without affecting the time of death (see Figure 11.2).

Length Bias

Because of variations in tumor growth rates, a greater proportion of the cancers detected by screening will have longer sojourn times. A tumor with a longer sojourn time may also be less aggressive and less life-threatening. This bias toward detection of slower growing, potentially less-lethal cancers is referred to as *length bias* (see Figure 11.3). This form of potential bias complicates the comparison of outcomes between cancers detected by screening and those found outside the screening program because the cancers most likely to escape detection may be the very cancers that have the greatest likelihood of mortality. Thus, survival differences associated with screening simply may be due to screening being more likely to identify the cases with the lowest potential for causing death.

Overdiagnosis

An overdiagnosed cancer is one that never would have become known to the patient if she or he had not undergone screening, because (i) the cancer is nonprogressive, and thus non-life-threatening, or (ii) because the patient was destined to die from some other cause before the cancer would have caused symptoms [6]. In the first case, although some tumors may have histologic features that are associated with slow growth and favorable prognosis, there are no features that clearly distinguish a progressive cancer from a nonprogressive one. Thus, overdiagnosis of nonprogressive cancers cannot be determined in any individual case, and only can be estimated in aggregate by comparing the cumulative incidence in a screened and unscreened group after a long duration of follow-up. In the second case, overdiagnosis occurs due to advancing the time of diagnosis in a patient who dies from

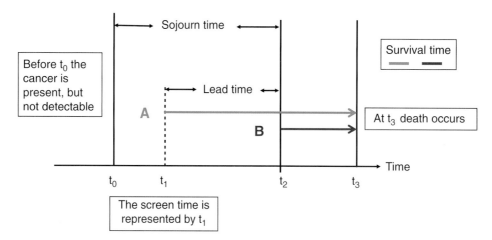

Figure 11.2 Cancer survival, lead time, and lead time bias. In this example, there are two hypothetical patients, A and B. Their cancers are undetectable before t_0; asymptomatic but detectable by screening at t_1 between t_0 and t_2; and detectable with symptoms after t_2. The lead time gained = $(t_2 - t_1)$. At t_3 death occurs for both hypothetical patients, A and B, but patient A appears to have longer survival because screening advanced the time of diagnosis.

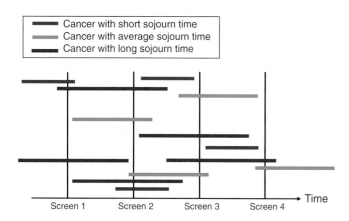

Figure 11.3 The relationship between sojourn time and length bias in cancer screening. Cancers that are intersected by the vertical lines (screening events) are screen detected, while those not intersected are missed by screening. Note that some cancers with long sojourn times are detectable at consecutive screening rounds.

another cause within what would have been the duration of sojourn time. Because screening may detect nonprogressive and nonlife threatening cancers, survival statistics for screen-detected cancers may be inflated by cancers that, by definition, posed no risk of death. While the concept of overdiagnosis generates considerable discussion as a harm of screening, estimates of overdiagnosis are highly susceptible to methodological assumptions, especially those that neglect factors that influence incidence rates in screened and unscreened populations over time.

Patient Self-Selection

In general, adults who are more likely to engage in preventive care (such as screening) are generally more health conscious (nonsmoker, etc.), more alert to the signs and symptoms of disease, more adherent to treatment, and generally healthier [7, 8]. These differences also may influence survival rates, although evidence to date suggests that this bias has only a modest influence on differences in outcomes in screened and unscreened populations [9].

Research Designs for the Evaluation of Screening

Investigators have used different approaches to study the efficacy and effectiveness of cancer screening, including various observational designs, case-control studies, and RCTs. Each of these designs has strengths and limitations, but among all study designs, measuring the efficacy of screening is best accomplished with a prospective RCT. However, RCT methodology is not in itself assurance of unbiased study findings. Indeed, some RCTs of screening have been stunning failures due to poor planning, execution, or simply bad luck. It is important to evaluate each study on the inherent strengths and weakness of its design. No single study design can provide all the answers needed for the evaluation of screening efficacy and effectiveness.

Randomized Controlled Trials

In an RCT the biasing effects of self-selection, lead-time bias, length bias, and overdiagnosis are largely overcome by random assignment to either an experimental group invited to receive screening or a control group not invited to screening [10]. Generally, the experimental group is invited to one or more rounds of screening, after which there is a period of follow-up sufficient to observe a difference in the disease-specific death rates in the invited versus control group. Likewise, a valid end-point in an RCT of a screening test that also is intended to detect precursor lesions would be the incidence rate of invasive cancer. A mortality end-point measured from randomization date is not subject to the biasing effects of lead-time, length bias, or overdiagnosis bias. However, even randomized designs cannot entirely eliminate section bias since some patients in the group invited to screening will opt not to participate but would undergo screening once the value of the test is established, and some individuals randomized to usual care may seek screening outside of the trial, and may benefit from the same intervention that is offered to the invited group. When these rates of nonadherence and contamination are excessive, outcome measures may be seriously biased.

Some have proposed that all-cause mortality is a preferable end-point in RCTs due to possible biases in assignment of cause of death in experimental and control groups [11] and it is not uncommon to see reports in the literature or systematic reviews cite the effect of a screening test on both disease-specific and all-cause mortality, as if the latter was a superior indicator of efficacy due to the elimination of all possible bias. It is not. An emphasis on all-cause mortality is both overcautious and impractical for several reasons. First, cause-of-death committees routinely build safeguards into the process of death ascertainment, such as blind review, so that assignment to the invited versus control group is unknown, as well as a blinded consensus process that referees disputes about the underlying cause of death between multiple reviewers. Although some level of misallocation may occur, there is little evidence that the rate of error approaches a level that would measurably bias the determination of outcomes [12]. Second, there is little reason to expect a single intervention designed to contribute to reduced mortality from one cause to reduce mortality from all causes. The goal of specific preventive health measures is to prevent premature death from one or several related causes. Third, all-cause mortality is an inefficient end-point, especially when the cancer in question represents a small percentage of overall mortality (as is the case for any single cause of death), and thus, achieving a statistically significant difference in all-cause mortality would require study sizes that dwarf the already very large study sizes required for RCTs of screening [13]. That said, one aspect of all-cause mortality that is relevant for investigation in the follow-up period is whether deaths in the intervention group cluster in another cause of mortality, which may indicate an adverse effect of therapy.

An RCT of screening evaluates the effect of an invitation to screening rather than exposure to screening, that is, the end results are evaluated based on an intention-to-treat analysis to hold known and unknown biases in check. Thus, mortality rates in the invited group are compared with the control group mortality rates regardless of exposure to screening. While this may seem counterintuitive, simply evaluating end results based on exposure to screening will reintroduce the selection bias that randomization is intended to overcome. While noncompliance to the invitation to screening in the experimental group, and contamination in the control group (i.e., participation in screening outside of the trial), will influence the magnitude of the observed outcome, if nonadherence rates are modest it is an acceptable trade-off for keeping biases in check. Statistical methods have been developed to remove this bias and more closely measure the effect of exposure to screening [14], but the primary analysis always will be based on intention-to-treat. Additional consideration in the design and interpretation of RCTs to evaluate cancer screening tests include the importance of avoiding the temptation to evaluate outcomes based on age at diagnosis versus age at randomization [15]; and being aware that the duration of screening and the various options for follow-up protocols, including whether the control group is offered a single round of screening during the last screening round, will influence the magnitude of the estimate of the efficacy of screening [16].

Observational Studies

Case-Control Studies

Retrospective case-control studies can provide useful evidence on screening effectiveness. Case-control studies identify "cases" based on an outcome of interest (incidence, diagnosis of advanced disease, mortality, etc.), and compare them with "controls", who do not have that outcome, based on that exposure of interest, in this instance, exposure to screening. The advantage of this approach is that it is low-cost and can provide evidence more quickly than prospective studies when the screening procedure is already in clinical use [17]. The apparent ease and simplicity of case-control studies belies their complexity and vulnerability to bias and confounding from uncontrolled factors. When compared with RCTs, case-control studies typically show more favorable results associated with screening because a case-control study typically measures the effect of exposure (not invitation) to screening.

Trend Studies

Although examination of trends in incidence and mortality rates after the introduction of screening is intuitively appealing, trend analysis is subject to a number of biases. This approach has been especially common in the evaluation of modern mammography screening [18]. One common error is to begin the evaluation period immediately following the introduction of screening, which inherently assumes that the entire target population was immediately screened, whereas the first round of screening can often last 2–3 years. A second problem results from contamination in the postscreening period from deaths attributable to cases diagnosed prior to the introduction of screening. These deaths can have a substantial influence on mortality trends a decade or more after screening begins. Tabar *et al.* observed that as much as 50% of all breast cancer deaths within 10 years after screening is introduced are attributable to cases diagnosed before screening was introduced [19]. Third, long follow-up is necessary to observe the benefits of screening, and commonly these studies are limited by inadequate follow-up. Finally, because trend studies typically do not have data on exposure to screening, it is not possible to draw credible conclusions about the influence of screening on mortality or trends in stage at diagnosis.

Incidence-based Mortality Studies

Incidence-based mortality (IBM) studies are a form of trend study with the important distinction that the evaluation of the effects of screening are restricted to cohorts with known exposure or absence of exposure to screening. In an IBM analysis, only cases and controls diagnosed after the introduction of screening, and accordingly, only deaths from cancer in this group are included in the analysis, while cases diagnosed prior to the introduction of screening and associated deaths are censored. Further, IBM studies are able to adjust for the time required to introduce screening once a policy of inviting the public to screening is in place, and can measure both the effect of invitation and exposure to screening. IBM studies are methodologically superior to ordinary trend studies [18].

Measures of Screening Performance

A screening test should distinguish those who may have a detectable cancer from those who very likely do not. The emphasis on likelihood is based on the distinction between a screening test, which should be simple and low-cost, from the more complex and extensive additional testing and procedures that occur after an abnormal screening test result. Based on the results of the screening test, those who may have cancer then undergo more definitive testing to determine if the screening test result is a *true positive* or a *false positive*. Those with normal screening test results ultimately will be determined to have had either a *true negative* or *false negative* result. Historically, screening tests have been distinguished from diagnostic tests in this continuum, although this distinction technically is misleading. Any additional evaluation following a positive screening test should be considered part of the screening continuum since the majority of adults with positive screening tests ultimately are determined with additional testing to not have cancer, and technically none of the additional testing truly is diagnostic. A diagnostic process only occurs when a pathologist examines tissue acquired with a biopsy and renders a decision about the presence or absence of malignancy. Thus, while additional focused imaging studies following a positive mammography exam, or a colonoscopy following a positive stool blood test, can rule out the likelihood of malignancy, they should not be thought of as diagnostic, but rather as "problem-solving" examinations and part of the screening continuum.

The primary measures used to evaluate the performance of a screening test are sensitivity, specificity, positive predictive values (PPV) and negative predictive value (NPV). In addition, increasingly the absolute benefit of a screening test may be expressed in terms of the number needed to invite (NNI), which is a nebulous concept since it does not measure an outcome associated with exposure to screening [20] or more appropriately the number needed to screen (NNS) to prevent one death.

Sensitivity and Specificity

Sensitivity measures the likelihood that the test will have a positive result when applied to a person who truly has the disease. Test sensitivity is measured with the results from a single screening test, whereas program sensitivity reflects the testing at specified intervals over time (for example, an annual stool blood test over a period of several years). Test specificity is the probability of a negative result when applied to a person who does not have the disease. The conventional formulas for calculating sensitivity and specificity, PPV and NPV are shown in Table 11.2.

A certain degree of inaccuracy in screening is inevitable, although high sensitivity and high specificity are desirable. A test that has poor sensitivity will miss cancers, possibly leading to false reassurance and delays in diagnosis. A test with poor specificity will raise suspicion of disease in adults who do not have cancer, leading to further testing, anxiety, and, for some, invasive procedures. Tests that result in false positive determinations should not be described collectively as "unnecessary", since the false positive rate combines the truly necessary workups with those that might have been avoided with more accurate tests, more accurate interpretation, or better attention to quality. It is

Table 11.2 Measures of screening performance.

Screening test results	Disease status		
	Yes	No	Total
Positive	a	b	a + b
Negative	c	d	c + d
Total	a + c	b + d	

True positive results = a.
True negative results = d.
False negative results = c.
False positive results = b.
Test sensitivity = true positives/true positives + false negatives, or: a/(a + c).
Test specificity = true negatives/true negatives + false positives, or: d/(d + b).
Positive predictive value (PPV) = true positives/true positives + false positives, or: a/(a + b).
Negative predictive value (NPV) = false negatives/false negatives + true negatives, or: d/(c + d).

important to acknowledge that the inherent nondiagnostic features of a screening test mean that false positive test results are an expected cost of testing the many to find the few.

Positive and Negative Predictive Values

The PPV is the probability that a subject with a positive screening result actually has the disease. The NPV is the probability that an individual with a negative screening test result truly is disease free. The NPV is a quantification of the reassurance value of a negative test. While sensitivity and specificity are properties of the test itself, predictive value is also a function of the risk of the disease in the population being screened.

Number Needed to Screen to Prevent One Death

Disease-specific death rates in the study and control groups can be used to estimate how many patients would have to be screened to save one life compared with usual care. However, the interpretation of the NNS requires careful attention to detail, since this statistic often can be misleading. First, in the evaluation of RCT data, what is described as the NNS often is the NNI, a largely useless measure since it does not reflect the rate of exposure to screening in the invited group, or exposure to screening (contamination) in the control group [20]. Second, the NNS is highly sensitive to the duration of follow-up. Premature estimation of the NNS will result in an artificially inflated estimate if there has not been sufficient time for deaths to accumulate in the control group. Third, the NNS is influenced by the effectiveness of the screening and the prevalence of disease in the group undergoing screening, so as expected, the NNS will be higher in younger versus older cohorts. Finally, it is useful to express NNS in terms of the number of screening rounds, and the duration of follow-up after screening stops to fully measure the effectiveness of the exposure to screening.

Cost Effectiveness

There are two basic approaches to the evaluation of costs and outcomes related to screening: cost-benefit analysis (CBA) and cost-effectiveness analysis (CEA). In CBA, which is less commonly applied in the evaluation of screening, benefits and costs are expressed in monetary terms for a particular health outcome [21]. If costs exceed benefits, the intervention is judged to be not cost-beneficial and therefore not justified. In contrast, CEA is focused on the unit or net cost of achieving a particular health-related outcome [22]. In cancer screening, CEA can be expressed in terms of the cost to detect one cancer, prevent one death, add a year of life, add a quality-adjusted year of life, or most commonly, the marginal cost per year of life saved (MCYLS). The marginal costs of screening are the costs incurred by implementing a screening program minus the costs of case detection and management in the absence of screening.

The Acceptability of the Screening Test

A screening test's potential to reduce disease burden is highly dependent on adherence with recommended screening intervals and follow-up procedures. Low participation rates in cancer screening may be due to low acceptance by providers and the target population, but more attributable to suboptimal rates of referral to screening, and adherence to the referral, and the latter may be influenced by complexity, logistics, and costs. Apart from having health insurance, the single most important factor related to screening participation is a recommendation from an individual's healthcare provider [23].

Common Screening Tests

In this section we address screening tests that are commonly recommended for the early detection of cancer according to some of principles outlined in Table 11.1, and discuss screening recommendations from the American Cancer Society (ACS) and the United States Preventive Services Taskforce (USPSTF).

Breast Cancer

Long before the first experimental evidence demonstrated the efficacy of screening in reducing mortality, breast cancer was understood as a progressive disease with more favorable prognosis when it was diagnosed early in its natural history. In the early twentieth century, this awareness led clinicians to promote palpation in the office setting, but also self-examination so that women might identify symptoms earlier and seek clinical evaluation. Today, the principal screening test for breast cancer is mammography.

Screening Tests
Mammography
Mammography is an X-ray examination of the breasts to detect abnormalities that may be breast cancer. Mammography has evolved from general purpose X-ray equipment to dedicated film-screen units, and now in the United States (US) and in most breast cancer screening programs around the world, to full-field digital mammography units that capture the images electronically with solid state detectors [24]. Digital mammography has been shown to provide improved accuracy in pre- or perimenopausal women younger than 50 years who have dense

breasts [25–27]. Likewise, newer digital breast tomosynthesis systems (also known as 3D mammography) have shown improved sensitivity and specificity [28].

A screening examination involves two views of each breast: a craniocaudal (CC) view and a mediolateral oblique (MLO) view. Prior to taking the X-ray, a radiologic technologist positions a woman's breast on the image receptor and then applies pressure with a compression paddle to reduce breast thickness and motion, which enhances image quality [29]. Women with positive examinations commonly only undergo additional, problem solving imaging including special mammography views with full-field digital mammography or digital breast tomosynthesis to examine an area of suspicion, and less frequently with ultrasound, or magnetic resonance imaging (MRI) when mammography or ultrasound are judged to not be informative. Abnormalities that cannot be resolved with additional imaging generally will proceed to ultrasound- or radiographically-directed core needle or fine needle biopsy, or surgical excision.

Physical Examinations—Clinical Breast Examination and Breast Self-Examination
Clinical breast examination (CBE) involves visual inspection and physical palpation of the breasts by a trained examiner [30], while breast self-examination (BSE) involves a woman's periodic, systematic visual and physical palpation of her breasts [31].

Relative and Absolute Benefits of Screening
Mammography
Data from the nine RCTs of mammography screening, and meta-analysis results, are shown in Table 11.3, indicating a 20–21% reduction in breast cancer mortality associated with an invitation to screening [12, 32–39].

This summary point estimate is not a good reflection of the effectiveness of modern mammography for a number of reasons. In the RCTs, nonadherence with the randomization assignment diminishes the degree to which the results of an intention-to-treat analysis approximate a measure of effectiveness, that is, the benefit of actually attending screening. Also, there have been considerable improvements over the years in mammography technology and protocols that improved the effectiveness of screening. Further, differences in RCT outcomes largely can be explained by the degree to which the aggregate rate of advanced disease was reduced in the invited group compared with the control group, which is evident in the strong association in the individual trials between the risk of being diagnosed with an advanced breast cancer and the risk of dying from breast cancer [40]. Thus, while meta-analyses of the RCT data confirm that there are statistically significant age-specific and overall mortality reductions associated with an invitation to screening, individual RCTs and the evaluation of outcomes among women attending modern, organized mammography screening programs indicate that mortality reductions associated with exposure to screening are roughly twice as high, or greater, than estimates from meta-analysis [41–43]. The IARC's in-depth review of both RCTs and observational studies in 2015 concluded that the breast cancer mortality reduction provided by mammography is approximately 40% [44].

Table 11.3 The randomized controlled trials of breast cancer screening.

Trial	Year	Age group	Follow-up (years)	Breast cancer death		Person–years		RR	95% CI	Reference
				Screen	Control	Screen	Control			
HIP	1963	40–64	18	180	236	483,275	487,164	0.77	0.63, 0.93	[33]
MMST1	1976	45–69	19.2	161	198	360,000	362,000	0.82	0.66, 1.01	[12]
Two County	1977	40–49	29	351	367	1,632,492	1,200,887	0.70	0.61, 0.81	[34]
Edinburgh	1979	45–64	14	156	167	301,155	276,363	0.86	0.69, 1.07	[35]
CNBSS1&2	1980	40–59	25	180	171	968,676	968,432	1.05	0.85, 1.30	[36]
Stockholm	1981	40–64	11	66	45	473,153	239,460	0.74	0.51, 1.08	[37]
Gothenburg	1982	39–59	10	63	112	237963	324895	0.77	0.56, 1.05	[38]
UK Age Trial	1991	40–41	0–10	83	219	532,747	1,058,322	0.75	0.58, 0.97	[39]
Fixed-effect								0.797	0.74, 0.86	
Random-effect								0.803	0.73, 0.88	

Test for heterogeneity: $Q = 10.572$ ($P = 0.158$).

The UK Independent Review Panel and the Nordic Cochrane Institute each estimated a 20% and 19% (respectively) reduction in breast cancer deaths associated with an invitation to screening [45, 46] but then differed nearly 10-fold in their estimate of the number of women who needed to be invited (NNI) to screening to save one life (1/250 vs 1/2000, respectively). The USPSTF estimated age-specific estimates of the NNI for women aged 40–49 and 60–69, with a range from 1,904 to 377, respectively [47]. Each of these, in turn, is different from the estimates from the EUROSCREEN Working Group, which estimated a NNS of 96 women from observational data, [48, 49]. Closer examination reveals that each measure of absolute risk differs in terms of the reference population, mortality benefit, duration of screening and follow-up, rate of uptake, and whether invitation or exposure to screening is being compared. When standardized to a common scenario, that is, the recent UK Independent Panel report's estimate of the effect of screening women aged 50–69 in the UK every 3 years over a 20-year period (with 77% uptake) on breast cancer mortality from ages 55–79, the NNS ranged from 96–257, reducing a 20-fold difference in estimates of absolute benefit to about a 2.5-fold-difference [50]. When evaluating estimates of the NNS, it is important to scrutinize the underlying parameters of the estimate.

Clinical Breast Examination and Breast Self-Examination

Early evidence from several of the mammography RCTs demonstrated independent contributions of CBE to early detection, and thus, for many years, CBE was recommended as a stand-alone exam for women under age 40, and in combination with mammography for women age 40 years and older. However, in women aged 20–39, CBE contributes very little to breast cancer detection since incidence is very low in this age group, and for women 40 years and older, where mammography screening is recommended, CBE has only a very small independent contribution to breast cancer detection (2–6%), while also contributing to false positive outcomes [51]. The sensitivity of CBE also is poor, especially for smaller tumors, detecting fewer than 50% of breast cancers in women ages 40 years and older [52].

As was the case with CBE, BSE also was promoted for many years. However, evidence supporting the value of BSE in reducing breast cancer mortality has always been limited, and eventually results from two RCTs of BSE training [53, 54] failed to provide compelling evidence of the efficacy of BSE in reducing deaths from breast cancer. Each also observed that BSE was associated with a higher false positive rate compared with the control group. However, in low and middle resource countries where mammography may not be feasible, CBE and BSE may be the only method of breast cancer screening available to women, and it is presently being evaluated as a method for downstaging palpable breast cancer [55, 56]. In these settings it may be the case that undergoing CBE and being taught BSE also achieves an important contribution to raising awareness about symptoms of breast cancer and the importance of prompt reporting to the healthcare provider. Finally, as is the case with all screening tests, mammography is imperfect; thus, all women undergoing regular screening need to be alert to breast changes and should report them promptly. Well woman exams at all ages are a good opportunity to reinforce this message.

Screening Outcome Measures

The sensitivity and specificity of mammography fall within acceptable parameters and vary somewhat by age, with sensitivity, specificity, and PPV improving incrementally with increasing age [57]. For example, in the US Breast Cancer Surveillance Consortium (BCSC), overall sensitivity was 84.4%, with lower sensitivity for women aged 40–44 (73.4%) versus women aged 70–74 (83.3%), while overall specificity was 90.8%, which also was lower in women aged 40–44 (87.7%) versus women aged 70–74 (93.3%) [57]. The rate of abnormal interpretations is higher for first screening mammograms, and varies by age in single screening rounds, from 12% among women aged 40–49 to 6.5% in women aged 80–89 [58]. False negative rates are somewhat higher in younger women compared with older women, and range across all ages from 1.0–1.5 per 1,000 [58, 59].

Limitations and Adverse Outcomes

The sensitivity of mammography is strongly influenced by mammographic breast density, with sensitivity as high as 98% in women with predominantly fatty breasts, and as low as 48% in women with extremely dense breasts [60, 61]. Ultrasonic imaging has been used for many years in women with a suspicious abnormality that is not easily or fully seen on the mammogram, or to image an area of the breast with dense fibroglandular tissue. Studies of supplemental ultrasound as an adjunct to screening mammography for women with mammographically dense breasts have demonstrated a significant improvement in the cancer detection rate [62]. However, the improvement in sensitivity comes at a significant cost to the false positive rate, and this and resource issues have limited the use of supplemental ultrasound in the screening setting.

Adverse outcomes associated with mammography screening include false negatives, recall for additional imaging and biopsy that ultimately prove to be a benign finding, anxiety associated with the screening process and false positive findings [63], and overdiagnosis [64]. False positives do result in anxiety, but for the large majority of women it is brief and temporary [63]. To the extent that overdiagnosis associated with mammography screening exists, it represents a significant harm since women will undergo treatment unnecessarily. The range of estimates of overdiagnosis in breast cancer screening varies widely, ranging from 0 to over 50%, although extreme estimates result from failure to adjust for known confounders such as inadequate follow-up, lead-time, and incidence trends [6]. Credible estimates range from 0 to 10%, with a higher fraction of overdiagnosis attributable to ductal carcinoma *in situ* lesions. For purposes of patient communication, the percent of breast cancers that may be overdiagnosed is less important in informed decision making than the lifetime risk of being overdiagnosed. The UK Independent Review estimated that the risk of overdiagnosis from the RCTs applied to a period of screening every 3 years over a 20-year period was slightly above 1% [45].

Screening Recommendations

Screening guidelines for breast cancer are based on age-specific recommendations that differ by age to start screening, the screening interval, the age to stop screening, and recommendations for adults at higher than average risk (see Table 11.4) [65, 66]. The ACS recommends that women should have the opportunity to begin annual screening between the ages of 40 and 44 years; women aged 45–54 with an average risk of breast cancer should undergo annual screening mammography; women age 55 years and older should transition to biennial screening or have the opportunity to continue screening annually. Women should continue screening mammography as long as their overall health is good and they have a life expectancy of 10 years or more [66]. The USPSTF recommends that women aged 50–74 should undergo biennial screening mammography. Women between the ages of 40 and 49 who place a higher value on the potential benefit than the potential harms of screening may make an individual decision to begin biennial screening before age 50. The USPSTF found insufficient evidence to recommend for or against screening after age 74, but concluded that decisions about screening after age 74 should be individualized [65].

The ACS recommends that women at significantly higher risk for breast cancer due to known mutation carrier status, or who have a first degree relative who has tested positive for a BRCA mutation, or are affected by rarer high risk genetic syndromes, or who have an approximately 20–25% lifetime risk based on pedigree analysis of both the maternal and paternal lineage should begin annual mammography and MRI at age 30, or earlier as determined by shared decision making [67]. MRI and mammography screening also should begin earlier (age 25, or 8 years after radiation, whichever comes last) for women who have been treated for cancer at a younger age with radiation to the chest [68].

Colorectal Cancer

The goal of screening for colorectal cancer is both the detection of early-stage adenocarcinomas and the detection and removal of potentially precancerous lesions, in particular adenomatous and serrated polyps [69, 70]. Serrated polyps are often referred to as flat polyps since they may not protrude from the wall of the colon. Reduction in colorectal cancer morbidity and mortality through screening is achieved through a combination of (i) a more favorable stage at diagnosis of occult disease and (ii) the removal of precursor lesions, which can contribute to disease prevention.

Polyps are common in adults over age 50. Since the majority of polyps will not develop into adenocarcinoma, histology, morphology, and size determine their clinical importance as precursor lesions [71, 72]. The most common and clinically important polyps are adenomatous polyps, which represent about one-half to two-thirds of all colorectal polyps. The adenoma–carcinoma sequence is thought to be the common pathway to colorectal cancer [73]. However, there are alternative routes to colorectal cancer carcinogenesis, of which the serrated

Table 11.4 ACS and USPSTF guidelines for breast cancer screening in average risk women.

Recommendation	ACS	USPSTF
Breast self-exam (BSE)	Not recommended	Against clinicians teaching BSE
Clinical breast exam (CBE)	Not recommended	Insufficient evidence
Mammography	40–44: opportunity for informed decision; annual screening for women who chose to begin screening 45–54: annual screening 55+: biennial screening, with option to continue annual screening 75+: continue screening as long as health is good and life expectancy 10+ years	40–49: individual decision; biennial screening for women who chose to begin screening Ages 50–74: biennial screening Ages 75+: insufficient evidence

neoplasia pathway may be the most important and may account for 10–30% of all colorectal adenocarcinomas [74]. Incidental hyperplastic polyps and mucosal tags are not believed to have clinical significance in the development of colorectal cancer.

The evidence for the importance of colorectal polyps in the development of colorectal cancer is largely indirect but is nonetheless convincing. First, adenomas and colorectal cancers have similar anatomic distribution, and the average age at which polyps begin to appear precedes the age-incidence curve of colorectal cancer [75], with an estimated dwell time of about 10 years for an adenomatous polyp <1 cm to become an invasive lesion [76]. Second, there is a strong association between polyp size and the grade of dysplasia [77]. Third, epidemiologic evidence has shown a lower incidence of colorectal cancer among individuals who have had large adenomatous polyps removed compared with the general population, and this protection only extends to the area of the bowel that has been examined [78].

Screening Tests for Colorectal Cancer

Screening methods for colorectal cancer fall into two general categories: (1) fecal occult blood tests (FOBT), which include guaiac-based FOBT (gFOBT), immunochemical-based FOBT (fecal immunochemical tests, or FIT), and a multitarget FOBT test that combines a FIT with a stool DNA test (mtsDNA); and (2) the structural exams, which include colonoscopy, flexible sigmoidoscopy (FSIG), and computed tomography colonography (CTC). Double contrast barium enema (DCBE) also provides a radiographic image of the entire bowel, but is used so rarely today that it will not be discussed [79]. These tests vary in terms of the degree of underlying evidence supporting their use, efficacy, costs, cost-effectiveness, and acceptability among patients and referring physicians. In the US, FSIG and DCBE are rarely performed, and low sensitivity variants of FOBT are not recommended [80]. Nevertheless, except for low-sensitivity FOBT, any one of the tests listed above has the potential to reduce incidence and mortality from colorectal cancer significantly if applied in a program of regular screening.

Stool Tests (gFOBT, FIT, and mtsDNA tests)

Stool blood tests aim to detect the presence of occult blood in stool, which may derive from colorectal cancer or larger adenomas. The most common stool blood tests in use today are gFOBTs, which detect blood in the stool through the pseudoperoxidase activity of heme or hemoglobin, whereas FIT, and the immunochemical assay in a mtsDNA test, react only to human hemoglobin, which make FITs specific only to bleeding in the large bowel. Because bleeding from cancers or large polyps may be intermittent, the proper use of stool blood tests requires annual testing, with the collection of one or more samples of stool from one or several bowel movements, depending on manufacturer's recommendations [81]. All positive stool tests must be followed up with colonoscopy to complete the screening process. Repeating the stool test, or referring the patient for an alternative test, such as FSIG, is not appropriate.

gFOBT

The performance of gFOBT is highly dependent on following a recommended protocol [82], that is, specimens should be collected over a 3-day period from three successive bowel movements, with two samples from each bowel movement placed on each test card. Once samples from three separate bowel movements have been collected, the gFOBT cards should be returned according to the provider's instructions for processing. Annual testing following this regimen is required to achieve the program sensitivity observed in the RCTs.

Serious shortcoming with gFOBTs include the wide range of performance between products, nonadherence with manufacturer's recommendations, and errors in test interpretation. For example, in a comparison with an early version of sDNA, Imperiale *et al.* showed that one of the most common gFOBT variants used in clinical practice (Hemoccult II) had only 13% sensitivity for colorectal cancer, and only 14% sensitivity for advanced neoplasia when used according to the manufacturer's recommendations [83]. Some false negatives may have been attributable to poor test development and interpretation. Sensitivity is degraded further when gFOBT is not used according to the manufacturer's recommendations. Nadel *et al.* reported results from a national survey of primary care providers, in which more than half of physicians reported using both in-office gFOBT and the take-home method, and 25% reported in-office testing as the only method of stool testing they used with their patients [84]. Collins *et al.* demonstrated that single sample in-office gFOBT following digital rectal examination had only 10% sensitivity for cancer, and only 4.9% sensitivity for advanced neoplasia [85]. Leading guideline development groups strongly recommend against in-office gFOBT [80, 86], and also recommend that only high sensitivity FOBT be used for CRC screening, which, in the US, essentially leaves only one gFOBT (Hemoccult SENSA) as an acceptable choice for screening. In two prospective studies, the sensitivity of a single Hemoccult SENSA for colorectal cancer ranged from 61.5 to 79.4%, and the specificity ranged from 86.7 to 96.4% [82, 87].

FIT

Because FIT is more specific for human blood than guaiac-based tests and because the globin portion of hemoglobin is digested in the upper GI tract, it is more specific for lower gastrointestinal bleeding and thus more specific for CRC [88]. In comparison to gFOBT, most variants of FIT require fewer samples or less direct handling of stool. The greater ease of a single sample FIT performed at home has been shown to improve adherence with testing and test completion [89, 90].

Like gFOBTs, FITs are produced by different manufacturers and differ in terms of specimen collection technique, number of samples, and performance. Qualitative FITs have a fixed cutoff set by the manufacturer, for the amount of human hemoglobin, whereas quantitative FIT allow for adjustable cutoffs which can be set to achieve higher or lower sensitivity. In a review of the performance of FIT variants from 19 studies, pooled sensitivity was 0.79 for CRC, and specificity was 0.94. Single sample FIT variants demonstrated similar performance to multiple sample FITs [91] which is an important observation since adherence with screening is higher when only a single sample is required [89].

mtsDNA

A newer approach to testing stool aims to detect both occult blood and DNA markers. Because colorectal polyps and malignancies exfoliate cells into the lumen, it is possible to examine the stool for an array of DNA markers associated with colorectal cancer. At the time of writing, the only sDNA test available is a mtsDNA test produced by Exact Sciences (Cologuard), which utilizes a multiple marker panel that includes quantitative molecular assays for KRAS mutations, aberrant *NDRG4* and *BMP3* methylation, and β-actin DNA (as an internal reference of DNA quantity and integrity), plus a hemoglobin immunoassay, which is intended to detect advanced lesions not identified by the marker panel [92]. Unlike gFOBT or FIT, mtsDNA requires a large sample of stool, and collection kits are designed to collect all the stool from a single bowel movement.

Imperiale *et al.* compared the mtsDNA test with an FIT in patients scheduled for colonoscopy [92]. Among 9,989 participants in the evaluation cohort, the sensitivity of mtsDNA exceeded that of FIT for detection of cancer (92.3% vs 73.8%) and advanced neoplasia (42.4% vs 23.8%). The specificity of the mtsDNA and FIT was 89.8% and 96.4%, respectively, among participants with negative colonoscopy results.

Structural Exams – Direct Visualization of the Bowel

Structural exams such as colonoscopy, FSIG, and CTC have the advantage of providing direct visualization of the portion of the bowel that is examined, thus generally providing greater test sensitivity for CRC and adenomatous polyps compared with FOBT, and also allowing for wider screening intervals (5 or 10 years). However, these tests are more expensive, and require patients to undergo bowel cleansing, each of which has been shown to be a barrier to adherence to screening recommendations.

Colonoscopy

Colonoscopy has a unique advantage among all screening tests for colorectal cancer in that direct visualization of the entire large bowel (terminating at the cecum) is possible, and clinically significant adenomas can be identified and removed during the examination. The modern colonoscope is far more complex than a flexible sigmoidoscope since it must be capable of air insufflation, irrigation, suction, and the passage of biopsy forceps and polypectomy snares [93]. Like sigmoidoscopes, the tip of the instrument is equipped with a small video camera and light to provide high-resolution visualization of the wall of the bowel. Patients generally are placed on a liquid diet one or more days before the examination, followed by either ingestion of oral lavage solutions or saline laxatives to stimulate bowel movements until the bowel is clean. Proper bowel preparation is a critical element in the accuracy and cost-effectiveness of screening with colonoscopy [94]. Split-dose bowel preparation, where the bowel preparation begins the night before the exam and is completed very early on the morning of the exam has been shown to be superior to taking the entire dose the evening before the exam [95]. It is common for the patient to receive either anesthesia or a mild sedative prior to the procedure [96] but it is not essential for those who tolerate the procedure with only mild discomfort [97]. Colonoscopy is commonly done in a hospital or stand-alone surgical center. The examination is more complicated than FSIG, with higher risk of complications, mostly due to the effects of sedation, biopsy, or polypectomy [98–100]. A skilled operator can complete an uncomplicated examination in approximately 30 min.

The performance of colonoscopy is influenced by variability in the distribution of adenomas in the distal and proximal colon, the sensitivity of the test for precancerous lesions with varying morphological appearances, the quality of bowel cleansing, failure to reach the cecum, and other quality assurance measures related to the examination and the examiner. Some studies suggest that colonoscopy is less effective in reducing incidence and mortality related to lesions in the proximal colon compared with the distal colon [101, 102] although it is not clear whether less favorable outcomes related to the proximal versus distal colon are a function of disease natural history, greater quality challenges, or both. Colonoscopy has often been described as the "gold standard", for CRC screening, due both to being a direct visualization technology and being the reference examination for comparing the performance of other CRC screening tests. However, both tandem studies, and more recent investigations comparing CTC with colonoscopy show that some cancers and large adenomas are missed during colonoscopy. Specificity measures commonly are not reported. The sensitivity of colonoscopy for CRC per lesion (versus per patient) ranged from 50% to 100%; per lesion sensitivity for adenomas ≥ 10 mm ranged from 89.8% to 97.6%; and per lesion sensitivity for adenomas ≥ 6 mm ranged from 75.8% to 90.4% [103–105].

Colonoscopy quality indicators include adequacy of the bowel preparation, the endoscopic withdrawal time, the cecal intubation rate and, most important, the adenoma detection rate (ADR). The ADR is defined as the proportion of patients undergoing screening colonoscopy that had one or more adenomas detected. Gastrointestinal organizations recommend a target composite ADR of ≥ 25% (for men, ≥ 30%; for women, ≥ 20%) [106]. Studies have demonstrated a strong correlation between the average ADR recorded for an individual endoscopist and the likelihood of interval cancers among the patients served by that endoscopist [107, 108]. In spite the clinical importance of this measure, wide variations in the ADR between individual endoscopists persist [109]. The importance of having a high ADR cannot be overemphasized. In one study, each 1% increase in the ADR was associated with a 5% decrease in the risk of a fatal interval colorectal cancer [107].

Flexible Sigmoidoscopy

Flexible sigmoidoscopy is a relatively simple procedure to examine the distal colon that requires minimal preparation prior to the examination [110]. The common sigmoidoscope used today is flexible and about 60 cm in length, allowing for examination of somewhat less than half of the colon. Operator visualization is achieved through either fiberscope or videoscope. Patient preparation involves a saline laxative enema 1 to 2 hours before the examination, and the test is generally performed without sedation. A skilled examiner can complete the examination in less than 10 minutes. If the test is positive, the patient should be referred for colonoscopy. Complications during flexible sigmoidoscopy are rare, but similar to colonoscopy include perforations and bleeding [111]. In the US, very few adults report having undergone recent screening with FSIG.

CT Colonography

CT colonography or "virtual colonoscopy", is an imaging procedure that uses computer programming to combine multiple helical CT scans to create two- or three-dimensional images of the interior of the colon. These images can be rotated for different views and even combined for a complete, "virtual" view of the colon that can be viewed in a manner that simulates the insertion and withdrawal of a colonoscope. As with colonoscopy, patients must undergo bowel cleansing prior to the examination. In addition to screening, indications for CT colonography include incomplete colonoscopy, screening in elderly or frail adults, and patients with a contraindication for sedation.

Evaluation of CT colonography typically has used study designs in which patients first underwent a CT exam, which was then followed by optical colonoscopy with the examiner blinded to the CT exam findings. Back to back evaluations of CT have demonstrated sensitivities for large adenomas and cancer equivalent to colonoscopy [103, 112]. Sensitivity is lower for lesions ≤ 6 mm, although these lesions are regarded as clinically less significant and raise questions as to whether or not there is actual value in test sensitivity for lesions that pose no real threat in the near term.

Relative and Absolute Benefits of CRC Screening

Direct evidence on the efficacy of screening derives from prospective RCTs of gFOBT and FSIG, and indirect evidence supporting the other screening tests is consistent with these findings. Six large RCTs evaluating the efficacy of screening for CRC with gFOBT (specifically, Hemoccult II) have been conducted in Europe and the US [113–118]. In the US Minnesota trial, which has the longest follow-up among the six RCTs, the most recent follow-up (30 years) showed a 32% mortality reduction associated with annual screening; a 22% reduction in mortality associated with biennial screening [113]. In a subsequent analysis of Minnesota trial data with 18 years of follow-up, Mandel *et al.* also observed a 20% reduction in incidence in the group invited to annual screening, and an 18% reduction in incidence in the group invited to biennial screening, likely attributable to detection and removal of advanced neoplasia [119]. There are no RCTs that have evaluated the efficacy of high sensitivity stool tests for the reduction of incidence and mortality for CRC, although modeling results suggest that their performance would be superior [120].

Four RCTs have successfully evaluated the efficiency of one or two rounds of CRC screening with FSIG, with each demonstrating a reduction in deaths and CRC incidence associated with detection and treatment of cancers and adenomas in the distal colon [114, 121–123]. In the United Kingdom Flexible Sigmoidoscopy Screening Trial (UKFSST), Atkin *et al.* observed a 31% reduction in CRC deaths, and a 23% reduction in CRC incidence.

There are no RCTs that have measured the efficacy of colonoscopy or CTC to reduce incidence and mortality, although indirect evidence and modeling provide confidence that each is effective in achieving that dual goal [120]. In a case-control study of 32,702 veterans, patients who had undergone colonoscopy with polypectomy were significantly less likely to develop colorectal cancer (odds ratio, 0.48; 95% CI, 0.35–0.66) [124]. Zauber *et al.* studied the long-term effect of colonoscopic polypectomy on colorectal cancer mortality in the National Polyp Study and observed 53% fewer colorectal cancer deaths associated with colonoscopic polypectomy compared with the expected rate in the general population [72].

Among 88,902 participants in the Nurses' Health Study and the Health Professionals Follow-up Study followed over a period of 22 years, those who underwent negative colonoscopy were 56% less likely to develop colorectal cancer and 68% less likely to die from colorectal cancer compared with participants who did not undergo colonoscopy [102].

Limitations and Adverse Outcomes

Harms associated with CRC screening mostly are associated with the structural examinations, either as primary screening tests, or when utilized in the continuum of screening in asymptomatic adults who have a positive stool test. There is little evidence that there is any overdiagnosis of invasive disease associated with colorectal cancer screening, except for overdiagnosis that would occur if an adult with serious life-limiting comorbidity were to inappropriately undergo screening and be diagnosed with colorectal cancer. Harms associated with flexible sigmoidoscopy and colonoscopy include perforations or bleeding associated with the procedure. There is little evidence of harms associated with CTC, although concerns have been raised about radiation exposure from multiple procedures, and the identification of extracolonic findings that may require invasive procedures to reconcile.

Screening Recommendations

Most organizations recommend that average-risk adults should be regularly screened for colorectal cancer beginning at age 50 although there are some differences in recommended options for regular surveillance (Table 11.5).

ACS recommendations for average risk individuals include annual high sensitivity FOBT (guaiac or immunochemical), mtsDNA every 3 years, flexible sigmoidoscopy every 5 years, annual FOBT and flexible sigmoidoscopy every 5 years after initial screening with both tests, or total colon examination with colonoscopy every 10 years, and CTC every 5 years. For individuals undergoing screening tests other than colonoscopy, all positive test results must be followed up with colonoscopy.

Many primary care providers regard a FOBT as an ineffective test for colorectal cancer screening [125, 126]. Although there is a wide range of performance within and between stool testing variants, it is important to recognize that annual, high sensitivity FOBT when used according to manufacturer's recommendations is associated with long-term outcomes that are very similar to colonoscopy performed every 10 years [127]. Since individuals vary in their preferences for invasive versus noninvasive testing, it is important for clinicians to offer at least the option for colonoscopy or high sensitivity FOBT to ensure high rates of adherence to colorectal cancer screening. Adherence with screening recommendations has been shown to be higher when patients are offered a choice between FOBT and colonoscopy [128].

Adults at high risk for colorectal cancer generally are recommended to begin colonoscopy earlier and undergo screening more frequently [80, 129–131]. Higher-risk individuals include those with a personal history of adenomatous polyps or colorectal cancer, a family history of adenomatous polyps or colorectal cancer, a family history of familial adenomatous polyposis, a family history of hereditary nonpolyposis colorectal cancer, or a personal history of inflammatory bowel disease.

Table 11.5 ACS and USPSTF guidelines for colorectal cancer screening in average risk adults ages 50 years and older.

Recommendation	ACS	USPSTF
High sensitivity guaiac-based fecal occult blood tests (gFOBT) or fecal immunochemical tests (FIT)	Annual testing: stool sampled from regular bowel movements with adherence to manufacturer's recommendation for collection techniques and number of samples is recommended. **FOBT with the single stool sample collected on the clinician's fingertip during a digital rectal examination is not recommended.** "Throw in the toilet bowl" FOB tests also are not recommended. In comparison with guaiac-based tests for the detection of occult blood, immunochemical tests are more patient-friendly, and are likely to be equal or better in sensitivity and specificity. There is no justification for repeating FOBT in response to an initial positive finding; patients with positive findings should be referred to colonoscopy.	Annual
Multitarget stool DNA test (aka, MT-sDNA, or FIT-DNA)	Every 3 years, per manufacturer's recommendations	Every 1, or 3 years
Flexible sigmoidoscopy	Every 5 years, FSIG can be performed alone, or consideration can be given to combining FSIG performed every 5 years with a highly sensitive gFOBT or FIT performed annually.	Every 5 years, or Every 10 years when combined with annual FIT
Colonoscopy	Every 10 years	Every 10 years
Computed tomography colonoscopy (CT-Colonography, or CTC)	Every 5 years. Positive tests must be followed up with a colonoscopy.	Every 5 years
Age to stop screening	Screening should continue as long as an individual is in good health and has a life expectancy of at least 10 years	Age 85 Age >76–85: Individual decision. Taking into account the patient's overall health and prior screening history

Cervical Cancer

The long-term downward trend in cervical cancer incidence and mortality in many of the world's regions is a measure of the success of the Papanicolaou (Pap) test at detecting cervical cancer and precursor lesions, that is, cervical intraepithelial neoplasia (CIN) [132]. Since the introduction of the Pap smear, the control of cervical cancer has evolved due to understanding of the role of human papilloma virus (HPV) in its etiology [133], with demonstration of the role of HPV vaccines in the prevention of high risk HPV infection [134], and the use of HPV testing as a co-test as well as a stand-alone screening test [135]. The goal of cervical cancer screening principally is the detection of CIN in order to prevent its progression to invasive disease. Although cancer registries commonly do not collect data on precursor lesions, a recent report from a large healthcare plan showed a prevalence of cytologic abnormalities (CIN 2+) of 7.1% among women 21 years of age and older undergoing screening, with the prevalence decreasing with increasing age [136].

Screening for cancer of the cervix, specifically precancerous lesions, is effective in reducing both the incidence and mortality from cervical cancer. Cervical cancer is characterized by a long sojourn time, with potentially cancerous lesions progressing through a succession of identifiable stages prior to becoming invasive disease. If precursor lesions are detected, a variety of treatment options can prevent the progression to invasive disease. Age-specific incidence data available from NCI's Surveillance, Epidemiology, and End Results (SEER) program and from cross-sectional studies of small geographic areas or clinic populations are consistent with the following observations: (i) the prevalence of precursor dysplastic lesions is greater among younger women compared with older women; (ii) a significant proportion of premalignant lesions will regress, especially in younger women; (iii) carcinoma *in situ* (CIN) of the cervix peaks in the mid-30s; and (iv) the incidence of invasive disease peaks in the mid-forties, remaining relatively constant among White women and continuing to rise among African American women [137].

Screening and Diagnostic Methods

The Pap test is the most widely used cancer-screening test in the world. At the most basic level, the test involves the collection of epithelial cells from the cervical squamocolumnar junction, or transformation zone, sampling both the ectocervix and endocervix. Historically, cervical cytology specimens were smeared onto a glass slide, but in many countries the conventional smear has been replaced with liquid-based preparations (LBP), which use similar specimen collection techniques. However, instead of placing the sample on a glass slide, the sample is suspended in a fixative solution, after which it is dispersed, filtered, and then distributed on a glass slide in a monolayer. The process results in fewer unsatisfactory slides because there are fewer artifacts (blood, mucus, etc.) and because cells are not overlapping, which overcomes some of the quality assurance challenges associated with the conventional smear.

An adequate Pap test requires optimal sample collection, which depends both on patient preparation, and the collection and preparation of the specimen. Women should be counseled to avoid intercourse, douching, use of intravaginal medications, or tampons at least 48 h prior to the examination. Optimal sample collection and preparation begins with attention to details of proper specimen labeling, and accompanying patient clinical history (age, date of last menstrual period, history of prior abnormal Pap tests, current pregnancy, use of hormonal contraceptives, intrauterine device, or use of menopausal hormonal therapy). Specimens should be collected with an extended tip spatula; studies comparing specimen collection devices have shown that the widely used Ayre spatula performs poorly based on the frequency of inadequate smears and diminished ability to detect lesions [138, 139]. Likewise, cotton swabs should not be used due to similar performance issues. Additional specimen collection devices, including brushes and brooms, may be used depending on the clinical appearance of the cervix to ensure complete sampling of the transformation zone. If two specimen devices are used, the exocervical sample should be obtained first followed by the endocervical sample. Specimens collected for LBP should be immediately immersed in the liquid medium, whereas specimens collected for a conventional smear should be smeared on the slide followed by immediate fixation [140]. A Pap test is judged to be unsatisfactory if there is scant cellularity (<5,000 well-visualized/well preserved squamous or squamous metaplastic cells from a patient without clinical considerations that account for low cellularity) [141] or if more than 75% of the cells are obscured. An unsatisfactory Pap test should be repeated within 2–4 months.

Even under the best of circumstances, the Pap smear has a significant error rate. Sampling error is estimated to account for about two-thirds of false-negative tests whereas errors in interpretation account for the remaining third [142]. A technology assessment of cervical cytology by the Duke University Center for Clinical Health Policy Research concluded that conventional smear screening had specificity of 98% but sensitivity of only 51% [142]. While LBP has a lower rate of unsatisfactory slides, studies have not demonstrated that LBP has greater accuracy [143].

After decades of evolving cervical cytology reporting systems, the Bethesda System was developed in 1988 to provide a standard for cytopathology reports. It was last updated in 2014 (Table 11.6) [144].

Because it is well established that persistent cervical infection with high-risk HPV genotypes is necessary for the development of cervical cancer and its immediate precursor lesion, CIN grade 3 (CIN3), HPV testing is increasingly finding applications for co-testing, primary screening, surveillance, and risk stratification. Epidemiologic studies have shown that nearly 100% of cervical cancer cases test positive for HPV [145]. HPV type 16 (HPV16) is the most carcinogenic HPV genotype, followed by HPV18, and each account for approximately 55–60% and 10% respectively of all cervical cancers [145–147]. Approximately 10 other HPV genotypes cause the remaining 25% to 35% of cervical cancers [148]. There currently are five FDA approved HPV assays for the detection of high risk HPV, which use different technologies to identify genetic DNA from HPV or, depending on the test, are specific for between 2 and 14 high risk HPV types [149].

There are four common approaches to using HPV testing for cervical cancer screening, including: (1) screening with HPV test alone; (2) co-testing, combining a Pap test with an HPV test; (3) HPV testing with cytology triage for women with positive HPV test results (reflex cytology); and (4) Pap testing with HPV triage of women with positive HPV test results

Table 11.6 The 2001 Bethesda System.

Specimen Type	Indicate conventional smear (Pap smear) versus liquid-based versus other
Specimen Adequacy	
Satisfactory for evaluation	Describe presence or absence of endocervical/transformation zone component and any other quality indicators, e.g., partially obscuring blood, inflammation, etc.
Unsatisfactory for evaluation	Specimen rejected/not processed (*specify reason*), or Specimen processed and examined, but unsatisfactory for evaluation of epithelial abnormality because of (*specify reason*)
Interpretation/result (optional)	Negative for intraepithelial lesion or malignancy
Squamous Cell	Atypical squamous cells: • Of undetermined significance (ASC-US) • Cannot exclude HSIL (ASC-H) Low grade squamous intraepithelial lesion (LSIL) • Encompassing: HPV/mild dysplasia/CIN 1 High grade squamous intraepithelial lesion (HSIL) • Encompassing: moderate and severe dysplasia, CIS/CIN 2 and CIN 3 • With features suspicious for invasion (*if invasion is suspected*) Squamous cell carcinoma
Glandular Cell	Atypical • Endocervical cells (NOS *or specify in comments*) • Endometrial cells (NOS *or specify in comments*) • Glandular cells (NOS *or specify in comments*) Atypical • Endocervical cells, favor neoplastic • Glandular cells, favor neoplastic Endocervical adenocarcinoma *in situ* Adenocarcinoma • Endocervical • Endometrial • Extrauterine • Not otherwise specified
Other Malignant Neoplasms	Specify
Educational Notes and Suggestions (Optional)	Suggestions should be concise and consistent with clinical follow-up guidelines published by professional organizations (references to relevant publications may be included).

(reflex HPV) [143]. HPV testing, whether as a stand-alone test or co-testing with the Pap test, measurably improves the sensitivity of cervical cancer screening by approximately 40–50% compared with cytology alone, although at a cost of diminished specificity [150, 151].

Relative and Absolute Benefit

There has never been a randomized trial of the efficacy of screening for cancer of the cervix, principally because cytologic screening was an accepted part of medical care before the randomized trial with a mortality end-point had become the standard by which the efficacy of a screening test is evaluated [152].

However, observational evidence from trends in incidence and mortality as well as opportunities for natural experiments have been accepted as evidence for the efficacy of cervical cancer screening. Widely cited evidence for the contribution of cytologic screening to reducing cervical cancer mortality is the long-term decline in the death rate from cervical cancer in the US coincident with the introduction of the Pap smear [153]. Further, evaluations of cervical cancer screening rates in five Nordic countries [154–158] compared mortality rates before and after the introduction of cytologic screening between two time periods (1963–1967 and 1978–1982); cervical cancer mortality reductions between 8 and 73% were observed. In Norway, where participation rates were lowest, mortality remained comparatively unchanged whereas in Iceland, which organized an aggressive screening program that had high rates of participation, the mortality reduction (73%) was greatest among the five countries [154, 156, 158]. Similar temporal changes have been observed in countries that introduced cervical cancer screening more recently [159]. Numerous examples of case-control studies have also shown a benefit from cervical cancer screening [160, 161].

Pooled analysis of four European RCTs compared HPV-based screening for cervical cancer with cytology-based screening, with cervical cancer precursors and invasive cervical cancer as the end-points. With approximately 1.2 million women years of observation with a median follow-up of 6.5 years, the investigators reported that HPV-based screening provides 60–70% greater protection against invasive cervical cancer versus cytology alone [162].

Limitations and Adverse Outcomes

Pap testing has limited sensitivity, although with regular testing program sensitivity is reasonable for a disease that has a long sojourn time. Co-testing with HPV tests and cervical cytology measurably improves sensitivity, but at a cost of diminished specificity. Harms associated with cervical cancer screening include short-term anxiety associated with positive test results, and for women who undergo colposcopy and biopsy, harms include pain, bleeding, and infection. Potential harms associated with treatment of CIN include procedure-related harms, such as pain, bleeding, infection, etc., and longer term effects such as weakening of the cervix leading to increased risk of pre-term birth [143].

Screening Recommendations

In 2012, the ACS, the American Society for Colposcopy and Cervical Pathology (ASCCP), and the American Society for Clinical Pathology (ASCP) issued a joint guideline for cervical cancer screening based on a systematic evidence review and using a collaborative process that included 25 organizations [148]. Similar recommendations were released in 2012 by the USPSTF [163]. The screening guideline recommends surveillance strategies and options based on a woman's age, screening history, risk factors, and her choice of screening tests. Of particular note, women under age 21 years should not be screened regardless of their age of sexual initiation, and women at any age should not be screened annually by any screening method (Table 11.7).

Age 21 was chosen as the age to begin screening because cervical cancer is rare in women younger than 21. Testing adolescents leads to unnecessary evaluation and potentially to avoidable treatment of preinvasive cervical lesions that have a high probability of eventual regression within the long lead time period. Because treatment is associated with reproductive problems, screening before age 21 was judged to represent a net harm. While annual screening is associated with slightly higher

Table 11.7 ACS and USPSTF guidelines for cervical cancer screening in average risk women ages 21 years and older.

Recommendation	ACS	USPSTF
Women aged 21–65	Cervical cancer screening should begin at age 21 years. For women ages 21–29 years, screening should be done every 3 years with conventional or liquid-based Pap tests For women ages 30–65 years, screening should be done every 5 years with both the HPV test and the Pap test (preferred), or every 3 years with the Pap test alone (acceptable)	The USPSTF recommends screening for cervical cancer in women aged 21–65 years with cytology (Pap smear) every 3 years or, for women aged 30–65 years who want to lengthen the screening interval, screening with a combination of cytology and HPV testing every 5 years
Women <30	The ACS recommends against screening for cervical cancer with HPV testing, alone or in combination with cytology, in women younger than age 30 years, or with any method before age 21	The USPSTF recommends against screening for cervical cancer with HPV testing, alone or in combination with cytology, in women younger than age 30 years, or with any method before age 21
Women >65	Women aged older than 65 years who have had ≥3 consecutive negative Pap tests or ≥2 consecutive negative HPV and Pap tests within the last 10 years, with the most recent test occurring in the last 5 years, should stop cervical cancer screening. Women with a history of CIN2 or a more severe diagnosis should continue to follow routine screening recommendations for women ages 30–65 for at least 20 years, even if screening extends beyond age 65 years	The USPSTF recommends against screening for cervical cancer in women older than age 65 years who have had adequate prior screening and are not otherwise at high risk for cervical cancer
Women who have had a hysterectomy	Women who have had a total hysterectomy should stop cervical cancer screening	The USPSTF recommends against screening for cervical cancer in women who have had a hysterectomy with removal of the cervix and who do not have a history of a high-grade precancerous lesion (cervical intraepithelial neoplasia [CIN] grade 2 or 3) or cervical cancer

sensitivity, this improvement is gained at the high cost of many unnecessary evaluations and treatments. The rationale for screening women aged 21–29 every 3 years was based on comparisons of outcomes associated with 1, 2, and 3 year screening. As noted above, annual testing results in slightly greater benefit, but a considerable excess of harms, while little difference in benefit was observed in 2- versus 3-year screening intervals [148]. For women aged 30–65, the same logic of Pap testing every 3 years holds. The guidelines also endorse co-testing with the Pap test and an HPV test every 5 years, which is preferred over screening with the Pap smear alone. Evidence shows that the combination of HPV testing and cytology results in increased detection of prevalent CIN3, and in subsequent rounds a decrease in CIN 3+ and invasive cancer. The greater sensitivity of co-testing also results in longer sojourn times, and the opportunity to extend the screening interval. After age 65, women with a history of adequate prior negative screening findings, and no history of CIN 2+ within the past 20 years can stop screening. Once screening is discontinued it should not resume for any reason, even if a woman reports having a new sexual partner. Additional details for managing cervical cancer screening in women with abnormal findings, or with a different risk, are detailed in the guideline [148].

The recommendations in Table 11.7 were developed for women at average risk and do not apply to women with a history of cervical cancer, women who were exposed *in utero* to diethylstilbestrol, women who are immunocompromised by organ transplantation, chemotherapy, or chronic corticosteroid treatment, or women who are positive for the human immunodeficiency virus, for which the original guideline manuscript should be consulted for further guidance [148].

Lung Cancer

In the 1990s, the potential for an early detection strategy took a favorable turn through investigations of low dose, thoracic CT (LDCT) imaging [164] which demonstrated considerably greater sensitivity for the detection of small pulmonary nodules and cancers compared with chest X-ray (CXR) [165].

Screening and Diagnostic Methods

LDCT is the only screening test that has been shown to reduce lung cancer mortality in current and former cigarette smokers at higher than average risk for lung cancer [166]. Use of conventional CXR for lung cancer screening is not appropriate and is not recommended. The screening process requires identification of adults who are current or former smokers who meet eligibility criteria based on age, pack year smoking history, the number of years since cessation (if former smokers), and overall good health; some organizations have expanded eligibility to include other risk factors (see below). Adults who meet eligibility criteria should undergo a process of informed decision making about the benefits, limitations, and potential harms associated with lung cancer screening. Those who elect to undergo lung cancer screening should be screened annually.

The American College of Radiology (ACR) and the Society of Thoracic Radiology (STR) [167] recommend that LDCT of the chest for lung cancer screening should be performed without the use of intravenous contrast medium utilizing multidetector

helical (spiral) technique during a single breath-hold, and should include axial images acquired and viewed at ≤ 2.5-mm slice thickness, with reconstruction intervals equal to or less than the slice thickness, or at smaller (≤1.0-mm) acquisition slice thicknesses and reconstruction intervals to allow for better characterization of small lung nodules. The screening protocol should be developed to obtain diagnostic-quality images with the lowest possible patient radiation exposure. Attention to exposure levels is important because positive findings are common, and patients with positive test results are likely to require additional surveillance, resulting in repeated, shorter-interval CT examinations.

Nodules identified on the examination should be described with respect to their size, attenuation (soft tissue, type of calcification, fat), opacity (i.e., solid, ground glass or nonsolid, or containing both solid and ground-glass components), and margins (smooth, lobulated, or spiculated). If prior imaging studies are available, they should be reviewed so that change from previous exams can be assessed and referenced. Computer-assisted nodule detection and volumetric assessment of nodule size and growth are useful tools for evaluation. The interpreting radiologist should recommend the appropriate management and follow-up based on the findings, and should use a structured reporting system [168]. Whichever guideline is chosen for management of screen-detected lung nodules, it should be noted on the radiology report [169, 170].

Relative and Absolute Benefit

In the 1970s and 1980s four prospective trials of lung cancer screening were carried out, using combinations of chest X-ray and sputum cytology [171–175]. All were methodologically limited at inception in their ability to demonstrate a benefit from screening [164, 176] and none showed a significant reduction in lung cancer mortality associated with an invitation to screening, although some results were suggestive of a survival benefit [164, 176–178].

Promising results from observational studies of LDCT led to the initiation of RCTs in Europe and the US [179], of which the largest was the US National Lung Screening Trial (NLST) [166]. The NLST randomized 53,454 adults aged 55–74 at high risk for lung cancer to either, invitation to three rounds of annual LDCT screening or invitation to three rounds of annual CXR. Participants were current or former smokers (quit ≤15 years) who had at least a 30 pack year history of smoking and were in reasonably good health. In 2010, the NCI announced that the study had observed 20% fewer lung cancer deaths in the LDCT arm compared with the CXR arm, and that there was no evidence that adverse events associated with lung cancer screening were sufficiently common to question the balance of benefits and harms [180]. Similar European RCTs are still underway at the time of writing [181, 182].

Limitations and Adverse Outcomes

LDCT will not detect all lung cancers, and detection of a cancer by LDCT does not guarantee that death from lung cancer will be avoided. Harms associated with LDCT screening include anxiety associated with abnormal testing results, additional imaging tests and biopsy associated with false positive results; in rare instances, serious harms including hospitalizations, and

Table 11.8 ACS and USPSTF guidelines for lung cancer screening with LDCT in current and former smokers aged 55–74.[1]

Recommendation	ACS	USPSTF
Adults aged 55–74/80	Clinicians with access to high-volume, high quality lung cancer screening and treatment centers should initiate a discussion about annual lung cancer screening with apparently healthy patients aged 55–74 years who have at least a 30 pack-year smoking history, and who currently smoke or have quit within the past 15 years A process of informed and shared decision making with a clinician related to the potential benefits, limitations, and harms associated with screening for lung cancer with LDCT should occur before any decision is made to initiate lung cancer screening Smoking cessation counseling remains a high priority for clinical attention in discussions with current smokers, who should be informed of their continuing risk of lung cancer. Screening should not be viewed as an alternative to smoking cessation	The USPSTF recommends annual screening for lung cancer with low-dose computed tomography (LDCT) in adults aged 55–80 years who have a 30 pack-year smoking history and currently smoke or have quit within the past 15 years. Screening should be discontinued once a person has not smoked for 15 years or develops a health problem that substantially limits life expectancy or the ability or willingness to have curative lung surgery

[1] The ACS recommends against screening for lung cancer in adults with chest X-ray for adults at any level of risk.

death, albeit very rare, can result from diagnostic evaluations in patients without and with lung cancer. Other harms include investigations for incidental findings outside of the lung field (which also may prove to be beneficial), radiation risk from multiple follow-up exams, and overdiagnosis, although current studies are not sufficiently mature to estimate overdiagnosis.

Lung cancer screening with LDCT has a relatively high rate of identification of benign, noncalcified nodules. In a systematic review, the average nodule detection rate per round of screening was 20% [183]. In the LDCT arm of the NLST, 27.3% of NLST study subjects experienced a positive test result in the first round of screening, and over three screening rounds 39.1% of individuals experienced at least one abnormal CT scan [166]. The recall rate tends to decline in subsequent rounds [183], and in the NLST it declined between the second and third screening round because stable nodules were no longer considered positive [166]. The majority of individuals with abnormal LDCT test results required only additional imaging to determine if one or more nodules were growing. Among those who required further evaluation, only 2.7% underwent invasive procedures [166] and the rate of complications resulting from a diagnostic procedure following a positive screening test also was relatively low and considerably higher in patients with a diagnosis of lung cancer versus those whose abnormality was determined to be benign (11.2% vs 0.06%, respectively) [166]. One study reported that indeterminate lung cancer screening test results increased anxiety, but that anxiety diminished over time, a finding similar to what has been observed in breast cancer screening [184].

Screening Recommendations

Recommendations from the ACS [185], the USPSTF [186], and other organizations that have issued lung cancer screening guidelines mostly are consistent with the NLST protocol [166] with respect to identifying a high risk group of current and former smokers as the target group for screening (Table 11.8) [187].

Some recommendations, such as those from the National Comprehensive Cancer Network, recommend lung cancer screening among current and former smokers with fewer pack years of smoking beginning at age 50 if they have one or more risk factors (family history, occupational exposures, etc.) in addition to smoking history [169]. The ACS lung cancer screening

guideline emphasizes that clinicians with access to high-volume, high quality lung cancer screening and treatment centers should ascertain the smoking status and smoking history of their patients aged 55–74 (Table 11.8), and should initiate a discussion about lung cancer screening with those patients who have at least a 30 pack-year smoking history, currently smoke or have quit within the past 15 years, and are in relatively good health. Core elements of this discussion should include the benefits, uncertainties, and harms associated with screening for lung cancer with LDCT (Table 11.9). Adults who choose to be screened should follow the NLST protocol of annual LDCT screening until they reach age 74. CXR should not be used for cancer screening.

Table 11.9 Key discussion points for the process of shared decision making related to screening for early lung cancer detection with low dose helical CT.

- Benefit: screening with LDCT has been shown to reduce the risk of dying from lung cancer substantially;
- Limitations: LDCT will not detect all lung cancers or all lung cancers early, and not all patients who have a lung cancer detected by LDCT will avoid death from lung cancer;
- Harms: there is a significant chance of a false positive result, which will require additional periodic testing, and in some instances, an invasive procedure to determine whether an abnormality is lung cancer or some non-lung related incidental finding. Less than one in 1,000 patients with a false positive result experience a major complication resulting from a diagnostic workup. Death within 60 days of a diagnostic evaluation has been documented, but is rare and most often occurs in patients with lung cancer.

Helping individuals clarify their personal values can facilitate effective decision making

- Individuals who value the opportunity to reduce their risk of dying from lung cancer and who are willing to accept the risks and costs associated with having a LDCT and the relatively high likelihood of the need for further tests, even tests that have the rare but real risk of complications and death, may opt to be screened with LDCT every year.
- Individuals who place greater value on avoiding testing that carries a high risk of false positives and a small risk of complications, and who understand and accept that they are at a much higher risk for death from lung cancer than from screening complications, may opt not to be screened with LDCT.

Of particular importance is that current smokers should be informed of their continuing risk of lung cancer and referred to smoking cessation programs. Screening should not be viewed as an alternative to smoking cessation.

Prostate Cancer

Prostate cancer is the most common cancer diagnosed in men. Prostate cancer screening has been a contentious and challenging issue due to limited data on the efficacy of screening, and the inability to distinguish truly life-threating disease from that which is not. Prostate cancer is often described as a disease a man is more likely to die "with" than "from". Not only are competing causes of death important, owing to the older average age at prostate cancer diagnosis, but prostate cancer treatment commonly results in significant quality-of-life diminishing harms that presently leave questions about the balance of benefits to harms unresolved.

Screening and Diagnostic Methods

The principal methods for early prostate cancer detection are the digital rectal examination (DRE), the prostate-specific antigen (PSA) blood test, and transrectal ultrasonography (TRUS).

Digital Rectal Examination

For the detection of symptoms of prostate cancer, palpation should begin at the apex of the prostate and continue to the base to assess the size and consistency of the gland. Palpable asymmetry of the prostate gland and, particularly, hard nodular areas may indicate presence of prostate cancer.

A principal limitation of DRE is that most advanced, palpable cancers and many clinically important cancers are in regions of the gland that are inaccessible to digital palpation. Although results are highly correlated with PSA levels, the DRE often is recommended as one component of prostate cancer screening because: (i) it may detect cancers missed by other tests [188] including potentially aggressive cancers at lower than conventional PSA cut-offs ($\geq 4\,ng/ml$) [189]; (ii) it is a low-cost procedure; and (iii) it has value in evaluating other prostate abnormalities such as benign prostatic hyperplasia or acute prostatitis [190].

PSA

PSA is a glycoprotein enzyme secreted by the epithelial cells of the prostate gland. It is organ specific; in men with healthy prostates, PSA is present in low concentration in serum, but in men with prostate disorders, including cancer, PSA may be elevated.

The principal strengths of the PSA test are its sensitivity, reasonable cost, and high patient acceptance. The principal drawback of the test is its imperfect specificity, since common conditions such as benign prostatic hyperplasia and prostatitis can cause borderline or markedly abnormal test results. Conversely, the high sensitivity of the test, depending on cut-off levels, may result in considerable overdiagnosis of small indolent cancers that might require no treatment, and of relatively indolent cancers that would not become life threatening in an older male. Further, while a threshold for an abnormal PSA in men older than 50 years of $\geq 4.0\,ng/ml$ was established in the early 1990s [191], it is now understood that there is no level of PSA below $4.0\,ng/ml$ for which there is certainty a patient does

not have prostate cancer [192]. These test features have led to harsh criticism of PSA, which some have argued may be misplaced. As Vickers *et al.* have shown, PSA measures at age 60 are 90% accurate at predicting prostate cancer death within 25 years [193]. In a separate commentary, Vickers and Lilja assert that PSA is a good predictor of high grade disease, and the fact that it does not do well at distinguishing between low-grade cancer and no cancer at all does not mean that the PSA has no clinical value [194]; rather, they argue, it means there is a need to develop better markers to distinguish aggressive from indolent disease. Work presently is underway to improve the specificity of PSA, that is, using PSA derivatives and additional kallikrein markers to improve the performance characteristics of the PSA test [195], the use of the Prostate Health Index, which is a mathematical algorithm that combines total PSA, free PSA, and [-2] proPSA [196], urinary gene expression signatures [197], and other approaches. However, to date none have sufficient data to replace, or routinely supplement, PSA screening in order to reduce overdetection and overtreatment of indolent disease [198].

TRUS

TRUS uses a small rectal probe placed against the prostate gland to image the entire gland. Due to poor sensitivity of greyscale TRUS in the detection of prostate cancer and specificity of sonographic abnormalities, it is not used in screening. Rather, TRUS-guided acquisition of multiple biopsies from specific locations has become the standard approach to diagnose prostate cancer in men with either an abnormal DRE, PSA or both [199]. Likewise, using TRUS for measuring gland volume and evaluating other morphological features associated with malignancy provide useful information and should be documented. The limitations of TRUS have led to experimental work with color and power Doppler, elastography, and fusion MRI biopsy techniques, where MRI performed before the biopsy procedure is used to guide ultrasound guided biopsy [199, 200].

Additional tests are required to characterize the aggressiveness of prostate cancer for purposes of management and risk stratification. A 5-point Gleason grade is used to categorize prostate cancer architecture from very well differentiated to undifferentiated, and a Gleason score is calculated by adding the two most common Gleason grades from the cores, ensuring that the worst score is included. A Gleason score can range from 2 to 10, with a score of ≤ 6 indicating a low-risk tumor (indolent, well-differentiated); a score of 7 is an intermediate risk tumor; and a score of 8–10 is judged to be a clinically aggressive tumor [201].

Relative and Absolute Benefit

PSA became widely used for screening following its commercial introduction as a test for monitoring prostate cancer patients [202]. This pattern of use resulted in a marked increase in prostate cancer incidence rates in the US from the late 1980s until 1992 [137], and a subsequent decline – a classic pattern of rise and fall in incidence consistent with the detection of a sizable prevalence of occult disease that potentially would have been detected subsequently if screening had not taken place. Over the reminder of the decade, the incidence rate rose to "catch up" with the earlier incidence trend [137]. Following the increase in incidence in the US, prostate cancer mortality began to fall and has declined in the US since 1993 [137]. The explanation for this decline in mortality remains unresolved, with some arguing that the decline was attributable in part to screening, while others argued it was entirely attributable to improvements in therapy [203, 204]. However, the decline in deaths was associated with a marked decline in the detection of cancers at advanced stage, providing support for the argument that screening was an important factor [203].

Disparate findings from two large RCTs of prostate cancer screening still have not led to consensus about whether prostate cancer screening is efficacious in reducing prostate cancer mortality. In the Prostate, Lung, Colorectal, and Ovarian (PLCO) RCT [205] investigators concluded that an invitation to prostate cancer screening was not associated with a reduction in prostate cancer mortality (RR = 1.09, 95% CI, 0.87–1.36), whereas the European Randomized Study of Prostate Cancer Screening (ERSPC) observed a statistically significant reduction in prostate cancer mortality associated with an invitation to screening (RR = 0.80, 95% CI, 0.65–0.98) [206]. These results have not changed appreciably with additional follow-up, leaving us with two RCTs with very different outcomes. Each trial has been criticized for limitations in methodology and reporting. In particular, the PLCO has been criticized for very high rates of pre-trial exposure to PSA testing, and very high rates of control group contamination (>50%), while the ERSPC has been criticized for the fact that the results depended on statistically significant mortality reductions in only two of seven participating centers. In the Goteborg RCT, one of the participating centers in the ERSPC where the trial was established and underway before joining the ERSPC, the investigators observed a prostate cancer mortality reduction of nearly 50% associated with an invitation to screening [207]. With considerably greater follow-up, the authors concluded that screening for prostate cancer was associated with a reduction in prostate cancer mortality, but cautioned that the potential for significant overdiagnosis and overtreatment still was substantial. Etzioni and Thompson have concluded that careful scrutiny of the outcomes of the two trials strongly suggests a clinically significant benefit from screening, and what is left to do is optimize implementation of screening to maximize benefit and minimize harm [208].

Limitations and Harms

Both DRE and PSA have limitations in sensitivity and specificity, especially as presently used in screening. While sensitivity of PSA improves with lower cut-off levels, and when used in combination with DRE, improved sensitivity diminishes specificity. Further, additional tests are required to characterize the aggressiveness of prostate cancer for purposes of management and risk stratification. The PSA test itself is not associated with any significant harms, and attending screening also has not been shown to result in psychological distress, although men with positive findings do experience some distress, as expected, while waiting for biopsy results [209]. In the ERSPC, only 6% of men with positive PSA screening results reported high levels of anxiety [210].

Complications associated with a prostate biopsy include hematuria, rectal bleeding, hematospermia, urinary tract infection, and acute urinary retention, although the overall, serious complication rate is very low [211]. Complications requiring hospitalization are very uncommon (0.3%) [199].

There are significant concerns about overdiagnosis and over-treatment of prostate cancer, and concerns as well that too often men who are diagnosed with prostate cancer are counseled to, or not dissuaded from, immediately choosing radical therapy, especially given the uncertainty about whether the disease truly is life threatening and associated side effects associated with radical prostatectomy. Two alternatives to immediate radical therapy, observation and active surveillance, are increasingly replacing immediate treatment for men who are elderly or frail with limited longevity, or men with potentially indolent cancers who choose to defer treatment until the disease clearly reveals that it is progressive. Both active surveillance and observation involve monitoring no less often than every 6 months; patients in active surveillance may undergo periodic prostate biopsies, and will proceed to curative treatment if there is any indication of disease progression; in contrast, patients in observation are monitored until symptoms develop or are imminent, as suggested by very elevated PSA levels (>100 ng/ml), at which point they will should begin palliative androgen deprivation therapy [201].

Screening Recommendations

The current ACS guideline for the early detection of prostate cancer was published in 2010 [212] and states that men who have at least a 10-year life expectancy should have an opportunity to make an informed decision with their healthcare provider about whether to be screened for prostate cancer with serum PSA, with or without DRE, after receiving information about the benefits, risks, and uncertainties associated with prostate cancer screening (see Table 11.10). Most leading organizations endorse informed or shared decision making for prostate cancer screening. In 2012 the USPSTF recommended against prostate cancer screening [213], but in 2017 issued a draft update of the 2012 prostate cancer screening recommendation that reverses the previous recommendation by endorsing shared decision making regarding PSA-based screening for prostate cancer for men ages 55–69 [214]. The USPSTF draft recommendation recommends against PSA-based screening for men age 70 years and older.

Prostate cancer screening should not occur without an informed decision-making process (Table 11.11). Men at average risk should receive this information beginning at age 50. Men at higher risk, including African American men and men with a family member (father or brother) diagnosed with prostate cancer before age 65, should receive this information beginning at age 45. Men at appreciably higher risk (multiple family members diagnosed with prostate cancer before age 65) should receive this information beginning at age 40. Men should either receive this information directly from their healthcare providers or be referred to reliable and culturally appropriate sources. Patient decision aids are helpful in preparing men to decide whether to be tested [215]. For men who are unable to decide, the screening decision can be left to the discretion of the healthcare provider, who should factor into the decision his or her knowledge of the patient's general health preferences and values. Asymptomatic men who have less than a 10-year life expectancy based on age and health status should not be offered prostate cancer screening.

For men who choose to be screened for prostate cancer after a process of shared or informed decision making: (i) screening is recommended with the PSA with or without the DRE (DRE is recommended along with PSA for men with hypogonadism, due to reduced sensitivity of PSA); (ii) for men whose PSA is less

Table 11.10 ACS and USPSTF guidelines for prostate cancer screening.

Recommendation	ACS	USPSTF
Average risk men aged 50+	Prostate-specific antigen test (PSA) with or without digital rectal examination (DRE)	The USPSTF recommends against prostate-specific antigen (PSA)-based screening for prostate cancer
	Men who have at least a 10-year life expectancy should have an opportunity to make an informed decision with their healthcare provider about whether to be screened for prostate cancer, after receiving information about the potential benefits, risks, and uncertainties associated with prostate cancer screening. Prostate cancer screening should not occur without an informed decision making process	
	Men at higher risk, including African-American men and men with a family member (father or brother) diagnosed with prostate cancer before age 65, should receive this information beginning at age 45. Men at appreciably higher risk (multiple family members diagnosed with prostate cancer before age 65) should receive this information beginning at age 40	

Table 11.11 Core elements of the information to be provided to men to assist with their decision about prostate cancer screening.

Prostate cancer is an important health concern for men:

- Screening with the prostate-specific antigen (PSA) blood test alone or with both the PSA and digital rectal exam (DRE) detects cancer at an earlier stage than if no screening is performed
- Prostate cancer screening may be associated with a reduction in the risk of dying from prostate cancer. However, evidence is conflicting and experts disagree about the value of screening
- For men whose prostate cancer is detected by screening, it is currently not possible to predict which men are likely to benefit from treatment. Some men who are treated may avoid death and disability from prostate cancer. Others who are treated would have died of unrelated causes before their cancer became serious enough to affect their health or shorten their lives
- Depending on the treatment selected, treatment of prostate cancer can lead to urinary, bowel, sexual, and other health problems. These problems may be significant or minimal, permanent or temporary
- The PSA and DRE may have false positive or false negative results, meaning men without cancer may have abnormal results and get unnecessary additional testing, and clinically significant cancers may be missed. False positive results can lead to sustained anxiety about prostate cancer risk
- Abnormal results from screening with the PSA or DRE require prostate biopsies to determine whether or not the abnormal findings are cancer. Biopsies can be painful, may lead to complications like infection or bleeding, and can miss clinically significant cancer
- Not all men whose prostate cancer is detected through screening require immediate treatment, but they may require periodic blood tests and prostate biopsies to determine the need for future treatment
- In helping men to reach a screening decision based on their personal values, once they understand the uncertainties, risks, and potential benefits, it can be helpful to provide reasons why some men decide for or against undergoing screening. For example:
  - A man who chooses to be screened might place a higher value on finding cancer early, might be willing to be treated without definite expectation of benefit, and might be willing to risk injury to urinary, sexual, and/or bowel function
  - A man who chooses not to be screened might place a higher value on avoiding the potential harms of screening and treatment, such as anxiety or risk of injury to urinary, sexual, or bowel function

than 2.5 ng/ml, screening intervals can be extended to every 2 years. Screening should be conducted yearly for men whose PSA level is 2.5 ng/ml or higher; and (iii) a PSA level of 4.0 ng/ml or higher has historically been used to recommend referral for further evaluation or biopsy, which remains a reasonable approach for men at average risk for prostate cancer. For PSA levels between 2.5 and 4.0 ng/ml, healthcare providers should consider an individualized risk assessment that incorporates other risk factors for prostate cancer, particularly for high-grade cancer, which may be used for a referral recommendation [212]. Factors that increase the risk of prostate cancer include African American race, family history of prostate cancer, increasing age, and abnormal DRE. A prior negative biopsy lowers risk. Statistical models are available that merge this information to achieve an estimate of a man's overall risk of prostate cancer, and, more specifically, his risk of high grade prostate cancer [216]. If prostate cancer is found, men should receive appropriate counseling about treatment options, ideally from an interdisciplinary treatment team. Avoiding radical therapy in men with a low likelihood of having rapidly progressive prostate cancer improves the balance of benefits and harms of therapy.

Conclusion

The cancers that have been described in this chapter are those for which there are data supporting regular screening, or for which shared decision making is endorsed. Other cancers for which there is compelling evidence that an early detection strategy may be efficacious are currently under investigation, such as screening for ovarian cancer [217] while other cancers do not have sufficient or compelling data to support regular screening or alternative approaches such as self-exams. No matter how compelling or intuitive an early detection strategy may appear, in the absence of confirming, experimental evidence, population-based screening cannot be recommended.

Achieving the full potential of cancer screening is more likely in organized care-delivery systems, within which each of the key steps that need to occur is governed by rules, roles, relationships, and oversight. While a system is no guarantee that a screening program will achieve its fullest potential, without systems, achieving that potential is much less likely. High quality screening requires high rates of: (i) standardized, timely and routine risk assessment in order to identify and properly triage adults at high risk; (ii) competent discussions with the target population about what to expect from screening; (iii) reminder and outreach systems to ensure that the target population receives regular screening at recommended intervals; (iv) systems to ensure timely workups of adults with positive findings, and to avoid delays in diagnosis and treatment; (v) centralized assessment of the technical quality of screening to ensure that every screening examination has a high probability of meeting a minimum standard of quality and accuracy; (vi) registries and routine review of screening outcomes to provide health professionals involved in screening with the opportunity to assess their performance; (vii) centralized data linking patient information, screening history, and screening outcomes in order to measure the effectiveness of screening programs and identify opportunities to improve the process to achieve better outcomes. Tools exist to support primary care providers to build a system to support their own patient panel [218] but other elements listed above, such as programs to ensure the quality of screening, depend on centralized organization, such as is common in Europe. In the US, integrated care delivery systems have the opportunity and obligation to develop these kinds of comprehensive systems.

References

1 Shapiro S. Screening for secondary prevention of disease. In: HK Armenian, S Shapiro (eds) *Epidemiology and Health Services*. New York: Oxford University Press, 1998:183–206.

2 Andrews J, Guyatt G, Oxman AD, *et al*. GRADE guidelines: 15. Going from evidence to recommendations: the significance and presentation of recommendations. *J Clin Epidemiol* 2013;66(7):719–25.

3 Wilson JMG, Jungner G. *Principles and Practice of Screening for Disease*. Geneva: World Health Organization, 1968.

4 Smith RA. Screening fundamentals. *Monogr Natl Cancer Inst* 1997;22:15–22.

5 Duffy SW, Chen HH, Tabar L, Day NE. Estimation of mean sojourn time in breast cancer screening using a Markov chain model of both entry to and exit from the preclinical detectable phase. *Stat Med* 1995;14:1531–43.

6 Puliti D, Duffy SW, Miccinesi G, *et al*. Overdiagnosis in mammographic screening for breast cancer in Europe: a literature review. *J Med Screen* 2012;19(Suppl 1):42–56.

7 Sutton S, Wardle J, Taylor T, *et al*. Predictors of attendance in the United Kingdom flexible sigmoidoscopy screening trial. *J Med Screen* 2000;7:99–104.

8 Dugue PA, Lynge E, Rebolj M. Mortality of non-participants in cervical screening: register-based cohort study. *Int J Cancer* 2014;134:2674–82.

9 Odgaard-Jensen J, Vist GE, Timmer A, *et al*. Randomisation to protect against selection bias in healthcare trials. Cochrane Database Syst Rev 2011:MR000012.

10 Prorok P, Chamberlain J, Day N, Hakama M, Miller A. UICC Workshop on the evaluation of screening programs for cancer. *Int J Cancer* 1984;34:1–4.

11 Black WC, Haggstrom DA, Welch HG. All-cause mortality in randomized trials of cancer screening. *J Natl Cancer Inst* 2002;94:167–73.

12 Nystrom L, Andersson I, Bjurstam N, *et al*. Long-term effects of mammography screening: updated overview of the Swedish randomised trials. *Lancet* 2002;359:909–19.

13 Gail MH, Katki HA. Re: all-cause mortality in randomized trials of cancer screening. *J Natl Cancer Inst* 2002;94:862; author reply 5–6.

14 Cuzick J, Edwards R, Segnan N. Adjusting for non-compliance and contamination in randomized clinical trials. *Stat Med* 1997;16:1017–29.

15 Prorok PC, Hankey BF, Bundy BN. Concepts and problems in the evaluation of screening programs. *J Chronic Dis* 1981;34:159–71.

16 Duffy SW, Smith RA. A note on the design of cancer screening trials. *J Med Screen* 2015;22(2):65–8.

17 Cronin KA, Weed DL, Connor RJ, Prorok PC. Case-control studies of cancer screening: theory and practice. *J Natl Cancer Inst* 1998;90:498–504.

18 Moss SM, Nystrom L, Jonsson H, *et al*. The impact of mammographic screening on breast cancer mortality in Europe: a review of trend studies. *J Med Screen* 2012;19 Suppl 1:26–32.

19 Tabar L, Vitak B, Tony HH, *et al*. Beyond randomized controlled trials: organized mammographic screening substantially reduces breast carcinoma mortality. *Cancer* 2001;91:1724–31.

20 Tabar L, Vitak B, Yen MF, *et al*. Number needed to screen: lives saved over 20 years of follow-up in mammographic screening. *J Med Screen* 2004;11:126–9.

21 Garber AM, Weinstein MC, Torrance GW, Kamlet MS. *Theoretical foundations of cost-effectiveness analysis. In: MR Gold, JE.Siegel, LB Russell, MC Weinstein (eds), Cost-Effectiveness in Health and Medicine*. New York: Oxford University Press, 1996.

22 Eisenberg JM. Clinical economics. A guide to the economic analysis of clinical practices. *JAMA* 1989;262:2879–86.

23 Fenton JJ, Cai Y, Weiss NS, *et al*. Delivery of cancer screening: how important is the preventive health examination? *Arch Intern Med* 2007;167:580–5.

24 Smith RA, Duffy SW, Tabar L. Breast cancer screening: the evolving evidence. *Oncology (Williston Park)* 2012;26:471–5, 9–81, 85–6.

25 Pisano ED, Hendrick RE, Yaffe MJ, *et al*. Diagnostic accuracy of digital versus film mammography: exploratory analysis of selected population subgroups in DMIST. *Radiology* 2008;246:376–83.

26 Stout NK, Lee SJ, Schechter CB, *et al*. Benefits, harms, and costs for breast cancer screening after US implementation of digital mammography. *J Natl Cancer Inst* 2014;106:dju092.

27 Kerlikowske K, Hubbard RA, Miglioretti DL, *et al*. Comparative effectiveness of digital versus film-screen mammography in community practice in the United States: a cohort study. *Ann Intern Med* 2011;155:493–502.

28 Friedewald SM, Rafferty EA, Rose SL, *et al*. Breast cancer screening using tomosynthesis in combination with digital mammography. *JAMA* 2014;311:2499–507.

29 Burnside ES, Park JM, Fine JP, Sisney GA. The use of batch reading to improve the performance of screening mammography. *Am J Roentgenol* 2005;185:790–6.

30 McDonald S, Saslow D, Alciati MH. Performance and reporting of clinical breast examination: a review of the literature. *CA Cancer J Clin* 2004;54:345–61.

31 *How to perform breast self-examination*. Johns Hopkins University, 2015. Available at: http://www.hopkinsmedicine. org/healthlibrary/conditions/breast_health/how_to_ perform_a_breast_self-examination_bse_85,P00135/ (accessed 25 May 2017).

32 Marmot MG, Altman DG, Cameron DA, *et al*. The benefits and harms of breast cancer screening: an independent review. *Br J Cancer* 2013;108:2205–40.

33 Shapiro S. Periodic screening for breast cancer: the HIP Randomized Controlled Trial. Health Insurance Plan. *J Natl Cancer Inst* 1997;22:27–30.

34 Tabar L, Vitak B, Chen TH, *et al*. Swedish two-county trial: impact of mammographic screening on breast cancer mortality during 3 decades. *Radiology* 2011;260(3):658–63.

35 Alexander FE, Anderson TJ, Brown HK, *et al*. 14 years of follow-up from the Edinburgh randomised trial of breast-cancer screening [see comments]. *Lancet* 1999;353:1903–8.

36 Miller AB, Wall C, Baines CJ, *et al*. Twenty five year follow-up for breast cancer incidence and mortality of the Canadian National Breast Screening Study: randomised screening trial. *BMJ* 2014;348:g366.

37 Frisell J, Lidbrink E. The Stockholm Mammographic Screening Trial: risks and benefits in age group 40–49 years. *J Natl Cancer Inst* 1997;89(22):49–51.

38 Bjurstam N, Bjorneld L, Warwick J, *et al*. The Gothenburg Breast Screening Trial. *Cancer* 2003;97:2387–96.

39 Moss SM, Wale C, Smith R, *et al*. Effect of mammographic screening from age 40 years on breast cancer mortality in the UK Age trial at 17 years' follow-up: a randomised controlled trial. *Lancet Oncol* 2015;16:1123–32.

40 Tabar L, Yen AM, Wu WY, *et al*. Insights from the breast cancer screening trials: how screening affects the natural history of breast cancer and implications for evaluating service screening programs. *Breast J* 2015;21:13–20.

41 Broeders M, Moss S, Nystrom L, *et al*. The impact of mammographic screening on breast cancer mortality in Europe: a review of observational studies. *J Med Screen* 2012;19 Suppl 1:14–25.

42 Coldman A, Phillips N, Wilson C, *et al*. Pan-Canadian study of mammography screening and mortality from breast cancer. *J Natl Cancer Inst* 2014;106(11).

43 Hofvind S, Ursin G, Tretli S, Sebuodegard S, Moller B. Breast cancer mortality in participants of the Norwegian Breast Cancer Screening Program. *Cancer* 2013;119:3106–12.

44 Lauby-Secretan B, Scoccianti C, Loomis D, *et al*. Breast-cancer screening – viewpoint of the IARC Working Group. *N Engl J Med* 2015;372:2353–8.

45 Independent UK Panel on Breast Cancer Screening. The benefits and harms of breast cancer screening: an independent review. *Lancet* 2012;380:1778–86.

46 Gotzsche PC, Jorgensen KJ. Screening for breast cancer with mammography. *Cochrane Database Syst Rev* 2013;6:CD001877.

47 Nelson HD, Tyne K, Naik A, *et al*. Screening for breast cancer: an update for the U.S. Preventive Services Task Force. *Ann Intern Med* 2009;151:727–37, W237–42.

48 Paci E. Summary of the evidence of breast cancer service screening outcomes in Europe and first estimate of the benefit and harm balance sheet. *J Med Screen* 2012;19 Suppl 1:5–13.

49 Paci E, Broeders M, Hofvind S, Puliti D, Duffey S, GROUP atEW. *European breast cancer service screening outcomes: a first balance sheet of the benefits and harms Cancer Epidemiol Biomarkers Prev* 2014;23(7):1159–63.

50 Duffy SW, Chen TH, Smith RA, Yen AM, Tabar L. Real and artificial controversies in breast cancer screening: a perspective article. *Breast Cancer Management* 2013;2:519–28.

51 Bancej C, Decker K, Chiarelli A, *et al*. Contribution of clinical breast examination to mammography screening in the early detection of breast cancer. *J Med Screen* 2003;10:16–21.

52 Oestreicher N, White E, Lehman CD, *et al*. Predictors of sensitivity of clinical breast examination (CBE). *Breast Cancer Res Treat* 2002;76:73–81.

53 Semiglazov VF, Moiseyenko VM, Bavli JL, *et al*. The role of breast self-examination in early breast cancer detection (results of the 5-years USSR/WHO randomized study in Leningrad). *Eur J Epidemiol* 1992;8:498–502.

54 Thomas DB, Gao DL, Self SG, *et al*. Randomized trial of breast self-examination in Shanghai: methodology and preliminary results (see comments). *J Natl Cancer Inst* 1997;89:355–65.

55 Pinotti JA, Barros AC, Hegg R, Zeferino LC. Breast cancer control programme in developing countries. *Eur J Gynaecol Oncol* 1993;14:355–62.

56 Sankaranarayanan R, Ramadas K, Thara S, *et al*. Clinical breast examination: preliminary results from a cluster randomized controlled trial in India. *J Natl Cancer Inst* 2011;103:1476–80.

57 National Cancer Institute-funded Breast Cancer Surveillance Consortium co-operative agreement (U01CA63740 UC, U01CA86082, U01CA63736, U01CA70013, U01CA69976, U01CA63731, U01CA70040). Performance Measures for 1,838,372 Screening Mammography Examinations from 2004 to 2008 by Age – based on BCSC data through 2009. National Cancer Institute, 2014.

58 Nelson HD, O'Meara ES, Kerlikowske K, Balch S, Miglioretti D. Factors associated with rates of false-positive and false-negative results from digital mammography screening: an analysis of registry data. *Ann Intern Med* 2016;164:226–35.

59 Hofvind S, Ponti A, Patnick J, *et al*. False-positive results in mammographic screening for breast cancer in Europe: a literature review and survey of service screening programmes. *J Med Screen* 2012;19 Suppl 1:57–66.

60 Kerlikowske K, Carney PA, Geller B, *et al*. Performance of screening mammography among women with and without a first-degree relative with breast cancer. *Ann Intern Med* 2000;133:855–63.

61 Boyd NF, Guo H, Martin LJ, *et al*. Mammographic density and the risk and detection of breast cancer. *N Engl J Med* 2007;356:227–36.

62 Berg WA, Blume JD, Cormack JB, *et al*. Combined screening with ultrasound and mammography vs mammography alone in women at elevated risk of breast cancer. *JAMA* 2008;299:2151–63.

63 Nelson HD, Pappas M, Cantor A, *et al*. Harms of Breast Cancer Screening: Systematic Review to Update the 2009 U.S. Preventive Services Task Force Recommendation. *Ann Intern Med* 2016;164:256–67.

64 Kopans DB, Smith RA, Duffy SW. Mammographic screening and "overdiagnosis". *Radiology* 2011;260:616–20.

65 Siu AL, Force USPST. Screening for Breast Cancer: U.S. Preventive Services Task Force Recommendation Statement. *Ann Intern Med* 2016;164:279–96.

66 Oeffinger KC, Fontham ETH, Etzioni R, *et al*. Breast Cancer Screening for Women at Average Risk: 2015 Guideline Update from the American Cancer Society. *JAMA* 2015;314(15):1599–614.

67 Saslow D, Boetes C, Burke W, *et al*. American Cancer Society guidelines for breast screening with MRI as an adjunct to mammography. *CA Cancer J Clin* 2007;57:75–89.

68 Mulder RL, Kremer LC, Hudson MM, *et al*. Recommendations for breast cancer surveillance for female survivors of childhood, adolescent, and young adult cancer given chest radiation: a report from the International Late Effects of Childhood Cancer Guideline Harmonization Group. *Lancet Oncol* 2013;14:e621–9.

69 Arends MJ. Pathways of colorectal carcinogenesis. *Appl Immunohistochem Mol Morphol* 2013;21:97–102.

70 Strum WB. Colorectal adenomas. *N Engl J Med* 2016;374:1065–75.

71 Bond JH. Colon polyps and cancer. *Endoscopy* 2003;35:27–35.

72 Zauber AG, Winawer SJ, O'Brien MJ, *et al*. Colonoscopic polypectomy and long-term prevention of colorectal-cancer deaths. *N Engl J Med* 2012;366:687–96.

73 Ahnen DJ. The American College of Gastroenterology Emily Couric Lecture – the adenoma-carcinoma sequence revisited: has the era of genetic tailoring finally arrived? *Am J Gastroenterol* 2011;106:190–8.

74 Szylberg L, Janiczek M, Popiel A, Marszalek A. Serrated polyps and their alternative pathway to the colorectal cancer: a systematic review. *Gastroenterol Res Pract* 2015;2015:573814.

75 Stryker S, Wolff B, Culp C, Libbe S, Ilstrup D, MacCarty R. Natural history of untreated colonic polyps. *Gastroenterology* 1987;93:1009–13.

76 Winawer SJ, Fletcher RH, Miller L, *et al*. Colorectal cancer screening: clinical guidelines and rationale (see comments) (published errata appear in Gastroenterology 1997 Mar;112(3):1060 and 1998 Mar;114(3):625). *Gastroenterology* 1997;112:594–642.

77 O'Brien M, Winawer S, Zauber A, *et al*. The National Polyp Study. Patient and polyp characteristics associated with high-grade dysplasia in colorectal adenomas. *Gastroenterology* 1990;98:371–9.

78 Winawer SJ, Zauber AG. Colonoscopic polypectomy and the incidence of colorectal cancer. *Gut* 2001;48:753–4.

79 Johnson CD, MacCarty RL, Welch TJ, *et al*. Comparison of the relative sensitivity of CT colonography and double-contrast barium enema for screen detection of colorectal polyps. *Clin Gastroenterol Hepatol* 2004;2:314–21.

80 Levin B, Lieberman DA, McFarland B, *et al*. Screening and surveillance for the early detection of colorectal cancer and adenomatous polyps, 2008: a joint guideline from the American Cancer Society, the US Multi-Society Task Force on Colorectal Cancer, and the American College of Radiology. *CA Cancer J Clin* 2008;58:130–60.

81 Weinberg DS, Schoen RE. In the clinic. Screening for colorectal cancer. *Ann Intern Med* 2014;160.

82 Allison JE, Sakoda LC, Levin TR, *et al*. Screening for colorectal neoplasms with new fecal occult blood tests: update on performance characteristics. *J Natl Cancer Inst* 2007;99:1462–70.

83 Imperiale TF, Ransohoff DF, Itzkowitz SH, Turnbull BA, Ross ME. Fecal DNA versus fecal occult blood for colorectal-cancer screening in an average-risk population. *N Engl J Med* 2004;351:2704–14.

84 Nadel MR, Berkowitz Z, Klabunde CN, *et al*. Fecal occult blood testing beliefs and practices of U.S. primary care physicians: serious deviations from evidence-based recommendations. *J Gen Intern Med* 2010;25:833–9.

85 Collins JF, Lieberman DA, Durbin TE, Weiss DG. Accuracy of screening for fecal occult blood on a single stool sample obtained by digital rectal examination: a comparison with recommended sampling practice. *Ann Intern Med* 2005;142:81–5.

86 Screening for prostate cancer: U.S. Preventive Services Task Force recommendation statement. *Ann Intern Med* 2008;149:185–91.

87 Levi Z, Birkenfeld S, Vilkin A, *et al*. A higher detection rate for colorectal cancer and advanced adenomatous polyp for screening with immunochemical fecal occult blood test than guaiac fecal occult blood test, despite lower compliance rate. A prospective, controlled, feasibility study. *Int J Cancer* 2011;128:2415–24.

88 Young GP, Symonds EL, Allison JE, *et al*. Advances in Fecal Occult Blood Tests: the FIT revolution. *Digest Diseases Sci* 2015;60:609–22.

89 Chubak J, Bogart A, Fuller S, Laing SS, Green BB. Uptake and positive predictive value of fecal occult blood tests: a randomized controlled trial. *Prev Med* 2013;57:671–8.

90 Robertson DJ, Lee JK, Boland CR, *et al*. Recommendations on Fecal Immunochemical Testing to Screen for Colorectal Neoplasia: A Consensus Statement by the US Multi-Society Task Force on Colorectal Cancer. *Gastroenterology* 2017;152(5):1217–37.

91 Lee JK, Liles EG, Bent S, Levin TR, Corley DA. Accuracy of fecal immunochemical tests for colorectal cancer: systematic review and meta-analysis. *Ann Intern Med* 2014;160:171.

92 Imperiale TF, Ransohoff DF, Itzkowitz SH, *et al*. Multitarget stool DNA testing for colorectal-cancer screening. *N Engl J Med* 2014;370:1287–97.

93 Lightdale CJ. Modern colonoscopy continues to evolve and improve. *Gastrointest Endosc Clin N Am* 2015;25:xiii–xiv.

94 Sharara AI, Abou Mrad RR. The modern bowel preparation in colonoscopy. *Gastroenterol Clin North Am* 2013;42:577–98.

95 Altawil J, Miller LA, Antaki F. Acceptance of split-dose bowel preparation regimen for colonoscopy by patients and providers. *J Clin Gastroenterol* 2014;48:e47–9.

96 Childers RE, Williams JL, Sonnenberg A. Practice patterns of sedation for colonoscopy. *Gastrointest Endosc* 2015;82:503–11.

97 Takahashi Y, Tanaka H, Kinjo M, Sakumoto K. Sedation-free colonoscopy. *Dis Colon Rectum* 2005;48:855–9.

98 Cobb WS, Heniford BT, Sigmon LB, *et al*. Colonoscopic perforations: incidence, management, and outcomes. *Am Surg* 2004;70:750–7; discussion 7–8.

99 Chukmaitov A, Bradley CJ, Dahman B, *et al*. Association of polypectomy techniques, endoscopist volume, and facility type with colonoscopy complications. *Gastrointest Endosc* 2013;77:436–46.

100 Cooper GS, Kou TD, Rex DK. Complications following colonoscopy with anesthesia assistance: a population-based analysis. *JAMA Intern Med* 2013;173:551–6.

101 Brenner H, Chang-Claude J, Seiler CM, Rickert A, Hoffmeister M. Protection from colorectal cancer after colonoscopy: a population-based, case-control study. *Ann Intern Med* 2011;154:22–30.

102 Nishihara R, Wu K, Lochhead P, *et al*. Long-term colorectal-cancer incidence and mortality after lower endoscopy. *N Engl J Med* 2013;369:1095–105.

103 Pickhardt PJ, Choi JR, Hwang I, *et al*. Computed tomographic virtual colonoscopy to screen for colorectal neoplasia in asymptomatic adults. *N Engl J Med* 2003;349:2191–200.

104 Johnson CD, Chen MH, Toledano AY, *et al*. Accuracy of CT colonography for detection of large adenomas and cancers. *N Engl J Med* 2008;359:1207–17.

105 Zalis ME, Blake MA, Cai W, *et al*. Diagnostic accuracy of laxative-free computed tomographic colonography for detection of adenomatous polyps in asymptomatic adults: a prospective evaluation. *Ann Intern Med* 2012;156:692–702.

106 Rex DK, Schoenfeld PS, Cohen J, *et al*. Quality indicators for colonoscopy. *Gastrointest Endosc* 2015;81:31–53.

107 Corley DA, Jensen CD, Marks AR, *et al*. Adenoma detection rate and risk of colorectal cancer and death. *N Engl J Med* 2014;370:1298–306.

108 Kaminski MF, Regula J, Kraszewska E, *et al*. Quality indicators for colonoscopy and the risk of interval cancer. *N Engl J Med* 2010;362:1795–803.

109 Millan MS, Gross P, Manilich E, Church JM. Adenoma detection rate: the real indicator of quality in colonoscopy. *Dis Colon Rectum* 2008;51:1217–20.

110 von Karsa L, Patnick J, Segnan N, *et al*. European guidelines for quality assurance in colorectal cancer screening and diagnosis: overview and introduction to the full supplement publication. *Endoscopy* 2013;45:51–9.

111 Singh H, Penfold RB, De Coster C, *et al*. Predictors of serious complications associated with lower gastrointestinal endoscopy in a major city-wide health region. *Can J Gastroenterol* 2010;24:425–30.

112 Laghi A, Rengo M, Graser A, Iafrate F. Current status on performance of CT colonography and clinical indications. *Eur J Radiol* 2013;82:1192–200.

113 Shaukat A, Mongin SJ, Geisser MS, *et al*. Long-term mortality after screening for colorectal cancer. *N Engl J Med* 2013;369:1106–14.

114 Scholefield JH, Moss SM, Mangham CM, Whynes DK, Hardcastle JD. Nottingham trial of faecal occult blood testing for colorectal cancer: a 20-year follow-up. *Gut* 2012;61:1036–40.

115 Malila N, Palva T, Malminiemi O, *et al*. Coverage and performance of colorectal cancer screening with the faecal occult blood test in Finland. *J Med Screen* 2011;18:18–23.

116 Lindholm E, Brevinge H, Haglind E. Survival benefit in a randomized clinical trial of faecal occult blood screening for colorectal cancer. *Br J Surg* 2008;95:1029–36.

117 Kronborg O, Jorgensen OD, Fenger C, Rasmussen M. Randomized study of biennial screening with a faecal occult blood test: results after nine screening rounds. *Scand J Gastroenterol* 2004;39:846–51.

118 Faivre J, Dancourt V, Lejeune C, *et al*. Reduction in colorectal cancer mortality by fecal occult blood screening in a French controlled study. *Gastroenterology* 2004;126:1674–80.

119 Mandel JS, Church TR, Bond JH, *et al*. The effect of fecal occult-blood screening on the incidence of colorectal cancer. *N Engl J Med* 2000;343:1603–7.

120 Zauber AG, Lansdorp-Vogelaar I, Knudsen AB, *et al*. *Evaluating Test Strategies for Colorectal Cancer Screening-Age to Begin, Age to Stop, and Timing of Screening Intervals: A Decision Analysis of Colorectal Cancer Screening for the U.S. Preventive Services Task Force from the Cancer Intervention and Surveillance Modeling Network (CISNET)*. Rockville (MD): Agency for Healthcare Research and Quality, 2009.

121 Atkin WS, Edwards R, Kralj-Hans I, *et al*. Once-only flexible sigmoidoscopy screening in prevention of colorectal cancer: a multicentre randomised controlled trial. *Lancet* 2010;375:1624–33.

122 Schoen RE, Pinsky PF, Weissfeld JL, *et al*. Colorectal-cancer incidence and mortality with screening flexible sigmoidoscopy. *N Engl J Med* 2012;366:2345–57.

123 Segnan N, Armaroli P, Bonelli L, *et al*. Once-only sigmoidoscopy in colorectal cancer screening: follow-up findings of the Italian Randomized Controlled Trial – SCORE. *J Natl Cancer Inst* 2011;103:1310–22.

124 Muller AD, Sonnenberg A. Prevention of colorectal cancer by flexible endoscopy and polypectomy. A case-control study of 32,702 veterans (see comments). *Ann Intern Med* 1995;123:904–10.

125 Brown T, Lee JY, Park J, *et al*. Colorectal cancer screening at community health centers: a survey of clinicians' attitudes, practices, and perceived barriers. *Prev Med Rep* 2015;2:886–91.

126 Zapka J, Klabunde CN, Taplin S, *et al*. Screening colonoscopy in the US: attitudes and practices of primary care physicians. *J Gen Intern Med* 2012;27:1150–8.

127 Zauber AG, Lansdorp-Vogelaar I, Knudsen AB, *et al*. Evaluating test strategies for colorectal cancer screening: a decision analysis for the U.S. Preventive Services Task Force. *Ann Intern Med* 2008;149(9):659–69.

128 Inadomi JM, Vijan S, Janz NK, *et al*. Adherence to colorectal cancer screening: a randomized clinical trial of competing strategies. *Arch Intern Med* 2012;172:575–82.

129 Lieberman DA, Rex DK, Winawer SJ, *et al.* Guidelines for colonoscopy surveillance after screening and polypectomy: a consensus update by the US Multi-Society Task Force on Colorectal Cancer. *Gastroenterology* 2012;143:844–57.

130 Stoffel EM, Mangu PB, Gruber SB, *et al.*, American Society of Clinical Onoclogy, European Society of Clinical Oncology. Hereditary colorectal cancer syndromes: American Society of Clinical Oncology Clinical Practice Guideline endorsement of the familial risk-colorectal cancer: European Society for Medical Oncology Clinical Practice Guidelines. *J Clin Oncol* 2015;33:209–17.

131 Giardiello FM, Allen JI, Axilbund JE, *et al.* Guidelines on genetic evaluation and management of Lynch syndrome: a consensus statement by the US Multi-society Task Force on colorectal cancer. *Am J Gastroenterol* 2014;109:1159–79.

132 Koss LG. The Papanicolaou test for cervical cancer detection. A triumph and a tragedy (see comments). *JAMA* 1989;261:737–43.

133 Wheeler CM. The natural history of cervical human papillomavirus infections and cervical cancer: gaps in knowledge and future horizons. *Obstet Gynecol Clin North Am* 2013;40:165–76.

134 Apter D, Wheeler CM, Paavonen J, *et al.* Efficacy of human papillomavirus 16 and 18 (HPV-16/18) AS04-adjuvanted vaccine against cervical infection and precancer in young women: final event-driven analysis of the randomized, double-blind PATRICIA trial. *Clin Vaccine Immunol* 2015;22:361–73.

135 Cuzick J, Myers O, Hunt WC, *et al.* Human papillomavirus testing 2007–2012: co-testing and triage utilization and impact on subsequent clinical management. *Int J Cancer* 2015;136:2854–63.

136 Wright TC, Jr., Stoler MH, Behrens CM, *et al.* The ATHENA human papillomavirus study: design, methods, and baseline results. *Am J Obstet Gynecol* 2012;206:46 e1– e11.

137 Howlander N, Noone A, Krapcho M, *et al. SEER Cancer Statistics Review, 1975–2012.* Bethesda: National Cancer Institute, 2015.

138 Martin-Hirsch P, Lilford R, Jarvis G, Kitchener HC. Efficacy of cervical-smear collection devices: a systematic review and meta-analysis. *Lancet* 1999;354:1763–70.

139 Kaur P, Kushtagi P. Plastic spatula with narrow long tip provides higher satisfactory smears for Pap test. *J Cytol* 2013;30:159–61.

140 Davey DD, Cox JT, Austin RM, *et al.* Cervical cytology specimen adequacy: patient management guidelines and optimizing specimen collection. *J Low Gen Tract Dis* 2008;12:71–81.

141 Birdsong G, Davey DD. Specimen adequacy. In: R Nayar R, DC Wilbur (eds), *The Bethesda System for Reporting Cervical Cytology: Definitions, Criteria, and Explanatory Notes,* 3rd edn. New York: Springer, 2015:1–29.

142 Agency for Health Care Policy and Research. Evidence Report on Evaluation of Cervical Cytology. Rockville: Agency for Health Care Policy and Research, 1999. Report No.: AHCPR Pub. No. 99-E009.

143 Vesco KK, Whitlock EP, Eder M, *et al. Screening for Cervical Cancer: A Systematic Evidence Review for the U.S. Preventive Services Task Force.* Evidence Synthesis No. 86. Rockville, MD: Agency for Healthcare Research and Quality, May 2011.

144 Nayar R, Wilbur DC. *The Bethesda System for Reporting Cervical Cytology: Definitions, Criteria, and Explanatory Notes,* 3rd edn. New York: Springer, 2015.

145 Walboomers JM, Jacobs MV, Manos MM, *et al.* Human papillomavirus is a necessary cause of invasive cervical cancer worldwide. *J Pathol* 1999;189:12–9.

146 Munoz N, Bosch FX, de Sanjose S, *et al.* Epidemiologic classification of human papillomavirus types associated with cervical cancer. *N Engl J Med* 2003;348:518–27.

147 de Sanjose S, Quint WG, Alemany L, *et al.* Human papillomavirus genotype attribution in invasive cervical cancer: a retrospective cross-sectional worldwide study. *Lancet Oncol* 2010;11:1048–56.

148 Saslow D, Solomon D, Lawson HW, *et al.* American Cancer Society, American Society for Colposcopy and Cervical Pathology, and American Society for Clinical Pathology screening guidelines for the prevention and early detection of cervical cancer. *J Low Gen Tract Dis* 2012;16:175–204.

149 Cytopathology And More, 2012. Available from: http://www.captodayonline.com/Archives/0112/0112k (accessed 25 May 2017).

150 Petry KU, Menton S, Menton M, *et al.* Inclusion of HPV testing in routine cervical cancer screening for women above 29 years in Germany: results for 8466 patients. *Br J Cancer* 2003;88:1570–7.

151 Mayrand MH, Duarte-Franco E, Rodrigues I, *et al.* Human papillomavirus DNA versus Papanicolaou screening tests for cervical cancer. *N Engl J Med* 2007;357:1579–88.

152 Morrison A. *Screening in Chronic Disease.* New York: Oxford University Press, 1992.

153 Gardner JW, Lyon JL. Efficacy of cervical cytologic screening in the control of cervical cancer. *Prev Med* 1977;6:487–99.

154 Laara E, Day NE, Hakama M. Trends in mortality from cervical cancer in the Nordic countries: association with organised screening programmes. *Lancet* 1987;1:1247–9.

155 Hakama M, Magnus K, Petterson F, Storm H, Tulinius H. Effect of organized screening on the risk of cervical cancer in the Nordic countries. In: AB Miller, J Chamberlain, NE Day, M Hakama, PC Prorok (eds), *Cancer Screening.* Cambridge: Cambridge University Press, 1991.

156 Johannesson G, Geirsson G, Day N. The effect of mass screening in Iceland, 1965–74, on the incidence and mortality of cervical carcinoma. *Int J Cancer* 1978; 21:418–25.

157 Hakama M. Effect of population screening for carcinoma of the uterine cervix in Finland. *Maturitas* 1985;7(1):3–10.

158 Magnus K, Langmark F, Andersen A. Mass screening for cervical cancer in Ostfold county of Norway 1959–77. *Int J Cancer* 1987;39:311–6.

159 Sriplung H, Singkham P, Iamsirithaworn S, Jiraphongsa C, Bilheem S. Success of a cervical cancer screening program: trends in incidence in songkhla, southern Thailand, 1989–2010, and prediction of future incidences to 2030. *Asian Pac J Cancer Prev* 2014;15:10003–8.

160 Olesen F. A case-control study of cervical cytology before diagnosis of cervical cancer in Denmark. *Int J Epidemiol* 1988;17:501–8.

161 Macgregor JE, Campbell MK, Mann EM, Swanson KY. Screening for cervical intraepithelial neoplasia in north east Scotland shows fall in incidence and mortality from invasive cancer with concomitant rise in preinvasive disease. *BMJ* 1994;308:1407–11.

162 Ronco G, Dillner J, Elfstrom KM, *et al*. Efficacy of HPV-based screening for prevention of invasive cervical cancer: follow-up of four European randomised controlled trials. *Lancet* 2014;383:524–32.

163 Moyer VA. Screening for cervical cancer: U.S. Preventive Services Task Force recommendation statement. *Ann Intern Med* 2012;156:880–91, W312.

164 Strauss G, Dominioni L. Varese meeting report. *Lung Cancer* 1999;23:171–2.

165 Henschke CI, McCauley DI, Yankelevitz DF, *et al*. Early Lung Cancer Action Project: overall design and findings from baseline screening. *Lancet* 1999;354:99–105.

166 National Lung Screening Trial Research Team. Reduced Lung-Cancer Mortality with Low-Dose Computed Tomographic Screening. *N Engl J Med* 2011;365(5):395–409.

167 Kazerooni EA, Austin JH, Black WC, *et al*. ACR-STR practice parameter for the performance and reporting of lung cancer screening thoracic computed tomography (CT): 2014 (Resolution 4). *J Thorac Imaging* 2014;29:310–6.

168 Lung CT Screening Reporting and Data System (Lung-RADS) American College of Radiology, 2014. Available from: http://www.acr.org/Quality-Safety/Resources/LungRADS (accessed 25 May 2017).

169 Lung Cancer Screening. National Comprehensive Cancer Network, 2016. http://www.nccn.org/professionals/physician_gls/pdf/lung_screening.pdf (https://www.nccn.org/professionals/physician_gls/f_guidelines.asp#site for access information).

170 Naidich DP, Bankier AA, MacMahon H, *et al*. Recommendations for the management of subsolid pulmonary nodules detected at CT: a statement from the Fleischner Society. *Radiology* 2013;266:304–17.

171 Fontana RS, Sanderson DR, Woolner LB, *et al*. Screening for lung cancer. A critique of the Mayo Lung Project. *Cancer* 1991;67:1155–64.

172 Berlin NI. Overview of the NCI cooperative early lung cancer detection program. In: L Dominioni, G Strauss (eds), *International Conference on Prevention and Early Diagnosis of Lung Cancer*. Varese, Italy, 1998:11–4.

173 Frost JK, Ball WC, Jr., Levin ML, *et al*. Early lung cancer detection: results of the initial (prevalence) radiologic and cytologic screening in the Johns Hopkins study. *Am Rev Respir Dis* 1984;130:549–54.

174 Kubik A, Polak J. Lung cancer detection. Results of a randomized prospective study in Czechoslovakia. *Cancer* 1986;57:2427–37.

175 Melamed MR, Flehinger BJ, Zaman MB, *et al*. Screening for early lung cancer. Results of the Memorial Sloan–Kettering study in New York. *Chest* 1984;86:44–53.

176 U.S. Preventive Services Task Force. Lung cancer screening: recommendation statement. *Ann Intern Med* 2004;140:738–9.

177 Fontana RS. The Mayo Lung Project: a perspective. *Cancer* 2000;89:2352–5.

178 Kubik A, Haerting J. Survival and mortality in a randomized study of lung cancer detection. *Neoplasma* 1990;37:467–75.

179 Field JK, Smith RA, Duffy SW, *et al*. The Liverpool Statement 2005: priorities for the European Union/United States spiral computed tomography collaborative group. *J Thorac Oncol* 2006;1:497–8.

180 Statement concerning the lung cancer screening trial. National Cancer Institute, 2010. http://www.health.harvard.edu/cancer/transcript-of-national-cancer-institute-press-briefing-about-the-trial-using-ct-scans-to-screen-for- (accessed 11 June 2017).

181 Horeweg N, Scholten ET, de Jong PA, *et al*. Detection of lung cancer through low-dose CT screening (NELSON): a prespecified analysis of screening test performance and interval cancers. *Lancet Oncol* 2014;15:1342–50.

182 Field JK, Baldwin D, Brain K, *et al*. CT screening for lung cancer in the UK: position statement by UKLS investigators following the NLST report. *Thorax* 2011;66:736–7.

183 Bach PB, Mirkin JN, Oliver TK, *et al*. Benefits and harms of CT screening for lung cancer: a systematic review. *JAMA* 2012;307:2418–29.

184 Byrne MM, Weissfeld J, Roberts MS. Anxiety, fear of cancer, and perceived risk of cancer following lung cancer screening. *Med Decis Making* 2008;28:917–25.

185 Wender R, Fontham ETH, Barrera E, *et al*. American Cancer Society Lung Cancer Screening Guidelines. *CA Cancer J Clin* 2013;63(2):107–17.

186 Moyer VA, Force USPST. Screening for lung cancer: U.S. Preventive Services Task Force recommendation statement. *Ann Intern Med* 2014;160:330–8.

187 Smith RA, Manassaram-Baptiste D, Brooks D, *et al*. Cancer screening in the United States, 2015: a review of current American cancer society guidelines and current issues in cancer screening. *CA Cancer J Clin* 2015;65:30–54.

188 Schroder FH, van der Maas P, Beemsterboer P, *et al*. Evaluation of the digital rectal examination as a screening test for prostate cancer. Rotterdam section of the European Randomized Study of Screening for Prostate Cancer. *J Natl Cancer Inst* 1998;90:1817–23.

189 Okotie OT, Roehl KA, Han M, *et al*. Characteristics of prostate cancer detected by digital rectal examination only. *Urology* 2007;70:1117–20.

190 Basler JW, Thompson IM. Lest we abandon digital rectal examination as a screening test for prostate cancer (editorial; comment). *J Natl Cancer Inst* 1998;90:1761–3.

191 Catalona WJ, Smith DS, Ratliff TL, *et al*. Measurement of prostate-specific antigen in serum as a screening test for prostate cancer (published erratum appears in N Engl J Med 1991 Oct 31;325(18):1324) (see comments). *N Engl J Med* 1991;324:1156–61.

192 Thompson IM, Pauler DK, Goodman PJ, *et al*. Prevalence of prostate cancer among men with a prostate-specific antigen level < or =4.0 ng per milliliter. *N Engl J Med* 2004;350:2239–46.

193 Vickers AJ, Cronin AM, Bjork T, *et al*. Prostate specific antigen concentration at age 60 and death or metastasis from prostate cancer: case-control study. *BMJ* 2010;341:c4521.

194 Vickers AJ, Lilja H. PSA is dead, long live PSA. *Eur Urol* 2012;61:467–8; discussion 9–70.

195 Bryant RJ, Lilja H. Emerging PSA-based tests to improve screening. *Urol Clin North Am* 2014;41:267–76.

196 Loeb S, Catalona WJ. The Prostate Health Index: a new test for the detection of prostate cancer. *Ther Adv Urol* 2014;6:74–7.

197 McKiernan J, Donovan MJ, O'Neill V, *et al*. A novel urine exosome gene expression assay to predict high-grade prostate cancer at initial biopsy. *JAMA Oncol* 2016;2(7):882–9.

198 Patel HD, Chalfin HJ, Carter HB. Improving prostate cancer screening and diagnosis: health policy and biomarkers beyond PSA. *JAMA Oncol* 2016;2(7):867–8.

199 Harvey CJ, Pilcher J, Richenberg J, Patel U, Frauscher F. Applications of transrectal ultrasound in prostate cancer. *Br J Radiol* 2012;85 Spec No 1:S3–17.

200 Bjurlin MA, Meng X, Le Nobin J, *et al*. Optimization of prostate biopsy: the role of magnetic resonance imaging targeted biopsy in detection, localization and risk assessment. *J Urol* 2014;192:648–58.

201 Prostate Cancer. National Comprehensive Cancer Network, 2017. https://www.nccn.org/professionals/physician_gls/pdf/prostate.pdf (accessed 11 June 2017).

202 Stamey TA, Yang N, Hay AR, *et al*. Prostate-specific antigen as a serum marker for adenocarcinoma of the prostate. *N Engl J Med* 1987;317:909–16.

203 Tarone RE, Chu KC, Brawley OW. Implications of stage-specific survival rates in assessing recent declines in prostate cancer mortality rates. *Epidemiology* 2000;11:167–70.

204 Etzioni R, Legler JM, Feuer EJ, *et al*. Cancer surveillance series: interpreting trends in prostate cancer – part III: quantifying the link between population prostate-specific antigen testing and recent declines in prostate cancer mortality. *J Natl Cancer Inst* 1999;91:1033–9.

205 Andriole GL, Crawford ED, Grubb RL, 3rd, *et al*. Mortality results from a randomized prostate-cancer screening trial. *N Engl J Med* 2009;360:1310–9.

206 Schroder FH, Hugosson J, Roobol MJ, *et al*. Screening and prostate-cancer mortality in a randomized European study. *N Engl J Med* 2009;360:1320–8.

207 Hugosson J, Carlsson S, Aus G, *et al*. Mortality results from the Goteborg randomised population-based prostate-cancer screening trial. *Lancet Oncol* 2010;11:725–32.

208 Etzioni RD, Thompson IM. What do the screening trials really tell us and where do we go from here? *Urol Clin North Am* 2014;41:223–8.

209 Dale W, Bilir P, Han M, Meltzer D. The role of anxiety in prostate carcinoma: a structured review of the literature. *Cancer* 2005;104:467–78.

210 Carlsson S, Aus G, Wessman C, Hugosson J. Anxiety associated with prostate cancer screening with special reference to men with a positive screening test (elevated PSA) – results from a prospective, population-based, randomised study. *Eur J Cancer* 2007;43:2109–16.

211 Loeb S, Vellekoop A, Ahmed HU, *et al*. Systematic review of complications of prostate biopsy. *Eur Urol* 2013;64:876–92.

212 Wolf AM, Wender RC, Etzioni RB, *et al*. American Cancer Society guideline for the early detection of prostate cancer: update 2010. *CA Cancer J Clin* 2010;60:70–98.

213 Moyer VA. Screening for prostate cancer: U.S. Preventive Services Task Force recommendation statement. *Ann Intern Med* 2012;157:120–34.

214 U.S. Preventive Services Task Force. Draft Recommendation Statement: Prostate Cancer: Screening. U.S. Preventive Services Task Force. April 2017. https://www.uspreventiveservicestaskforce.org/Page/Document/draft-recommendation-statement/prostate-cancer-screening1 (accessed 29 September 2017).

215 Ilic D, Jammal W, Chiarelli P, *et al*. Assessing the effectiveness of decision aids for decision making in prostate cancer testing: a systematic review. Psychooncology 2015. doi: 10.1002/pon.3815.

216 Louie KS, Seigneurin A, Cathcart P, Sasieni P. Do prostate cancer risk models improve the predictive accuracy of PSA screening? A meta-analysis. *Ann Oncol* 2015;26:848–64.

217 Jacobs IJ, Menon U, Ryan A, *et al*. Ovarian cancer screening and mortality in the UK Collaborative Trial of Ovarian Cancer Screening (UKCTOCS): a randomised controlled trial. *Lancet* 2016;387:945–56.

218 How to Increase Colorectal Cancer Screening Rates in Practice: A Primary Care Clinician's Evidenced-Based Toolbox and Guide. American Cancer Society, 2015. Available at: http://nccrt.org/about/provider-education/crc-clinician-guide/ (accessed 25 May 2017).

Section 2

Cancer Biology

12

The Principles and Drivers of Cancer

Charles Saxe and William C. Phelps

American Cancer Society, Atlanta, Georgia, USA

Architectural complexity in living tissue comes from the bricks themselves, the individual cells …on occasion, a cell may choose to go its own way … It is then that we see the much-feared chaos that we call cancer.

Robert Weinberg, One Renegade Cell [1]

Introduction – The Causal Chain of Cancer

Many scientific historians consider the modern era of cancer research to have begun in the nineteenth century with the work of Rudolf Virchow, establishing the cell as the fundamental building block of all living organisms, and thus the primary focus of the study of cancer. For both cancer biologists working in laboratories and for clinicians taking care of patients, the cancer cell is the primary unit of disease.

Whether studying molecules, cells, or tumors in animal models or humans, for much of the twentieth century, the fundamental question being pursued was what drives cancer cells to grow beyond normal mechanisms of control. In the latter half of the century, attention was focused on the nucleus and our genes. In the 1980s and 1990s, scientists discovered cancer genes which can be broadly divided into oncogenes and tumor suppressor genes commonly thought of as the accelerators and brakes in a cell. Studies in animal and human cells demonstrated that mutations to oncogenes result in gains of function that contribute to uncontrolled growth, whereas mutations in tumor suppressor genes cause loss of function that inactivates their normal role in the arrest of cell growth. As we approached the twenty-first century, it was apparent that cancer progression requires mutations in *both* kinds of cancer genes.

In 2000, an important conceptual framework was published by Robert Weinberg and Douglas Hanahan called the "Hallmarks of Cancer" [2], which attempts to organize the myriad traits acquired by cancer cells into six functional groups, or hallmarks. This framework was updated in 2011 [3] to incorporate much of the last decade of astounding progress in understanding the collection of the more than 100 diseases called cancer.

Today's cancer research looks beyond the mutations of single cells to incorporate the enabling role of angiogenesis, the impact of the microenvironment surrounding a cancer cell, both the positive and negative influences of immune components, and the potential role of cancer stem cells in recurrence and metastasis. This chapter is arranged according to a more conventional scheme from least to greatest complexity – from genes to cells to tumors. Such a simple organization is best considered, however, in the context of the hallmarks of cancer, which focuses on the acquisition of traits that promote cancer growth and spread.

Endogenous Alteration to DNA

Point Mutations

The integrity of nuclear DNA is paramount to the life of a cell. Any alteration of the cells' DNA is potentially lethal to the cell and perhaps the entire organism. Paradoxically, the mutability of DNA enables genetic variation, immunological responsiveness, and species evolution, while at the same time allowing for the deleterious accumulation of damage that can lead to cancer. It has been estimated that the average rate of damage to a person's DNA is about 800 events per hour [4] primarily due to errors made during DNA replication. Most of the damage is corrected by the repair processes active in all cells, so that most DNA damage never becomes a heritable mutation. Unrepaired mutations may have little effect on the cell if they occur in the vast noncoding regions of the genome, or if they are genetically silent causing no heritable phenotypic change in a gene product. Also, since somatic eukaryotic cells are diploid, mutations may initially arise as heterozygous and recessive. One of the common chromosomal changes associated with progression to cancer is loss of heterozygosity where a mutation is duplicated through mitotic recombination, resulting in genotypic homozygosity and phenotypic expression. Fortunately only a small minority of DNA mutations remains unrepaired leading to heritable changes in cells which result in a growth advantage. Though rare, this is often an important step in malignant transformation.

Mammalian cells encode three different DNA polymerases which are involved in replication of chromosomal DNA; polymerases α, ε, and δ [5]. The fidelity of the polymerase machinery is very high but not infallible. Under normal conditions, the error rate for mammalian DNA replication is thought to be 10^{-6}–10^{-8} [6]. Thus, each time a human cell divides it must faithfully duplicate 3 billion base pairs of DNA introducing the possibility for creation of thousands of changes in the genome with each cell division. However, many of the nucleotides that are initially misincorporated are repaired immediately by proofreading enzymes attached to the synthetic apparatus. Furthermore, with sophisticated postreplication repair functions, the actual accumulation of mutations is estimated to be less than 1 in a billion nucleotides [7]. Indeed, newborn children are thought to carry fewer than 100 new mutations relative to their parents [8].

During DNA synthesis, polymerase complexes can simply insert the wrong base at the wrong position in a growing strand. If one purine is substituted for another (e.g., adenine in place of a guanine), this causes a transition. If the mistake is not detected and corrected, replication of both strands would result in replacement of the original A:T pair with G:C. Alternatively, if a purine is substituted for a pyrimidine (or vice versa), this causes a transversion and when replicated, this would result in substitution of G:C for C:G or A:T for T:A. Such nucleotide point mutations can occur both randomly and through chemical modification by mutagens (see below). Mistakes during DNA replication can also include insertions or deletions of one or more extra bases due to slippage of the polymerase complex [9] which can stutter within areas of the genome rich in repeated sequences.

Chemical Modifications

With respect to cancer initiation or progression, the most important sources of endogenous chemical modifications that result in DNA damage are hydrolysis, oxidative damage, and covalent DNA adduct formation. These forms of damage can arise as a consequence of normal, endogenous metabolic activity.

The most common form of damage to DNA is hydrolysis of the glycosidic bond connecting the nucleobase to the sugar phosphate backbone of the DNA strand. It has been estimated that perhaps 10,000 abasic sites (locations in DNA without any purine or pyrimidine base) are created each day in human cells [10]. Most of such potential mutations are removed by the DNA repair system using the complementary strand as a guide. However, when unrepaired sites are encountered by the DNA polymerase machinery, there is a preference for generic insertion of adenine [11] opposite the abasic site potentially introducing a change in the DNA sequence.

Oxidative damage occurs as a result of reactive oxygen species (ROS), which can be created during normal metabolism and as a consequence of exposure to carcinogenic chemicals or radiation. Mitochondrial electron transport chains important for cellular energy production, and the cellular peroxisomes that are critical to lipid biosynthesis, are two important sources of reactive oxygen molecules. The most important ROS molecules in cells include superoxide (O_2^-), singlet oxygen ($^1O_2$), hydroxyl radicals (OH), and hydrogen peroxide (H_2O_2) all of which are highly reactive, causing DNA oxidation and damage. Under conditions of cellular stress, the levels of dangerous ROS can rise dramatically. Oxidative damage of DNA varies from single or double-stranded breaks to base gaps in sequence. Cells encode a number of defense mechanisms to counter the endogenous production of ROS including antioxidant chemicals (e.g., ascorbic acid, polyphenols, or glutathione), as well as several enzymatic systems (catalase, peroxidase, and superoxide dismutase). When the production of ROS exceeds the counter capacity of antioxidants, oxidative stress ensues and DNA damage can accumulate. One of the most oxidized bases found in DNA under conditions of oxidative stress is 8-oxo-deoxyguanosine (8-oxo-dG) which will mis-pair with adenine rather than cytosine resulting in a GC to TA transversion [12].

The inappropriate addition of chemical adducts to DNA can occur due to the presence of endogenous chemical agents. For example, normal metabolites of estrogen can cause both oxidative damage to DNA through generation of free radicals, as well as promoting the formation of DNA adducts. Incomplete catabolism of estrogen can lead to the generation of catechol estrogen quinones, which can form covalent adducts with cellular DNA on purines, resulting in single-stranded breaks [13]. Another common reactive molecule in cells is s-adenosylmethionine (SAM), which can methylate DNA, typically on guanine and adenine residues. Of course, the primary role of methylation of DNA is not mutagenic but instead is used in epigenetic regulation of expression [14]. Although the underlying DNA sequence remains unchanged, the ability of the DNA to be transcribed to mRNA and translated to protein is reduced. Methyl groups are added to cytosine at CpG sites and when clustered, are associated with a reduced level of transcription around that site.

Exogenous Factors Affecting DNA

Chemicals, Light, Radiation

Following the landmark discovery of the structure of DNA in the 1950s, many chemical carcinogens were evaluated for their ability to bind and disrupt DNA [15]. Over the course of the next decade of work, it became apparent that there was a correlation between the DNA binding capacity of a chemical and its mutagenic activity. In the early 1970s, on the basis of this concept, Bruce Ames developed an important biological assay for mutagenicity based upon the ability to rapidly detect frameshift or point mutations in DNA using *Salmonella typhimurium* [16]. Today, the Ames test is broadly used as a primary screen for chemicals which may be potentially carcinogenic.

DNA-disrupting mutagens can be direct carcinogens. Highly electrophilic compounds with a strong affinity for negatively charged DNA such as ethylene oxide or nitrogen mustards (which are both alkylating agents) can form covalent DNA adducts. Nucleophilic (proton seeking) or less reactive compounds, including aromatic chemicals and heterocyclic amines, require chemical or enzymatic conversion to the actual carcinogen, and are therefore called indirect carcinogens. Aflatoxins are toxic, mutagenic, and carcinogenic [17]. They are naturally occurring toxins produced as secondary metabolites by the soil fungi, *Aspergillus flavus*, which is commonly found to contaminate improperly stored foods. Ingestion of the toxin from contaminated food (e.g., corn, nuts, and dried fruits) is associated with liver damage and hepatocellular carcinoma [18]. Aflatoxin is metabolized in the liver through the activity of cytochrome P450-dependent monooxygenase to epoxides, which can bind both protein and DNA. The aflatoxin epoxide can form adducts at guanine residues leading to characteristic mutations in key regulatory genes such as *p53* [19].

Smoking effectively delivers a mixture of some 5000 compounds to the lungs and other tissues including 73 compounds which are deemed carcinogens [20]. Either directly or indirectly through metabolism of compounds in smoke, electrophilic mutagens (e.g., epoxides) are delivered to cells, leading to the formation of DNA adducts. If unrepaired, these result in mutations that can promote the development of cancer. Multiple studies have shown that mutations in the *KRAS* and *TP53* genes are commonly found in the lung epithelium of smokers and in lung tumors [21–23]. Perhaps the most direct evidence for carcinogenicity using individual compounds from tobacco smoke is for NNK (4-(methyl nitrosamino)-1-(3-pyridyl)-1-butanone) and PAH (polycyclic aromatic hydrocarbons) which have been shown to readily induce lung tumors in animals [24, 25]. Both compounds are considered genotoxic carcinogens that are enzymatically activated into DNA binding electrophiles [26]. *TP53* mutations can be found in the majority of human lung cancers, and the spectrum of these mutations is different when comparing smokers to nonsmokers [27]. Mutational signatures (including a preponderance of G > T and C > A transversions) that have been observed in lung cancer reflect the imprint of damage from chemicals in smoke [28]. This effectively makes the connection in the causal chain between smoking, mutagens in smoke, and somatically acquired DNA damage in lung tumor cells.

Epidemiological evidence has suggested that environmental factors play an important role in the incidence and distribution of cancer around the world [29]. Rigorous identification of cancer-causing chemicals in the environment is difficult in part because of the 20–30 year-long delay commonly seen between exposure and the appearance of cancer. There has been considerable debate over the years about whether safe doses or thresholds of carcinogens can be defined. Rigorously distinguishing between endogenous and exogenous DNA damage can be challenging in part because some exogenous mutagens can also be produced endogenously (e.g., reactive aldehydes), and similar types of damage (e.g., 8-oxo-dG) can be induced by both exogenous chemicals and endogenous metabolism. Thus, any approximation of the relative contributions of exogenous exposure and endogenous factors in mutagenesis of DNA is only a best estimate.

Ionizing radiation (high energy electromagnetic waves and particles) can damage biological systems at an atomic level through displacement of electrons. Probably the most familiar forms of such radiation are X-rays and gamma rays. It has been estimated that 80% of human exposure to ionizing radiation is from natural sources while the remainder results from intentional medical exposure [30]. It has been estimated that an exposure of a cell to 1 Gy of ionizing radiation will result in 40 double-stranded DNA breaks, 1000 single-stranded breaks, 1000 base oxidations, and 150 DNA-protein cross-links. For comparison, the typical therapeutic dose for cancer treatment ranges between 20 and 100 Gy, and a typical X-ray dose for diagnostic use is about 10,000-fold less [31].

Infectious Diseases

Viruses take advantage of a wide range of properties across their varied host cells. Once inside a susceptible cell, viruses often modify the activity of the cell (e.g., turn off cellular DNA replication) to favor virus replication. Since most viruses require actively dividing cells to replicate, they have developed a variety of strategies to stimulate or maintain host cells in an actively dividing state to create an environment conducive to particle production. Malignant transformation of an infected host cell is generally not thought to be a favorable event for the virus since virus particles are typically not produced by cancer cells. For a virus, a cancer cell represents a dead-end state which is no longer useful for virus spread. As a result, one could say that tumor viruses cause cancer more by accident than design yet they do so through the common hallmarks associated with all cancers [32].

Although virus or bacterial infection may be required for some types of cancer (e.g., cervical carcinoma and Kaposi sarcoma) and strongly associated with others, infection alone does not induce cancer as other extrinsic cofactors or genetic alterations are required. A useful though imperfect conceptual classification is to divide these agents into direct versus indirect carcinogens [33]. Direct cancer-causing infectious agents (e.g., HPV, EBV) encode gene products that directly contribute to cell transformation, and are present and expressed in all cells of the cancers they cause. In contrast, indirect agents don't necessarily encode transforming properties; instead, cancer may arise due to persistent infection and chronic inflammatory tissue damage over several decades (e.g., hepatocellular or gastric cancer).

In terms of lives affected, the most important human tumor virus family is the human papillomavirus. Papillomaviruses are small DNA viruses that exclusively infect mucosal or cutaneous epithelial cells, and are best known as the causative agent of benign skin and genital warts. Almost 200 different types of HPVs have been described, and a subset of about two dozen types (high risk HPVs) is associated with genital and oral cancers.

The early functions of viruses drive cellular proliferation within an actively differentiating epithelium. To alter normal cell cycle control, the high-risk HPV E6 protein ("E" indicating expression early in the HPV life cycle) interacts with the p53 protein and HPV E7 interacts with the retinoblastoma protein (Rb). These two viral proteins stimulate cell proliferation, and are selectively retained and expressed in all HPV-associated genital and oral cancers [34]. In spite of the very high prevalence of HPV infection in the sexually active population, most infections resolve on their own within a few years, and only a small fraction will progress to cancer. Malignant progression appears to require persistent infection with an ongoing inflammatory response, potentially interacting with the effects of one or more cofactors such as smoking or estrogen [32].

For many decades, SV40 (simian virus) was among the most important tools available to cell and molecular biologists for the study of eukaryotic DNA replication, transcriptional and translational control, RNA splicing, as well as cellular transformation. A virus related to SV40 is the most recently discovered human tumor virus. In 2008, Patrick Moore and Yuan Chang were able to link a rare but lethal form of human skin cancer to a previously undescribed virus they named MCPyV (Merkel cell polyomavirus) [35]. There are about 1500 cases per year of Merkel cell carcinoma in the United States with few treatment options available [36].

A proportion of people infected with either hepatitis B (HBV) or hepatitis C (HCV) will develop a chronic infection, which puts them at significant risk for hepatocellular carcinoma (HCC). Infection with one of these two viruses accounts for more than 80% of liver cancer around the world. Under most circumstances, HCC develops following several decades of chronic viral infection, liver damage, inflammation, and cirrhosis [37]. HBV is a small DNA virus which, following infection of hepatocytes, integrates into the host genome leading to cellular transformation. By contrast, HCV is a positive-stranded RNA virus that does not integrate into the host genome, although it causes significant disruption to signal transduction pathways in infected cells. During chronic HBV or HCV infection, the host immune system responds to viral antigens on infected cells, leading to a persistent cycle of hepatocyte damage and repair. Cellular proliferation associated with repair increases risk of replicative errors and provides a favorable environment for the accumulation of oncogenic mutations. Other risk factors commonly associated with HCC such as alcohol consumption or exposure to aflatoxins may act to accelerate the rate of DNA mutation occurring as a result of immune-mediated damage [38].

Epstein Barr virus (EBV) is a DNA virus in the herpesvirus family. Infection of adolescents is commonly associated with the mild flu-like symptoms of mononucleosis. EBV associated cancers such as Burkitt's lymphoma and nasopharyngeal carcinoma, however, show a pronounced geographic distribution. Taken together with the knowledge that nearly all adults are seropositive for EBV, understanding the causal chain in these cancers is complex and believed to be associated with a variety of genetic, environmental or dietary cofactors [39]. The causal role of EBV in lymphoid malignancies is thought to derive from the ability of the virus to efficiently infect and immortalize B lymphocytes rendering them capable of indefinite growth. EBV carcinogenesis requires the activity of two major viral proteins: LMP (latent membrane protein) and EBNA (Epstein-Barr nuclear antigen). EBNA-1 has been shown to affect antigen processing in infected cells and cause down-regulation of apoptosis. Perhaps of greater importance in EBV-related cancers is the LMP-1 protein, which is primarily responsible for proliferation of infected B-cells [40]. LMP-1 is expressed on the membranes of infected cells and appears to mimic the activities of a constitutively activated TNF (tumor necrosis factor) receptor, CD40.

Another member of the herpesvirus family is Kaposi's sarcoma virus (KSHV) or human herpesvirus 8 (HHV-8). KSHV causes Kaposi's sarcoma, a cancer of endothelial cells [41]. Prior to the human immunodeficiency virus (HIV) epidemic beginning in the 1980s, Kaposi's sarcoma was uncommon and associated with elderly men of Mediterranean or African descent. HIV infection and the resulting damage to the immune system are believed to enable KSHV infection and cancer. The most important latent proteins associated with KSHV transformation appear to be LANA which is functionally analogous to EBV EBNA, and v-FLIP which plays a similar role to the EBV LMP protein. LANA appears to play a number of important roles including perturbation of the p53 and Rb pathways and promotion of chromosomal instability. The KSHV v-FLIP protein, like LMP, interferes with the TNFα-induced apoptotic pathway [42].

The first described and perhaps most extensively studied cancer virus, Rous sarcoma virus (RSV) provided the touchstone discovery for the highly productive search for murine and avian transforming retroviruses. RSV is an acutely transforming retrovirus which, during integration into the host cell genome, captures a protooncogene into the viral genome. The recombinant retrovirus can efficiently transform naïve cells through stable integration of the passenger protooncogene in the newly infected cells. The ability of murine and avian retroviruses to capture cellular proto-oncogenes was greatly exploited during the 1970s and 1980s to identify many of the most important oncogenes being studied today (e.g., *RAS*, *ABL*, *EGFR*, *VEGFR*, *HER-2/NEU*).

In spite of the plethora of RNA tumor viruses infecting animals, there are no known examples of acutely transforming human retroviruses. The best known human retrovirus, HIV, specifically infects and destroys immune cells. Although HIV infection does not directly cause cancer, it causes profound immunodeficiency, which secondarily increases the incidence of other viral-associated cancers (e.g., cervical cancer and Kaposi's sarcoma). Like HIV, HTLV-1 (human T-cell leukemia virus type 1) is a human retrovirus associated with cancer – adult T-cell leukemia (ATL). HTLV-1 shares a number of structural features with other retroviruses, although infection with HTLV-1 (unlike HIV) does not lead to immune suppression. Very often, infection with HTLV-1 will lead to an asymptomatic carrier state with a 3–5% lifetime risk for development of ATL several decades after infection [43]. As with all retroviruses, by virtue of reverse transcription, the viral genome is integrated into the host cell DNA. HTLV-1 does not appear to carry an obvious viral or cellular protooncogene; instead the viral protein, Tax, induces a polyclonal proliferation of infected T-cells effectively establishing a premalignant state [44].

Roughly half the world's population is thought to have the gram negative, spiral-shaped bacteria, *Helicobacter pylori* colonizing their upper gastrointestinal tract. *H. pylori* was identified in the 1980s by the pioneering work of Barry Marshall and Robin Warren who formulated and proved the iconoclastic theory that a bacterial infection in the acidic environment of the stomach might be the cause of gastric ulcers [45]. If left untreated 1–3% of those infected are expected to progress to gastric cancer resulting in about 1 million new cases each year around the world [46].

There are two important pathogenic factors associated with *H. pylori* infection: the cytotoxin-associated antigen (CagA) and vacuolating cytotoxin A (VacA). Epidemiological evidence suggests that CagA-positive strains of *H. pylori* are specifically associated with the risk for development of gastric cancer [47]. The CagA protein is inserted into the cell membrane of gastric epithelial cells where it becomes phosphorylated by the host cellular c-Src/Lyn kinases triggering a change in the shape of the epithelial cells facilitating bacterial attachment [48]. VacA becomes associated with lipid rafts in the host cell membranes leading to the formation of large, intracellular vacuoles. Infection is sensed by Toll-like and Nod-like receptors, which triggers an inflammatory response including release of pro-inflammatory cytokines (e.g., IL-6, IL-17A, TNFα, IFNϒ), and recruitment of neutrophils, macrophages and lymphocytes [49]. Persistent bacterial infection and chronic inflammation play important roles in carcinogenesis through induction of tissue repair and oxidative DNA damage. In addition, both genetic [50] and environmental [51] factors appear to influence risk for development of stomach cancer.

DNA Repair

Mechanisms of Repair

All cellular organisms from bacteria to plants to humans encode a sophisticated collection of functionally redundant enzymatic machinery to repair damage to their genomes. The life of every cell is entirely dependent upon the structural integrity of its DNA and access to the encoded information. Cancer can arise by increasing the rate or type of DNA damage or by impairing the ability of the cell to repair damage. It has become increasingly apparent in the past few years that cancer is commonly associated with inactivating mutations or epigenetic silencing of DNA repair systems. Indeed, many of the inherited mutations discovered to be associated with an elevated risk of cancer are in genes that normally function in DNA repair [52].

There are at least five multicomponent systems arrayed to repair different types of DNA lesions. As discussed above, damage to DNA can be caused by a wide range of normal cellular process, as well as a host of exogenous insults resulting from external exposures. This damage can result in modification to DNA including single or double-stranded breaks in the double helix. Chemical modifications and single-stranded breaks are more common and more easily repaired using the complementary strand as a template. By contrast, double-stranded breaks are potentially catastrophic as the coding and regulatory information inherent in the linear sequence can be lost (Table 12.1).

The simplest form of DNA repair is a single-component pathway called direct reversal which does not require a template for repair, nor does it require hydrolysis of the phosphodiester backbone. Direct reversal is commonly used to repair O-methyl guanine modifications by the enzyme, MGMT (methyl guanine methyltransferase). A particularly common lesion associated with DNA alkylation is the addition of the O^6 methyl group to guanine, which can lead to mis-pairing with thymine instead of cytosine. MGMT will facilitate transfer of the methyl group from the DNA strand to a cysteine residue on the protein, restoring the guanine base on the DNA. Its importance is underscored by the observation that knock-out mice deficient in MGMT are hypersensitive to alkylating agents like temozolomide [53], and epigenetic silencing of the MGMT gene is common in cancer [54].

To repair single-stranded DNA damage, cells are equipped with three mechanisms of repair: base excision repair (BER), nucleotide excision repair (NER), and mismatch repair (MMR).

Table 12.1 DNA damage and repair.

DNA damage		DNA repair	Common mutant genes in cancer
Single stranded	O-methylguanine	Methyl guanine methyltransferase (MGMT)	*MGMT*[1]
	Replication errors Base mismatches Base insertions Base deletions	Mismatch repair (MMR)	*MSH1, MSH6* (colon) *MLH1* *PMS2*
	Abasic sites 8-Oxo-guanine SS breaks	Base excision repair (BER)	*MUTYH* (colon)
	Bulky adducts Pyrimidine dimers	Nucleotide excision repair (NER)	*XP* family (skin)
	Abasic sites Bulky adducts Pyrimidine dimers	Translesional synthesis (TLS)	*FANC* family (leukemia, liver) *XPV* (skin)
Double stranded	Double-strand breaks Inter-strand crosslinks	Homologous recombination (HR)	*BRCA1, BRCA2* (breast, ovarian) *MRE11* (breast) *BLM* *WRN* (sarcoma) *FANC* family (leukemia, liver) *RECQL4* (osteosarcoma) *ATM*
		Nonhomologous end-joining (NHEJ)	*NBS* (lymphoma) *WRN* (sarcoma) *ATM*

[1] Promoter methylation rather than inactivating mutation.

Since damage is restricted to only one strand, these systems each use the complementary strand as a template for the repair process.

The BER pathway [55] is used to repair small, single-stranded lesions which have not caused major structural disruption to the DNA. Nucleotide base deamination, oxidation, or some forms of alkylation are typically repaired using the BER system. The first step in repair is mediated by a specific DNA glycosylase (11 different genes in humans), which is responsible for recognition of the lesion and cleavage of the N-glycosidic bond to remove the defective base leaving an abasic site in the DNA. The abasic site is removed by an AP (apurinic/apyrimidinic) endonuclease which cleaves the phosphodiester backbone 5' to the baseless site. The broken link in the chain is then repaired by DNA polymerase (in humans, pol ß is dominant) and DNA ligase (in humans DNA ligase I or III and XRCC1) using the undamaged complementary strand as the instructive blueprint. This final step overlaps with conventional single-stranded break repair. The importance of the repair system is underscored by the observation that attempts to make homozygous deletions in transgenic mice in polymerase β, DNA ligase III, or XRCC1 result in embryonic lethality [56–58].

The NER system is responsible for the repair of bulky, helix-distorting chemical lesions such as those arising from tobacco smoke, platinum-based cancer drugs, and ultraviolet light [59]. In mammalian cells, there are at least nine proteins involved in NER together with a number of important cofactors (e.g., ERCC1). Xeroderma pigmentosum (XP) is a rare autosomal disease with up to a 10,000-fold increase in the risk of skin cancers and a 50-fold increase in brain and CNS cancers [60]. XP is caused by a deficiency in NER due most commonly to mutations in the XPA gene, which is critical for DNA damage recognition. In addition to mutations in XPA, there are at least several other forms of the disease affecting different genes that are important to NER. At a mechanistic level, NER is divided into two subpathways, global genome (GG-NER) and transcription-coupled (TC-NER), which differ in part by their locations. GG-NER can repair damage anywhere in the genome while TC-NER is associated exclusively with actively transcribed strands of genes.

The MMR system recognizes and repairs insertions or deletions that arise during DNA replication [61]. Mismatched bases (e.g., C:T or A:G) cause distortions in the double helix that are recognized as sites for repair. MMR machinery must distinguish the newly replicated DNA strands that might contain errors. In eukaryotes, the lagging strand in newly synthesized DNA contains nicks which must be sealed by DNA ligase, and it is thought that the nicks provide a signal for proofreading functions including MMR. Excision of mismatched bases, insertions, or deletions normally involves removal of as much as a few thousand bases prior to template directed repair synthesis. Mutations in the component genes of MMR are associated with instability in size and repetition of microsatellite DNA – short tandem repetitive DNA sequences. Lynch syndrome, also known as hereditary nonpolyposis colon cancer, is a hereditary condition caused by mutation in one of four MMR genes (MLH1, MSH2, MSH6, and PMS2), resulting in predisposition to colorectal and endometrial cancer [62].

Double-stranded breaks in DNA are particularly hazardous to a cell's viability. Two important mechanisms exist to repair double-stranded breaks in DNA: nonhomologous end joining (NHEJ) and homologous recombination (HR). In general, HR is thought to be a more accurate process.

The canonical NHEJ pathway requires the end-joining DNA binding proteins Ku (Ku70/Ku80 heterodimer) and the XRCC4-DNA ligase IV complex among other factors. The pathway is essential for genomic stability although paradoxically, NHEJ is generally considered an error prone process [63]. Further, it is NHEJ that facilitates immunoglobulin V(D)J gene rearrangements which are required for immune diversity [64]. Double-stranded breaks in DNA are rapidly bound by the Ku proteins which are present in cells at high concentration and have a very high affinity for DNA ends. The Ku/DNA complex subsequently becomes a scaffold for assembly of the remaining members of the repair complex which process and re-ligate the ends of the DNA. By contrast with HR, NHEJ can re-ligate the ends of broken DNA with little or no homology. Mutations of Ku in mouse models results in genomic instability and significant chromosomal rearrangements [65]. When coupled to *p53* mutations, the mice rapidly developed lymphomas [66]. No spontaneous mutations in the Ku genes have been discovered in humans thus far; however, patients with mutations in DNA ligase IV (LIG4 syndrome) are radiosensitive and predisposed to multiple myeloma [67].

Unlike NHEJ, HR requires extensive DNA sequence homology to facilitate repair, and is restricted to certain times during the cell cycle when sister chromatids (identical copies) or the homologous chromosome are condensed and proximal. The initial step in HR involves creation of a 3' single-strand by the MRN complex followed by loading of the Rad51 protein on the single strand to form a helical nucleoprotein filament. The nucleoprotein complex facilitates homologous base pairing and strand invasion or exchange of homologous duplex DNA templates forming so-called Holliday structures which were originally associated with DNA recombination. DNA polymerase extends the 3' end of the damaged strand using the template from the duplex of the sister chromatid. HR repair is thought to be quite adaptable to effect repair of many forms of double-stranded damage and may involve as many as 200 different factors under different conditions [68].

An important step in the understanding of the genetic basis for hereditary breast and ovarian cancer was made in the 1990s with the discovery of the *BRCA1* and *BRCA2* genes [69–71]. Studies to understand the normal activities of *BRCA1* and *2* connected the mutations to defects in DNA repair, specifically in homologous recombination which causes affected cells to accumulate unrepaired chromosomal defects [72, 73]. The BRCA1 protein plays a critical role in the sensing of DNA damage and helps to provide a platform for assembly of important factors for the initial steps in HR. In contrast, BRCA2 does not appear to be involved in the sensing of DNA damage, instead being more involved in effector functions in HR through interaction with *Rad51* and with *PALB2* (another gene associated with hereditary breast cancer). The extension of the concept of synthetic lethality to cancer treatment owes it origins to the recognition that cancer cells harboring mutations in HR (e.g., *BRCA1* and *BRCA2* mutations) are hypertensive to killing by drugs which inactivate other DNA repair pathways [74].

Finally, when considering repair of DNA, it is important to note a cell's choice is more than binary – repair or die. In the event that DNA damage cannot be repaired and a DNA replication fork is stalled, an alternative path forward includes synthesis over or around the affected region. Normal replicative DNA polymerases are replaced with a system for translesional DNA synthesis (TLS) which includes specialized polymerases with much larger active sites to accommodate damaged or distorted DNA [75]. Unfortunately, the concession is that TLS is an error prone process resulting in an increase in mutation. There has been recent interest for inhibition of TLS polymerase for cancer therapy, which might interfere with the emergence of drug resistance resulting from enhanced mutation induced by the chemotherapeutic agent (e.g., platinum drugs) [76].

Telomerase

Cancer is much more common in aging populations and there are a number of molecular pathways and features that link cellular aging and malignant progression. The discovery of the role of telomerase in cancer helped to resolve a molecular paradox inherent in the activity of DNA polymerases used to replicate our chromosomal DNA. The "end replication problem" is a result of the fact that replicative DNA polymerases are constitutionally unable to synthesize a new template all the way to the template end. As a consequence, with each succeeding cell division, the ends of chromosomes are progressively lost. Telomeres are the ends of chromosomes which are composed of repeated DNA sequence elements which form binding sites for protein complexes called shelterin [77]. The enzyme telomerase was discovered in the mid-1980s [78], and was soon shown to possess an unusual RNA directed, DNA polymerase activity or reverse transcription normally associated with retroviruses. The complete structure of the telomerase complex at the ends of chromosomes also contains, in addition to the enzyme (TERT), a short RNA template and a protein factor, dyskerin, which functions to add short DNA sequence repeats to the ends of chromosomes. Most adult cells have lost the expression of telomerase, and thus the gradual shortening of chromosomes is thought to represent a physical clock that counts down during cellular aging. As chromosomes become too short, cells age and die. By contrast, embryonic stem cells retain the capacity to express telomerase and thus are resistant to this form of molecular aging. Immortalized cancer cells and most cancers [79] have also been found to express telomerase and the introduction of a constitutively expressed *TERT* gene will immortalize primary cells [80]. On the basis of these and many other studies, induction of telomerase to repair and protect chromosomal DNA ends has become one of the hallmarks of cancer cells.

The Drivers of Cancer

Overview

Ultimately, what distinguishes a cancer cell is the ability to grow under conditions where normal cells cannot. In addition, cancer cells pass on this unrestrained growth potential to their offspring thus providing a long-term growth advantage to the cancer cell and its progeny. That growth advantage may be due to a

number of factors: the ability to grow in the absence of growth signals (often the result of activating mutations in *oncogenes*); insensitivity to growth inhibiting signals (the result of loss of a *tumor suppressor* gene); unlimited cell division; the ability to evade cell death signals; acquisition of their own, unique, vasculature; the ability to invade surrounding tissue and metastasize to distant sites in the body. Each of these hallmarks involves the loss of normal coordination of a number of integrated processes. These processes are regulated by interconnected signaling pathways. It is therefore no surprise that oncogenes and tumor suppressors work largely through disruption of 12 signaling pathways [81, 82].

The advent of whole exomic (protein encoding) and genomic DNA sequencing has provided a wealth of new information about the nature of mutations associated with cancer. For example, many solid tumors harbor between 40 and 60 independent genes in which mutations are found that are predicted to affect the function of their protein products [82]. Based on several lines of evidence, it is clear that the majority of these mutations play little or no role in initiating or maintaining the cancer cell phenotype. This has led to the concept of *passenger* and *driver* mutations [83]. A driver mutation in the cellular context is one whose expression confers a growth advantage to the cell that expresses it. There are a limited number of genes in which such mutations occur. Though the exact number is not known, there is a consensus building around 140 such genes with estimates varying from <150 to as many as 300–400. Any given tumor can express from as few as one (e.g., medulloblastoma) to as many as eight (e.g., some breast cancers) drivers.

As it is important to distinguish between driver and passenger mutations, it is also important to distinguish driver mutations from driver genes. A number of mutations are found in driver genes, but only a subset of those mutations actually provides the growth advantage that defines a driver mutation. These are the driver mutations. The others, while still in driver genes, do not have the same effect on cellular behavior and are therefore defined as passenger mutations.

There is further delineation of the driver genes that promote cancer formation. These genes fall into three major categories: genes involved in DNA repair, which have been discussed earlier in the chapter, oncogenes, and tumor suppressor genes.

Oncogenes

An oncogene is the mutated form of a normal cellular gene designated a *proto-oncogene*. The role of oncogenes can be described as accelerators of cell growth and division. Mutations in oncogenes encode proteins that enable cells to grow in the absence of the signals that are normally required to regulate growth, and they often affect either autocrine (a cell secretes a chemical messenger that binds to receptors on the same cell) or paracrine signaling (a cell secretes a chemical messenger that binds to receptors on a nearby cell). Oncogenes were originally identified from studies of tumor-forming viruses. The first oncogenic virus was identified by Peyton Rous in 1911 [84]. In 1976, the tumor-inducing component of that virus was identified and became the first oncogene, *src* (sarcoma gene) [85].

Oncogene mutations can result in hyperactivation of the protein or misregulation in time and/or space of the activity of the normal protein. Characteristically, they act in a dominant fashion in that a mutation in a single allele leads to cellular transformation and tumor growth. The mutations can be the result of single base changes that increase protein activity or increase its stability, regulatory mutations that increase the expression levels or alter the timing of expression (e.g., promoter mutations), gene or chromosomal amplifications, or chromosomal translocations that result in a fused and altered protein. Oncogenes affect cell proliferation, cell survival, or both. Oncogenes are the altered form of normal cell regulatory genes and are often growth factor receptors (e.g., platelet derived growth factor receptor) or protein kinases (e.g., src), or components of specific signal transduction pathways critical for growth regulation (e.g., ras, raf, APC, *patched*, Stat3, myc) [82].

Tumor Suppressor Genes

The first evidence for the existence of tumor suppressor genes came from studies in which tumor and normal cells were fused to form hybrid cells, which were found to be less tumorigenic than the tumor-generating parent. The interpretation was that the normal cell provided something that suppressed tumorigenesis, and which was missing from the tumor cell [86]. This meant that some tumor-forming mutations were recessive, loss of function mutations, unlike the dominant mutations of oncogenes. Subsequent studies established that loss of a specific chromosome from the hybrid cell could restore tumor-formation ability. This led to the idea that tumor formation could be suppressed by the presence of one wild type copy of a gene and to the identification of *RB1* (the retinoblastoma gene) as the first tumor suppressor gene [87, 88].

Though it is an oversimplification, the normal function of tumor suppressors can be viewed as putting the brakes on cell growth and division. They do this in a number of ways. They are often negative regulators of oncogenes; they can play a role in cell cycle checkpoint regulation or checkpoints for DNA damage and spindle assembly; and they can stimulate apoptosis [89].

Cell Death and its Resistance in Cancer Cells

The number of cells in an organism is tightly regulated by a finely tuned balance between cell growth/division and cell death. This balance is necessary not only to maintain tissue homeostasis, but is important in creating and maintaining organ size and shape, and for a number of critical developmental processes like heart development and removing webbing between developing digits.

There are a number of ways that cells die. One that is a particular focus of cancer biologists is the process of apoptosis or "programmed cell death". Apoptosis is a genetically programmed means for a cell to "commit suicide". This mechanism is used during developmental morphogenesis, to regulate cell numbers and to rid the organism of damaged cells (e.g., DNA-damaged cells) [90]. Because of the latter two uses in particular, it plays a significant role in tumor suppression, and many tumor suppressor genes function in the control of apoptosis. It is little wonder that evasion of cell death is one of the defining hallmarks of cancer [3].

Cells dying via an apoptotic pathway have morphologically unique characteristics: they shrink in size; their plasma membrane loses its underlying architecture causing the membranes to "bleb" on the cell surface; their nucleus changes shape, and their DNA is fragmented. Another important characteristic of apoptotic cells is that, unlike cells undergoing necrosis (the other major type of cell death), their membranes remain intact, cell contents remain enclosed and cells do not rupture. Consequently, there is a minimal inflammatory response and the dead cells are generally engulfed by neighboring cells or local macrophages.

There are two distinct pathways by which cells can be induced to undergo apoptosis. One, the so-called extrinsic pathway, is mediated by extracellular signals acting through a family of cell surface receptors. Collectively these "death receptors" are called the tumor necrosis factor (TNF) receptor family, and include receptors such as CD95/FAS, TNF-R1 and TRAIL-R1. Extracellular ligands that are recognized by these receptors include FasL, TNF-α, and TRAIL. Upon ligand binding, the death receptors trimerize and recruit the protein FADD. FADD is an adaptor protein that in turn recruits procaspase-8 to form the death-inducing signaling complex. This complex facilitates the cleavage and activation of caspase-8 (an initiator caspase), which in turn activates the effector caspases, 3, 6, and 7 (executioner caspases) [91]. This caspase-activating cascade results in the cleavage of a number of downstream protein targets, ultimately leading to apoptosis.

The other apoptosis pathway, the intrinsic pathway, requires intracellular signals (e.g., oxidative stress, DNA damage) and is mediated by changes in the outer mitochondrial membrane, via the actions of the Bcl-2 family of proteins. The Bcl-2 protein family is defined by containing one or more Bcl-2 homology (BH) domains and is functionally divided into pro-apoptotic and anti-apoptotic family members. Mechanistically, the intracellular signals induce a subset of pro-apoptotic proteins, the BH3-only family members (e.g., BID, BIM, BAD and NOXA). Activation of BH-3 only proteins induces either binding and inhibition of anti-apoptotic family members (e.g., BCL-2, BCL-X_L, and MCL-1), or the oligomerization and activation of the pro-apoptotic proteins BAX and BAK. This latter process itself is inhibited by binding of BAX and BAK by anti-apoptotic family members [92]. The activation of BAX or BAK results in their insertion into the outer mitochondrial membrane, oligomerization, and subsequent outer membrane permeabilization. This results in the release of proteins, including cytochrome c, that activate a caspase cascade and result in apoptotic cell death [93, 94].

The founding member of the BCL family, *BCL-2*, was first identified as a proto-oncogene present as an overexpressed gene within a chromosomal translocation in B-cell lymphoma. The pro-apoptotic family members largely appear to function as classical tumor suppressors, though BAX functions in a more complex manner. It has also been recently reported that the tumor suppressor Rb1 can interact with the pro-apoptotic protein, BAX, at the mitochondrial membrane, and induce mitochondrial membrane leakage and apoptosis. Rb1 alone can also be targeted to mitochondria and can induce apoptosis [95]. This suggests potentially new directions by which therapeutics targeting apoptosis can be designed.

Therapeutic targeting of the apoptotic pathways is a major focus of current cancer therapy. Many chemotherapeutics cause DNA damage, with the intent to induce apoptosis through the intrinsic pathway. Other chemotherapeutics trigger the immune system to produce TNF, thus stimulating apoptosis through the extrinsic pathway. Many tumors, however, have defects in one or more apoptotic pathways and are inherently resistant to chemotherapy. As stated earlier, mutations in the *p53* pathways are present in many tumors and contribute to apoptosis-mediated chemotherapy resistance. These mutations are largely "loss-of-function" mutations, but "gain-of-function" mutations also exist. Likewise, down-regulation of pro-apoptotic members of the *BCL-2* family or up-regulation of anti-apoptotic family members is associated with chemotherapy resistance. Increasing knowledge of the details of these pathways is leading to more and better strategies for combatting chemotherapy resistance.

Cancer drug targeting for induction of apoptosis largely focuses on the BCL-2 family of proteins, in particular BCL-X_L. Hematological cancers in which BLC-2 is overexpressed (e.g., lymphocytic leukemias) have shown the greatest sensitivity to apoptosis-inducing drugs such as ABT-263. In general, these agents have limited use because of the high toxicity that result from the off-target effects of inhibiting BCL-X_L in platelets. Recent work [96] suggests there is still great promise for this approach. By designing more selective BCL-2 inhibitors, Souers *et al*. identified an agent that has high selectivity for BCL-2, is much less toxic than earlier generation BCL-2 inhibitors, and seems to stimulate significant tumor apoptosis in both animal and human studies. Further success is indicated by the recent FDA approval of BH3 mimetics from the treatment of 17p-deleted chronic lymphocytic leukemia [97]. In a variation on the theme, recent studies in epithelial tumors have investigated a combination treatment of a *MEK* inhibitor and a BCL-X inhibitor [98]. In human cell lines, mouse xenographs of human *KRAS*-mutant cancer cells, and a *Kras* mouse model, significant tumor regression was observed. Though toxicity studies were not complete in these reports, the overall approach seems to be viable and likely to provide direction for other combination studies focused on *RAS* mutations and apoptosis inhibition.

Anoikis defines another form of apoptosis. It is induced when cells lose attachment to the extracellular matrix (ECM) or adhere to matrix or cells in an inappropriate location. It was first described in 1994 and represents a normal, physiological mechanism for maintaining tissue integrity [99]. Study of anoikis has become a significant research area as it is believed to represent a new set of targets for therapy [100].

Other, nonapoptotic mechanisms of cell death also play roles in cancer. One of particular importance and the focus of much current research is autophagy ("self-eating"), more precisely macroautophagy. Autophagy is a fundamental process of degrading and recycling cytosolic components and involves engulfing this material and trafficking it to the lysosome [101, 102]. Excess autophagy can lead to nonapoptotic cell death. Autophagy is also used as a survival response to cellular starvation conditions and it is this aspect that most directly relates to cancer progression. Inhibition of mTOR (mammalian target of rapamycin) with rapamycin activates the autophagy pathway. Autophagy can also be activated by the tumor suppressor *PTEN*

through inhibition of PI3K (phosphoinositide 3-kinase) which itself phosphorylates and activates AKT. AKT in turn can stimulate mTOR activity. The connection is that many cancers are mutant for *PTEN*. The inactivation of *PTEN* leads to the continuous activation of the mTOR complex, which blocks autophagy. Strategies to stimulate one or more autophagic pathways, including the mTOR pathway, are making their way into the clinic.

Induction of Angiogenesis

Angiogenesis is the process by which new blood vessels are formed from already extant ones. It is fundamentally a developmental mechanism of generating new vasculature. It involves a process referred to as "sprouting" whereby individual endothelial cells, in response to extracellular signals, degrade components of the ECM, and migrate to fuse with an existing vessel. These endothelial tubes and their attendant pericytes generate vessels that are loosely constructed and are described as "leaky". This characteristic is essential for allowing the passage of tumor cells into the circulation during metastasis. Because of the enormous energy requirements of a growing solid tumor, angiogenesis is essential for its growth and subsequent metastasis.

Based on ground breaking work by Algire and colleagues [103], Judah Folkman proposed in 1971 that blocking tumor angiogenesis could be the key to stopping or even reversing tumor growth [104]. At the time this was a new and controversial concept but has subsequently led to the creation of antiangiogenic therapies, an entire category of cancer treatments. This approach was initiated with the monoclonal antibody, bevacizumab (Avastin), and now, with greater understanding of the processes that regulate angiogenesis, is a major focus of new treatment options. The control of angiogenesis is based on the notion of an "angiogenic switch" that controls a balance between angiogenesis inducers and suppressors [105].

Growth factors are a major category of angiogenesis inducers (also referred to as proangiogenic factors). These can be either nonspecific growth factors such as EGF (epidermal growth factor), FGF (fibroblast growth factor), and PDGF (platelet-derived growth factor) that affect many kinds of cells, or vascular endothelial-specific growth factors. There are three families of angiogenesis-specific inducers and their receptors. These are the vascular endothelial growth factors (VEGFs) and receptors (VEGFRs), the ephrins and ephrin receptors, and angiopoietins and Tie receptors. The role of VEGF proteins is in initiating angiogenesis and the roles of the ephrins and angiopoietins is more in the maturation of the new vessels. There are five known VEGF isoforms (VEGFA-E) and three VEGFRs (VEGFR1-3). Signaling via VEGFA and VEGFR2 is the most well-characterized mechanism of VEGF induction. Binding of VEGFA to VEGFR2 leads to activation of the RAS-Raf-MAPK pathway, much like that of other growth factors. It also leads to activation of PI3K and AKT. This in turn leads to inhibition of apoptosis and also increased vascular permeability via increased levels of nitric oxide generated by AKT stimulation of nitric oxide synthase. Expression of the *VEGF* genes is regulated by a variety of oncogeneic proteins (e.g., EGFR and Src) and tumor suppressors (e.g., *p53*). They are also regulated by the oxygen-sensing protein, hypoxia-inducible factor-1 (HIF-1). This protein is made of two subunits one of which, HIF-1α, is degrading under normoxic conditions and stabilized under hypoxic conditions. When tumor growth outpaces the existent vasculature, HIF-1α is stabilized; the HIF-1 protein can then act in the nucleus to activate a number of genes, most notably *VEGF*. That in turn leads to increased angiogenesis allowing further expansion of the tumor.

Angiogenesis can be "switched off" by inhibitors such as angiostatin, endostatin, thrombospondin-1-2, and *p53*. Angiostatin and endostatin are proteolytic cleavage products of larger proproteins and can be generated by the activities of matrix metalloproteinases that are present in the tumor microenvironment. Increased expression of thrombspondin-1 is, in part, regulated by binding of *p53* to its promoter. Thus, mutations in *p53* lead to decreased levels of thrombospondin-1 and an increase in angiogenesis.

Even with all of the new knowledge regarding the mechanisms that control angiogenesis, antiangiogenesis therapies have had limited use in the clinic. However, new approaches are on the horizon and there is every reason to believe antiangiogenic therapies will become part of the arsenal available to oncologists in the future [106].

Tumor blood vessel formation may also occur by at least two other mechanisms. Circulating endothelial progenitor cells can be incorporated into new vasculature and are known to contribute to colon cancer and some lymphomas [107]. Vascular mimicry is a process in which tumor cells themselves behave as endothelial cells and form channels and a neovasculature. This is seen in metastatic uveal and cutaneous melanoma [108].

Tissue Invasion and Metastasis

The process by which tumor cells leave the primary site and spread to sites throughout the body is referred to as metastasis. While metastasis is an inherently inefficient process and only a small subset of cells in a primary tumor have the potential to form metastases, it is the leading cause of cancer-related deaths, with at least two-thirds of cancer patients having metastasis at the time of diagnosis and it being responsible for upwards of 90% of cancer patient mortality. Invasion and metastasis are what distinguishes benign from malignant neoplasms [3, 109]. Metastasis is not the result of random or nonspecific events. There is a predictable sequence of events (often referred to as the metastatic cascade) that define the metastatic process. These steps include: (i) disruption of the basement membrane; (ii) detachment of the metastatic cell from the body of the tumor; (iii) invasion of the underlying ECM; (iv) entry into the vascular system (intravasation); (v) transport through the vasculature; (vi) arrest and adhesion to the inner surface of the blood or lymphatic vessel; (vii) exit from the vasculature (extravasation); (viii) colonization of the new tissue and proliferation. While many of the molecular details are yet to be worked out regarding metastasis, much information now exists with respect to each of these processes. A brief discussion follows about some of the steps in the cascade. For more complete discussions, several current reviews are recommended [110, 111].

The initial stages of metastasis involve the detachment of tumor cells, either as individuals or small clusters, and migration towards the tumor-induced vasculature. The cell–cell junctions maintained largely by E-cadherin must be disrupted and in this context E-cadherin acts as a tumor suppressor [112, 113]. This is followed by degradation of the basement membrane, which is largely composed of type IV collagen. This in turn allows the movement of tumor cells through the basement membrane and into the extracellular matrix, which is composed of proteins like collagen, fibronectin, laminin, and proteoglycans like chondroitin sulfate proteoglycans. The invasion of the surrounding tissues is mediated by the activities of serine and matrix metalloproteases, which are secreted by the tumor cells. The same classes of proteases are used during the intravasation process (see below; [114, 115]. Also secreted by the tumor cells is colony-stimulating factor-1 (CSF-1). Macrophages near the vessels have CSF-1 receptors on their surfaces, which when bound by ligand induce production and secretion of EGF. EGF acts as a chemoattractant to the tumor cells which contain EGF receptors (EGFR). Stimulation of EGFR results in increased secretion of CSF-1, thus creating a positive feedback loop that results in the movement of tumor cells and macrophage towards the nearby vasculature. Impressive intravital staining experiments have demonstrated this to be a major mechanism of breast tumor cells migration towards vessels [116]. Much of this process (large parts of which are not discussed here) is reminiscent of events that occur during normal embryogenesis. This has led to the idea that cancer cell metastasis is a form of recapitulating the epithelial–mesenchymal transition mechanism of early embryonic development [117, 118].

As described above, the vasculature induced by tumor cells is abnormal and displays loose cell–cell junctions. This allows tumor cells to readily pass through the vessel walls and enter the circulation, the process of intravasation. Once inside the vessel the tumor cells travel singly or in clusters with platelets and lymphocytes. It is thought that these clusters protect the tumor cells from the shear forces generated in the circulation. These cells are disseminated throughout the body. Escape from the blood or lymphatic vessels is the process of extravasation. While much of this is a reversal of intravasation, there are significant differences. Extravasation involves adhesion of the tumor cell to the inner surface of the vessel. It is well established that different tumor types preferentially metastasize to different organs. This can in part be explained by circulating tumor cells landing at the first organ downstream of the original tumor site (the so-called first-pass organ theory). However, this does not fully explain the nonrandom distribution of metastatic cells. The first explanation of this phenomenon was put forward by Paget in 1889 [119, 120] with the "seed and soil" concept which proposes that certain organs or tissues provide particularly favorable environments for colonization and growth of specific tumor types. Evidence for this concept was first provided experimentally by Fidler *et al.* (reviewed in [121]). Several mechanisms are involved in this process. First it is, in part, mediated by binding to selectin proteins, particularly E-selectin. It also involves recognition by the tumor cells of chemokines secreted by distant stromal cells. A major player is CXC-chemokine ligand 12 (CXCL12) [122], which is thought to attract specific tumor cells expressing the G-protein coupled chemokine receptors CXCR4 and CXCR7. This signaling results in the tumor cells adhering to specific sites on the endothelial cells, extravasating out of the vasculature, then migrating and adhering to the ECM at the new, secondary, site. From there it is the interaction with the tumor microenvironment that determines whether tumor cells grow, die, or become quiescent. A recent finding demonstrates that one of the preferred sites for some tumor metastases is the original tumor. This is thought to contribute to tumor heterogeneity.

A novel class of genes, the metastasis suppressor genes, has received much recent attention. First described by Patricia Steeg *et al.* in 1988 [123, 124], the common characteristic of these genes is that their expression blocks metastasis from a primary tumor but may have little or no effect on growth of that tumor. Many, however, do effect growth at a secondary tumor site. Reduced expression results in increased rates of metastasis and thus they are analogous to tumor suppressors. There are now more than 30 known metastasis suppressors and they are found both intracellularly and in the ECM. The precise function of many is not known although it is clear they affect many different steps in the metastasis cascade. They include adhesion proteins like E and N-cadherin, Rho-GTPase-activating proteins like DLC1, G-protein coupled receptors like KISS1R, and transcriptional regulators like CRSP3 (reviewed in [125]). This list has recently expanded to include metastatasis-suppressor microRNAs like miR-203 [126].

The Tumor Microenvironment

While much of the focus on tumor formation and progression has been on the role(s) of oncogenes and tumor suppressor genes expressed in the neoplastic cells, it has become increasingly clear that the environment in which these cells reside is also critical. The ECM and the stromal cells surrounding the neoplastic cells constitute the tumor microenvironment (TME), and the interactions between the TME and neoplastic cells affect virtually everything defining the hallmarks of cancer [3]. This importance has been highlighted in two recent reviews [127, 128]. Upwards of 300 proteins contribute to the TME. These include cell adhesion molecules, serine and metalloproteases, growth factors, and structural proteins (e.g., collagen), and are contributed by both the neoplastic and stromal cells. It includes a variety of cell types, including tumor-associated macrophages and other immune cells, endothelial cells and pericytes of the neovasculature, and a group of cells broadly defined as cancer-associated fibroblasts. The TME provides the nutritional and metabolic requirements needed for the tumor to survive and grow. As discussed above, it provides the cells and extracellular signaling molecules to stimulate and guide metastasis. It is the "soil" that provides the environment metastatic cells use to define their secondary growth sites.

Neovascular cells play roles beyond the chemotactic one mentioned above. These include limiting apoptosis, modulating energy metabolism, and specifically generating abnormal vessels that are essential for the process of intravasation. Much of this is accomplished through VEGF/VEGFR2 signaling (reviewed in [128]).

The immune cell contribution is extensive; they provide growth factors (e.g., EGF, TGF-β, and TNF-α), and are one of the sources of proteases (e.g., metalloproteases, serine proteases, cysteine proteases) that degrade and remodel the ECM to allow tumor growth, invasion, and metastasis.

The cancer-associated fibroblasts also play many roles. They help stimulate tumor growth by secreting mitogenic factors such as insulin-like growth factor-1, hepatocyte growth factor and stromal-derived factor-1. By secreting ECM molecules and ECM-modifying proteases, they play a role in changing the TME from one present around relatively normal cells to that which promotes tumor growth. They play an important role in stimulating angiogenesis (reviewed in [128]).

It should also be pointed out that each of the general stromal cell types described above may play a role in supporting the growth and maintenance of cancer-stem cells, a topic beyond the scope of this chapter.

The TME has become a major focus of new therapies. As the details become available regarding the composition, specificity, and function of different components of the TME, it appears that new sources of biomarkers and targets for novel therapies are near at hand. It is the continued exploration of the fundamental biology underlying cancer growth and metastasis that is providing the best hopes for improved prevention, detection, and treatment of cancer and for improving the lives of cancer patients.

Conclusion

Our understanding of the underlying cell and molecular biology of cancer has grown exponentially in the last decade. We have a more sophisticated view of how DNA damage and misregulation drive not only the initiation but the maturation of the cancerous state. We know more about the signals that control a cell's ability to grow in the absence of positive cues and to ignore growth-inhibiting cues. We understand much more about how angiogenesis is stimulated and how it is used to not only nourish growing tumors but facilitate metastasis. And finally, we are slowly growing to appreciate the importance of tumor stroma and the role the tumor microenvironment plays in cancer development. All of this knowledge is leading to more and better strategies to prevent, detect and treat cancer. And more is on the way.

References

1 Weinberg RA. *One Renegade Cell*. New York: Basic Books, 1998.

2 Hanahan D, Weinberg RA. The hallmarks of cancer. *Cell* 2000;100(1):57–70.

3 Hanahan D, Weinberg RA. Hallmarks of cancer: the next generation. *Cell* 2011;144(5):646–74.

4 Vilenchik MM, Knudson AG, Jr. Inverse radiation dose-rate effects on somatic and germ-line mutations and DNA damage rates. *Proc Natl Acad Sci USA* 2000;97(10):5381–6.

5 Garg P, Burgers PM. DNA polymerases that propagate the eukaryotic DNA replication fork. *Crit Rev Biochem Mol Biol* 2005;40(2):115–28.

6 Kunkel TA. DNA replication fidelity. *J Biol Chem* 2004; 279(17):16895–8.

7 McCulloch SD, Kunkel TA. The fidelity of DNA synthesis by eukaryotic replicative and translesion synthesis polymerases. *Cell Res* 2008;18(1):148–61.

8 Roach JC, Glusman G, Smit AF, *et al*. Analysis of genetic inheritance in a family quartet by whole-genome sequencing. *Science* 2010;328(5978):636–9.

9 Viguera E, Canceill D, Ehrlich SD. Replication slippage involves DNA polymerase pausing and dissociation. *EMBO J* 2001;20(10):2587–95.

10 Lindahl T. Instability and decay of the primary structure of DNA. *Nature* 1993;362(6422):709–15.

11 Jackson AL, Loeb LA. The contribution of endogenous sources of DNA damage to the multiple mutations in cancer. *Mutat Res* 2001;477(1–2):7–21.

12 Suzuki T, Kamiya H. Mutations induced by 8-hydroxyguanine (8-oxo-7,8-dihydroguanine), a representative oxidized base, in mammalian cells. *Genes Environ* 2016;39:2.

13 Yue W, Santen RJ, Wang JP, *et al*. Genotoxic metabolites of estradiol in breast: potential mechanism of estradiol induced carcinogenesis. *J Steroid Biochem Mol Biol* 2003;86(3–5): 477–86.

14 Gao X, Reid MA, Locasale JW. Metabolic interactions with cancer epigenetics. *Mol Aspects Med* 2017;54:50–57.

15 Wheeler GP, Skipper HE. Studies with mustards. III. In vivo fixation of C14 from nitrogen mustard-C14H3 in nucleic acid fractions of animal tissues. *Arch Biochem Biophys* 1957;72(2):465–75.

16 McCann J, Choi E, Yamasaki E, Ames BN. Detection of carcinogens as mutagens in the salmonella/microsome test: assay of 300 chemicals. *Proc Natl Acad Sci USA* 1975;72 (12):5135–9.

17 Magnussen A, Parsi MA. Aflatoxins, hepatocellular carcinoma and public health. *World J Gastroenterol* 2013;19(10):1508–12.

18 Van Rensburg SJ, Cook-Mozaffari P, Van Schalkwyk DJ, *et al*. Hepatocellular carcinoma and dietary aflatoxin in Mozambique and Transkei. *Br J Cancer* 1985;51(5):713–26.

19 Hsu IC, Metcalf RA, Sun T, *et al*. Mutational hotspot in the p53 gene in human hepatocellular carcinomas. *Nature* 1991; 350(6317):427–8.

20 Hecht SS. Lung carcinogenesis by tobacco smoke. *Int J Cancer* 2012;131(12):2724–32.

21 Denissenko MF, Pao A, Tang M, Pfeifer GP. Preferential formation of benzo[a]pyrene adducts at lung cancer mutational hotspots in P53. *Science* 1996;274(5286):430–2.

22 Rodenhuis S, van de Wetering ML, Mooi WJ, *et al*. Mutational activation of the K-ras oncogene. A possible pathogenetic factor in adenocarcinoma of the lung. *N Engl J Med* 1987;317(15):929–35.

23 Ding L, Getz G, Wheeler DA, *et al*. Somatic mutations affect key pathways in lung adenocarcinoma. *Nature* 2008;455(7216):1069–75.

24 Hecht SS. Biochemistry, biology, and carcinogenicity of tobacco-specific N-nitrosamines. *Chem Res Toxicol* 1998;11(6):559–603.

25 Smith LE, Denissenko MF, Bennett WP, *et al*. Targeting of lung cancer mutational hotspots by polycyclic aromatic hydrocarbons. *J Natl Cancer Instit* 2000;92(10):803–11.

26 Weng Y, Fang C, Turesky RJ, *et al*. Determination of the role of target tissue metabolism in lung carcinogenesis using conditional cytochrome P450 reductase-null mice. *Cancer Res* 2007;67(16):7825–32.

27 Pfeifer GP, Denissenko MF, Olivier M, *et al*. Tobacco smoke carcinogens, DNA damage and p53 mutations in smoking-associated cancers. *Oncogene* 2002;21(48):7435–51.

28 Pleasance ED, Stephens PJ, O'Meara S, *et al*. A small-cell lung cancer genome with complex signatures of tobacco exposure. *Nature* 2010;463(7278):184–90.

29 Doll R, Peto R. The causes of cancer: quantitative estimates of avoidable risks of cancer in the United States today. *J Natl Cancer Instit* 1981;66(6):1191–308.

30 *Sources and Effects of Ionizing Radiation*. New York: United Nations, 2010.

31 Ward JF. DNA damage produced by ionizing radiation in mammalian cells: identities, mechanisms of formation, and reparability. *Prog Nucl Acid Res Mol Biol* 1988;35:95–125.

32 Mesri EA, Feitelson MA, Munger K. Human viral oncogenesis: a cancer hallmarks analysis. *Cell Host Microbe* 2014;15(3):266–82.

33 zur Hausen H. Oncogenic DNA viruses. *Oncogene* 2001; 20(54):7820–3.

34 Galloway, DA, Laimins, LA, Human papillomaviruses: shared and distinct pathways for pathogenesis. *Curr Opin Virol* 2015; 14:87–92.

35 Feng H, Shuda M, Chang Y, Moore PS. Clonal integration of a polyomavirus in human Merkel cell carcinoma. *Science* 2008;319(5866):1096–100.

36 Liu W, MacDonald M, You J. Merkel cell polyomavirus infection and Merkel cell carcinoma. *Curr Opin Virol* 2016;20:20–27.

37 Guidotti LG, Chisari FV. Immunobiology and pathogenesis of viral hepatitis. *Ann Rev Pathol* 2006;1:23–61.

38 Arzumanyan A, Reis HM, Feitelson MA. Pathogenic mechanisms in HBV- and HCV-associated hepatocellular carcinoma. *Nature Rev Cancer* 2013;13(2):123–35.

39 Klein G. Burkitt lymphoma – a stalking horse for cancer research? *Semin Cancer Biology* 2009;19(6):347–50.

40 Raab-Traub N. Novel mechanisms of EBV-induced oncogenesis. *Curr Opin Virol* 2012;2(4):453–8.

41 Moore PS, Chang Y. The conundrum of causality in tumor virology: the cases of KSHV and MCV. *Semin Cancer Biology* 2014;26:4–12.

42 Giffin L, Damania B. KSHV: pathways to tumorigenesis and persistent infection. *Adv Virus Res* 2014;88:111–59.

43 Panfil AR, Martinez MP, Ratner L, Green PL. Human T-cell leukemia virus-associated malignancy. *Curr Opin Virol* 2016;20:40–46.

44 Matsuoka M, Jeang KT. Human T-cell leukaemia virus type 1 (HTLV-1) infectivity and cellular transformation. *Nature Rev Cancer* 2007;7(4):270–80.

45 Marshall BJ, Warren JR. Unidentified curved bacilli in the stomach of patients with gastritis and peptic ulceration. *Lancet* 1984;1(8390):1311–5.

46 Backert S, Neddermann M, Maubach G, Naumann M. Pathogenesis of Helicobacter pylori infection. *Helicobacter* 2016;21(Suppl 1):19–25.

47 Huang JQ, Zheng GF, Sumanac K, Irvine EJ, Hunt RH. Meta-analysis of the relationship between cagA seropositivity and gastric cancer. *Gastroenterology* 2003;125(6):1636–44.

48 Higashi H, Tsutsumi R, Muto S, *et al*. SHP-2 tyrosine phosphatase as an intracellular target of Helicobacter pylori CagA protein. *Science* 2002;295(5555):683–6.

49 Wilson KT, Crabtree JE. Immunology of Helicobacter pylori: insights into the failure of the immune response and perspectives on vaccine studies. *Gastroenterology* 2007;133(1):288–308.

50 El-Omar EM, Carrington M, Chow WH, *et al*. Interleukin-1 polymorphisms associated with increased risk of gastric cancer. *Nature* 2000;404(6776):398–402.

51 Haenszel W, Kurihara M. Studies of Japanese migrants. I. Mortality from cancer and other diseases among Japanese in the United States. *J Natl Cancer Instit* 1968;40(1):43–68.

52 Bhattacharjee S, Nandi S. Choices have consequences: the nexus between DNA repair pathways and genomic instability in cancer. *Clin Transl Med* 2016;5:45.

53 Glassner BJ, Weeda G, Allan JM, *et al*. DNA repair methyltransferase (Mgmt) knockout mice are sensitive to the lethal effects of chemotherapeutic alkylating agents. *Mutagenesis* 1999;14(3):339–47.

54 Esteller M, Hamilton SR, Burger PC, Baylin SB, Herman JG. Inactivation of the DNA repair gene O6-methylguanine-DNA methyltransferase by promoter hypermethylation is a common event in primary human neoplasia. *Cancer Res* 1999;59(4):793–7.

55 Dianov GL, Hubscher U. Mammalian base excision repair: the forgotten archangel. *Nucleic Acids Res* 2013;41(6):3483–90.

56 Sobol RW, Horton JK, Kuhn R, *et al*. Requirement of mammalian DNA polymerase-beta in base-excision repair. *Nature* 1996;379(6561):183–6.

57 Gao Y, Katyal S, Lee Y, *et al*. DNA ligase III is critical for mtDNA integrity but not Xrcc1-mediated nuclear DNA repair. *Nature* 2011;471(7337):240–4.

58 Tebbs RS, Thompson LH, Cleaver JE. Rescue of Xrcc1 knockout mouse embryo lethality by transgene-complementation. *DNA Repair* 2003;2(12):1405–17.

59 Le May N, Egly JM, Coin F. True lies: the double life of the nucleotide excision repair factors in transcription and DNA repair. *J Nucleic Acids* 2010;2010.

60 DiGiovanna JJ, Kraemer KH. Shining a light on xeroderma pigmentosum. *J Invest Dermatol* 2012;132(3):785–96.

61 Larrea AA, Lujan SA, Kunkel TA. SnapShot: DNA mismatch repair. *Cell* 2010;141(4):730 e1.

62 Martin-Lopez JV, Fishel R. The mechanism of mismatch repair and the functional analysis of mismatch repair defects in Lynch syndrome. *Fam Cancer* 2013;12(2):159–68.

63 Budman J, Chu G. Processing of DNA for nonhomologous end-joining by cell-free extract. *EMBO J* 2005;24(4):849–60.

64 Alt FW, Zhang Y, Meng FL, Guo C, Schwer B. Mechanisms of programmed DNA lesions and genomic instability in the immune system. *Cell* 2013;152(3):417–29.

65 Smith GC, Jackson SP. The DNA-dependent protein kinase. *Genes Dev* 1999;13(8):916–34.

66 Lim DS, Vogel H, Willerford DM, *et al*. Analysis of ku80-mutant mice and cells with deficient levels of p53. *Mol Cell Biol* 2000;20(11):3772–80.

67 Ben-Omran TI, Cerosaletti K, Concannon P, Weitzman S, Nezarati MM. A patient with mutations in DNA Ligase IV: clinical features and overlap with Nijmegen breakage syndrome. *Am J Med Gen* 2005;137A(3):283–7.

68 Allen C, Ashley AK, Hromas R, Nickoloff JA. More forks on the road to replication stress recovery. *J Mol Cell Biol* 2011;3(1):4–12.

69 Hall JM, Lee MK, Newman B, *et al*. Linkage of early-onset familial breast cancer to chromosome 17q21. *Science* 1990;250(4988):1684–9.

70 Miki Y, Swensen J, Shattuck-Eidens D, *et al*. A strong candidate for the breast and ovarian cancer susceptibility gene BRCA1. *Science* 1994;266(5182):66–71.

71 Wooster R, Neuhausen SL, Mangion J, *et al*. Localization of a breast cancer susceptibility gene, BRCA2, to chromosome 13q12-13. *Science* 1994;265(5181):2088–90.

72 Jasin M. Homologous repair of DNA damage and tumorigenesis: the BRCA connection. *Oncogene* 2002;21(58):8981–93.

73 Venkitaraman AR. Functions of BRCA1 and BRCA2 in the biological response to DNA damage. *J Cell Sci* 2001;114:3591–8.

74 Ashworth A. A synthetic lethal therapeutic approach: poly(ADP) ribose polymerase inhibitors for the treatment of cancers deficient in DNA double-strand break repair. *J Clin Oncol* 2008;26(22):3785–90.

75 Sale JE, Lehmann AR, Woodgate R. Y-family DNA polymerases and their role in tolerance of cellular DNA damage. *Nature Rev Mol Cell Biol* 2012;13(3):141–52.

76 Waters LS, Minesinger BK, Wiltrout ME, *et al*. Eukaryotic translesion polymerases and their roles and regulation in DNA damage tolerance. *Microbiol Mol Biol Rev* 2009;73(1):134–54.

77 Doksani Y, de Lange T. The role of double-strand break repair pathways at functional and dysfunctional telomeres. *Cold Spring Harb Perspect Biol* 2014;6(12):a016576.

78 Greider CW, Blackburn EH. Identification of a specific telomere terminal transferase activity in Tetrahymena extracts. *Cell* 1985;43(2):405–13.

79 Shay JW, Bacchetti S. A survey of telomerase activity in human cancer. *Eur J Cancer* 1997;33(5):787–91.

80 Hahn WC, Counter CM, Lundberg AS, Beijersbergen RL, Brooks MW, Weinberg RA. Creation of human tumour cells with defined genetic elements. *Nature* 1999;400(6743):464–8.

81 Weinberg RA. *The Biology of Cancer*, 2nd edn. New York: Garland Science, 2013.

82 Vogelstein B, Papadopoulos N, Velculescu VE, *et al*. Cancer genome landscapes. *Science* 2013;339(6127):1546–58.

83 Pon JR, Marra MA. Driver and passenger mutations in cancer. *Ann Rev Pathol* 2015; 10:25–50.

84 Rous P. A sarcoma of the fowl transmissible by an agent separable from the tumor cells. *J Exp Med* 1911;13(4):397–411.

85 Stehelin D, Varmus HE, Bishop JM, Vogt PK. DNA related to the transforming gene(s) of avian sarcoma viruses is present in normal avian DNA. *Nature* 1976;260(5547):170–3.

86 Harris H. Cell fusion and the analysis of malignancy. *Proc Royal Soc London Series B* 1971;179(1054):1–20.

87 Knudson AG, Jr, Meadows AT, Nichols WW, Hill R. Chromosomal deletion and retinoblastoma. *N Engl J Med* 1976;295(20):1120–3.

88 Friend SH, Bernards R, Rogelj S, *et al*. A human DNA segment with properties of the gene that predisposes to retinoblastoma and osteosarcoma. *Nature* 1986;323(6089):643–6.

89 Sherr CJ. Principles of tumor suppression. *Cell* 2004; 116(2):235–46.

90 Kerr JF, Wyllie AH, Currie AR. Apoptosis: a basic biological phenomenon with wide-ranging implications in tissue kinetics. *Br J Cancer* 1972;26(4):239–57.

91 Ashkenazi A. Targeting death and decoy receptors of the tumour-necrosis factor superfamily. *Nature Rev Cancer* 2002;2(6):420–30.

92 Cheng EH, Wei MC, Weiler S, *et al.* BCL-2, BCL-X(L) sequester BH3 domain-only molecules preventing BAX- and BAK-mediated mitochondrial apoptosis. *Mol Cell* 2001;8(3):705–11.

93 Danial NN, Korsmeyer SJ. Cell death: critical control points. *Cell* 2004;116(2):205–19.

94 Okada H, Mak TW. Pathways of apoptotic and non-apoptotic death in tumour cells. *Nature Rev Cancer* 2004;4(8):592–603.

95 Hilgendorf KI, Leshchiner ES, Nedelcu S, *et al.* The retinoblastoma protein induces apoptosis directly at the mitochondria. *Genes Dev* 2013;27(9):1003–15.

96 Souers AJ, Leverson JD, Boghaert ER, *et al.* ABT-199, a potent and selective BCL-2 inhibitor, achieves antitumor activity while sparing platelets. *Nature Med* 2013;19(2):202–8.

97 FDA approves new drug for chronic lymphocytic leukemia in patients with a specific chromosomal abnormality. Available at: http://www.fda.gov/NewsEvents/ Newsroom/ PressAnnouncements/ucm495253.htm (accessed 28 May 2017).

98 Corcoran RB, Cheng KA, Hata AN, *et al.* Synthetic lethal interaction of combined BCL-XL and MEK inhibition promotes tumor regressions in KRAS mutant cancer models. *Cancer Cell* 2013;23(1):121–8.

99 Frisch SM, Francis H. Disruption of epithelial cell-matrix interactions induces apoptosis. *J Cell Biol* 1994;124(4): 619–26.

100 Buchheit CL, Weigel KJ, Schafer ZT. Cancer cell survival during detachment from the ECM: multiple barriers to tumour progression. *Nature Rev Cancer* 2014;14(9):632–41.

101 Cuervo AM. Autophagy: many paths to the same end. *Mol Cell Biochem* 2004;263(1–2):55–72.

102 Cuervo AM. Autophagy: in sickness and in health. *Trends Cell Biol* 2004;14(2):70–7.

103 Algire GH, Chalkley HW, Earle WE, *et al.* Vascular reactions of normal and malignant tissues in vivo. III. Vascular reactions' of mice to fibroblasts treated in vitro with methylcholanthrene. *J Natl Cancer Instit* 1950;11(3):555–80.

104 Folkman J. Tumor angiogenesis: therapeutic implications. *N Engl J Med* 1971;285(21):1182–6.

105 Baeriswyl V, Christofori G. The angiogenic switch in carcinogenesis. *Semin Cancer Biol* 2009;19(5):329–37.

106 Lin Z, Zhang Q, Luo W. Angiogenesis inhibitors as therapeutic agents in cancer: Challenges and future directions. *Eur J Pharmacol* 2016;793:76–81.

107 Rafii S, Lyden D, Benezra R, Hattori K, Heissig B. Vascular and haematopoietic stem cells: novel targets for anti-angiogenesis therapy? *Nature Rev Cancer* 2002;2(11):826–35.

108 Folberg R, Hendrix MJ, Maniotis AJ. Vasculogenic mimicry and tumor angiogenesis. *Am J Pathol* 2000;156(2):361–81.

109 Reddy BY, Lim PK, Silverio K, *et al.* The microenvironmental effect in the progression, metastasis, and dormancy of breast cancer: a model system within bone marrow. *Int J Breast Cancer* 2012;2012:721659.

110 Reymond N, d'Agua BB, Ridley AJ. Crossing the endothelial barrier during metastasis. *Nature Rev Cancer* 2013; 13(12):858–70.

111 Nguyen DX, Bos PD, Massague J. Metastasis: from dissemination to organ-specific colonization. *Nature Rev Cancer* 2009;9(4):274–84.

112 Jeanes A, Gottardi CJ, Yap AS. Cadherins and cancer: how does cadherin dysfunction promote tumor progression? *Oncogene* 2008;27(55):6920–9.

113 van Roy F. Beyond E-cadherin: roles of other cadherin superfamily members in cancer. *Nature Rev Cancer* 2014;14(2):121–34.

114 Chabottaux V, Ricaud S, Host L, *et al.* Membrane-type 4 matrix metalloproteinase (MT4-MMP) induces lung metastasis by alteration of primary breast tumour vascular architecture. *J Cell Mol Med* 2009;13(9B):4002–13.

115 Frohlich C, Klitgaard M, Noer JB, *et al.* ADAM12 is expressed in the tumour vasculature and mediates ectodomain shedding of several membrane-anchored endothelial proteins. *Biochem J* 2013;452(1):97–109.

116 Wyckoff JB, Wang Y, Lin EY, *et al.* Direct visualization of macrophage-assisted tumor cell intravasation in mammary tumors. *Cancer Res* 2007;67(6):2649–56.

117 Mani SA, Guo W, Liao MJ, *et al.* The epithelial-mesenchymal transition generates cells with properties of stem cells. *Cell* 2008;133(4):704–15.

118 Nakaya Y, Sheng G. EMT in developmental morphogenesis. *Cancer Lett* 2013;341(1):9–15.

119 Paget S. The distribution of secondary growths in cancer of the breast. *Lancet* 1889;133:571–3.

120 Venkitaraman AR. Chromosome stability, DNA recombination and the BRCA2 tumour suppressor. *Curr Opin Cell Biol* 2001;13(3):338–43.

121 Talmadge JE, Fidler IJ. AACR centennial series: the biology of cancer metastasis: historical perspective. *Cancer Res* 2010;70(14):5649–69.

122 Teicher BA, Fricker SP. CXCL12 (SDF-1)/CXCR4 pathway in cancer. *Clin Cancer Res* 2010;16(11):2927–31.

123 Steeg PS, Bevilacqua G, Kopper L, *et al.* Evidence for a novel gene associated with low tumor metastatic potential. *J Natl Cancer Inst* 1988;80(3):200–4.

124 Steeg PS, Bevilacqua G, Pozzatti R, Liotta LA, Sobel ME. Altered expression of NM23, a gene associated with low tumor metastatic potential, during adenovirus 2 Ela inhibition of experimental metastasis. *Cancer Res* 1988;48(22):6550–4.

125 Hurst DR, Welch DR. Metastasis suppressor genes at the interface between the environment and tumor cell growth. *Int Rev Cell Mol Biol* 2011;286:107–80.

126 Michel CI, Malumbres M. microRNA-203: tumor suppression and beyond. *Microrna* 2013;2(2):118–26.

127 Fang H, Declerck YA. Targeting the tumor microenvironment: from understanding pathways to effective clinical trials. *Cancer Res* 2013;73(16):4965–77.

128 Hanahan D, Coussens LM. Accessories to the crime: functions of cells recruited to the tumor microenvironment. *Cancer Cell* 2012;21(3):309–22.

Section 3

Diagnosis

13

Imaging in Oncology

Andreas G. Wibmer, Andreas M. Hötker, Maura Miccò, David M. Panicek, and Hedvig Hricak

Memorial Sloan-Kettering Cancer Center, New York, New York, USA

Introduction

Imaging has emerged as an essential diagnostic tool in oncology. Its value has been shown for screening, diagnosis, staging, treatment selection, treatment response assessment and post-treatment surveillance, as well as in the workup of suspected treatment-related complications. Thanks to rapid advances in conventional, cross-sectional, nuclear medicine, and molecular imaging methods, imaging can provide morphological, metabolic, and functional information. In addition, interventional radiologic techniques allow image-guided diagnosis and minimally invasive, lesion-targeted therapies. Imaging is therefore contributing increasingly to risk-adapted, personalized cancer treatment.

Technical Principles

Conventional Radiography (X-rays, Plain Films)

X-rays are a form of electromagnetic radiation characterized by an extremely short wavelength, shorter than that of light. Because of their short wavelength, they are able to penetrate materials that absorb or reflect light. X-rays can be produced in an X-ray tube by focusing a beam of high-energy electrons onto a target that is most commonly made of tungsten. The rays penetrate the human body and produce a two-dimensional image of internal structures. A radiograph (e.g., chest X-ray) is a photographic record produced by the passage of X-rays onto a film, where they cause a chemical reaction that leads to image production. As the X-rays pass through human tissues, some of them are absorbed, thereby reducing (attenuating) the amount of remaining rays. The degree of X-ray attenuation depends on the nature of the tissue and its thickness. Tissues of high density and/or high atomic number elements (e.g., bone) cause more X-ray attenuation and are shown on the plain film as lighter grey or white areas. Less dense tissues (e.g., fat or air) cause less X-ray attenuation and appear darker on the plain film. These characteristics result in good contrast between structures with markedly different densities (e.g., lungs and soft tissue in chest X-rays). However, the contrast between different soft tissue structures (e.g., muscle and blood vessels) is poor. One method for improving the distinction between soft tissues is to administer exogenous contrast material (e.g., barium) to outline or fill hollow viscera. Intravenous iodinated contrast material has also been used to improve visualization of the kidneys, collecting systems and urinary bladder.

Mammography is one of the most demanding X-ray exams to perform and interpret. The breast consists of glandular soft tissue with relatively small differences in density. Thus, mammography requires very high image quality for the detection of small pathological changes, and mammographic equipment is tailored to provide high tissue contrast and fine spatial resolution. In addition, physical compression of the breast is used to flatten and thus better delineate the breast parenchyma.

Fluoroscopy is a radiographic technique that depicts the anatomy and motion of internal structures (such as esophagus, stomach, bowel, and diaphragm) in real time by using a constant stream of X-rays (applied intermittently, to reduce radiation exposure).

Advantages of radiography: simple; fast; low radiation dose; low cost.

Limitations: insensitive; often produces nonspecific findings.

Computed Tomography (CT)

CT is a cross-sectional imaging technique in which a radiation source (X-ray tube) rotates around the patient, sending X-rays through the patient to reach specialized detectors on the opposite side. The amount of X-rays penetrating the body (minus those absorbed by each tissue encountered) is measured by the detectors. The resultant data is analyzed by a computer and displayed as a grey-scale image. The computer determines the attenuation (differences in X-ray absorption of tissues related to different anatomic numbers) for each small volume of body tissue (voxel) and assigns a Hounsfield unit (HU). The CT image is a representation of the different tissue densities. Minor differences in density are sufficient to allow accurate display of anatomy and differentiation between organs, provide evidence of pathology, and enable identification of specific materials such as fat or calcium. The relative density may be also measured electronically, using the Hounsfield unit scale, which ranges from −1000 (air), to 0 (water), to +1000 (cortical bone).

The earliest clinical CT scanners took many minutes to produce a series of images. Technological advances allowed helical (spiral) CT scanners, which appeared in the early 1990s, to image a continuous volume of the body, rather than individual, discrete sections. Modern helical CT machines, referred to as multidetector-row CT (MDCT), or multislice CT (MSCT) machines, currently obtain 16–256 images simultaneously, enabling a large volume of the body to be scanned in seconds; the multiple fan beams produce accurate, high-quality three-dimensional (3D) image data sets and allow multiplanar reconstructions. These advances have allowed applications such as CT colonography (virtual colonoscopy), cardiac CT, and CT angiography to gain wide clinical acceptance. CT is also useful for needle guidance during percutaneous biopsy (CT-guided biopsy).

Iodinated contrast material is often administered intravenously at CT to: better differentiate normal structures from abnormal ones; increase the visibility of and characterize pathological tissue; and fill blood vessels. MDCT with intravenous contrast media can directly image a tumor located anywhere in the body as an "enhancing mass", demonstrating tumor margins and relationships with surrounding organs, tumor blood supply, and the internal structure or "texture" of the tumor (Figure 13.1).

The intensity and pattern of enhancement may help to narrow the differential diagnosis.

Contrast material, such as barium or an iodinated agent, is often given orally (and sometimes rectally) for abdominal and pelvic CT to facilitate differentiation of bowel from masses, to evaluate the wall thickness and lumen of the bowel, and to detect and delineate fistulous connections with bowel. Although the newer, nonionic contrast agents are generally well tolerated, adverse reactions can occur (ranging from urticaria, sneezing, and dyspnea to, rarely, anaphylaxis). Premedication with steroids can help prevent most subsequent reactions in patients who have had an adverse reaction, although the use of alternative imaging methods should be considered.

Advantages of CT: cross-sectional display; moderate soft tissue contrast; moderate spatial resolution.

Limitations: ionizing radiation dose; expensive.

Magnetic Resonance Imaging (MRI)

MRI is currently the most versatile imaging technology available. It uses the magnetic properties of spinning hydrogen atoms to generate intrinsic contrast between different tissues. This cross-sectional imaging technique applies a strong, external, unidirectional magnetic field to an area inside a large, powerful magnet, into which the patient is placed. Most current medical MRI scanners have field strengths of 1.5 or 3.0 Tesla (1.5 T or 3 T), which are about 30,000 to 60,000 times the strength of the earth's magnetic field, respectively. When placed within this strong external magnetic field, a fraction of the hydrogen atoms

(a)

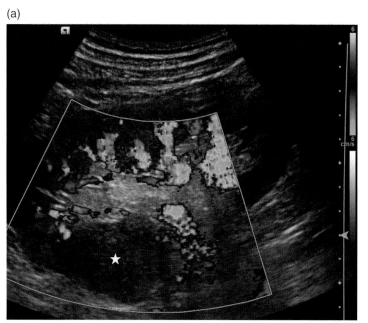

(b)

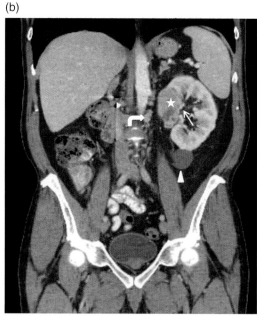

Figure 13.1 A 61-year-old male with clear cell renal carcinoma (pathological stage T3b). The patient had previously undergone right radical nephrectomy for tumor. (a) Longitudinal, color-encoded transabdominal Doppler ultrasound of the left kidney shows a 4-cm tumor in the posterior renal cortex (star). Note the hypovascularity of the tumor compared to normal renal cortical parenchyma, recognizable by the lack of Doppler signal within the tumor. (b) Coronal contrast-enhanced CT shows that the renal tumor (star) is in direct contact with renal sinus fat (arrow). Such contact is associated with a high probability of muscular venous branch invasion, which was histologically proven in this case. An enlarged, enhancing paraaortic mass is suspicious for lymph node metastasis (curved arrow). An incidental simple cyst in the lower pole of the left kidney (arrowhead) shows a thin wall, homogeneous water-like attenuation, and no contrast enhancement.

within the patient align in a direction either parallel or antiparallel to it. The majority of the atoms aligns in a single direction parallel to the field, in a phenomenon known as longitudinal magnetization. A second magnetic field, known as the radiofrequency pulse (RF pulse) and transmitted by radiofrequency coils, is intermittently applied at right angles to the original external field. The RF waves momentarily deflect the hydrogen atoms, modifying their spin orientation. (Gradient coils can be also used to produce variations to the magnetic field.) When the RF pulse is turned off, the atoms return to their original precession or orientation (the direction parallel to the original external field), emitting radiowave "echoes" (RF signal) in the process. The signal used to create MR images is derived from the energy released by atoms precessing from different energy states. This exchange of energy is called "resonance" and involves two processes: T1 relaxation (longitudinal relaxation) and T2 relaxation (transverse relaxation). The emissions are detected by RF receiver coils, which are applied around the body part or region of interest. Receiver coils are available in various shapes and sizes, tailored for the examination of particular body parts.

Computer analysis of MR signals is used to produce the MR images. Images display the different resonance characteristics of the various tissues. MR signal depends on inherent properties of the tissues and structures being examined, such as their proton density and chemical environments. The time between the excitation of the hydrogen atoms by the external RF pulse and the detection of the radiowave echoes from the same atoms represents the "echo time" (TE). The "repetition time" (TR) represents the interval between each successive RF pulse emitted by the MRI scanner. By modifying the duration and amplitude of the RF pulse, as well as the timing and repetition of its application, different imaging sequences can be obtained that are somewhat analogous to the different "stains" used in pathology. By manipulating TR and TE, the basic T1-weighted or T2-weighted imaging sequences are produced; the former use short TR and short TE, and the latter, long TR and long TE. A tissue with a long T1 and T2 (like water) is dark in the T1-weighted image and bright in the T2-weighted image. A tissue with a short T1 and an intermediate T2 (like fat) is bright in the T1-weighted image and gray in the T2-weighted image. General categories of MR imaging sequences include spin echo, inversion recovery, and gradient-recalled echo (gradient echo).

Because MRI – without using ionizing radiation – provides superb contrast between different tissues, many MRI exams can be performed without the injection of intravenous contrast material. Anatomical details can be better appreciated on T1-weighted images, whereas contrast between soft tissues (e.g., tumor and adjacent organs) is clearer on T2-weighted images. The MRI acquisition process allows the generation of multiple adjacent planar images as well as 3D volume images of the body region being studied (Figure 13.2).

Another MR technique, diffusion-weighted imaging (DWI), is sensitive to the random Brownian motion (diffusion) of water molecules within tissue. Areas of reduced water-molecule diffusion appear on DWI as relatively high (bright) signal. Cytotoxic edema is characterized by restricted diffusion of water molecules, and DWI is currently the most sensitive imaging test available for the diagnosis of acute cerebral infarction. Neoplastic tissues are characterized by increased cellularity, and the consequent reduction of the extracellular space is reflected as an area of restricted diffusion on DWI. This MRI sequence shows promise in characterizing pathological tissue without the injection of intravenous contrast media. Other functional dynamic sequences include perfusion imaging (which allows quantitative analysis of organ vascularity as regional blood volume and blood flow) and spectroscopy (which allows quantitative analysis of metabolites or cellular elements within normal or pathological tissue). All of these functional techniques improve the diagnostic accuracy and specificity of MRI.

Gadolinium (Gd) is a paramagnetic element that shortens the T1 relaxation time of the tissue or material within which it is present, thus increasing the signal seen on T1-weighted images. Various formulations of chelated Gd are used as intravenous MRI contrast agents. Although these agents are generally well tolerated, some patients exhibit adverse reactions to them; most reactions are relatively minor, but on rare occasions, they can be fatal. In the late 1990s, nephrogenic systemic fibrosis (NSF) was reported as a rare complication after administration of Gd-based contrast media, mostly occurring in patients with end-stage renal failure and on dialysis. Before contrast administration, each patient's renal function is now evaluated to assess the risk of NSF, generally using estimated glomerular filtration rate (eGFR) as the metric. This policy and the availability of refined, chemically more stable contrast agents have resulted in the virtual elimination of this complication after 2009. Oral contrast agents have been used in MRI to delineate bowel more clearly, but none has been found to be ideal; currently, oral contrast is rarely administered. Antiperistaltic agents, however, are often used to decrease (involuntary) bowel motion during scanning.

It is important to understand that there are several important contraindications to the MRI process, related to the interactions between the strong magnetic fields and certain ferromagnetic materials (such as some cerebral aneurysm clips, or metallic foreign objects in or near the eye) and implanted electronic devices (such as most cardiac pacemakers). Patients must be carefully screened for the presence of such items to prevent them from experiencing serious injury. The environment in which the MRI is performed must also be meticulously monitored by personnel familiar with numerous safety issues related to working in a strong magnetic field.

Severely anxious or claustrophobic patients may have difficulty tolerating the scan times involved in MRI and may require sedation or, in some cases, general anesthesia.

Although scanning during pregnancy has not been proven to produce any adverse effects on the mother or fetus, alternative imaging techniques should be explored first. Also, Gd-based contrast agents should be avoided during pregnancy.

Advantages of MRI: sensitive; high contrast; no ionizing radiation.

Limitations: expensive; complex; long scan times (motion leads to artifacts); claustrophobia; some contraindications to scanning.

Ultrasound (US)

US is a cross-sectional imaging technique that uses sound waves with a frequency greater than the upper limit of the human

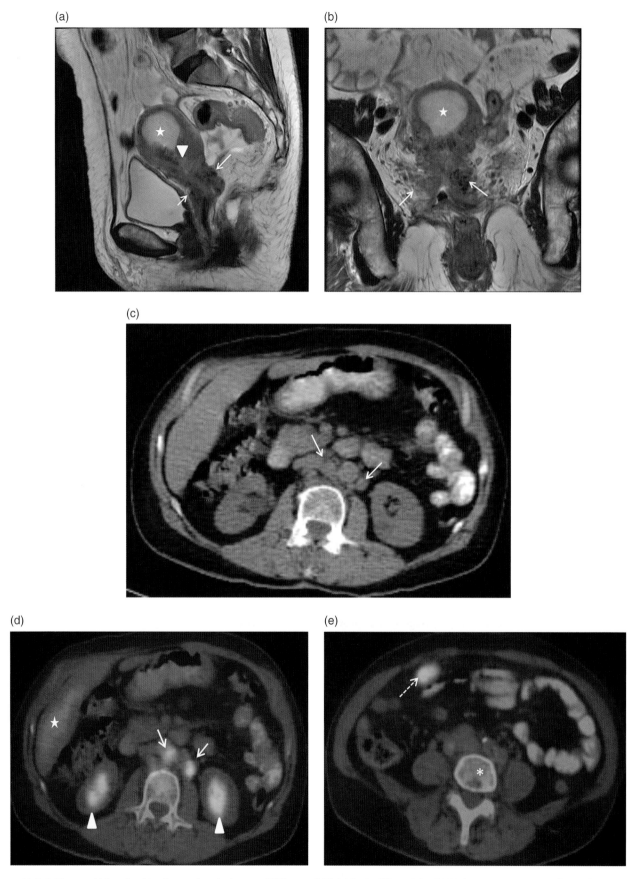

Figure 13.2 A 53-year-old female with advanced cervical cancer (FIGO stage IVB). (a) Sagittal T2-weighted MRI demonstrates a cervical mass (arrows) with extension into the lower uterine segment (arrowhead) and a distended endometrial cavity (star). (b) Coronal T2-weighted MRI demonstrates bilateral parametrial invasion (arrows) and distended endometrial cavity (star). (c) Axial CT image with oral contrast demonstrates subcentimeter left para-aortic and aortocaval lymph nodes (arrows). (d, e) Axial fused FDG PET and CT images demonstrate abnormal FDG tracer uptake in left para-aortic and aortocaval lymph nodes consistent with metastatic involvement (arrows) and in a right anterior peritoneal tumor implant (dashed arrow). The fused images also show physiologic tracer accumulation in the liver (star) and bone marrow (asterisk), as well as excreted tracer in the renal collecting systems bilaterally (arrowheads).

hearing range (from the Latin *ultra*, meaning "beyond"). US works on a principle similar to that of marine sonar, which emits pulses of sound and listens for echoes that come back from objects that reflect those sound waves (e.g., the bottom of the sea). The time interval from the emission of the sound pulse to the perception of the echo is directly related to the distance between the sonar and the reflecting object. In the case of medical US, the sound waves are both emitted and received by hundreds of piezo crystals that are aligned in a hand-held transducer. The sound waves penetrate the body and are partially reflected at the boundary of differing tissue interfaces. The amount of reflection depends on a physical property of each tissue type, the impedance (from the Latin *impedare*, meaning "to hinder"). Tissues with high impedance (e.g., the air-filled lung) strongly hinder the transmission of US waves, while tissues with low impedance (e.g., bones, stones, calcifications) hinder transmission only to a minor degree. The greater the difference in impedance between two adjacent tissue types, the greater the amount of reflection of US waves at their boundary.

A medical US scanner electronically combines two variables – distance and intensity of reflection – and produces two-dimensional gray-scale images. The amount of reflection produced by a distinct tissue is called its *echogenicity*. Pathologies are depicted when they obliterate normal tissue boundaries and/or have a different echogenicity than the normal surrounding tissue.

Modern US scanners work in a real-time manner and allow dynamic examinations of moving organs (e.g., the heart). Movements of liquids (e.g., blood) can be visualized by the application of Doppler US, which works on the same principle as a radar gun. In both techniques, the wave-reflecting objects are moving towards or away from the transducer (e.g., a blood cell for Doppler US, or a car for radar). As a consequence, the frequency of the reflected wave is shifted depending on the relative direction of motion and the velocity of the reflecting object. The US scanner detects this frequency shift and displays the information as a graph or as a color overlay on the gray-scale image. In oncologic imaging, Doppler US scans facilitate the detection and characterization of pathologies and provide information about their blood supply (Figure 13.1). Although used only in specialized circumstances, US contrast media, consisting of gas-filled microbubbles with a high degree of echogenicity, can be administered intravenously and enhance the echogenicity of tissues in which they accumulate (e.g., focal liver lesions).

The spatial resolution of an US image depends mainly on the frequency of the applied US waves; higher frequencies result in higher resolution. However, high-frequency US waves can only penetrate superficial structures. The deeper the organ of interest, the longer the required wavelength and the lower the spatial resolution. Only the superficial aspects of tissues with impedance substantially different from the impedance of their surrounds, such as bone or lung, can be visualized at US. The presence of overlying gas, such as in the gastrointestinal tract, or a large body habitus can also strongly impair the quality of an US examination. Endoscopic US, which is performed with an US transducer located at the tip of an endoscope, overcomes this limitation by allowing the transducer to be placed close to the region of interest. It is used for examining an inner body surface (e.g., the esophageal or rectal wall) or adjacent organs (e.g., the pancreas or perigastric lymph nodes).

Advantages of US: no ionizing radiation; inexpensive; readily available; portable.

Limitations: dependent on operator expertise; inability to penetrate through gas/air, extensive fat, or bone.

Nuclear and Molecular Imaging Techniques

Nuclear and molecular imaging techniques display the distribution of radiopharmaceuticals in the body. A radiopharmaceutical molecule consists of two parts: a radionuclide (i.e., a radioactive atomic nucleus) and a pharmaceutical compound. The biochemical nature of a pharmaceutical compound determines its uptake, distribution, and excretion in the body. The radionuclide is utilized for tracking and localizing the molecule, as the emitted radiation can be detected by radiosensitive imaging devices. Many tumors differ from healthy tissue in their molecular and/or metabolic properties. For example, relative to healthy tissues, most tumors demonstrate increased glucose metabolism, defined as the "Warburg" phenomenon. If glucose molecules are injected intravenously in a patient with cancer, a substantial portion of the molecules will be taken up and metabolized by tumor cells. By labeling glucose molecules with a radioactive substance prior to injection, one can observe their accumulation in tumor cells. This allows the detection and localization of many neoplastic lesions.

The following paragraphs discuss the three most widely-distributed nuclear and molecular imaging techniques used in oncology: bone scintigraphy, single-photon emission computed tomography (SPECT), and positron-emission tomography (PET). Other nuclear imaging techniques, such as thyroid scans, parathyroid scans, myocardial perfusion scans, pulmonary ventilation and perfusion scans, and hepatobiliary scans, are based on the same principle of radiopharmaceutical uptake assessment and are thoroughly described elsewhere [1].

Bone Scintigraphy (Bone Scan)

Bone scintigraphy, which can be used to detect and localize bone metastases, involves the use of the radiopharmaceutical ^{99m}m-technetium methylene diphosphonate (^{99m}Tc-MDP). After intravenous injection, ^{99m}Tc-MDP is distributed throughout the body and accumulates in structures and tissues based on their relative blood supply and the presence of bone production or repair. A few hours after receiving the injection, the patient is placed in front of a gamma camera that detects gamma rays emitted from the radionuclides. The acquired two-dimensional whole-body images and higher-resolution "spot views" of small portions of the body depict areas of uptake, including "hot spots" of relatively increased MDP uptake, and "cold" (photopenic) areas of relatively decreased uptake. MDP accumulation can also occur in non-neoplastic processes that induce high bone turnover (e.g., traumatic fractures and degenerative joint disease), resulting in false positive results.

Advantages of bone scintigraphy: provides whole-body images; relatively inexpensive.

Limitations: not sensitive to fast-growing lytic tumors; low specificity.

Single-Photon Emission Computed Tomography

In contrast to conventional scintigraphy, the gamma camera in single-photon emission computed tomography (SPECT) acquires not just one image from one angle, but multiple two-dimensional images from different angles. The acquired information is processed by a computer that performs a tomographic reconstruction, resulting in 3D information about the distribution of the radiopharmaceutical. The SPECT examinations most frequently performed in oncology are 3D bone scans.

SPECT/CT is a SPECT device with a built-in CT scanner, allowing simultaneous acquisition of functional information (from SPECT) and anatomical information (from CT).

Advantages of SPECT: can be used for whole-body imaging; provides 3D information.

Limitations: low temporal and spatial resolution; inability to quantify processes; few suitable radiopharmaceuticals currently available.

Positron Emission Tomography (PET) and PET/CT

PET relies on the injection of an agent labeled with an unstable, positron-emitting radionuclide (most commonly ^{18}F), whose atomic nucleus emits a positron that collides with its antiparticle, an electron. This results in an annihilation event, in which the masses of both particles are completely transformed into energy, according to the energy–mass equivalence rule. This energy is released in the form of two photons (high-energy gamma rays), which diverge from the point of annihilation in nearly perfectly opposite directions. The PET device contains a ring of gamma detectors that detect the emitted photons. If the positron decay has occurred in the center of the detector ring, both photons will be detected at the same time by two opposing detectors, as both photons travel at the same speed. Photons from eccentrically-located decays will still be detected by opposite detectors, but at slightly different time points, as one photon must travel further than the other. This time difference can be used to calculate the location of the decay.

The most widely used radiopharmaceutical in PET imaging is ^{18}F-fluoro-deoxyglucose (^{18}F-FDG). Similarly to unlabeled glucose, this molecule is taken up in relatively large concentrations by many malignant tumors (the Warburg phenomenon). In contrast to normal glucose, ^{18}F-FDG does not undergo glycolysis but remains trapped in the cell cytoplasm; it therefore accumulates in cells that have intense glucose metabolism (e.g., brain, heart muscle, and malignant cells) (Figure 13.2). Unlike normal glucose, ^{18}F-FDG does not undergo tubular reabsorption after primary glomerular filtration. It is thus rapidly excreted by the kidneys, and a high concentration of ^{18}F-FDG appears physiologically in the urinary tract (Figure 13.2).

PET provides metabolic information but is hindered by relatively low spatial resolution, providing only coarse anatomical detail. The accuracy of PET is increased by the use of scanners that coregister PET with anatomical CT images (or, only recently, with MRI). PET/CT scanners combine the functional and metabolic information obtained from PET with the detailed cross-sectional anatomy captured by CT in the same examination (Figure 13.2). Quantification of the relative accumulation of FDG in a volume of tissue (which can expressed through metrics such as the standardized uptake value [SUV]) allows some functional characterization of tissue (benign versus malignant solid tissue, such as in a solitary pulmonary nodule), assessment of tumor metabolism, evaluation of response to treatment, and detection of recurrent tumor.

Advantages of PET/CT: provides fused anatomic and metabolic information; allows whole-body scanning.

Limitations: limited availability; expensive; complex; ionizing radiation emitted by both the PET and CT components.

Imaging in Different Clinical Settings

Screening

The prognosis and appropriate treatment of cancer in a specific patient typically are related to the tumor stage at initial diagnosis. An underlying premise in screening is that early detection of cancerous tissue before the patient is symptomatic, and before the tumor has spread beyond its site of origin, can lead to a better patient outcome. However, the benefits of radiological screening examinations are required to outweigh any potential harm to the patient (e.g., from ionizing radiation, and harm from overdiagnosis and overtreatment). An in-depth discussion of screening in oncology can be found in Chapter 11.

Diagnosis and Staging

General

Patients are referred to a radiology department for various reasons, such as the need to investigate a suspicious finding further, or to undergo staging after initial diagnosis of a neoplasm. The referring physician and the radiologist are responsible for selecting the most appropriate imaging modality for initial staging, which depends on the tumor type and organ to be examined. In patients with contraindications to certain modalities (e.g., some cardiac pacemakers in patients for MRI), switching to another imaging modality might be necessary.

The extent of required preoperative staging is usually laid out in guidelines from organizations such the National Comprehensive Cancer Network for the United States. The workup depends on both tumor type and stage, which can influence the choice of modality, the exact parameters for the examination, and the anatomical region(s) that need(s) to be imaged. Specific recommendations for imaging of various tumor types can be found in other chapters in this book.

Radiology also plays an important role in the initial differential diagnosis of a suspicious lesion when its histology is still unknown. Though some lesions can be clearly identified and characterized by imaging only, others may need to be evaluated using US-, CT- or MRI-guided biopsy.

Communication between radiologists and referring physicians is of critical importance throughout the disease course for a given patient. This includes both the provision of the relevant medical history by the referring physician as well as a written report by the radiologist that includes all relevant findings and their interpretation in the context of clinical issues related to the specific type of cancer.

Local Staging

The components of local staging of a primary tumor depend on tumor type and location. For most tumors, the size of the primary tumor (which is often important for determining T stage in the TNM classification) is measured. The exact position of the primary tumor relative to nearby vessels (including anatomical variants of those vessels) or other structures needs to be assessed, as does the presence or lack of infiltration of adjacent organs (Figures 13.1 and 13.2). In certain tumors that are treated surgically, this evaluation is of critical importance to determine the optimal surgical approach, as some findings might indicate the need for neoadjuvant treatment (e.g., radio-chemotherapy) and follow-up re-staging before attempted resection. Regional lymphatic nodes are evaluated for signs of metastatic involvement, as such involvement may change the therapeutic approach considerably. The most common signs of metastatic nodal involvement include enlargement (e.g., short-axis diameter >1.0 cm), contrast enhancement and central necrosis on any imaging modality; however, the specificity of most imaging techniques for this purpose is low, as normal-sized nodes may harbor small metastatic deposits, and enlarged nodes may be inflammatory or reactive yet not contain tumor (Figure 13.2).

Distant Metastasis

Due to its ability to quickly scan large portions of the body and its wide availability, CT is the imaging modality most commonly used to search for distant metastases. However, depending on the location of the suspected lesions, other imaging modalities might be preferable. For example, in the search for brain metastases, contrast-enhanced MRI has superior sensitivity compared to contrast-enhanced CT. This is especially true in the detection of small, asymptomatic metastases (which might change the therapeutic approach) and leptomeningeal involvement. Consequently, MRI of the brain is part of the basic diagnostic workup in patients with lung cancer, even if no neurological symptoms are apparent, and in any patient with suspicious neurological symptoms. However, if MRI is not available or is contraindicated, contrast-enhanced CT is a viable alternative.

The detection of lung metastases is best performed with CT, as it provides the highest spatial resolution. A commonly encountered dilemma is the differential diagnosis of small pulmonary nodules. About half of all smokers are found to have small pulmonary nodules on CT [2], and such nodules are found in cancer patients as well. Their distinction from lung metastasis can be especially challenging in the absence of signs of benignity, such as central calcification (although calcifications also can occur in lung metastases of some tumors, such as osteosarcoma) or intralesional fat (diagnostic of hamartoma). The etiology of such a nodule can sometimes only be determined by biopsy or serial follow-up imaging.

As the liver is one of the organs with the highest incidence of metastases, the accurate evaluation of suspicious hepatic lesions is of great importance. MRI provides the highest sensitivity, specificity, and accuracy in the detection and classification of liver metastases – especially if an organ-specific contrast agent is used. In that case, the accuracy of MRI in the liver even supersedes that of CT or PET [3]. Additionally, MRI helps differentiate benign lesions (such as cysts or hemangiomas) from malignant lesions. US can be used to characterize a hepatic lesion as solid or cystic. Although US does not require the use of ionizing radiation, its accuracy is highly dependent on operator experience.

CT is used to detect and evaluate lymph nodes for possible involvement by tumor. MRI, including DWI, is an alternate modality for assessing lymph nodes. Newer MRI contrast agents containing ultra-small superparamagnetic iron oxide particles have achieved good results in differentiating benign from malignant lymph nodes in several studies, but the agents are currently not available in the United States for routine clinical use. PET/CT also can be used to evaluate lymph nodes.

Bone scintigraphy has been the standard procedure in the detection of bone metastasis for many years. Radiography and CT can also demonstrate bone metastases if they produce lytic or (reactive) blastic changes in the bone; marrow metastases are rarely evident with these modalities, however. More recently, MRI has proven to be more sensitive and specific in the detection of bone metastasis, as it directly demonstrates tumor deposits replacing normal marrow. The development of more rapid, whole-body MRI protocols for evaluation of the bone marrow has made MRI an attractive alternative modality.

Assessment of Response to Therapy

For many years, changes in the products of bidimensional measurements of individual tumor deposits served as a surrogate for tumor response to therapy (WHO criteria [4]). In 2000, the *Response Evaluation Criteria In Solid Tumors* (RECIST [5]) were published, followed by an updated version, RECIST 1.1., in 2009 [6]. RECIST is now used more widely in clinical trials than any other set of response criteria. RECIST calls for target lesions to be defined and measured on the baseline scan; the measurements are then compared to those from subsequent follow-up scans. The longest diameters of all target lesions (up to five lesions per patient in RECIST 1.1, with a maximum of two per organ) are summed and compared to the smallest sum in the study as a reference. The change in the target lesions during therapy is then characterized as stable disease (SD), partial response (PR, $\geq$30% decrease in the sum of target lesions), complete response (CR) or progressive disease (PD, $\geq$20% increase in the sum of diameters, or any new metastasis identified on follow-up scans). Although RECIST requires only unidimensional measurement of lesions, its accuracy for treatment response assessment has not been proven to be inferior to that of bidimensional criteria (such as the WHO criteria).

Although RECIST has been found to reliably characterize a patient's response to treatment in many solid tumors, certain limitations have been identified. Most notably, the effect of some chemotherapeutic agents (especially molecularly-targeted therapies) does not necessarily result in a change in tumor size. Additionally, it can be challenging to differentiate residual tumor from fibrosis in patients treated with radiotherapy.

To overcome these and other limitations, various other criteria systems have been developed, based on tumor-specific and treatment-specific issues. Some examples include the Cheson criteria for lymphoma, Choi criteria for gastrointestinal stromal tumor [7], EASL/mRECIST for hepatocellular carcinoma [8], and RECICL for ablative therapies of liver tumors [9]. Also, several other imaging techniques are currently being investigated to supplement conventional, morphological imaging data with quantitative functional information that characterizes the local microenvironment. For example, PET/CT can assess the magnitude of change in SUV; diffusion-weighted MRI can measure the change in tumor cellularity; MR spectroscopy can directly evaluate the concentration of certain metabolites that correlate with tumor growth or necrosis; and dynamic contrast-enhanced MRI can quantify a tumor's microcirculation and therapy-induced change. Additionally, these techniques can be used to differentiate between scar tissue and viable tumor – a distinction that is often difficult to make using conventional imaging alone.

Assessing the success or failure of newer interventional ablative therapies, such as radiofrequency ablation, cryoablation, or laser ablation, requires the use of different response assessment criteria. Whereas the usual goal of medical therapies for cancer is to shrink or, ideally, eliminate a tumor, the goal of ablative therapies is to destroy the tumor deposit as well as a rim of surrounding normal tissue. Thus, the size of the ablation zone at postprocedure imaging should be at least 1 cm larger than the tumor ablated.

Follow-up

Follow-up imaging examinations are usually performed at specified intervals (e.g., between cycles of chemotherapy, or after neoadjuvant chemotherapy but before surgical resection) to estimate the effect of treatment, or after completion of curative treatment to evaluate for local recurrence or new distant metastasis. These examinations need to be compared to prior exams to assess for change in the size or number of lesions, as well as for the development of tumor necrosis. Typically, the same imaging modality is used for each follow-up study to facilitate such comparison. Additionally, the use of consistent imaging protocols at follow-up is preferred, as changes in contrast rate or contrast phase can significantly change the apparent size of a lesion.

To aid the comparison of metastasis across different examinations at different time points, software solutions have been developed that automatically assess lesions (e.g., by automatically registering the images of two studies and providing volumetric measurements of tumor deposits).

In general, the time interval between follow-up assessments is specified in local or national guidelines and is also modified based on the biologic aggressiveness of the tumor in a given patient. The interval between two follow-up examinations might be changed for a clinical indication as well, such as if a patient reports new symptoms and the possibility of a new metastasis or treatment-related toxicity needs to be evaluated. It is also important to remember that patients with cancer are susceptible to the full range of noncancerous conditions experienced by all people, so that all new findings should not reflexively be assumed to represent cancer.

Radiation Protection

Several medical imaging techniques are based on the application of ionizing radiation (e.g., X-rays in radiographs and CT, or gamma-rays in PET). Ionizing radiation is characterized by its ability to liberate electrons from an atom or molecule, thereby 'ion-izing' it and altering its chemical properties. This results in the separation of chemical bonds within biological molecules, which in turn can cause damage to biological systems.

Radiobiology, which investigates the effects of radiation on living things, differentiates between *deterministic* and *stochastic* effects of ionizing radiation. Deterministic effects (from the Latin *determinare*, meaning "to predefine") are dose-dependent and predictable. They reliably occur above a threshold dose, and their severity depends on the applied dose. Acute radiation syndrome is an example of a deterministic radiation effect. It occurs within 24 h of exposure to a very high dose of ionizing radiation and is caused by damage to cell membranes and molecular structures. Depending on the dose, this syndrome consists of cutaneous ('radiation burn') and gastrointestinal symptoms (e.g., vomiting), blood disorders (e.g., low blood cell counts, bleeding), or neurological effects. It should be noted that doses high enough to have deterministic effects are not encountered in oncologic imaging, where low doses and low dose rates are typically utilized.

Stochastic effects (from the Ancient Greek στοχαστικός meaning "presumably"), on the other hand, occur with a certain degree of probability. The probability of a stochastic effect increases with the applied dose, but the severity of the effect is independent of the dose. Radiation-induced cancer and teratogenesis (i.e., abnormal physiological development) are the most serious examples of stochastic effects of ionizing radiation. Quantitative data on stochastic effects of ionizing radiation on human health is limited, as its collection requires large-scale epidemiological studies that allow mathematical compensation for multiple confounding factors such as smoking, environment, lifestyle, etc. [10–12]. The relevance of *in vitro* and animal studies is limited by the varying degrees of radiation resistance among species. The most solid data available on this issue, which has derived from Japanese atomic bomb survivors, showed that the lifetime risk for cancer begins to increase with a dose of 150 milliSievert (mSv) or more [13]. The doses applied in medical imaging depend on the specific imaging parameters used as well as patient size; they can range from 0.02 mSv for a chest X-ray, to approximately 12 mSv for a CT angiogram of the heart, and potentially up to about 25 mSv for a CT of the chest, abdomen, and pelvis. As a basis for comparison, individuals in the United States are exposed to an average of about 6 mSv per year from natural background radiation [14]. Recent, large, population-based studies appear to show an increased risk of cancer in patients who underwent CT during childhood or adolescence [15, 16]. Other studies found no association between fetal exposure to ionizing radiation (CT or radionuclide imaging) and the risk of childhood cancer [17]. Such mixed results are to be expected at the low radiation doses utilized for imaging. Indeed, acute doses less than 150 mSv may be too small to allow epidemiological detection of excess cancers given the background of naturally occurring cancers; it is also possible that the mechanisms of action for many biological effects of radiation exposure at low doses may differ from those occurring at higher doses [18]. The establishment and use of risk coefficients to estimate public health determinants from individual or population exposures must be considered in the context of various epidemiological and methodological uncertainties: uncertainties caused by the low statistical power and precision of studies of radiation risk; uncertainties in modeling radiation risk data and generalizing risk estimates across different populations and dose rates; and uncertainties caused by the reliance on observational rather than experimental data [19]. While recognizing these uncertainties, proper *justification* of radiation use as well as *optimization* of radiation protection must be performed for the prudent protection of both patients and staff [20].

The primary aim of radiation protection is to provide an appropriate standard of protection for people and the environment without unduly limiting the beneficial practices that require radiation exposure. Medical imaging radiation sources are used deliberately to provide diagnostic information for the care of patients and are designed to be used in a controlled manner. Under the principle of justification, medical imaging is only prescribed or performed when it will result in more good than harm – that is, when the diagnostic information provides a benefit that exceeds the potential risks. Several professional societies have developed referral guidelines and appropriateness criteria to assist in the justification step (e.g. American College of Radiology [21]; or European Commission [22]). For patients with cancer, the benefits of appropriately justified procedures far outweigh the low individual risks. When a justified imaging examination is ordered, it must be carried out using dose reduction and optimization techniques that ensure the dose used is as low as reasonably achievable (ALARA) while allowing sufficient imaging quality to provide the needed diagnostic information. Medical physicists and other imaging professionals can provide valuable assistance in this process.

References

1 Giussani A. *Imaging in Nuclear Medicine*. New York: Springer, 2013.

2 MacMahon H, Austin JH, Gamsu G, *et al.* Guidelines for management of small pulmonary nodules detected on CT scans: a statement from the Fleischner Society. *Radiology* 2005;237(2):395–400.

3 Hammerstingl R, Huppertz A, Breuer J, *et al.* Diagnostic efficacy of gadoxetic acid (Primovist)-enhanced MRI and spiral CT for a therapeutic strategy: comparison with intraoperative and histopathologic findings in focal liver lesions. *Eur Radiol* 2008;18(3):457–67.

4 Miller AB, Hoogstraten B, Staquet M, Winkler A. Reporting results of cancer treatment. *Cancer* 1981;47(1):207–14.

5 Therasse P, Arbuck SG, Eisenhauer EA, *et al.* New guidelines to evaluate the response to treatment in solid tumors. European Organization for Research and Treatment of Cancer, National Cancer Institute of the United States, National Cancer Institute of Canada. *J Natl Cancer Inst* 2000;92(3):205–16.

6 Eisenhauer EA, Therasse P, Bogaerts J, *et al.* New response evaluation criteria in solid tumours: revised RECIST guideline (version 1.1). *Eur J Cancer* 2009;45(2):228–47.

7 Choi H, Charnsangavej C, Faria SC, *et al.* Correlation of computed tomography and positron emission tomography in patients with metastatic gastrointestinal stromal tumor treated at a single institution with imatinib mesylate: proposal of new computed tomography response criteria. *J Clin Oncol* 2007;25(13):1753–9.

8 Bruix J, Sherman M, Llovet JM, *et al.* Clinical management of hepatocellular carcinoma. Conclusions of the Barcelona-2000 EASL conference. European Association for the Study of the Liver. *J Hepatol* 2001;35(3):421–30.

9 Kudo M, Kubo S, Takayasu K, *et al.* Response Evaluation Criteria in Cancer of the Liver (RECICL) proposed by the Liver Cancer Study Group of Japan (2009 Revised Version). *Hepatol Res* 2010;40(7):686–92.

10 National Research Council (U.S.). Committee to Assess Health Risks from Exposure to Low Level of Ionizing Radiation. *Health risks from exposure to low levels of ionizing radiation: BEIR VII Phase 2*. Washington, D.C.: National Academies Press, 2006.

11 United Nations. Scientific Committee on the Effects of Atomic Radiation. Sources and effects of ionizing radiation: United Nations Scientific Committee on the Effects of Atomic Radiation: UNSCEAR 2006 report to the General Assembly, with scientific annexes. New York: United Nations, 2008.

12 Valentin J. Low-dose extrapolation of radiation-related cancer risk. *Ann ICRP* 2005;35(4):1–140.

13 Preston DL, Ron E, Tokuoka S, *et al.* Solid cancer incidence in atomic bomb survivors: 1958–1998. *Radiat Res* 2007;168(1):1–64.

14 Schauer DA, Linton OW. NCRP Report No. 160, Ionizing radiation exposure of the population of the United States, medical exposure – are we doing less with more, and is there a role for health physicists? *Health Phys* 2009;97(1):1–5.

15 Miglioretti DL, Johnson E, Williams A, *et al.* The use of computed tomography in pediatrics and the associated radiation exposure and estimated cancer risk. JAMA Pediat 2013:1–8.

16 Mathews JD, Forsythe AV, Brady Z, *et al.* Cancer risk in 680 000 people exposed to computed tomography scans in childhood or adolescence: data linkage study of 11 million Australians. *BMJ* 2013;346:f2360.

17 Ray JG, Schull MJ, Urquia ML, *et al.* Major radiodiagnostic imaging in pregnancy and the risk of childhood malignancy: a population-based cohort study in Ontario. *PLoS Med* 2010;7(9):e1000337.

18 Dauer LT, Brooks AL, Hoel DG, *et al.* Review and evaluation of updated research on the health effects associated with low-dose ionising radiation. *Radiat Prot Dosimetry* 2010; 140(2):103–36.

19 NCRP. NCRP Report No. 164 – Uncertainties in Internal Radiation Dose Assessment National Council on Radiation Protection and Measurements, 2009.

20 ICRP Publication 105. Radiation protection in medicine. *Ann ICRP* 2007;37(6):1–63.

21 ACR. ACR Appropriateness Criteria®, 2016 Release. Available from: http://www.acr.org/Quality-Safety/Appropriateness-Criteria (accessed 28 May 2017).

22 Environment ECD-Gft. Referral guidelines for imaging. European Commission; 2000, Available from: https://health.gov.mt/en/forms/Documents/radiation_protection.pdf (accessed 28 May 2017).

14

The Pathologic Evaluation of Neoplastic Diseases

John D. Pfeifer[1] and Mark R. Wick[2]

[1] *Washington University Medical Center, St. Louis, Missouri, USA*
[2] *University of Virginia Health System, Charlottesville, Virginia, USA*

Introduction

Pathology is a dynamic facet of medical practice, in which specialists who are skilled at laboratory analysis actively contribute to the care of patients. Many areas of anatomic pathology and clinical pathology/laboratory medicine, including surgical pathology, cytopathology, hematopathology, blood banking, clinical chemistry, and microbiology, are regularly involved in the precise definition of disease and in the monitoring of therapeutic results. Even the autopsy can be included in this statement, because its aim is to serve as a "quality assurance" measure to be used in a prospective educational manner by clinicians.

The pathologist's understanding of oncologic disorders has progressed far beyond the recognition of abnormal tissues with the microscope, although that activity still retains paramount importance. Today, the laboratory specialist plays an integral role in eliminating incorrect differential diagnostic considerations, determining prognostic factors, evaluating treatment outcomes, and otherwise supporting the multidisciplinary care of oncology patients. Technologic advances have enlarged the scope of such activities significantly, but they must be utilized and integrated with other studies prudently, in the context of their strengths and weaknesses [1].

This chapter briefly summarizes the general activities of pathologists in this setting, and presents a practical introduction to the diverse analyses they perform that have an impact on patients with malignant neoplasms.

Interactions Between Clinicians and Pathologists

To utilize the services of pathologists optimally, clinicians must be familiar with the strengths and limitations of the technical procedures employed in the laboratory. Oncologists and surgeons are not merely consumers of pathologic data; rather, they should be interactive participants in the generation of such information. Much of what the anatomic pathologist is able to

say about any given case is dependent on receipt of pertinent clinical facts, prompt and proper submission of specimens, and physical adequacy of the tissue sample itself. A rapid and confident pathologic diagnosis is assured only when those factors receive proper attention.

It is wise, and advisable, for clinicians to consult with the pathology laboratory before scheduling selected invasive diagnostic procedures that will yield pathologic specimens. A discussion may then take place on the best means of obtaining the tissue, the possible need for intraoperative pathologic consultation, special processing requirements, and the role, if any, of adjunctive laboratory analyses in diagnosis and prognosis. For example, if lymphoma is suspected in a patient with lymphadenopathy, it is better to undertake an excisional lymph node biopsy instead of fine needle aspiration; conversely, the latter procedure usually yields adequate tissue in cases of probable metastatic carcinoma. In addition, karyotyping, selected genotypic analyses, biochemical assays, and certain immunohistochemical studies can be performed only on fresh tissue, and they are precluded if the specimen is placed in fixative solution before dispatch to the pathology laboratory.

Definitions of Tumor Types

Current tumor classification systems encompass a multitude of terms that are based on biologic behavior, cellular function, histology, embryonic origin, and anatomic location as well as eponyms (Table 14.1). Nomenclature is important because it is how pathologists communicate a diagnosis, and because specific tumor designations carry well-defined clinical implications.

Neoplasms (literally "new growths") may be benign or malignant. They consist of the proliferating tumor cells themselves and a supportive stroma containing connective tissue and blood vessels. An abundant stromal collagenous response to a neoplasm (most often to a malignant one) is called *desmoplasia*.

The most important features used to define a tumor as benign or malignant are the empirically known biologic behavior and

Table 14.1 Nomenclature pertaining to neoplastic diseases.

Origin of cell or tissue	Benign	Malignant
Tumors of epithelial origin		
Squamous cells	Squamous cell papilloma	Squamous cell carcinoma
Basal cells	–	Basal cell carcinoma
Glandular or ductal epithelium	Adenoma	Adenocarcinoma
	Cystadenoma	Cystadenocarcinoma
Transitional cells	Transitional cell papilloma	Transitional cell carcinoma
Bile duct epithelium	Bile duct adenoma	Cholangiocarcinoma
Liver cells	Hepatocellular adenoma	Hepatocellular carcinoma
Melanocytes	Nevus	Malignant melanoma
Renal epithelium	Renal tubular adenoma	Renal cell carcinoma
Skin adrenal glands		
Sweat glands	Sweat gland adenoma	Sweat gland carcinoma
Sebaceous glands	Sebaceous gland adenoma	Sebaceous gland carcinoma
Tumors of mesenchymal origin		
Hematopoietic–lymphoid tissue	–	Leukemias, lymphomas, Hodgkin's disease, multiple myeloma
Neural and retinal tissue		
Nerve sheath	Neurilemoma, neurofibroma	Malignant peripheral nerve sheath tumor
Nerve cells	Ganglioneuroma	Neuroblastoma
Retinal cells (cones)	–	Retinoblastoma
Connective tissue		
Fibrous tissue	Fibroma, fibromatosis	Fibrosarcoma
Fat	Lipoma	Liposarcoma
Bone	Osteoma	Osteogenic sarcoma
Cartilage	Chondroma	Chondrosarcoma
Muscle		
Smooth muscle	Leiomyoma	Leiomyosarcoma
Striated muscle	Rhabdomyoma	Rhabdomyosarcoma
Endothelium and related tissues		
Blood vessels	Hemangioma	Angiosarcoma, Kaposi's sarcoma
Lymph vessels	Lymphangioma	Lymphangiosarcoma
Synovium	–	Synovial sarcoma
Mesothelium	–	Malignant mesothelioma
Meninges	Meningioma	Malignant meningioma
Other origins		
Uncertain	–	Ewing sarcoma/peripheral neuroectodermal tumor
Renal analage	–	Wilm's tumor
Germ cells	Mature cystic teratoma (in women, dermoid cyst)	Seminoma (dysgerminoma), embryonal carcinoma, endodermal sinus tumor
Trophoblast	Hydatideiform mole	Choriocarcinoma

Source: adapted from Lieberman MW, Lebovite RM, Neoplasia. In: I Damjanov, J Linder (eds), Anderson's Pathology, 10th edn. St Louis: Mosby, 1996:517.
Note: This list is not exhaustive but is intended to provide an introduction to tumor nomenclature.

the microscopic appearance. Generally, benign neoplasms are innocuous and slow-growing, while malignant lesions often exhibit more rapid proliferation, invade adjacent tissues, and metastasize. Benign neoplasms usually have a bland microscopic appearance, while malignant neoplasms often manifest mitotic activity, abnormal nuclear chromatin, cellular pleomorphism, and areas of necrosis. However, exceptions to these generalizations abound. Benign neoplasms can kill the patient if inopportunely located (e.g., an ependymoma blocking the aqueduct of Sylvius, or uterine intravascular leiomyomatosis eventually obstructing the right heart), and some can metastasize (e.g., benign giant cell tumor of bone). Malignant neoplasms, on the other hand, may have a bland, mature cellular microscopic appearance, as seen in small lymphocytic lymphoma.

Malignant neoplasms of epithelial origin are called *carcinomas*. For example, if predominantly glandular or ductal, they are termed *adenocarcinomas*; if derived from a stratified squamous epithelium, *squamous cell carcinomas*. Neoplasms originating in a specific organ may be named accordingly; thus, hepatocellular carcinoma or adrenocortical carcinoma. Malignant neoplasms of mesenchymal origin are designated *sarcomas* (if differentiating toward fat cells, *liposarcoma*; toward fibrous tissue, *fibrosarcoma*; smooth muscle, *leiomyosarcoma*; blood vessels, *angiosarcoma*; and so on). Malignant tumors do not necessarily have benign counterparts, and the converse also applies.

Modifying adjectives used in diagnosis often reflect prognostic information, as in "poorly differentiated adenocarcinoma". Neoplasms with biologically ambiguous names are referred to with a precise modifier, e.g., malignant versus benign schwannoma. Nonspecific anatomic names generally should be avoided; as an illustration of this point, "bronchogenic carcinoma" is vague and could refer to squamous cell carcinoma, adenocarcinoma, small-cell neuroendocrine carcinoma, or other tumor types.

Neoplasms of the hematopoietic system usually have no benign analogues. Consequently, the terms leukemia and lymphoma, together with appropriate adjectives (e.g., *chronic myelogenous leukemia; follicular lymphoma; mantle-zone lymphoma*), always refer to malignant proliferations. Similarly, *melanoma* is always used to describe a malignant melanocytic neoplasm.

Finally, time-honored but idiosyncratic eponyms remain in diagnostic usage. These are employed in reference to such neoplasms as Ewing sarcoma (primitive neuroectodermal tumor), Warthin tumor (a benign lesion of the salivary glands), and Brenner tumor (a neoplasm with both benign and malignant forms derived from the surface epithelium of the ovary).

Macroscopic Examination of Tissue Specimens

As a discipline, pathology had its beginnings in the postmortem gross (i.e., macroscopic) examination of diseased tissues. Even before the microscope had come into general use, several disorders were well recognized at a macroscopic level, including malignant melanoma and various carcinomas. In the current rush to introduce new and ever-more molecular techniques to diagnostic medicine, it is tempting to forget that the trained observer's eyes and tactile senses are crucial to good surgical and pathologic practice.

The pathologist grossly examines all resected tumors submitted to the laboratory with several objectives in mind. First, the presence of representative tissue is confirmed, and the suitability of the specimen for further study is judged. Second, margins of excision are labeled with indelible ink (which can be recognized microscopically) to retain the orientation of the specimen for subsequent histologic analysis (including assessment of the adequacy of surgical margins). Third, the specimen is opened and sectioned by the pathologist, at which time notes are made on the consistency, color, and extent of the neoplastic growth. By integration of documented macroscopic characteristics with knowledge of the clinical findings, a differential diagnosis may be reached at this stage and appropriate samples taken to resolve it. For example, a soft tissue tumor of the retroperitoneum may have the gross appearance of a liposarcoma; however, to confirm that interpretation definitively, prosected tissues are placed in special fixative and examined later with the microscope and possibly other modalities of study. Not uncommonly, macroscopic features alone are sufficient to suggest a final diagnosis (Figure 14.1).

It is imperative that the pathologist examine the entire resected tumor before it is subdivided by the surgeon for other purposes (e.g., before a portion of a neoplasm is sent directly from the operating room to a research laboratory for investigational purposes). When careful inspection of the lesional borders is important, it is a disservice to patient care to violate the tissue margins before they can be adequately examined pathologically. For example, a malignant rather than a benign diagnosis is rendered in cases of follicular thyroid lesions if they penetrate the capsular boundaries; obviously, receipt of a "partial" specimen in the gross pathology laboratory after tissue had already been collected for tissue banking, special studies, or research could prevent proper examination of such a lesion.

Anatomic orientation of excised tissues should be a routine part of the information submitted to the pathology department. This allows for the precise localization of a tumor that is present at the margin of resection.

Histologic Study of Human Malignancies

In the hands of individuals who are well-trained in morphologic diagnosis, the light microscope continues to serve as the cornerstone of surgical pathology. With the proviso that the tissue processing requirements outlined above have been met, the simple use of the hematoxylin and eosin staining method on paraffinembedded tissue sections is sufficient to make the final diagnosis for the great majority (~90%) of malignant neoplasms. That is an important point to remember, because the added indiscriminate application of nonmorphological studies, as described subsequently, would be completely unnecessary and potentially confounding in such cases. It should be noted, however, that certain clinical procedures (e.g., vigorous compression of tissue specimens during endoscopic biopsy or extensive use of electrical or thermal cautery during resection) have the potential to interfere with diagnosis because they markedly compromise microscopic anatomy.

(a)

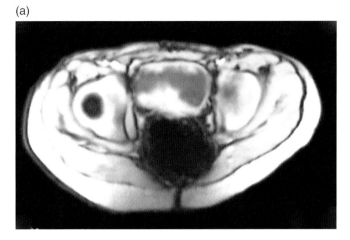

(b)

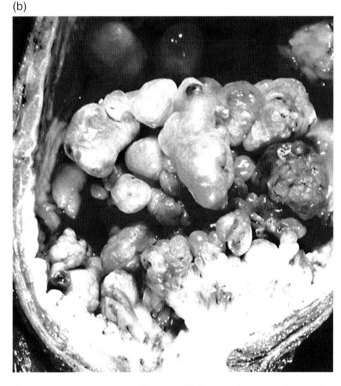

Figure 14.1 Imaging studies of a child with hematuria show an intravesical mass (a). The resected tumor manifests a multiply polypoid "grape cluster"-like appearance (b), which is contextually diagnostic of botryoid embryonal rhabdomyosarcoma.

For the morphologic features of a tissue to be optimally visualized by routine light microscopy, the specimen must undergo proper preparation and processing [2]. First, a minimum period of fixation in formalin (or an alternative mordant) is required; after fixation, the pathologist completes the gross examination of the specimen and excises the slices of the tissue which will be subjected to further processing to produce the stained sections on glass slides that are required for histopathologic diagnosis. Routine processing of tissue in practice, therefore, requires at least an overnight time interval. If special studies are warranted for diagnosis (such as routine immunohistochemistry, flow cytometry, or *in situ* hybridization), additional time is obviously needed for them.

Once stained microscopic slides have been obtained, the pathologist employs knowledge of histology and cytology to recognize changes that are related to neoplasia and other diseases. Tissue growth patterns, the degree of cellular differentiation, and details relating to prognosis, such as adequacy of surgical excision, are assessed. Ideally, a firm diagnosis of cancer would always be possible by brief examination of routinely processed tissue on glass slides. Unfortunately, that is an unrealistic expectation, and sometimes there is no substitute for experience, painstaking analysis, and consultation among laboratory physicians on a difficult case.

There are several potential reasons for diagnostic uncertainty in the morphological interpretation of biopsy or resection specimens. An important example relates to the natural history of any given pathologic process. A biopsy may be obtained at a time when a neoplastic lesion is not fully developed and therefore lacks dispositive histologic features [3]. In addition, treatments such as irradiation or chemotherapy often alter the pathologic characteristics of the tissue [4, 5]. Other lesions that cause a great deal of consternation are the so-called "borderline" or "minimal deviation" malignancies. These proliferations, which can be epithelial, mesenchymal, or melanocytic in nature, are characterized by microscopic features which differ only modestly from those of benign neoplasms or reactive processes [6].

In the course of arriving at a diagnosis, the pathologist will often discuss pertinent findings with the responsible clinician. Ultimately, a written report is issued for all specimens. Documentation is made of the tumor type (and grade, if applicable), as well as information that can be used by oncologists to assign a stage to the lesion in cases of malignancies [7]. Pathologists may be familiar with the biologic attributes of some tumors that even experienced oncologists have not encountered. Under those circumstances, a comment may be included in the tissue report regarding the expected behavior of the lesion, together with pertinent literature citations and recommendations for therapy.

Staging and Grading

Determination of tumor stage and grade not only offers important prognostic information but also allows for comparison of therapeutic results using various cooperative and research treatment protocols. Tumor grading is based primarily on the degree of differentiation of the malignant cells (including morphology of individual cells, and arrangement or architecture of cells forming the neoplasms) and secondarily through estimation of the rate of growth as indicated by the mitotic rate (Figures 14.2 and 14.3). Because the correlation between histologic appearance and biologic behavior is imperfect, grading criteria vary greatly for different neoplasms. Nonetheless, all grading criteria attempt to describe the extent to which the tumor cells resemble their normal tissue counterparts. Accurate grading is complicated by variations in differentiation from area to area in large tumors, as well as by site-related considerations and changes in tumor biology with time.

Tumor stage is based on the size of the primary lesion and the presence of lymph nodal or hematogenous metastasis. The major staging systems in use are the TNM classification

(a)

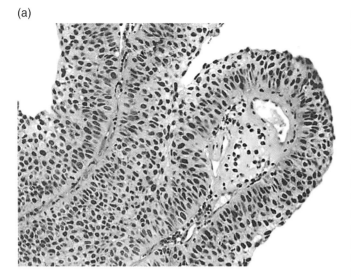

(b)

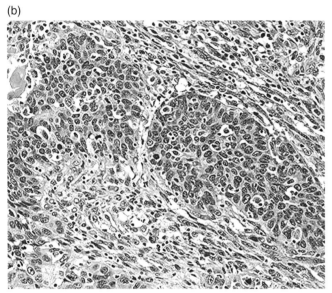

Figure 14.2 Well-differentiated papillary noninvasive urothelial carcinoma shows minimal morphological differences from hyperplastic, non-neoplastic urothelium (a). Poorly differentiated urothelial carcinoma with sarcomatoid (spindle-cell) features has little microscopic resemblance to normal urothelium (b).

(for primary *T*umor size, presence and extent of lymph *N*ode involvement, and distant *M*etastasis) and the AJCC (American Joint Committee on Cancer) system, which divides tumors into stages 0 to IV [8].

Frozen Section Examination

Surgeons regularly request that pathologists perform an intraoperative consultation of a tissue specimen, which can involve gross examination only, cytopathologic evaluation, or microscopic examination. The term "frozen section" (FS) is synonymous with an intraoperative microscopic consultation. A sample of fresh tissue obtained during a surgical procedure is rapidly frozen by the pathologist. Histologic sections are then prepared using a cryostat (refrigerated microtome), fixed briefly, stained with hematoxylin and eosin, and examined microscopically. The entire procedure, including thorough histologic study, usually can be accomplished within 15 min. Proper interpretation requires a complete gross examination of the tissue prior to sectioning, and a well-trained pathologist with experience. Informative, interactive communication with the surgeon and an adequate clinical history are also essential.

As with all diagnostic procedures, FS consultation has specific indications. In general, these include the identification of a particular tissue for the surgeon, demonstration of the presence and nature of a pathologic lesion, definition of the adequacy of surgical margins or the extent of disease, and a determination that the excised material is sufficient for diagnosis. Frozen sections should *not* be used merely to satisfy the curiosity of the surgeon, or to compensate for inadequate preoperative evaluation of the patient. Similarly, FS is not as accurate as formal pathologic interpretation of fixed tissue, and therefore FS should not be regarded merely as a rapid means for communicating a diagnosis to the patient and his or her family members.

Although histopathologic interpretation of cryostat sections is technically limited and more difficult than diagnosis using fixed paraffin-embedded tissues, frozen sections are well-regarded as a useful means of intraoperative consultation. The accuracy of FS diagnosis is commonly reported to be 94–98%, but these figures vary depending on the tissue type and the clinical reason for consultation [9, 10]. For example, if the clinical differential diagnosis is that of lymphoma versus a reactive lymphoproliferative lesion, FS is often incapable of making that distinction. Similarly, the evaluation of large thyroid or thymic tumors for capsular invasion, or of *in situ* intraductal mammary proliferations, is not recommended by FS because of inherent contextual errors attached to the process in these settings.

It should be obvious that FS diagnoses often have a significant influence on the nature and extent of the surgical procedure being performed. Hence, they must be utilized prudently by both surgeons and pathologists alike.

Cytopathology

Cytopathology is the science and practice of morphologic examination of individual cells and small groups of cells for the purpose of diagnosis. Suitable specimens are collected in one of three basic ways: exfoliation from an epithelial surface (e.g., cervical smears obtained with a spatula or brush; bronchial washings or brushings [Figure 14.4]); aspiration of fluid from body cavities (e.g., cerebrospinal fluid obtained by lumbar puncture, ascites sampled by paracentesis); and fine needle aspiration of "solid" lesions of the breast, thyroid, salivary glands, lung, and other organs (Figure 14.5). The cytologic preparation is then spread on a glass slide, fixed, and stained by a variety of methods. In most instances, the Papanicolaou or DiffQuik stains yield the greatest clarity of nuclear detail. Special investigations also may be carried out on cytologic specimens (e.g., immunocytochemistry, static cytometry, and

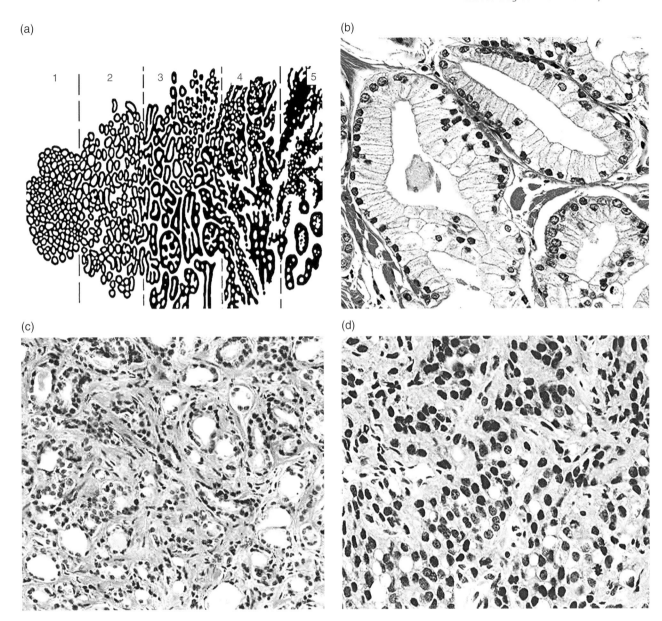

Figure 14.3 Gleason scoring of prostatic carcinoma is done by observing the range of microscopic growth patterns in the tumor, which are segregated into five groups (a). The first and second most dominant patterns are summed to yield the Gleason "score" (e.g., 3 + 4, 4 + 5, etc.). Gleason pattern 1 and 2 tumors are well differentiated (b); pattern 3 lesions are moderately differentiated (c); and pattern 4 and 5 neoplasms are poorly differentiated (d).

molecular genetic testing), but these must be anticipated before sample procurement because special provisions for such analyses may be needed.

Although generalizations are difficult, the cytomorphologic evaluation of a possible malignancy is predicated on specific features of the cytoplasm and nucleus in the lesional cells. Malignant cells show consistent aberrations in nuclear structure including dyskaryosis (coarse or dense granularity, hyperchromasia, abnormally large nucleoli) and anisonucleosis (marked variation in nuclear shape and size); mitotic abnormalities may also be present (Figure 14.6). Anisocytosis, or pronounced variation in cellular size or shape, is seen in malignancies as well. The volumetric nuclear-to-cytoplasmic ratio is increased; most malignant cells have an oversized

nucleus that displaces all but a small peripheral zone of cytoplasm. Intercellular cohesion is likewise abnormal; however, carcinomas do retain enough cell-to-cell adhesion to make their cytologic attributes dissimilar to those of lymphomas and other mesenchymal neoplasms. Because reactive and reparative cellular changes (due to inflammation, infection, irradiation, or cytotoxic chemotherapy) can easily be confused with malignant proliferations, a complete clinical history is essential for accurate cytopathological diagnosis.

Cytology has a high degree of reliability when morphologic interpretations are performed by experienced, well-trained individuals [11, 12]. Nonetheless, one should always consider the value of confirming the diagnosis by conventional biopsy, if possible, prior to definitive treatment.

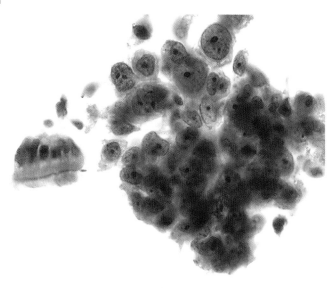

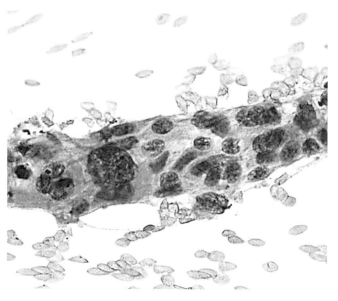

Figure 14.4 This bronchial brushing cytology specimen shows a cluster of highly atypical epithelioid cells that are three-dimensional and show prominent nucleoli. The image is that of adenocarcinoma. A fragment of non-neoplastic bronchial epithelium is seen for comparison at the far left of the photograph.

Figure 14.6 A broad range of nuclear sizes, shapes, and densities is represented in this fine needle aspiration specimen from an adenosquamous carcinoma of the lung.

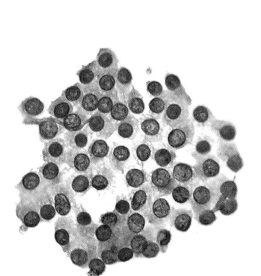

Figure 14.5 Fine-needle aspiration of a thyroid mass yielded this specimen, in which cohesive, cytologically monotonous cells are present with nuclear grooves. The image is diagnostic of papillary thyroid carcinoma.

Special Slide-Based Procedures

In approximately 10% of all oncology cases, routinely assessed microscopic features of neoplasms may be insufficiently conclusive for a firm and final diagnosis. For example, amelanotic malignant melanomas, large-cell non-Hodgkin lymphomas, and anaplastic carcinomas can be maddeningly similar histologically, often mandating the use of immunohistochemical studies to distinguish them from one another (Figure 14.7). Similarly, spindle-cell sarcomas of soft tissue can resemble one

another so markedly that adjuvant analyses may be necessary for a final diagnosis (Figure 14.8). Of course, such evaluations require additional time for implementation and interpretation. These techniques merit further discussion, because they are used commonly and provide extremely useful information.

Immunohistochemistry

Practical immunohistochemistry is currently based on an indirect, antibody-enzyme method known in common parlance as the "immunoperoxidase" procedure. In this technique, frozen or rehydrated deparaffinized tissue sections, or cytologic smears, are overlaid with a specific, well characterized primary antibody directed at an antigen of diagnostic value. After controlled incubation and subsequent removal of the primary reagent, a second antibody with generic specificity for the first is exposed to the tissue sections. The latter antibody may be labeled with biotin, providing a "bridge" for the subsequent binding of an avidin-biotin horseradish peroxidase complex that completes the immunochemical assembly. The peroxidase enzyme can then be used to catalyze an oxidation-reduction reaction in the presence of a dye that is precipitated at the site of antibody binding. After a counterstaining procedure designed to highlight morphologic details, the presence of the antigen of interest can be visualized at a light microscopic level within the tissue section (Figure 14.9) [13–15].

With few exceptions, these antigenic determinants are not absolutely tissue or tumor specific. Therefore, the pathologist must employ panels of primary antibodies in the study of malignant tumors, building an antigenic "fingerprint" that eventually allows for a final interpretation. A sampling of commonly assessed antigens is listed in Table 14.2. Based on the relative tissue specificities of these antigens, algorithms can be constructed that enable the resolution of differential diagnostic problems with histologically similar neoplasms [16].

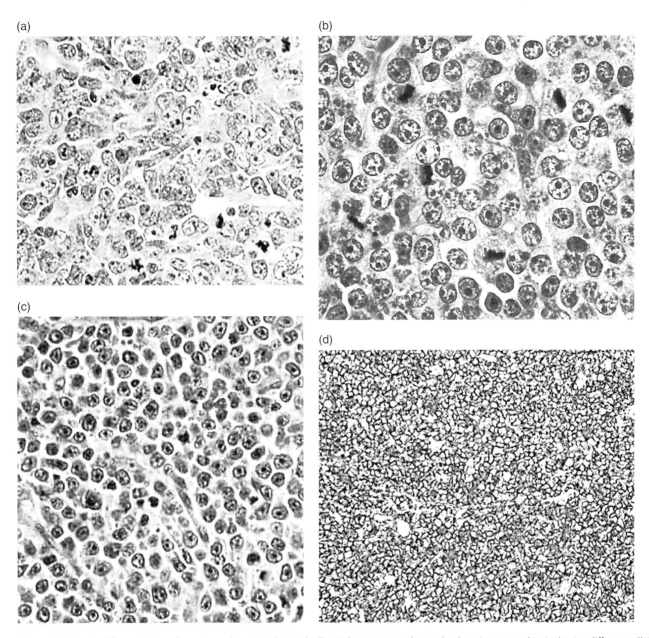

Figure 14.7 Poorly differentiated malignant neoplasms can be markedly similar to one another under the microscope, despite having different cellular lineages. As examples, poorly differentiated sinonasal carcinoma (a), amelanotic sinonasal melanoma (b), and sinonasal large-cell non-Hodgkin lymphoma (c) are shown here, the histologic images of which are mutually superimposable. Special studies are necessary to separate them diagnostically; for example, an immunostain for CD45 (leukocyte common antigen) is shown in (d) in large-cell lymphoma

Some immunohistochemical assays also are obtained to aid with prognosis and treatment. As an example, immunohisto-chemical detection of overexpressed Her-2 oncoprotein (or *HER2* gene amplification, detected by *in situ* hybridization, as described below) in breast cancer cells is associated with a response to trastuzumab and related drugs [17]. Other studies have concluded that immunohistochemical markers of cell pro-liferation (e.g., MIB-1) may also represent potential prognostic tools [18].

It must be emphasized that immunohistochemistry is clearly incapable of distinguishing benign from malignant tumors. Its purpose is principally to distinguish between microscopic "look-alikes" that have differing prognoses or which require

dissimilar treatments. Another use for antibody-enzyme stain-ing methods is the localization of clinically important tumor markers within tissue sections, as discussed below.

In situ Hybridization

Two advances have allowed for a wide application of *in situ* hybridization (ISH) technology to diagnostic pathology, specifi-cally, the labeling of DNA probes by nonradioactive methods, and the development of techniques that permit the direct rec-ognition of endogenous nucleic acids in paraffinembedded tis-sue sections or cytological smears. The use of ISH has several diagnostic advantages. Small tissue fragments and archival

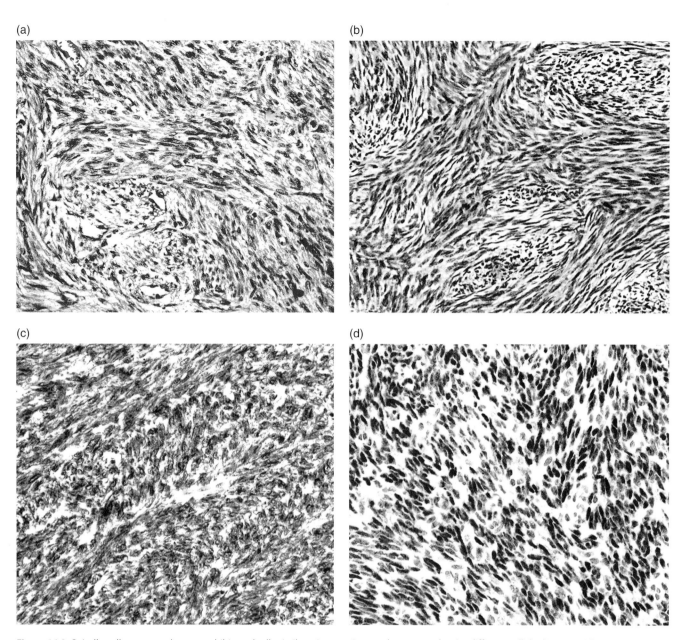

Figure 14.8 Spindle-cell sarcomas also may exhibit markedly similar microscopic growth patterns, despite different cellular lineages. A leiomyosarcoma is shown in (a), and a monophasic synovial sarcoma is depicted in (b). Their histological appearances are virtually identical. However, immunostains for desmin (a myogenic marker) are positive in leiomyosarcoma (c) and others for transducin-like enhancer protein of split 1 (TLE1) are reactive in monophasic synovial sarcoma (d). Those findings are mutually exclusive.

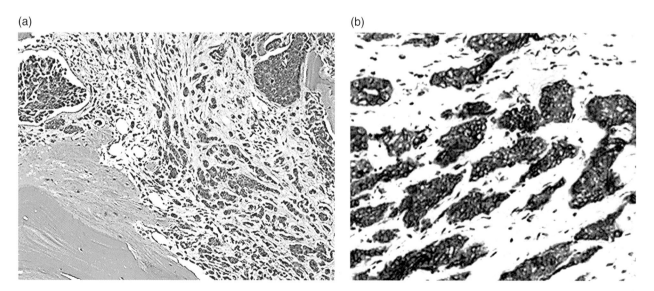

Figure 14.9 Metastatic carcinoma is present in this bone biopsy (a); the patient previously had no history of malignancy, and, therefore, the source of the tumor was unknown. Immunostaining for prostate-specific antigen (b) establishes the identity of the lesion as metastatic prostatic adenocarcinoma.

Table 14.2 Selected antigenic moieties of diagnostic value in practical immunohistochemistry.

Antigen	Predominant distribution	Common diagnostic uses
Cytokeratin	Epithelial cells	Distinction of carcinoma from lymphoma or melanoma
Cytokeratin isoforms	Epithelial cells	Determination of primary site of metastatic carcinoma (pattern of expression of various isoforms is related to site of origin)
Epithelial membrane antigen	Epithelial cells	Distinction of carcinoma from melanoma
Leukocyte common antigen	Leukocytes	Distinction of lymphoma from carcinoma or melanoma
Desmin	Myogenous cells	Identification of smooth muscle or skeletal muscle tumors
Muscle specific actin	Myogenous cells	Identification of smooth muscle or skeletal muscle tumors
Prostate specific antigen	Prostatic epithelium	Identification of metastatic prostatic carcinoma
Calcitonin	Parafollicular thyroid epithelium	Distinction of medullary thyroid carcinoma from other thyroid tumors
Carcinoembryonic antigen	Endodermally derived epithelium	Identification of gastrointestinal and lung adenocarcinomas; distinction of adenocarcinomas from mesothelioma
Placental alkaline phosphatase	Placental tissue and germ cell tumors	Identification of possible germ cell and trophoblastic tumors
Alpha-fetoprotein	Neoplastic hepatocytes and selected germ cell tumors	Identification of hepatocelluar carcinoma, endodermal sinus tumor, and other germ cell tumors
β-Human chorionic gonadotropin	Placental tissue; trophoblastic and germ cell tumors	Identification of trophoblastic differentiation in germ cell tumors
CA-125	Müllerian epithelium	Identification of possible female genital tract carcinomas
CA-19-9	Alimentary tract epithelium	Identification of possible gastrointestinal and pancreatic carcinomas
Gross cystic disease fluid protein 15	Mamary epithelium and apocrine glands	Identification of metastatic breast carcinoma
Estrogen receptor and progesterone receptor	Mammary epithelium	Identification of metastatic breast carcinoma; prediction of clinical response to homornal therapy in breast carcinoma
HMB-45	Melanocytic cells	Identification of melanoma
Chromogranin-A	Neuroendocrine cells	Identification of neuroendocrine carcinomas
Synaptophysin	Neuroendocrine cells	Identification of neuroendocrine carcinomas and neuroectodermal tumors
CD31	Vascular endothelium	Identification of vascular neoplasms
CD34	Vascular endothelium and some soft tissue tumors	Identification of vascular neoplasms, solitary fibrous tumors, dermatofibrosarcoma protuberans
ErbB-2 (gene product of *HER2/neu*)	Epithelium	Level of expression can provide prognostic information for breast carcinomas

material can be used with this method, and the reaction product is localized to specific cells (or even subcellular compartments), allowing for simultaneous evaluation of the histologic image and the ISH result [19–22].

For ISH, direct or indirect labeling of nucleic acid probes with fluorescent marker molecules (fluorescein), chromogenic enzymes (horseradish peroxidase or alkaline phosphatase) (Figure 14.10), or electron-opaque plastic spheres, is used to detect and localize target nucleic acid sequences [20, 21]. ISH has been confirmed as a useful procedure for the diagnosis of some neoplasms, and assessment of the likely response to specific treatments. One of the most significant advantages of chromosome ISH is its application to interphase cells, in which context it is referred to as interphase fluorescent *in situ*

hybridization (interphase FISH). Interphase FISH analysis is a straightforward and remarkably versatile technique that can be performed on sections of formalin-fixed paraffin-embedded (FFPE) tissue and cytology preparations. It has several major advantages over conventional cytogenetics in that it can be performed on nondividing cells; the technique thus facilitates detection of molecular abnormalities even in neoplasms with low proliferation rates. The fact that interphase FISH can be performed on tissue sections that preserve tumor architecture provides a major advantage in that it makes it possible to evaluate genotype-phenotype correlations of specific cells. In surgical pathology, the technique is used primarily to detect somatic cancer-associated alterations with known diagnostic, prognostic, or therapeutic implications.

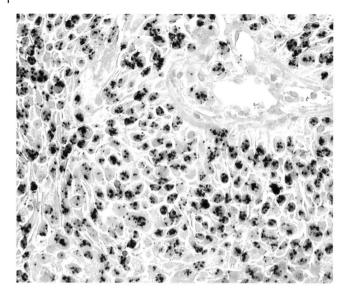

Figure 14.10 This uterine cervical squamous carcinoma has been studied by chromogenic *in situ* hybridization for human papillomavirus type 18. The tumor cells show a positive integration signal (blue) in virtually all the neoplastic cells.

Currently, the most versatile interphase FISH probes are gene-specific probes that target distinct chromosomal regions of interest. The testing is clinically useful when a particular cytogenetic alteration (deletion, gain, amplification, translocation) is a sensitive and specific marker for a single tumor type, either as a diagnostic biomarker (as in many hematopoietic malignancies) or as a prognostic biomarker helping to predict which tumors will be aggressive or indolent (*HER-2/neu* amplification testing in breast cancer). The use of interphase FISH to detect tumor-associated chromosomal translocations is par-

ticularly useful as an ancillary diagnostic aid in hematopoietic and soft tissue malignancies (Figure 14.11). Multiple unique sequence probes, each labeled with a different fluorophore, are often used in the same assay to permit more detailed analysis of genetic abnormalities.

Evaluation of Tumor Markers in Tissue and Biofluids

A "tumor marker" is a biochemical indicator of the presence of a neoplastic proliferation. In clinical usage, this term refers to a molecule that can be detected in serum, plasma, or other body fluids; in the setting of the pathologic evaluation of neoplasms, the term usually refers to molecules that can be detected in cytology specimens or tumor sections by immunohistochemistry. No tumor marker is specific; virtually all of them are present in the serum at low levels in the normal physiologic state or in non-neoplastic diseases, and any given marker may be seen in conjunction with a variety of neoplasms. Tumor markers can be divided into two broad categories: tumor-derived moieties and tumor-associated (or host-response) markers.

Tumor-derived markers include: oncofetal antigens (alpha-fetoprotein [AFP] and carcinoembryonic antigen [CEA]); hormones (human chorionic gonadotropin [hCG], human placental lactogen, antidiuretic hormone, parathyroid hormone, calcitonin, insulin-like growth factors, catecholamine metabolites); tissue-specific proteins (immunoglobulins, prostate-specific antigen [PSA], gross cystic disease fluid protein-15); enzymes (gamma-glutamyl transpeptidase); isoenzymes (prostatic acid phosphatase [PAP], placental alkaline phosphatase [PLAP], neuron-specific enolase [NSE]); oncogene products (*src, N-myc, H-ras*); various polyamines; sialic acid; and glycolipids.

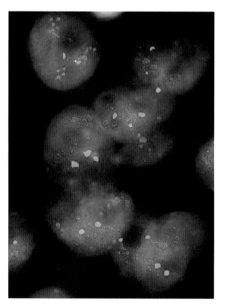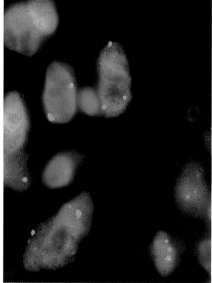

Figure 14.11 Examples of gene amplification detected by fluorescent *in situ* hybridization. Right panel: glioblastoma with epidermal growth factor receptor (EGFR) amplification in a so-called "double minute" pattern with small individual red signals (the green signal represents a centromeric probe for chromosome 7 while the red signal is the gene specific probe for EGFR). Left panel: invasive breast cancer with *HER-2/neu* amplification showing numerous red gene signals and considerably fewer green CEP17 signals (the green signal represents a centromeric probe for chromosome 17 while the red signal is the gene specific probe for Her2/neu; in this example, the *HER-2/neu* to CEP17 signal ratio is >2.0).

Figure 14.12 Example of the classification of a lymphoma by flow cytometry (see Table 14.3). (a) Section of spleen from a 61-year-old woman showing effacement of the parenchyma by large malignant lymphocytes. (b) Scattergram of the malignant infiltrate obtained by flow cytometry. Note the presence of two gated regions corresponding to small lymphoctyes and large lymphocytes (arbitrarily labeled *R1* and *R3*, respectively). The results of multiparametric analysis of the cells within region R3 when combined with the morphology of the tumor are diagnostic of large cell lymphoma, B cell type.

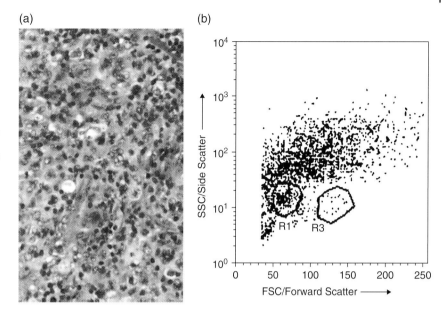

(a)

(b)

Tumor-associated (host-response) markers are most often used together with tumor-derived markers. For example, in concert with NSE levels, serum ferritin levels in neuroblastoma have been shown to correlate with stage of disease and response to therapy. Other host-response markers include interleukin-2, tumor necrosis factor, immune complexes, acute phase reactants (C-reactive protein, alpha 2-macroglobulin), and enzymes (lactic dehydrogenase, creatine kinase BB isoenzyme, glutamate dehydrogenase).

Flow Cytometry

Flow cytometry allows for the rapid quantitative measurement of cellular characteristics such as size, surface marker expression, and DNA content. Briefly, for flow cytometry, a monodispersed cell sample is stained with appropriate fluorochromes and passed through a flow chamber designed to align the stream of cells so that they are individually struck by a focused laser beam. The scattered light and fluorescent emissions are separated according to wavelength by appropriate filters and mirrors, and directed to detectors which convert the emissions into electronic signals that are analyzed and stored for future display by a computer. The data are displayed as a frequency histogram (number of cells versus fluorescent energy) for single-parameter analysis or as a scattergraph for multiparametric evaluation. The principle of "gating" (the placement of electronic windows around areas in the frequency distribution so that the computer analyzes data only on cells falling within the windows) can be used to take full advantage of multiparametric analysis [23].

The fluorochromes used to stain cells in flow cytometry include compounds that bind stoichiometrically to DNA, that label both DNA and RNA but fluoresce at different wavelengths for each, or that can be attached covalently to antibodies against cell surface antigens. Simultaneous multiparametric analysis is possible using two or more fluorochromes that emit at different wavelengths.

In vivo "single cell suspensions", such as peripheral blood or bone marrow, can be analyzed easily by flow cytometry. Solid tissues, including lymph nodes and solid tumors, require additional preparation (usually gentle enzymatic, detergent, or mechanical treatment) to achieve a monodispersed sample. Methods also have been developed for analysis of archival tissue that has been formalin fixed and embedded in paraffin [23].

Surface Marker Analysis

The role of cell surface antigen analysis in the diagnosis of lymphoid and other hematopoietic malignancies is well established. Multiparametric evaluation with a panel of monoclonal antibodies against surface antigens (Figure 14.12 and Table 14.3) facilitates classification of different subtypes of lymphoma and leukemia, and has become a routine facet of diagnosis.

DNA Measurements

Although many flow cytometric studies have examined DNA ploidy as a prognostic factor, several variables complicate its interpretation. For example, very few, if any, malignant tumors have a chromosomal complement that is normal in number and structure. "Diploid range" malignancies, therefore, actually represent a heterogeneous group of lesions with chromosomal abnormalities below the level of resolution of flow cytometry. Furthermore, some tissues, such as liver, normally contain tetraploid and even octaploid populations. It is therefore difficult to arrive at summary statements regarding the correlation of flow cytometric data with prognosis.

Cytogenetics

Specific chromosomal abnormalities are consistently associated with certain malignant neoplasms, and specific aberrations often have diagnostic and prognostic relevance [24, 25]. Although the application of molecular biology techniques to the detection of such aberrations has much greater sensitivity (see below), in many situations routine karyotypic analysis of a

Table 14.3 Example of the use of selected monoclonal antibodies for the classification of a lymphoma by flow cytometry.

Antibody (cluster designation)	Specificity	Percentage of positive cells in gated regions of Figure 14.12[1]	
		R1	R3
T cell markers			
CD3	Pan T cell	58	8
CD4	Helper-inducer T cell subset	26	7
CD8	Cytotoxic-suppressor T cell subset	26	7
B cell markers			
CD19	B cells	14	93
HLA-DR	B cells, activated T cells (major histocompatibility complex class II antigen)	62	100
Anti-IgM	B cell subset (immunoglobulin heavy chain isotype M)	2	38
Anti-lambda	B cell subset (lambda light chain)	13	68

[1] The staining pattern is diagnostic only for the region of the scattergram containing the large atypical lymphocytes (the gated region labeled *R3*). The cells in the R3 region stain positive for HLA-DR, CD19, and lambda immunoglobulin light chain, consistent with a monoclonal B cell population (see Figure 14.12).

tumor is still the best procedure available to probe chromosome structure. Specific abnormalities are best characterized in leukemias and lymphomas, although typical abnormalities have also been described in nonhematopoietic tumors. For example, it has become apparent that many malignant soft tissue tumors contain consistent chromosome aberrations (Table 14.4). The most common structural changes are balanced translocations, deletions, and gene amplifications.

The Philadelphia chromosome, present in most cases of chronic myeloid leukemia, is the classic example of a balanced translocation; because cases lacking the Ph chromosome have a less favorable prognosis, karyotypic analysis can provide clinically relevant information in chronic myeloproliferative disorders. The karyotypic manifestations of gene amplification include homogeneously staining regions of single chromosomes and "double minutes", which are small paired extrachromosomal chromatin fragments; the study of homogeneously staining regions and double minutes in neuroblastoma resulted in the demonstration of a strong correlation between stage, prognosis, and amplification of the *N-myc* oncogene.

Molecular Biologic Techniques

Molecular biologic techniques have become an integral part of the evaluation of many malignancies, facilitated in recent years with the development of high-throughput molecular technologies and global initiatives such as the human genome project. Molecular techniques used in diagnostic tumor biology are based on the fact that cancer is a genetically determined disease which occurs largely as a result of DNA mutations in oncogenes (overexpression), tumor suppressor genes (loss of function), and a wide variety of other genes involved in cell cycle control,

apoptosis, and intracellular metabolism. These mutations are either germline, somatic, or a combination of the two. Fresh or snap frozen tissue is preferred for the extraction of both RNA and DNA; however, in recent years the methodologies for extraction of nucleic acids from FFPE tissues have been greatly improved.

Molecular pathology allows for the establishment of a more definitive diagnosis and classification of neoplasms based on specific mutational profiles, provides prognostic information, and is used to direct therapy (increasingly through the demonstration of mutations that are the targets of specific drugs). However, it is important to recognize that, as with all other lab tests, the analytic sensitivity and specificity of molecular approaches is not perfect due to the intrinsic biologic variability of disease. Because only a subset of cases of a specific disease harbors the characteristic mutation, since more than one genetic abnormality can be associated with a specific tumor, since more than one tumor can share the same mutation, and so on, even a molecular test with perfect analytic performance will have a lower sensitivity and specificity when used for clinical analysis of patient samples.

From a practical standpoint, this lack of diagnostic specificity for many diseases and tumor types provides a cautionary note against attempts to interpret molecular test results in the absence of the clinical history and without knowledge of the histopathologic features of the case. The lack of diagnostic specificity also ensures that cases will arise in which there is a lack of concordance between the diagnosis suggested by the genetic findings and traditional histopathology [26]. The debate over the best approach to resolve the ambiguity presented by these cases reflects the fundamental impact of molecular genetics on the classification of disease as well as the power of morphology as the historical standard of pathologic diagnosis by which new methods of classification must

Table 14.4 Examples of chromosomal translocations in hematopoietic and soft tissue/bone tumors.

Tumor	Translocations	Involved genes
Chronic myeloid leukemia	t(9;22) (q34;9-11)	*ABL/BCR*
Burkitt lymphoma	t(8;14) (q24;q23)	*C-MYC/IgH*
Mantle cell lymphoma	t(11;14) (q13;q32)	*CCND1/IgH*
Follicular lymphoma	t(14;18) (q32;q21)	*IgH/BCL-2*
Alveolar rhabdomyosarcoma	t(2;13) (q35;q14)	*PAX3/FKHR*
	t(1;13) (p36;q14)	*PAX7/FKHR*
Ewing tumor/PNET	t(21;22) (q24;q12)	*EWSR1/FLI1*
	t(21;22) (q22;q12)	*EWSR1/ERG*
	t(7;22) (p22;q12)	*EWSR1/ETV1*
	t(17;22) (q12;q12)	*EWSR1/E1AF*
	t(2;22) (q33;q12)	*FEV/EWSR1*
Clear cell sarcoma	t(12;22) (p12;q12)	*ATF1/EWSR1*
Congenital fibrosarcoma and mesoblastic nephroma	t(12;15) (p13;q25)	*ETV6/NTRK3*
Extraskeletal myxoid chondrosarcoma	t(9;22) (q22;q12)	*EWSR1/TEC*
	t(9;17) (q22;q11)	*RBP56/TEC*
	t(9;15) (q22;q21)	*TEC/TCF12*
Myxoid liposarcoma	t(12;16) (q13;p11)	*TLS (FUS)/CHOP*
	t(12;22) (q13;q12)	*EWSR1/CHOP*
Desmoplastic round cell tumor	t(11;22) (p13;q12)	*WTI/EWSR1*
Synovial sarcoma	t(X;18) (p11;q11)	*SYT-SSX1*
		SYT-SSX2

be measured. In these cases with discordant molecular and histopathologic features, the most prudent approach is to acknowledge the presence of the discrepancy, and in consultation with the patient's treating physicians, reappraise all the clinical data, pathological findings, and therapeutic implications.

Microarray Analysis

Microarrays consist of an ordered arrangement of DNA molecules (known as features) linked to a solid matrix support. Because each DNA feature has been mapped to a specific region of the genome, measurement of the number of nucleic molecules in the test sample bound at each feature (usually achieved by labeling the test sample with a fluorophore, and then measuring the fluorescent signal for each feature) provides information on the presence, gain, or loss of the corresponding allele or chromosomal region. The resolution of microarray analysis is in theory limited only by the number of features in the array, and commercially available oligonucleotide arrays (utilizing probes that are 25–75 bp long) provide a high level of probe coverage

across the genome with a resolution of a few kilobases. Microarray testing can be performed on a variety of specimen types including peripheral blood lymphocytes, bone marrow, and FFPE tissue, and techniques have been developed for copy number analysis, gene expression analysis, DNA sequencing, and DNA methylation analysis [27, 28].

Copy Number Analysis

There are two general strategies for array-based measurement of copy number changes, namely comparative genomic hybridization (CGH) and single nucleotide polymorphism (SNP) analysis.

CGH can be used to survey the entire genome for chromosomal deletions and amplifications [29]. For a typical CGH test, genomic DNA from the tumor sample is labeled with a green fluorophore, and genomic DNA from a paired normal tissue sample is labeled with a red fluorophore. The green and red probes are mixed, and then used in a single hybridization; regions where the ratio deviates significantly from the expected one-to-one relationship are areas where there has been a change in DNA copy number in the tumor versus the paired normal tissue; regions where the green to red ratio is significantly greater than one are areas of chromosomal gain (amplifications), and regions where the green to red ratio is significantly lower than one are areas of chromosomal loss (deletions). The resolution of microarray-based CGH (aCGH) is in theory limited only by the number of features in the array, and often has a higher sensitivity than conventional cytogenetic analysis.

SNP analysis employs microarrays in which the features included on the array have been selected based on the frequency of the SNP within various populations (to provide epidemiologic information across ethnic groups), the SNP's association with specific diseases or phenotypes, and chromosomal location. SNP testing is performed by comparing signal intensities from the assay substrate (derived from the DNA of the patient sample) to that of a reference in order to determine relative gains and losses.

Gene Expression Analysis

An emerging area in the field of tumor markers and prognostication is transcriptional profiling via microarray analysis [30]. In this method, gene expression rather then DNA copy number is measured. Microarray analysis of mRNA and miRNA has many applications, but clinically most applications are focused on the level of mRNA abundance (which is generally related to the level of gene expression at the protein level).

RNA profiling can subclassify histologically indistinguishable tumors (including lymphomas, carcinomas, and sarcomas) into biologically relevant subtypes or subgroups with signatures that predict subsequent prognosis, both for specific tumor types and more globally [31, 32]. Several commercial assays are now available for analysis of clinical samples based on these observations. However, clinically predictive gene expression signatures are not always reproducible across multiple studies of the same tumor type [33], a result that is likely explained by the use of differing and nonstandardized microarray platforms, the examination of patient cohorts that are not matched for clinical and treatment parameters, and the relatively complex phenotype of survival which can be dependent upon many variables in addition to tumor molecular signatures.

Several studies have demonstrated that gene expression profiles can define the cell lineage of a tumor, including of metastases of unknown origin, and that this diagnosis is 80–90% accurate based upon thorough retrospective analysis of clinical data [34, 35].

Polymerase Chain Reaction

Polymerase chain reaction (PCR) is a very sensitive method for the detection of specific nucleic acid sequences based on the exponential *in vitro* amplification of a segment of DNA. The method requires a pair of oligonucleotide primers, usually about 20 nucleotides in length, that complement both ends of each strand of a target sequence. The target DNA must first be denatured by heating and the reaction mixture cooled to allow the complementary sequences of the primers to anneal to their target. Heat resistant Taq-DNA polymerase synthesizes new strands of DNA based on the nucleotide template between the primers. This cycle is then repeated, usually 20 to 30 times, resulting in exponential amplification of the target sequence. Thus, within a few hours, 10^8–10^9 copies of the target DNA sequence can easily be produced. PCR can be performed on virtually all types of pathological specimens including fresh tissue, FFPE tissue, cytological fluids, and laser microdissected sections [36].

PCR and its variants have many advantages. First, very few target cells are required, allowing for diagnostic use on limited biopsy or cytological samples. Second, while fresh tissue is the best source of DNA (and RNA), PCR can also be performed on FFPE tissues. Third, the technique is simple, quick, and inexpensive; most PCR amplifications can be performed in only a few hours. Fourth, the method has very high sensitivity and specificity; when optimized, PCR can detect one abnormal cell in a background of at least 10^5 normal cells [37], and can even be used to analyze single copy genes from individual cells [38]. Fifth, PCR makes phenotype–genotype correlations possible; as traditionally performed on a tissue fragment or tissue section, PCR provides only an indirect correlation of morphology and genetic abnormalities. However, more precise phenotypic–genotypic analysis is achieved by collecting individual cells by manual microdissection, laser capture microdissection, flow cytometry, or even immunomagnetic methods [39, 40].

However, PCR does have some limitations in routine use. Although the extreme sensitivity of PCR underlies its clinical utility, it also greatly increases the risk of erroneous test results due to cross-contamination of samples, especially contamination due to PCR product carryover [41]. In fact, PCR is so sensitive that it amplifies target DNA and RNA sequences from cellular debris as well as viable cells [42]; consequently, the significance of PCR-based detection of tumor derived nucleic acids in lymph nodes and peripheral blood can be uncertain.

The number of PCR applications in diagnostic contemporary surgical pathology is enormous and a comprehensive listing is beyond the scope of this chapter. However, some of its major uses include: identification of chromosomal translocations for diagnostic purposes and for the detection of minimal residual disease after treatment; detection of gene amplifications such as *HER2*, *N-myc*; identification of point mutations at any genetic locus including in oncogenes and tumor suppressor genes; and determination of lymphoma clonality via immunoglobulin and T-cell receptor gene rearrangements.

PCR Variants

Many variants of PCR have been developed to suit specific needs in the evaluation of neoplasms.

Multiplex PCR is a technique in which two or more different sets of primers are added to the same PCR mixture [43]; this allows for analysis of multiple DNA target sequences from one sample.

Reverse-transcriptase PCR (RT-PCR) is a modification based on the unique ability of a reverse transcriptase enzyme to make a DNA copy (cDNA) from a target mRNA molecule [44]. RT-PCR is especially useful for identification of fusion transcripts that are formed from translocations whose breakpoints are scattered over large regions of DNA; in these situations, although the DNA translocation products may vary, the chimeric RNA transcribed from the translocated chimeric gene remains constant from case to case (Figure 14.13).

Quantitative PCR (Q-PCR) is used to enumerate the number of molecules in the test sample that contained the target sequence. The technique employs real-time measurements of DNA accumulation (which is why the technique is sometimes referred to as real-time PCR) as the PCR progresses to provide a precise estimate of the initial concentration of the target sequence. Q-PCR can be applied to fresh as well as FFPE tissue, and phenotype–genotype correlations are possible through analysis of specific cell populations collected via microdissection, laser capture microdissection, and so on. Q-PCR can also be used to measure mRNA abundance via simple modifications of RT-PCR.

DNA Sequence Analysis

Many molecular tests performed to evaluate tumor specimens focus on somatic or acquired DNA alterations in the cells of the disease process. Because PCR-based approaches are quick, reliable, and sensitive, PCR has become a central technology for much of clinical DNA sequence analysis, via both direct and indirect approaches. The development of massively parallel, high throughput sequencing methods (collectively known as next generation sequencing methods) has had a profound impact on the breadth of testing that can be performed in routine clinical practice.

PCR-Based Sequence Analysis

Direct DNA sequencing by the dye terminator cycle sequencing method (so-called Sanger sequencing after the method's inventor) is currently used for most routine DNA sequence analyses performed to identify one (or at most several) mutations (Figure 14.14).

Indirect identification of normal and/or mutant alleles at a specific locus can substitute for direct determination of specific

Figure 14.13 Example of molecular genetic analysis of Ewing sarcoma/peripheral neuroectodermal tumor (ES/PNET) arising in the kidney of a 60-year-old woman. (a) Hematoxylin and eosin stained section of the tumor. (b) Reverse transcriptase polymerase chain reaction (RT-PCR) of formalin-fixed paraffin-embedded tissue demonstrates the presence of an *EWSR1-FLI1* gene fusion transcript that is characteristic of ES/PNET. Lane 1, molecular size markers; lane 2, positive control RT-PCR product from an ES/PNET cell line (*EWSR1* exon 7 to *FLI1* exon 5 fusion); lane 3, renal tumor (*EWSR1* exon 7 to *FLI1* exon 8 fusion); lane 4, negative control.

(a)

(b)

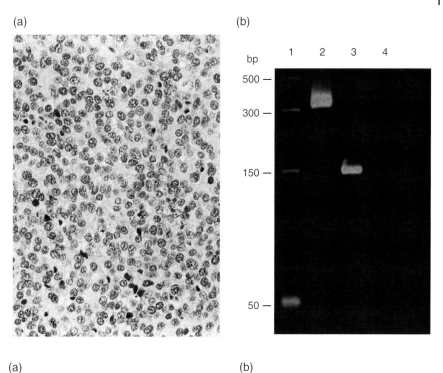

Figure 14.14 Example of the use of Sanger sequencing to characterize the genotype of a gastrointestinal stromal tumor (GIST). (a) Hematoxylin and eosin stained section of the tumor. (b) DNA was extracted from formalin-fixed paraffin embedded sections of the tumor, and direct DNA sequence analysis of the *KIT* gene was performed. The computer-generated base sequence (top) inferred from the automated sequencing electropherogram (bottom) is shown; comparison with the wild-type *KIT* sequence demonstrates a six base deletion that changes codons 552 through 554 but maintains the gene's open reading frame, a mutation characteristic of GIST.

(a)

(b)

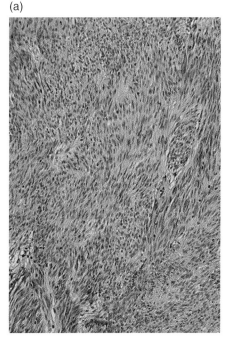

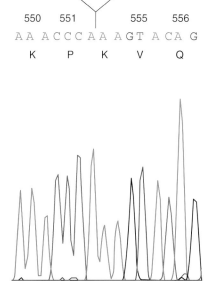

nucleotide sequences in many clinical settings. Virtually all of the indirect methods are PCR based and can be applied to a broad range of specimen types. Examples of indirect methods include the technique of allelic discrimination by size which is based on the fact that alleles that vary by small insertions or deletions can be distinguished based on the size of the PCR product after gel electrophoresis. Similarly, the technique of restriction fragment length polymorphism analysis is commonly used for the identification of base pair mutations which result in altered size fragments following treatment with specific restriction enzymes, hence the name restriction fragment length polymorphism analysis [45]; mutations that either create or destroy a restriction endonuclease site can easily be

distinguished by a two step process that involves DNA digestion with the restriction endonuclease followed by gel electrophoresis to size fractionate the digested DNA.

Next Generation Sequencing

The high throughput of massively parallel sequencing methods (also known as next generation sequencing methods, or simply NGS), coupled with their low cost and high accuracy, makes them well suited for analysis of cancer specimens in clinical settings where diagnosis or choice of therapy requires the information about the presence of mutations in several different areas of the same gene, and/or in several different genes [46]. The rapid, widespread adoption of NGS methods is because NGS can be used to comprehensively evaluate multiple genetic loci when only a limited quantity of DNA is available for testing; there is an increasing number of targeted therapies (which requires analysis of an ever-increasing number of genes), while ever smaller tissue specimens are available for testing (a result of current trends to shift from large excisional biopsies to needle or aspiration biopsies for diagnosis). NGS methods are well matched with the emerging paradigm of personalized medicine.

Identifying the landscape of mutations in a cancer specimen, rather than a single mutation, has several direct clinical applications. First, the pattern of mutations itself can be diagnostic in cases in which traditional histopathologic examination is not definitive [47]. Second, the mutations can predict the efficacy of a particular drug for that tumor (Figure 14.15), for example, alterations in exon 19 of *EGFR* in patients with nonsmall cell lung cancer who are responsive to treatment with gefitinib [48];

other somatic mutations predict resistance to therapy with tyrosine kinase inhibitors, such as *KRAS* mutations in lung cancer [49]. Third, mutations can provide prognostic information on the risk of disease progression or relapse. For example, an internal tandem duplication in the *FLT3* gene is associated with poor prognosis in acute myeloid leukemia while mutations in nucleophosmin (*NPM1*) are associated with a favorable prognosis [50].

Input DNA used in clinical NGS testing can be derived from a variety of patient sample sources including peripheral blood, bone marrow aspirate specimens, buccal swabs, surgical resections, needle biopsies, and fine needle aspirations; cell free DNA (cfDNA, especially circulating tumor DNA) is an emerging test substrate [51]. For solid tumors the most frequently available specimen type is FFPE tumor tissue, and it is reassuring that FFPE specimens as well as fresh tumor samples are both amenable to NGS analysis.

(a)

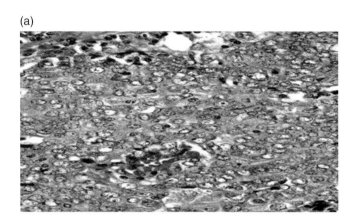

(b)

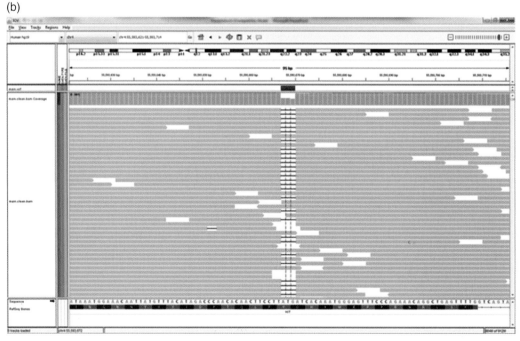

Figure 14.15 Example of the use of DNA sequence analysis of a panel of 50 genes by next generation sequencing to identify unexpected sequence changes that suggest the use of a targeted therapy. The thymic carcinoma in this patient (a) was no longer responsive to standard therapies; next generation sequence testing identified a 3 bp deletion of KIT resulting in p.D579del (b), a deletion known to be responsive to tyrosine kinase inhibitor therapy with imatinib in other tumor types. The patient was treated with imatinib as part of a clinical trial, with a resulting decrease in tumor size that lasted over 2 years.

The computerized algorithms used to evaluate the massive data sets generated by NGS tests, to identify differences between the tumor's sequence and a reference sample, are referred to as bioinformatics pipelines. Given the intrinsic genomic instability of malignancies and their often complicated intratumoral heterogeneity, maximum clinical utility of NGS of cancer specimens can only be achieved using a bioinformatics pipeline designed to detect the different types of sequence changes (single nucleotide variants, small insertions and deletions, copy number variants, and structural variants) at allele frequencies that are physiologically relevant. Sensitive and specific identification of the four main classes of variants requires an optimized assay design and computational approach for each [52, 53].

An increasing number of resources are being created to support the task of sequence variant identification, and equally importantly, the process of variant annotation [54]. Variant annotation is the description of the relationships between identified variants and clinical phenotypes such as disease diagnosis (i.e., tumor type), response to specific drug treatments, clinical trials focused on that variant–disease association, and so on. Annotation of variants is important because even with NGS tests optimized for clinically relevant sensitivity and specificity, the majority of variants identified currently fall into the category of variants of unknown significance.

NGS assays that target a panel of genes (from several genes, to several hundred genes), the exome, or the entire genome have been developed. However, as with all lab tests, the utility of the various assays is extremely dependent on the clinical setting.

Targeted Gene Panels

Panels for acquired mutations in cancer specimens focus on genes that are considered clinically actionable in that there is well-established literature providing evidence for their diagnostic, predictive, and/or prognostic value. The panels may be quite narrow (e.g., only a few dozen genes) based on the specific cancer being evaluated such as colon adenocarcinoma, lung adenocarcinoma, or gastrointestinal stromal tumor, or much broader (e.g., hundreds of genes) based on recurrently mutated genes across multiple cancer types [55–57]. In general, since clinical utility has been defined for only a few thousand different mutations in a few hundred genes, sequence analysis in routine clinical practice focuses on panels of genes with well documented roles in diagnosis, prognosis, or prediction of response to therapy.

Exomes and Whole Genomes

Exome and genome sequencing are often applied to the study of cancer as a discovery tool in the investigative setting. Exome or genome sequencing is helpful for detection of copy number variations and is especially well-suited to detection of structural variants, which often involve noncoding DNA breakpoints.

Summary

This overview has briefly covered a number of conventional and recent techniques available to the pathologist for use in the evaluation of neoplastic diseases. Knowledge of the potential uses and abuses of these procedures is important to the clinician and helps ensure that patient care is not hindered through the omission or misapplication of pertinent studies. We cannot stress too greatly the cooperation required between pathologist and oncologist in the diagnosis of cancer and management of oncology patients.

References

1 Marchevsky AM, Wick MR. Evidence-based medicine, medical decision analysis, and pathology. *Hum Pathol* 2004;35:1179–88.

2 Wick MR, Mills NC, Brix WK. Tissue procurement, processing, and staining techniques. In: MR Wick (ed.) *Diagnostic Histochemistry*. Cambridge: Cambridge University Press, 2008:1–27.

3 Ackerman AB, Ragaz A. *Lives of Lesions*. New York: Lea & Febiger, 1984.

4 Petraki CD, Sfikas CP. Histopathological changes induced by therapies in the benign prostate and prostate adenocarcinoma. *Histol Histopathol* 2007;22:107–18.

5 Helpap B, Koch V. Histological and immunohistochemical findings of prostatic carcinoma after external or interstitial radiotherapy. *J Cancer Res Clin Oncol* 1991;117:608–14.

6 Henson DE, Albores-Saavedra J. *Pathology of Incipient Neoplasia*, 3rd edn. Oxford: Oxford University Press, 2001.

7 Valenstein PN. Formatting pathology reports: applying four design principles to improve communication and patient safety. *Arch Pathol Lab Med* 2008;132:84–94.

8 Edge S, Byrd DR, Compton CC, *et al.* (eds) *AJCC Cancer Staging Manual*, 7th edn. New York: Springer, 2011.

9 da Silva RD, Souto LR, Matsushita Gde M, Matsushita Mode M. Diagnostic accuracy of frozen section tests for surgical diseases. *Rev Col Bras Cir* 2011;38:149–54.

10 Winther C, Graem N. Accuracy of frozen section diagnosis: a retrospective analysis of 4785 cases. *APMIS* 2011;119:259–62.

11 Adams J, Wu HH. The utility of fine-needle aspiration in the diagnosis of primary and metastatic tumors to the lung: a retrospective examination of 1,032 cases. *Acta Cytol* 2012;56:590–5.

12 Factor R, Layfield LJ. Intraprocedural evaluation of fine-needle aspiration smears: how good are we? *Diagn Cytopathol* 2012;40:760–3.

13 Miller RT, Swanson PE, Wick MR. Fixation and epitope retrieval in diagnostic immunohistochemistry: a concise review with practical considerations. *Appl Immunohistochem Mol Morphol* 2000;8:228–35.

14 Taylor CR, Levenson RM. Quantification of immunohistochemistry – issues concerning methods, utility and semiquantitative assessment II. *Histopathology* 2006;49:411–24.

15 Kalyuzhny AE. *Immunohistochemistry: Essential Elements and Beyond*. New York: Springer, 2015.

16 Wick MR. Immunohistochemical approaches to the diagnosis of undifferentiated malignant tumors. *Ann Diagn Pathol* 2008;12:72–84.

17 Sauter G, Lee J, Bartlett JM, *et al.* Guidelines for human epidermal growth factor receptor-2 testing: biologic and methodologic considerations. *J Clin Oncol* 2009;27:1323–33.

18 Li LT, Jiang G, Chen Q, *et al.* Ki67 is a promising molecular garget in the diagnosis of cancer. *Mol Med Reports* 2015;11:1566–72.

19 Moelans CB, de Weger RA, Van der Wall E, van Diest PJ. Current technologies for HER2 testing in breast cancer. *Crit Rev Oncol Hematol* 2011;80:380–92.

20 Gruver AM, Peerwani Z, Tubbs RR. Out of the darkness and into the light: bright field in situ hybridisation for delineation of ERBB2 (HER2) status in breast carcinoma. *J Clin Pathol* 2010;63:210–19.

21 Lambros MB, Natrajan R, Reis-Filho JS. Chromogenic and fluorescent in situ hybridization in breast cancer. *Hum Pathol* 2007;38:1105–22.

22 Reis-Filho JS, de Landér Schmitt FC. Fluorescence in situ hybridization, comparative genomic hybridization, and other molecular biology techniques in the analysis of effusions. *Diagn Cytopathol* 2005;33:294–9.

23 Koss LG, Czerniak B, Herz F, Wersto RP. Flow cytometric measurements of DNA and other cell components in human tumors: a critical appraisal. *Hum Pathol* 1989;20:528–48.

24 Gersen SL, Keagle MB (eds) *The Principles of Clinical Cytogenetics*, 3rd edn. New York: Springer, 2013.

25 Rooney D (ed.) *Human Cytogenetics: Malignancy and Acquired Abnormalities*, 3rd edn. Oxford: Oxford University Press, 2001.

26 Hill DA, O'Sullivan MJ, Zhu X, *et al.* Practical application of molecular genetic testing as an aid to the surgical pathologic diagnosis of sarcomas: a prospective study. *Am J Surg Pathol* 2002;26:965–77.

27 Bertucci F, Viens P, Tagett R, *et al.* DNA arrays in clinical oncology: promises and challenges. *Lab Invest* 2003; 83:305–16.

28 Ahrendt SA, Halachmi S, Chow JT, *et al.* Rapid p53 sequence analysis in primary lung cancer using an oligonucleotide probe array. *Proc Natl Acad Sci USA* 1999;96:7382–7.

29 Pinkel D, Albertson DG. Comparative genomic hybridization. *Annu Rev Genomics Hum Genet* 2005;6:331–54.

30 Quackenbush J. Microarray analysis and tumor classification. *N Engl J Med* 2006;354:2463–72.

31 Beane J, Spira A, Lenburg ME. Clinical impact of high-throughput gene expression studies in lung cancer. *J Thorac Oncol* 2009;4:109–118.

32 Lu J, Getz G, Miska EA, *et al.* MicroRNA expression profiles classify human cancers. *Nature* 2005;435:834–8.

33 Reid JF, Lusa L, De Cecco L, *et al.* Limits of predictive models using microarray data for breast cancer clinical treatment outcome. *J Natl Cancer Inst* 2005;97:927–30.

34 Ojala KA, Kilpinen SK, Kallioniemi OP. Classification of unknown primary tumors with a data-driven method based on a large microarray reference database. *Genome Med* 2011;3:63.

35 Xu Q, Chen J, Ni S, *et al.* Pan-cancer transcriptome analysis reveals a gene expression signature for the identification of tumor tissue origin. *Mod Pathol* 2016;29:546–56.

36 Liu H, Huang X, Zhang Y, *et al.* Archival fixed histologic and cytological specimens including stained and unstained materials are amenable to RT-PCR. *Diagn Mol Pathol* 2002;11:222–7.

37 Kohler S, Galili N, Sklar JL, *et al.* Expression of bcr-abl fusion transcripts following bone marrow transplantation for Philadelphia chromosome-positive leukemia. *Leukemia* 1990;4:541–7.

38 Hahn S, Zhong XY, Holzgreve W. Single cell PCR in laser capture microscopy. *Methods Enzymol* 2002;356:295–301.

39 Persson A, Backvall H, Ponten F, *et al.* Single cell gene mutation analysis using laser-assisted microdissection of tissue sections. *Methods Enzymol* 2002;356:334–43.

40 Yaremko ML, Kelemen PR, Kutza C, *et al.* Immunomagnetic separation can enrich fixed solid tumors for epithelial cells. *Am J Pathol* 1996;148:95–104.

41 Kwok S, Higuchi R. Avoiding false positives with PCR. *Nature* 1989;339:237–8.

42 Yamamoto N, Kato Y, Yanagisawa A, *et al.* Predictive value of genetic diagnosis for cancer micrometastasis: histologic and experimental appraisal. *Cancer* 1997;80:1393–8.

43 Edwards MC, Gibbs RA. Multiplex PCR: advantages, development and applications. *PCR Methods Appl* 1994;3:S65–S75.

44 Salomon RN. Introduction to reverse transcriptase polymerase chain reaction. *Diag Mol Pathol* 1995;4:2–3.

45 Blomek B, Shields PG. Laboratory methods for the determination of genetic polymorphisms in humans. *IARC Sci Publ* 1999;148:133–47.

46 Kulkarni S, Pfeifer JD (eds) *Clinical Genomics: A Practical Guide to Clinical Next Generation Sequencing.* Amsterdam: Elsevier, 2015.

47 Sehn JK, Hagemann IS, Pfeifer JD, *et al.* Diagnostic utility of targeted next-generation sequencing in problematic cases. *Am J Surg Pathol* 2014;38:534–41.

48 Lynch TJ, Bell DW, Sordella R, *et al.* Activating mutations in the epidermal growth factor receptor underlying responsiveness of non-small-cell lung cancer to gefitinib. *New Engl J Med* 2014;350:2129–39.

49 Campos-Parra AD, Zuloaga C, Manriquez ME *et al.* KRAS Mutation as the biomarker of response to chemotherapy and EGFR-TKIs in patients with advanced non-small cell lung cancer: clues for its potential use in second-line therapy decision making. *Am J Clin Oncol* 2015;38:33–40.

50 Estey EH. Acute myeloid leukemia: update on risk-stratification and management. *Am J Hematol* 2013;88:318–27.

51 Elahimali YI, Khaddour H, Sarkissyan M, *et al.* The clinical utilization of circulating cell free DNA (CCFDNA) in blood of cancer patients. *Int J Mol Sci* 2013;14:18925–58.

52 Duncavage EJ, Abel HJ, Szankasi P, *et al.* Targeted next generation sequencing of clinically significant gene mutations and translocations in leukemia. *Mod Pathol* 2012;25:795–804.

53 O'Rawe J, Jiang T, Sun G, *et al.* Low concordance of multiple variant-calling pipelines: practical implications for exome and genome sequencing. *Genome Med* 2013;5:28.

54 http://www.ncbi.nlm.nih.gov/clinvar/docs/datasources/ (accessed 30 May 2017).

55 Cottrell CE, Al-Kateb H, Bredemeyer AJ, *et al*. Validation of a next-generation sequencing assay for clinical molecular oncology. *J Mol Diagn* 2014;16:89–105.

56 Pritchard CC, Salipante SJ, Koehler K, *et al*. Validation and implementation of targeted capture and sequencing for the detection of actionable mutation, copy number variation, and gene rearrangement in clinical cancer specimens. *J Mol Diagn* 2014;16:56–67.

57 http://foundationone.com/learn.php - 2 (accessed 30 May 2017).

15

Cancer Staging

Frederick L. Greene[1] and Lauren A. Kosinski[2]

[1] *UNC School of Medicine, Chapel Hill, North Carolina, USA*
[2] *The Seed House, Chestertown, Maryland, USA*

Introduction

The concept of cancer staging is inherently important to all who practice clinical medicine. Staging provides a framework for discussion with our patients and with each other. It is designed to stratify patients into groups that have similar outcomes. To achieve this, a common nomenclature and rules that are valid for solid tumors at all cancer sites has been created. This process will be discussed later in the chapter.

Since the mid-1980s, the Tumor (T), Node (N) and Metastasis (M) system has been considered the worldwide strategy for the staging of adult solid malignancy [1, 2]. The categorization of tumor features and identification of prognostic groupings is vital for planning clinical trials to assess treatment strategies whether they are surgical, pharmacologic, or radiation based. In addition, staging enables meaningful comparison of outcomes across large and diverse populations. Without a staging system, the stratification of most solid tumors would be garbled, and the difficulties making rational treatment recommendations would only be amplified in the increasingly complex domain of multimodal therapy. The creation of a uniform staging system and recognition of the power of data generated from its application was key to the development of the National Cancer Data Base (NCDB) in the late 1980s as a major undertaking by the American College of Surgeons Commission on Cancer and the American Cancer Society [3].

The TNM classification was developed by Pierre Denoix, a surgeon working in Paris in the 1940s and 1950s, and is based on the anatomic extent of cancer [4]. In 1987, the American Joint Committee on Cancer (AJCC) in the United States (US) joined in a collaborative effort with the UICC (Union for International Cancer Control) to promulgate the TNM classification throughout the world [2]. The AJCC working with the UICC serves as the oversight organization for the staging of cancer in the US and, since the 1970s, has participated with the UICC in the formulation and modernization of the TNM system. The reporting and updating of the TNM system has progressed through eight published editions; the eighth edition was introduced in 2017 for dissemination and eventual use in the management of cancer patients beginning January 1, 2018 [5]. These publications reflect the collaborative work and close relationship of the two groups. The most important challenge facing the continued application of TNM staging is the ability to interface the current taxonomy with the numerous nonanatomic prognostic factors currently in use or under study. Ongoing collaborative efforts by the UICC and AJCC are geared to blending or aligning nonanatomic prognostic factors with the traditional anatomic foundation of the TNM system. Although the anatomic system, TNM, is recommended worldwide for adult solid tumors, there are other staging systems that have had traditional use for hematologic and pediatric tumors. This chapter will focus on the current use of TNM and associated prognostic factors used for most adult solid tumors.

Characteristics of the TNM System

Although the TNM classification is an anatomical system, the ability to group TNM categories into prognostically related stages is based on a generalized pattern of *biological behavior*: progression of tumor growth. A solid tumor first grows locally in overall size and extent. At some sites such as the colon and rectum, the depth of tumor penetration through the bowel wall is most relevant, and at other sites such as primary breast cancer, tumor diameter determines T category. Metastases to regional lymph nodes (N-category) usually precede systemic metastasis (M category). Finally, metastases develop past these nodal basins either into nonregional lymph nodes or into a variety of solid organs.

The spread of tumors – regionally and especially systemically – has typically been the most important prognostic factor, but not the only one. A helpful broad definition of a prognostic factor is *a variable that can explain some of the heterogeneity associated with the expected course and outcome of a disease* [6]. Since individual solid tumors of a given type and stage may be biologically unique, the variability of tumor growth may be the result of multiple prognostic factors operating at the same tumor site and type. In the TNM system, such factors that have been recognized as influencing prognosis but that cannot be expressed in terms of T, N, or M status have been incorporated as prognostic factors. Although it has not yet been determined how to modify the TNM stage by these factors, elucidation of a defined weight for each would be expected to generate a refined assessment of outcome and enhanced therapeutic groupings.

Application of Prognostic Factors

The American Cancer Society estimates that approximately 1.7 million new cancer cases will be diagnosed in 2017 [7]. Of these, approximately 1.5 million will be solid tumors occurring in adults and, therefore, suitable for staging using the TNM system. The clinician's role begins with the selection of appropriate diagnostic tests for a specific site and tumor type. Without knowledge of a specific tumor's prognostic factors, it would be impossible to choose a proper imaging modality, serum marker, or other clinical assessment that would give relevant information. Prognostic factors also allow for tailoring an optimal treatment plan for each patient. In the era of multimodal therapy, selection of appropriate preoperative or postoperative chemoradiation is based on knowledge of the clinical or pathological stage of the cancer. The TNM stage is but one prognostic factor that allows for optimal treatment planning. Once treatment has been chosen, these factors also allow for the prediction of outcome for the individual patient. The tailored assessment refines expectations of prognosis and can help determine appropriate follow-up intervals and methods for monitoring patients based on the biologic features of their cancer. These factors are further used to give patients and their caregivers an educational perspective relative to the short-term and long-term outcomes of their malignancy.

Rating Prognostic Factors

The scheme developed to determine the clinical significance of potential prognostic factors starts with the review of published studies. Level I prognostic factors have a statistically significant impact on outcome and are critical for the management of the patient in terms of tumor growth and oncologic outcome. Level II factors may be independent as a prognostic factor. Many factors may not reach this benchmark since they do not retain prognostic value when combined with other factors. The final level (Level III) deals with clinical relevance. A factor must be proven to have a significant impact on the prognosis of a given patient and to serve as a major clinical determinant for care. The reporting of tumor markers and prognostic studies has been codified by Altman *et al.* who have published the Reporting Recommendations for Tumor Marker Prognostic Studies (REMARK) [8]. The 20-item checklist (Figure 15.1) developed by these authors was based on the concept that unified reporting of tumor markers that potentially could be utilized in staging and clinical diagnostics should conform to rigid criteria to allow others to assess the usefulness of the data and to judge the results. As newer tumor markers are incorporated into

anatomical and molecular cancer staging, this strategy will assume an even greater importance.

Prognostic factors can be organized into three groups [9]:

- Tumor-related factors
- Host-related factors
- Environmental-related factors.

This organization sets the stage for a systematic approach to assessing prognosis that goes far beyond the behavior and growth patterns of individual tumors: it also includes noncancer influences that, in the long run, may be more important than prognostic factors reflecting tumor biology itself.

Tumor-Related Prognostic Factors

The identification of the tumor-related prognostic factors begins with an assessment by the pathologist of the morphology, grade, and growth pattern of an individual cancer. Determination of the anatomic extent of the tumor (TNM status) occurs in two phases. The first phase is a clinical assessment based on physical exam and imaging studies. The second phase is the pathologic assessment that occurs after surgical resection (and often neoadjuvant therapy). The pathologist describes the tumor's extent based on gross and microscopic features of a resected specimen. Pathological staging has historically been more precise than clinical staging and has been regarded as more reliable for predicting prognosis, but this is in flux in an era of neoadjuvant therapy. Recently, the inclusion of tumor markers has enhanced the ability of the pathologist to give vital information for clinical decision making. One example is the use of serum markers in staging of testicular cancer. Although many of these molecular markers are not included in the TNM staging strategy, the future use of proliferative indices and genetic as well as molecular markers has great potential. Another dimension of tumor-related factors but less well delineated than pathological factors is the overall effect that tumors have on patients. This is manifest by clinical symptoms and performance status.

One of the inherent difficulties in updating the TNM system is the decision of what to include from the recent peer-reviewed literature. In breast cancer alone, consideration of at least 80 prognostic variables was undertaken during the review of this site for the sixth editions of the *AJCC Cancer Staging Manual* [10] and the UICC *TNM Classification of Malignant Tumours* [11]. Obviously not all of these variables have the same importance. Each must be judged on the basis of clinical impact and the likelihood of being an independent variable, which can stand alone as a prognosticator of outcome. Using breast cancer as an example, the customary prognostic parameters of lymph nodes status, tumor size, histologic grade, and overall pathologic TNM are traditionally strong prognostic factors. It is certainly recognized that the steroid receptor status (estrogen receptor/progesterone receptor) is important in the assessment of patient outcomes and treatment planning, but this factor as yet has not been intertwined in the overall staging strategy.

Patient-Related Prognostic Factors

Although the factors relating to tumors have an important effect on the overall prognosis, it has been shown recently that patient characteristics may be as important as the biologic

Introduction

1. State the marker examined, the study objectives, and any pre-specified hypotheses.

Materials and Methods

Patients

2. Describe the characteristics (for example, disease stage or co-morbidities) of the study patients, including their source and inclusion and exclusion criteria.

3. Describe treatments received and how chosen (for example, randomized or rule-based).

Specimen characteristics

4. Describe type of biological material used (including control samples) and methods of preservation and storage.

Assay methods

5. Specify the assay method used and provide (or reference) a detailed protocol, including specific reagents or kits used, quality control procedures, reproducibility assessments, quantitation methods, and scoring and reporting protocols. Specify whether and how assays were performed blinded to the study endpoint.

Study design

6. State the method of case selection, including whether prospective or retrospective and whether stratification or matching (for example, by stage of disease or age) was used. Specify the time period from which cases were taken, the end of the follow-up period, and the median follow-up time.

7. Precisely define all clinical endpoints examined.

8. List all candidate variables initially examined or considered for inclusion in models.

9. Give rationale for sample size; if the study was designed to detect a specified effect size, give the target power and effect size.

Statistical analysis methods

10. Specify all statistical methods, including details of any variable selection procedures and other model-building issues, how model assumptions were verified, and how missing data were handled.

11. Clarify how marker values were handled in the analyses; if relevant, describe methods used for cutpoint determination.

Results

Data

12. Describe the flow of patients through the study, including the number of patients included in each stage of the analysis (a diagram may be helpful) and reasons for dropout. Specifically, both overall and for each subgroup extensively examined report the number of patients and the number of events.

13. Report distributions of basic demographic characteristics (at least age and sex), standard (disease-specific) prognostic variables, and tumor marker, including numbers of missing values.

Analysis and presentation

14. Show the relation of the marker to standard prognostic variables.

15. Present univariable analyses showing the relation between the marker and outcome, with the estimated effect (for example, hazard ratio and survival probability). Preferably provide similar analyses for all other variables being analyzed. For the effect of a tumor marker on a time-to-event outcome, a Kaplan–Meier plot is recommended.

16. For key multivariable analyses, report estimated effects (for example, hazard ratio) with confidence intervals for the marker and, at least for the final model, all other variables in the model.

17. Among reported results, provide estimated effects with confidence intervals from an analysis in which the marker and standard prognostic variables are included, regardless of their statistical significance.

18. If done, report results of further investigations, such as checking assumptions, sensitivity analyses, and internal validation.

Discussion

19. Interpret the results in the context of the pre-specified hypotheses and other relevant studies; include a discussion of limitations of the study.

20. Discuss implications for future research and clinical value.

Figure 15.1 The REMARK checklist for reporting of prognostic factors. *Source:* Altman 2012 [8]. ©Altman *et al.;* licensee BioMed Central Ltd 2012.

fingerprint of the tumor [9]. The effects of age, race, gender, level of education and socioeconomic status have been evaluated in multiple patient populations and are important variables for potential inclusion in outcome assessment. One of the newer concepts is the impact of comorbidities such as coronary artery disease, obesity, hypertension and diabetes mellitus on cancer stage-related outcome [12]. Some inherited conditions such as hereditary nonpolyposis colorectal cancer act as prognostic factors and have been shown to have important effects on outcome. Using microsatellite instability as a marker, the genetic mutation confers favorable outcome stage-for-stage compared to other sporadic colorectal cancers [13]. Most likely, the future documentation and stratification of these comorbidities may be important in the assessment of adult solid tumors. These comorbidities must be documented and entered into registry information in order to identify these important parameters and to compare large population groups relative to cancer and comorbid conditions.

Environment-Related Prognostic Factors

The third group of factors that may play a significant role in the outcome of cancer patients is related to the overall environment surrounding the patient. One of these important determinants may be the experience of the physician caring for the patient. The importance of both surgeon and hospital experience is demonstrated in certain cancers by volume/outcome studies and is associated with both short- and long-term survival [14]. Not only is 30-day mortality following major surgical extirpation an important criterion, but 5-year survival may be related to the initial management by the surgeon, medical oncologist, and radiation oncologist. Log kill is an important concept in cancer care, but not all "log kills" are equal. For example, in rectal cancer, specimen integrity improves with focused training in total mesorectal excision and has direct correspondence with local cancer recurrence risk [15, 16]. In multimodal therapy, the combined experience of the management team may play a significant role in cancer prognosis. Likewise, the healthcare system in which the patient is treated is relevant. Early access to care, appropriate diagnostic studies, and screening for initial or early recurrence of cancer have an important place in determining prognosis. Ethnicity has been regarded as the most important concept in the development of certain cancers, but this may be outweighed by socioeconomic status in some cases [17]. Continued evaluation of these environmentally-related prognostic factors will be important in the future. Awareness of new environmental influences will emerge and may take precedence as we look at the cancer-related health of the entire society.

Managing Change

The re-evaluation of data is an absolute necessity to assure appropriate, up-to-date staging of any cancer site even though revisions present problems for data registries and for those designing clinical trials that may span a significant time period. Cancer outcomes based on stage groups can only be determined by analyzing registries and robust data sets. This is illustrated by a major change in breast cancer staging introduced in the sixth edition of the *AJCC Cancer Staging Manual* [10] and the UICC *TNM Classification of Malignant Tumours* [11] relating to the number of positive axillary lymph nodes. In this staging strategy, N1 reflects involvement of one to three nodes while N2 encompasses patients having four to nine axillary nodes involved. Patients with 10 or more axillary nodes are placed into an N3 category. Supraclavicular nodal involvement was designated as M1 in the fifth edition of the AJCC [18] and UICC [19] staging publications. Using large data sets, it was recognized that women with supraclavicular nodal involvement had the same outcomes as women with multiple node involvement in the axilla. A consequence of grouping women with supraclavicular nodal involvement into the M1 category was to exclude these patients from trials treating locoregional disease even though they had survival patterns similar to women with advanced local disease. Following these analyses, supraclavicular node-positive patients reverted to the N3 category, placing them in groups that can be assessed for local disease. These concepts have been carried forward in the seventh [20] and eighth editions of the breast cancer staging strategy [5].

Another example of staging system modification dealing with breast cancer involves the classification of sentinel lymph nodes, which has become important in the management of patients with breast cancer. A strategy for sentinel node documentation was needed. The notation for a sentinel node should be the N designation followed by "(sn)". This indicates that only the sentinel node was reported and that a full axillary dissection was not performed. Similarly, while it is not recommended that routine internal mammary node dissection be accomplished, a strategy for denoting internal mammary nodes that contain both microscopic and macroscopic disease was developed to quantify internal mammary nodes. The overall concept is that if pathologic or clinical data are important, there should be a methodology to incorporate these data points into the hospital-based registry.

As is true for breast cancer, the staging strategies for melanoma have benefited by the analysis of large data sets [21]. The results have indicated that not only is the absolute thickness of cutaneous melanoma relevant, but also the presence or absence of ulceration on the surface of the melanoma and mitotic rate (number of mitoses /mm^2) are significant variables that must be incorporated into the T category. This is now a standard determinant for melanoma staging introduced in the sixth and seventh editions of the *AJCC Cancer Staging Manual* [10, 20] and the UICC *TNM Classification of Malignant Tumours* [22].

Residual Tumor Classification

In addition to the traditional TNM, one of the strongest predictors of outcome is residual cancer following traditional surgical resection [23]. A strategy for denoting residual tumor has been developed to distinguish that a patient may have no residual disease (R0), microscopic residual tumor (R1), or macroscopic residual tumor (R2). The amount of cancer remaining after surgery may dictate further therapeutic interventions such as adjuvant radiotherapy and is an important prognostic factor relating to overall patient well-being. Surgeons must document the possibility of residual disease in the operative note and be vigilant assessing patients following resection. The pathologist reports whether microscopic disease is present at resection margins, and this must be reported as a critical determinant of patient outcome.

Isolated Tumor Cells Versus Micrometastases

Additions to the TNM system preferably are derived because of analysis of large datasets or information derived from groups within a clinical trial setting. Frequently, concepts are introduced to create a dynamic process to follow a site-specific factor. One such factor recognized in modern pathologic assessment is that smaller and smaller malignant cell clusters can be identified using immunohistochemical or routine hematoxylin and eosin staining [24]. While the overall significance of these isolated tumor cells (ITC) remains an enigma, it is important to define these clusters when visualized in lymph nodes. The definition of the ITC is any cell or small cluster of cells ≤ 0.2 mm and is denoted with the suffix (i-) or (i+). This is in comparison to micrometastases that are > 0.2 mm and extend up to 2 mm. Any cell group greater than 2 mm would be considered a macrometastasis. The designation (i+), however, would still define a pN0 lymph node, since the long-term prognosis of the ITC is unclear. Similarly, in the future, as polymerase chain reaction (PCR) is used to identify smaller and smaller cell clusters, a designation "(mol+)" for this technology was introduced in the sixth edition of the *AJCC Cancer Staging Manual* [10] and the UICC *TNM Classification of Malignant Tumours* [11]. There is little doubt that in the future these new techniques will be applied to the routine assessment of lymph nodes, bone marrow, and other sites, if they are shown to be clinically relevant. In other words, the full impact of detecting one out of a million or 10 million malignant cells is yet to be determined.

Staging and Large Data Sets

One of the outstanding achievements of the American College of Surgeons Commission on Cancer has been the establishment of the NCDB, developed in the late 1980s in association with the American Cancer Society [3]. This was based on patient data accrual from the hospitals that are currently accredited by the Commission on Cancer. Approximately 29 million patient entries have been made to date, which is a credit to the vigilance of hospital registrars who collect the data related to cancer patients. This data set is now being used to analyze individual sites and has been valuable in creating new staging strategies. The strength of the NCDB is that it provides information on patterns of care throughout the US. Included are patients with both rare and common malignancies. The NCDB contains appropriate TNM staging information, as well as treatment characteristics, patient demographics, and survival relative to treatment and stage. Data items that enable comparison of populations are continually being modified and supplemented as the importance of new variables emerge. One of the many distinguishing features of the NCDB compared to other oncologic outcomes data registries is the inclusion of specific surgical and pathologic details of patient care. These items include the surgical procedure, size of the surgical margin, number of regional lymph nodes obtained, and information related to residual tumor. In addition, the various treatment modalities and follow-up findings are included.

Currently there are important elements that do not appear in the NCDB data sets. These include provider data, estimates of patient satisfaction and quality of life, and more complete comorbidity information. Plans are being made to include these vital data in the NCDB since many of these – especially comorbidity – seem to be important in outcome assessment. Since data collection for the NCDB began in the late 1980s, a follow-up period of 20–25 years is available for many of the cases. Using NCDB data and the assessment of over 50,000 patients with stage III colon cancer [25], a revision of the staging strategies in the sixth edition of TNM has shown that there are three distinct subsets of patients with node-positive colon cancer with 5-year outcomes that are statistically different and that should be recorded separately in the outcome assessment of patients. Stage IIIA, which included approximately 11% of patients in the NCDB group, is characterized as having T1/2, N1 involvement. Stage IIIB includes approximately 60% of patients and is characterized as T3/4, N1. Stage IIIC includes approximately 29% of patients and is characterized by tumors that have N2 nodal involvement (four or more nodes involved in the mesentery). These three groups have a 5-year observed survival rate, which is separate and distinct. This same strategy was used to analyze approximately 6,000 patients with rectal cancer [26]. Three distinct subgroups were also observed in these patients. This strategy for the staging of colorectal cancer has been updated in the seventh and eighth editions of TNM and a new stage, IIC (T4bN0), has been introduced to highlight the importance of the new criterion, T4b [20].

Literature Review

One of the significant challenges to maintaining the currency of the staging system is to keep up with the voluminous literature published in peer-reviewed publications that deal with current and future staging concepts as well as new markers for cancer staging. Beginning in 2002, the UICC began an initiative to have expert panels review and catalogue TNM-relevant articles regarding most types of solid tumor sites [27]. This process of continuous review has been embraced by the site-specific staging task forces of the AJCC and has proved quite beneficial in the development of changes in TNM that will be included in the future publications of both the UICC and AJCC. This review process has also laid the foundation for a methodology for those wishing to make proposals for improvement or modification of the various TNM strategies. This approach also functions in an important archival role for researchers interested in having a common resource for literature review on staging strategies and methodology.

Staging and Neoadjuvant Therapy

Since development of the TNM strategy in the late 1940s and 1950s, treatment of cancer has evolved into the use of multimodality therapy that is interwoven into a matrix involving surgical extirpation, radiation, and chemotherapy. Over the last decade, the concept of preoperative chemoradiation has been applied to a variety of tumors. Currently these cancers are being treated with nonsurgical modalities after initial histologic confirmation and careful clinical staging. The incorporation of neoadjuvant therapy is a much more recent innovation than the initial designation of group staging in the TNM system and presents the challenge of incorporating temporal factors in the staging system.

The complete response to neoadjuvant therapy has also been defined as one of the most robust prognostic indicators in tumors amenable to preoperative therapy [28]. A complete pathologic response to drug or radiation therapy for carcinomas of the rectum and breast portend a much better outcome than in those patients who do not respond to neoadjuvant therapy. Using proper prefixes to identify the point at which assessments are made [29], the traditional categories T0, N0 and M0 fit well when there is no discernable tumor remaining after initial chemotherapy, radiation or use of both modalities.

When creating a new stage grouping, it is important to ensure that this designation would be applicable to any site which might be treated with neoadjuvant therapy and that the designation has prognostic significance in the likelihood of either a complete clinical (CR) and/or pathologic (PR) response. Currently these strategies are utilized for breast, rectal, head and neck, pancreatic and other gastrointestinal malignancies. There is growing evidence that at some tumor sites (such as anus and rectum) the reliability of clinical determination of complete response may be reliable enough to obviate surgical resection [28].

An educational process must accompany the introduction of any new staging definitions both to raise awareness of and to ensure comprehension of the terms or grouping. Education is also vital for implementation of new definitions; staging forms must be updated and distributed and proper collection of the data must be validated. It is anticipated that clinical scenarios resulting in T0, N0, M0 outcomes will be even more prevalent as newer and more targeted neoadjuvant regimens are developed.

The Future

Cancer staging is one of the primary activities in oncology practice and research. Knowledge of the extent of disease is required to characterize the disease prior to selecting treatment. The fundamental criteria for stratification of malignancies are the diagnosis, classified according to the ICD-O coding system, including the presenting site and the histologic type, and the assessment of anatomic disease extent.

There are multiple uses of the TNM classification and although there is a continuing conflict between those who desire a stable classification for the purpose of reporting long-term outcomes and those who want a classification to be clinically useful and reflect the current treatment strategies, overall the system is immeasurably useful and constitutes the foundation of clinical decision making and clinical practice guidelines. Those who would prefer the classification to remain unchanged include the cancer registries and the health services researchers. For the assessment of cancer outcomes over long periods of time, changes in classification are counterproductive. On the other hand, clinicians prefer a fluid classification that is relevant to their contemporary clinical practice and helpful in identifying appropriate treatment options [30]. It is widely accepted that the anatomic extent of disease is not the sole factor that needs to be considered in reaching treatment decisions and predicting the outcome. There are numerous nonanatomic prognostic factors that affect the course of the disease, response to treatment and the ultimate prognosis. These factors will be included into future iterations of TNM staging.

The staging and prognosis of most solid adult cancers are based on a careful assessment of prognostic factors related to the tumor, patient, and environment. While the most robust of these prognostic factors is reflected in the anatomic TNM staging system which itself reflects understanding of solid tumor biology, other characteristics including newer molecular markers and response to therapy will continually be added to this effort. Using these global prognostic factors, clinicians will be able to structure a more refined diagnostic and interventional approach for the management of cancer and to assess the outcome and prognosis of cancer using a more evidenced-based taxonomy. These strategies are dependent on new pathologic and imaging strategies, which are based on the molecular and biologic characteristics of tumors. Our ability to enhance data collection with new methods of medical informatics will allow a full assessment of patient populations and the ability to compare these populations across large sectors of society internationally. We cannot accomplish these goals without the future application of technology that allows full analysis of large amounts of data and the possibility of incorporating solutions using principles of artificial intelligence.

A major challenge today is to develop a staging system that can express both anatomic and nonanatomic prognostic factors while maintaining the pure anatomic extent of disease data. Combining these under the traditional TNM stage grouping, though convenient, carries the risk of "diluting" the anatomic data. An approach that has been adopted in the seventh edition [20] of TNM defines 2 stage groupings: "Anatomical Stage Grouping", includes the purely anatomic disease components (T, N, and M), and the heading "Anatomical/Prognostic Stage Grouping" combines the anatomical T, N, and M components with other prognostic factors such as tumor grade, histologic type, patient age, and serum tumor markers, among others. This strategy has been continued and further modified in the *AJCC Cancer Staging Manual*, eighth edition [5].

These are challenging times for all of us in clinical medicine who take care of cancer patients. We must constantly remember that our staging strategy is in fact our "language of cancer" [31]. We must constantly refine the templates related to this language. The art of staging and the application of prognostic variables echo the words of Charcot who wrote, "Disease is very old and nothing about it has changed. It is we who change as we learn what was formerly imperceptible".

References

1 Greene FL, Sobin LH. A worldwide approach to the TNM staging system: collaborative efforts of the AJCC and UICC. *J Surg Oncol* 2009;99:269–72.

2 Hutter RVP. At last – worldwide agreement on the staging of cancer. *Arch Surg* 1987;122:1235–9.

3 Winchester DP, Stewart AK, Phillips JL, *et al.* The National Cancer Data Base: past, present, and future. *Ann Surg Oncol* 2010;17:4–7.

4 Denoix PF. French Ministry of Public Health National Institute of Hygiene. Monograph No.4, Paris, 1954.

5 Amin MB, Edge SB, Greene FL, *et al.* (eds) *AJCC Cancer Staging Manual*, 8th edn. New York: Springer Nature, 2017.

6 Tannock IF, Hill RP (eds) *The Basic Science of Oncology*, 3rd edn. New York: McGraw-Hill, 1998.

7 Siegel RL, Miller KD, Jemal A. Cancer statistics, 2017. *CA Cancer J Clin* 2017;67(1):7–30.

8 Altman DG, McShane LM, Sauerbrei W, *et al.* Reporting recommendations for tumor marker prognostic studies (REMARK); explanation and elaboration. *BMC Med* 2012;10:51–90.

9 Gospodarowicz MK, O'Sullivan B, Sobin L (eds) *Prognostic Factors in Cancer*, 3rd edn. New York: John Wiley & Sons, Inc., 2006.

10 Greene, FL, Page DL, Fleming ID, *et al.* (eds) *AJCC Cancer Staging Manual*, 6th edn. New York: Springer, 2002.

11 Sobin LH, Wittekind C (eds) *TNM Classification of Malignant Tumours*, 6th edn. New York: Wiley-Liss, 2002.

12 Piccirillo JF, Feinstein AR. Clinical symptoms and comorbidity: significance or the prognostic classification of cancer. *Cancer* 1996;77:834–42.

13 Al-Sohaily S, Biankin A, Leong R, *et al.* Molecular pathways in colorectal cancer. *J Gastro Hepatol* 2012;27:1423–31.

14 Begg CB, Cramer LD, Hoskins WJ, Brennan MF. Impact of hospital volume on operative mortality for major cancer surgery. *JAMA* 1998;280:1747–51.

15 Bernstein TE, Endreseth BH, Romundstad P, Wibe A. Circumferential resection margin as a prognostic factor in rectal cancer. *Br J Surg* 2009;96:1348–57.

16 Nagtegaal ID, Quirke P. What is the role for the circumferential margin in the modern treatment of rectal cancer? *J Clin Oncol* 2008;26:303–12.

17 Freeman HP. Poverty, culture and social injustice: determinants of cancer disparities. *CA Cancer J Clin* 2004;54:72–7.

18 Fleming ID, Cooper JS, Henson DE, *et al.* (eds) *AJCC Cancer Staging Manual*, 5th edn. Philadelphia: Lippincott-Raven, 1997.

19 Sobin LH, Wittekind C (eds) *TNM Classification of Malignant Tumours*, 5th edn. New York: Wiley-Liss, 1997.

20 Edge SB, Byrd DR, Compton CC, *et al.* (eds) *AJCC Cancer Staging Manual*, 7th edn. New York: Springer, 2009.

21 Balch CM, Soong SJ, Gershenwald JE, *et al.* Prognostic factors analysis of 17,600 melanoma patients: validation of the American Joint Committee on Cancer melanoma staging system. *J Clin Oncol* 2001;19:3622–34.

22 Gospodarowicz MK, Wittekind C, Sobin LH (eds) *TNM Classification of Malignant Tumours*, 7th edn. Hoboken: John Wiley & Sons, Inc., 2009.

23 Wittekind C, Compton CC, Greene FL, Sobin LH. TNM residual tumor classification revisited. *Cancer* 2002;94:2511–16.

24 Singletary SE, Greene FL, Sobin LH. Classification of isolated tumor cells: clarification of the 6th edition of the AJCC Cancer Staging Manual. *Cancer* 2003;98:2740–1.

25 Greene FL, Stewart AK, Norton HJ. A new TNM staging strategy for node-positive (stage III) colon cancer: an analysis of 50,042 patients. *Ann Surg* 2002;236:416–21.

26 Greene FL, Stewart AK, Norton HJ. New tumor-node-metastasis staging strategy for node-positive (stage III) rectal cancer: an analysis. *J Clin Oncol* 2004;22:1778–84.

27 Gospodarowicz MK, Miller D, Groome PA, *et al.* The process for continuous improvement of the TNM classification. *Cancer* 2004;100:1–5.

28 Kosinski LA, Habr-Gama A, Ludwig K, Perez, R. Shifting concepts in rectal cancer management: a review of contemporary primary rectal cancer treatment strategies. *CA Cancer J Clin* 2012;62:173–202.

29 Brierley JD, Greene FL, Sobin LH, *et al.* The "y" symbol: an important classification tool for neoadjuvant cancer treatment. *Cancer* 2006;106:2526–7.

30 Boffa DJ, Greene FL. Reacting to changes in staging designations in the 7th edition of the AJCC staging manual. *Ann Surg Oncol* 2011;18:1–3.

31 Greene FL, Sobin LH. The TNM system: our language for cancer care. *J Surg Oncol* 2002;80:119–20.

Section 4

Treatment Modalities

16

Surgical Oncology Overview

M. Andrew Sicard[1] and Benjamin D. Li[2]

[1] *Surgical Associates of Opelousas, Opelousas, Louisiana, USA*
[2] *MetroHealth Cancer Center, Cleveland, Ohio, USA*

Introduction

We have witnessed enormous progress in cancer care in the past 100 years. One could argue that this progress started with safe surgical resection of solid tumors with tumor-free margins. This act represented the first and most dramatic impact on a patient's clinical outcome. Today, the importance of surgery in treating solid tumors has not diminished; it is, however, complemented by a multidisciplinary approach that has further improved cancer outcome.

What we do to treat cancer has grown exponentially since the first mention of surgery as a treatment for cancer was recorded in the Edwin Smith Papyrus around 1600 BC [1]. Cancer treatment has evolved along with our understanding of tumor biology. Also, improved surgical techniques and technology, along with the addition of chemotherapy, radiation therapy, hormonal manipulation therapy, target-specific therapy, biologics, and now, pharmacogenomics, have all added to the oncologist's armamentarium. However, a basic tenet of surgical oncology remains for solid tumors: surgical resection of a cancer with a tumor-free margin represents the best potential for cure when the disease is locally confined.

The nineteenth century was a time of great surgical importance. Milestones of this century include two key elements: Lister's development of aseptic technique and Morton and Longs' introduction of general anesthesia [2]. These advances allowed for the growth and development of surgery. For example, in 1867 Charles Moore, in his article "On the influence of inadequate operations on the theory of cancer", theorized that a complete operation for breast cancer involves removal of the entire breast [3]. This "removal of the entire breast" cannot be readily accomplished, with any degree of patient acceptance or reasonable outcome, without anesthesia and aseptic technique. Moore's idea of local control of cancer and the potential for systemic implications likely influenced many surgeons, most notably, William Halsted [4].

Halsted popularized the radical mastectomy by combining the teachings of his mentors into one definitive operation [4].

This surgery involved en bloc resection of the breast, pectoralis major, pectoralis minor and the axillary contents. Halsted believed that removing all the tissue in one piece was of utmost importance "lest the wound become infected by the division of tissue invaded by the disease" [5]. This rather deforming operation often resulted in some disability to his patients, which he stated to be "of very little importance as compared with [their] li[ves]" [5]. Halsted demonstrated that local recurrence was drastically reduced as a result of his operation [5]. Thus, the idea of local control resulting in cancer cure, by complete removal of the primary cancer, was established as a surgical principle.

The "Halstedian Theory" (cancer spreads by direct extension to other tissues) remained the theory of choice by a majority of physicians well into the twentieth century [6]. This idea led to other forms of radical cancer surgeries, such as the hemipelvectomy for sarcoma, the radical prostatectomy and the radical hysterectomy. However, the extent of surgical resection and the success rate of cure in solid tumors necessarily reached a finite limit. Despite the growth of more radical approaches, cure rates for cancer remained limited and did not correlate with the radical nature of the surgeries. As the understanding of tumor biology evolved, the notion that local resection had limited impact on distant dissemination, and thus survival, was appreciated.

The distant dissemination theory is not new; during the Halsted era, Stephen Paget, an English Surgeon, was establishing the "Seed and Soil" hypothesis. He postulated that tumor cells (seed) preferentially metastasized to certain organs (soil) [7]. However, this theory was not widely accepted until years later when it was confirmed by research.

Clinical trials by the National Surgical Adjuvant Breast and Bowel Project (NSABP) group, spearheaded by Bernard Fisher, played a critical role in the paradigm shift of the surgeons' approach to cancer treatment. The 1971 B-04 trial was a landmark study credited for beginning the end of the era of more and more radical surgery [8]. Results from this study showed that patients with operable breast cancer undergoing radical mastectomy had no better outcome than those who underwent total mastectomy [9]. The subsequent NSABP B-06 trial established that segmental mastectomy, lumpectomy with tumor-free margin, with whole breast irradiation is not inferior to total mastectomy for stage I and II breast cancer [10]. In a relatively short period of time, the surgical treatment of breast cancer evolved from the radical resection of an organ and the underlying musculature, to an organ-preserving procedure with adjuvant radiation therapy to obtain local control. This resulted in a more cosmetically appealing outcome, without compromising on local or systemic control of disease.

When discussing cancer treatments, surgical oncologist Blake Cady famously stated, "Biology is King. Selection is Queen. Technical maneuvers are the Prince and Princess" [11]. Though local control can be obtained by surgical resection, patients most frequently succumb to the disease due to systemic dissemination. To lower the risk for systemic recurrence, adjuvant systemic therapy, initially consisting of cytotoxic agents (discussed in Chapter 18), evolved.

In breast cancer, the idea of using cytotoxic agents to treat potential systemic disease in the adjuvant setting, thereby reducing the risk for cancer recurrence and cancer-related death after definitive surgery, was explored by the NSABP trial group and the Milan National Cancer Institute, amongst others [12–14]. The success of these trials laid the foundation for the use of chemotherapy in the adjuvant setting for control of potential systemic disease where no clinically detectable disease is evident [12].

Today, multimodal therapy for cancer treatment continues to grow. Definitive surgery is often complemented by radiation therapy, given preoperatively or postoperatively, to increase the chance for organ preservation and/or improved local control. Chemotherapy, given before surgery (neoadjuvant), after (adjuvant), or perioperatively has become the standard of care for a variety of solid tumors. Additionally, endocrine/hormonal manipulation (discussed in Chapter 19), immunotherapy (discussed in Chapter 20) and target-specific small molecules agents (discussed in Chapter 21) have all found their unique roles in cancer treatment. Though cancer treatments continue to evolve, definitive surgical treatment still remains critical in the care of patients with solid tumors. Moreover, the surgeon continues to play a central role in the treatment and management of most patients who present with a solid tumor.

In this chapter, we will explore the surgeon's role in the treatment and management of cancer. This begins with the diagnosis of cancer and continues with the staging of the extent of disease, resection with curative intent, management of metastatic disease, surgical palliation, plastic and reconstructive surgery, surgical prophylaxis, and access surgery. We will also highlight the use of the minimally invasive approach and the role of robotics in cancer surgery.

Diagnosis

Before any treatment can be initiated, an accurate diagnosis must be established. With very rare exceptions, tissue diagnosis is paramount in therapeutic decision making. Methods of obtaining tissue vary depending on cancer type, location, and patient selection. The goal of any biopsy is to obtain an adequate amount of tissue for a pathologist to make an accurate diagnosis (discussed in Chapter 14), in the least invasive manner, while avoiding jeopardizing future surgical management.

Surface lesions are easily accessible and amenable to excisional or incisional biopsies. For example, cutaneous lesions can usually easily be biopsied either by punch or excisional techniques. Similarly, lesions located on mucosal surfaces (gastrointestinal, respiratory, urothelial, etc.) can be sampled by using endoscopic techniques.

Fine-needle aspiration (FNA) is often used when lesions are deeper (e.g., breast masses, lymph nodes, thyroid nodules, etc.). FNA can also be performed on palpable or nonpalpable lesions, with the aid of imaging modalities including mammography, CT, and ultrasound. The aspirate from the lesion can then be examined morphologically to determine if neoplastic cells are present. The advantage of this technique is that it is quick and less invasive than an open biopsy. However, cytological samples typically provide very limited information regarding tumor architecture [15], may not provide sufficient material for some ancillary tests, and have a higher rate of nondiagnostic results, due in part to sampling error.

Core needle biopsy (CNB) can be performed in a clinic setting similar to FNA. In contrast, CNB preserves the tumor structural characteristics in relation to surrounding tissue. However, like FNA, there is a higher rate of sampling error compared to open biopsy. Sensitivity and specificity rates vary for both FNA and CNB depending on the examiner, the quality of the sample, and the site being examined. However, for many patients, CNB is adequate for diagnosis, with open biopsies reserved for those with nondiagnostic workups.

An open incisional biopsy allows a surgeon to obtain an adequate piece of tissue for accurate diagnosis under direct vision, thereby minimizing sampling error. In a larger lesion, such as a soft tissue mass suspicious for sarcoma, proper planning is necessary to avoid contamination of the tissue plane, as well as potential for compromising the future surgical resection. For example, if there is a soft tissue neoplasm on an extremity, the skin incision for the open biopsy should be placed longitudinally along the muscle belly of the extremity. On subsequent definitive resection, the scar, biopsy site, tumor, and underlying muscle involvement may be resected en bloc, with tumor-free margins. Also, hemostasis is of utmost importance with sarcoma biopsy, as inadequate hemostasis can lead to inadvertent dissemination of tumor cells into the local area.

Excisional biopsies, like incisional biopsies, provide pathologists with tissue to make a diagnosis. Excisional biopsies also have the benefit of being definitive surgeries in some instances. If adequate margins are taken at the time of biopsy, further intervention may not be necessary. As with incisional biopsies, surgeons should be cognizant of possible future surgical procedures. For example, when excising a breast mass, the surgeon should ensure that if a mastectomy is necessary, the biopsy incision can be incorporated in the definitive surgery. In some solid tumors (i.e., pancreatic, ovarian, and testicular tumors) routine biopsy may not be recommended prior to definitive treatment [16–18]. Thus, with knowledge of biopsy methods and tumor characteristics, surgeons can determine which lesions need to be biopsied and how to obtain tissue safely and effectively so that patients can be properly diagnosed and treatment initiated.

Staging

Cancer staging is a critical component in cancer treatment planning. Information garnered from a patient's history, physical examination, imaging studies, and biopsies are used to stage the patient. Staging is either determined clinically or pathologically. Clinical staging (cTNM) is based upon information gathered during history and physical examination or from imaging modalities. Pathological staging (pTNM) is derived from evaluation of actual tissue from a primary tumor, regional lymph node or metastatic lesion. The most often used staging system for solid tumors of adults is the tumor, node and metastasis (TNM) system of the American Joint Committee on Cancer (AJCC) and the Union for International Cancer Control (UICC). This is further explored in Chapter 15.

The surgeon's role in staging has changed significantly over the years. Improved imaging, such as computed tomography (CT) and positron emission tomography (PET) scans have decreased the need for more invasive methods of staging, for example, in Hodgkin lymphoma. Forty years ago, patients with Hodgkin lymphoma frequently underwent staging laparotomies, which involved splenectomy, liver biopsy and para-aortic lymph node biopsy [19]. Studies in the 1990s revealed that there was no significant difference in survival in patients who did or did not receive staging laparotomy prior to initiation of treatment [20]. Today with improved imaging and treatment modalities, staging laparotomy in Hodgkin lymphoma is of historical significance only [19].

Similarly, the role of surgery in nodal staging is evolving in solid tumors. For example, interest in selective lymph node biopsy for patients with melanoma led to the development of sentinel node biopsy. In brief, the sentinel node is the first echelon node that drains a tumor (and therefore, most likely to be involved if the cancer has spread to any lymph nodes). Sentinel node biopsy uses a radiotracer (Tc-labeled sulfur colloid) and/or isosuflan blue dye (Lymphazurin) to locate the first echelon nodes. The sentinel node(s) is then identified intraoperatively by using a gamma probe and the blue color for removal and pathologic evaluation. The success of the Multicenter Selective Lymphadenectomy Trial group (MSLT), comparing sentinel lymph node (SLN) biopsy to conventional complete regional node dissection, has resulted in the common use of SLN biopsy in melanoma with intermediate thickness for nodal staging [21].

The use of sentinel node biopsy instead of a complete axillary node dissection (ALND) has also been applied to breast cancer. In the NSABP-32 trial, the authors demonstrated that the overall survival, disease-free survival, and regional control were statistically equivalent between patients with negative SLN biopsy compared to those who were node-negative by ALND [22]. This study has allowed patients with SLN-negative disease to avoid ALND. SLN biopsy has now become the standard nodal staging technique for breast cancer patients without palpable axillary lymph nodes.

The majority of SLN biopsy research and application has revolved around breast cancer and melanoma. However, the usefulness of this technology has been applied in other areas including colon cancer. In colon cancer, the use of sentinel node identification has been advocated to identify the first draining nodes so that these nodes may be analyzed with increased pathologic scrutiny [23]. Use of this method has been shown to result in pathologic upstaging when compared to standard staging techniques [23]. Whether the identification of these micrometastases results in prolonged survival is yet to be demonstrated. As such, adoption of this technique in colon cancer has not gained the same widespread acceptance as in melanoma or breast cancer

However, there may be a continued need for en bloc nodal dissection in certain solid tumors. For example, en bloc gastrectomy with extended nodal dissection for gastric cancer may be associated with a better clinical outcome, if morbidity and mortality from nodal dissection can be avoided, compared to inadequate nodal sampling [24]. As our understanding of tumor biology improves, and effective multimodal therapies for solid tumors continue to grow, the role of surgical staging will continually change to accommodate advances in cancer treatment.

Surgery with Curative Intent

Despite the advances in surgical technique, critical care, and multimodal therapy, the primary goal for surgical resection of cancer with curative intent remains complete removal of the primary tumor and en bloc resection of adjacent tissue and/or organ(s), when necessary, to achieve a tumor-free resection margin. However, the availability of multimodal therapy has impacted the extent of resection needed and increased the pool of patients for whom resection would be helpful.

The amount of tumor-free margin required differs for various cancer types. For example, in cutaneous melanoma, tumor-free surgical margins are dependent on depth of invasion, as determined by Breslow thickness [25, 26]. Based on data obtained by the Intergroup Melanoma Committee and the World Health Organization Melanoma Program, melanoma less than 1 mm in depth requires a 1 cm surgical resection margin. In contrast, intermediate thick melanoma, more than 1 mm but less than 4 mm, requires a 2 cm margin [27, 28].

In some cancer, the advent of adjuvant therapy has resulted in less extensive surgery. Based on the findings of NSABP B-06 trial, the standard of care for most breast cancer is now breast conserving surgery, with a tumor-free margin, and breast irradiation. Patients undergoing breast conservation therapy (BCT) alone were found to have a higher rate of in-breast recurrence if breast irradiation is omitted [10].

Another example is the use of external beam radiation or brachytherapy in the treatment of extremity sarcomas. Historically, patients stricken with extremity sarcomas were often relegated to radical compartmental resection or amputation [29]. However, with the use of adjuvant radiation therapy, limb sparing surgery, when a tumor-free resection margin can be achieved without sacrifice of function, is possible with equivalent disease-free survival and overall survival when compared to amputation [29].

The role of chemotherapy prior to definitive surgery (neoadjuvant chemotherapy) has also impacted surgery. For example, in patients with a relatively large breast cancer with a relatively small breast (volume of disease >30% of breast), BCT with postoperative radiation therapy (XRT) may result in a cosmetically unacceptable outcome. The use of neoadjuvant chemotherapy, where primary tumor size reduction can be achieved for up to 70% of patients, may allow for effective BCT in patients who would otherwise require a mastectomy [30].

Additionally, the combined use of chemotherapy and XRT has increased the pool of patients who are potential candidates for surgical resection with curative intent, as well as increase the likelihood of organ preserving surgery. Three examples of this are: (i) Inflammatory breast cancer (IBCA); (ii) locally advanced rectal cancer; and (iii) locally advanced esophageal cancer. Prior to systemic chemotherapy, radical mastectomy for IBCA alone resulted in 5-year survival of <5% [31]. Combining neoadjuvant chemotherapy (and *HER2*-directed therapy) with postoperative systemic therapy plus XRT and modified radical mastectomy for IBCA patients has resulted in 5-year survival of >50% [32, 33]. Similarly, preoperative chemotherapy plus XRT has increased the rate for surgical resection with tumor-free margin in locally advanced rectal cancer and esophageal cancer [34–36]. Additionally, preoperative chemotherapy and radiation has increased the rate of sphincter preserving rectal resection (low anterior resection) in patients who otherwise would have required an abdominoperineal resection [36].

Management of Metastatic Disease

Surgical treatment for metastatic disease can be controversial and sometimes viewed as a futile effort. However, even when disease has disseminated beyond local disease, careful selection of patients for resection of isolated tumor metastasis can improve prognosis and lengthen median survival [37–39]. For example, a subset of patients with limited liver metastasis from colorectal cancer who undergo liver lesion resection have seen 5-year survival rates up to 58% compared to 11% for chemotherapy alone [40, 41]. However, survival benefit is more likely in patients who are free of extrahepatic disease and when liver resection results in removal of all liver metastasis [41]. Thus, patient selection is very important. Studies suggest that preoperative imaging, such as a PET scan, may help select patients most likely to benefit from liver resection (58% 5-year survival compared to historical 30% without a PET scan) [41].

Another example where metastasectomy appears helpful is in isolated lung metastasis from sarcoma. The lungs are the most common site of metastasis in sarcoma. The efficacy of systemic chemotherapy for the treatment of sarcoma pulmonary metastasis is limited [42, 43]. In patients with isolated sarcoma metastasis 3-year survival rates approach 46% with complete resection of the lesion(s), compared to 17% without resection [37]. The combination of recent progress in systemic treatments of metastatic disease, diagnostic imaging to accurately distinguish oligometastatic disease from more widely disseminated disease, and molecular profiling to assist in selection of patients likely to benefit from metastasectomy or surgical ablation is expanding the role of surgery in improving outcomes who were previously not considered as surgical candidates [44–46].

Surgery also has a role to play in disseminated disease confined within an anatomic cavity, as in peritoneal carcinomatosis. Peritoneal carcinomatosis is a form of disease spread seen in a variety of malignancies of intra-abdominal origin, including appendiceal, colorectal, gastric, and ovarian cancers. The mode

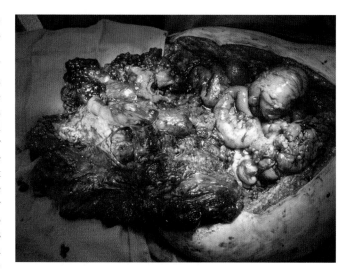

Figure 16.1 Example of peritoneal carcinomatosis with heavy disease burden present within the abdominal cavity.

of dissemination is thought to be transperitoneal seeding, with tumor implants covering the peritoneal and visceral lining of the abdominal cavity and visceral organs. As a result, there can be an extensive amount of tumor involvement of the peritoneal cavity (Figure 16.1).

Cytoreductive surgery is the process by which peritoneal disease is resected and/or ablated to minimal residual disease. Resections are frequently classified as R0 (microscopic tumor clearance), R1 (residual microscopic disease), or R2 (gross residual tumor). The aim of cytoreductive surgery is to achieve at least an R1 resection. R2 resection is generally thought to be less than effective.

The use of intraoperative hyperthermic intraperitoneal chemotherapy (HIPEC) complements the aim of cytoreductive surgery. In HIPEC, chemotherapy is delivered directly into the peritoneal cavity to treat any microscopic residual disease in an effort to reduce the risk for intraperitoneal implantation and/or recurrence [47]. Intraperitoneal chemotherapy has the theoretical advantage of a higher local concentration of a chemotherapeutic, usually mitomycin C or cisplatin, while minimizing systemic toxicity [47, 48]. The agents are delivered at hyperthermic temperatures, 39°–42°C, to potentiate their cytotoxic effects [47, 48]. With successful cytoreduction (R0/R1 resection) plus HIPEC, 5-year survival rates are reported to be as high as 50% [47, 49, 50]. In comparison to systemic chemotherapy, one study reveals improvement of median survival from 12.6 to 22.3 months with cytoreduction and HIPEC [51]. Several studies have analyzed the benefit of cytoreduction and HIPEC (Table 16.1) and will be further discussed in a later chapter.

Palliation

The natural course for cancer can be relentless. About half of the patients diagnosed with solid tumors will die from the sequelae of their disease. In bowel malignancies, some patients may require surgical intervention for the relief of symptoms secondary to tumor progression. Disease progression can lead to bowel obstruction, fistula formation, bleeding, malnutrition,

Table 16.1 Selected results from cytoreduction and hyperthermic intraperitoneal chemotherapy for peritoneal carcinomatosis literature.

Author	Date	Patients (n)	Chemotherapy	Overall survival
Fujimura [52]	1999	25	Multiple	55% at 1 year 26% at 3 years
Beaujard [43]	2000	83	MMC	Small granulations 41% at 3 years Bulky disease 10% at 1 year
Cavaliere [54]	2000	40		−61.4% at 2 years Median survival 30 months
Elias [55]	2001	64	MMC	60.1% at 3 years 27.4% at 5 years
Loggie [56]	2000	84	MMC	Median survival 14.3 months
Piso [57]	2001	17	Cisplatin	75% at 4 years
Shen [58]	2003	109	MMC	61% at 1 year 33% at 3 years Median survival 16 months
Sugarbaker [49]	1999	385	MMC	86% at 5 years with complete cytoreduction 20% at 5 years with incomplete cytoreduction
Jeung [59]	2002	49	5-FU	Median survival 12 months
Yonemura [60]	2005	107	MMC, Etoposide, Cisplatin	Median survival 11.5 months
Roviello [50]	2006	59	MMC/Cisplatin	50.8% 5 year survival

MMC, mitomycin C; 5-FU, 5-Flourouracil.

and pain. Surgery, such as bowel diversion, venting ostomies and wound management, may relieve pain and suffering. The surgeon is tasked with selecting patients who may benefit from such surgeries. Judicious patient selection is important, to avoid unnecessary surgery for end-stage patients who may otherwise be better served with less invasive intervention, such as endoscopic intestinal stenting, somatostatin analogs, or pain medication for effective symptom relief [61–64]. Patients with widespread disease burden and a very limited lifespan may perhaps be more optimally served by hospice care.

An example where palliative resection of primary tumor may be beneficial is in stage IV breast cancer patients with painful, bleeding, or infected locally advanced disease in the breast (Figure 16.2). Although not curative, palliative mastectomy may play a role for symptom relief and quality of life improvement. In a subset of patients, palliative mastectomy may impact on an improvement in median survival [65].

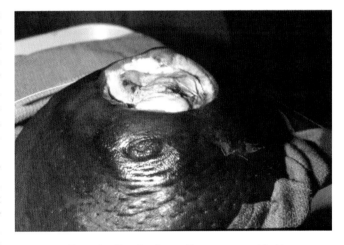

Figure 16.2 Example of locally advanced breast cancer with skin involvement and necrosis present.

Reconstructive and Plastic Surgery

Reconstructive and plastic surgery is an important part of oncologic surgery. The aim is to improve the quality of life of cancer patients, be it functional and/or cosmetic. The term, oncoplastic surgery, refers to the application of reconstructive and plastic surgery to oncology. Perhaps the most common type is breast reconstruction following simple or partial mastectomy. The purpose of oncoplastics in breast surgery is to avoid asymmetry and disfigurement. Plastic surgeons employ various methods for tissue expansion, autologous (advancement flaps and free flaps) or prosthetic, together with breast reduction

surgery techniques, to obtain optimal symmetry and cosmetic results [66]. In patients requiring simple mastectomy, skin sparing or nipple sparing techniques may be an option [67]. The preservation of skin allows for more cosmetically appealing reconstructions. Importantly, with any reconstruction, oncologic principles are not compromised. Tumor size, location, distance from the nipple and mulifocality are all factors, which must be considered prior to cosmesis [68].

Another example of where surgical reconstruction is critical is in the care of patients after radical resection for head and neck cancer. Composite resection of locally advanced head and neck malignancy often results in loss of function, including speech and ability to eat, or compromise in airway. Surgical reconstruction after ablative surgery can restore functional and esthetic loss and improve patient quality of life [69].

Surgical Prophylaxis

Although surgery cannot correct an inherited genetic defect that predisposes a patient to certain malignancies, removal of an end organ prior to cancer development has been effective in reducing future morbidity and mortality. With advancements in DNA testing for germ line mutations, prophylactic surgery prior to the development of certain cancers may be possible, thereby impacting a patient's long-term survival. This strategy, termed surgical prophylaxis, has been found to be beneficial for a number of genetically dependent malignancies. This includes patients with mutations in the *RET* gene (medullary thyroid carcinoma) [70], *BRCA1* gene (breast [71] and ovarian cancer [72]), and the APC gene (familial adenomatous polyposis syndrome) [73, 74]. Patient selection is crucial and must be weighed against subsequent postsurgical sequelae, including the development of secondary malignancies. Important factors to consider include lifetime risk for developing the specific cancer, a reliable way to identify at-risk patients for surgery, and a sensitive way to screen patients for de novo cancer after surgery [74].

Information on familial cancer syndromes can be found in Chapter 5: however, a brief discussion follows. Medullary thyroid carcinoma (MTC) develops in nearly 100% of patients with the *RET* oncogene mutation, seen in patients with MEN 2A, 2B and familial MTC [74, 75]. Prophylactic thyroidectomy prior to development of MTC in these patients is critical, as treatment for advanced MTC is largely ineffective [74]. *BRCA* mutations are associated with development of breast and ovarian cancers. *BRCA 1* mutation increases the lifetime risk for breast cancer from 3.8% to approximately 55–85% [74, 76, 77]. Likewise, ovarian cancer risk is increased from 1.5% to 15–65% [76, 77]. Prophylactic oophorectomies and mastectomies have been successful in reducing the risk of cancer development in patients with inherited *BRCA* mutations [74, 78]. Patients with *APC* gene mutation (familial adenomatous polyposis) have a 90% or greater chance of developing colorectal cancer, usually preceded by polyposis of the large intestine [74]. Patients identified by family screening for polyposis have better survival rates (87–94%) when compared to symptomatic patients with cancer at the time of colectomy (41%) [73, 79]. *APC* gene mutations are also associated with development of extracolonic tumor manifestations (desmoid tumors and periampullary adenocarcinoma) which are not as successfully salvaged by additional surgery, illustrating the limitations of surgical prophylaxis [73].

Access Surgery

Intravenous administration of systemic chemotherapy can be very distressing for patients. Access to veins can often be challenging, especially when repeated access has resulted in vein loss secondary to sclerosis. Central venous access, via tunneled catheters, port-a-catheters, or peripherally inserted central catheters can be far less distressing when systemic therapy needs to be administered for a prolonged period. In addition, when properly managed, central venous access can also be used for blood draws. Surgeons may elect to access the central venous system in a variety of ways, including internal jugular and subclavian vein access, via the Seldinger technique (percutaneous), or by cephalic vein cutdown. It is generally preferable not to access the femoral vein due to the higher incidence of infectious and thrombotic complications [80].

Surgical access for regional perfusion of chemotherapy is another example of access surgery. Regional chemotherapy allows for high concentrations of chemotherapeutics to be delivered to cancer cells while reducing systemic toxicity. Examples of access surgery for regional chemotherapy are hepatic artery infusion and isolated limb perfusion.

In hepatic artery infusion, the theoretical advantage of this chemotherapy administration technique, to treat liver colorectal metastasis, comes from the observation that metastatic lesions derive most of their blood supply from the hepatic artery while the portal circulation feeds hepatocytes. This allows a higher dose of chemotherapeutic agent(s) delivery to the metastases, but limits hepatic and systemic toxicity [81]. In hepatic artery infusion, an infusion pump is placed subcutaneously and connected to a catheter placed directly into the hepatic artery. Care must be taken to avoid inadvertent catheterization of the gastroduodenal artery, which will result in infusion of the stomach and small bowel with high dose chemotherapy and the subsequent complications.

In isolated limb perfusion, regional chemotherapy is administered to a confined extremity, such as in extremity melanoma and sarcoma. Intraoperatively, the major arterial and venous inflow and outflow are cannulated, allowing for connection to an oxygenated extracorporeal circuit. Systemic circulation is minimized by applying a tourniquet proximally. Chemotherapeutic agent(s) can then be infused, for example melphalan in the case of melanoma, in an attempt to control regional disease not amenable to limb salvage surgery [82].

Recent Surgical Technical Innovations

For the remainder of this chapter, two relatively new technical innovations in surgery will be discussed. The next section will discuss minimally invasive surgery (MIS) in cancer, specifically on colorectal cancer, as data for MIS in colorectal cancer is perhaps most mature. The second section is devoted to the application of robotic-assisted surgery in cancer. This is a more recent addition to the armamentarium of surgical oncology; as such, it is a rapidly evolving field with less data. However, the application of robotics-assisted surgery in urologic oncology is more developed and will be discussed briefly.

Minimally Invasive Surgery

Minimally invasive surgery (MIS) is a broad term to cover any procedure that is less invasive than standard open surgery, performed for the same purpose. MIS encompasses a wide spectrum of approaches, ranging from standard multiport

Table 16.2 Comparison of laparoscopic colectomy versus open colectomy randomized controlled trials.

Trial	Date	Open			Laparoscopic			Conclusions
		n	Complications (%)	LOS	*n*	Complications (%)	LOS	
COST[84]	2004	432	85(20)	6	433	92(21)	5*	No survival/recurrence advantage for laparoscopic colectomy. Laparoscopic colectomy is a safe alternative to open colectomy.
CLASICC[85]	2005	268	85(32)	11	526	172(33)	9*	In the short-term, laparoscopic surgery is as effective as open surgery for colon cancer. Laparoscopic LAR not yet justified due to impaired short-term results.
COLOR[86]	2005	621	110(20)	9.3	627	111(21)	8.2*	Although patients undergoing laparoscopic colon resection have longer duration of surgery, they have shorter LOS, less blood loss and tolerate oral fluid intake earlier. No difference in short-term oncologic outcomes.

COST, Clinical Outcome of Surgical Therapy Study; CLASICC, Conventional versus Laparoscopic-Assisted Surgery in Patients with Colorectal Cancer Trial; COLOR, Colon Cancer Laparoscopic or Open Resection Trial; LAR, low anterior resection; LOS, length of postoperative hospital stay in days.
* Indicates statistically significant difference <0.05.

laparoscopic surgery, to single port laparoscopic surgery, to "no" incision surgery via endoscopic approach. The common goal is to have a less visible scar, with the primary intent to reduce postoperative pain and hospital stay while increasing patient satisfaction. Surgical oncologists use minimally invasive approaches to stage, palliate, and cure cancer while attempting to follow previously established oncologic principles.

The role of MIS for palliation and staging continues to evolve. For example, biliary and bowel obstructions can be relieved using laparoscopic or endoscopic means, by stenting or bypass, with increased patient comfort and ease, and without open surgery [83]. Likewise, mediastinoscopy and laparoscopy provide means to obtain biopsy accurately for tissue diagnosis and staging of patients, thereby improving patient selection for neoadjuvant therapy, staged surgery with curative intent, or palliative therapy.

In MIS with curative intent, the most mature data demonstrating equivalent cancer outcome between open surgery and MIS is in colorectal cancer. Initially, concerns for MIS for colorectal cancer revolved around proper oncologic resections, that is, adequate lymphadenectomy, achieving a tumor-free surgical margin, and risk for port site metastasis. Advocates for MIS argued that there would be marked improvement as measured by decreased hospital stay, less pain, and a better quality of life. Three separate randomized controlled trials have addressed these concerns (Table 16.2). Results from these trials confirmed that oncologic outcomes for open versus laparoscopic colon resection were equivalent [2, 84–86]. Importantly, as a result of these studies, MIS for colon cancer has been endorsed by the American Society of Colon and Rectal Surgeons (ASCRS) as well as the Society of American Gastrointestinal Endoscopic Surgeons (SAGES) [2]. Of note, the authors of the Conventional versus Laparoscopic-Assisted Surgery in Patients with Colorectal Cancer (CLASICC) Trial did not suggest routine laparoscopic rectal resections for rectal cancer due to higher rates of positive circumferential resection margins (though not significant) and worse short-term outcomes [85].

Laparoscopic surgery for the treatment of cancer has been described for multiple organ systems including the esophagus, pancreas, adrenal glands, stomach and liver [2]. However, randomized clinical trials comparing open versus MIS are not likely to be available for all visceral organs, and organ-specific limitations, such as the observation of a higher risk for failure in rectal cancer as reported in the CLASSICC trial, may impact outcomes.

Robot-Assisted Surgery

Robot-assisted surgery, when added to MIS, offers the additional advantages of camera stability, three-dimensional views, wristed instruments, and elimination of parallax [87, 88]. The improved degree of freedom, especially in a confined space, is particularly attractive when applied to pelvic surgery. Thus, it is not surprising that the gynecologic oncologist and the urologic oncologist were the first to apply robot-assisted MIS to their armamentarium. As such, the most mature data examining robotic-assisted surgery compared to MIS alone or open surgery is perhaps in the prostate cancer literature.

The robot-assisted laparoscopic prostatectomy (RALP) is now a commonly performed surgery and exceeds the number of open and laparoscopic radical prostatectomies [89]. Through meta-analysis, robotic prostatectomy has been reported to be associated with shorter length of stay, fewer readmissions, fewer ureteral injuries, and fewer deep vein thrombosis events when compared to open and laparoscopic prostatectomies [89, 90]. Regarding surgical margins, RALP is considered comparable or superior to open prostatectomy and laparoscopic resection [89–91]. Preservation of urinary and sexual function is of high importance in patients undergoing radical prostatectomy [89]. Randomized controlled trials and meta-analyses of observational studies have generally found RALP to be comparable or superior to laparoscopic radical prostatectomy or open prostatectomy regarding urinary continence and erectile function [92–94].

In surgical oncology, robot-assisted surgery is being evaluated by a number of surgeons to assess the cost–benefit ratio of this technology. An example is in robotic-assisted adrenalectomy where outcomes have been found to be similar to patients undergoing laparoscopic resection [95, 96]. However, the cost of robotic-assisted adrenalectomy was determined by one study to be 2.3 times higher than that of laparoscopic adrenalectomy [96]. For robotic adrenalectomy and other robotic oncologic resections, randomized controlled trials are needed to determine potential benefit to counterbalance higher costs. Paradoxically, advantages of robotic surgery may only become apparent with more surgeon experience, which may not be possible due to potential funding issues.

Robot-assisted colorectal MIS surgeries, including low anterior resections, right and left hemicolectomies and abdominoperineal resections, have been performed and analyzed [89]. Unfortunately, studies at this time are limited to meta-analysis and systematic reviews. With this in mind, when compared to laparoscopic colectomy, current literature suggests that short-term outcomes (length of stay, estimated blood loss, conversion to open) are similar [89, 97, 98]. However, the cost of robotic-assisted colorectal surgery is significantly higher than open and laparoscopic means ($14,080 vs $9,120 and $8,386, respectively; $P < 0.01$) [99]. Before conclusions can be made regarding robotic-assisted colorectal surgery, long-term results of randomized controlled trials, including a current ongoing multicenter trial (ROLARR trial) [100], are needed. Furthermore, role, cost effectiveness, and efficacy of robot-assisted surgery for cancer remains to be fully defined.

Summary

Surgery in cancer care has evolved rapidly in the past 100 years. In solid tumors, the surgeon continues to play a critical role in many aspects of the treatment and diagnosis. This includes first and foremost, the role of complete surgical resection of a primary tumor with potential for cure (curative intent) when disease is confined locally. This is now complemented by a multidisciplinary approach to optimize clinical outcome with adjuvant therapy, be it radiation therapy for locoregional control, or systemic therapy, such as chemotherapy, hormonal manipulation or biologics to reduce the risk for systemic recurrence. A surgeon's role in cancer care involves obtaining tissue for diagnosis, staging the extent of the malignancy, selecting and performing the proper surgery with curative intent, determining the need for neoadjuvant versus adjuvant therapy to improve outcome, managing the presentation of an isolated metastatic lesion, providing surgical palliation, improving functional and cosmetic outcome, performing surgical prophylaxis prior to malignant transformation, or helping our colleagues with access surgery for delivery of systemic therapy.

References

1 Papac R. Origins of cancer therapy. *Yale J Biol Med* 200;74(6):391–8.

2 Rosenberg SA. Principles of surgical oncology. In: VT Devita (ed.) *Principle and Practice of Oncology*, 8 edn. Philadelphia: Lippincott Williams and Wilkins, 2008: 283–4.

3 Moore CH. On the influence of inadequate operations on the theory of cancer. *Roy Med Chir Soc Lond* 1867;1:244–80.

4 Cotlar, AM, Dubose JJ, Rose DM. History of surgery for breast cancer: radical to the sublime. *Curr Surg* 2003;60(3):329–37.

5 Halsted, WS. The results of radical operations for the cure of carcinoma of the breast performed at the Johns Hopkins Hospital from June, 1889 to January, 1894. *Johns Hopkins Hosp Reports* 1894 Jul;4:297–327.

6 Bland CS. The Halsted mastectomy: present illness and past history. *West J Med* 1981;134:549–55.

7 Langley RR, Fidler IJ. The seed and soil hypothesis revisited—the role of tumor-stroma interactions in metastasis to different organs. *Int J Cancer* 2011;128:2527–35.

8 National Surgical Adjuvant Breast and Bowel Project. Over 50 years of Clinical Trial History. Available from: http://www.nsabp.pitt.edu (accessed 31 May 2017).

9 Fisher B, Montague E, Redmon C, *et al*. Comparison of radical mastectomy with alternative treatments for primary breast cancer: a first report of results from a prospective randomized clinical trial. *Cancer* 1977;39(6 Suppl):2827–39.

10 Fisher B, Bauer M, Margolese R, *et al*. Five-year results of a randomized clinical trial comparing total mastectomy and segmental mastectomy with or without radiation in the treatment of breast cancer. *N Engl J Med* 1985;312(11):665–73.

11 Cady B. Basic principles in surgical oncology. *Arch Surg* 1997;132(4):338–46.

12 Devita VT, Chu E. A history of cancer chemotherapy. *Cancer Res* 2008;68(21):8643–53.

13 Fisher B, Carbone P, Economou SG, *et al*. 1-Phenylalanine mustard (L-PAM) in the management of primary breast cancer. A report of early findings. *N Engl J Med* 1975; 292(3):117–22.

14 Bonadonna G, Brusamolino E, Valegussa P, *et al*. Combination chemotherapy as an adjunct treatment in operable breast cancer. *N Engl J Med* 1976;294(8):405–10.

15 Willems SM, van Deurzen CH, van Diest PJ. Diagnosis of breast lesions: fine-needle aspiration cytology or core needle biopsy? *A review. J Clin Pathol* 2012;65(4):287–92.

16 Olumi AF, Richie JP. Urologic surgery. In: CM Townsend, RD Beauchamp, BM Evers, *et al*. (eds) *Sabiston Textbook of Surgery*, 17th edn. Philadelphia: Saunders, 2004:2283–318.

17 Steer ML. Exocrine pancreas. In: CM Townsend, RD Beauchamp, BM Evers, *et al*. (eds) *Sabiston Textbook of Surgery*, 17th edn. Philadelphia: Saunders, 2004:1643–78.

18 Bakkum-Gomez JN, Richardson DL, Seamon LG, *et al*. Influence of intraoperative capsule rupture on outcomes in stage in epithelial ovarian cancer. *Obstet Gynecol* 2009;113(1):11–17.

19 Gospodarowicz, MK. Hodgkin's lymphoma – patients' assessment and staging. *Cancer J* 2009;15(2):138–42.

20 Carde P, Hagenbeek A, Hayat M, *et al*. Clinical staging versus laparotomy and combined modality with MOPP versus ABVD in early-stage Hodgkin's disease: the H6 twin randomized

trials from the European Organization for Research and Treatment of Cancer Lymphoma Cooperative Group. *J Clin Oncol* 1993;11(11):2258–72.

21 Morton DL, Thompson JF, Essner R, *et al.* Validation of the accuracy of intraoperative lymphatic mapping and sentinel lymphadenectomy for early-stage melanoma: a multicenter trial. *Ann Surg* 1999;230(4):453–65.

22 Krag DN, Anderson SJ, Julian TB, *et al.* Sentinel-lymph-node resection compared with conventional axillary-lymph-node dissection in clinically node-negative patients with breast cancer: overall survival findings from the NSABP B-32 randomised phase 3 trial. *Lancet Oncol* 2010;11(10):927–33.

23 Stojadinovic A, Nissan A, Protic M, *et al.* Prospective randomized study comparing sentinel lymph node evaluation with standard pathologic evaluation for the staging of colon carcinoma: results from the United States Military Cancer Institute Clinical Trials Group Study G1-01. *Ann Surg* 2007;245(6):846–57.

24 Hartgrink HH, van de Velde CJ, Putter H, *et al.* Extended lymph node dissection for gastric cancer: who may benefit? Final results of the randomized Dutch gastric cancer group trial. *J Clin Oncol* 2004;22(11):2069–77.

25 Edge SB, Carducci M, Byrd DR (eds) *AJCC Cancer Staging Manual*, 7th edn. New York: Springer-Verlag, 2009.

26 Breslow A. Tumor thickness, level of invasion and node dissection in stage I cutaneous melanoma. *Ann Surg* 1975;182(5):572–5.

27 Balch CM, Urist MM, Karakousis CP, *et al.* Efficacy of 2-cm surgical margins for intermediate-thickness melanomas (1 to 4 mm): results of a multi-institutional randomized surgical trial. *Ann Surg* 1993;218(3):262–9.

28 Veronesi U, Cascinelli N. Narrow excision (1-cm margin): a safe procedure for thin cutaneous melanoma. *Arch Surg* 1991;126(4):438–41.

29 Morrison BA. Soft tissue sarcomas of the extremity. *BUMC Proceedings* 2003;16(3):285–90.

30 Wolmark N, Wang J, Mamounas E, Fisher, B. Preoperative chemotherapy in patients with operable breast cancer. Nine-year results from NSABP B-18. *J Natl Cancer Inst Monogr* 2001;30:96–102.

31 Baldini E, Gardin G, Evangelista G, *et al.* Long-term results of combined-modality therapy for inflammatory breast cancer. *Clin Breast Cancer* 2004;5(5):358–63.

32 Harris EE, Schultz D, Bretsch H, *et al.* Ten-year outcome after combined modality therapy for inflammatory breast cancer. *Int J Radiat Oncol Biol Phys* 2003;55(5):1200–18.

33 Tsai CJ, Li J, Gonzalez-Angulo AM, *et al.* Outcomes after multidisciplinary treatment of inflammatory breast cancer in the era of neoadjuvant HER2-directed therapy. *Am J Clin Oncol* 2015;38(3):242–7.

34 Urba SG, Orringer MB, Turrisi A, *et al.* Randomized trial of preoperative chemoradiation versus surgery alone in patients with locoregional esophageal carcinoma. *J Clin Oncol* 2001;19(2):305–13.

35 Bannon JP, Marks GJ, Mohiuddin M, *et al.* Radical and local excisional methods of sphincter-sparing surgery after high-dose radiation for cancer of the distal 3 cm of the rectum. *Ann Surg Oncol* 1995;2(3):221–7.

36 Janjan NJ, Khoo VS, Abbruzzese J, *et al.* Tumor downstaging and sphincter preservation with preoperative chemoradiation in locally advanced rectal cancer: the M. D. Anderson Cancer Center experience. *Int J Radiat Onc Biol Phys* 1999; 44(5):1027–38.

37 Billingsley KG, Burt ME, Jara E, *et al.* Pulmonary metastases from soft tissue sarcoma: analysis of patterns of diseases and postmetastasis survival. *Ann Surg* 1999;229(5):602–10.

38 Fong Y, Fortner J, Sun RL, *et al.* Clinical score for predicting recurrence after hepatic resection for metastatic colorectal cancer: analysis of 1001 consecutive cases. *Ann Surg* 1999;230(3):309–18.

39 Kato T, Yasui K, Hirai T, *et al.* Therapeutic results for hepatic metastasis of colorectal cancer with special reference to effectiveness of hepatectomy: analysis of prognostic factors for 763 cases recorded at 18 institutions. *Dis Colon Rectum* 2003;46(suppl):S22–31.

40 Ferrarotto R, Pathak P, Maru D, *et al.* Durable complete responses in metastatic colorectal cancer treated with chemotherapy alone. *Clin Colorectal Cancer* 2011; 10(3):178–82.

41 Fernandez FG, Drebin JA, Linehan DC, *et al.* Five-year survival after resection of hepatic metastases from colorectal cancer in patients screened by positron emission tomography with F-18 fluorodeoxyglucose (FDG-PET). *Ann Surg* 2004;240(3):438.

42 Lanza LA, Putnam JB Jr, Benjamin RS, Roth JA. Response to chemotherapy does not predict survival after resection of sarcomatous pulmonary metastases. *Ann Thorac Surg* 1991;51(2):219–24.

43 Jablons D, Steinberg SM, Roth J, *et al.* Metastasectomy for soft tissue sarcoma. Further evidence for efficacy and prognostic indicators. *J Thorac Cardiovasc Surg* 1989;97(5):695–705.

44 Reyes DK, Pienta KJ. The biology and treatment of oligometastatic cancer. *Oncotarget* 2015;6(11):8491.

45 Franklin JM, Sharma RA, Harris AL, Gleeson FV. Imaging oligometastatic cancer before local treatment. *Lancet Oncol* 2016;17(9):e406–14.

46 Gomez DR, Blumenschein GR, Lee JJ, *et al.* Local consolidative therapy versus maintenance therapy or observation for patients with oligometastatic non-small-cell lung cancer without progression after first-line systemic therapy: a multicentre, randomised, controlled, phase 2 study. *Lancet Oncol* 2016;17(12):1672–82.

47 Esquivel J. Cytoreductive surgery for peritoneal malignancies—development of standards of care for the community. *Surg Oncol Clin N Am* 2007;16(3):653–66.

48 Stewart IV JH, Shen P, Levine EA. Intraperitoneal hyperthermic chemotherapy for peritoneal surface malignancy: current status and future directions. *Ann Surg Oncol* 2005;12(10):765–77.

49 Sugarbaker PH, Chang D. Results of treatment of 385 patients with peritoneal surface spread of appendiceal malignancy. *Ann Surg Oncol* 1999;6(8):727–31.

50 Roviello F, Marrelli D, Neri A, *et al.* Treatment of peritoneal carcinomatosis by cytoreductive surgery and intraperitoneal hyperthermic chemoperfusion (ICHP): postoperative outcome and risk factors for morbidity. *World J Surg* 2006;30(11):2033–40.

51 Verwaal VJ, van Ruth S, de Bree E, *et al.* Randomized trial of cytoreduction and hyperthermic intraperitoneal chemotherapy versus systemic chemotherapy and palliative surgery in patients with peritoneal carcinomatosis of colorectal cancer. *J Clin Oncol* 2003;21(20):3737–43.

52 Fujimura T, Yonemura Y, Fujita H, *et al.* Chemohyperthermic peritoneal perfusion for peritoneal dissemination in various intra-abdominal malignancies. *Int Surg* 1999;84(3):60–6.

53 Beaujard AC, Glehen O, Caillot JL, *et al.* Intraperitoneal chemohyperthermia with mitomycin C for digestive tract cancer patients with peritoneal carcinomatosis. *Cancer* 2000;88(11):2512–19.

54 Cavaliere F, Perri P, Di Filippo F, *et al.* Treatment of peritoneal carcinomatosis with intent to cure. *J Surg Oncol* 2000;74:41–4.

55 Elias D, Blot F, El Otmany A, *et al.* Curative treatment of peritoneal carcinomatosis arising from colorectal cancer by complete resection and intraperitoneal chemotherapy. *Cancer* 2001;92(1):71–6.

56 Loggie BW, Fleming RA, McQuellon RP, *et al.* Cytoreductive surgery with intraperitoneal hyperthermic chemotherapy for disseminated peritoneal cancer of gastrointestinal origin. *Am Surg* 2000;66(6):561–8.

57 Piso P, Bektas H, Werner U, *et al.* Improved prognosis following peritonectomy procedures and hyperthermic intraperitoneal chemotherapy for peritoneal carcinomatosis from appendiceal carcinoma. *Eur J Surg Oncol* 2001;27(3):286–90.

58 Shen P, Levine EA, Hall J, *et al.* Factors predicting survival after intraperitoneal hyperthermic chemotherapy with mitomycin C after cytoreductive surgery for patients with peritoneal carcinomatosis. *Arch Surg* 2003;138(1):26–33.

59 Jeung HC, Rha SY, Jang WI, *et al.* Treatment of advanced gastric cancer by palliative gastrectomy, cytoreductive therapy and postoperative intraperitoneal chemotherapy. *Br J Surg* 2002;89(4):460–6.

60 Yonemura Y, Kawamura T, Bandou E, *et al.* Treatment of peritoneal dissemination from gastric cancer by peritonectomy and chemohyperthermic peritoneal perfusion. *Br J Surg* 2005;92(3):370–5.

61 Mystakidou K, Tsilika E, Kalaidopoulou O, *et al.* Comparison of octreotide administration vs conservative treatment in the management of inoperable bowel obstruction in patients with far advanced cancer: a randomized, double-blind, controlled clinical trial. *AntiCancer Res* 2002;22(2B):1187–92.

62 Tilney, HS, Lovegrove RE, Purkayastha S, *et al.* Comparison of colonic stenting and open surgery for malignant large bowel obstruction. *Surg Endosc* 2007;21(2):225–33.

63 Foster D, Shaikh MF, Gleeson E, *et al.* Palliative surgery for advanced cancer: identifying evidence-based criteria for patient selection: case report and review of literature. *J Palliat Med* 2016;19(1):22–9.

64 Folkert IW, Roses RE. Value in palliative cancer surgery: a critical assessment. *J Surg Oncol* 2016;114(3):311–15.

65 Blanchard D, Kay PB, Shetty SG, Elledge RM. Association of surgery with improved survival in stage IV breast cancer patients. *Ann Surg* 2008;247(5):732–8.

66 Anderson BO, Masetti R, Silverstein MJ. Oncoplastic approaches to the partial mastectomy: an overview of volume displacement techniques. *Lancet Oncol* 2005;6(3):145–57.

67 Gerber B, Krause A, Dieterich M, *et al.* The oncological safety of skin sparing mastectomy with conservation of the nipple-areola complex and autologous reconstruction: an extended follow-up Study. *Ann Surg* 2009;249(3):461–8.

68 Spear SL, Hannan CM, Willey SC. Nipple-sparing mastectomy. *Plas Reconstr Surg* 2009;123(6):1665–73.

69 Mucke T, Wolff KD, Wagenpfeil S, *et al.* Immediate microsurgical reconstruction after tumor ablation predicts survival among patients with head and neck carcinoma. *Ann Surg Oncol* 2010;17:287–95.

70 Wells SA Jr, Chi DD, Toshima K, *et al.* Predictive DNA testing and prophylactic thyroidectomy in patients at risk for multiple endocrine neoplasia type 2A. *Ann Surg* 1994;220(3):237–47.

71 Meijers-Heijboer H, van Geel B, van Putten WL, *et al.* Breast cancer after prophylactic bilateral mastectomy in women with a BRCA1 or BRCA2 mutation. *N Engl J Med* 2001;345(3):159–64.

72 Rebbeck TR, Lynch HT, Neuhausen SL, *et al.* Prophylactic oophorectomy in carriers of BRCA1 or BRCA2 mutations. *N Engl J Med* 2002;346(21):1616–22.

73 Heiskanen I, Luostarinen T, Jarvinen HJ, *et al.* Impact of screening examinations on survival in familial adenomatous polyposis. *Scand J Gastroenterol* 2000;35(12):1284–7.

74 You YN, Lakhani VT, Wells Jr SA. The role of prophylactic surgery in cancer prevention. *World J Surg* 2007;31(3):450–64.

75 Skinner MA, Moley JA, Dilley WG, *et al.* Prophylactic thyroidectomy in multiple endocrine neoplasia type 2A. *N Engl J Med* 2005;353(11);1105–13.

76 Ford D, Easton DF, Stratton M, *et al.* Genetic heterogeneity and penetrance analysis of the BRCA1 and BRCA2 genes in breast cancer families. *Am J Hum Genet* 1998;62(3):676–89.

77 Struewing JP, Hartge P, Wacholder S, *et al.* The risk of cancer associated with specific mutations of BRCA1 and BRCA2 among Ashkenazi Jews. *N Engl J Med* 1997;336(20):1401–8.

78 Kauff ND, Domchek SM, Friebel TM, *et al.* Risk-reducing salpingo-oophorectomy for the prevention of brca1- and brca2-associated breast and gynecologic cancer: a multicenter, prospective study. *Clin Oncol* 2008;26(8):1331–7.

79 Bertario L, Presciuttini S, Sala P, *et al.* Causes of death and postsurgical survival in familial adenomatous polyposis: results from the Italian Registry. Italian Registry of Familial Polyposis Writing Committee. *Semin Surg Oncol* 1994;10(3):225–34.

80 Merrer J, De Jonghe B, Golliot F, *et al.* Complications of femoral and subclavian venous catheterization in critically ill patients: a randomized controlled trial. *JAMA* 2001;286(6):700–7.

81 Kemeny NE, Melendez FD, Capanu M, *et al.* Conversion to resectability using hepatic artery infusion plus systemic chemotherapy for the treatment of unresectable liver metastases from colorectal carcinoma. *J Clin Oncol* 2009;27(21):3465–71.

82 Krementz ET, Carter RD, Sutherland CM, *et al.* Regional chemotherapy for melanoma. A 35-year experience. *Ann Surg* 1994;220(4):520–35.

83 Yim HB, Jacobson BC, Saltzman JR, *et al.* Clinical outcome of the use of enteral stents for palliation of patients with malignant upper GI obstruction. *Gastrointest Endosc* 2001;53(3):329–32.

84 Clinical Outcomes of Surgical Therapy Study Group. A comparison of laparoscopically assisted and open colectomy for colon cancer. *N Engl J Med* 2004;350(20):2050–9.

85 Guillou PJ, Quirke P, Thorpe H, *et al.* CLASICC Trial Group. Short-Term endpoints of conventional versus laparoscopic-assisted surgery in patients with colorectal cancer ulticenter randomized controlled trial. *Lancet* 2005;365(9472):1718–26.

86 Veldkamp R, Kuhry E, Hop WC, *et al.* COlon cancer Laparoscopic or Open Resection Study Group (COLOR). Laparoscopic surgery versus open surgery for colon cancer: short-term outcomes of a randomized trial. *Lancet Oncol* 2005;6(7):477–84.

87 Lanfranco AR, Castellanos AE, Desai JP, *et al.* Robotic surgery: a current perspective. *Ann Surg* 2004;239(1):14–21.

88 Griffen FD, Sugar JG. The future of robotics: a dilemma for general surgeons. *Bull Am Coll Surg* 2013;98(7):9–15.

89 Yu HY, Friedlander DF, Patel S, *et al.* The current status of robotic oncologic surgery. *CA Cancer J Clin* 2013;63(1):45–56.

90 Tewari A, Sooriakumaran P, Bloch DA, *et al.* Positive surgical margin and perioperative complication rates of primary surgical treatments for prostate cancer: a systematic review and meta-analysis comparing retropubic, laparoscopic, and robotic prostatectomy. *Eur Urol* 2012;61(1):541–8.

91 Koch MO. Robotic versus open prostatectomy: end of the controversy. *J Urol* 2016;196:9–10.

92 Asimakopoulos AD, Pereira Fraga CT, Annino F, *et al.* Randomized comparison between laparoscopic and robot-assisted nerve-sparing radical prostatectomy. *J Sex Med* 2011;8(5):1503–12.

93 Ficarra V, Novara G, Rosen RC, *et al.* Systematic review and meta-analysis of studies reporting urinary continence recovery after robot-assisted radical prostatectomy. *Eur Urol* 2012;62(3):405–17.

94 NCCN Clinical Practice Guidelines in Oncology. Prostate Cancer Version 1.2017. nccn.org (accessed 3 May 2017).

95 Brunaud L, Bresler L, Ayav A, *et al.* Robotic-assisted adrenalectomy: what advantages compared to lateral transperitoneal laparoscopic adrenalectomy? *Am J Surg* 2008;195(4):433–8.

96 Brunaud L, Ayav A, Zarnegar R, *et al.* Prospective evaluation of 100 robotic-assisted unilateral adrenalectomies. *Surgery* 2008;144(6):995–1001.

97 Leong QM, Kim SH. Robot-assisted rectal surgery for malignancy: a review of current literature. *Ann Acad Med Singapore* 2011;40(10):460–6.

98 Antoniou SA, Antoniou GA, Koch OO, *et al.* Robot-assisted laparoscopic surgery of the colon and rectum. *Surg Endosc* 2012;26(1):1–11.

99 Kim NK, Kang J. Optimal total mesorectal excision for rectal cancer: the role of robotic surgery from an expert's view. *J Korean Soc Coloproctol* 2010;26(6):377–87.

100 Collinson FJ, Jayne DG, Pigazzi A, *et al.* An international, multicentre, prospective, randomised, controlled, unblinded, parallel-group trial of robotic-assisted versus standard laparoscopic surgery for the curative treatment of rectal cancer. *Int J Colorectal Dis* 2012;27(2):233–41.

17

Radiotherapy

Curtiland Deville, Jr.[1], Gaurav Shukla[2], Ramesh Rengan[3], and Charles R. Thomas, Jr.[4]

[1] *Johns Hopkins University School of Medicine, Baltimore, Maryland, USA*
[2] *Thomas Jefferson University, Philadelphia, Pennysylvania, USA*
[3] *University of Washington, Seattle, Washington, USA*
[4] *Oregon Health and Science University, Portland, Oregon, USA*

Historical Viewpoint

The field of radiotherapy has evolved significantly since 1895, when X-rays were first described by Wilhelm Conrad Roentgen. The first patient cure with radiation was reported in 1899 for treatment of a basal cell epithelioma [1]. For a historical review of this field see references [2–5].

Radiation Physics

Radiation oncology as a field uses energy in the form of ionizing radiation delivered to a target for cure or palliation. A basic understanding of the physical properties of radiation is critical to understand what this radiation is, how it is produced, and how it reacts with tissue.

Electromagnetic Spectrum

Ionizing radiation used in radiotherapy includes both electromagnetic waves and particulate (i.e., particle) radiation. Electromagnetic radiation is energy that is transmitted at the speed of light through oscillating electric and magnetic fields. Electromagnetic waves are part of a broad spectrum that includes radio waves, microwaves, visible light, X-rays, and gamma rays (Figure 17.1). Although electromagnetic radiation is generally described as waves, radiation can also be described as photons or particles with packets of energy. A photon has a wavelength (λ), frequency (ν), and energy $E = h\nu$, where h is Planck's constant of proportionality (6.626×10^{-34} Joule seconds). Substituting for the frequency (ν), this equation becomes $E = hc/\lambda$, where c is the speed of light. The electromagnetic spectrum ranges from wavelengths of 10^5 m for radio waves to 10^{-12} for X-rays and cosmic rays. As energy varies inversely with wavelength, X-rays have a much greater energy than radio waves, which allows X-rays to be deeply penetrating and able to treat deep-seated tumors externally.

Types of Radiation

In radiotherapy, X-rays and gamma rays are the electromagnetic radiation used. These two types of radiation possess the same general properties, differing only in their source and energy.

When the radiation source is at a distance from the target (generally 80–100 cm), the term *teletherapy* is used. Teletherapy allows for a more uniform dose across the target volume. X-rays are produced outside of the nucleus by machines called linear accelerators when energetic, charged particles (usually electrons) impinge on a target and react with either atomic nuclei or orbital electrons. Particulate radiation includes electrons, protons, neutrons, alpha particles, negative pi-mesons, and heavy ions. Due to cost and size constraints, heavy particle radiation research is conducted at a limited number of institutions worldwide, although use is expanding.

When the distance between the radiation source and the target is short, the term *brachytherapy* is used, and generally refers to radiation inserted or implanted into the patient. In brachytherapy, radiation sources include radioactive nuclei that decay and emit positively charged alpha particles, positively charged beta particles, or negatively charged beta particles with a gamma ray. Clinically, alpha particles and beta particles are absorbed locally, and the gamma ray is generally responsible for deposition of radiation dose. Brachytherapy allows for a rapid falloff in dose away from the target volume, as predicted by the inverse square law (see Modalities in Radiotherapy, Brachytherapy section).

Radioactive Decay

The atomic nucleus contains protons and neutrons in usually stable configurations. If unstable, the isotope undergoes spontaneous transformations, that is disintegrations, to attempt to reach a more stable state. This process is called radioactive decay, and the species that undergo these transformations are generally called radioactive. A gamma ray (photon) is released during the decay, which can be used clinically for teletherapy

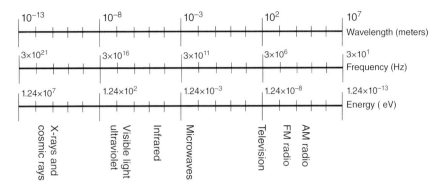

Figure 17.1 The electromagnetic spectrum extending over several orders of magnitude and identifying some of the more commonly noted regions of the spectrum.

(Cobalt-60), or more commonly, brachytherapy (see Modalities in Radiotherapy, Brachytherapy section).

Cobalt-60 has previously been in the United States (US) and continues to be globally an important isotope in external beam radiotherapy. Cobalt machines are considered the first clinical practical megavoltage machines [6]. The radioactive decay of Cobalt-60 releases 1.2 MeV gamma rays. Below 250 keV, maximum dose deposition is at the skin surface while above, it is at some distance below, allowing a "skin-sparing effect". The development of Cobalt-60 machines revolutionized external beam radiotherapy as they were simple in design and mechanically reliable, unlike the limited machines producing comparable MeV beams at the time (e.g., van de Graaf). They allowed for delivery of higher doses of radiation safely, without the limiting skin desquamation that was the hallmark of kilovoltage radiotherapy. Cobalt machines remain in widespread use across the developing world, but in the US have been entirely replaced by linear accelerators.

X-ray Production

Radiotherapy is most commonly delivered with beams of X-rays produced by directing highly accelerated electrons into a target. Modern radiation therapy machines are called linear accelerators. They use microwaves to accelerate electrons at very high energies. These electrons strike a target, usually tungsten, to produce mainly bremsstrahlung, "breaking energy", X-rays. This X-ray beam is "flattened" by a flattening filter to produce a more uniform dose and "collimated" by a collimator so that the beam size can be selected. The beam is then directed at the target volume within the patient. Alternatively, the electron beam can be used directly. In this scenario, rather than striking the target, the electrons strike a scattering foil that spreads out the electron beam, which is then directed to a superficial target.

Interaction with Matter

In tissue, gamma rays and X-rays may interact in several ways, including coherent scattering, photoelectric effect, Compton effect, pair production, and photodisintegration.

The dominant reaction varies with the energy of the radiation in use and composition of the matter. At the energies commonly used in radiotherapy, the dominant reaction is the Compton effect, in which a photon interacts with a loosely bound orbital electron (Figure 17.2). Part of the energy of the *incident* photon is transferred to the electron as kinetic energy. This Compton electron then may interact with other electrons in the surrounding tissue. The remaining energy is carried away by another *scattered* photon, which is less energetic than the original photon. The probability of Compton interactions essentially is independent of the atomic number of the target tissue, depending rather on the electron density of the target tissue. Thus, the amount of radiation absorbed is roughly the same whether the target is bone or soft tissue. In contrast, diagnostic X-rays are of lower energy and react predominantly by the photoelectric effect. In the photoelectric effect, a photon interacts with a tightly bound inner shell electron, resulting in complete absorption of the photon's energy and ejection of the electron from the orbit. The vacancy caused by the removal of the inner orbit electron must be filled by an outer orbit electron resulting in a *characteristic* X-ray. The photoelectric effect is highly dependent on atomic number; therefore, bone and soft tissue appear fairly different on a diagnostic X-ray film. Coherent scattering occurs with low-energy X-rays when a photon is scattered from an electron with a resultant change in direction, but no change in energy. As no energy is transferred it is not significant in therapeutic radiation, or diagnostic radiology; it plays a role in X-ray crystallography. Pair production occurs at higher energies and predominates at about 25 MeV. It occurs when at sufficiently high photon energies, a photon interacts with power nuclear forces and produces an electron-positron pair. Photodisintegration occurs at very high energies when X-rays deposit so much dose into the nucleus that it partially disintegrates with emission of neutrons from the nucleus.

Ionization

Radiation may be directly or indirectly ionizing. Charged particles are *directly ionizing*: if they have sufficient energy, they may directly disrupt the atomic or molecular structure of the material through which they pass and produce chemical and biological changes. Electromagnetic radiation (i.e., photons) and neutrons are *indirectly ionizing*: when they are absorbed in tissue, they give up their energy to produce fast-moving charged

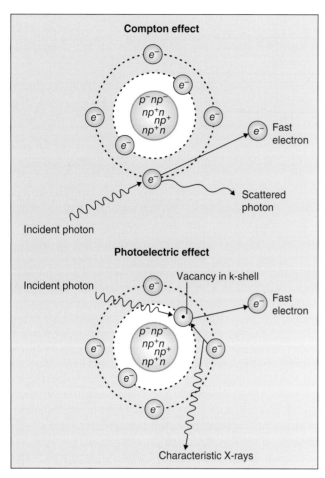

Figure 17.2 X-ray interactions in matter: the Compton effect and the photoelectric effect. The first step in the absorption of a photon of X-rays or gamma rays is the conversion of the energy of the photon into the kinetic energy of an electron or electron-positron pair. At higher energies, when the energy of the incident photon greatly exceeds the binding energy of the bound electrons in the atoms of the absorber, Compton scatter dominates. Part of the photon energy is given to the electron as kinetic energy, whereas the photon is deflected and has reduced energy. At lower energies, when the binding energy of the bound electrons of the atoms of the absorber is not small compared to the photon energy, the photoelectric effect is most important. The photon disappears completely as it interacts with a bound electron. The electron is ejected with kinetic energy equal to the photon energy, less the energy required to overcome the electron bond. The vacancy caused by the removal of the electron must be filled by an electron dropping from an outer orbit, giving rise to a photon of characteristic radiation. *Source:* Cox JD, Ang KK (eds) Radiation Oncology: Rationale, Technique, Results, 8th edn St Louis: Mosby, 2003:5. Reproduced with permission of Elsevier.

particles that then inflict the damage. In the case of electromagnetic radiation, fast-recoil electrons are produced. Neutrons give up their energy to yield fast-recoil protons, alpha particles, and heavier nuclear fragments.

Linear Energy Transfer

Linear energy transfer (LET) refers to the energy transferred per unit track of radiation, or how often a type of radiation will cause ionizations within the tissue through which it travels. X-rays, gamma rays, and electrons, most commonly used clinically in either tele- or brachytherapy, are relatively sparsely

ionizing, and therefore, low LET radiation. Neutrons and other heavy particles interact with the nucleus of an atom rather than with the orbital electrons. Heavy particles dislodge various lower energy showers of densely ionizing protons, neutrons, and others and deposit a large amount of energy over a short distance. This high LET radiation produces many ionizations in its path and is densely ionizing. This will become important when discussing the biologic effects of radiation on tissues (see Radiation Biology section).

Dose Deposition

The absorbed dose from an X-ray beam is the measure of energy deposited by the beam and absorbed by the target. Currently, the unit of absorbed dose is the Gray (Gy) defined as the Joules of energy absorbed in a kilogram of tissue (J/kg), which is equal to 100 rad. As X-rays pass through tissue there is an initial skin sparing and "build-up region" of increasing dose due to the forward moving photons interacting with electrons of the target tissue. There is eventually an area at a certain depth where the number of electrons entering from superficial interactions is exactly equal to the amount leaving that plane, which is termed D_{max} and represents the depth of the maximum number of ionization events. Beyond the D_{max}, the photon beam is "attenuated" as it interacts with tissue and there are fewer photons to travel forward and deposit dose. The beam's energy is the most important determinant on its depth dose and D_{max} in tissue (Figure 17.3). Beam energies produced by linear accelerators are typically in the 4–18 MeV range and depth dose increases with energy. In other words, an 18 MeV beam would have more skin sparing and a deeper D_{max} than a 4 MeV beam. Unlike photons, electrons travel relatively short distances in tissue. As they have much less mass compared to the interacting nuclei, they lose a large fraction of their energy as they travel through tissue leading to less skin sparing and more superficial dose, which makes them clinically useful in treating superficial targets such as skin cancer or in intraoperative radiation therapy (IORT). Other factors affecting the D_{max} are the field size and the tissue density. With larger field sizes there is greater scattering of photons within the field. Lung tissue being less dense allows for great photon transmission. Finally, machine components such as collimators, blocks to spare normal tissue and wedges and compensators, used to shape the field, also affect the delivered dose. All of these factors must be taken into account when determining the dose delivered to a target.

Radiation Biology Interactions and Considerations

Understanding of the biological effects of radiation at the cellular level continues to evolve. It was not until 1922 that radiation oncology became an accepted clinical field. At first, the practice of radiation oncology grew using clinical observations for guidance. The field of molecular biology, which would unearth details of cellular pathways governing cell division, repair, and death, rapidly accelerated in the second half of the twentieth century, leading to a concomitant rise in the area of

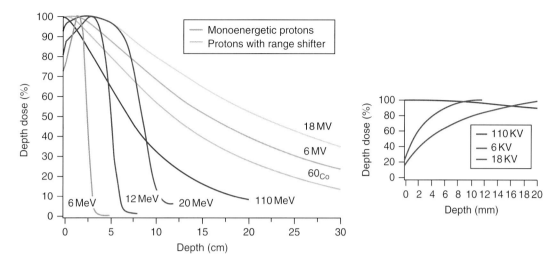

Figure 17.3 Percentage depth-dose curves for a variety of radiation types used in clinical radiation therapy. These include X-rays and γ-rays (110 kV to 18 MV) and various energies of electrons (6–20 MeV). The inset shows the pattern of absorption at shallow depths and provides an illustration of the skin-sparing effect of photons. *Source:* Abeloff M, Armitage J, Niederhuber J, Kastan M, McKenna W (eds) Abeloff's Clinical Oncology, 4th edn. Philadelphia: Churchill Livingstone, 2008:423. Reproduced with permission of Elsevier.

radiobiology. At its essence, radiation involves the deposition of energy via physical interactions into cells (see Radiation Physics section). This leads to ionizations that interact with critical cell structures. The breakage of bonds in these structures triggers many pathways within the cell. If enough damage accumulates, the end result is cell death. This section will elaborate on the complexities of this process, addressing the classic 4Rs of radiation biology: repair, repopulation, reassortment, and reoxygenation.

Interactions with Biologic Materials

While it is not certain that radiation leads to cell killing solely due to effects on DNA, there are abundant data that suggest that DNA is a critical structure in the process. DNA damage after radiation correlates strongly with cell lethality [7] and cells lacking DNA repair capabilities are particularly radiosensitive [8]. Two types of DNA damage have been characterized. *Direct* damage occurs when radiation is absorbed by DNA itself, leading to ionization of its comprising atoms and subsequent damage to the structure. *Indirect* damage occurs when radiation interacts with other molecules in the cell, such as water, leading to the formation of hydroxyl radicals and other oxygen free radicals – all of which can survive long enough to enter the cell nucleus and interact with DNA. Because water is so much more plentiful in the cell than is DNA, it is thought that this indirect pathway is the major mechanism of DNA damage.

Cell Survival Curves

Irradiation of tissues exposes millions of cells to some dose of energy. Each cell may receive a sufficient dose to cause irreparable damage (leading to cell death), or may recover from a sublethal dose. Further, the damage that each cell undergoes may not lead to cell death immediately; it may take hours, days, or even multiple irregular cell divisions before the cell dies. However large the number of cells surviving in a population allows for the generation of cell survival curves (Figure 17.4(a)), which show the relationship between the dose of radiation received and the proportion of surviving cells. These studies have been performed on normal tissue cultures as well as tumor cells, leading to curves characteristic for each cell type. When drawn on a semilog plot, the survival curves typically have a flat "shoulder" at low doses, with a gradually steepening angle downward as dose increases; at higher doses, cell lethality is exponentially related to dose. Many mathematical models have been derived to approximate the empirically obtained curves. The most influential of these is the linear quadratic model, which closely approximates cell behavior at clinically relevant doses [9]. The model proposes that cell death in response to radiation follows two potential events – one related linearly to dose, and one quadratically: $S = \exp(-(\alpha D + \alpha D^2))$, where S represents the fraction of surviving cells in a population after exposure to dose D (Figure 17.4(b)). The parameters α and β (and their ratio, α/β differ for different tissues. Tissues with high ratios tend to exhibit early cell death (and acute effects), while tissues with low ratios tend to exhibit late toxicity. Empirically derived values for these parameters helped lead to the concept of altering the delivery schedule, or fractionation, of radiation better to take advantage of tissue characteristics in differentially killing tumor while attempting to preserve the surrounding local tissue.

Cellular Repair

Single-strand DNA breaks are typically repaired relatively easily, using the opposite template strand, and thus contribute little toward the cell killing process. Double-strand breaks, however, are thought to be the major lesion in leading to cell death [10]. Cells have at least two modes of repair for double-strand breaks. The first, homologous repair, utilizes the undamaged sister chromatid or homologous chromosome as template to fill in missing DNA sequences. By using the template, this method has relatively high fidelity. The second, nonhomologous end joining, simply takes blunt ends of damaged DNA and rejoins

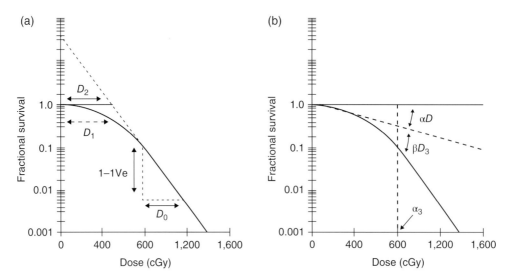

Figure 17.4 Cell survival curve and the linear quadratic model. (a) Typical survival curve for mammalian cells exposed to radiation (X-rays or gamma rays) of low linear energy transfer (low-LET). The curve is described by the initial slope $D1$, the final slope $D0$, and some expression of the width of the shoulder (either n, the extrapolation number, or $D0$, the quasi-threshold dose). (b) Typical survival curve for mammalian cells exposed to low-LET radiation, expressed in terms of the linear-quadratic model. In this model, two components contribute to cell killing: one is proportional to dose (αD), and the other is proportional to the square of the dose (βD^2). The ratio at which these two components are equal is the ratio of α/β. *Source:* Lenhard Jr R, Osteen R, Gansler T (eds) The American Cancer Society's Clinical Oncology, 1st edn. Williston, VT: Blackwell Publishing, Inc., 2001:170.

them. Without a template, this method is susceptible to chromosomal aberrations and mutagenesis. These methods are far less successful than the single-strand break repair methods. Cancer cells that are unable to repair their DNA damage after radiation eventually die by apoptosis, permanent cell cycle arrest, or mitotic catastrophe, depending on the particular signaling cascades including perturbation of the microenvironment that are initiated after the damage takes place.

The shoulder of the cell survival curve is thought to relate to the cell's ability to repair itself after radiation damage, known as *sublethal repair*. It is known that two doses of radiation given separately over time are less effective in cell killing than the sum of the doses given at the same time. The interval between doses has an effect as well, suggesting that repair has measurable kinetics reflected in each tissue's α/β ratio; tissues with high values (e.g., skin and bowel) respond acutely to radiation because they are less able to repair themselves than tissues with lower values (e.g., spinal cord and kidney), which tend to exhibit late effects rather than acute ones. The cell's condition and microenvironment during and after radiation may also influence whether that cell dies. Cells that are not proliferating (either due to poor environmental conditions or simply because they are out of the cell cycle) appear relatively resistant to radiation damage as compared with cells undergoing division [11]. It is thought that the resting cells have more time to repair this *potentially-lethal* DNA damage than their dividing counterparts. Both the sublethal and potentially-lethal damage repair mechanisms appear to require about 6 h in a clinical setting, which helps govern fractionation of radiation doses (see below).

Dose Rate Effects

Survival of cells has been shown to increase as the dose rate decreases [12]. As treatment time to deliver a dose lengthens, cells are able to repopulate in the tissue, potentially leading to diminished cell death. This concept has effects on the severity of acute toxicities as well as late toxicities after radiation. Overall treatment time is also related to cell repopulation; as this value increases, acute toxicity (and also tumor cell kill) decreases as a result.

Cell Cycle Effects

The radiosensitivity of cells changes as a function of the stage in the cell cycle. Cells in late G2 and in mitosis are the most sensitive (Figure 17.5). Cells in mid-to-late S phase and early G2 are most resistant. Cells in late G1 and early S phase are moderately sensitive, while cells in mid G1 are moderately resistant. Hence, preferential killing of cells in radiosensitive stages occurs, with relative accumulation of cells in radioresistant stages. It is hypothesized that the variations in sensitivity due to stage are related to changes in vulnerability and reparability of DNA during different stages [13]. Radiation also has effects on cell progression through the cycle, causing blocks in the G2-to-M phase and G1-to-S phase transitions. The G1 block is *p53* dependent, but because most tumors are *p53* deficient, the G2 block is more critical in leading to cell killing.

Fractionation

The concepts described above form, in part, the biologic basis for the fractionation of radiation dose into smaller divisions. Fractionation allows for normal tissues to undergo sublethal repair mechanisms between doses and for cells in relatively radioresistant stages of the cell cycle to reassort into more radiosensitive stages. In a clinical setting, it appears that approximately 6 h are needed for the repair mechanisms to be optimized in healthy tissues. As described above, early-responding tissues are responsible for acute radiation toxicity, and prolongation of the total treatment time can act to limit the severity of the acute

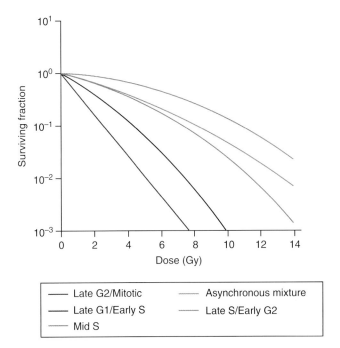

Figure 17.5 Cell cycle and radiosensitivity. Cells are most sensitive to radiation during late G2 and M phases, moderately sensitive during late G1 and S phases, and most resistant in mid S and early G2 phases. *Source:* Hoppe R, Phillips T. Leibel and Phillips Textbook of Radiation Oncology, 3rd edn. Philadelphia: Elsevier Saunders, 2010. Reproduced with permission of Elsevier.

effects. Late-responding tissues, however, typically show superior sublethal repair mechanisms and thus do not show significant acute toxicity. One consequence of this impact is that late-responding tissues (and indeed, these include many normal organs relative to tumor cells) will be preferentially spared by fractionation of dose. The reasons for this preferential acute radioresistance are not clear, though the increased prevalence of terminally differentiated cells in those tissues (in G0 resting phase) may play a role.

However, the interval between fractions should not be so long as to allow for cancer cell repopulation. Thus, the formulation of a treatment schedule is an optimization issue, often varying uniquely for different types and locations of disease. Standard fractionation in the US has historically ranged from 1.8 to 2.0 Gy per day, delivered 5 days per week, though this protocol emerged as much from considerations of patient/staff convenience and cost/equipment considerations as it did from biologic principles. Relatively more recent research has looked at alternate fractionation methods with promising results (Table 17.1):

- *Accelerated fractionation* refers to reducing the overall duration of total therapy (i.e., the number of days/weeks). The actual number of fractions, size of each fraction, and the total dose delivered may or may not be reduced; the goal is to complete the therapy sooner to reduce the risk of tumor cell repopulation.
- *Hyperfractionation* refers to increasing the number of fractions of treatment without changing the total treatment time. While patients receive a smaller dose per fraction, the increased number of fractions permits escalation to a larger total dose without increasing risk of late normal tissue toxicity.
- *Hypofractionation*, refers to decreasing the total number of fractions while delivering a larger dose per fraction. Historically this technique was reserved for palliation in patients having life expectancies that warranted the immediate benefit of larger doses over the risk of late toxicity. However, in the image-guided radiation therapy (IGRT) era, with the ability to better exclude normal tissues, there may be a benefit for hypofractionation in the curative setting. Clinical trials, particularly in brain, breast, lung, and prostate cancer have shown encouraging results and present increasingly acceptable, alternative dose regimens [14].

Oxygenation

The cell's environment can play a role in its response to radiation. The major microenvironmental factor is oxygen [15]. Decreased levels of oxygen (hypoxia) in tissue lead to a decreased response to radiation, while normal levels of oxygenation, such as those seen in normal tissues, are radiosensitizing. This effect is thought to be related to the indirect

Table 17.1 Examples of fractionation regimens.

		Week 1	2	3	4	5	6	7	Dose (Gy)	Fraction no.	Total dose (Gy)
Standard fractionation		|||||	|||||	|||||	|||||	|||||	|||||	|||	2.0	33	66
Accelerated fractionation	a.m.	|||||	|||||	|||||	|||||				1.6	42	67.2
	p.m.	|||||	|||||	|||||	|||||						
Accelerated boost	a.m.	|||||	|||||	|||||	|||||	|||||	|||||		1.8	40	69
	p.m.					|||||	|||||		1.5		
Hyperfractionation	a.m.	|||||	|||||	|||||	|||||	|||||	|||||	|||||	1.15	70	80.5
	p.m.	|||||	|||||	|||||	|||||	|||||	|||||	|||||	1.15		
Hypofractionation		|||||	|||||	|||||	|||||	|||||			2.5	25	62.5

method of DNA damage, in which radiation energy leads to the creation of oxygen radical species that then react with DNA molecules. The presence of oxygen also inhibits the repair of damaged molecules, which are typically facilitated by reduction reactions that are blocked by the presence of oxygen via the formation of irreversible peroxides. Oxygenation becomes important in tumor cell killing because tumors typically outgrow their blood supply, rendering significant amounts of tissue hypoxic as compared to normal tissue [16]. Tumors contain necrotic areas surrounded by chronically hypoxic foci, just out of the reach of sufficient vascular supply; these foci are largely radioresistant and theoretically limit the efficacy of radiation treatment. However, as tumor cells die in response to treatment, surviving cells in previously hypoxic areas may move back into the range of vascular supply, allowing them to reoxygenate and regain their radiosensitivity.

Radiosensitizers and Radioprotectors

For more than three decades, clinicians have administered chemotherapeutic agents in concert with radiation to take advantage of their synergistic effects. These include: antimetabolites (e.g., 5-fluorouracil, gemcitabine), which inhibit DNA synthesis during early S phase, prolonging that radiosensitive cell cycle period; platinums (including cisplatin and carboplatin), which cause inter- and intrastrand DNA crosslinks, leading to DNA strand breaks during attempted repair; and taxanes (paclitaxel and docetaxel), which stabilize microtubules, leading to prolongation of the radiosensitive G2 and M phases. All have been shown to increase cell killing when delivered concurrently with radiation, depending on the disease site.

Molecularly targeted agents are a promising area of research for radiosensitization, as they are potentially less toxic than chemotherapeutic agents and are often not sufficiently efficacious when given alone. The epidermal growth factor receptor (EGFR) is perhaps the most established target; antibodies (cetuximab) and molecular inhibitors (erlotinib) have been developed and are being tested in clinical trials. DNA damage response pathways are another target, with Chk1 inhibitors showing sensitization benefit in tumor cell cultures [17].

Methods to increase the partial pressure of oxygen in tumors to increase radiosensitivity have been explored, including hyperbaric oxygen therapy or administration of erythropoietin during treatment, but these have had mixed results without conferring a generalizable benefit. Nitroimidazoles, which may potentiate the effect of free radicals, have had some success in improving radiosensitivity in animal models, but have yet to show effect in humans, perhaps due to the inability of these agents to adequately diffuse into poorly vascularized hypoxic tissues. New methods to overcome the hypoxia problem are emerging. Tirapazamine, a prodrug, becomes activated into a cytotoxin under hypoxic conditions, with the possibility of a synergistic effect with radiation [18]. Radioprotection is also being explored, with the goal of differential sparing of normal tissues. Compounds containing sulfhydryls (e.g., amifostine), which may act as free radical scavengers, may confer some benefit in reducing toxicity in head and neck cancers and are being explored for use in other sites.

Clinical Sequelae, Toxicity, and Survivorship

An understanding of *radiation toxicity* is critical for members of the healthcare team and patient because normal tissues are affected adversely by radiation. The goals should be well defined prior to its onset. Patients being treated with curative intent may accept a certain risk of undesirable side effects if the end goal is to eradicate disease and prolong survival. Theoretically, they should receive the highest possible dose to the tumor to maximize the potential for tumor control while minimizing the incidence of severe toxicity. On the other hand, patients with incurable disease receiving palliative treatment to improve quality of life may be less willing to endure iatrogenic side effects.

All organs have a threshold for toxicity, though they are difficult to quantify precisely due to the interaction of many factors, It is clear that the total dose delivered and the volume of the organ exposed to radiation are two important factors. Tumor localization, dose rate, fractionation, the use of radiosensitizers and/or radioprotectors, and the choice of modality can also be modulated. Other types of treatment (medical and/or surgical) may be utilized to further manage undesirable side effects. Still, while technological advances in radiation delivery have significantly improved this optimization problem, the balancing act between the risk of complications and the potential for cure remains. Radiation toxicities can be subdivided into acute and late effects. Acute effects are those observed during or immediately following a course of radiation, while late effects do not appear until at least 3–6 months after the conclusion of therapy. Much effort has been made to better relate irradiated organ doses to clinical toxicities. Table 17.2 shows the Quantitative Analyses of Normal Tissue Effects in the Clinic (QUANTEC) summary for approximate dose/volume data correlated to outcome for several organs following conventional fractionation [19]. It is important to note that QUANTEC values are generally derived from conventional fractionation schemes and 3D conformal techniques; with the increasing use of intensity modulated radiation therapy (IMRT) and hypofractionated approaches, the normal tissue complication probability (NTCP) models will likely undergo re-evaluation and modification. Acute effects typically occur in tissues with high α/β ratios (see above) that require rapid cell turnover in the healthy state, such as skin and mucosa. Skin erythema and desquamation are commonly observed, as are oral mucositis, esophagitis, pneumonitis, and hematopoietic cytopenia (again depending on the areas being irradiated). Acute effects are self-limiting, typically resolving within the weeks after treatment concludes, and are thus generally managed symptomatically. Two acute side effects of radiation may occur despite the fact that they do not involve tissues with high rates of cell turnover: nausea and fatigue. The mechanisms for these side effects remain uncertain. Plasma levels of inflammatory cascade cytokines such as TGF-β, TNF-α, and IL-6 appear to be related to the risk of developing acute effects. In the future, these biomarkers may allow for individualization of therapy to reduce that risk.

Occasionally, acute effects can be so severe that they lead to late effects; these are termed "late consequential" effects. A common example is fibrosis and dysphagia following chemoradiation in head and neck cancer. The mucosa is denuded for a prolonged duration during treatment, leading to ulceration. However, late effects can also occur in the absence of

Table 17.2 QUANTEC summary: approximate dose/volume/outcome data for several organs following conventional fractionation.

Critical structure	Maximum dose	Toxicity rate	Toxicity endpoint
Brain	<60 Gy	<3%	Symptomatic necrosis
	72 Gy	5%	
	90 Gy	10%	
Brainstem	<54 Gy	<5%	Neuropathy or necrosis
Brainstem (1 cm^3 point dose)	<64 Gy	<5%	Neuropathy or necrosis
Optic nerve/chiasm	<55 Gy	<3%	Optic neuropathy
	55–60 Gy	3–7%	
	>60 Gy	>7–20%	
Spinal cord	50 Gy	0.2%	Myelopathy
	60 Gy	6%	
	69 Gy	50%	
Larynx	<66 Gy	<20%	Vocal dysfunction
Lung	V20 < 30%	<20%	Symptomatic pneumonitis
Esophagus	V35 < 50%	<30 %	Grade 2+ esophagitis
	V50 < 40%	<30%	
	V70 < 20%	<30%	
Heart (pericardium)	V30 < 46%	<15%	Pericarditis
	V25 < 10%	<1%	Long-term cardiac mortality
Liver	<32 Gy	<5%	RILD (in normal liver function)
	<42 Gy	<50%	RILD (in normal liver function)
	<28 Gy	<5%	RILD (in Child-Pugh A or HCC)
	<36 Gy	<50%	RILD (in Child-Pugh A or HCC)
Kidney (bilateral)	V12 < 55%	<5%	Clinical dysfunction
	V20 < 32%	<5%	
	V23 < 30%	<5%	
	V28 < 20%	<5%	
	<28 Gy	<50%	
Stomach	<45 Gy	<7%	Ulceration
Rectum	V50 < 50%	<10%	Grade 3+ toxicity
	V60 < 35%	<10%	
	V65 < 25%	<10%	
	V70 < 20%	<10%	
	V75 < 15%	<10%	
Bladder	<65 Gy	<6%	Grade 3+ toxicity

Source: Marks *et al.* [19]. Reproduced with permission of Elsevier.

acute effects; these are termed "true late" effects and can occur in virtually any organ that receives radiation. They include fibrosis, fistula formation, and long-term organ damage. The mechanisms for late effects are likely multifactorial and not clearly understood; most hypotheses involve some combination of direct cell depletion in the organ and a loss of functional vasculature supplying that organ. Examples include radiation myelitis, radiation-induced brachial plexopathy, and radiation-induced bowel obstruction. Finally, radiation treatment can lead to secondary cancers likely related to DNA damage and mutagenesis.

Attempts at standardizing toxicity documentation have evolved over the past few decades. Grading scales documented by the healthcare provider include the Common Terminology Criteria for Adverse Events and the Radiation Therapy Oncology Group (RTOG)/ European Organisation for Research and Treatment of Cancer scale [20]. Patient-reported outcomes are also increasingly being evaluated in clinical and research settings, such as the International Prostatic Symptom Scale evaluating urinary function and bother [21]. Long-term morbidity and functional concerns are increasingly important with more long-term survivors. The concept of survivorship has evolved to address this concern. The Institute of Medicine recently advised the mandate of providing patients with treatment summaries and survivorship plans of care to provide better understanding and anticipation of the potential long-term sequelae of complex cancer therapies, such as effects on fertility, mobility, and function [22].

Radiotherapy Processes: Indication, Planning, and Delivery

Clinical Indication

Radiotherapy plays an important role across a wide variety of tumors and sites. Upwards of two-thirds of cancer patients will undergo radiotherapy during the course of their disease [23]. The indication for radiotherapy is generally made in a multidisciplinary setting with input from the entire therapeutic team, which may include physicians – surgical, medical, gynecologic, orthopedic, pediatric, and radiation oncologists, pathologists, diagnostic radiologists – and extended team members – nursing, social work, nutrition, dental, pain management, interventionalists, and other physician extenders.

The indication for radiotherapy is first defined as curative or palliative. In the curative setting treatment may be primary, also referred to as definitive or radical, and in some cases referred to as organ preservation (e.g., laryngeal, bladder, and cervical cancers [24]). If the tumor persists or recurs locally, surgical "salvage" may be offered if feasible.

Radiotherapy may also occur as an adjuvant treatment to reduce the risk of recurrence. This most commonly occurs in combination with surgery as either postoperative therapy, for example lumpectomy followed by radiotherapy in breast conservation therapy, or preoperative, "neoadjuvant", therapy, as with limb salvage for soft tissue sarcoma where preoperative radiotherapy is offered with resection in avoidance of amputation. The aim of combining treatments is to improve the chances of cure by reducing locoregional recurrence while preserving organ function.

Concurrent or sequential systemic and/or targeted therapies may be offered depending on the treatment site, related to aforementioned synergistic effects. These have been demonstrated in large, multi-institutional, cooperative group randomized trials in the treatment of central nervous system, head and neck, lung, gastrointestinal, genitourinary, and gynecologic malignancies [25], importantly leading to significant increases in survival over radiotherapy alone, despite anticipated increases in acute and late morbidity. Novel targeted therapies, such as cetuximab, are similarly showing synergistic effects with radiotherapy and are increasingly being studied as concurrent therapy [26].

Regarding noncurative treatment, radiotherapy is the most common method to palliate tumor-related symptoms. Common indications include the treatment of bone metastases that are causing pain or concerning for impending fracture in a weight-bearing bone. Treatment may be delivered as one fraction ($8\,Gy \times 1$) or other hypofractionated regimens ($3\,Gy \times 10$ fractions, $4\,Gy \times 5$ fractions) to provide rapid pain relief [27]. Radiation remains the main treatment modality for the relief of symptoms in patients with progressive and incurable cancers. It often is employed to stop bleeding or relieve obstruction (e.g., of airway, bowel), and to relieve pain. Other common indications include early intervention for spinal cord compression, brain metastases, or superior vena cava syndrome.

The prescription dose will be dependent on the treatment intent in addition to the disease characteristics, staging studies, extent of disease definable on diagnostic studies or suspected based on known disease patterns, and the available treatment modalities. The dose-limiting factor usually is one or more normal structures in the region. A plan must then be devised to treat this entire region to the dose desired for each region while keeping the volume of normal tissue below its tolerance dose.

Simulation

Successful outcomes are critically dependent on treatment planning methods and techniques. Treatment planning is dependent on imaging and immobilization techniques. The patient is brought for a treatment planning session, often referred to as a *simulation*, where the treatment position will be "simulated" and established to ensure precise reproducibility with each treatment. The patient is positioned in a manner that ensures optimal tumor targeting with protection of normal tissues and organs at risk, strict reproducibility, and comfort to ensure compliance. This is generally achieved with the patient lying flat in the supine or prone position, although there are some other treatment delivery techniques which may utilize a lateral decubitus, seated, or even standing position (e.g., total skin electron beam radiation). Commercially available immobilization devices are often used, such as foam knee supports, vacuumed bags for limbs, body casts, or thermoplastic head masks. These are made and/or indexed at the simulation and are kept for use throughout the entire radiation course for each patient. Children under age 5, or any patient unable to keep still alone in the treatment room may require general anesthesia for simulation and each fraction of radiotherapy.

Mostly now historical, conventional simulators were fluoroscopy units designed to reproduce the geometry of treatment machines. Fluoroscopy was used to outline the boundaries of the field, with plain film X-rays being taken to include the general outline of the area to be treated. Although fluoroscopic simulators still exist today, since the introduction of computed tomography (CT), mostly three-dimensional (3D) treatment planning systems now are available to permit more accurate or more conformal delivery of radiation treatment. 3D treatment planning systems use CT data, which can often be augmented by fusion with other radiologic modalities such as positron emission tomography (PET) and magnetic resonance imaging (MRI). The CT data set is acquired at 1.5–5 mm intervals depending on the treatment site. The most common and efficient method is to use a CT simulator to set up the radiation fields combining the processes of obtaining CT images and field design. Modern techniques include 4D acquisition, which can record and account for motion and is particularly useful for thoracic and abdominal malignancies. CT images of the patient are transferred directly to a computer system that allows the physician to outline the tumor volume and critical structures on individual CT slices. Additional data from MRI scanning or PET imaging can be fused with images obtained in the CT simulator to improve the accuracy of planning. This produces an accurate 3D representation of both the tumor that is to be treated and normal tissues that are to be avoided during the delivery of radiation. At the conclusion of the simulation, the treatment isocenter is defined. Most modern radiation treatments are *isocentric*, meaning that there is one point around which the treatment machine gantry, the couch, and the collimator in the head of the treatment machine rotate. Laser lights in the simulator and the treatment room are used to assist in the positioning of the patient relative to the isocenter. Permanent skin marks, that is India ink tattoos, are generally used to correspond to the laser light coordinates.

Treatment Planning

Next, the target volumes and organs at risk are delineated consistent with International Commission on Radiation Units and Measurements (ICRU) standards [28]. Careful review of the clinical data must be done to delineate the tissue to be treated. The volume to be treated is defined as the *target volume* and is created by adding three components together. First, the *gross tumor volume* (GTV) is delineated. The GTV consists of all known detectable disease, including any abnormal lymph nodes. This volume refers to the total volume of tumor detectable by diagnostic staging procedures such as CT, MRI, PET, and endoscopy. The *clinical target volume* (CTV) encompasses the gross tumor volume plus regions considered to harbor potential microscopic disease and other areas at risk for spread, such as draining lymphatic regions. Multiple CTVs, that is CTV 1, CTV 2...may be defined if various dose levels are to be targeted, for example in the treatment of elective regional lymph nodes, which do not receive the full dose of radiation. The *planning target volume* (PTV) includes a margin around the clinical target volume to allow for internal target motion (e.g., peristalsis, coughing, respiration, etc.), and setup uncertainty. Finally, a margin must be added to account for the physical characteristics of radiation such as the penumbra (the edge of the beam where dose falls off rapidly). If a gross total surgical resection has occurred with no residual detectable tumor, a GTV cannot be defined, and the initial target delineated is a CTV. Finally, the adjacent organs at risk (OAR) are delineated. The RTOG has now defined several publicly available contouring atlases across body sites to aid in consistent and systematic target volume delineation in the modern era of advanced imaging in treatment planning [29].

Once the target volumes and OARs have been defined, a desired prescription dose is determined with dose volume targets established for the GTV, CTV, and PTV, and OAR constraints set, which are provided to the medical physicist and/or treatment planning dosimetrists. Next, treatment planning involves selecting the angles, energy, number, and weighting of beams to deliver the planned dose with the most optimal normal tissue sparing. 3D treatment planning has allowed for more complex treatment as the doses to the tumor and normal organs can be evaluated more accurately with often better estimation of the possible toxicity based on dose-volume exposures, which have been correlated to treatment outcome. The treatment plan is evaluated in part by assessing the plotted dose–volume histogram (DVH),

which shows the dose delivered throughout the volume of the tumor and each normal organ in the radiation field (Figure 17.6). Systematic analyses have been performed across treatment sites to attempt to correlate DVHs with clinical toxicity and were recently summarized in the QUANTEC [18]. Similarly, some data is available on organ tolerance and injury (see section on Radiation Toxicity). It is generally undesirable to treat an organ beyond its known tolerance. However, occasionally there may be instances where an organ is intentionally dosed close to or even beyond its tolerance, particularly in the case where tumor location necessitates and/or function may be spared in the contralateral organ, and/or the organ exists in parallel (as opposed to series). In a serial organ, like the spinal cord, failure of any component of the organ will cause failure of the entire organ distal to the site of exposure. In a parallel organ, such as the lung or kidney, the patient might be able to tolerate loss of part of the organ's function without significant clinical detriment provided certain volume considerations are not exceeded.

Normal tissues and organs at risk can be protected and shielded within radiation beams in various ways. The first "blocks" were manually placed pieces of lead or depleted uranium that were inserted in the radiation field to block the structures below them. With the discovery of a low-melting-point alloy of lead, it became possible to create complex blocks that were custom made for each patient and that followed the divergent properties of the beam to shield organs defined on the simulation films more accurately [30]. More recently, with modern linear accelerators, the time-consuming production and cumbersome, manual-labor usage of custom blocks have been largely replaced by the use of *multileaf collimators* (MLC). The MLC system uses 5–10 mm "leaves" that actually are partitioned jaws of the collimator in the head of the treatment machine. These leaves can be moved in from the edges of the field to block the radiation field and effectively shape the beam as desired.

IGRT

Once treatment planning is completed, digitally reconstructed radiographs (DRRs) are produced from the CT data to represent the treatment fields. *Beam's eye views* also are valuable to the radiation therapists delivering the treatment, since they offer a radiographic representation of the orientation of each beam. Verification of the treatment position is generally performed and the patient begins the course of radiotherapy. Each day, the patient is positioned by the radiation therapists in the exact position in which the simulation and verification were done. To account for variability in target position from fraction to fraction, so-called "interfraction" motion, in the modern era, the reproducibility of the patient's treatment position is monitored on an often, daily basis by the use of portal images taken with on-board imaging while the patient is in the treatment position, referred to as image-guided radiotherapy. Current techniques include kilovoltage or megavoltage imaging compared to the simulation DRR, and cone beam CT compared to the simulation CT. This imaging may sometimes be used in conjunction with implanted fiducial markers. Radiofrequency transponders are also commercially available, which may provide real-time target tracking and provide information on "intrafraction" motion,

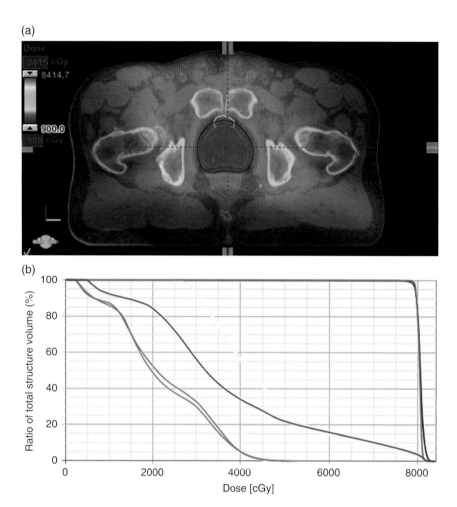

Figure 17.6 Typical prostate IMRT treatment plan using volumetric modulated arc therapy showing conformal avoidance of the rectum (brown), bladder (yellow), and femoral heads (orange and green), while delivering the dose prescription (79.2 Gy) to the clinical (magenta) and planning (navy) target volumes. (a) Axial cross-section with dose color wash. (b) Corresponding dose-volume histograms of the target volumes and organs-at-risk.

which may occur during treatment due to internal organ motion. Generally, a threshold is set, whereby treatment is interrupted if the target moves beyond that threshold. Emerging, but limited evaluation of IGRT techniques suggests improvements in the therapeutic ratio of therapy with the potential for improved tumor control and toxicity profiles. Most notably IGRT techniques are credited for allowing reduction in PTV margins, exposing less normal tissues to high doses of radiation, and further dose escalation to target volumes.

Modalities in Radiotherapy

Technological advances have allowed for continued improvements in techniques to deliver radiotherapy. The most common modalities and techniques that will be reviewed include: brachytherapy, radionuclide therapy, 3D conformal radiotherapy, IMRT, stereotactic radiosurgery, particle therapy, and neutron therapy.

Brachytherapy

Brachytherapy involves the placement of radioactive sources inside or adjacent to the tumor (see Radiation Physics, Radioactive Decay section). Numerous isotopes have been used therapeutically (Table 17.3). It is most commonly used in the treatment of

prostate and cervical cancers, although there are applications in sarcomas, head and neck cancers, and elsewhere. Since the start of the twenty-first century, image guidance has been a point of emphasis [31] in improving the accuracy of source placement via CT, MRI, and/or ultrasound, which improves local control while reducing normal tissue toxicity. Brachytherapy can be subdivided into interstitial, intracavitary, and intravascular methods:

- *Interstitial* brachytherapy involves the placement of sealed sources into the tissue itself. The sources are typically iridium-192 wire or iodine-125 seeds. They may be temporary (e.g., in soft-tissue sarcoma or in oral cavity squamous cell carcinoma), or they may be permanent (e.g., in prostate cancer).
- *Intracavitary* brachytherapy places the radiation source into a body cavity rather than into the tissue. The most common type of intracavitary brachytherapy is for treatment of gynecologic cancer, though it can be utilized in the nasopharynx or rectum.
- *Intravascular* brachytherapy utilizes the vasculature to deliver radioactive sources inside a catheter to a specific anatomic target using fluoroscopic guidance. Recently, this technique has been employed in the treatment of primary hepatocellular cancers and colorectal metastases to the liver via administration of yttrium-90 microspheres through the hepatic artery. It has also been used for treatment of coronary artery stenosis with strontium-90.

Table 17.3 Therapeutic isotopes.

Isotope	Half-life average	Energy (keV)
Photon		
^{226}Ra	1620 y	830
^{137}Cs	30 y	662
^{198}Au	2.7 d	412
^{192}Ir	73.8 d	370
^{125}I	60 d	28
^{103}Pd	16.97 d	21

Isotope	Half-life	Maximum energy (keV)
Beta		
^{32}P	14.3 d	1710
^{90}Sr/^{90}Y	28.5 y/2.7 d	550/2280
^{188}W/^{188}Re	69.4 d/17 h	350/2120
^{186}Re	3.8 d	1070
^{62}Zn/^{62}Cu	9.3 h/9.7 min	660/2930
^{133}Xe	5.2 d	360
^{131}I	8.0 d	600
^{89}Sr	50.5 d	1495
^{166}Ho	26.8 h	1850

Source: Cox JD, Ang KK (eds) Radiation Oncology: Rationale, Technique, Results, 8th edn. St Louis: Mosby, 2003: 6. Reproduced with permission of Elsevier.

To reduce the exposure of the medical staff, the radiation is administered via remote afterloading, in which the implant is connected by sealed tubes to an external source. This system is then triggered to deliver the radiation after the staff has left the shielded treatment room. High dose rate methods, which can be performed on an outpatient basis, are largely replacing low dose rate methods due to the latter's need for hospital admission.

Systemic Targeted Radionuclide Therapy

Another type of internal radiation known as systemic targeted radionuclide therapy may use antibodies or other carriers to deliver radiation selectively to cancer cells while sparing normal tissues. While the biggest advances in molecular engineering have occurred in the last 25 years, this technique has been utilized for over 50 years in treatment of thyroid cancer. Radiolabeled iodine-131 is administered into the bloodstream and because it is selectively taken up and concentrated in the thyroid, it is remarkably efficacious with little side effects other than hypothyroidism and increased risk of secondary malignancy [32]. Hematologic malignancies may express antigens that are potential targets for radioimmunotherapy, or delivery of selective radiation via conjugation to monoclonal antibodies. For example, nearly all B cell lymphomas express CD20, and two agents (tositumomab and ibritumomab tiuxetan) have been developed which target this antigen, with promising response rates [33]. Radioimmunotherapy has shown limited success in the realm of solid tumors, due to severe bone marrow toxicity, poor tumor penetration, and the development of an immune

response to the monoclonal antibodies utilized thus far. Some tumors that express somatostatin receptors appear to be susceptible to peptide receptor radiation therapy, in which somatostatin analogs (e.g., octreotide) are labeled with radioactive sources (e.g., yttrium-90 or lutetium-177) [34]. Radium-223, an alpha emitter that selectively targets bone metastases with alpha particles, shows growing potential with improved survival in the setting of castrate-resistant prostate cancer and bone metastases [35].

Three-dimensional conformal radiation therapy

In three-dimensional conformal radiation therapy (3DCRT), the area of high dose is shaped to the tumor volume while minimizing the dose to the surrounding tissues by using a set of fixed radiation beams with Cerrobend block shielding of normal tissue as previously described, which stop the transmission of photons to those areas desired to be shielded. The development of the linear accelerator offered the ability to deliver shaped beams from multiple angles as it rotated around the patient to deliver a homogenous dose to a target. In this "forward treatment planning", the beam orientation, shape, size, modifiers, and so on are defined first, followed by the calculation of dose that results from this design. Changes to achieve better dose distribution are made by modifying the beam weighting, adding or subtracting beams, and so forth, until the desired dose distribution is achieved.

IMRT

The introduction of the MLC, whereby the machine shapes the beams rather than requiring additional beam-shaping devices such as Cerrobend blocks, made conformal radiation therapy significantly easier. The MLCs, which can move continuously during treatment, allow for the modulated intensity of each beam deliberately to deliver nonuniform doses to varying parts of the treatment field, and ultimately deliver a desired, composite dose distribution to a target and normal tissues. This technology forms the basis for IMRT [36]. Although the treatment can be delivered by standard modern linear accelerators, planning is significantly more labor intensive than conventional radiation therapy and requires the use of more sophisticated modeling software for optimization [37]. Physicist and physician, assisted by sophisticated computer software, evaluate dozens or hundreds of treatment plans that have been "inverse planned" to optimize the dose to the tumor [38]. An important concept used for most IMRT is that of inverse planning, in contrast to the forward planning that is used for most conventional treatment planning. In inverse treatment planning, the desired dose distribution is stated first, followed by computer optimization to adjust beam intensities to attempt to achieve that dose distribution. Optimization includes stating the dose that the tumor and areas at risk should receive, as well as dose limits to normal tissues. These parameters are based on maximizing the probability of tumor control and minimizing the toxicity profiles of the various normal tissues and organs. Because normal tissues have different tolerances, different organs will have different thresholds. After the computer optimizes the dose distribution, the physician may choose what is deemed to be an optimal plan by evaluating the dose distribution and the DVHs (see Figure 17.6). Currently, multiple IMRT delivery techniques are available, including dynamic (sliding window) MLC IMRT, static (step and shoot) IMRT, dynamic conformal arc therapy (DCAT), intensity-modulated arc therapy (IMAT), volumetric modulated arc therapy (VMAT), tomotherapy IMRT, and finally, non-MLC based robotic linac IMRT. Detailed explanation of these is beyond the scope of this chapter; only the latter three are reviewed here.

Tomotherapy uses a narrow slit beam in a manner analogous to a CT scanner [39]. An MLC system is attached to a conventional low-energy megavoltage linear accelerator, and treatment is delivered to a narrow slice of the patient using arc rotation. The beam intensity is varied by interposing the leaves of the collimator in and out of the radiation beam path as the gantry rotates around the patient. Tomotherapy can be integrated with diagnostic CT systems, permitting real-time treatment monitoring and image-guidance, although true-adaptive radiotherapy is not yet commonplace [40]. VMAT treats a patient using one or more arcs, with the MLC defined aperture constantly changing, as well as the rotation speed and the dose rate. VMAT is delivered using a conventional linear accelerator and treats the entire tumor volume at once, unlike tomotherapy, which treats slice by slice [41]. VMAT is also more efficient than conventional IMRT, in that the treatment is delivered over all gantry angles, rather than at a number of specific angles [42]. Finally, robotic linac IMRT involves the placement of a linear accelerator mounted on an industrial robot arm. In this approach, the robot arm provides the ability to aim small beamlets of radiation with any orientation relative to the target volume, thus potentially giving this form of IMRT more flexibility than any of those previously discussed. The treatment plan is thus determined by the trajectory of the robot and the dose delivered at each orientation. This approach was first used as a stereotactic radiosurgery device in the late 1990s [43]. Subsequently, the use of this device (commercially known as Cyberknife®) for sophisticated IMRT was proposed. There are currently several commercially available devices to deliver stereotactic radiotherapy to extracranial sites, sometimes referred to as stereotactic body radiotherapy [44].

Extensive dosimetric studies have verified that IMRT provides superior dose distribution over conventional 3DCRT, but limited clinical data, including sparse randomized trials, exist across various treatment sites, to indicate whether this dosimetric benefit translates into clinical meaningful outcomes [45]. IMRT can be used to enhance the therapeutic ratio via dose escalation and/ or reduction in normal tissue toxicity. Among the cancer sites investigated using IMRT to escalate total dose are breast, head and neck, intracranial, prostate, and gynecologic malignancies [46–50]. It is anticipated that favorable dose distributions should result in decreased toxicity, yet no definitive, randomized study has demonstrated the clinical impact of IMRT in reducing toxicity to normal tissues. Because the dose distributions made possible by IMRT's planning and treatment delivery are superior to conventional conformal 3D plans, improvements in clinical outcomes are expected, although the relative long-term benefits and safety of IMRT in many sites remain to be demonstrated. As with all novel technologies there may be estimated and unknown adverse sequelae [51]. For IMRT, specific concerns include the increased difficulty in verifying treatment, and delivery and dose

relative to 3DCRT, which delivers a homogenous dose. Factors such as organ motion may have a greater impact. Finally, as more beams are added, treatment time increases, then, although less normal tissue will be treated to tolerance doses, the volume of normal tissue that receives some integral dose of radiation (e.g., scattered radiation), in fact, increases, as does the total-body integral dose of radiation, and may relate to issues such as secondary malignancy.

Particle Therapy

Particle beam therapy utilizes subatomic particles instead of X-rays or gamma rays to deliver the dose of radiation. The development and application of particle radiation therapy has gained accelerated interest and has been motivated by its physical and radiobiologic characteristics. The physical property allows for precise dose localization and superior depth dose distribution with heavy charged particles such as protons. The potential radiobiologic advantage for heavier charge particles, such as carbon and helium, are that high LET radiation deposits more dose along its path than conventional X-rays, which are low LET. High-LET radiation is more damaging to hypoxic cells and less cell cycle dependent, and there is less repair of induced damage. Because protons are 1800 times heavier than electrons, accelerating and delivering them to the patient requires higher energies and heavier magnets than photon linear accelerators that employ electron accelerators. Thus, heavy ion particle accelerators are significantly more costly to build and maintain.

Proton Therapy

Although protons have a slightly higher linear energy transfer than X-rays, they are not generally considered high linear energy transfer particles. Their advantage over X-rays is the physical dose distribution. When a heavy, charged particle, such as a proton, passes through tissue, the dose it deposits increases slowly with depth, then reaches a sharp increase at its maximum depth of penetration, called the Bragg peak (Figure 17.7). The maximum depth of penetration can be adjusted by varying the energy of the proton beam or by adding or removing compensating material placed in the path of the beam. Clinically, the Bragg peak is often spread out using specialized filters to achieve the dose deposition pattern desired, but still with the desirable sharp dose fall-off at the deep edge of the beam. Using multiple beams or varying compensators, it is possible to design a conformal 3D dose distribution [52] (Figure 17.8). Proton therapy has often been used for tumors in close proximity to critical normal structures, such as orbital, paranasal sinus, and CNS tumors, including pediatric medulloblastoma requiring craniospinal irradiation [53]. In the treatment of uveal melanoma for example, organ-sparing avoidance of enucleation has been found for a larger majority of patients in separate single institution series [54] in this malignancy that had been difficult to treat with photons due to toxicity to normal structures of the eye. Tumors involving the skull base, such as chordoma or chondrosarcoma are difficult to manage as a result of their proximity to critical neural structures. While maximum surgical resection is the mainstay of therapy, complete resections are difficult and adjuvant radiotherapy is commonly utilized. Tumoricidal doses >70 Gy RBE (relative biological effectiveness) for gross disease

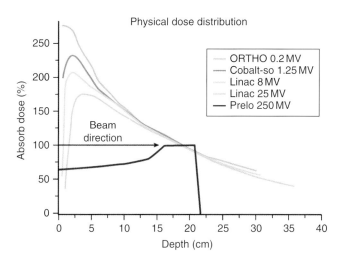

Figure 17.7 Depth-dose distributions for a proton beam compared with other photon beams. The dose for the proton beam is limited for the entrance tissues, reaches a Bragg peak at the desired depth, then displays an extremely sharp fall-off. *Source:* Abeloff M, Armitage J, Niederhuber J, Kastan M, McKenna W (eds) Abeloff's Clinical Oncology, 4th edn. Philadelphia: Churchill Livingstone, 2008:443. Reproduced with permission of Elsevier.

cancer, modeling studies have shown that three-dimensional conformal therapy using protons spares normal tissues better than IMRT in the low-to-mid dose range [58]. To date, clinical studies have shown only limited differences, if any, in toxicity profiles [59]. A randomized trial is currently underway [60]. Protons may have benefits in treating prostate cancer for the two following reasons. First, there is the expected reduction in normal tissue integral dose, which may be important in preventing radiation-induced second malignancies, particularly in younger men [61]. Secondly, escalation of dose to focal lesions within the prostate may be more feasible with protons compared with X-ray therapy. Finally in NSCLC, improvements in treatment-related toxicity, mainly esophagitis and pneumonitis, are sought, particularly in the setting of mediastinal involvement and concurrent chemotherapy [62] and a randomized comparison with photons is ongoing [63].

Not without controversy [64] due to higher cost of delivery relative to other radiotherapy techniques, the availability of proton therapy as a standard treatment modality is anticipated to become more widespread, with increasing numbers of centers worldwide and emerging technologies making the delivery less costly [65].

have been difficult to apply with photon therapy alone, but shown to be feasible and to improve outcomes with proton therapy [55].

There is increasing interest in application of proton therapy across the body to take advantage of its physical properties and dose distribution. Sites of study include hepatocellular carcinoma (HCC), prostate cancer, gastrointestinal malignancies, head and neck cancer, and non-small-cell lung cancer (NSCLC). Radiation has traditionally held a minor role in treating HCC, as the liver is a highly radiosensitive structure. There has been interest in using the normal tissue sparing properties of charged particle irradiation to deliver high doses of radiation to HCC, particularly in the setting of portal vein thrombus and other patients that may be poor operative candidates, especially in area where it is more endemic [56, 57]. In men with prostate

Neutron Therapy

The most compelling benefit of neutron radiation therapy over photon therapy was noted for unresectable salivary gland carcinomas where a phase III RTOG/MRC trial showed a significant local control advantage of neutrons over photons (56% vs 17%), but no overall survival advantage due to distant metastases [66]. As these tumors are considered relatively less radiosensitive tumors, neutron therapy was also investigated enthusiastically for sarcomas of the bone, cartilage, and soft tissue, with some encouraging outcomes in unresectable disease [67]. Nonetheless, given its often less desirable dose distributions than charged particle therapy and potential for causing late toxicity [68], interest in neutron therapy has waned with no active clinical studies. It is used selectively in certain specialist centers, which still have capability, generally for the aforementioned sites.

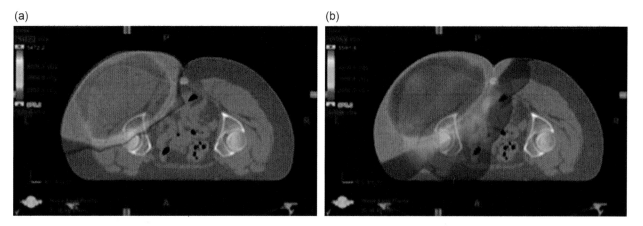

Figure 17.8 Color wash dose distributions comparing intensity modulated radiotherapy (IMRT) with photons (b) and uniform scanning proton therapy (a) for a patient with a gluteal soft tissue sarcoma, with a preoperative prescription dose of 50.0 Gy (RBE). Note the reduction in integral dose with the proton plan, particularly to the abdominopelvic organs.

Conclusion

Since its inception at the end of the nineteenth century, radiotherapy has played a primary role in cancer management. Today, radiation oncology is a rapidly evolving field sitting at the nexus of imaging, oncology, physics, and biology. Technological developments in imaging and treatment delivery units, and improved understanding of cancer biology and pathway targets, will continue to advance the field through the twenty-first century and the era of personalized medicine increasing cell kill and reducing normal tissue toxicity, further enhancing the therapeutic ratio of treatment.

References

1 Perez CA, Brady L (eds) *Principles and Practice of Radiation Oncology*, 3rd edn. Philadelphia: Lippincott Williams & Wilkins, 1997.

2 Rossi HH, Kellerer AM. Roentgen. *Radiat Res* 1995;144(2): 124–8.

3 del Regato JA. The American Radium Society: its diamond jubilee. *Am J Clin Oncol* 1991;14(2):93–100.

4 Giroud F. *Marie Curie: A Life*. New York: Holmes and Meier, 1986.

5 del Regato JA. Fractionation: a panoramic view. *Int J Radiat Oncol Biol Phys* 1990;19(5):1329–31.

6 Johns HE. The physicist in cancer treatment and detection. *Int J Radiat Oncol Biol Phys* 1981;7(6):801–8.

7 Nunez MI, McMillan TJ, Valenzuela MT, *et al.* Relationship between DNA damage, rejoining and cell killing by radiation in mammalian cells. *Radiother Oncol* 1996;39:155–65.

8 Dikomey E, Dahm-Daphi J, Brammer I, *et al.* Correlation between cellular radiosensitivity and non-repaired double-strand breaks studied in nine mammalian cell lines. *Int J Radiat Biol* 1998;73:269–78.

9 Kellerer AM, Rossi HH. The theory of dual radiation action. *Curr Top Radiat Res Q* 1972; 8:85.

10 Powell S, McMillan TJ. DNA damage and repair following treatment with ionizing radiation. *Radiother Oncol* 1990;19:95–108.

11 Phillips R, Tolmach L. Repair of potentially lethal damage in x-irradiated HeLa cells. *Radiation Res* 1966;29:413–22.

12 Hall EJ, Bedford JS. Dose rate: its effect on the survival of HeLa cells irradiated with gamma rays. *Radiat Res* 1964; 22:305–15.

13 Warters RL, Lyons BW. Variation in radiation-induced formation of DNA double-strand breaks as a function of chromatin structure. *Radiat Res* 1992; 130:309–18.

14 Ko EC, Forsythe K, Buckstein M, Kao J, Rosenstein BS. Radiobiological rationale and clinical implications of hypofractionated radiation therapy. *Cancer Radiother* 2011;15(3):221–9.

15 Palcic B, Skarsgard LD. Reduced oxygen enhancement ratio at low doses of ionizing radiation. *Radiat Res* 1984;100:328.

16 Tomlinson R, Gray L. The historical structure of some human lung cancers and the possible implications for radiotherapy. *Br J Cancer* 1955; 9:539–42.

17 Dai Y, Grant S. New insights into checkpoint kinase 1 in the DNA damage response signaling network. *Clin Cancer Res* 2010;16(2):376–83.

18 Rischin D, Peters L, Hicks R, *et al.* Phase I trial of concurrent tirapazamine, cisplatin, and radiotherapy in patients with advanced head and neck cancer. *J Clin Oncol* 2001;19:535–42.

19 Marks LB, Yorke ED, Jackson A, *et al.* Use of normal tissue complication probability models in the clinic. *Int J Radiat Oncol Biol Phys* 2010;76(3 Suppl):S10–9.

20 Trotti A, Byhardt R, Stetz J, *et al.* Common toxicity criteria: version 2.0. an improved reference for grading the acute effects of cancer treatment: impact on radiotherapy. *Int J Radiat Oncol Biol Phys* 2000;47(1):13–47.

21 Barry MJ, Coffey DC, Fitzpatrick J, *et al.* Recommendations of the International Consensus Committee concerning patient evaluation for research studies. In: ATK Cockett, Y Aso, C Chatelain, *et al.* (eds) *Proceedings of the International Consultation on Benign Prostatic Hyperplasia (BPH)*. Channel Islands: Paris Scientific Communication International, 1991: 279–81.

22 Hewitt M, Greenfield S, Stovall E. *From Cancer Patient to Cancer Survivor: Lost in Transition*. Washington: The National Academies, 2006.

23 Introduction to Radiation Oncology. ASTRO. https://www. astro.org/uploadedFiles/_MAIN_SITE/Patient_Care/ Patient_Education/Content_Pieces/RTforGeneralPublic.ppt.

24 Thariat J, Hannoun-Levi JM, Sun Myint A, *et al.* Past, present, and future of radiotherapy for the benefit of patients. *Nat Rev Clin Oncol* 2013;10(1):52–60.

25 Salama JK, Vokes EE. New radiotherapy and chemoradiotherapy approaches for non-small-cell lung cancer. *J Clin Oncol* 2013;31(8):1029–38.

26 Bonner JA, Harari PM, Giralt J, *et al.* Radiotherapy plus cetuximab for locoregionally advanced head and neck cancer: 5-year survival data from a phase 3 randomised trial, and relation between cetuximab-induced rash and survival. *Lancet Oncol* 2010;11(1):21–8.

27 Hartsell WF, Scott CB, Bruner DW, *et al.* Randomized trial of short- versus long-course radiotherapy for palliation of painful bone metastases. *J Natl Cancer Inst* 2005;97(11):798–804.

28 Prescribing, Recording and Reporting Photon Beam Therapy (Supplement to ICRU Report 50). ICRU Report 62. Bethesda, MD: International Commission on Radiological Units and Measurements, 1999: pp ix, 52.

29 Radiation Therapy Oncology Group Contouring Atlases. http://www.rtog.org/CoreLab/ContouringAtlases.aspx (accessed 1 June 2017).

30 Korba A, Zivznuska FR, Purdy JA, *et al.* Pseudoblocks and portal localization. *Radiology* 1977;122:260–1.

31 Merrick GS, Butler WM, Wallner KE, *et al.* Variability of prostate brachytherapy pre-implant dosimetry: a multi-institutional analysis. *Brachytherapy* 2005;4:241.

32 Kassis AI, Adelstein SJ. Radiobiologic principles in radionuclide therapy. *J Nucl Med* 2005; 46(Suppl 1):4S–12S.

33 Witzig TE, Fishkin P, Gordon LI, *et al*. Treatment recommendations for radioimmunotherapy in follicular lymphoma: a consensus conference report. *Leuk Lymphoma* 2011;52(7):1188–99.

34 Gabriel M. Radionuclide therapy beyond radioiodine. *Wien Med Wochenschr* 2012;162(19–20):430–9.

35 Parker C, Nilsson S, Heinrich D, *et al*. Alpha emitter radium-223 and survival in metastatic prostate cancer. *N Engl J Med* 2013;369(3):213–23.

36 Webb S. *Intensity-Modulated Radiation Therapy*. Bristol: Institute of Physics Publishing, 2000.

37 Miles EA, Clark CH, Urbano MT, *et al*. The impact of introducing intensity modulated radiotherapy into routine clinical practice. *Radiother Oncol* 2005;77:241–6.

38 MRT Collaborative Working Group. Intensity-modulated radiotherapy: current status issues of interest. *Int J Radiat Oncol Biol Phys* 2001;51:880–914.

39 Mackie TR, Holmes T, Swerdloff S, *et al*. Tomotherapy: a new concept for the delivery of dynamic conformal radiotherapy. *Med Phys* 1993;20(6):1709–19.

40 Lu W, Olivera GH, Chen Q, Chen ML, Ruchala KJ. Automatic re-contouring in 4D radiotherapy. *Phys Med Biol* 2006; 51(5):1077–99.

41 Palma DA, Verbakel WF, Otto K, Senan S. New developments in arc radiation therapy: a review. *Cancer Treat Rev* 2010; 36(5):393–9.

42 Bedford JL, Warrington AP. Commissioning of volumetric modulated arc therapy (VMAT). *Int J Radiat Oncol Biol Phys* 2009;73:537.

43 Schweikard A, Adler JR. Robotic radiosurgery with noncylindrical collimators. *Comput Aided Surg* 1997; 2:124.

44 Arcangeli S, Scorsetti M, Alongi F. Will SBRT replace conventional radiotherapy in patients with low-intermediate risk prostate cancer? *A review. Crit Rev Oncol Hematol* 2012;84(1):101–8.

45 Shih HA, Harisinghani M, Zietman AL, *et al*. Mapping of nodal disease in locally advanced prostate cancer: rethinking the clinical target volume for pelvic nodal irradiation based on vascular rather than bony anatomy. *Int J Radiat Oncol Biol Phys* 2005;63(4):1262–9.

46 Hurkmans CW, Cho BC, Damen E, *et al*. Reduction of cardiac lung complication probabilities after breast irradiation using conformal radiotherapy with or without intensity modulation. *Radiother Oncol* 2002;62:163–71.

47 Chao KS. Protection of salivary function by intensity-modulated radiation therapy in patients with head neck cancer. *Semin Radiat Oncol* 2002;12:20–5.

48 Pirzkall A, Debus J, Haering P, *et al*. Intensity modulated radiotherapy (IMRT) for recurrent, residual, or untreated skull-base meningiomas: preliminary clinical experience. *Int J Radiat Oncol Biol Phys* 2003;55:362–72.

49 Zelefsky MJ, Fuks Z, Leibel SA. Intensity-modulated radiation therapy for prostate cancer. *Semin Radiat Oncol* 2002;12:229–37.

50 Kavanagh BD, Schefter TE, Wu Q, *et al*. Clinical application of intensity-modulated radiotherapy for locally advanced cervical cancer. *Semin Radiat Oncol* 2002;12:260–71.

51 Glatstein E. Intensity-modulated radiation therapy: the inverse, the converse, the perverse. *Semin Radiat Oncol* 2002;12:272–81.

52 Suit H. The Gray Lecture 2001: coming technical advances in radiation oncology. *Int J Radiat Oncol Biol Phys* 2002; 53:798–809.

53 Allen AM, Pawlicki T, Dong L, *et al*. An evidence based review of proton beam therapy: the report of ASTRO's emerging technology committee. *Radiother Oncol* 2012;103(1):8–11.

54 Egger E, Zografos L, Schalenbourg A, *et al*. Eye retention after proton beam radiotherapy for uveal melanoma. *Int J Radiat Oncol Biol Phys* 2003;55:867–80.

55 Torres MA, Chang EL, Mahajan A, *et al*. Optimal treatment planning for skull base chordoma: photons, protons, or a combination of both? *Int J Radiat Oncol Biol Phys* 2009;74(4):1033–9.

56 Hong TS, Wo JY, Yeap BY, *et al*. Multi-institutional phase II study of high-dose hypofractionated proton beam therapy in patients with localized, unresectable hepatocellular carcinoma and intrahepatic cholangiocarcinoma. *J Clin Oncol* 2016;34(5):460–8.

57 Mizumoto M, Okumura T, Hashimoto T, *et al*. Proton beam therapy for hepatocellular carcinoma: a comparison of three treatment protocols. *Int J Radiat Oncol Biol Phys* 2011; 81(4):1039–45.

58 Trofimov A, Nguyen PL, Coen JJ, *et al*. Radiotherapy treatment of early-stage prostate cancer with IMRT and protons: a treatment planning comparison. *Int J Radiat Oncol Biol Phys* 2007;69(2):444–53.

59 Fang P, Mick R, Deville C, *et al*. A case-matched study of toxicity outcomes after proton therapy and intensity-modulated radiation therapy for prostate cancer. *Cancer* 2015;121(7):1118–27.

60 Proton Therapy vs IMRT for Low or Low-Intermediate Risk Prostate Cancer. http://clinicaltrials.gov/ct2/show/NCT01617161 (accessed 1 June 2017).

61 Fontenot JD, Lee AK, Newhauser WD. Risk of secondary malignant neoplasms from proton therapy and intensity-modulated x-ray therapy for early-stage prostate cancer. *Int J Radiat Oncol Biol Phys* 2009;74(2):616–22.

62 Bush DA, Slater JD, Shin BB, *et al*. Hypofractionated proton beam radiotherapy for stage I lung cancer. *Chest* 2004; 126(4):1198–203.

63 Image-Guided Adaptive Conformal Photon Versus Proton Therapy. http://clinicaltrials.gov/show/NCT00915005 (accessed 1 June 2017).

64 Suit H, Kooy H, Trofimov A, *et al*. Should positive phase III clinical trial data be required before proton beam therapy is more widely adopted? *No. Radiother Oncol* 2008;86(2): 148–53.

65 Hede K. Research groups promoting proton therapy "lite". *J Natl Cancer Inst* 2006;98(23):1682–4.

66 Douglas JG, Lee S, Laramore GE, *et al*. Neutron radiotherapy for the treatment of locally advanced major salivary gland tumors. *Head Neck* 1999;21:255–63.

67 Laramore GE, Griffith JT, Boespflug M, *et al*. Fast neutron radiotherapy for sarcomas of soft tissue, bone, cartilage. *Am J Clin Oncol* 1989;12:320–6.

68 Cohen L, Saroja KR, Hendrickson FR, *et al*. Neutron irradiation of human pelvic tissues yields a steep dose-response function for late sequelae. *Int J Radiat Oncol Biol Phys* 1995; 32:367–72.

18

Cytotoxic Chemotherapy

R. Donald Harvey and Fadlo R. Khuri

Winship Cancer Institute, Emory University School of Medicine, Atlanta, Georgia, USA

Introduction

Since the origin of "chemotherapy" in 1907, initiated and named by the German biochemist Paul Ehrlich during his search for a cure for syphilis, this term has evolved to describe all drugs used in neoplastic diseases. Drugs with different mechanisms, from mechlorethamine to vemurafenib, can generically be called chemotherapy, without regard to chemical, efficacy, or safety differences. Despite this lack of specificity, clinicians typically consider chemotherapy as cytotoxic agents separately from small molecule inhibitors, monoclonal antibodies, hormonal therapy, and immunomodulating agents.

Chemotherapy can be traced back to World War I, where nitrogen mustard gas was used in chemical warfare with the effect of skin blistering and pulmonary damage. Upon exposure, soldiers also had reductions in circulating lymphocytes. Following a ban on chemical weapons by the Geneva Protocol of 1925, pharmacologists Louis Goodman and Alfred Gilman created the more stable nitrogen mustard, with preclinical and clinical trial activity in leukemia and lymphoma [1–3]. Subsequently, development and use of antifolates and the rational synthesis of 5-fluorouracil ushered in broader use of chemotherapy for cancer [4]. From this, additional single agents and combinations evolved to the point where childhood acute lymphocytic leukemia (ALL), germ cell cancers, Hodgkin lymphoma (HL), and other cancers can be cured with conventional cytotoxic chemotherapy. While adverse effects such as nausea, vomiting, diarrhea, alopecia, mucositis, and myelosuppression are seen, supportive care improvements including antiemetic agents and colony-stimulating factors have increased dose intensity and improved quality of life, allowing more patients to continue to receive effective therapy. This chapter is intended to provide a global overview of cytotoxic chemotherapy and its use.

The Scientific Basis for Cytotoxic Chemotherapy Use in Cancer

Knowledge of cancer regulation/dysregulation and the tumor microenvironment has expanded rapidly. Cells progress through multiple stages in transformation to malignancy. As DNA becomes mutated and cells evade death signals, they are increasingly susceptible to DNA-damaging agents and interruption of signaling and division. Normal neighboring cells become recruited to create a tumor stroma, leading to a number of the hallmark capabilities of cancer cells described by Hanahan and Weinberg as well as creating protected niches for drug delivery evasion [5]. The evolving field of cancer stem cells has implications for treatment, as increasing tumor heterogeneity (both genetic and phenotypic) translates into needs for more complex, rational drug regimens and formulations that account for cellular and anatomic location differences.

Despite evolving understanding, fundamental laws still govern the use of cytotoxic chemotherapy. Skipper's laws are based on experiments with L1210 murine leukemia lines at the Southern Research Institute [6]. The first is that doubling time of the fraction of cells in proliferation is constant. Functionally, a fixed population of cells will increase in number until death of the host occurs. The second is that a fixed concentration of chemotherapy, alone or in combination, will kill a fixed percentage of cells regardless of the tumor burden, requiring repeated administration for cure. Recovery periods between chemotherapy cycles are driven by toxicity, and cancer cells can repopulate during rests. The understanding of a concentration–time–effect relationship for cytotoxic chemotherapy from these laws has led to modern day evaluations of approaches such as dose-dense regimens and high-dose conditioning regimens with autologous stem cell support (SCT). Adding to Skipper's laws is that cancers grow at differing rates, depending on the total cell volume.

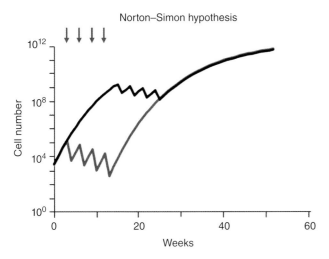

Figure 18.1 The Norton–Simon hypothesis [9]. The repeated administration of chemotherapy (arrows) leads to tumor volume regression that is proportional to the rate of growth. Minimizing the time between therapies will increase the likelihood of continued cell death across heterogeneous cell types. *Source:* Charles Schmidt. The Gompertzian View: Norton Honoured for Role in Establishing Cancer Treatment Approach. J Natl Cancer Inst 2004;96(20):1492–3. Reproduced with permission of Oxford University Press.

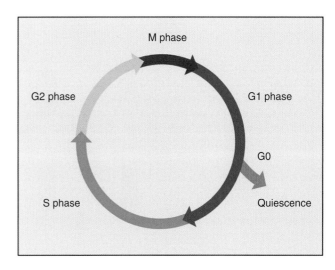

Figure 18.2 The cell cycle. Cells progress through a cycle that consists of phases for growth (G1, S, and G2) and division (M), and they become quiescent when they exit this cycle (G0). The lines depict the relative length of time in each phase, and conventional cytotoxic chemotherapy works in each portion of the cycle, except G0, depending on mechanism of action. *Source:* National Institute of General Medical Sciences, Crabtree and Company. http://images.nigms.nih.gov/index.cfm?event=viewDetail& imageID=2499.

Known as Gompertzian growth, cancer cell collections grow in sigmoidal fashion, with the slowest rates at both the earliest and latest times in their life cycle (inception and death) [7]. Although Gompertzian growth doesn't account for tumor biology differences, treatment effects, and the development of resistance, it has value in treatment considerations across the patient continuum, from prevention and early detection to advanced disease. Because Skipper's laws and Gompertzian growth apply only to the fraction of actively proliferating cells, the optimal time to intervene in cancer is at the earliest point, when the fraction not in a growth phase is minimal. This is borne out in laboratory and patient survival data, where, in the majority of instances, treatment is most successful for cure at early stages. The middle portion of the sigmoidal curve is, paradoxically, when one sees the maximum treatment response, as the highest numbers of cells are in growth phase and most susceptible. Norton and Simon took Gompertzian growth further and showed that tumor cell population and size at any point depends on all drug treatment up to and including that time, and that drug effect is not only a concentration–time effect, since relationships may not be linear [8]. Put simply, the Norton–Simon hypothesis is that *tumor volume regression is proportional to the rate of growth* (Figure 18.1) [9]. The application is that a large tumor volume with a small growth fraction will have a reduced cell kill for a given chemotherapy dose or regimen. From this, the clinical notion that chemotherapy should be given with minimal time between cycles and that regimens be sequential and non-cross-resistant to eradicate all populations was created.

Principles of Cytotoxic Chemotherapy Pharmacology

Reproductive capacity of normal and cancerous cells is governed by external growth factors and receptors that communicate to the nucleus via signal transduction, with a number of

discrete steps. Taking advantage of the disparity in cell cycle activity of normal versus malignant cells forms the basis for how conventional cytotoxic agents are used (Figure 18.2).

The cell cycle was described in 1951 by Howard and Pelc [10]. The two broad phases of cell replication are interphase (growth, nutrient acquisition, DNA replication) and mitotic phase (cell constituent replication, final daughter cell division). More specifically, cells go through G_1, S, and G_2 phases during interphase. The G_1 (G meaning gap) phase is controlled by multiple cyclin-dependent kinases (CDKs) at various checkpoints as well as the *p53* gene, and is when cells expand and metabolic activity increases following nutrient gathering. After entering G_1, cells are committed to completing replication. Amino acid and energy consumption escalates, as does synthesis of ribonucleic acid (RNA), certain proteins required for DNA replication, and functional organelles (e.g., ribosomes, mitochondria). G_1 duration is highly variable depending on complexity of cell function, and lasts 2–3h to days. In G_1, as mentioned earlier, progression of cells to the S phase is regulated by CDKs, which also govern other transition points. The S phase is that period during which DNA synthesis occurs, and many chemotherapeutic agents work here to interrupt critical steps in cellular division. Following DNA synthesis, cells transition to G_2 to prepare for mitosis with rapid growth in cell volume, protein synthesis, and, as the cell progresses to the prophase of mitosis, chromatin conversion into chromosomes. If DNA was synthesized incorrectly, the cell will undergo apoptosis, also known as programmed cell death.

During the mitotic (M) phase, the cell first undergoes constituent reorganization, including chromosome contraction, cytoskeleton reformation to mitotic spindles, and dissolution of nuclear envelopes. M phase is described by prophase (chromosome contraction), metaphase (chromosome organization), anaphase (chromosome splitting), and telophase (chromosome unwinding to chromatin). All are geared toward cytokinesis and

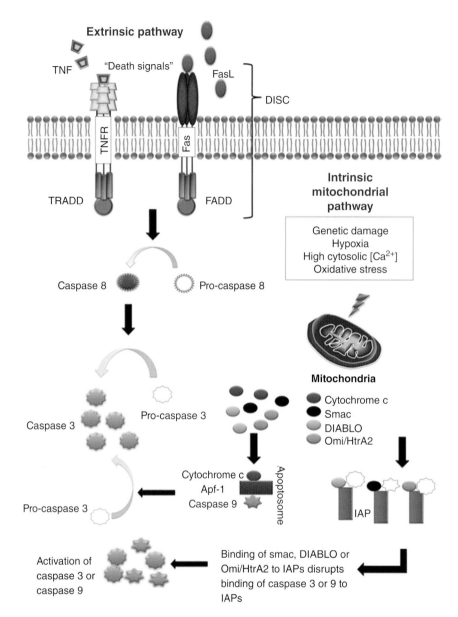

Figure 18.3 Intrinsic and extrinsic pathways of apoptosis [13]. Both pathways of apoptosis activate caspases, which initiate and execute the apoptotic function. Caspase 3 catalyzes nuclear apoptosis, and caspase 9 is critical for the apoptosome, which further activates caspase 3. Other downstream caspases induce cleavage of protein kinases, cytoskeletal proteins, DNA repair proteins and inhibitory subunits of endonucleases. They also alter cytoskeleton integrity and cell cycle signaling, which cause morphological changes and eventual phagocytosis. *Source:* adapted from Figure 1, page 3 at http://www.jeccr.com/content/pdf/1756-9966-30-87.pdf. Open access journal.

division. During M phase cancer cells are most sensitive to chemotherapy. However, it is also the shortest portion, encompassing only 10% of the total cell cycle due to cyclins that drive division [11]. Cells can enter G_0 following mitosis, a resting phase with no replication. Quiescence continues until the cell is signaled to enter G_1 and initiate replication. The ratio of cells in any phase other than G_0 to those in G_0 is called the growth fraction [12].

Following chemotherapy, cells in growth phase can undergo death through a number of paths, depending on the mechanism of action of the anticancer agent. Apoptosis is most relevant to conventional cytotoxic chemotherapy and has two phases, initiation and execution comprised of the intrinsic (mitochondrial) and extrinsic (death receptor) pathways (Figure 18.3).

Three general changes occur: (i) caspase activation; (ii) DNA and protein breakdown; and (iii) membrane changes and recognition by phagocytic cells [13]. Mechanisms of apoptosis triggering are vague; however, some drug classes (e.g., taxanes) initiate death by cell cycle arrest. Specifically, taxanes inactivate the antiapoptotic protein bcl-2, leading to increased cell death susceptibility. Cells may avoid apoptosis through multiple mechanisms, including reduced caspase activity, reduction in death receptor signaling, and changing ratios of proapoptotic and antiapoptotic proteins. Promoting cancer cell apoptosis is an ongoing, active sector of drug development.

A fundamental principle of chemotherapy efficacy is the susceptibility of a cancer cell initially and over time, or mechanisms of potential resistance. Resistance may be intrinsic (present prior to therapy, e.g., anthracyclines in colorectal cancer) or acquired (declining sensitivity over time, e.g., methotrexate in certain non-Hodgkin lymphomas [NHL]). Physiologic barriers also contribute to resistance, for example the blood–brain barrier prevents many active agents from entering the central nervous system (CNS) to treat primary and metastatic disease. Individual variability in drug metabolism and transporters (pharmacogenetics) also contribute to relative resistance.

Similarly to bacteria, cancer cells may evolve to resistance when heterogeneous populations are exposed to subtherapeutic chemotherapy concentrations, triggering mutations leading to survival and/or selection of mutated populations that evade death. The tumor suppressor gene *TP53* is often altered following carcinogenic DNA damage, leading to increased protein production and delays in progression through cell cycles, thus allowing time for DNA repair mechanisms to engage in cancer cells [14]. *TP53* is inactivated in many cancers and loss leads to additional genetic alterations and resistance. It is important to note that genetically resistant cells are always resistant, regardless of cell cycle phase, while cells not in the susceptible phase of the cycle are always effectively resistant [15]. Drug-specific mechanisms of resistance are many, and are categorized as decreased uptake, increased extrusion, decreased activation, increased deactivation, decreased formation of drug-target complexes, and increased repair of drug-induced damage [16]. Methotrexate resistance is a comprehensive example of resistance development, as it enters cells through identified transporters (reduced folate carriers, SLC19A1), must be activated (polyglutamation), forms a bond with a target enzyme for activity (dihydrofolate reductase), and is actively excreted (ATP-binding cassette B1 [ABCB1]). For genetically acquired resistance, prevention depends on maximizing cell kill proportion to prevent mutation development, which may emerge in as few as 100 cells. The Goldie–Coldman hypothesis is based on this concept, and states that overcoming resistance requires giving multiple active agents concurrently over the shortest timeframe possible [17]. Subsequent application has led to terms like dose density and dose intensity, which incorporate a measure of time into treatment (e.g., mg/m^2/week). Dose dense therapy in breast cancer may potentially improve disease outcomes, including overall survival, validating further investigation of this approach [18].

Because cytotoxic chemotherapy works across the cell cycle and is susceptible to resistance mechanisms, it is rational to combine agents of differing classes to maximize cell kill rate, prevent/avoid resistance, and avoid overlapping toxicities. Initially, as an example, alkylating agents were given alone. However, this is generally ineffective, with few notable exceptions (cladribine in hairy cell leukemia). When building an anticancer regimen, principles include: (i) each drug must have known single agent activity; (ii) agents should have differing mechanisms of action and resistance; (iii) agents should have minimal overlapping toxicity; and (iv) each drug and the regimen should optimize dose and schedule. All of these principles are found in a common regimen, R-CHOP (rituximab, cyclophosphamide, doxorubicin [hydroxydaunorubicin], vincristine [Oncovin®], prednisone) used in NHL, which incorporates a monoclonal antibody, alkylating agent, topoisomerase inhibitor, mitotic spindle inhibitor, and corticosteroid. Toxicities, mechanisms of action and resistance pathways of each agent are unique, and all have single agent activity.

Practical Aspects of Chemotherapy Administration

Taking advantage of pharmacology principles is optimal. However, one is often faced with practical challenges in care. Chemotherapy-induced toxicity (e.g., in bone marrow, nerves, heart, lungs) may necessitate dose reductions or other changes. Chemotherapy clearance may also be compromised in renal or hepatic dysfunction, causing increased exposure with added toxicity. Elderly patients may have age-related organ function decline with altered pharmacokinetics. Regimens that require daily patient visits can disrupt schedules and make treatment completion difficult, and methods of payment for therapies may drive agent selection, route, or frequency.

Routes and schedules of chemotherapy incorporate drug physicochemical properties, cell cycle activity, adverse events, and tumor biology. The intravenous (IV) route is used for many agents due to delivery and formulation. Agents are given by IV push or bolus (<10 min) or infusion (10 min or longer), and infusion duration may alter activity and adverse events. Fluorouracil, when given IV bolus, causes mucositis and myelosuppression, whereas when given as a 48-h infusion, diarrhea predominates, and activity is superior in advanced colorectal cancer [19]. Doxorubicin by prolonged infusion (>6 h) has a lower risk of cardiomyopathy, with no change in response or survival [20]. In select cases, such as paclitaxel, 96-h infusion regimens were investigated based on resistance and activity concerns. However, subsequent evaluations showed no benefit over 3-h infusions [21]. The increasing availability of oral agents increases convenience, and, pharmacokinetically, simulates a prolonged infusion. While oral drugs increase simplicity, concerns of adherence and frequency of clinician communication arise, since patients are more independent. Additional, but less common, routes of chemotherapy administration include intraperitoneal (e.g., carboplatin/paclitaxel in ovarian cancer), intrathecal (e.g., methotrexate, cytarabine in ALL), and intraarterial (e.g., doxorubicin in hepatically-guided embolization).

Timing of chemotherapy delivery may be changed based on likelihood of treatment success. Administering agents prior to surgical resection, called neoadjuvant or induction therapy, follows a number of pharmacology principles. It may be used with known metastases (colorectal) and/or large primary cancers to reduce disease burden prior to surgery. Other benefits include: immediate treatment of systemic disease; *in vivo* assessment of tumor responsiveness; improved surgical outcomes; and conversion from large inoperable masses to resectable, increasing cure rates [22]. Neoadjuvant regimens are limited in cycle number (e.g., four) to minimize toxicity and perform timely definitive surgery. The alternative to neoadjuvant treatment is adjuvant therapy, given after resection with or without radiation. It is employed in cancers with high recurrence rates, including breast, stage II–III non-small cell lung (NSCLC), colorectal, and stage III melanoma. Like neoadjuvant treatment, adjuvant chemotherapy treats micrometastatic disease that does not appear on radiographic evaluation but is suspected to be present based on tumor biology (size, site, extent of lymph node involvement). Not all patients and cancers, however, have clear benefit for systemic treatment beyond surgery and/or radiation, and risk assessment tools can be used to decide optimal treatment. For example, Adjuvant! Online is a validated benefit–risk tool for breast, NSCLC, and colon cancer that provides recurrence risk and survival probabilities from clinical and biological data [23].

Combined chemotherapy/radiation is referred to as multimodality therapy or chemoradiotherapy and is used to maximize cell kill in radiosensitive cancers. Examples of use include laryngeal, stage III NSCLC, esophageal, and rectal cancers [24–27]. The benefit is based on tumor biology, as chemotherapy may improve blood supply to the tumor bed, increasing the activity of radiation. Many drugs are radiation sensitizers (e.g., cisplatin, fluorouracil, paclitaxel), causing synergistic cell kill compared with single modalities.

Classes of Agents (Table 18.1)

The sections that follow are an overview of general classes of cytotoxic chemotherapy agents. For more detailed information, the reader is encouraged to review specific agents.

Alkylating Agents

Alkylating agents are the largest, most diverse group of cytotoxic chemotherapy agents. The first class was nitrogen mustards, specifically mechlorethamine. The mechanism of action is direct DNA damage through covalent binding at guanine bases, with subsequent apoptosis. All produce reactive intermediates that bind to multiple cellular components. Some (e.g., busulfan) may be called bifunctional, meaning they can cross-link opposing guanine bases, leading to greater activity. Alkylating agents are non-cell cycle specific (i.e., cells do not have to be in a certain phase of growth to be susceptible)

allowing for intermittent dosing, and have a steep dose–response–toxicity curve, with myelosuppression as the dose-limiting toxicity. Many (busulfan, cyclophosphamide, melphalan, carmustine) are incorporated into high-dose regimens for conditioning prior to autologous and allogeneic SCT.

Within alkylating agents, further subclassification is necessary. The nitrogen mustards mechlorethamine, chlorambucil, melphalan, cyclophosphamide, ifosfamide, and bendamustine were the first group. Each has unique activity and adverse event profiles, and three (chlorambucil, melphalan, cyclophosphamide) are available orally.

Cyclophosphamide (PO [per oram], IV) and ifosfamide (IV) are oxazaphosphorine prodrugs, with multiple intermediate and final metabolites. One metabolite, acrolein, is produced by both agents, but is more clinically significant with ifosfamide, as molar amounts produced following ifosfamide administration are much higher than those with cyclophosphamide at equivalent doses [28]. Acrolein is toxic to urothelial cells and can cause hemorrhagic cystitis with higher concentrations and longer bladder residence times. Patients should urinate frequently after dosing with either agent. Adequate hydration (≥2 additional L/day) prevents hemorrhagic cystitis with cyclophosphamide; however, the chemoprotectant mesna must be used with all doses of ifosfamide. Mesna binds and inactivates acrolein, and is given at a minimum intravenous dose of 60% of the ifosfamide dose, based on specific regimens [29]. Mesna can cause false positive ketonuria, important when monitoring urinalysis results for hematuria following ifosfamide administration [30]. The ifosfamide metabolite chloracetaldehyde, similar to chloral hydrate, is also produced in a dose-dependent fashion. Chloracetaldehyde readily crosses the blood–brain barrier, and can lead to somnolence and encephalopathy hours to days after ifosfamide initiation. Frequently, patients receive other agents that may cause CNS depression (e.g., lorazepam for nausea), so attributing causality can be difficult. Risk factors include reduced renal function, low albumin, concurrent aprepitant, and prior cisplatin therapy [31, 32]. Reversal agents including methylene blue, thiamine, and dexmedetomidine have been

Table 18.1 Cytotoxic chemotherapy and cell cycle activity.

Class	Cell cycle phase of activity	Example agents	Comment(s)
Alkylating agents	All	Busulfan, melphalan, mechlorethamine, cyclophosphamide, ifosfamide, temozolomide, procarbazine, dacarbazine, cisplatin, carboplatin, oxaliplatin, bendamustine	Dose-limiting toxicity with majority of agents is myelosuppression. Steep dose-response curve allows use in stem cell support.
Antimetabolites	S	Methotrexate, pemetrexed, pralatrexate, fluorouracil, capecitabine, cytarabine, fludarabine, azacytidine, decitabine, gemcitabine	Toxicity and efficacy due to disease burden, dose, and bolus versus continuous infusions (e.g., fluorouracil).
Microtubule targeting agents	M	Vincristine, vinblastine, vinorelbine, paclitaxel, docetaxel, ixabepilone, eribulin	All cause neurotoxicity as a dose-limiting effect. Vinca alkaloids are fatal if given intrathecally.
Topoisomerase inhibitors	G2/S	Irinotecan, topotecan, etoposide	Etoposide associated with secondary leukemia development.
Antitumor antibiotics	All	Bleomycin, doxorubicin, idarubicin, epirubicin	All fluoresce and may cause chronic cardiotoxicity (anthracyclines) or pulmonary toxicity (bleomycin).

used with moderate success. However, most cases resolve spontaneously [33, 34]. Ifosfamide is activated by the cytochrome P450 (CYP) 3A4 pathway, while cyclophosphamide is primarily metabolized through the CYP2B6 route, making interactions more likely with ifosfamide. Cyclophosphamide bioavailability is 70–85% following oral dosing [35].

Melphalan (L-phenylalanine mustard) (PO, IV) is rapidly degraded after IV admixture, and must be given within 1 h of reconstitution, usually over 15–30 min. The oral formulation has erratic bioavailability (25–89%), and is losing favor in multiple myeloma treatment due to more effective and tolerable therapies [36, 37]. Although not solely cleared renally, melphalan tolerability and neutropenia are worse in patients with moderate to severe renal dysfunction, necessitating dose reduction [38]. Additionally, mucositis, diarrhea, and nausea and vomiting are common with high doses (140–200 mg/m^2). Rarely, melphalan causes pulmonary fibrosis. However, like busulfan, fibrosis is more likely with prolonged low dose exposure. Despite these limitations, high dose melphalan remains the preferred conditioning in autologous SCT for multiple myeloma. Bendamustine (IV), another nitrogen mustard, was FDA approved for chronic lymphocytic leukemia (CLL) in 2008, but synthesized in 1963 [39]. Metabolism is through CYP1A2, and the majority of parent drug (94–96%) is bound to albumin. Toxicities of bendamustine equate to other nitrogen mustards, with myelosuppression being dose-limiting and nausea and vomiting occurring in 13%.

The second class of alkylating agents are nitrosoureas, including carmustine, lomustine, and streptozocin. As a class, they are lipophilic and cross the blood–brain barrier readily. However, the only commonly used agent is carmustine (BCNU), available intravenously and in a biodegradable polymer wafer for local placement in brain tumors. Carmustine is incorporated into autologous SCT regimens with etoposide, cytarabine and melphalan (BEAM), and must be given over 1–2 h to prevent toxicity from the diluent, ethanol. Myelosuppression may be prolonged, with count recovery taking as long as 8 weeks. Like other agents in the class, carmustine can rarely cause pulmonary fibrosis.

Hydrazine and triazine alkylating agents include procarbazine (PO), dacarbazine (IV), and temozolomide (PO, IV). Procarbazine is used in Hodgkin lymphoma and some CNS tumors. It is highly emetogenic, and has monoamine oxidase (MAO) inhibitor properties, meaning patients should eat diets low in tyramine-containing foods (e.g., red wine, aged cheeses) to prevent hypertensive crises, and concurrent medications should be screened for potential interactions. Because of azoospermia, infertility, and an increased incidence of secondary leukemia in the MOPP (mechlorethamine, Oncovin® [vincristine], procarbazine, prednisone) regimen, procarbazine and MOPP are avoided in young patients with Hodgkin lymphoma. Dacarbazine, however, is critical in the treatment of Hodgkin lymphoma, and is part of ABVD (Adriamycin® [doxorubicin], bleomycin, vinblastine, dacarbazine) as one of the preferred initial regimens in advanced stage disease. Although they share similar structures, dacarbazine is also active in melanoma, whereas procarbazine is not. Some references recommend dose reduction in patients with creatinine clearances (CrCL) <60 mL/min. However, this should be done judiciously when the goal is cure (e.g., Hodgkin lymphoma) [38]. Dacarbazine is a substrate of CYP1A2 and CYP2E1. Temozolomide is active in

melanoma and CNS tumors, alone and with radiation. Along with myelosuppression, temozolomide may predispose patients to *Pneumocystis jirovecii* pneumonia (PCP), and risk is increased with corticosteroids or longer dosing regimens, necessitating prophylaxis with trimethoprim-sulfamethoxazole in all patients. Increased activity of the enzyme MGMT (O-6-methylguanine-DNA methyltransferase) in glioblastoma is associated with temozolomide resistance. Patients with decreased MGMT are more likely to benefit from combination radiation therapy and temozolomide, and determination of MGMT status may help select therapy [40, 41].

Busulfan (PO, IV) is the only alkane sulfonate agent in the class. Previously, it was used for management of chronic myeloid leukemia; however, bcr-abl-targeted tyrosine kinase inhibitors have replaced it. Today, busulfan, like melphalan, is primarily used in SCT conditioning. In combination with cyclophosphamide or fludarabine, it is one of the most common agents used in preparative regimens for allogeneic SCT. Pharmacokinetically guided and intravenous dosing of busulfan have reduced the incidence of sinusoidal obstruction syndrome (formerly veno-occlusive disease), and both are commonly employed [42]. Goal exposure is an area-under-the-concentration time curve (AUC) of 900–1350 µM-min with every 6 h dosing or an AUC of 5000–6000 µM-min with daily administration [43]. Intravenous busulfan has greatly reduced exposure variability compared to oral, making the benefits of AUC targeting with the IV formulation for toxicity prevention less clear. High dose busulfan can also induce seizures, necessitating prophylaxis with antiepileptic agents, preferably levetiracetam due to lack of hepatic interactions [44].

The platinums cisplatin, carboplatin, and oxaliplatin are diverse, highly active IV anticancer agents. Each reacts with water to form a nucleophilic complex, with subsequent DNA-platinum adduct formation [45]. The prototype is cisplatin, which in combination with other drugs produces cure rates of 85% in testicular cancer, compared to 10% prior to its use [46]. Other cancers that respond alone and in combination include lung, ovarian, cervical, head and neck, and bladder. Historically, nausea and vomiting were dose limiting with cisplatin. However, antiemetics including a corticosteroid, 5-HT$_3$ antagonist, and neurokinin-1 antagonist have drastically reduced the frequency and severity. Cisplatin is renally cleared and nephrotoxic, necessitating dose reduction in renal dysfunction and adequate hydration with normal saline-containing fluids before (1–2 L) and after. Other measures, including administration of mannitol, furosemide, and 3% saline do not provide greater benefit than fluids alone in renal prophylaxis [47]. Nephrotoxicity is cumulative, and early manifestations include hypokalemia and hypomagnesemia [48]. Single doses >100 mg/m^2 provide no more efficacy than lower doses, with greater risk of nephrotoxicity. Extending infusion times may reduce incidence and severity of nephrotoxicity. Dividing cisplatin doses over multiple days (e.g., 20 mg/m^2 × 5) reduces toxicities, but potential negative effects on efficacy have not been fully evaluated in all cancers [49]. Neurologic damage including peripheral neuropathy and ototoxicity may be encountered with cumulative cisplatin, and increasing exposure adds to risk. All pediatric patients should have baseline and periodic neurologic and hearing assessment, with adult patients followed closely from initiation of therapy. Carboplatin is a renally cleared platinum used in lung, ovarian, melanoma, refractory lymphomas, and head and neck cancer. Although renally cleared, it is not nephrotoxic, and causes myelosuppression more frequently than cisplatin. Nausea, vomiting, and neurotoxicity are also less common with carboplatin. Due to renal clearance and thrombocytopenia, Calvert *et al.* established a pharmacodynamic relationship between exposure (AUC), glomerular filtration rate (GFR), and risk of thrombocytopenia, resulting in the dosing equation [50]:

$$\text{Dose (mg)} = \text{target AUC} \times (\text{GFR} + 25)$$

Goal AUC varies based on disease and partner agents and modalities, with examples of an AUC of 2 weekly in radiation sensitization, and an AUC of 4–7 in combination with other drugs (e.g., AUC 6 with paclitaxel for some cancers, both given every 21 days). Patients on hemodialysis are assumed to have GFR = 0, meaning dose = target AUC × 25. Dosing should occur on a nondialysis day, with dialysis occurring 12–24 h following dosing [51]. Increasing target AUC leads to increasing likelihood of reduction of platelet counts from baseline values, e.g., an AUC of 8 was associated with nadir platelet counts of 15–26% of pretreatment values. Most clinicians cap GFR/CrCL at 125–130 mL/min using the Cockcroft–Gault estimation method. However Calvert used radionuclide measurement of GFR with ^{51}CrEDTA originally, and newer estimations (e.g., Modification of Diet in Renal Disease [MDRD]). may yield different results. All platinum agents may cause a delayed hypersensitivity reaction; the greatest amount of data is with carboplatin. A type I IgE-mediated reaction may occur following six cycles and is an anaphylactic reaction, with hypotension, flushing, urticaria, chest tightness, and dyspnea seen [52]. Incidence varies, with rates as high as 27%, with the highest rates seen in ovarian cancer patients following more than seven cycles. Acute treatment should include epinephrine, diphenhydramine, and corticosteroids. Desensitization protocols have been described and permit continued therapy when risk–benefit ratios are favorable. An important drug interaction with carboplatin includes increased myelosuppression when given before paclitaxel, likely due to reduced paclitaxel clearance. Oxaliplatin is the third platinum agent, originally approved for colorectal cancer, with activity in lymphomas and pancreas, esophageal, and gastric cancers. Unlike cisplatin and carboplatin, no adjustments are needed for renal or hepatic dysfunction [53, 54]. A unique neurotoxicity, a cold-induced peripheral, perioral, and/or pharyngolaryngeal dysesthesia, occurs in up to 92% [55]. Counseling should mention gloves upon exposure to cold and avoiding cold beverages during treatment. A peripheral sensory neuropathy (reversible within 3–4 months after discontinuation) may also be seen in increasing incidences with cumulative doses >1000 mg/m^2. Ototoxicity and myelosuppression occur, but less frequently than with cisplatin and carboplatin, respectively.

Antimetabolites

The antimetabolites are a broad category, but generally classified into folate antagonists and pyrimidine or purine antagonists. All antimetabolites have low molecular weights and act in the S phase of the cell cycle.

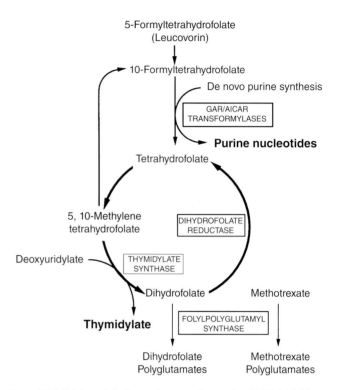

Figure 18.4 Folate metabolism and enzymatic reactions [104]. Inhibition of dihydrofolate reductase leads to depletion of intracellular reduced folate reserves, and accumulation of dihydrofolate. Increased amounts of dihydrofolate polyglutamates and can inhibit another key enzyme in DNA synthesis, thymidylate synthase. These effects in concert lead to reduced DNA synthesis in cancer cells following dihydrofolate reductase inhibition with antifolates. *Source:* Takimoto 1996 [104]. Reproduced with permission of Alphamed Press.

Folate antagonists include methotrexate (IV, PO), pemetrexed (IV), and pralatrexate (IV). All are renally cleared, cause myelosuppression and mucositis, and inhibit the enzyme dihydrofolate reductase (DHFR) (Figure 18.4). Methotrexate (amethopterin) is the prototypical antifolate, and since 1950, has been incorporated into acute leukemia, lymphoma, sarcoma, and breast, bladder, and head and neck cancer treatment as well as graft-versus-host disease (GVHD) prevention in allogeneic SCT [56]. The dose range is broad; with effectiveness in GVHD at 5–15 mg/m^2 versus osteosarcoma, where up to 12 g/m^2 weekly is used. Methotrexate has reasonable oral bioavailability up to 40 mg/m^2 (42%). However, above this it declines to <25% [57]. Preservative-free methotrexate (5–15 mg) can be given directly into the CNS, alone or with cytarabine and/or hydrocortisone. For clinical and interventional purposes, methotrexate is commonly broken into low, intermediate, and high dose categories. Low and intermediate dose (<50 and 50–500 mg/m^2) regimens can be given as an outpatient, do not require leucovorin rescue (unless unexpected toxicity is seen), and do not require additional hydration or urinary alkalinization. Doses above 500 mg/m^2 change the properties and toxicity profile of methotrexate and may require such interventions. All dose ranges should be considered for reduction in renal dysfunction, typically with CrCL <60 mL/min [38]. Because of its acidic properties, methotrexate should only be given in high dose regimens with confirmed urinary alkalinization (a urine pH of 7 or higher) to prevent crystallization and promote excretion. This is achieved with the addition of sodium bicarbonate (e.g., 100 mEq/L) or acetate to IV fluids with 5% dextrose in water, with a goal of 2–4 L/m^2 daily (~125–150 mL/hour in adults). Another convenient approach is the use of acetazolamide 500 mg PO QID prior to treatment initiation, in combination with IV fluids, which increases urine pH to 7.5 within two doses in the majority of patients [58]. Once alkalinization is established and renal function verified, infusions of 4–24 h duration are used for high dose administration. Methotrexate moves freely into multiple spaces, including the CNS, peritoneum, pericardium, and pleura, with consequences for treatment and toxicity. High doses reach CNS concentrations of 3–10% of systemic values, and leeching into large volume extravascular spaces creates delayed elimination due to a reservoir effect, prolonging the need for leucovorin rescue. Optimally, any effusion is drained prior to initiation. Leucovorin, a tetrahydrofolate derivative and cofactor for thymidylate synthase (TS) and other purine and pyrimidine synthesis steps, bypasses DHFR and can therefore rescue normal cells from the toxic effects of methotrexate. It is hepatically metabolized, orally bioavailable up to 50 mg, and does not cross the blood–brain barrier. Leucovorin or levoleucovorin (at 50% of planned or calculated leucovorin doses) should be initiated after all high dose methotrexate to prevent myelosuppression and mucositis. Leucovorin initiation timing varies based on regimen, but enough time should elapse to allow for methotrexate to inhibit DHFR. Many protocols specify 24 h after methotrexate initiation; however, original data shows efficacy as late as 42 h [59]. Once begun, leucovorin dosing should follow serum methotrexate concentrations, with many nomograms available. Pharmacist consultation should be sought prior to all high dose methotrexate to help guide use and leucovorin rescue dosing and schedule. Leucovorin should continue until methotrexate values are below 0.1 µM (10^{-7} M) at 72 h, with some centers continuing below 0.01 µM. Early identification of patients out of risk has also been successful, with patients having values <5 µM at 24 h considered low risk [60]. When patients demonstrate excessive concentrations and delayed methotrexate clearance with rising creatinine, aggressive intervention with high leucovorin doses and alkalinized IV fluids should occur. Glucarpidase (carboxypeptidase G2) is a recombinant enzyme that rapidly hydrolyzes the carboxyl terminal glutamate residue into inactive metabolites and lowers methotrexate concentrations. Doses of 50 units/kg reduce values by 98% within 30 min, with a sustained effect [61]. If glucarpidase is used, leucovorin should be continued, but not given 2 h before or after glucarpidase. Adverse effects aside from myelosuppression and mucositis include dermatitis, tumor lysis syndrome, arachnoiditis and encephalopathy (more common with concurrent intrathecal administration). Transaminitis and pulmonary fibrosis occur with chronic administration of low doses. Guidelines for dosing in hepatic dysfunction are vague, but consideration of dose reductions with serum bilirubin >3 mg/dL and avoidance with >5 mg/dL is reasonable. Significant interactions include trimethoprim-sulfamethoxazole, probenecid, NSAIDs, amiodarone, and, potentially, levetiracetam and proton pump inhibitors – all delay clearance and should be discontinued and avoided during treatment.

Pemetrexed is an antifolate that inhibits TS and glycinamide ribonucleotide formyltransferase. It has activity in mesothelioma and non-squamous NSCLC as well as bladder, ovarian, and cervical cancers. Like methotrexate, it accumulates in pleural spaces, and has dermatologic and myelosuppressive adverse events. However, leucovorin rescue is not needed [62]. Patients receiving pemetrexed should receive dexamethasone to prevent rash and daily folate with vitamin B12 prior to therapy and every three cycles to minimize myelosuppression.

Pralatrexate was FDA approved in 2009 for relapsed or refractory T-cell lymphoma, and it inhibits both DHFR and folylpolyglutamyl synthetase, depleting thymidine pools through inhibition of single carbon transfers. Patients should also be given B12 and folate prior to and during therapy to minimize myelosuppression, but do not require dexamethasone. Pralatrexate is renally cleared, similarly to methotrexate and pemetrexed.

Pyrimidine antagonists act as false bases by interacting with TS, incorporating into DNA (thymine, cytosine) and RNA (cytosine, uracil) in place of nucleic acids. They substitute for thymine and cytosine in DNA. The prototype is 5-fluorouracil (5-FU) (IV, topical), synthesized in the 1950s as a false base in place of uracil [63]. Like other pyrimidine antagonists, fluorouracil is converted intracellularly through phosphorylation to active metabolites, including fluorodeoxyuridine monophosphate (FdUMP), fluorodeoxyuridine triphosphate, and fluorouridine triphosphate. These inhibit TS and prevent RNA synthesis. Fluorouracil is degraded by dihydropyrimidine dehydrogenase (DPD), with more than 80–90% catabolism in the liver, which has high concentrations of DPD [64]. Administering leucovorin prior to fluorouracil increases activity by stabilizing the bond between FdUMP and TS by the reduced folate cofactor N5, N10-methylenetetrahydrofolate [65]. Fluorouracil has varying effects and toxicities given as an IV bolus compared to lower bolus doses followed by 2 day infusions (the preferred strategy in colorectal cancer). It has activity in breast, pancreas, anal, esophageal, head and neck, and hepatobiliary cancers and is also used as a radiosensitizer. Toxicities include diarrhea, mucositis, myelosuppression (more common with bolus), and palmar–plantar erythrodysesthesia, or hand–foot syndrome. Rarely (1–5%), chest pain with EKG changes may be seen, thought to be secondary to a vasospastic angina [66]. Clinical features include first cycle appearance, potentially greater incidence with continuous infusion (72%), progression to myocardial infarction (22%), response to antianginal therapy (68%), and high likelihood of recurrence with rechallenge. Previous history of cardiovascular disease does not appear to be predictive of occurrence. Fluorouracil is not eliminated by the CYP system; however, warfarin interactions have been described, and may occur following multiple cycles [67, 68].

An oral prodrug of fluorouracil, capecitabine, is converted to fluorouracil in a multistep process: (i) conversion in the liver by carboxylesterase to 5′-deoxy-5-fluorocytidine (5′-DFCR); (ii) 5′DFCR conversion in the liver and tumor tissues by cytidine deaminase to 5′-deoxy-5-fluorouridine (5′-DFUR); and (iii) conversion of 5′DFUR to 5-FU in tumor cells by thymidine phosphorylase, present in relatively higher amounts in cancer than normal tissues. It approximates fluorouracil given by continuous infusion, with efficacy in many similar cancers, including breast, colorectal, pancreatic, esophageal, and hepatobiliary. Mucositis, myelosuppression, and chest pain may also be seen. However, more pronounced toxicities of palmar–plantar erythrodysesthesia (median onset 79 days, 54–60%, grade 3 11–17%)

and diarrhea (median time to onset 34 days, 47–57%, grade 3/4 14–16%) occur [69]. Unlike fluorouracil, capecitabine must be reduced in renal dysfunction, with 75% of planned doses with CrCL 30–50 mL/min, and recommendations to avoid use with CrCL <30 mL/min [70]. Initial dosing in hepatic impairment is not defined, but patients who develop grade 3 or higher bilirubin (more than three times upper limit of normal [ULN)]) should be held until less than three times ULN. Recent retrospective data suggests concurrent proton pump inhibitors may diminish capecitabine efficacy in colorectal and gastroesophageal cancer patients, potentially due to diminished absorption; however, prospective pharmacokinetic evaluations are needed for confirmation [71, 72].

Gemcitabine (2′, 2′-Difluoro-2′-Deoxycytidine) (IV) is a deoxycytidine analogue synthesized in 1986 as an antiviral [73]. Initial approval was in pancreas cancer, but it has efficacy in lymphomas, soft tissue sarcomas and lung, breast, ovarian, bladder, and hepatobiliary cancers. Like other agents in the class, it is a prodrug that requires phosphorylation prior to incorporation into DNA, and is deactivated by deoxycytidine kinase. It disrupts RNA processing and translation through direct incorporation. Toxicity and pharmacokinetics, specifically tissue distribution, differ with short (30 min) infusions versus prolonged (100 min or more), with increasing accumulation [74]. Fixed dose rate infusions of $10 \, mg/m^2/min$ have been used to increase intracellular concentrations of the triphosphate form, but with more hematologic toxicity [75]. Adverse events include myelosuppression (more commonly thrombocytopenia), with rare events of pulmonary toxicity (pneumonitis, fibrosis), hepatic failure, and hemolytic-uremic syndrome. Gemcitabine is also a potent radiosensitizer.

Pyrimidine antimetabolites are active in leukemias and lymphomas, with the most experience being with cytarabine (IV, IT [liposomal]). It is an analogue of deoxycytidine and must be triphosphorylated to be active prior to inclusion in DNA. The active form also inhibits several DNA polymerases, which in turn impair DNA elongation and repair. Cytarabine is active in all acute leukemias and some NHL subtypes, is given with other agents as conditioning for autologous SCT, and may be given intrathecally as conventional cytarabine or as a liposomal formulation. It rapidly distributes into tissues and crosses the blood–brain barrier readily. In acute myeloid leukemia (AML), induction therapy is given as a continuous infusion of $100 \, mg/m^2$ IV daily for 7 days (total dose = $700 \, mg/m^2$) with an anthracycline for 3 days, when disease burden is highest. In contrast, optimal consolidation for AML is $3 \, g/m^2$ IV every 12 h on days 1, 3, and 5 (total dose = $18 \, g/m^2$). Cytarabine adverse events and clearance are dependent on dose and schedule. Myelosuppression is disease-dependent, as count recovery following induction therapy can take up to 4–6 weeks. At induction doses, myelosuppression is the only frequent adverse event. With doses above $1 \, g/m^2$, cytarabine enters the CNS and ocular spaces, increasing potential for cerebellar toxicity (ataxia, lethargy, confusion) and conjunctivitis. All patients receiving high doses should have monitoring for cerebellar toxicity, including gait and finger-to-nose assessments daily and for 24 h after completion. Risk factors include age >60, creatinine >1.5 mg/dL, concurrent intrathecal use and total doses of >30 g [76, 77]. Consideration should be given to reduction in renal dysfunction with high

doses, as well as patients whose serum creatinine increases by 0.5 mg/dL or more during treatment. Cerebellar toxicity is reversible when detected early. Conjunctivitis can be prevented with frequent use of saline or corticosteroid eye drops beginning with initiation and continuing for 48 h after the last dose. In high doses, cytarabine can rarely cause pericarditis.

Azacytidine (IV, SQ) and decitabine (IV) are antimetabolites classified as DNA methyl transferase inhibitors, or hypomethylating agents. Both are active in myelodysplastic syndromes and acute leukemias and require phosphorylation. Neither has clear guidance in the setting of renal or hepatic dysfunction.

Purine antagonists also act as false bases for DNA incorporation, by substituting for guanine, adenosine, and adenine. Agents in this class include mercaptopurine (6-MP) (PO), thioguanine (6-TG) (PO), fludarabine (IV, PO outside the US), cladribine (IV), pentostatin (IV), clofarabine (IV), and nelarabine (IV). Some, for example fludarabine, also inhibit DNA polymerase α and ribonucleotide reductase.

The first purine antagonists were mercaptopurine and thioguanine, sulfur-substituted analogues of the purine bases hypoxanthine and guanine, respectively. Mercaptopurine is inactive in parent form, and undergoes conversion via three routes: (i) phosphorylation to the active monophosphate forms (6-thioguanine nucleotides) by hypoxanthine-guanine phosphoribosyltransferase (HGPRT) in the liver and gastrointestinal tract: (ii) inactivation by xanthine oxidase; and (iii) inactivation by thiopurine methyltransferase (TPMT). Azathioprine (IV, PO), a prodrug of mercaptopurine, is converted in the liver, likely through glutathione-S-transferase. Patients who are homozygous for TPMT deficiency (0.3% of the population) are at increased risk for profound myelosuppression with azathioprine and mercaptopurine [78]. Pharmacogenetic testing may be warranted in patients beginning treatment. Mercaptopurine and thioguanine are used in ALL during induction and maintenance phases and cause myelosuppression, nausea, vomiting, diarrhea, and mucositis. However, these are routinely manageable. Hepatotoxicity may also be seen, with elevations in transaminases and bilirubin. Mercaptopurine and thioguanine should be taken in the evening on an empty stomach to maximize absorption, and bioavailability is 50% and 14–46%, respectively. A critical drug interaction with allopurinol occurs with azathioprine and mercaptopurine and is due to impaired mercaptopurine catabolism. If used with allopurinol, a 25–33% empiric dose reduction should be employed. Interactions with trimethoprim-sulfamethoxazole have also been reported, with greater than expected neutropenia [79]. In renal dysfunction (CrCL <50 mL/min), a 50% dose reduction, with subsequent increase based on nadir neutrophil counts, is reasonable. Consideration of reduction in hepatic dysfunction is also warranted. Measurement of 6-thioguanine nucleotides in red blood cells has been utilized to assess adherence and understand toxicity and resistance. However, substantial methodological differences in laboratory techniques is a concern for standardizing reference ranges and guiding therapy [80].

Fludarabine is a prodrug purine antagonist, rapidly converted to 2-fluoro-ara-adenosine (F-ara-A), which enters cells and is converted to the active triphosphate metabolite F-ara-ATP prior to DNA incorporation. It is used in chronic lymphocytic leukemia (CLL), AML, follicular NHL, Waldenstrom's macroglobulinemia, and as conditioning in allogeneic SCT. Unlike other purine antagonists, it causes profound lymphopenia (CD4 and CD8 reductions) in the T cell lineage along with myelosuppression. Patients are at risk for the opportunistic infections such as PCP, fungal infections, and herpes viruses, and should receive appropriate prophylaxis. Autoimmune hemolytic anemia has been reported, as well as neurotoxicity, which is very rare in patients receiving $\leq$30 mg/m^2/day for 5 days. Fludarabine is renally cleared, an important consideration in the elderly CLL population, and recommendations for reductions with CrCL as high as 80 mL/min have been made, although most reduce when values are below 50 mL/min or after toxicity [81].

Cladribine, pentostatin, and nelarabine are other purine antagonists with preferential activity for T cells, cause profound myelosuppression and immunosuppression, and are renally cleared. Cladribine and pentostatin are both highly active in hairy cell leukemia. Cladribine frequently requires only one course of treatment in many cases of hairy cell leukemia, and is active in CLL and low grade NHL. Unlike cladribine, pentostatin inhibits adenosine deaminase and has been used in GVHD treatment. Clofarabine was FDA approved for refractory pediatric ALL, but it also has activity in adults and AML. Pharmacology is similar to other agents. However, it has been associated with a capillary leak syndrome – prophylactic corticosteroids (e.g., hydrocortisone 100 mg/m^2 IV days 1–3) are recommended in combination with hydration to prevent a systemic inflammatory reaction. Nelarabine is a potent antimetabolite and ara-G prodrug used exclusively in T cell ALL. It crosses the blood–brain barrier well, and is associated with severe neurotoxicity evolving from somnolence to seizures, with a higher incidence in patients with a history of intrathecal treatment.

While hydroxyurea (PO) is classified as an antimetabolite, it works primarily against RNA as a ribonucleotide reductase inhibitor. The antitumor effect of hydroxyurea is limited to head and neck cancer as a radiosensitizer and is also used to reduce blood counts quickly in myeloproliferative disorders. Because it inhibits protein translation, it has a rapid on/off effect of 48–72 h and is readily titrated. Beyond blood count reduction, hydroxyurea also causes a megaloblastosis (a potential marker of adherence) and may cause rash. Dose reductions may be necessary in patients with CrCL <50 mL/min. However, if short courses are used reductions are not needed [38].

Microtubule Targeting Agents

Targeting the cell cycle in M phase is a rational approach to anticancer therapeutics, since cells are highly vulnerable during mitosis. Many agents in the class are derived from plant sources (e.g., vincristine from periwinkle, paclitaxel from the Pacific yew tree) and have complex chemical structures. Initially, plant-sourced agents were used and contributed to a greater understanding of mechanisms of action, leading to more refined medicinal chemistry and subclassification. The vinca alkaloids were the first to be described. All possess a basic nucleus of catharanthine and vindoline, with alterations on the vindoline nucleus creating different agents. They all interact with tubulin, disrupting assembly into microtubules that leads to mitosis arrest in metaphase. All vinca alkaloids are vesicants (extravasation can cause blistering and tissue necrosis), hepatically

cleared, and uniformly fatal if given intrathecally. They include vincristine (IV), vinblastine (IV), and vinorelbine (IV, PO in Europe). Each has unique activity and adverse event profiles, ranging from myelosuppression (no risk with vincristine, dose-limiting toxicity with vinorelbine) to neurotoxicity (highest with vincristine). Similarly, anticancer activity is variable. Vincristine has activity in ALL, lymphomas, neuroblastoma, and Wilms tumor. It is widely distributed into tissues, but does not cross the blood–brain barrier. Clearance is through CYP3A4; it is a p-glycoprotein substrate, with a half-life of over 40 h. All vincristine doses should be prepared in a small volume IV bag to prevent confusion with IT syringe administration of other clear solutions such as cytarabine. Frequently, doses are capped at 2 mg. However, justification for this routine practice is questionable, as neurotoxicity is rarely associated with single doses and many clinical trials did not cap doses [82]. Neurotoxicity is cumulative and therapy-limiting, with peripheral sensory deficits being most common. Patients should undergo interviews and symptom-directed physical examinations to identify evolving neuropathy. Initially, paresthesias develop that may progress to loss of deep tendon reflexes without intervention. Autonomic neuropathy may occur, with constipation and urinary retention occasionally seen. Dose reduction with bilirubin >3 mg/dL should be considered based on the goal of chemotherapy.

Vinblastine, in contrast to vincristine, has activity in bladder cancer and germ cell tumors, and is myelosuppressive. Like vincristine, it is active in lymphomas, is cleared through CYP3A4, and should be dose-reduced with elevated bilirubin. It is a minor inhibitor of CYP3A4 and CYP2D6. Neurotoxicity patterns are similar. However, the frequency and severity is less than that seen with vincristine.

Vinorelbine is the least neurotoxic of the vinca alkaloids due to specificity for mitotic over axonal microtubules, but is also the most myelosuppressive [83]. It has activity in lung, breast, cervical and ovarian cancers, as well as lymphomas and soft tissue sarcomas. Dose adjustments are more conservative, and are recommended for bilirubin $\geq$2 mg/dL [70].

Taxanes are a unique class of microtubule-targeting agents that bind to α- and β-tubulin, stabilizing microtubules against depolymerization and disassembly [84, 85]. Microtubules formed in the presence of taxanes are more stable than normal, and therefore disrupt cell division dynamics during interphase. Discovery of paclitaxel (IV), the reference agent in the class, was by a National Cancer Institute program that screened thousands of plant species. The bark of the Pacific yew tree, or *Taxus brevifolia*, was initially used to isolate paclitaxel. However, synthetic methods are used today [86]. Because it is a natural product, the rates and severity of hypersensitivity reactions during infusion initially limited use; however, premedication regimens using corticosteroids, diphenhydramine, and H$_2$ antagonists (e.g., ranitidine) have reduced the incidence from over 40% to 1–3% [87]. The dilution vehicle for paclitaxel, polyoxyethylated castor oil (Cremophor® EL), has been implicated in hypersensitivity reactions, and limits single dose ceilings for paclitaxel [88]. Initial development was focused on longer (96 h) infusions with the goal of maximizing cell kill by prolonged exposure to the greatest number of cells in the shortest portion of the cell cycle. However, similar activity has been seen with 3-h infusions every 21 days and hourly infusions weekly [21]. Paclitaxel activity is broad, with routine use in adenocarcinoma of unknown primary, melanoma and Kaposi's sarcoma as well as lung, breast, ovarian, cervical, esophageal, head and neck, bladder cancers, and others. It is hepatically cleared by CYP2C8 and CYP3A4, and dose reduction should be considered with bilirubin ≥1.25 times the upper limit of normal. It is widely distributed, with a terminal half-life of 15–50 hours, and clearance is linearly correlated with length of infusion [89]. A significant drug interaction with carboplatin may occur, so paclitaxel should be given prior to carboplatin to reduce severity of myelosuppression. Alopecia and cumulative neurotoxicity are prevalent, and some patients may experience myalgias for 2–3 days after infusion, relieved by NSAIDs. Rarely, bradycardia and arrhythmias occur during infusion. A newer formulation of paclitaxel, nanoparticle albumin-bound paclitaxel (nab-paclitaxel) does not require the use of polyoxyethylated castor oil as a vehicle, can be given over 30 min, and doesn't require premedication. Nab-paclitaxel is active in NSCLC, pancreatic, ovarian, and breast cancer with weekly and every 3 weeks dosing.

Docetaxel (IV) is the second agent in the class, and is similar in mechanism to paclitaxel, although it has activity in patients with prostate cancer as well as cancers previously treated with paclitaxel [90]. It is formulated in polysorbate 80, hepatically cleared by CYP3A4, requires dose adjustment with hepatic dysfunction (elevated transaminases and alkaline phosphatase), and is given over 1 h. Like paclitaxel, myelosuppression and neuropathy are common. However, docetaxel requires premedication only with dexamethasone the day before, during, and after to prevent fluid retention and hypersensitivity reactions. It may also rarely cause nail bed changes and hyperlacrimation.

The most recent addition to the class is cabazitaxel (IV), an agent with activity in docetaxel-treated prostate cancer. Like paclitaxel, it requires a three drug premedication regimen and is cleared by CYP3A4 and CYP2C8. It also requires dose adjustment in hepatic impairment. Unlike the other taxanes, it is not a substrate for multidrug resistance proteins [91].

Newer microtubule inhibitor agents include the epothilone ixabepilone (IV) and the halichondrin B derivative eribulin (IV), as well as inhibitors of the kinesin spindle protein in development. Both ixabepilone and eribulin are active in breast cancer, cause myelosuppression and neuropathy, and require dose adjustment in hepatic impairment. Ixabepilone is a CYP3A4 substrate, while eribulin is excreted in bile unchanged.

Topoisomerase Inhibitors

Topoisomerase enzymes regulate the winding of DNA, and either bind to single or double-stranded segments, cutting the phosphate backbone of DNA for replication. The enzyme topoisomerase I catalyzes relaxation of supercoiled DNA in all phases of replication, transcription, and recombination. It induces a single strand break, allowing release of DNA torsional strain with transcription of the DNA sequence for new cells to form. Topoisomerase II unwinds strands and actively inserts new DNA strands into the helix, and anneals the break prior to chromosome formation. More recently, the anthracyclines, anthracenedione, and antitumor antibiotics have been shown to inhibit topoisomerase II [92, 93].

Topoisomerase I inhibitors include the camptothecin analogues irinotecan (CPT-11) (IV) and topotecan (IV, PO). Both are derivatives of camptothecin, an extract from the Chinese tree *Camptotheca accuminata* [94]. They exist as equilibrium lactone and carboxylate species, with the closed-ring active lactone predominating at acidic pH. Irinotecan is a prodrug, with carboxylesterases creating the active metabolite SN-38, which exerts activity by stabilizing topoisomerase I-DNA complexes leading to DNA strand breaks. It is cell cycle nonspecific, with activity in colorectal, pancreas, gastric, esophageal, and lung cancers. SN-38 metabolism is modulated by the enzyme system UGT1A1, and germline genetic variability in enzyme expression has been linked to neutropenia severity after treatment [95]. The resulting moiety, SN-38 glucuronide (SN-38G), is excreted in bile, and may be converted back to SN-38 by intestinal bacterial glucuronidases. Severe diarrhea can be seen with increased intestinal SN-38 concentrations, either due to decreased SN-38G production or increased intestinal cleavage. The use of lower irinotecan doses abrogates the original observations of severe neutropenia and diarrhea seen in development. However, intrapatient variability in UGT1A1 genotype and activity can cause toxicities with lower doses. Homozygosity of the genotype UGT1A1*28, also known as Gilbert syndrome, is associated with the most severe toxicities, and patients with bilirubin ≥1.5 mg/dL should be considered for empiric reductions. Irinotecan exposure may be also influenced by smoking status, with chronic smokers producing lower amounts of SN-38. Diarrhea may occur in two distinct phases, an acute cholinergic diarrhea (<24 h), prevented by atropine, and SN-38-mediated diarrhea, which requires aggressive antidiarrheals (e.g., loperamide 4 mg orally every 4 h). Myelosuppression, as mentioned, may also limit therapy with weekly and every 3 week dosing.

Topotecan has activity in ovarian, SCLC, and cervical cancer, and is given either daily for 5 days or weekly. It is renally cleared, and should be reduced in patients with CrCL <40 mL/min, although dose-limiting myelosuppression may still occur. Unlike irinotecan, topotecan crosses the blood–brain barrier, and up to 30% of systemic concentrations may reach the CNS.

Classic topoisomerase II inhibitors include the epipodophyllotoxins etoposide (VP-16) (IV, PO) and teniposide (IV), the latter solely used in pediatric ALL. Both are associated with increased risks of secondary AML, characterized by the genetic alteration of t(11;23), with a short latency period of 1–3 years following exposure [96]. Etoposide is active in SCLC, germ cell tumors, lymphomas, and is commonly used in conditioning for autologous SCT. It is orally bioavailable, and doses should be twice those given intravenously (i.e., 50% bioavailability). The vehicle for etoposide is polysorbate 80, and it will precipitate at concentrations >0.4 mg/mL. Higher doses (e.g., 60 mg/kg) may be given as undiluted drug. However, hypotension and metabolic acidosis become concerns. Renal clearance requires dose adjustments in patients with CrCL <50 mL/min. Common toxicities include myelosuppression, stomatitis, and, rarely, hypersensitivity reactions. The formulation etoposide phosphate (IV) is also available, which has improved solubility. Teniposide also causes myelosuppression, stomatitis, and rare hypersensitivity reactions, and both agents are CYP3A4 substrates.

Antitumor Antibiotics

This class of cytotoxic chemotherapy agents is a catchall for agents derived from bacterial sources. Many were isolated from *Streptomyces* species with large chemical structures that fluoresce brightly. Mechanisms of action include direct intercalation into DNA, generation of oxygen free radicals, topoisomerase II inhibition, and DNA crosslinking, or combinations of each. All agents are given IV and include the anthracyclines (doxorubicin, pegylated liposomal doxorubicin, daunorubicin, liposomal daunorubicin, idarubicin, and epirubicin), the anthracenedione mitoxantrone, dactinomycin, bleomycin, and mitomycin. Other commonalities (except bleomycin) include vesicant properties, hepatic/biliary clearance, myelosuppression, alopecia, and radiation recall. There are also significant chronic toxicities, including cardiac (anthracyclines) and pulmonary (bleomycin).

The anthracycline class is the broadest, with doxorubicin being the prototypical and most commonly used agent. Doxorubicin intercalates DNA, inhibits topoisomerase II and DNA-dependent RNA polymerase, produces oxygen free radicals, and is specific for the S phase. Activity is broad, with thyroid, breast and bladder cancers, sarcoma, and lymphomas all sensitive. It is widely distributed and hepatically cleared, with an active metabolite doxorubicinol. Doxorubicin, like all agents in the class, can cause cardiotoxicity, classified as acute (EKG abnormalities, arrhythmias, rare pericarditis) and chronic (biventricular heart failure). Acute toxicity is relatively infrequent. Chronic toxicity is dose-limiting and requires monitoring of all patients with assessment of ejection fraction prior to treatment and periodically thereafter. It is likely caused by oxygen free radical generation, although cardiac-based topoisomerase II may contribute [97]. Risk factors include cumulative doses $\geq$550 mg/m^2, IV bolus injection (as opposed to prolonged infusions of $\geq$6 h), concurrent cardiotoxic agents (e.g., trastuzumab), mediastinal radiation, advanced age, and pre-existing cardiac disease, notably hypertension [20, 98, 99]. There is significant variability in dose as a predictor of cardiotoxicity, with guidelines suggesting capping lifetime exposure to 450–550 mg/m^2. Other adverse events include urine discoloration and photosensitivity. The pegylated liposomal doxorubicin (PLD) formulation is active in myeloma, breast and ovarian cancer, Kaposi's sarcoma, and others. The liposomal form stays in circulation longer than the conventional agent. Unique to PLD is palmar–plantar erythrodysesthesia (hand–foot syndrome), which can occur in up to 50% of patients. Cardiotoxicity with PLD is potentially lower than with conventional doxorubicin, as patients treated up to 500 mg/m^2 had lower rates of heart failure. However, additional comparative data are needed [100].

Daunorubicin and idarubicin are anthracyclines used in acute leukemias, but have similar clinical pharmacology and adverse event profiles to doxorubicin. Idarubicin is more potent, with doses of approximately one-fifth that of daunorubicin in induction for AML.

Epirubicin is a topoisomerase II inhibitor with activity in breast, esophageal, and gastric cancers. Cumulative doses of less than 900 mg/m^2 are recommended to prevent chronic cardiotoxicity (seven to nine cycles of therapy for breast cancer

when used in combination with fluorouracil and cyclophosphamide). However, patients should be risk stratified individually.

Mitoxantrone was initially thought to be less cardiotoxic that doxorubicin. However, data are unclear on this benefit [101]. It is a topoisomerase II inhibitor and is active in lymphomas, AML, and prostate cancer.

The other agents in this class include dactinomycin, mitomycin, and bleomycin. Dactinomycin is used in pediatric sarcomas, germ cell tumors, Wilms tumors, and gestational trophoblastic disease, and is eliminated through bile and urine unchanged with a half-life of 36 h. Mitomycin is active in bladder and anal cancers, and primarily acts via DNA crosslinking, similar to alkylating agents. It is also given intravesically for superficial bladder cancer. Metabolism is rapid, with no adjustments needed in hepatic or renal dysfunction. Myelosuppression with mitomycin may be substantially delayed, with recovery taking up to 7–8 weeks. It rarely causes a severe hemolytic uremic syndrome with subsequent renal failure. Bleomycin is active in germ cell tumors and lymphomas, particularly Hodgkin lymphoma, and is dosed in units of activity, where 1 unit = 1 mg. It has also been used as a sclerosing agent in patients with malignant pleural effusions; however, talc is preferred due to efficacy and cost. Bleomycin is renally cleared, and dose adjustments are required with CrCL <50 mL/min. It may rarely cause hypersensitivity, and test dosing has been recommended, although since test dosing may not predict subsequent reactions, this practice is questionable [102]. Pulmonary toxicity is a significant concern, and patients should have pulmonary function testing with a focus on alveolar diffusion of gases, measured by the diffusion capacity of carbon monoxide (D$_{LCO}$), prior to therapy. If D$_{LCO}$ is <35% of baseline at any time, therapy should be stopped. Risk factors include age >70, chest radiation, and total doses of >400 units. Although evidence is largely anecdotal, many clinicians avoid concurrent and subsequent high fractions of inspired oxygen (FiO$_2$) in patients with hypoxemia due to bleomycin or other causes, for fear of worsening pulmonary damage. Toxicity may evolve to fibrosis from interstitial pneumonitis, and is thought to be due to a lack of hydrolases in lung tissue [103]. Bleomycin may also cause rash and fever in 50% of patients.

Conclusion

The translation of cell cycle biology to effective clinical pharmacology continues to evolve, based on new insights and rational drug design. For example, inhibitors of CDKs continue to be evaluated in early phase trials with the hope that an additional class of cytotoxic agents will become incorporated into routine treatment. Novel approaches to microtubule inhibition (e.g., kinesin spindle protein inhibitors) also continue to evolve. Despite new approaches to drug design based on molecular biology, it is likely conventional cytotoxic chemotherapy will never be relegated to a niche role in treatment, based on an established track record of use and success in many cancers. For this reason, clinicians need to be aware of the clinical pharmacology, activity, and adverse events associated with their use.

References

1 Goodman LS, Wintrobe MM, Dameshek W, *et al.* Landmark article Sept. 21, 1946: nitrogen mustard therapy. Use of methyl-bis(beta-chloroethyl)amine hydrochloride and tris(beta-chloroethyl)amine hydrochloride for Hodgkin's disease, lymphosarcoma, leukemia and certain allied and miscellaneous disorders. By Louis S. Goodman, Maxwell M. Wintrobe, William Dameshek, Morton J. Goodman, Alfred Gilman and Margaret T. McLennan. *JAMA* 1984;251(17):2255–61.

2 Gilman A. The initial clinical trial of nitrogen mustard. *Am J Surg* 1963;105:574–8.

3 Spurr CL, Jacobson LO, *et al.* The clinical application of a nitrogen mustard compound methyl bis (beta-chloroethyl) amine to the treatment of neoplastic disorders of the hemopoietic system. *Cancer Res* 1947;7(1):51.

4 Heidelberger C, Chaudhuri NK, Danneberg P, *et al.* Fluorinated pyrimidines, a new class of tumour-inhibitory compounds. *Nature* 1957;179(4561):663–6.

5 Hanahan D, Weinberg RA. Hallmarks of cancer: the next generation. *Cell* 2011;144(5):646–74.

6 Skipper HE. Historic milestones in cancer biology: a few that are important in cancer treatment (revisited). *Semin Oncol* 1979;6(4):506–14.

7 Laird AK. Dynamics of tumor growth. *Br J Cancer* 1964;13:490–502.

8 Simon R, Norton L. The Norton-Simon hypothesis: designing more effective and less toxic chemotherapeutic regimens. *Nat Clin Pract Oncol* 2006;3(8):406–7.

9 Schmidt C. The Gompertzian view: Norton honored for role in establishing cancer treatment approach. *J Natl Cancer Inst* 2004;96(20):1492–3.

10 Steel GG. Autoradiographic analysis of the cell cycle: Howard and Pelc to the present day. *Int J Radiat Biol Relat Stud Phys Chem Med* 1986;49(2):227–35.

11 Lilly MA, Duronio RJ. New insights into cell cycle control from the Drosophila endocycle. *Oncogene* 2005;24(17):2765–75.

12 Hunter T, Pines J. Cyclins and cancer. II: Cyclin D and CDK inhibitors come of age. *Cell* 1994;79(4):573–82.

13 Wong RS. Apoptosis in cancer: from pathogenesis to treatment. *J Exp Clin Cancer Res* 2011;30:87.

14 Smith ML, Chen IT, Zhan Q, *et al.* Interaction of the p53-regulated protein Gadd45 with proliferating cell nuclear antigen. *Science* 1994;266(5189):1376–80.

15 Bruce WR, Meeker BE, Valeriote FA. Comparison of the sensitivity of normal hematopoietic and transplanted lymphoma colony-forming cells to chemotherapeutic agents administered in vivo. *J Natl Cancer Inst* 1966;37(2):233–45.

16 Giaccone G, Pinedo HM. Drug resistance. *Oncologist* 1996;1(1 & 2):82–7.

17 Goldie JH, Coldman AJ. A mathematic model for relating the drug sensitivity of tumors to their spontaneous mutation rate. *Cancer Treat Rep* 1979;63(11–12):1727–33.

18 Bonilla L, Ben-Aharon I, Vidal L, *et al.* Dose-dense chemotherapy in nonmetastatic breast cancer: a systematic review and meta-analysis of randomized controlled trials. *J Natl Cancer Inst* 2010;102(24):1845–54.

19 de Gramont A, Bosset JF, Milan C, *et al.* Randomized trial comparing monthly low-dose leucovorin and fluorouracil bolus with bimonthly high-dose leucovorin and fluorouracil bolus plus continuous infusion for advanced colorectal cancer: a French intergroup study. *J Clin Oncol* 1997;15(2):808–15.

20 van Dalen EC, van der Pal HJ, Caron HN, Kremer LC. Different dosage schedules for reducing cardiotoxicity in cancer patients receiving anthracycline chemotherapy. *Cochrane Database Syst Rev* 2006;(4):CD005008.

21 O'Neil BH, Socinski MA. 96-hour paclitaxel infusions: at least 93 hours too long. *Cancer Invest* 2003;21(4):660–2.

22 Gralow JR, Burstein HJ, Wood W, *et al.* Preoperative therapy in invasive breast cancer: pathologic assessment and systemic therapy issues in operable disease. *J Clin Oncol* 2008;26(5):814–9.

23 Olivotto IA, Bajdik CD, Ravdin PM, *et al.* Population-based validation of the prognostic model ADJUVANT! for early breast cancer. *J Clin Oncol* 2005;23(12):2716–25.

24 Wong R, Malthaner R. Combined chemotherapy and radiotherapy (without surgery) compared with radiotherapy alone in localized carcinoma of the esophagus. *Cochrane Database Syst Rev* 2001;(2):CD002092.

25 O'Rourke N, Roque I Figuls M, Farre Bernado N, Macbeth F. Concurrent chemoradiotherapy in non-small cell lung cancer. *Cochrane Database Syst Rev* 2010 2010;(6):CD002140.

26 Sauer R, Liersch T, Merkel S, *et al.* Preoperative versus postoperative chemoradiotherapy for locally advanced rectal cancer: results of the German CAO/ARO/AIO-94 randomized phase III trial after a median follow-up of 11 years. *J Clin Oncol* 2012;30(16):1926–33.

27 Bernier J, Domenge C, Ozsahin M, *et al.* Postoperative irradiation with or without concomitant chemotherapy for locally advanced head and neck cancer. *N Engl J Med* 2004;350(19):1945–52.

28 Fleming RA. An overview of cyclophosphamide and ifosfamide pharmacology. *Pharmacotherapy* 1997;17(5 Pt 2):146–54.

29 Hensley ML, Hagerty KL, Kewalramani T, *et al.* American Society of Clinical Oncology 2008 clinical practice guideline update: use of chemotherapy and radiation therapy protectants. *J Clin Oncol* 2009;27(1):127–45.

30 Ben Yehuda A, Heyman A, Steiner-Salz D. False positive reaction for urinary ketones with mesna. *Drug Intell Clin Pharm* 1987;21(6):547–8.

31 David KA, Picus J. Evaluating risk factors for the development of ifosfamide encephalopathy. *Am J Clin Oncol* 2005;28(3):277–80.

32 Howell JE, Szabatura AH, Hatfield Seung A, Nesbit SA. Characterization of the occurrence of ifosfamide-induced neurotoxicity with concomitant aprepitant. *J Oncol Pharm Pract* 2008;14(3):157–62.

33 Bernard PA, McCabe T, Bayliff S, Hayes D, Jr. Successful treatment of ifosfamide neurotoxicity with dexmedetomidine. *J Oncol Pharm Pract* 2010;16(4):262–5.

34 Pelgrims J, De Vos F, Van den Brande J, *et al.* Methylene blue in the treatment and prevention of ifosfamide-induced encephalopathy: report of 12 cases and a review of the literature. *Br J Cancer* 2000;82(2):291–4.

35 Stewart DJ, Morgan LR, Jr, Verma S, Maroun JA, Thibault M. Pharmacology, relative bioavailability, and toxicity of three different oral cyclophosphamide preparations in a randomized, cross-over study. *Invest New Drugs* 1995;13(1):99–107.

36 Ehrsson H, Eksborg S, Osterborg A, Mellstedt H, Lindfors A. Oral melphalan pharmacokinetics—relation to dose in patients with multiple myeloma. *Med Oncol Tumor Pharmacother* 1989;6(2):151–4.

37 Woodhouse KW, Hamilton P, Lennard A, Rawlins MD. The pharmacokinetics of melphalan in patients with multiple myeloma: an intravenous/oral study using a conventional dose regimen. *Eur J Clin Pharmacol* 1983;24(2):283–5.

38 Kintzel PE, Dorr RT. Anticancer drug renal toxicity and elimination: dosing guidelines for altered renal function. *Cancer Treat Rev* 1995;21(1):33–64.

39 Tageja N, Nagi J. Bendamustine: something old, something new. *Cancer Chemother Pharmacol* 2010;66(3):413–23.

40 Hegi ME, Diserens AC, Gorlia T, *et al.* MGMT gene silencing and benefit from temozolomide in glioblastoma. *N Engl J Med* 2005;352(10):997–1003.

41 Stupp R, Mason WP, van den Bent MJ, *et al.* Radiotherapy plus concomitant and adjuvant temozolomide for glioblastoma. *N Engl J Med* 2005;352(10):987–96.

42 McCune JS, Holmberg LA. Busulfan in hematopoietic stem cell transplant setting. *Expert Opin Drug Metab Toxicol* 2009;5(8):957–69.

43 Russell JA, Tran HT, Quinlan D, *et al.* Once-daily intravenous busulfan given with fludarabine as conditioning for allogeneic stem cell transplantation: study of pharmacokinetics and early clinical outcomes. *Biol Blood Marrow Transplant* 2002;8(9):468–76.

44 Eberly AL, Anderson GD, Bubalo JS, McCune JS. Optimal prevention of seizures induced by high-dose busulfan. *Pharmacotherapy* 2008;28(12):1502–10.

45 Rosenberg B, VanCamp L, Trosko JE, Mansour VH. Platinum compounds: a new class of potent antitumour agents. *Nature* 1969;222(5191):385–6.

46 Einhorn LH. Treatment of testicular cancer: a new and improved model. *J Clin Oncol* 1990;8(11):1777–81.

47 Morgan KP, Buie LW, Savage SW. The role of mannitol as a nephroprotectant in patients receiving cisplatin therapy. *Ann Pharmacother* 2012;46(2):276–81.

48 Schilsky RL, Anderson T. Hypomagnesemia and renal magnesium wasting in patients receiving cisplatin. *Ann Intern Med* 1979;90(6):929–31.

49 von der Maase H, Andersen L, Crinò L, Weinknecht S, Dogliotti L. Weekly gemcitabine and cisplatin combination therapy in patients with transitional cell carcinoma of the urothelium: A phase II clinical trial. *Ann Oncol* 1999;10(12):1461–5.

50 Calvert AH, Newell DR, Gumbrell LA, *et al.* Carboplatin dosage: prospective evaluation of a simple formula based on renal function. *J Clin Oncol* 1989;7(11):1748–56.

51 Janus N, Thariat J, Boulanger H, Deray G, Launay-Vacher V. Proposal for dosage adjustment and timing of chemotherapy in hemodialyzed patients. *Ann Oncol* 2010;21(7):1395–403.

52 Markman M, Kennedy A, Webster K, *et al.* Clinical features of hypersensitivity reactions to carboplatin. *J Clin Oncol* 1999;17(4):1141.

53 Synold TW, Takimoto CH, Doroshow JH, *et al.* Dose-escalating and pharmacologic study of oxaliplatin in adult cancer patients with impaired hepatic function: a National Cancer Institute Organ Dysfunction Working Group study. *Clin Cancer Res* 2007;13(12):3660–6.

54 Takimoto CH, Remick SC, Sharma S, *et al.* Dose-escalating and pharmacological study of oxaliplatin in adult cancer patients with impaired renal function: a National Cancer Institute Organ Dysfunction Working Group Study. *J Clin Oncol* 2003;21(14):2664–72.

55 Argyriou AA, Cavaletti G, Briani C, *et al.* Clinical pattern and associations of oxaliplatin acute neurotoxicity: a prospective study in 170 patients with colorectal cancer. *Cancer* 2013;119(2):438–44.

56 Meyer LM, Miller FR, Rowen MJ, Bock G, Rutzky J. Treatment of acute leukemia with amethopterin (4-amino, 10-methyl pteroyl glutamic acid). *Acta Haematol* 1950;4(3):157–67.

57 Teresi ME, Crom WR, Choi KE, Mirro J, Evans WE. Methotrexate bioavailability after oral and intramuscular administration in children. *J Pediatr* 1987;110(5):788–92.

58 Shamash J, Earl H, Souhami R. Acetazolamide for alkalinisation of urine in patients receiving high-dose methotrexate. *Cancer Chemother Pharmacol* 1991;28(2):150–1.

59 Bleyer WA. Methotrexate: clinical pharmacology, current status and therapeutic guidelines. *Cancer Treat Rev* 1977;4(2):87–101.

60 Evans WE, Pratt CB, Taylor RH, Barker LF, Crom WR. Pharmacokinetic monitoring of high-dose methotrexate. Early recognition of high-risk patients. *Cancer Chemother Pharmacol* 1979;3(3):161–6.

61 Widemann BC, Balis FM, Kim A, *et al.* Glucarpidase, leucovorin, and thymidine for high-dose methotrexate-induced renal dysfunction: clinical and pharmacologic factors affecting outcome. *J Clin Oncol* 2010;28(25):3979–86.

62 Brandes JC, Grossman SA, Ahmad H. Alteration of pemetrexed excretion in the presence of acute renal failure and effusions: presentation of a case and review of the literature. *Cancer Invest* 2006;24(3):283–7.

63 Longley DB, Harkin DP, Johnston PG. 5-fluorouracil: mechanisms of action and clinical strategies. *Nat Rev Cancer* 2003;3(5):330–8.

64 Diasio RB, Harris BE. Clinical pharmacology of 5-fluorouracil. *Clin Pharmacokinet* 1989;16(4):215–37.

65 Rustum YM. Biochemical rationale for the 5-fluorouracil leucovorin combination and update of clinical experience. *J Chemother* 1990;2 Suppl 1:5–11.

66 Saif MW, Shah MM, Shah AR. Fluoropyrimidine-associated cardiotoxicity: revisited. *Expert Opin Drug Saf* 2009; 8(2):191–202.

67 Davis DA, Fugate SE. Increasing warfarin dosage reductions associated with concurrent warfarin and repeated cycles of 5-Fluorouracil therapy. *Pharmacotherapy* 2005;25(3):442–7.

68 Magagnoli M, Masci G, Castagna L, Morenghi E, Santoro A. High incidence of INR alteration in gastrointestinal cancer

patients treated with mini-dose warfarin and 5-fluorouracil-based regimens. *Ann Oncol* 2006;17(1):174–6.

69 Hoff PM, Ansari R, Batist G, *et al.* Comparison of oral capecitabine versus intravenous fluorouracil plus leucovorin as first-line treatment in 605 patients with metastatic colorectal cancer: results of a randomized phase III study. *J Clin Oncol* 2001;19(8):2282–92.

70 Superfin D, Iannucci AA, Davies AM. Commentary: oncologic drugs in patients with organ dysfunction: a summary. *Oncologist* 2007;12(9):1070–83.

71 Chu MP, Hecht JR, Slamon D, *et al.* Association of proton pump inhibitors and capecitabine efficacy in advanced gastroesophageal cancer: secondary analysis of the TRIO-013/LOGiC Randomized Clinical Trial. JAMA Oncol 2016 Oct 13.

72 Sun J, Ilich AI, Kim CA, et al. Concomitant administration of proton pump inhibitors and capecitabine is associated with increased recurrence risk in early stage colorectal cancer patients. *Clin Colorectal Cancer* 2016;15(3):257–63.

73 Bianchi V, Borella S, Calderazzo F, *et al.* Inhibition of ribonucleotide reductase by 2'-substituted deoxycytidine analogs: possible application in AIDS treatment. *Proc Natl Acad Sci USA* 1994;91(18):8403–7.

74 Grimison P, Galettis P, Manners S, *et al.* Randomized crossover study evaluating the effect of gemcitabine infusion dose rate: evidence of auto-induction of gemcitabine accumulation. *J Clin Oncol* 2007;25(36):5704–9.

75 Ko AH, Dito E, Schillinger B, *et al.* Phase II study of fixed dose rate gemcitabine with cisplatin for metastatic adenocarcinoma of the pancreas. *J Clin Oncol* 2006;24(3):379–85.

76 Mayer RJ, Davis RB, Schiffer CA, *et al.* Intensive postremission chemotherapy in adults with acute myeloid leukemia. Cancer and Leukemia Group B. *N Engl J Med* 1994;331(14):896–903.

77 Smith GA, Damon LE, Rugo HS, Ries CA, Linker CA. High-dose cytarabine dose modification reduces the incidence of neurotoxicity in patients with renal insufficiency. *J Clin Oncol* 1997;15(2):833–9.

78 Lennard L, Van Loon JA, Weinshilboum RM. Pharmacogenetics of acute azathioprine toxicity: relationship to thiopurine methyltransferase genetic polymorphism. *Clin Pharmacol Ther* 1989;46(2):149–54.

79 Rees CA, Lennard L, Lilleyman JS, Maddocks JL. Disturbance of 6-mercaptopurine metabolism by cotrimoxazole in childhood lymphoblastic leukaemia. *Cancer Chemother Pharmacol* 1984;12(2):87–9.

80 Armstrong VW, Shipkova M, von Ahsen N, Oellerich M. Analytic aspects of monitoring therapy with thiopurine medications. *Ther Drug Monit* 2004;26(2):220–6.

81 Martell RE, Peterson BL, Cohen HJ, *et al.* Analysis of age, estimated creatinine clearance and pretreatment hematologic parameters as predictors of fludarabine toxicity in patients treated for chronic lymphocytic leukemia: a CALGB (9011) coordinated intergroup study. *Cancer Chemother Pharmacol* 2002;50(1):37–45.

82 McCune JS, Lindley C. Appropriateness of maximum-dose guidelines for vincristine. *Am J Health Syst Pharm* 1997;54(15):1755–8.

83 Gregory RK, Smith IE. Vinorelbine—a clinical review. *Br J Cancer* 2000;82(12):1907–13.

84 Jordan MA, Toso RJ, Thrower D, Wilson L. Mechanism of mitotic block and inhibition of cell proliferation by taxol at low concentrations. *Proc Natl Acad Sci USA* 1993;90(20):9552–6.

85 Rao S, Orr GA, Chaudhary AG, Kingston DG, Horwitz SB. Characterization of the taxol binding site on the microtubule. 2-(m-Azidobenzoyl)taxol photolabels a peptide (amino acids 217-231) of beta-tubulin. *J Biol Chem* 1995;270(35):20235–8.

86 Rowinsky EK, Donehower RC. Paclitaxel (taxol). *N Engl J Med* 1995;332(15):1004–14.

87 Weiss RB, Donehower RC, Wiernik PH, *et al.* Hypersensitivity reactions from taxol. *J Clin Oncol* 1990;8(7):1263–8.

88 Sparreboom A, Baker SD, Verweij J. Paclitaxel repackaged in an albumin-stabilized nanoparticle: handy or just a dandy? *J Clin Oncol* 2005;23(31):7765–7.

89 Sonnichsen DS, Relling MV. Clinical pharmacokinetics of paclitaxel. *Clin Pharmacokinet* 1994;27(4):256–69.

90 Verweij J, Clavel M, Chevalier B. Paclitaxel (Taxol) and docetaxel (Taxotere): not simply two of a kind. *Ann Oncol* 1994;5(6):495–505.

91 Beltran H, Beer TM, Carducci MA, *et al.* New therapies for castration-resistant prostate cancer: efficacy and safety. *Eur Urol* 2011;60(2):279–90.

92 Kasahara K, Fujiwara Y, Sugimoto Y, *et al.* Determinants of response to the DNA topoisomerase II inhibitors doxorubicin and etoposide in human lung cancer cell lines. *J Natl Cancer Inst* 1992;84(2):113–8.

93 Boland MP, Fitzgerald KA, O'Neill LA. Topoisomerase II is required for mitoxantrone to signal nuclear factor kappa B activation in HL60 cells. *J Biol Chem* 2000;275(33):25231–8.

94 Wall ME, Wani MC, Natschke SM, Nicholas AW. Plant antitumor agents. 22. Isolation of 11-hydroxycamptothecin from Camptotheca acuminata Decne: total synthesis and biological activity. *J Med Chem* 1986;29(8):1553–5.

95 Innocenti F, Undevia SD, Iyer L, *et al.* Genetic variants in the UDP-glucuronosyltransferase 1A1 gene predict the risk of severe neutropenia of irinotecan. *J Clin Oncol* 2004;22(8):1382–8.

96 Winick NJ, McKenna RW, Shuster JJ, *et al.* Secondary acute myeloid leukemia in children with acute lymphoblastic leukemia treated with etoposide. *J Clin Oncol* 1993;11(2):209–17.

97 Zhang S, Liu X, Bawa-Khalfe T, *et al.* Identification of the molecular basis of doxorubicin-induced cardiotoxicity. *Nat Med* 2012;18(11):1639–42.

98 Von Hoff DD, Layard MW, Basa P, *et al.* Risk factors for doxorubicin-induced congestive heart failure. *Ann Intern Med* 1979;91(5):710–7.

99 Hershman DL, McBride RB, Eisenberger A, *et al.* Doxorubicin, cardiac risk factors, and cardiac toxicity in elderly patients with diffuse B-cell non-Hodgkin's lymphoma. *J Clin Oncol* 2008;26(19):3159–65.

100 Safra T, Muggia F, Jeffers S, *et al.* Pegylated liposomal doxorubicin (doxil): reduced clinical cardiotoxicity in patients

reaching or exceeding cumulative doses of 500 mg/m2. *Ann Oncol* 2000;11(8):1029–33.

101 Smith LA, Cornelius VR, Plummer CJ, *et al.* Cardiotoxicity of anthracycline agents for the treatment of cancer: systematic review and meta-analysis of randomised controlled trials. *BMC Cancer* 2010;10:337.

102 Lam MS. The need for routine bleomycin test dosing in the 21st century. *Ann Pharmacother* 2005;39(11):1897–902.

103 Sleijfer S. Bleomycin-induced pneumonitis. *Chest* 2001;120(2):617–24.

104 Takimoto CH. New antifolates: pharmacology and clinical applications. *Oncologist* 1996;1(1):68–81.

19

Hormonal Therapy for Cancer

Amelia B. Zelnak[1] and Bradley C. Carthon[2]

[1] *Atlanta Cancer Care, Northside Hospital Cancer Institute, Atlanta, Georgia, USA*
[2] *Winship Cancer Institute, Emory University School of Medicine, Atlanta, Georgia, USA*

Historical Background of Hormonal Therapy for Breast Cancer

Beatson first observed the role of estrogen deprivation in treatment of breast cancer in 1895 after observing the regression of advanced breast cancer following oophorectomy. In 1900, Boyd reported tumor regression in approximately one-third of premenopausal patients who underwent bilateral oophorectomy as treatment for advanced breast cancer. The major advancement in endocrine therapy of breast cancer resulted from an understanding of estrogen action and the successful development of antiestrogens. The nonsteroidal estrogen diethylstilbestrol (DES) was discovered in the 1930s. Jensen and Jacobson observed in 1962 that radiolabeled estradiol localized to estrogen target tissues and proposed that an estrogen receptor (ER) must be present in these tissues to regulate response to estradiol. The ER was subsequently identified and ER assays were developed to predict which breast cancer patients would respond to hormonal therapy [1].

In 1958 Lerner, Holthaus, and Thompson reported the biologic properties of the first nonsteroidal antiestrogen, MER-25 [2]. MER-25 had low potency and was associated with unacceptable central nervous system side effects. A successor compound, clomiphene, was a more potent antiestrogen and demonstrated modest activity in the treatment of advanced breast cancer [3]. Harper and Walpole demonstrated that tamoxifen had antiestrogenic and antifertility properties.[4]. Tamoxifen was evaluated in a number of clinical scenarios, but ultimately was developed for the treatment of breast cancer [5].

The first successful use of tamoxifen in treating advanced breast cancer was reported in 1971, with 10 of 46 patients (22%) demonstrating response to therapy [6]. These results were similar to those with DES; however, tamoxifen was much better tolerated. Tamoxifen, became the endocrine therapy of choice for advanced breast cancer in the 1970s. In 1986, tamoxifen was approved for adjuvant treatment of postmenopausal women with node-positive breast cancer. In 1990, tamoxifen was approved as adjuvant treatment for pre- and postmenopausal women with node-negative disease [7].

Aromatase inhibitors (AIs) prevent the peripheral conversion of androstenedione into estrogen, resulting in decreased levels of circulating estrogen [8, 9]. AIs are not effective in the management of premenopausal breast cancer patients in whom the ovaries are the main source of estrogen. Non-selective AIs, such as aminoglutethimide, were poorly tolerated by patients and have been replaced by newer AIs developed in the 1990s, such as anastrozole, letrozole, and exemestane. The selective AIs have proven to be extremely active drugs for postmenopausal women with all stages of hormone-sensitive breast cancer [10].

General Therapeutic Strategies for Metastatic Breast Cancer

Approximately two-thirds of breast cancers express hormone receptors, either ER or progesterone receptor (PR), or both. The likelihood of expressing ER and/or PR increases with age and postmenopausal status. The decision to choose one endocrine therapy over another must take into consideration the comparative efficacy, ease of administration, potential side effects, and menopausal status of the patient. The hormone receptor status of a tumor determines the likelihood that a patient will respond to endocrine therapy. Of patients with tumors positive for both ER and PR, 75–80% will respond to first-line endocrine therapy [11]. The response rates to endocrine therapy are lower for ER-positive, PR-negative tumors and ER-negative, PR-positive tumors at 25–30% and 40–45% respectively [11, 12]. Patients with very low levels or ER and PR expression may still derive benefit from endocrine therapy [13]. Patients whose tumors do not express either ER or PR typically do not benefit from endocrine therapy.

Multiple clinical trials have been performed in postmenopausal women with metastatic breast cancer comparing selective AIs to tamoxifen [14, 15]. Compared to tamoxifen, AIs had equivalent or longer time to progression depending on the study, and the side-effect profile favors AIs. Based upon these results, AIs are now used routinely in the first-line treatment of metastatic breast cancer in postmenopausal women. A subset of patients who respond to first-line endocrine therapy will respond to subsequent hormonal maneuvers at the time of progression. Up to 25% of patients will have objective tumor responses to AIs after initial treatment with tamoxifen [16–18], and up to 20% of patients will respond to fulvestrant after tamoxifen [19, 20].

Current Hormonal Therapies for Breast Cancer

Selective Estrogen Receptor Modulators (SERM)

Tamoxifen

Tamoxifen is a SERM that is currently FDA-approved for the treatment of all stages of hormone-responsive breast cancer and for breast cancer prevention in high-risk women. Tamoxifen inhibits breast cancer cell growth by competitive antagonism of estrogen at the ER [6]. Tamoxifen showed equivalent efficacy to androgens or high-dose estrogens in postmenopausal women, with a more favorable toxicity profile.

Estradiol binds to the nuclear ER, which then produces a change in shape to fully expose the DNA-binding domain on the protein complex. The activated receptor complex then dimerizes and binds to an estrogen response element (ERE) located in the promoter region of estrogen-responsive genes. Once bound to the ERE, the ER acts as an anchor for other transcription factors or associated proteins that, when assembled and associated with RNA polymerase, produce a transcription complex. The estrogen-responsive gene is then transcribed and subsequently translated to proteins that are involved in either growth responses or differentiation responses (e.g., PR synthesis).

Type I antiestrogens, like tamoxifen, appear to form a receptor complex that is incompletely converted to the fully activated form [21]. As a result, the expression of estrogen-responsive genes is not activated [22]. Tamoxifen also potentially inhibits tumor growth through mechanisms not mediated by the ER. Tamoxifen has been shown to inhibit protein kinase C and calmodulin-dependent cyclic adenosine monophosphate (cAMP) phophodiesterase, inhibit angiogenesis, and to decrease the synthesis of breast cancer mitogens [23–25].

With the daily oral administration of one 20 mg tablet or two 10 mg tablets of tamoxifen, steady-state plasma concentrations are reached after approximately 4 weeks. Tamoxifen is metabolized by the hepatic cytochrome P450 2D6 and is excreted primarily by the biliary system. Its major metabolites, endoxifen (4-hydroxy-N-desmethyl-tamoxifen) and 4-hydroxytamoxifen, remain active and bind to the estrogen receptor with higher affinity than tamoxifen [26, 27]. Analysis of CYP2D6 polymorphisms in large randomized trials has shown that CYP2D6 phenotypes of reduced enzyme activity were not associated with a worse breast cancer outcome on tamoxifen [28, 29]. Due to the lack of association seen between CYP2D6 genotype and tamoxifen response, CYP2D6 testing is not currently recommended.

Tamoxifen has antiestrogenic effects on some tissues including the breast and has estrogenic effects elsewhere in the body. This complex mechanism of action results in side effects of treatment which are both beneficial and detrimental. In postmenopausal women treated with tamoxifen, studies have shown an increase in bone density [30, 31]. The NSABP P-1 chemoprevention trial demonstrated fewer osteoporotic fracture events in women who received 5 years of tamoxifen compared to placebo. However, the results did not reach statistical significance [32].

Tamoxifen has been shown to have beneficial effects on the lipid profile by lowering total cholesterol, mainly due to its effect on low-density lipoprotein (LDL) cholesterol [33]. Tamoxifen also lowers fibrinogen, lipoprotein(a), and homocysteine, all factors that contribute to cardiovascular risk [34–36]. Extended follow-up of the Swedish tamoxifen adjuvant trial demonstrated reduced mortality from coronary heart disease in patients receiving 5 years of adjuvant tamoxifen, compared to those receiving 2 years of treatment [37]. Other studies of adjuvant tamoxifen have shown no cardiovascular benefit, with possible increased risk of cerebrovascular accidents [38].

Tamoxifen has been associated with an increased incidence of endometrial carcinoma in both treatment and prevention of breast cancer [32, 38, 39]. The relative risk of endometrial cancer in the tamoxifen-treated women from the NSABP P-1 prevention trial was 3.28. The increased risk was predominantly seen in women over the age of 50 with a relative risk of 5.33 compared to relative risk of 1.42 among women under 50. All the endometrial cancers seen in the tamoxifen-treated women were International Federation of Gynecology and Obstetrics (FIGO) stage I and of good prognosis. There was also an increased incidence of deep venous thrombosis in the tamoxifen-treated women in the NSABP P-1 trial. The relative risk of pulmonary embolism in the tamoxifen group was 2.15 [38].

Raloxifene

Raloxifene is another SERM that was initially developed as treatment for breast cancer. Raloxifene has a shorter half-life than tamoxifen, and has less estrogenic effects on the endometrium in preclinical models [40]. Raloxifene was evaluated in patients with tamoxifen-refractory metastatic breast cancer [41]. There were no partial or complete responders, with only one patient achieving a minor response, indicating significant cross-resistance between raloxifene and tamoxifen. Development of raloxifene as treatment for advanced breast cancer was discontinued after a study in the first-line setting showed lower than expected response rates [42].

Based on its estrogenic effects on bones, raloxifene was developed as a treatment for osteoporosis. Interestingly, the rate of breast cancers was significantly lower in patients treated with raloxifene for osteoporosis, compared to patients treated with placebo which led to its development as a breast cancer preventive [43]. Based on the results of the Study of Raloxifene and Tamoxifen (STAR) trial which showed similar efficacy between tamoxifen and raloxifene in preventing breast cancer in high risk women, raloxifene is currently approved for the prevention of breast cancer in postmenopausal women [44]. The incidence of endometrial cancer was lower in patients treated with raloxifene, compared to tamoxifen. Raloxifene was associated with a significantly reduced incidence of thromboembolic effects compared to tamoxifen, although there was no difference in the rate of cerebrovascular accidents. The rate of osteoporotic fractures was similar between the two groups.

Luteinizing Hormone-Releasing Hormone (LHRH) Agonists

Ovarian ablation has been shown to be effective in improving survival in premenopausal patients with metastatic breast cancer [45]. There are a number of methods by which ovarian ablation can be achieved: surgical oophorectomy, ovarian irradiation, or reversible chemical castration using LHRH agonists. Naturally occurring LHRH is a decapeptide with a short biologic half-life that is secreted in a pulsatile fashion from the hypothalamus into the portal circulation. LHRH causes the secretion of LH and FSH from the pituitary, which in turn stimulate the ovaries to synthesize and secrete estrogen [46]. LHRH agonists are synthetic peptides which bind to the gonadotropin-releasing hormone (GnRH) receptor and have a prolonged duration of action compared with the native protein [47]. Immediately after the initiation of therapy with one of the LHRH analogs in a premenopausal woman, plasma levels of estradiol and gonadotropins rise, but long-term use paradoxically suppresses ovarian function and plasma estradiol levels fall to castrate levels

Aromatase Inhibitors

In postmenopausal women, estrogen is synthesized predominantly from nonglandular sources when androgenic substrates produced by the adrenal glands are converted to estradiol by the aromatase enzyme [48]. Aromatase inhibitors (AIs) provide an effective means to suppress plasma estrogen levels in postmenopausal women. In menstruating women, where the ovaries are the predominant source of estrogen, these agents lead to upregulation of gonadotropins due to decreased feedback from estrogen, ultimately leading to increased ovarian stimulation [10, 48].

Clinical use of first- and second-generation AIs such as aminoglutethimide was limited by side effects associated with blocking synthesis of a number of steroidal hormones including cortisol, aldosterone, and thyroxine [49]. The increased specificity of newer generation AIs has resulted in a much improved side-effect profile [48]. AIs which are currently used in clinical practice fall into two different subclasses: steroidal and nonsteroidal. Exemestane is a steroidal (Type I) AI and anastrozole and letrozole are nonsteroidal (Type II) AIs. Exemestane forms covalent bonds near the active site of the enzyme leading to irreversible inhibition of the enzymatic activity. Nonsteroidal AIs bind reversibly and competitively inhibit the active site on the enzyme from binding to its natural substrate [50]. All three drugs are orally administered once a day (anastrozole 1 mg, letrozole 2.5 mg, exemestane 25 mg).

Aromatase inhibitors have been well-tolerated in clinical trials and have a different side-effect profile than tamoxifen due to their lack of partial estrogenic activity. The most common side effects seen with AIs are hot flashes, musculoskeletal pain, vaginal dryness, and headache. Musculoskeletal complaints can lead to treatment discontinuation, and intervention with increased exercise, nonsteroidal anti-inflammatory agents, or switching to an alternative antiestrogen may improve adherence. In contrast to tamoxifen, AIs have not been associated with an increased risk of endometrial cancer or thromboembolic disease. However, the profound suppression of estrogen levels by AIs has led to increased incidence of bone fractures and osteoporosis. All women who are initiated on an AI should be advised about daily calcium and vitamin D supplementation, smoking cessation, and the importance of exercise in maintaining good bone health [51, 52]. A baseline BMD should be obtained and monitored periodically while taking an AI. Women can be initiated on bisphosphonate or denosumab therapy to maintain or improve bone mineral density and reduce fracture risk based upon National Comprehensive Cancer Network Guidelines [52].

Fulvestrant

Fulvestrant is a steroidal analogue of 17-beta-estradiol. It binds to the estrogen receptor preventing receptor dimerization, and effectively downregulates the estrogen receptor in both preclinical and clinical studies [53]. Fulvestrant is the only available agent in this class, and is administered as an intramuscular injection. Early randomized trials compared the efficacy of fulvestrant given as a monthly 250 mg injection to anastrozole in women with advanced breast cancer whose disease has progressed on prior hormonal therapy. Combined analysis of two randomized trials including 851 patients showed equivalent time to progression, overall response, clinical benefit rate and duration of response [19, 20, 54]. It was on the basis of these trials that fulvestrant has been approved by the FDA for use in women with metastatic breast cancer which has progressed on previous hormonal therapy.

Pharmacokinetic studies of fulvestrant when given at the 250 mg monthly dose indicated that a steady state concentration was achieved in 3–6 months. Other dosing schedules where fulvestrant was given as a 500 mg loading dose on days 1, 14, and 28 have also been investigated, and steady-state concentrations are achieved by 1 month. A large, randomized phase 3 trial was conducted to compare the efficacy of the FDA-approved dosage of 250 mg every 28 days to 500 mg given on days 0, 14, 28, and then every 28 days thereafter. Based upon improved median progression-free survival and median overall survival, the FDA updated the fulvestrant approval, recommending the 500 mg loading and therapeutic dose schedule [55].

Megestrol Acetate (Megace)

Megestrol acetate (Megace) is an orally active progesterone derivative that can be used to treat advanced breast cancer. Progestins have several mechanisms of action that might explain the observed antitumor effect in advanced breast cancer. Treatment with progestins downregulates the expression of ER, rendering the cell less sensitive to the effects of estrogen. Progestins can also bind to androgen and glucocorticoid receptors that are expressed by some breast cancer cells, and this receptor binding may cause downstream events that inhibit growth [56]. Higher dosages of progestins are capable of suppressing the hypothalamic–pituitary–adrenal axis, resulting in inhibition of steroidogenesis, with a resulting fall in circulating estrogens [57]. Although clinical trials have demonstrated response to therapy in advanced breast cancer patients, the use of megestrol acetate in the clinic has been limited by side effects including weight gain. Weight gain is the most common side effect; less common side effects include hypertension, congestive heart failure, thrombophlebitis, and pulmonary embolism.

Current Hormonal Therapies for Prostate Cancer

Androgens are produced by Leydig cells within the testes, but also to a smaller degree within the adrenal gland, and in peripheral tissue such as the prostate and prostatic tumor cells. Androgens such as dehydroepiandrosterone and androstenedione are eventually converted to testosterone and its active form, dihydrotestosterone (DHT), which binds the androgen receptor. The hormone receptor complex is translocated from the cytoplasm into the cell nucleus, where it binds to DNA via androgen responsive elements. This binding initiates transcription of androgen responsive genes such as prostatic specific antigen (PSA) [58].

Huggins and Hodges demonstrated that inhibition of androgens led to regression of advanced prostate cancer [59]. Since that time, androgen deprivation has been the mainstay of treatment for metastatic prostate cancer that is not amenable to local therapy such as prostatectomy or radiation alone. Of note, in locally advanced or high risk prostate cancer, androgen deprivation is often used in concert with radiation therapy, as multiple trials have shown a benefit of combination therapy in that setting. Castration for metastatic disease can be accomplished by medical or surgical castration, either alone or in combination with an antiandrogen. Antiandrogens are utilized in the setting of a significant volume of disease in order to prevent symptoms associated with the initial testosterone surge that comes from the use of GnRH agonists such as leuprolide or goserelin [60]. Moreover, if men show PSA progression or fail to reach castrate levels of testosterone with primary androgen deprivation, combined androgen blockade with antiandrogens such as bicalutamide, flutamide, or nilutamide can be utilized as a secondary hormonal approach further to prevent androgen availability to cancer cells.

Inevitably, men will develop castration resistant prostate cancer (CRPC), defined as clinical signs of progression or change in PSA/imaging in the setting of castrate levels of testosterone (<50 ng/mL). There are multiple mechanisms by which castration resistance develop, including point mutations or amplification in the androgen receptor [61], activation of the receptor by alternate ligands [62], activation of alternative signaling pathways such as the PI3K/AKT pathway[63, 64] and alteration of apoptotic factors or androgen receptor cofactor imbalances [65]. Once men develop castration resistance, they require additional therapies that are able to overcome these mechanisms of resistance.

LHRH Agonists and Antagonists

Mechanism of action of LHRH agonists is similar in the treatment of breast and prostate cancer. LHRH agonists are synthetic peptides which bind to the GnRH receptor and have a prolonged duration of action [47]. In men, treatment with a LHRH agonist may cause an initial surge in LH and FSH and increase in testosterone before a subsequent drop in LH levels and castrate-levels of testosterone are achieved. This flare phenomenon can be prevented by the addition of an antiandrogen. Unlike GnRH agonists, antagonists, such as degaralix, do not lead to an initial testosterone surge and provide similar rates of treatment response [66]. GnRH antagonists are often used in situations where an initial testosterone flare may be especially notable, such as in the setting of high volume disease or when rapid therapeutic onset is needed.

Two separate phase III trials have shown an enhanced effect of androgen deprivation along with upfront cytotoxic chemotherapy in newly diagnosed hormone naïve metastatic prostate cancer. Both the CHAARTED study [67] and the STAMPEDE trial [68] compared androgen deprivation alone or in combination with docetaxel chemotherapy in men with metastatic prostate cancer. An overall survival benefit was noted in both trials for patients with metatstatic disease, particularly those with large amounts of disease. Additional studies examining the combination of novel agents with traditional androgen deprivation are ongoing in prostate cancer of all stages.

Antiandrogens

Nonsteroidal antiandrogens such as bicalutamide, flutamide, or nilutamide, are oral agents which bind to the androgen receptor, and inhibit binding of testosterone and other androgens from binding to the receptor. This prevents the activation and upregulation of androgen-responsive genes by the androgen receptor. The half-life of the agents range from about 5 h for flutamide, to about 2 days for nilutamide, and about 5–6 days for bicalutamide. Common side effects include gynecomastia, sexual dysfunction, vasomotor symptoms, liver enzyme abnormalities, osteoporosis, and gastrointestinal symptoms [69].

Prior studies have shown that men on combined androgen blockade for a prolonged period of time (median range 24–39 months) who demonstrate PSA increase, may benefit from antiandrogen withdrawal. Up to 40% of these men can have a decrease in PSA by removal of the antiandrogen [70, 71]. This may be due to alterations in the androgen receptor that enable antiandrogens actually to stimulate rather than inhibit signaling. Removing the antiandrogen may further enhance time of PSA suppression and should be considered in appropriate patients.

Ketoconazole

Ketoconazole blocks the synthesis of androgens in the adrenal gland by inhibiting the enzyme 17α-hydoxylase/17, 20-lyase (CYP17), and can also be used in the treatment of metastatic prostate cancer patients [72]. Ketoconazole can cause hepatotoxicity and hydrocortisone must be given concurrently due to potential development of adrenal insufficiency. While not used as frequently recently due to availability of newer agents with overall survival benefits, this agent may be considered in patients unable to afford or without access to more novel agents. There is some data that patients are still able to respond to newer 17, 20-lyase inhibitors after previously receiving ketoconazole [73].

Abiraterone

Abiraterone acetate (AA) is a cytochrome P45017, 20-lyase, 17a-hydroxylase (CYP 17) inhibitor which inhibits the conversion of cholesterol into testosterone and DHT. Due to its inhibition of the cholesterol biochemical pathway, AA must be given with prednisone to prevent adrenal insufficiency. The efficacy of abiraterone was demonstrated in a heavily pretreated population of patients who had received docetaxel chemotherapy where the AA cohort experienced an overall survival benefit [74]. This has also been examined in a separate trial for chemotherapy naïve CRPC patients, who also experienced and overall survival benefit [75]. The side effects of this agent included fluid retention, hypertension, and hypokalemia, all thought to be related to mineralocorticoid activity alteration.

Enzalutamide

Enzalutamide, previously known as MDV3100, works by not only inhibiting access of androgens to the androgen receptor (AR), but it also prevents translocation of the ligand-receptor complex into the nucleus, and inhibits the association of the AR-ligand complex to DNA [76]. Based on the strong results demonstrated in the AFFIRM trial, enzalutamide was recently granted FDA approval for the use in men with CRPC who have failed taxane-based chemotherapy [77]. Notable side effects included fatigue, diarrhea, and hot flashes. In addition, less than 1% of patients receiving enzalutamide experienced new-onset seizures, suggesting that in a few patients, the drug may lower a patient's seizure threshold. As with abiraterone, the activity of enzalutamide was subsequently investigated in chemotherapy naïve metastatic patients in the PREVAIL trial. This study compared enzalutamide verus placebo in the pre-chemotherapy castration resistant setting. This study was stopped early given a progression-free survival benefit, as well as an overall survival benefit of enzalutamide over placebo [78]. Enzalutamide is now FDA approved in the chemotherapy naïve CRPC setting.

Two recent randomized phase II trials compared the novel antiandrogen enzalutamide to bicalutamide in patients with both metastatic and nonmetastatic castration resistant prostate cancer. The STRIVE trial showed a progression-free survival benefit and decreased risk of death compared to bicalutamide in men with metastatatic or nonmetastatic disease [79]. The TERRAIN trial also showed a progression-free survival benefit of enzalutamide compared to bicalutamide in metastatic prostate cancer patients [80]. Despite the promising results of enzalutamide in this setting, cost of the agent may prevent usage in some patients. Bicalutamide or other antiandrogens remain a viable option in those instances.

Estrogens, Progestins, and Glucocorticoids

Estrogens are believed to work in prostate cancer patients due to their castration effect. DES has well-documented side effects such as gynecomastia and thrombotic complications and its use required prophylactic doses of anticoagulant therapy. Agents such as DES have had a marked decrease in use, due to newer agents that are more easily tolerated.

Progestins such as megace or medroxyprogesterone appear to also have marginal activity in metastatic CRPC patients. These agents, as noted above, have limitations such as weight gain, the most common side effect. Less common side effects include hypertension, congestive heart failure, thrombophlebitis, and pulmonary embolism. Glucocorticoids such as dexamethasone and prednisone also have modest activity as single agents. Of note, prednisone is often included as a part of other nonhormonal treatment trials, due to the historical activity of the agent alone. The glucocorticoids also can play a role in pain relief. These agents have the side effects of weight gain, osteoporosis, hyperglycemia, and mood effects. The use of these agents as monotherapy while less common, may be useful in patients for palliative effect, or in patients with nonoptimal performance status.

Endocrine Resistance

Endocrine resistance is a critical issue for patients with metastatic breast and prostate cancer. Some tumors harbor intrinsic resistance to endocrine agents and do not benefit from endocrine therapy; in the metastatic setting all tumors ultimately acquire resistance to endocrine therapy. The mechanisms underlying resistance are complex, and involve enhanced activation of signaling pathways. The addition of the mTOR inhibitor everolimus to exemestane in metastatic breast cancer patients who progressed or recurred after treatment with a nonsteroidal AI, showed improved progression free survival [81]. The addition of the cyclin dependent kinase 4/6 inhibitors palbociclib and ribociclib to first line therapy with letrozole has shown improved progression-free survival [82]. Multiple trials are ongoing to further investigate combinations of targeted agents with endocrine therapy in metastatic and early stage breast cancer [83].

Conclusions

Hormonal therapy remains a mainstay of therapy for endocrine-sensitive cancers such as breast and prostate cancer. Newer agents such as abiraterone and enzalutamide have been developed for prostate cancer in recent years, expanding the treatment options for these patients. FDA agents approved for initial use in the postchemotherapy setting have now been examined in chemotherapy naïve patients. This trend of examining hormonal-based therapies for earlier use in CRPC continues with other agents currently in clinical trials. These and additional hormonal-based agents will hopefully be approved for clinical use both in breast and prostate cancer patients in the next few years.

References

1 Jensen EV, Jordan VC. The estrogen receptor: a model for molecular medicine. *Clin Cancer Res* 2003;9(6):1980–9.

2 Lerner LJ, Holthaus FJ, Jr, Thompson CR. A non-steroidal estrogen antiagonist 1-(p-2-diethylaminoethoxyphenyl)-1-phenyl-2-p-methoxyphenyl ethanol. *Endocrinology* 1958;63(3):295–318.

3 Hecker E, Vegh I, Levy CM, *et al.* Clinical trial of clomiphene in advanced breast cancer. *Eur J Cancer* 1974;10(11):747–9.

4 Harper MJ, Walpole AL. A new derivative of triphenylethylene: effect on implantation and mode of action in rats. *J Reprod Fertil* 1967;13(1):101–19.

5 Jordan VC. Antiestrogenic and antitumor properties of tamoxifen in laboratory animals. *Cancer Treatment Rep* 1976;60(10):1409–19.

6 Cole MP, Jones CT, Todd ID. A new anti-oestrogenic agent in late breast cancer. An early clinical appraisal of ICI46474. *Br J Cancer* 1971;25(2):270–5.

7 Winer EP, Hudis C, Burstein HJ, *et al.* American Society of Clinical Oncology technology assessment on the use of aromatase inhibitors as adjuvant therapy for women with hormone receptor-positive breast cancer: status report 2002. *J Clin Oncol* 2002;20(15):3317–27.

8 Judd HL, Judd GE, Lucas WE, Yen SS. Endocrine function of the postmenopausal ovary: concentration of androgens and estrogens in ovarian and peripheral vein blood. *J Clin Endocrinol Metab* 1974;39(6):1020–4.

9 Richards JS, Hickey GJ, Chen SA, *et al.* Hormonal regulation of estradiol biosynthesis, aromatase activity, and aromatase mRNA in rat ovarian follicles and corpora lutea. *Steroids* 1987;50(4–6):393–409.

10 Smith IE, Dowsett M. Aromatase inhibitors in breast cancer. *N Engl J Med* 2003;348(24):2431–42.

11 Wittliff JL. Steroid-hormone receptors in breast cancer. *Cancer* 1984;53(3 Suppl):630–43.

12 McGuire WL, Chamness GC, Fuqua SA. Estrogen receptor variants in clinical breast cancer. *Mol Endocrinol* 1991; 5(11):1571–7.

13 Harvey JM, Clark GM, Osborne CK, Allred DC. Estrogen receptor status by immunohistochemistry is superior to the ligand-binding assay for predicting response to adjuvant endocrine therapy in breast cancer. *J Clin Oncol* 1999;17(5):1474–81.

14 Bonneterre J, Buzdar A, Nabholtz JM, *et al.* Anastrozole is superior to tamoxifen as first-line therapy in hormone receptor positive advanced breast carcinoma. *Cancer* 2001;92(9):2247–58.

15 Mouridsen H, Gershanovich M, Sun Y, *et al.* Superior efficacy of letrozole versus tamoxifen as first-line therapy for postmenopausal women with advanced breast cancer: results of a phase III study of the International Letrozole Breast Cancer Group. *J Clin Oncol* 2001;19(10):2596–606.

16 Buzdar A, Douma J, Davidson N, *et al.* Phase III, multicenter, double-blind, randomized study of letrozole, an aromatase inhibitor, for advanced breast cancer versus megestrol acetate. *J Clin Oncol* 2001;19(14):3357–66.

17 Buzdar AU, Jonat W, Howell A, *et al.* Anastrozole versus megestrol acetate in the treatment of postmenopausal women with advanced breast carcinoma: results of a survival update based on a combined analysis of data from two mature phase III trials. *Arimidex Study Group. Cancer* 1998;83(6):1142–52.

18 Kaufmann M, Bajetta E, Dirix LY, *et al.* Exemestane is superior to megestrol acetate after tamoxifen failure in postmenopausal women with advanced breast cancer: results of a phase III randomized double-blind trial. The Exemestane Study Group. *J Clin Oncol* 2000;18(7):1399–411.

19 Howell A, Robertson JF, Quaresma Albano J, *et al.* Fulvestrant, formerly ICI 182,780, is as effective as anastrozole in postmenopausal women with advanced breast cancer progressing after prior endocrine treatment. *J Clin Oncol* 2002;20(16):3396–403.

20 Osborne CK, Pippen J, Jones SE, *et al.* Double-blind, randomized trial comparing the efficacy and tolerability of fulvestrant versus anastrozole in postmenopausal women with advanced breast cancer progressing on prior endocrine therapy: results of a North American trial. *J Clin Oncol* 2002;20(16):3386–95.

21 Allan GF, Leng X, Tsai SY, *et al.* Hormone and antihormone induce distinct conformational changes which are central to steroid receptor activation. *J Biol Chem* 1992;267(27): 19513–20.

22 Tate AC, Greene GL, DeSombre ER, Jensen EV, Jordan VC. Differences between estrogen- and antiestrogen-estrogen receptor complexes from human breast tumors identified with an antibody raised against the estrogen receptor. *Cancer Res* 1984;44(3):1012–8.

23 Colletta AA, Benson JR, Baum M. Alternative mechanisms of action of anti-oestrogens. *Breast Cancer Res Treat* 1994; 31(1):5–9.

24 Jordan VC. Growth factor regulation by tamoxifen is demonstrated in patients with breast cancer. *Cancer* 1993;72(1):1–2.

25 Winston R, Kao PC, Kiang DT. Regulation of insulin-like growth factors by antiestrogen. *Breast Cancer Res Treat* 1994;31(1):107–15.

26 Stearns V, Johnson MD, Rae JM, *et al.* Active tamoxifen metabolite plasma concentrations after coadministration of tamoxifen and the selective serotonin reuptake inhibitor paroxetine. *J Natl Cancer Inst* 2003;95(23):1758–64.

27 Desta Z, Ward BA, Soukhova NV, Flockhart DA. Comprehensive evaluation of tamoxifen sequential biotransformation by the human cytochrome P450 system in vitro: prominent roles for CYP3A and CYP2D6. *J Pharmacol Exp Ther* 2004;310(3):1062–75.

28 Regan MM, Leyland-Jones B, Bouzyk M, *et al.* CYP2D6 genotype and tamoxifen response in postmenopausal women with endocrine-responsive breast cancer: the breast international group 1-98 trial. *J Natl Cancer Inst* 2012;104(6):441–51.

29 Rae JM, Drury S, Hayes DF, *et al.* CYP2D6 and UGT2B7 genotype and risk of recurrence in tamoxifen-treated breast cancer patients. *J Natl Cancer Inst* 2012;104(6):452–60.

30 Love RR, Mazess RB, Barden HS, *et al.* Effects of tamoxifen on bone mineral density in postmenopausal women with breast cancer. *N Engl J Med* 1992;326(13):852–6.

31 Kristensen B, Ejlertsen B, Dalgaard P, *et al*. Tamoxifen and bone metabolism in postmenopausal low-risk breast cancer patients: a randomized study. *J Clin Oncol* 1994;12(5):992–7.

32 Fisher B, Costantino JP, Wickerham DL, *et al*. Tamoxifen for prevention of breast cancer: report of the National Surgical Adjuvant Breast and Bowel Project P-1 Study. *J Natl Cancer Inst* 1998;90(18):1371–88.

33 Bruning PF, Bonfrer JM, Hart AA, *et al*. Tamoxifen, serum lipoproteins and cardiovascular risk. *Br J Cancer* 1988;58(4):497–9.

34 Love RR, Wiebe DA, Feyzi JM, Newcomb PA, Chappell RJ. Effects of tamoxifen on cardiovascular risk factors in postmenopausal women after 5 years of treatment. *J Natl Cancer Inst* 1994;86(20):1534–9.

35 Saarto T, Blomqvist C, Ehnholm C, Taskinen MR, Elomaa I. Antiatherogenic effects of adjuvant antiestrogens: a randomized trial comparing the effects of tamoxifen and toremifene on plasma lipid levels in postmenopausal women with node-positive breast cancer. *J Clin Oncol* 1996;14(2):429–33.

36 Anker G, Lonning PE, Ueland PM, Refsum H, Lien EA. Plasma levels of the atherogenic amino acid homocysteine in post-menopausal women with breast cancer treated with tamoxifen. *Int J Cancer* 1995;60(3):365–8.

37 Carstensen J. Prolonged tamoxifen therapy: effects on contralateral breast cancer, endometrial cancer and cardiovascular mortality. *Breast Cancer Res Treat* 2003;82(Abstract 425).

38 Fisher B, Costantino JP, Wickerham DL, *et al*. Tamoxifen for the prevention of breast cancer: current status of the National Surgical Adjuvant Breast and Bowel Project P-1 study. *J Natl Cancer Inst* 2005;97(22):1652–62.

39 Tamoxifen for early breast cancer: an overview of the randomised trials. Early Breast Cancer Trialists' Collaborative Group. *Lancet* 1998;351(9114):1451–67.

40 Black LJ, Goode RL. Uterine bioassay of tamoxifen, trioxifene and a new estrogen antagonist (LY 117018) in rats and mice. *Life Sci* 1980;26:1453–1458.

41 Buzdar AU, Marcus C, Holmes F, Hug V, Hortobagyi G. Phase II evaluation of Ly156758 in metastatic breast cancer. *Oncology* 1988;45(5):344–5.

42 Gradishar W, Glusman J, Lu Y, *et al*. Effects of high dose raloxifene in selected patients with advanced breast carcinoma. *Cancer* 2000;88(9):2047–53.

43 Cauley JA, Norton L, Lippman ME, *et al*. Continued breast cancer risk reduction in postmenopausal women treated with raloxifene: 4-year results from the MORE trial. Multiple outcomes of raloxifene evaluation. *Breast Cancer Res Treat* 2001;65(2):125–34.

44 Vogel VG, Costantino JP, Wickerham DL, *et al*. Effects of tamoxifen vs raloxifene on the risk of developing invasive breast cancer and other disease outcomes: the NSABP Study of Tamoxifen and Raloxifene (STAR) P-2 trial. *JAMA* 2006;295(23):2727–41.

45 Klijn JG, Beex LV, Mauriac L, *et al*. Combined treatment with buserelin and tamoxifen in premenopausal metastatic breast cancer: a randomized study. *J Natl Cancer Inst* 2000;92(11):903–11.

46 Schally AV. Aspects of hypothalamic regulation of the pituitary gland. *Science* 1978;202(4363):18–28.

47 Conn PM, Crowley WF, Jr. Gonadotropin-releasing hormone and its analogues. *N Engl J Med* 1991;324(2):93–103.

48 Santen RJ, Harvey HA. Use of aromatase inhibitors in breast carcinoma. *Endocr Relat Cancer* 1999;6(1):75–92.

49 Santen RJ, Worgul TJ, Lipton A, *et al*. Aminoglutethimide as treatment of postmenopausal women with advanced breast carcinoma. *Ann Intern Med* 1982;96(1):94–101.

50 Kudachadkar R, O'Regan RM. Aromatase inhibitors as adjuvant therapy for postmenopausal patients with early stage breast cancer. *CA Cancer J Clin* 2005;55(3):145–63.

51 Hillner BE, Ingle JN, Chlebowski RT, *et al*. American Society of Clinical Oncology 2003 update on the role of bisphosphonates and bone health issues in women with breast cancer. *J Clin Oncol* 2003;21(21):4042–57.

52 Gradishar WJ, Anderson BO, Balassanian R, *et al*. Breast Cancer Version 2.2017. NCCN Clinical Practice Guidelines in Oncology, 2017; nccn.org (accessed 23 August 2017).

53 Olufolabi AJ, Booth JV, Wakeling HG, *et al*. A preliminary investigation of remifentanil as a labor analgesic. *Anesth Analgesia* 2000;91(3):606–8.

54 Howell A, Pippen J, Elledge RM, *et al*. Fulvestrant versus anastrozole for the treatment of advanced breast carcinoma: a prospectively planned combined survival analysis of two multicenter trials. *Cancer* 2005;104(2):236–9.

55 Di Leo A, Jerusalem G, Petruzelka L, *et al*. Results of the CONFIRM phase III trial comparing fulvestrant 250 mg with fulvestrant 500 mg in postmenopausal women with estrogen receptor-positive advanced breast cancer. *J Clin Oncol* 2010;28(30):4594–600.

56 Teulings FA, van Gilse HA, Henkelman MS, Portengen H, Alexieva-Figusch J. Estrogen, androgen, glucocorticoid, and progesterone receptors in progestin-induced regression of human breast cancer. *Cancer Res* 1980;40(7):2557–61.

57 Alexieva-Figusch J, Blankenstein MA, Hop WC, *et al*. Treatment of metastatic breast cancer patients with different dosages of megestrol acetate; dose relations, metabolic and endocrine effects. *Eur J Cancer Clin Oncol* 1984;20(1):33–40.

58 Schmidt LJ, Tindall DJ. Androgen receptor: past, present and future. *Curr Drug Targets* 2013;14(4):401–7.

59 Huggins C. Effect of orchiectomy and irradiation on cancer of the prostate. *Ann Surg* 1942;115(6):1192–200.

60 Schulze H, Senge T. Influence of different types of antiandrogens on luteinizing hormone-releasing hormone analogue-induced testosterone surge in patients with metastatic carcinoma of the prostate. *J Urol* 1990;144(4):934–41.

61 Edwards J, Krishna NS, Grigor KM, Bartlett JM. Androgen receptor gene amplification and protein expression in hormone refractory prostate cancer. *Br J Cancer* 2003;89(3):552–6.

62 Sharifi N, McPhaul MJ, Auchus RJ. "Getting from here to there"—mechanisms and limitations to the activation of the androgen receptor in castration-resistant prostate cancer. *J Investig Med* 2010;58(8):938–44.

63 Antonarakis ES, Carducci MA, Eisenberger MA. Novel targeted therapeutics for metastatic castration-resistant prostate cancer. *Cancer Lett* 2010;291(1):1–13.

64 Sarker D, Reid AH, Yap TA, de Bono JS. Targeting the PI3K/AKT pathway for the treatment of prostate cancer. *Clin Cancer Res* 2009;15(15):4799–805.

65 Harris WP, Mostaghel EA, Nelson PS, Montgomery B. Androgen deprivation therapy: progress in understanding mechanisms of resistance and optimizing androgen depletion. *Nat Clin Pract Urol* 2009;6(2):76–85.

66 Klotz L, Boccon-Gibod L, Shore ND, et al. The efficacy and safety of degarelix: a 12-month, comparative, randomized, open-label, parallel-group phase III study in patients with prostate cancer. *BJU Int* 2008;102(11):1531–8.

67 Sweeney CJ, Chen YH, Carducci M, et al. Chemohormonal Therapy in metastatic hormone-sensitive prostate cancer. *N Engl J Med* 2015;373(8):737–46.

68 James ND, Sydes MR, Clarke NW, et al. Addition of docetaxel, zoledronic acid, or both to first-line long-term hormone therapy in prostate cancer (STAMPEDE): survival results from an adaptive, multiarm, multistage, platform randomised controlled trial. *Lancet* 2016;387(10024):1163–77.

69 Damber JE, Aus G. Prostate cancer. *Lancet* 2008;371(9625):1710–21.

70 Sartor AO, Tangen CM, Hussain MH, et al. Antiandrogen withdrawal in castrate-refractory prostate cancer: a Southwest Oncology Group trial (SWOG 9426). *Cancer* 2008;112(11):2393–400. E

71 Scher HI, Kelly WK. Flutamide withdrawal syndrome: its impact on clinical trials in hormone-refractory prostate cancer. *J Clin Oncol* 1993;11(8):1566–72.

72 De Coster R, Caers I, Coene MC, et al. Effects of high dose ketoconazole therapy on the main plasma testicular and adrenal steroids in previously untreated prostatic cancer patients. *Clin Endocrinol* 1986;24(6):657–64.

73 Dreicer R, Maclean D, Suri A, et al. Phase I/II Trial of Orteronel (TAK-700) – an investigational 17,20-lyase inhibitor – in patients with metastatic castration-resistant prostate cancer. *Clin Cancer Res* 2014;20(5):1335–44.

74 de Bono JS, Logothetis CJ, Molina A, et al. Abiraterone and increased survival in metastatic prostate cancer. *N Engl J Med* 2011;364(21):1995–2005.

75 Ryan CJ, Smith MR, de Bono JS, et al. Abiraterone in metastatic prostate cancer without previous chemotherapy. *N Engl J Med* 2013;368(2):138–48.

76 Scher HI, Beer TM, Higano CS, et al. Antitumour activity of MDV3100 in castration-resistant prostate cancer: a phase 1–2 study. *Lancet* 2010;375(9724):1437–46.

77 Scher HI, Fizazi K, Saad F, et al. Increased survival with enzalutamide in prostate cancer after chemotherapy. *N Engl J Med* 2012;367(13):1187–97.

78 Beer TM, Armstrong AJ, Rathkopf DE, et al. Enzalutamide in metastatic prostate cancer before chemotherapy. *N Engl J Med* 2014;371:424–33.

79 Penson DF, Armstrong AJ, Concepcion R, et al. Enzalutamide versus bicalutamide in castration-resistant prostate cancer: The STRIVE Trial. *J Clin Oncol* 2016;34(18):2098–106.

80 Shore ND, Chowdhury S, Villers A, et al. Efficacy and safety of enzalutamide versus bicalutamide for patients with metastatic prostate cancer (TERRAIN): a randomised, double-blind, phase 2 study. *Lancet Oncol* 2016;17(2):153–63.

81 Baselga J, Campone M, Piccart M, et al. Everolimus in postmenopausal hormone-receptor-positive advanced breast cancer. *N Engl J Med* 2012;366(6):520–9.

82 Finn RS, Crown JP, Lang I, et al. The cyclin-dependent kinase 4/6 inhibitor palbociclib in combination with letrozole versus letrozole alone as first-line treatment of oestrogen receptor-positive, HER2-negative, advanced breast cancer (PALOMA-1/TRIO-18): a randomised phase 2 study. *Lancet Oncol* 2015 Jan;16(1):25–35.

83 Hortobagyi GN, Stemmer SM, Burris HA, et al. Ribociclib as first-line therapy for HR-positive, advanced breast cancer. *N Engl J Med* 2016;375(18):1738–48.

20

Immunotherapy of Cancer

Diwakar Davar, Ahmad A. Tarhini, and John M. Kirkwood

University of Pittsburgh Medical Center, Pittsburgh, Pennsylvania, USA

Introduction

In this chapter, we review tumor immunogenicity and the role of the immune system in cancer before delineating approaches towards developing effective immunotherapies in the following categories: nonspecific immunostimulants; cytokines; inhibition of negative or augmentation of positive T-cell co-signaling; adoptive cellular therapy; and active immunization. We conclude by discussing the panoply of available immunotherapeutic options currently approved for use.

Tumor Immunogenicity

Tumor immunogenicity refers to the intrinsic host immune response elicited by tumors in the host where they arise. There is significant variation between the immune responses elicited by cancers of the same type in different individuals and among the different types of cancer. Tumor immunogenicity is determined by the intrinsic tumor antigenicity and by factors in the tumor microenvironment (TME), which includes host stromal cell responses.

Tumor-specific mutations result in the expression of a variety of proteins that are antigenic and elicit specific antitumor immune responses. These tumor antigens were originally divided into two broad categories: tumor-specific antigens (TSA) present only on tumor cells and not on others, and tumor-associated antigens (TAA) present mostly on tumor cells but found on some normal cells. This classification was imprecise as several putative TSAs were found to be expressed on normal cells as well.

Currently, tumor antigens are classified based on their structure and function and are divided into five groups based on the classification method proposed by van der Bruggen *et al.* [1] (see Table 20.1).

Role of the Immune System in Cancer

Tumor antigens elicit antitumor immune responses of several kinds in the host. However, these responses may be suppressed by factors within the TME, enabling the continued growth and proliferation of the malignant cells. Burnet and Thomas proposed the "cancer immunosurveillance" hypothesis that lymphocytes acting as sentinels recognized and destroyed continuously arising, transformed cells with malignant potential. The evolutionary advantage of such a system was not lost on proponents of this hypothesis who stated that [2, 3]:

> *"It is an evolutionary necessity that there should be some mechanism for eliminating or inactivating such potentially dangerous mutant cells and it is postulated that this mechanism is of immunological character."*

The increased frequency of malignancies in inherited and acquired immunodeficient states (severe combined immunodeficiency, HIV/AIDS) supported this hypothesis [4]. However, several observations undermined the immunosurveillance hypothesis including the progression of tumors that expressed non-self antigens and were recognized as foreign by the host immune system.

The "immunoediting theory" advanced the immunosurveillance hypothesis by attempting to explain this contradiction. This theory advances three phases of the relationship between tumors and the host immune system: elimination, equilibrium, and escape (three "Es") [5, 6]. The *elimination phase* of cancer immunoediting refers to the detection and elimination of tumor cells by effector arms of the immune system – akin to the process described in the initial immunosurveillance theory. This phase is designated complete when all the tumor cells are eliminated or incomplete if only a portion of tumor cells are eliminated. In the latter, a state of equilibrium develops in which the tumor cells continue to multiply, accruing mutations and increasing their antigenicity which then elicits a tumor-specific response that holds tumor growth in check – the *equilibrium phase*. Eventually, however, natural selection selects for tumor cells that resist, avoid, or suppress the antitumor immune response leading to tumor escape and unfettered tumor growth – *escape phase*.

Tumor escape results from tumor-induced tolerogenic mechanisms which can be classified according to either *anatomical location* (central [thymus or bone marrow] versus peripheral

Table 20.1 Tumor antigens [1].

Cancer-testis antigens (CT antigens)	CT antigens are normally expressed only in germline tissues that are immune sanctuaries. For example, the testis is an immunoprivileged site in which sperm, although immunogenic, are not recognized as foreign and subjected to immune attack. The blood–testis barrier in combination with altered cytokine expression (suppressed levels of proinflammatory cytokines and elevated levels of immunoregulatory cytokines) and the absence of MHC molecules on germline cells account for this phenomenon. CT antigens are primarily expressed in a variety of cancers but not in normal somatic tissues and elicit potent immune responses – making them desirable targets for cancer immunotherapy. ● Examples include MAGE-1, MAGE-2, MAGE-3, MAGE-12, BAGE, GAGE, NY-ESO-1, CML66, and CML88.
Differentiation antigens	Differentiation antigens refer to proteins that are differentially expressed in either a stage-specific or a tissue-specific fashion in cancer cells compared to normal tissue. Immunotherapy directed at differentiation antigens is likely to cause minimal damage to native tissues but may be handicapped by self-tolerance. ● Examples include tyrosinase and Melan-A/MART-1 antigens which are expressed at high levels in melanoma but not on other cells although normal melanocytes have low-level expression. Others include gangliosides (GM3, GM2, GD2, GD3) of which GM2 is the most antigenic.
Overexpressed antigens	These antigens are overexpressed in cancer cells compared to normal cells. ● Examples include: ALK and EGFR in lung adenocarcinoma; MUC-1 in colon, breast, ovarian, lung and pancreatic cancers; PRAME in acute and chronic leukemias, non-Hodgkin lymphoma and melanoma; and, WT-1 in the majority of acute leukemias.
Mutation and splice variant antigens	Any combination of genetic mutations, splice variations and alterations in post-transcriptional modification can result in functional differences in the expressed protein. ● Genetic mutations can be further subclassified as chromosomal translocations (BCR-ABL, ETV6-AML1, NPM1-ALK1, PML-RARA), internal tandem repeats (FLT3), substitutions (BRAF), alternative open reading frames (CDKN2A); and intron encoding (MUM1). ● Functionally, these mutated antigens have differential tissue expression – NY-CO-38, for example, has four splice variants, each of which has a different tissue expression.
Viral antigens	Oncoviruses refer to DNA or RNA viruses that are capable of causing cancer. Upon infection, oncoviruses express a variety of viral proteins that are subsequently expressed in infected human cells and are then presented to and recognized by the immune system. There are seven known oncoviruses, of which five are DNA viruses and two are RNA viruses: ● DNA viruses. Human papilloma virus (HPV) (cervical cancers and squamous cell carcinomas of the oropharynx and anogenital regions); Epstein-Barr virus (EBV) (Burkitt's lymphoma, Hodgkin's lymphoma, nasopharyngeal carcinoma, gastric cancer and post-transplantation lymphoproliferative disease); Merkel cell polyomavirus (Merkel cell carcinoma); Kaposi's sarcoma-associated herpesvirus (HHV-8) (Kaposi's sarcoma); and hepatitis B virus (HBV) (hepatocellular carcinoma). ● RNA viruses. Hepatitis C virus (HCV) (hepatocellular carcinoma); and human T-lymphotropic virus (HTLV-1) (adult T-cell leukemia).

tolerance) or *mechanism* (deletional versus non-deletional tolerance). The presence of tumor-specific T-cells that recognize non-mutated CT antigens provides evidence for central tolerance. However, T-cell tolerance in cancer largely occurs peripherally in the TME secondary to either *deletional mechanisms* (active elimination of reactive cells) or *non-deletional mechanisms* that prevent the generation of an antigen-specific response despite T-cell recognition secondary to either suboptimal activation (resulting in T-cell anergy) or T-cell suppression. T-cell anergy occurs when T-cell activation occurs in the absence of appropriate co-stimulation [7, 8]. Tumors directly or indirectly suppress T-cells by:

- Down-regulating major histocompatibility (MHC) molecules
- Increased expression of anti-apoptotic molecules such as FLIP and BCL-XL
- Expressing T-cell inhibitory ligands such as PD-L1/B7-H1, HLA-G, and HLA-E
- Expressing soluble factors that directly suppress T-cells including TGF-β, VEGF, IL-10, and gangliosides
- Expanding myeloid cell populations
- Altering levels of intracellular factors that suppress T-cells including IDO and E3 ubiquitin ligase.

At present, investigators are evaluating methods to manipulate the intra- and extracellular mechanisms that underpin T-cell tolerance to alter the TME, reduce tolerance, and stimulate immune responses to directly trigger tumor cell death.

Nonspecific Immunostimulants

With the success of the bacille de Calmette et Guérin (BCG) vaccination campaign following World War II, BCG was proposed as an anticancer therapy given early observations of a lower than expected incidence of cancer in patients with tuberculosis [9] but enthusiasm flagged until Coe and Feldman, in 1966, demonstrated that intravesical instillation of BCG elicited a delayed-type hypersensitivity response similar to that seen in the skin [10].

Successful treatment of primary bladder cancer and melanoma metastatic to the bladder wall led Morales to develop intravesical administration of BCG in patients with recurrent transitional cell carcinoma of the bladder [11]. Morales' therapy utilized intravesical as well as percutaneous administrations of BCG vaccine at weekly intervals for 6 weeks to reduce the risk of recurrence [11]. When tested prospectively in two randomized controlled trials against standard cystoscopy alone, Morales' protocol significantly reduced the recurrence rate and prolonged the time to recurrence – these data are summarized in Table 20.2 [11].

Table 20.2 Registration trials of immunotherapeutic agents in bladder cancer, melanoma, RCC, and prostate cancer.

Agent (FDA approval)	No. of patients (study reference)	Study design	Primary endpoint	Treatment arms	Responses	OS/PFS/RFS	HR (95% CI)
Bladder cancer							
Intravesical BCG (1990)	387 (Nijmegen study, 1993) [11]	TaT1 cancer	Recurrence	TICE BCG vs BCG-RIVM vs mitomycin C	Not reported	DFS at 2 years: 53% (TICE BCG) vs 62% (BCG-RIVM) vs 64% (MMC) [NS]	Not reported
	377 (SWOG 8795, 1995) [11]	TaT1 cancer at high risk of recurrence	Recurrence	TICE BCG vs mitomycin C	Not reported	DFS at 2 years: 57% (BCG) vs 45% (MMC) [S]	Not reported
Melanoma							
IFN-α2b (1996)	287 (E1684, 1996) [26]	Non-randomized, open-label stage II–III (T2–4N0M0/ TanyN + M0) melanoma (89% node positive)	RFS (later amended to OS)	HDI vs observation	N/A	Median RFS: 1.4 years (HDI) Median OS: 3.2 years (HDI)	RFS – 1.38 [S] OS – 1.22 [NS]
	642 (E1690, 2000) [27]	Non-randomized, open-label stage II–III (T2–4N0M0/ TanyN + M0) melanoma (74% node positive)	RFS	HDI vs LDI vs observation	N/A	Median RFS: 2.3 years (HDI) Median OS: 7.0 years (HDI)	RFS – 1.24 [NS] OS – Not reported
	774 (E1694, 2001) [28]	Non-randomized, open-label stage II–III (T2–4N0M0/ TanyN + M0) melanoma (77% node positive)	RFS and OS (co-primary endpoints)	HDI vs GMK vaccine	N/A	Median RFS: 3.1 years (HDI) Median OS: 3.8 years (HDI)	RFS – 1.22 [S] OS – 1.32 [S]
Pegylated IFN-α2b, Peginteron* (2011)	1256 (EORTC 18991, 2008 and 2012) [29]	Randomized, open-label stage III (TanyN + M0) melanoma (100% node positive)	RFS	Pegylated IFN-α2b vs observation	N/A	RFS – 3.0 months (IFN) vs 2.2 months (observation) [NS] DMFS – 47 months (IFN) vs 38 months (observation) [NS] OS – 47.8% (IFN) vs 46.4% (observation) [NS]	RFS – 0.87 (0.76–1.00) [NS] DMFS – 0.93 (0.81–1.07) [NS] OS – 0.96 (0.82–1.11) [NS]
IL-2 Aldesleukin, Proleukin* (1998)	283 total - 134 melanoma, 149 RCC (Rosenberg et al., 1994) [15]	Non-randomized, open-label, advanced metastatic melanoma and RCC	Regression, durability of response, OS	IL-2 720,000 IU/kg q8h. 15 doses per cycle with two cycles/course for up to five courses (high-dose IL-2, HD IL-2) No comparator	CR: melanoma 6.7% (9/134), RCC 6.7% (10/149) PR: melanoma 10.4% (14/134), RCC 13.4% (20/149) ORR: 18.7% (53/283)	OS rates: 3 years – 22% (melanoma), 34% (RCC) 5 years – 11% (melanoma), 23% (RCC)	Not reported
	270 (Atkins et al., 1999) [16]	Phase II non-randomized, open-label, advanced metastatic melanoma and RCC	Regression, durability of response, OS	HD IL-2 600,000– 720,000 IU/kg per dose. No comparator	CR: 6.3% (17/270) PR: 9.6% (26/270) ORR: 15.9% (26/270)	Median duration of response: 8.9 months Median PFS: 13.1 months	Not reported

RCC

Drug	Trial	Study description	Endpoint	Comparator	Response	OS/Efficacy	OS (HR comparison)
IL-2 Aldesleukin, Proleukin® (1992)	255 (Fyfe et al., 1995) [17]	Pooled results from seven non-randomized, open-label phase II trials in advanced RCC	OR	HD IL-2 No comparator	CR: 5% PR: 9% ORR: 14%	Median OS (all patients): 16.3 months Median OS (responders): not calculated as only 3/36 responding patients died Median duration of response (all responders): 20.3 months	Not reported
SC IFN-α2b + bevacizumab (2007)	649 (AVOREN, 2007 and 2010) [30]	Randomized, advanced RCC (MSKCC risk – intermediate [56%] and poor [9%]; predominantly clear cell; postnephrectomy 99%)	OS	SC IFN-α2b + bevacizumab vs SC IFN-α2b + placebo	ORR: SC IFN-α2b + bevacizumab: 31% ORR: SC IFN-α2b + placebo: 13%	Reported in 2007 and updated in 2010 Median OS in ITT: Bev + IFN-α 23.3 months vs IFN-α alone 21.3 months By MSKCC risk category: *Favorable* – Bev + IFN-α 35.1 months vs IFN-α + placebo 37.2 months *Intermediate* – Bev + IFN-α 22.6 months vs IFN-α + placebo 19.3 months *Poor* – Bev + IFN-α 6.0 months vs IFN-α + placebo 5.1 months	Median OS (Bev + IFN-α compared to IFN-α alone): Unstratified HR 0.91 (0.76–1.10) [NS] Stratified HR 0.86 (0.72–1.04) [NS] Median OS of pts receiving TKI subsequently (Bev + IFN-α compared to IFN-α alone): 0.80 (0.56–1.13) [NS]
	732 (CALGB 90206, 2008 and 2010) [31]	Non-randomized, open label, advanced RCC (MSKCC risk – intermediate [64%] and poor [10%]; predominantly clear cell; prior nephrectomy 85%)		SC IFN-α2b + bevacizumab vs SC IFN-α2b alone	SC IFN-α2b + bevacizumab: 25.5% (ORR) SC IFN-α2b alone: 13.1% (ORR)	Reported in 2008 and updated in 2010 Median OS: Bev + IFN-α 18.3 months vs IFN-α alone 17.4 months By MSKCC risk category: *Favorable* – Bev + IFN-α 32.5 months vs IFN-α alone 33.5 months *Intermediate* – Bev + IFN-α 17.7 months vs IFN-α alone 16.1 months *Poor* – Bev + IFN-α 6.6 months vs IFN-α alone 5.7 months	Median OS (Bev + IFN-α compared to IFN-α alone): stratified 0.86 (0.73–1.01) [NS]

(Continued)

Table 20.2 (Continued)

Agent (FDA approval)	No. of patients (study reference)	Study design	Primary endpoint	Treatment arms	Responses	OS/PFS/RFS	HR (95% CI)
Prostate Cancer							
Sipuleucel-T, Provenge® (2010)	225 (D9901 and D9902A combined analysis, 2009) [78]	Randomized, double blind, placebo-controlled, metastatic CRPC	Safety and efficacy	Sipuleucel-T infusion vs placebo	PSA response rate 4.8% (sipuleucel-T infusion) vs 0% (placebo)	Median OS: sipuleucel-T 23.2 months vs placebo 18.9 months [S] Median TTP: sipuleucel-T 11.1 months vs placebo 9.7 months [NS]	Placebo vs sipuleucel-T in OS: 1.50 (1.10–2.05) [S] Placebo vs sipuleucel-T in PFS: 1.26 (0.95–1.68) [NS]
	512 (IMPACT, 2010) [79]	Randomized, double blind, placebo-controlled, metastatic CRPC	OS	Sipuleucel-T infusion vs placebo	PSA response rate 2.6% (sipuleucel-T infusion) vs 1.3% (placebo)	Median OS: sipuleucel-T 25.8 months vs placebo 21.7 months [S] Median TTP: sipuleucel-T 3.7 months vs placebo 3.6 months [NS] Estimated probability of survival at 36 months: sipuleucel-T 31.7% vs placebo 23.0%	Sipuleucel-T vs placebo in OS: 0.78 (0.61–0.98) [S] Sipuleucel-T vs placebo in TTP: 0.95 (0.75–1.12) [NS]

APC, antigen-presenting cells; BCG, bacillus Calmette–Guérin; CALGB, Cancer and Leukemia Group B; CRPC, castrate resistant prostate cancer; CR, complete response; DTIC, dacarbazine; EORTC, European Organisation for Research and Treatment of Cancer; GM-CSF, granulocyte-macrophage colony-stimulating factor; GMK, G(M2) ganglioside conjugated to KLH (keyhole limpet hemocyanin); HDI, high dose IFN-α2b; ITT, intention to treat; LDI, low dose IFN-α2b; MMC, mitomycin C; MSKCC, Memorial Sloan Kettering Cancer Center; ORR, overall response rate; OS, overall survival; PA2024, prostate acid phosphatase fused to GM-CSF; PBMC, peripheral blood mononuclear cells; PFS, progression free survival; PR, partial response; PSA, prostate specific antigen; RCC, renal cell cancer; RFS, relapse free survival; TTP, time to progression.

Multiple randomized trials have evaluated other nonspecific immune stimulants including *Corynebacterium parvum*, levamisole, or combinations of these agents. These trials have generally produced negative or inconsistent results in small trials so are not part of the standard therapeutic armamentarium.

Cytokines

IL-2

IL-2 is a T-cell growth factor that was shown to have potent antitumor effects in a variety of murine tumor models [12]. Given the dose-dependent nature of responses that suggested increased efficacy with higher doses, investigators developed high-dose regimens in which IL-2 was administered by intravenous infusion every 8 h for up to 14 doses over a 5-day period with or without lymphokine-activated killer (LAK) cells [13, 14]. Despite modest antitumor response rates (16%) and a high incidence of grade III/IV toxicity requiring inpatient administration in specialized units with frequent monitoring, high-dose IL-2 (HD IL-2) as a single agent received United States Food and Drug Administration (FDA) approval primarily on the basis of durable responses in metastatic renal cell carcinoma (RCC) (1992) and metastatic melanoma (1998) [15–17] (see Table 20.2).

IL-2 has been conjugated with a variety of monoclonal antibodies (MoAb) creating a new class of agent termed "immunocytokines". Immunocytokines act primarily by initiating antibody-dependent cell-mediated cytotoxicity, and secondarily directly activating effector cells expressing cognate receptors, minimizing systemic toxicity. Several of these have been developed and are in clinical testing, including denileukin diftitox (DD, DAB$_{389}$ IL-2/Ontak®, Eisai), L19-IL2 and Hu14.18-IL2 (EMD273063).

DD is a fusion protein comprising IL-2 fused to the first 388 amino acids of diphtheria toxin. DD's clinical activity appears dependent on β-subunit (CD122) of high- and intermediate-affinity IL-2 receptors making it naturally selective for T-cell, B-cell and NK-cell malignancies. Following promising phase I/II trials, DD was evaluated in a phase III trial of cutaneous T-cell lymphoma with confirmed CD25 expression – based on the premise that DD preferentially bound to α-subunit of IL-2R.

It was subsequently found to bind the β-subunit (CD122) instead, but 30% of 71 patients had objective responses (20% partial response and 10% complete response) without significant differences in response rates or durations between the two dose levels (9 or 18 μg/kg/d) evaluated [18]. DD is FDA-approved for the treatment of patients with persistent or recurrent cutaneous T-cell lymphoma.

Hu14.18-IL2 (EMD273063) is an immunocytokine comprising a MoAb directed against GD2 – a disialoganglioside expressed on tumors of neuroectodermal origin including neuroblastoma and melanoma – conjugated to IL-2. The phase I study of Hu14.18-IL2 suggested that the agent was relatively well tolerated with a maximum-tolerated dose of 7.5 mg/m^2/d in melanoma patients [19]. A phase II study was initiated at one dose level below the maximum-tolerated dose in 14 patients with metastatic melanoma. No complete responses were reported though 1/14 patients had a partial response and 4/14 had stable disease [20]. A second National Cancer Institute (NCI) phase II trial has completed accrual though results have not been forthcoming (NCT00109863).

L19-IL2 is an immunocytokine that targets the alternatively-spliced extra-domain B of fibronectin. The first-in-human phase I study of L19-IL2 in patients with advanced malignancies comprised 33 patients (18 with advanced RCC) and reported disease stabilization in 17 patients (15 with RCC) [21]. The subsequent phase II study enrolled 32 advanced melanoma patients to receive L19-IL2/DTIC combination and reported an overall response rate (ORR) of 28% (eight of 29 patients) with more than 60% of patients alive at 12 months, although this was a nonrandomized phase IIa trial [22]. A randomized phase IIb trial has completed accrual but is not yet reported (NCT01055522). Cytokine combinations currently in phase III testing are summarized in Table 20.3.

IL-2 Combinations

Prior IL-2 containing combinations typically used lower doses of IL-2 in combination with chemotherapy (biochemotherapy) and were largely ineffective. Current combinations pending evaluation include high dose (HD) IL-2 with radiotherapy (SBRT/IL-2 - NCT01416831); molecularly targeted therapy including vemurafenib (PROCLIVITY-01[NCT01683188] and

Table 20.3 Ongoing Phase III trials of cytokines singly or in combination.

Agent (trade name, Sponsors)	Description	Tumor type	Study design/endpoints
Multikine® (CEL-SCI Corporation/Teva Pharmaceuticals Industries/ Orient Europharma)	Leucocyte interleukin (LI) – comprising IL-2, IL-1α, GM-CSF, IFN-α, and TNF-α	Previously untreated advanced oropharyngeal SCC given prior to SOC surgery and radiation or chemoradiation (NCT01265849)	Randomized, open-label phase III trial of Multikine® alone or in combination with cyclophosphamide, indomethacin and zinc (CIZ) compared to SOC alone (IT-MATTERS) Primary: 3-year OS
L19IL2/L19TNF (Philogen S.p.A.)	L-19 IL-2 in combination with L-19TNF	Previously untreated stage IIIB/IIIC resectable patients with injectable cutaneous, subcutaneous, or nodal melanoma (NCT02938299)	Randomized, open-label phase III trial of L19IL2/L19TNF followed by surgery vs surgery alone (Pivotal) Primary: RFS rate

GM-CSF, granulocyte-macrophage colony-stimulating factor; OS, overall survival; PFS, progression free survival; TNF, tumor necrosis factor.

COMBAT-1 [NCT01754376]), DTIC (NCT00553618) and low-dose TMZ (NCT01124734). Other ongoing combinations with immunotherapy include ipilimumab anti-CTLA4 blocking antibody (NCT01480323), vaccines (recMAGE-A3 + AS15 ASCI - NCT01266603) and VEGF-trap aflibercept (NCT01258855). NCT01480323 is a phase II study evaluating ipilimumab in combination with intratumoral IL-2 based on the hypothesis that intratumoral IL-2 induces melanoma-specific immune responses that may be potentiated by ipilimumab. Observations in murine models suggesting complete tumor eradication with L19–IL2 combined with CTLA-4 blockade (compared to L19–IL2 alone, L19–IL2/PD-1 blockade or L19–IL2/L19-TNF) are encouraging. A phase II NCI study of HD IL-2 combined with ipilimumab yielded complete response rate of 17% and 5-year survival rate of 25% – underscoring the potential of this combination [23].

Interferons

Interferons comprise a large group of structurally related molecules with diverse actions. Type 1 IFNs comprise IFN-α, IFN-β, IFN-ω, IFN-ε and IFN-κ – of which IFN-α, IFN-β and IFN-ω are most important clinically. Type 1 IFNs are primarily produced by dendritic cells (DC) responding to infectious insults and serve as a link between the adaptive and innate arms of our immune response. Type 1 IFNs collectively signal via the IFN-α receptor (IFN-αR) with downstream signaling mediated via the JAK/STAT pathway and IFN regulatory factor (IRF)-9 which binds the STAT1-STAT2 complex and migrates to the nucleus to regulate the expression of RNA-dependent protein kinases [24].

Among the various type 1 IFNs evaluated as cancer immunotherapy, IFN-α2b is the most extensively described, with potent activity against multiple malignancies. Its mechanism of action is thought to be immunomodulatory rather than purely cytotoxic or anti-angiogenic. Tumors inhibit native antitumor immunity through multiple mechanisms, including the recruitment of T-regulatory (Treg) cells within the TME, expression of inhibitory T-cell markers such as PD-L1, constitutive activation of STAT3, and elaboration of VEGF, IL-10 and TGFβ [25]. IFN-α administration up-regulates MHC Class I (HLA-ABC) and II (DR, DP, DQ) expression, improving the function of CD8+ and CD4+ tumor-infiltrating lymphocytes and aid in both T-cell recruitment and DC-mediated T-cell priming to reverse tumor-mediated immunosuppression.

IFN-α2b has regulatory approval for the adjuvant treatment of high-risk resected melanoma and advanced RCC. Adjuvant treatment with high-dose IFN-α2b (HDI) significantly and reproducibly improves relapse free survival (RFS), and to a lesser extent has improved overall survival, in up to 30% of treated patients [26–28]. European trials of pegylated IFN-α2b (PEG IFN) have demonstrated RFS improvements chiefly in microscopically node-positive patients without OS improvement [29].

Interferon Combinations

Subcutaneous IFN-α at intermediate dose-levels in combination with bevacizumab (SC IFN-α/bevacizumab) produces an ORR of 25–30% and improved progression-free survival (PFS) in metastatic RCC, as demonstrated in two separate phase III trials – AVOREN and CALGB 90206 – discussed in detail in a separate section below [30, 31]. Responses were primarily seen in patients with low-volume pulmonary and/or soft tissue metastases with excellent performance status (i.e. "favorable-risk" classification under the Memorial Sloan-Kettering Cancer Center (MSKCC) risk system). Unlike in melanoma, IFN-α has not demonstrated efficacy alone or in combination with other agents in the adjuvant setting and has no role in this paradigm.

Efforts to improve upon the benefit of IFN-α are being evaluated. In advanced RCC, a phase I/II trial of SC IFN-α/pazopanib (NCT01513187) and a phase II of IL-2/IFN-α/bevacizumab (NCT01274273) are both pending.

Immunotherapy Targeting T-cell Cosignaling Checkpoints

Activation of naïve T-cells is initiated through T-cell receptor (TCRs) recognition of cognate antigenic peptides presented in the context of MHC molecules located on antigen presenting cells (APCs). Although this step initiates the T-cell activation cascade, without subsequent synergistic cosignaling primed T-cells become immunologically inert (anergic). Following APC–TCR interaction, cosignaling receptors on the T-cell surface are reorganized to form the "immunological synapse" – an aggregate of specific molecules where T-cell activation is initiated and sustained [32]. Cosignaling is mediated by T-cell cosignaling receptors – cell surface molecules which belong to either the immunoglobulin or tumor necrosis factor receptor superfamilies – and transduce positive (costimulatory) or negative (coinhibitory) signals into T-cells. Cosignals can either *upregulate* the immune response such as the interaction between B7 on APCs and CD28 on CD4+ T-helper cells, or *downregulate* the immune response.

Immunotherapeutic agents targeting mediators of T-cell cosignaling are a major research focus following the success of clinical trials involving inhibitors of cytotoxic T lymphocyte antigen-4 (CTLA-4) and programmed death receptor 1 (PD-1, CD279) in advanced melanoma and other malignancies.

CTLA-4 Inhibition

CTLA-4 (also known as CD152) is a member of the B7-CD28 immunoglobulin superfamily and is expressed on the surface of CD4+ T-helper cells. Unlike the costimulatory signal between B7 and CD28, the B7/CTLA-4 interaction inhibits T-cell activation *directly* by competing with CD28 for binding sites on CD80/86 on APCs and *indirectly* by the dephosphorylation of TCR-proximal signaling moieties via secondary molecules such as PI3K, SHP-2, AP-1/AP-2 that access the YVKM motif on the cytoplasmic side of CTLA-4 [33]. CD4(+)CXCR5(+)Foxp3(+) regulatory T-cells contain intracellular CTLA-4 though its function here is less clear. Ipilimumab (Medarex Inc/Bristol-Myers Squibb) and tremelimumab (MedImmune/Pfizer) are two fully humanized CTLA-4 blocking MoAb that were evaluated in clinical trials.

Two separate phase III studies in the second line (against gp100 vaccine at 3 mg/kg dosage) and in first line (against dacarbazine and combined with dacarbazine at 10 mg/kg dosage) have revealed remarkably similar antitumor effects for ipilimumab [34, 35]. These have been reviewed by the FDA and European Medicines Agency resulting in regulatory approval for the treatment of metastatic melanoma. These results are summarized in Table 20.4. The 2010 MDX010-20 trial compared ipilimumab alone (3 mg/kg every 3 weeks for four doses) and ipilimumab plus an experimental gp100 peptide vaccine to a vaccine only arm in patients with metastatic melanoma in the second line setting. Subsequently the 2011 BMS-024 study compared ipilimumab (10 mg/kg every 3 weeks for four doses) plus dacarbazine (850 mg/m^2) to dacarbazine with placebo in previously untreated patients with metastatic melanoma [34, 35]. Although associated with only modest improvements in response rates (ORR 11–15%) and progression-free/overall survival endpoints, survival curves appeared to flatten after 3 years. A pooled analysis revealed that 21% of patients had durable long-term responses with no evidence of relapse at 10 years of follow-up [36].

Ipilimumab was also evaluated in the adjuvant setting in high-risk stage III melanoma. In EORTC 18071, European investigators compared ipilimumab (10 mg/kg every 3 weeks for four doses; then 10 mg/kg every 3 months for 3 years) to placebo. Toxicity was significant: 52% of patients requiring treatment discontinuation secondary to adverse events and five treatment-related deaths. However, ipilimumab did result in significantly improved progression-free survival (25% reduction in risk of progression) and overall survival (28% reduction in the risk of death) [37, 38]. Ipilimumab is being evaluated against standard HDI in an Eastern Cooperative Oncology Group study – E1609 (NCT01274338) – that includes two ipilimumab arms (3 mg/kg and 10 mg/kg) and will hence clarify how it compares to HDI and whether benefits are dose dependent.

Current investigational ipilimumab combinations in various stages of accrual include: inhibitors of immune checkpoints or checkpoint ligands (B7-H3 antagonist MGA271, NCT02381314); galectin inhibitor GR-MD-02 (NCT02117362); bi-specific antibodies (blinatumomab, NCT02879695); immune stimulants (intratumoral CAVATAK™, NCT02307149); TLR9 agonist MGN1703 and IMO-2125 (NCT02668770, NCT02644967); all-trans retinoic acid (NCT02403778); GM-CSF (NCT02009397, NCT02339571); angiogenesis inhibitor (bevacizumab, NCT01950390); targeted therapies (CDK inhibitor SGI-110, NCT02608437); multi-kinase inhibitor imatinib (NCT01738139); HDAC inhibitors panabinostat and entinostat and ACY241 (NCT02032810, NCT02453620, NCT02935790); radiation (NCT01565837, NCT02239900, NCT02115139, NCT02406183); chemotherapy (FOLFIRINOX, NCT01896869); chemoradiotherapy (NCT01711515).

Tremelimumab monotherapy (at 15 mg/kg intravenously every 90 days) was associated with an ORR of 6.6% in a phase II trial for patients with relapsed or refractory melanoma, where these were mostly durable and of more than 6 months duration [39, 40]. However, the phase III trial registration trial of tremelimumab against chemotherapy (temozolamide or dacarbazine) in previously untreated patients with advanced melanoma was negative – with similar response rates and overall survival in tremelimumab and chemotherapy treated patients resulting in study closure [41]. Given limited single-agent activity, ongoing tremelimumab evaluation primarily consists of combinations with PD-1/PD-L1 checkpoint inhibitors (NCT02588131,

NCT02537418, NCT02536794, NCT02754856, NCT02261220, NCT02519348, NCT02519348, NCT02794883). Additional combinations undergoing evaluation include CCR4 inhibitor KW-0761 (NCT02301130); CSF-1R inhibitor LY3022855 (NCT02718911); PARP inhibitor olaparin (NCT02953457); angiogenesis inhibitor MEDI3617 (NCT02141542); chemotherapy conditioning pre stem cell transplant (NCT02716805); chemotherapy (NCT02658214, NCT02879318); and radiation (NCT02311361, NCT02888743, NCT02639026, NCT02868632).

PD-1/PD-L1 Antagonism

Beyond CTLA-4, several other T-cell checkpoints and receptors are involved in negative regulatory feedback loops that may be associated with immune tolerance of tumor antigens: these include programed death 1 (PD-1), T-cell immunoglobulin and mucin-3 (TIM-3), lymphocyte activation gene-3 (LAG-3), CD160, BTLA, LAIR1, 2B4 and TIGIT [42]. Functional details of other immunoregulatory checkpoints are described elsewhere [42]. Of these checkpoints, programmed death-1 (PD-1, CD279) is the best characterized and agents targeting the PD-1/PD-L1 axis have been developed. Similar to CTLA-4, the PD-1 protein is a member of the B7-CD28 immunoglobulin superfamily and is expressed on *activated, but not resting* T-cells, B-cells, and myeloid cells. PD-1 has two ligands both of which are members of the B7 family: PD-L1 (B7-H1, CD274) expressed on T-cells and B-cells in response to receptor signaling and on macrophages and DCs and PD-L2 primarily expressed on DCs. The interaction between PD-1 and PD-L1 results in inhibition of T-cell proliferation, survival, and function. Thus, while CTLA-4 negatively regulates T-cell activation during the *initial* phase of antigen presentation, PD-1 regulates the *effector phase* of T-cell responses during long-term antigen exposure. PD-1 blockade has been shown to promote the generation of antigen-specific cytotoxic T-cells (CTL) and the increased survival of effector T-cells, and may overcome Treg-mediated suppression.

Initial glimpses of transformative potential of inhibitors of PD-1/PD-L1 came from phase I trials of the anti-PD-1 inhibitors nivolumab (BMS-936558, Bristol-Myers Squibb), pembrolizumab (lambrolizumab or MK-3475, Merck), and PD-L1 inhibitor BMS-936559 (Bristol-Myers Squibb). Response rates were significantly higher than those observed in prior trials of immunotherapy with cumulative response rates of 18% (BMS-936559) to 38% (pembrolizumab) [43–45]. Similar to trials involving the anti-CTLA-4 blocking antibody ipilimumab, immune-related response patterns were observed [46]. Unlike ipilimumab, however, responses were rapid, and observed in multiple tumor types besides the traditionally "immunogenic" tumors melanoma and RCC including non-small cell lung cancer (NSCLC), classical Hodgkin lymphoma, bladder cancer, head and neck squamous cell carcinoma (HNSCC) [47–63]. Responses were also durable – pooled analyses from several studies indicated that survival curves plateaued after 24–36 months. The unprecedented success of PD-1/PD-L1 checkpoint blockade has resulted in these agents gaining regulatory approval for multiple indications: nivolumab (melanoma, NSCLC, HNSCC, RCC and Hodgkin lymphoma); pembrolizumab (melanoma, NSCLC, HNSCC); and atezolizumab

Table 20.4 Registration trials of PD-1 and CTLA-4 inhibitors in melanoma, NSCLC, RCC, Hodgkin's lymphoma and SCCHN.

Agent (FDA Approval)	No. of patients (study reference)	Study design	Primary endpoint	Treatment arms	Overall response rates	OS/PFS/RFS	HR (95%CI)
Melanoma							
Ipilimumab (2011 – advanced melanoma; 2015 – adjuvant melanoma)	676 (Medarex MDX010-20) [34]	Randomized phase III, advanced previously treated melanoma, 3:1:1 randomization to receive ipilimumab/gp100, ipilimumab alone or gp100 alone	ORR, subsequently amended to OS	Ipilimumab 3 mg/kg q3 weeks (4 doses) + gp100 peptide vaccine vs ipilimumab 3 mg/kg q3 weeks (4 doses) alone vs gp100 vaccine alone	Ipilimumab alone: 10.9% Ipilimumab + gp100: 5.7% gp100 alone: 1.5%	OS rates (1/2 year): Ipilimumab alone: 45.6%/23.5% Ipilimumab + GP-100: 43.5%/21.6% GP-100 alone: 25.3%/13.7% OS duration: Ipilimumab alone: 10.1 months Ipilimumab + GP-100: 10.0 months GP-100 alone: 6.4 months PFS duration: Ipilimumab alone: 2.86 months Ipilimumab + GP-100: 2.76 months GP-100 alone: 2.76 months	Median OS: Ipilimumab (compared to GP-100 alone): 0.66 (0.51–0.87) [S] Ipilimumab/gp100 (compared to gp100 alone): 0.68 (0.55–0.85) [S] Median PFS: not reported
	502 (CA184-024) [35]	Randomized, double blind, advanced previously untreated melanoma, 1:1 randomization to receive ipilimumab/dacarbazine or dacarbazine alone	OS	Ipilimumab 3 mg/kg q3 weeks (four doses) + dacarbazine vs dacarbazine alone	Ipilimumab + DTIC: 33.2% (DCR), 15.2% (ORR) DTIC alone: 30.2% (DCR), 10.3% (ORR)	OS rates (1/2/3 year): Ipilimumab + DTIC: 47.3%/28.5%/20.8% DTIC alone: 36.3%/17.9%/12.2 OS duration: Ipilimumab + DTIC: 11.2 months DTIC alone: 9.1 months PFS duration: Ipilimumab + DTIC: 2.8 months DTIC alone: 2.6 months	Median OS: Ipilimumab/DTIC (compared to DTIC alone): 0.72 [S] Median PFS: Ipilimumab/DTIC (compared to DTIC alone): 0.76 [S]
	951 (EORTC 18071) [37, 38]	Randomized, double blind, stage IIIA-IIIC melanoma, 1:1 randomization to receive ipilimumab or matched placebo	RFS (OS secondary)	Ipilimumab 10 mg/kg q3 weeks (four doses) + ipilimumab 10 mg/kg q3 months (3 years) vs matched placebo	N/A	5 year OS rate: Ipilimumab: 65.4% Placebo: 54.4%	Median OS: Ipilimumab (compared to placebo): 0.72 [S] Median PFS: Ipilimumab (compared to placebo): 0.76 [S]

Drug (year)	Trial (ref)	Study design	Endpoint	Treatment	Response rate	PFS/OS rate	Median OS/PFS
Pembrolizumab (2014)	834 (KEYNOTE-006) [47]	Randomized phase III, open-label, ipilimumab-naïve, 1:1:1 randomization to receive pembrolizumab q3 or pembrolizumab q2 or ipilimumab	PFS, OS	Pembrolizumab 10 mg/kg q3 weeks vs pembrolizumab 10 mg/kg q2 weeks vs ipilimumab 3 mg/kg q3 weeks (four doses)	Pembrolizumab 10 mg/kg q3 weeks: 33% Pembrolizumab 10 mg/kg q2 weeks: 34% Ipilimumab 3 mg/kg q3: 12%	6 month PFS rate: Pembrolizumab 10 mg/kg q3 weeks: 46% Pembrolizumab 10 mg/kg q2 weeks: 47% Ipilimumab 3 mg/kg q3: 27% 1 year OS rate: Pembrolizumab 10 mg/kg q3 weeks: 68% Pembrolizumab 10 mg/kg q2 weeks: 74% Ipilimumab 3 mg/kg q3 weeks: 58%	Median OS: Pembrolizumab 10 mg/kg q3 weeks (compared to ipilimumab): 0.69 [S] Pembrolizumab 10 mg/kg q2 weeks (compared to ipilimumab): 0.63 [S] Median PFS: Pembrolizumab 10 mg/kg q3 weeks (compared to ipilimumab): 0.58[S] Pembrolizumab 10 mg/kg q2 weeks (compared to ipilimumab): 0.58 [S]
	540 (KEYNOTE-002) [48]	Randomized phase II, open-label, ipilimumab-refractory, 1:1:1 randomization to receive pembrolizumab 10 mg/kg or pembrolizumab 2 mg/kg or investigator-choice chemotherapy	PFS	Pembrolizumab 10 mg/kg q3 weeks vs pembrolizumab 2 mg/kg q3 weeks vs investigator-choice chemotherapy	Pembrolizumab 10 mg/kg q3: 25% Pembrolizumab 2 mg/kg q3: 21% Investigator-choice chemotherapy: 4%	6 month PFS rate: Pembrolizumab 10 mg/kg q3 weeks: 38% Pembrolizumab 2 mg/kg q3 weeks: 34% Investigator-choice chemotherapy: 16% 9 month PFS rate: Pembrolizumab 10 mg/kg q3 weeks: 29% Pembrolizumab 2 mg/kg q3 weeks: 24% Investigator-choice chemotherapy: 8%	Median OS: Not reported Median PFS: Pembrolizumab 10 mg/kg q3 weeks (compared to chemotherapy): 0.50 [S] Pembrolizumab 2 mg/kg q3 weeks (compared to chemotherapy): 0.57 [S]
Nivolumab (2015)	418 (CheckMate-066) [49]	Randomized phase III, placebo-controlled, Ipilimumab-naïve, 1:1 randomization to receive Nivolumab 3 mg/kg or Dacarbazine	OS	Nivolumab 3 mg/kg q2 weeks vs Dacarbazine 1000 mg/m^2 q3 weeks	Nivolumab: 40% Dacarbazine: 14%	1 year OS rate: Nivolumab: 73% Dacarbazine: 42%	Median OS: Nivolumab (compared to dacarbazine) 0.42 [S] Median PFS: Nivolumab (compared to dacarbazine) 0.43 [S]
	405 (CheckMate-037) [50]	Randomized phase III, open-label, ipilimumab-refractory, 1:1 randomization to receive nivolumab 3 mg/kg or investigator-choice chemotherapy	ORR (reported), OS (not reported)	Nivolumab 3 mg/kg q2 weeks vs investigator-choice chemotherapy (dacarbazine 1000 mg/m^2 q3 weeks or carboplatin AUC 6 with paclitaxel 175 mg/m^2 q3 weeks	Nivolumab: 38% Chemotherapy: 5%	6 month PFS rate: Nivolumab: 48% Chemotherapy: 34%	Median OS: Not reached Median PFS: Nivolumab (compared to chemotherapy)0.82 [NS]

(Continued)

Table 20.4 (Continued)

Agent (FDA Approval)	No. of patients (study reference)	Study design	Primary endpoint	Treatment arms	Overall response rates	OS/PFS/RFS	HR (95%CI)
Ipilimumab + nivolumab	945 (CheckMate-067) [51]	Randomized phase II, open-label, ipilimumab-naive, 1:1:1 randomization to receive nivolumab or nivolumab/ipilimumab or ipilimumab	PFS and OS	Nivolumab 3 mg/kg q2 weeks *vs* ipilimumab 3 mg/kg q3 weeks (four doses) with nivolumab 1 mg/kg q3 weeks (four doses) followed by nivolumab 3 mg/kg q2 weeks vs ipilimumab 3 mg/kg q3 weeks (four doses)	Nivolumab: 44% Nivolumab/ ipilimumab: 58% Ipilimumab: 19%	Not reported	Median OS: Not reached Median PFS: Nivolumab/ipilimumab (compared to ipilimumab): 0.42 [S] Nivolumab/ipilimumab (compared to nivolumab): 0.74 [S] Nivolumab (compared to ipilimumab): 0.57 [S]
Non-Small Cell Lung Cancer							
Pembrolizumab (second line) (2015)	305 (KEYNOTE-024) [52]	Randomized phase III, open-label, pre-treated, PD-L1 positive (>50% tumor cells PD-L1 positive), 1:1 randomization to receive pembrolizumab or platinum-based chemotherapy	PFS	Pembrolizumab 200 mg q3 weeks for 2 years vs platinum-based chemotherapy	Pembrolizumab: 45% Platinum-based chemotherapy: 28%	6 month PFS rate: Pembrolizumab: 62% Platinum-based chemotherapy: 50% 6 month OS rate: Pembrolizumab: 80% Platinum-based chemotherapy: 72%	Median OS: not reached Median PFS: Pembrolizumab (compared to chemotherapy): 0.50 [S]
Pembrolizumab (first line PD-L1 positive) (2016)	1034 (KEYNOTE-010) [53]	Randomized phase II/III, open-label, previously untreated, PD-L1 positive (>1% tumor cells PD-L1 positive), 1:1:1 randomization to receive pembrolizumab 10 mg/kg or pembrolizumab 2 mg/kg or docetaxel	PFS, OS	Pembrolizumab 2 mg/kg q3 weeks vs pembrolizumab 10 mg/kg q3 weeks vs docetaxel 75 mg/m^2 q3 weeks	ORR (all patients): Pembrolizumab 2 mg/kg q3: 18% Pembrolizumab 10 mg/kg q3: 18% Docetaxel: 18% ORR (50% tumor cells PD-L1 positive) Pembrolizumab 2 mg/kg q3: 30% Pembrolizumab 10 mg/kg q3: 29% Docetaxel: 8%	1 year OS rate: Pembrolizumab 10 mg/kg: 52% Pembrolizumab 2 mg/kg: 43% Docetaxel: 35%	Median OS (all patients): Pembrolizumab 10 mg/kg (compared to docetaxel): 0.61 [S] Pembrolizumab 2 mg/kg (compared to docetaxel): 0.71 [S] Median OS (>50% tumor cells PD-L1 positive): Pembrolizumab 10 mg/kg (compared to docetaxel): 0.50 [S] Pembrolizumab 2 mg/kg (compared to docetaxel): 0.54 [S] Median PFS: not reported

					ORR	OS/PFS rates	Median OS/PFS
Nivolumab (second line) (2015)	582 (CheckMate 057) [54]	Randomized phase III, open-label, previously treated; 1:1 randomization to receive Nivolumab 3 mg/kg or docetaxel	OS	Nivolumab 2 mg/kg q2 weeks vs docetaxel 75 mg/m² q3 weeks	Nivolumab: 19% Docetaxel: 12%	1 year OS rate: Nivolumab: 51% Docetaxel: 39% 1 year PFS rate: Nivolumab: 19% Docetaxel: 8%	Median OS (all patients): Nivolumab (compared to Docetaxel): 0.73 [S] Median PFS (all patients): Nivolumab (compared to docetaxel): 0.92 [NS]
Atezolizumab (second line) (2016)	850 (OAK) [55]	Randomized phase III, open-label, previously treated; 1:1 randomization to receive atezolizumab 1200 mg or docetaxel	OS	Atezolizumab 1200 mg q4 weeks vs docetaxel 75 mg/m² q3 weeks	Atezolizumab: 14% Docetaxel: 13%	OS/PFS rates: not reported	Median OS (all patients): Atezolizumab (compared to docetaxel): 0.74 [S] Median PFS: not reported
	287 (POPLAR) [56]	Randomized phase II, open-label, previously treated; 1:1 randomization to receive atezolizumab 1200 mg or docetaxel	OS	Atezolizumab 1200 mg q4 weeks vs docetaxel 75 mg/m² q3 weeks	Atezolizumab: 15% Docetaxel: 15%	OS/PFS rates: not reported	Median OS (all patients): Atezolizumab (compared to docetaxel): 0.69 [S] Median OS (PD-L1, PD-L2, PD-1, B7-1, CD8+ IFN-gamma signature > median expression): Atezolizumab (compared to docetaxel): 0.46, 0.39, 0.43, 0.45, 0.43 respectively [S] Median PFS (all patients): Atezolizumab (compared to docetaxel): 0.94 [NS]

Renal Cell Cancer

Nivolumab (second line) (2015)	821 (CheckMate 025) [57]	Randomized, phase III, open-label, previously treated, 1:1 randomization to receive nivolumab 3 mg/kg or everolimus	OS	Nivolumab 2 mg/kg q2 weeks vs everolimus 10 mg daily	Nivolumab: 25% Everolimus: 5%	OS/PFS rates: not reported	Median OS (all patients): Nivolumab (compared to everolimus): 0.73 [S] Median PFS (all patients): Nivolumab (compared to everolimus): 0.88 [NS]

Bladder Cancer

Atezolizumab (second line) (2016)	310 (IMvigor210) [58]	Non-randomized phase II, open-label, previously treated urothelial/bladder cancer	ORR and ORR by PD-L1 positivity in immune cells in the tumor microenvironment by immune histochemistry: IC0 (<1%), IC1 (≥1% but <5%), and IC2/3 (≥5%)	Atezolizumab 1200 mg q3 weeks	Atezolizumab (all patients): 15% Atezolizumab (IC0): 8% Atezolizumab (IC1): 10% Atezolizumab (IC1/2/3): 18% Atezolizumab (IC2/3): 26%	OS/PFS rates: not reported	Median OS (all patients): Atezolizumab (compared to docetaxel): 0.74 [S] Median PFS: not reported

(Continued)

Table 20.4 (Continued)

Agent (FDA Approval)	No. of patients (study reference)	Study design	Primary endpoint	Treatment arms	Overall response rates	OS/PFS/RFS	HR (95%CI)
Classical Hodgkin Lymphoma							
Nivolumab (second line) (2016)	23 (CheckMate 039) [59]	Non-randomized, phase IB, open-label, previously treated	ORR, safety	Nivolumab 1-3 mg/kg q2 weeks	Nivolumab: 87%	OS/PFS rates: not reported	Median OS/PFS: not reported
	240 (CheckMate 205) [60]	Non-randomized, phase II, open-label, previously treated	ORR, safety	Nivolumab 3 mg/kg q2 weeks	Nivolumab: 66%	6 month OS rate: Nivolumab: 99% 6 month PFS rate: Nivolumab: 77%	Median OS/PFS: not reported
HNSCC							
Pembrolizumab (2016)	174 (KEYNOTE-012) [61, 62]	Non-randomized, phase IB, open-label, previously treated	ORR, safety	Pembrolizumab 10 mg/kg q2 weeks	Pembrolizumab: 18%	6 month OS rate: Pembrolizumab: 59% 6 month PFS rate: Pembrolizumab: 23%	Not reported
Nivolumab (2016)	361 (CheckMate 141) [63]	Randomized phase III, open-label, previously treated, 2:1 randomization to receive nivolumab 3 mg/kg or chemotherapy	OS	Nivolumab 3 mg/kg q2 weeks *vs* investigator-choice chemotherapy	Nivolumab: 13% Chemotherapy: 6%	1 year OS rate: Nivolumab: 36% Chemotherapy: 17% 6 month PFS rate: Nivolumab: 20% Chemotherapy: 10%	Median OS (all patients): Nivolumab (compared to chemotherapy): 0.70 [S] Median PFS (all patients): Nivolumab (compared to chemotherapy): 0.89 [NS]

ORR, overall response rate; OS, overall survival; PFS, progression-free survival; RFS, relapse-free survival; S, significant; NS, not significant.

(NSCLC and bladder cancer) – these regulatory studies are summarized in Table 20.4.

Appreciation of the differential effects of CTLA-4 inhibition (proliferation of a subset of transitional memory T-cells) and PD-1 inhibition (increased CD8+ T-cell lytic activity and natural killer cell function) was supplanted by preclinical studies that revealed that combined CTLA-4 and PD-1 blockade resulted in non-overlapping changes in gene expression [64]. These studies supported the rationale for investigating dual PD-1/CTLA-4 checkpoint inhibition in the clinic. Following dose-finding phase I [65] and randomized phase II CheckMate-069 [66] studies, a randomized three-arm study (CheckMate-067) evaluated ipilimumab, nivolumab or ipilimumab/nivolumab combination in ipilimumab-naïve patients [51]. Although toxicity was considerable – requiring treatment discontinuation in 36% of treated patients – 58% of patients who received ipilimumab/nivolumab had objective responses (see Table 20.4).

Multiple companies have developed PD-1 and PD-L1 inhibitors, all of which are being tested in an avalanche of clinical trials using these agents singly or in combination in a host of diseases. These data are summarized in several excellent review articles [67, 68]. Ipilimumab/nivolumab combinations are being evaluated in multiple diseases including: CNS metastatic melanoma (NCT02320058 and NCT02939300); uveal melanoma (NCT01585194, NCT02626962); small cell lung cancer (NCT02046733, NCT02538666); second line EGFR mutant NSCLC (NCT02864251); pleural mesothelioma (NCT02899299); gastric/gastro-esophageal junction carcinoma (NCT02872116); gastrointestinal stromal tumor (NCT02880020); hepatocellular carcinoma (NCT01658878); microsatellite unstable colorectal carcinoma (NCT02060188); second line squamous lung cancer (NCT02785952); with 5-azacitidine for myelodysplastic syndromes (NCT02530463); with blinatumomab for refractory CD19+ B-cell ALL (NCT02879695); with brentuximab for refractory Hodgkin's lymphoma (NCT01896999); and with radiation therapy (NCT02866383, NCT02659540). In efforts to improve the toxicity profile of ipilimumab in combination, several studies are testing alternative schedules and/or lower doses of ipilimumab (1 mg/kg every 3, 6 or 12 weeks instead of 3 mg/kg every 3 weeks). These studies suggest that lower/less intense doses of ipilimumab result in lower incidence of Grade 3/4 adverse events with no compromise in antitumor efficacy.

Other Agents

Other T-cell cosignaling targets of interest are the *costimulatory checkpoints* (OX40, 4-1BB/CD137, TIM-1, glucocorticoid-induced TNFR-related protein [GITR], herpes virus entry mediator [HVEM], LIGHT) and the *co-inhibitory checkpoints* (B and T lymphocyte attenuator [BTLA], leukocyte-associated immunoglobulin-like receptor 1 [LAIR-1], TIM-3, T cell immunoreceptor with Ig and ITIM domains [TIGIT]) [42]. Agonistic antibodies to costimulatory checkpoints under investigation include anti-OX40 MoAb and anti-4-1BB MoAb (urelumab, BMS-663513, Bristol-Myers Squibb). Dose-finding first-in-human trials of these agents have been launched and are in various stages of completion.

Adoptive Cellular Therapy

Adoptive cell therapy (ACT) is premised on the *ex vivo* identification of antitumor T-lymphocytes, which are expanded *in vitro* and then subsequently reinfused into patients, usually accompanied by growth factors to stimulate their *in vivo* survival and expansion. A component of these therapies has been the use of chemotherapy or radiotherapy to reduce the lymphocyte population of the patient, to modulate the host suppressive environment, and create 'space' for the infused T-lymphocytes.

Tumors may directly suppress host immunity through a combination of tumor-derived soluble (VEGF, TGF-β, IL-10, indoleamine 2,3-dioxygenase [IDO]) and cell-associated inhibitory factors (PD-L1) together with tumor-initiated recruitment of host immunosuppressive cells (CD4 + CD25 + Foxp3+ Treg and myeloid-derived suppressor cells) that collectively contribute to a highly immunosuppressive TME. ACT aims to reverse tumor-mediated immunosuppression through the transfer of CD8+ T-cells which can be inhibited by CD4 + CXCR5 + Foxp3+ Tregs found in TME. The use of lymphodepleting regimens increases the efficacy of ACT *directly* by removing CD4 + CD25 + Foxp3+ Tregs and *indirectly* by removing cellular elements of the host immune system that compete for cytokines necessary for optimal CD8+ T-cell function ("cytokine sink" theory) [69, 70]. The three key elements of ACT are: (i) transfer of tumor-specific CD8+ T-cells, (ii) CD8+ T-cell stimulation through coadministration of T-cell growth/activation factors and (iii) host lymphodepletion to remove Tregs and cytokine sinks [71]. Early approaches utilizing autologous T-cells in combination with lymphodepletion and high-dose IL-2 was associated with objective responses in approximately 20–40% of selected patients with metastatic melanoma [72].

More recently, investigators have developed chimeric antigen receptor (CAR) modified T-cells. CARs consist of recombinant receptors that typically target molecules on the tumor surface – ideally ones that are highly tumor-specific and minimally expressed on healthy tissue. Unlike conventional TCRs including that found in autologous ACT, CARs recognize unprocessed antigens independent of copresentation with human leukocyte antigen (HLA) machinery. CARs comprise an extracellular antigen-recognition domain linked via transmembrane and spacer domains to an intracellular signaling domain that typically includes costimulatory domains and T-cell activation. CAR-modified T-cells are manufactured by isolating a patient-specific T-cell (typically through leucopharesis) and subsequent introduction of the CAR transgene using *in vitro*-transcribed mRNA species (typically through RNA electroporation) or viral-mediated transduction.

Primary clinical experience with CAR T-cells has been with hematological malignancies – including B-cell acute lymphoblastic leukemia (B-ALL) (targeting CD19), chronic lymphoblastic leukemia (CLL) (targeting CD19), multiple myeloma (targeting CD19), acute myelogenous leukemia (targeting CD33) and refractory CD20+ lymphoma (targeting CD19 or CD20) [73]. Experience with CD19-directed CAR for CLL/myeloma, CD19/20-directed CAR for lymphoma and CD33-directed CAR for AML are limited to small case series with encouraging results that require further validation. The experience with

CD19-directed CAR in B-ALL has been remarkable: high rates of initial remissions in heavily pretreated patients, although excitement was tempered by development of relapse in ~50% mediated by CD19-positive and CD19-negative blasts. Although CAR optimization (additional costimulatory domains, etc) may enhance CAR T-cell persistence and reduce CD19-positive relapse, CD19-negative relapse may require alternative strategies.

Targeting nonhematological malignancies with CAR T-cells has been confounded by several factors unique to solid tumors including: absence of unique tumor-associated antigens, limited persistence of CAR T-cells, diminished T-cell homing and immunosuppressive TME. Early studies have focused on neuroblastoma (targeting GD2 ganglioside) and HER2 positive osteosarcoma/Ewing's sarcoma (targeting HER2) [74, 75]. Toxicities unique to this modality include "on-target, off-tumor" toxicities, cytokine release syndrome (CRS) and neurologic toxicities – which require highly trained personnel well versed in the recognition and management of these syndromes and access to specialized reversal agents (such as IL-6R antagonist tocilizumab for CRS).

CAR-modified T-cell therapies represent a novel means of harnessing the power of the immune system to treat cancer. CAR-modified T-cells will likely enter the oncologic armamentarium soon, especially to treat relapsed/refractory B-ALL and other hematologic malignancies. However, before this modality can gain widespread acceptance, many biologic challenges require added additional evaluation including strategies to define target antigen(s), improve CAR T-cell therapy safety, improve CAR T-cell persistence and delineate optimal conditioning regimens. Challenges peculiar to solid tumors including tumor heterogeneity, antigen loss, and immunosuppressive TME have to be tackled. One germane issue that precludes more widespread evaluation of this modality is the difficulty associated with manufacturing high-quality clinical-grade CAR-modified T-cell products which limits access to a few tertiary centers with extensive experience.

Vaccine-Based Immunotherapy

Cancer vaccines aim to elicit durable antitumor effects that result in sustained clinical responses. Vaccines can be categorized based on the nature of the antigen(s) incorporated – whole cell, protein, peptide, recombinant virus, dendritic cell, and naked DNA. Cancer vaccines have been studied in the adjuvant, neoadjuvant and metastatic settings across a broad array of malignancies. These studies have largely failed to show any reproducible benefit either in relation to progression or survival. The gamut of metastatic cancer patients treated with cancer vaccines between 1995 and 2010 at the NCI have been reviewed in two separate publications [76, 77]. Overall, ORRs of 3–4% were noted with infrequent CRs.

Although these results diminished interest in cancer vaccines, the approach was validated a decade ago, as a dendritic cell based vaccine for men with castration-resistant prostate cancer (CRPC), Sipuleucel-T (Provenge, APC8015, Dendreon Corporation) reached positive results in regard to overall survival, and received FDA approval. This vaccine consists of autologous dendritic cells (DCs) extracted via leukapharesis and subsequently activated *ex vivo* by incubation with a recombinant fusion protein PA2024 consisting of prostatic acid phosphatase (PAP) fused to granulocyte–macrophage colony-stimulating factor (GM-CSF). A course of sipuleucel-T consists of three treatments, each administered 2 weeks apart with 3 days between leukapharesis and DC reinfusion. The registration phase III trial (D9902B/IMPACT) randomly assigned 512 patients to receive sipuleucel-T or placebo in a 2:1 ratio and reported improved OS (median 4.1 month increase with a 22% reduction in the relative risk of death). No impact upon PFS was noted [78]. Sipuleucel-T had earlier demonstrated benefit in relation to OS in two additional randomized phase III trials against placebo (D9901, D9902A) [79] (reviewed in Table 20.2).

Although the survival benefit and favorable toxicity profile are positive attributes, the lack of biomarkers that would allow assessment of response has confounded further development. A biomarker study involving samples from the pooled patients from all three sipuleucel-T trials (D9901, D9902A, D9902B) reported improved survival in patients with antigen-specific T-cell/DC immune responses [80]. If prospectively validated, this may guide further development of this modality. Ongoing research is aimed at assessing the benefit of sipuleucel-T combinations including: anti PD-1 CT-011 and cyclophosphamide (NCT01420965), IDO inhibitor indoximod (NCT01560923), ipilimumab (NCT01832870), and with stereotactic radiation therapy (NCT01818986).

GVAX (BioSante Pharmaceuticals) is a cancer vaccine prepared from multiple cell lines genetically modified to secrete GM-CSF and then irradiated. Although not mitotically active, the cells remain metabolically active. The GVAX prostate cancer vaccine utilized two different CRPC cell lines – PC-3 (bone metastatic CRPC) and LNCaP (lymph node metastatic CRPC with mutated androgenic receptors). Early phase trials indicated that the vaccine was well tolerated and immunogenic. GVAX was evaluated in two phase III trials in separate patient populations: as a single agent in asymptomatic chemotherapy-naïve patients with CRPC (VITAL-1) and in combination with docetaxel in symptomatic taxane-naïve patients with CRPC (VITAL-2) [81, 82]. In both studies, control patients received standard docetaxel and prednisone. Notably, both studies were prematurely terminated for futility analyses. In the adjuvant setting in melanoma, GVAX vaccination resulted in vaccine site immune infiltrates and immune-reactive profiles in circulating monocytes although the addition of low-dose cyclophosphamide affect numbers of circulating regulatory T-cells [83].

Currently, several trials are evaluating the GVAX approach with tumors other than CRPC. A phase II trial is comparing GVAX to placebo in high-risk MDS/AML patients following allogeneic stem cell transplantation (NCT01773395). Other trials are assessing whether adding low-dose cyclophosphamide to GVAX potentiates its activity by reducing immunomodulatory effects: utilizing the neoadjuvant approach in prostate cancer (NCT01696877) and pancreatic cancer (NCT00727441) and an adjuvant approach in combination with FOLFIRINOX/radiation in pancreatic cancer (NCT01595321).

MAGE-A3 is a CT antigen expressed in a wide variety of malignancies including 66% of melanoma. Unlike peptides which elicit MHC-restricted activity, MAGE-A3 vaccination elicits a broad range of T-cell responses. Recombinant MAGE-A3 was combined with a potent immunostimulant AS15 to form the MAGE-A3 antigen-specific cancer immunotherapeutic (MAGE-A3-ASCI). Early trials demonstrated that MAGE-A3-ASCI induced specific T-cell responses and resulted in durable clinical responses in advanced melanoma and high-risk resected NSCLC [84, 85]. In both trials, microarray gene expression profiling identified a genetic signature that predicted response and was subsequently independently validated [86, 87]. However, randomized phase III trials evaluating the role of adjuvant MAGE-A3-ASCI vaccination compared to placebo in advanced melanoma (DERMA) and NSCLC (MAGRIT) following resection were both negative [88].

Initial forays into cancer vaccination were largely unsuccessful – largely attributable to outmoded designs that failed to induce immune responses. Next generation vaccine approaches using novel idiotypes and innovative immune adjuvants were developed but phase III clinical trials have not been particularly successful (results summarized in Table 20.5). The success of checkpoint inhibitors underscores the importance of peripheral tolerance mechanisms and suggests potentials for combinations with vaccines. Further optimization of vaccination strategy will also require defining optimal balance of antigens/neoantigens and picking appropriate adjuvants.

Active Immunotherapeutic Options

Bladder Cancer: Immunostimulants for Adjuvant Disease

Patients with nonmuscle invasive bladder cancer are grouped into three categories of recurrence and progression. The 1-year/5-year *probabilities of recurrence* for low-risk, intermediate-risk and high-risk patients are 15%/31%, 24%/46%, 61%/78%. Commensurate 1-year/5-year *probabilities of progression* are 0.2%/0.8%, 1%/6%, 5–17%/17–45% respectively [89]. Low-risk patients are typically treated with transurethral resection of all visible bladder tumors (TURBT) followed by a single instillation of adjuvant intravesical chemotherapy, typically mitomycin C. In patients whose risk of recurrence is intermediate-to-high, adjuvant treatment consisting of either intravesical chemotherapy or Morales' BCG protocol consisting of intravesical instillations of reconstituted Theracys® (81 mg) or TICE® BCG (50 mg) is standard of care following TURBT. Level 1 evidence suggests that intravesical therapy increases disease-free and overall survival while reducing the need for subsequent cystectomy in these patients [90].

Prostate Cancer: Dendritic Cell-Based Immunotherapy

Metastatic prostate cancer is initially treated with chemical or surgical androgen deprivation (ADT). However, most men develop biochemical, radiographic and/or symptomatic progression despite castrate levels of testosterone (<50 ng/ml) after 12–24 months. In asymptomatic or minimally symptomatic CRPC patients, sipuleucel-T improved overall survival in a phase III trial [78]. Interestingly, no PFS improvement was noted and conventional markers of objective response including PSA and imaging indicated progression and confounded

efficacy assessment. Sipuleucel-T has demonstrated survival benefits against placebo in two additional randomized phase III trials (see Table 20.2) [79].

Melanoma: Cytokines for Adjuvant Disease

Although amenable to cure when discovered early, patients with deeper primary tumors (AJCC stage IIB-C) and those with regional lymph node or in-transit metastases (IIIB-C) have an increased risk of relapse and death.

HDI is approved for the adjuvant treatment of stage IIB/C and all stage III high-risk resected melanoma. The landmark phase III trials of adjuvant HDI are summarized in Table 20.2 [26–28]. Of the various dosing schedules and routes tested, only HDI (IV 20 MU/m^2 5 days a week for 4 weeks followed by SC 10 MU/m^2 3 days a week for 48 weeks) has demonstrated reproducible improvements in RFS across multiple trials among the 14 major studies performed worldwide to date. The improvements in both survival and relapse-free interval in two of these studies (compared to observation and GMK vaccine (GM2 ganglioside conjugated to keyhole limpet hemocyanin)) are the only survival improvements noted yet in adjuvant therapy trials.

The pegylated formulation of IFN-α was compared to observation in patients with node-positive resected melanoma (stage IIIA or greater) in a phase III EORTC trial. EORTC 18991 investigators found that 5 years of pegylated IFN-α2b improved RFS but not OS [29]. Although compliance was an issue, the incidence of grade 3/4 fatigue (24%) and depression (10%) in EORTC 18991 was similar to that seen in the HDI trials. Unplanned subset analyses suggested an outsized benefit for patients with ulcerated primaries and microscopic nodal metastases – for which the EORTC is conducting another study of the same regimen in this population.

Melanoma: Cytokines and Oncolytic Immunotherapeutic Vaccines for Metastatic Disease

HD IL-2 is dosed at 600,000 or 720,000 IU/kg/dose administered intravenously every 8 h for up to 14 consecutive doses over 5 days per cycle. Each course of therapy comprises two such cycles delivered 4 weeks apart and patients are typically treated with a single course of therapy with stable or responding patients receiving further courses. HD IL-2 is FDA-approved for advanced melanoma based on the results from two non-randomized phase II trials (summarized in Table 20.2) [15–17]. HD IL-2 is associated with complete responses in ~6% and partial responses in ~10% for an objective response rate in ~16% of treated patients. Significant toxicity, low response rates and high administrative costs have plagued this option despite the undeniable survival benefit in responding patients. Investigators have sought to identify either prognostic or predictive biomarkers to improve the therapeutic index of HD IL-2. Initial reports of an immune signature that appeared to predict responders have not been prospectively validated [91].

Talimogene laherparepvec (T-vec, OncoVEX$^{\text{GM-CSF®}}$, Amgen) is a novel oncolytic immunotherapeutic vaccine – which comprises an attenuated herpes simplex virus type 1 genetically modified to produce GM-CSF. In a phase III trial that compared intracutaneous T-vec to GM-CSF alone, patients who received T-vec had significantly greater durable response rates. Benefit

Table 20.5 Recently completed and ongoing Phase III trials of cancer vaccines.

Agent (trade name, sponsors)	Description	No. of patients (study reference)	Tumor type	Study design/ endpoints	Final results
Allovectin-7® (Vical/AnGes MC)	Plasmid/lipid complex containing the DNA sequences encoding HLA-B7 and ß2 microglobulin	390	Advanced melanoma	Randomized, single blinded, phase III of intralesional Allovectin-7® compared to dacarbazine or temozolamide Primary: ORR	Negative (details not reported)
Algenpantucel-L, HyperAcute® (NewLink Genetics Corporation)	Allogeneic whole pancreatic cells expressing α-galactosyl (αGal) epitopes that elicit complement-mediated lysis and antibody-dependent cell-mediated toxicity	722	Resected high-risk pancreatic cancer	Randomized open label phase III trial of algenpantucel-L gemcitabine with or without 5-flurouracil (5FU) chemoradiation *vs* gemcitabine with or without 5FU chemoradiation alone Primary: OS	Negative (details not reported)
		302	Borderline resectable or locally advanced unresectable pancreatic carcinoma (NCT01836432)	Randomized open label phase III trial of algenpantucel-L with FOLFIRINOX vs FOLFIRINOX alone Primary: OS	Pending
AGS-003, Arcelis® (Argos Therapeutics)	Autologous dendritic cells	450	Advanced RCC (NCT01582672)	Randomized open label phase III trial of AGS-003 vs sunitinib (ADAPT) Primary: OS	Pending
Belagenpumatucel-L, Lucanix® (NovaRx Corporation)	Genetically modified whole cell	270 [97]	Stage III/IV NSCLC currently in remission or stable disease	Randomized, double-blinded, placebo-controlled phase III trial of Lucanix maintenance therapy following platinum-based combination therapy vs placebo Primary: OS	OS HR (belagenpumatucel-L versus placebo): 0.94 [NS]
BiovaxID® (Biovest International/National Cancer Institute)	Autologous tumor derived immunoglobulin idiotype vaccine	177 [98]	Indolent follicular non-Hodgkin lymphoma (NHL) during first complete remission	Randomized, double blinded, phase III of FNHLId1 + GM-CSF compared to KLH + GM-CSF Primary: DFS	DFS HR (BiovaxID versus placebo) (177 randomized): 0.81 [NS] DFS HR (BiovaxID versus placebo) (117 treated randomized): 0.62 [S]
CDX-110 or **Rindopepimut** (Celldex Therapeutics)	Peptide vaccine targeting a novel junctional epitope of the EGFR deletion mutant EGFRvIII expressed in approximately 60–70% of patients with GBM	700	Newly diagnosed GBM	Randomized, double-blinded, placebo-controlled phase III trial of temozolamide + vaccine vs temozolamide + placebo (ACT-IV) Primary: OS	Negative (details not reported)
IMA901, (immatics biotechnologies GmbH)	Multi-peptide vaccine targeting ADF-1/2, APO-1, CCN-1, GUC-1, K67-1, MET-1, MUC-1, RGS-1 and MMP-1 with HBV-1 (as a marker peptide)	339 [99]	Advanced RCC	Randomized phase III of IMA901 plus sunitinib vs sunitinib alone in HLA-A*02 positive patients (IMPRINT) Primary: OS	Negative (details not reported)
L-BLP25 or BLP25 Liposome Vaccine, Stimuvax® (Oncothyreon/Merck KGaA)	Peptide vaccine targeting Mucin 1 (MUC1) antigen	285	Unresectable stage III NSCLC in Asian patients with objective response or stable disease following primary chemoradiation	Randomized double-blinded placebo-controlled phase III trial of L-BLP25 vs placebo following definitive chemoradiation (INSPIRE) Primary: OS	Negative (details not reported)

Agent	Description	N	Patient population	Trial design	Result
MAGE-A3 ASCI, GSK1572932A (GlaxoSmithKline)	Peptide vaccine targeting MAGE-A3 antigen – a tumor-associated antigen overexpressed in many carcinomas including melanoma (up to 76%), NSCLC (35–50%), bladder (30–58%) and liver (24–78%) – in combination with a proprietary immune-stimulant AS15 (QS21 saponin, TLR-4 agonist monophosphoryl lipid A and TLR-9 agonist CpG7909).	2278	Stage IB-IIIA NSCLC expressing MAGE-A3 genetic signature following complete surgical resection	Randomized, double-blinded, placebo-controlled phase III trial of adjuvant MAGE-A3 vs placebo (MAGRIT) Primary: DFS	Negative (details not reported)
		1351	Macroscopic lymph node positive melanoma (stage III B/C) expressing MAGE-A3 genetic signature following complete surgical resection	Randomized, double-blinded, placebo-controlled phase III trial of adjuvant MAGE-A3 vs placebo (DERMA) Primary: DFS	Negative (details not reported)
MVA-MUC-IL2 or **TG4010** (Transgene, Novartis)	Recombinant vaccine using vaccinia vector engineered to deliver the transgenes for human MUC1 antigen and human IL-2	1000	Advanced squamous or nonsquamous NSCLC (NCT01383148)	Randomized double-blinded placebo-controlled phase IIB/III trial of TG4010 immunotherapy vs placebo with concurrent chemotherapy (TIME) Primary: PFS (IIB) and OS (III)	Pending
Nelipepimut-S/E75, NeuVax® (Galena Biopharma)	Peptide vaccine containing the Her2-derived E75 peptide	700	T1-3 node-positive (stage IIA-IIIC) breast cancer following SOC treatment (surgery +/– chemo-radiation) in Her-2 negative HLA-A2/HLA-A3 patients (NCT01479244)	Randomized, double-blinded, placebo-controlled phase III trial of adjuvant NeuVax following SOC treatment for node-positive breast cancer vs placebo (PRESENT) Primary: DFS	Pending
PROSTVAC-VF/TRICOM® (Bavarian Nordic A/S)	Recombinant vaccine using vaccinia and fowlpox vectors engineered to deliver the transgenes for PSA and T-cell costimulatory molecules LFA-3, B7.1 and ICAM-1 (TRICOM)	1298	Asymptomatic or minimally symptomatic men with CRPC excluding men with rapid PSA doubling (<1 month) and metastases to areas other than bone or lymph nodes (NCT01322490)	Randomized, double-blinded, placebo-controlled phase III trial of PROSTVAC V/F vaccine alone or in combination with GM-CSF vs double placebo (PROSPECT) Primary: OS	Pending
Talimogene laherparepvec, OncoVEX^{GM-CSF} (Amgen)	Genetically attenuated HSV-1 strain modified to be tumor-specific (ICP34.5 deletion provides tumor-selective replication) and to secrete GM-CSF (insertion of coding sequence for human GM-CSF)	433 [92]	Unresectable stage IIIB-IV melanoma	Randomized open label phase III trial of talimogene laherparepvec (T-vec) vs GM-CSF alone 2:1 randomization Primary: durable response rate	ORR: T-vec 26.4% vs GM-CSF 5.7% OS HR (T-vec vs GM-CSF): 0.79 [NS]

CR, complete response; CRPC, castrate resistant prostate cancer; DFS, disease free survival; 5-FU, 5-flurouracil; GBM, glioblastoma multiforme; GM-CSF, granulocyte-macrophage colony-stimulating factor; HLA, human leucocyte antigen; NSCLC, non-small cell lung cancer; ORR, overall response rate; OS, overall survival; PFS, progression free survival; PR, partial response; RCC, renal cell cancer; RFS, relapse free survival; TTP, time to progression; SCC, squamous cell carcinoma; SOC, standard of care.

was commensurate to metastatic substage: M1a patients having significantly greater response and survival than M1b or M1c patients and led to regulatory approval for the treatment of stage IIIB/IIIC unresectable and stage IV melanoma [92]. Further evaluation of T-vec in combination with PD-1 checkpoint inhibitors is planned (NCT02965716).

RCC: Immunostimulants and Cytokines for Metastatic Disease

Before the advent of agents targeting specific molecular pathways such as mTOR and VEGF/PDGF, advanced RCC was primarily treated with immunotherapeutic modalities including interferon and HD IL-2 with modest results in unselected patients. HD IL-2 dosed as in melanoma was approved in 1992 for the treatment of advanced RCC on the basis of phase III trials conducted by the NCI. Although associated with low response rates and significant treatment-related toxicity, responses were persistent with a majority of complete responders remaining disease-free long-term [17].

Two large multicenter randomized trials – Avastin and Interferon in Renal Cancer (AVOREN) and Cancer and Leukemia Group B (CALGB 90206) – have evaluated the IFN-α/bevacizumab combination compared to IFN-α alone in the era predating the use of first-line targeted therapies [30, 31]. In both trials, IFN-α was dosed at 9×10^6 MU given thrice weekly with bevacizumab 10 mg/kg given fortnightly. Although the IFN-α/bevacizumab combination resulted in improved median PFS irrespective of the MSKCC risk category, neither study reported a significant survival improvement compared to the control group (although a nonsignificant survival benefit was noted in AVOREN). These results led to the approval of the IFN-α/bevacizumab combination for the first-line treatment of patients with metastatic RCC by the FDA in 2009. The results of the regulatory trials of HD IL-2 and the IFN-α/bevacizumab combination in metastatic RCC are summarized in Table 20.2.

The advent of agents directed against the hypoxia-inducible factor axis either via the vascular endothelial growth factor (VEGF) pathway or the mammalian target of rapamycin (mTOR) pathway has become a challenge. At present, there are seven targeted agents approved for the treatment of advanced RCC including the mTOR inhibitors (temsirolimus [Torisel®] and everolimus [Afinitor®]) and multityrosine kinase receptor inhibitors (TKIs: sunitinib [Sutent®], sorafenib [Nexavar®], axitinib [Inlyta®], pazopanib [Votrient®], Cabozantinib [Cabometyx®]) of which sunitinib, pazopanib and temsirolimus are approved for use in the first line. In the absence of survival data (except for temsirolimus in poor-risk patients) and biomarkers to guide selection, drug selection has largely been based on study eligibility criteria; line of therapy for which agent was approved; toxicity profile; underlying histology; and patient comorbidities.

Although HD IL-2 is potentially curative and approved for first line use in patients with good performance status there is no predictive or prognostic biomarker that allows the individualization of therapy. Although the IFN-α/bevacizumab combination is approved for use in first line on the basis of robust phase III data from two trials, it has largely been supplanted by TKIs (sunitinib, pazopanib) and the mTOR inhibitor temsirolimus in patients with predominantly clear-cell histology.

Immunotherapy Targeting T-cell Cosignaling Checkpoints: Melanoma, NSCLC, RCC, Classical Hodgkin Lymphoma, Bladder Cancer and HNSCC

Although the role of the immune system in suppressing tumor growth has been appreciated for over a century – it was James Allison who first recognized the importance of coinhibitory/costimulatory molecules in mediating antitumor immunity and demonstrated that antibody blockade of a T-cell inhibitory molecule (CTLA-4) enhanced antitumor immunity in murine models [93, 94]. Subsequent clinical trials validated this concept. CTLA-4 inhibitor ipilimumab is currently approved for the adjuvant treatment of resected stage III melanoma and for metastatic melanoma (both first and second line) based on the results of three randomized phase III trials – summarized in Table 20.4.

Similarly, fundamental work by Tasuko Honjo and colleagues utilizing mouse models of chronic infectious disease established PD-1 and its ligands PD-L1 and PD-L2 as negative regulators of effector T-cell function acting primarily in inflamed tissues [93, 94]. These studies spawned the development of antibodies that blocked either the receptor (PD-1) or its ligands (PD-L1) and demonstrated a remarkable ability to reverse attenuated immune responses even in chronically exhausted T-cells. Early dose-finding studies established a paradigm that is now common to trials involving checkpoint inhibitors: early (occasionally dramatic) responses in a variable fraction of treated patients including patients with "non-immunogenic" cancers. Two PD-1 blocking antibodies (pembrolizumab and nivolumab) and PD-L1 blocking antibody (atezolizumab) have garnered regulatory approval for multiple indications that are summarized in Table 20.4 including:

- Pembrolizumab: melanoma (first and second line); NSCLC (first and second line); HNSCC (second line)
- Nivolumab: melanoma (first and second line); classical Hodgkin lymphoma (second line); RCC (second line); HNSCC (second line); NSCLC (second line)
- Atezolizumab: NSCLC (second line); bladder cancer (second line)
- Nivolumab/ipilimumab combination: melanoma.

Tumor assessments in patients treated with checkpoint inhibitors are conducted at week 12, week 24, and every 3 months thereafter until progression is noted. Novel patterns of response – termed immune-related response criteria (irRC) – have been described in patients treated with both ipilimumab and PD-1 inhibitors and include a pattern in which eventual response is preceded by an initial increase in tumor burden. Patients with these response patterns require close clinical and radiographical monitoring to prevent inadvertent treatment discontinuation [46].

Treatment with checkpoint inhibitors is also associated with an unique spectrum of treatment-related toxicities termed immune-related adverse events (irAEs). These appear to arise from general immunologic enhancement and span a wide gamut of organ systems including dermatologic, gastrointestinal, hepatic, endocrine, and other less common inflammatory events. Management typically involves withholding the offending agent, supportive care and occasionally institution of oral or parenteral corticosteroids depending on the severity of the observed toxicity [95]. However, close monitoring is required as fatalities have been reported particularly with gastrointestinal toxicity for which institution of greater immunosuppression (TNFα inhibitors or mycophenolate) may be required in steroid-refractory patients.

Conclusion

The field of cancer immunotherapy has been completely transformed over the preceding decade with the advent of highly effective therapies that have produced remarkable results in a select group of patients. Efforts to improve the shoulder of response have focused on understanding the mechanistic basis underlying cancer immunity – elegantly outlined by Chen and Mellman in "The Cancer-Immunity Cycle" [96]:

1) Release of cancer cell antigens
2) Cancer antigen presentation
3) T-cell and APC priming and activation
4) T-cell traffic to tumors
5) T-cell infiltration of tumors
6) Recognition of cancer cells by T-cells in tumors
7) T-cell mediated cancer cell death.

At each step, various stimulatory and inhibitory factors affect antitumor immune responses and may be augmented or suppressed by tumor-specific and/or patient-specific factors. Each of these factors singly or in combination represent potential means by which antitumor immunity may be enhanced. Although it seems abundantly clear that patients with a pre-existing CD8+ T-cell infiltrate may require only PD-1 monotherapy to achieve durable remissions, how best to treat T-cell "non-inflamed" tumors remains unclear. The immune response is specific yet adaptable, durable and self-propagating. Although our understanding of the immune system is at best rudimentary and incomplete, its vast diversity may be the ultimate match for cancer's protean complexity.

Funding: This work was supported by Award Number P50 CA121973 from the National Cancer Institute. The content is solely the responsibility of the authors and does not necessarily represent the official views of the National Cancer Institute or the National Institutes of Health.

References

1 Van den Eynde BJ, van der Bruggen P. T cell defined tumor antigens. *Curr Opin Immunol* 1997;9(5):684–93.

2 Burnet M. Cancer; a biological approach. I. The processes of control. *Br Med J* 1957;1(5022):779–86.

3 Thomas L. On immunosurveillance in human cancer. *Yale J Biol Med* 1982;55(3-4):329–33.

4 Gatti RA, Good RA. Occurrence of malignancy in immunodeficiency diseases. A literature review. *Cancer* 1971;28(1):89–98.

5 Dunn GP, Old LJ, Schreiber RD. The three Es of cancer immunoediting. *Annu Rev Immunol* 2004;22:329–60.

6 Schreiber RD, Old LJ, Smyth MJ. Cancer immunoediting: integrating immunity's roles in cancer suppression and promotion. *Science* 2011;331(6024):1565–70.

7 Schwartz RH. T cell anergy. *Annu Rev Immunol* 2003;21:305–34.

8 Nurieva R, Wang J, Sahoo A. T-cell tolerance in cancer. *Immunotherapy* 2013;5(5):513–31.

9 Pearl R. Cancer and tuberculosis. *Am J Hygiene* 1929;9:97.

10 Coe JE, Feldman JD. Extracutaneous delayed hypersensitivity, particularly in the guinea-pig bladder. *Immunology* 1966;10(2):127–36.

11 Herr HW, Morales A. History of bacillus Calmette-Guerin and bladder cancer: an immunotherapy success story. *J Urol* 2008;179(1):53–6.

12 Rosenberg SA, Mulé JJ, Spiess PJ, *et al*. Regression of established pulmonary metastases and subcutaneous tumor mediated by the systemic administration of high-dose recombinant interleukin 2. *J Exp Med* 1985 May 1;161(5):1169–88.

13 Rosenberg SA, Lotze MT, Muul LM, *et al*. Observations on the systemic administration of autologous lymphokine-activated killer cells and recombinant interleukin-2 to patients with metastatic cancer. *N Engl J Med*;313(23):1485–92.

14 Rosenberg SA, Lotze MT, Muul LM, *et al*. A progress report on the treatment of 157 patients with advanced cancer using lymphokine-activated killer cells and interleukin-2 or high-dose interleukin-2 alone. *N Engl J Med* 1987;316(15):889–97.

15 Rosenberg SA, Yang JC, Topalian SL, *et al*. Treatment of 283 consecutive patients with metastatic melanoma or renal cell cancer using high-dose bolus interleukin 2. *JAMA* 1994;271(12):907–13.

16 Atkins MB, Lotze MT, Dutcher JP, *et al*. High-dose recombinant interleukin 2 therapy for patients with metastatic melanoma: analysis of 270 patients treated between 1985 and 1993. *J Clin Oncol* 1999;17(7):2105–16.

17 Fyfe G, Fisher RI, Rosenberg SA, *et al*. Results of treatment of 255 patients with metastatic renal cell carcinoma who received high-dose recombinant interleukin-2 therapy. *J Clin Oncol* 1995;13(3):688–96.

18 Prince HM, Duvic M, Martin A, *et al*. Phase III placebo-controlled trial of denileukin diftitox for patients with cutaneous T-cell lymphoma. *J Clin Oncol* 2010;28(11):1870–7.

19 King DM, Albertini MR, Schalch H, *et al*. Phase I clinical trial of the immunocytokine EMD 273063 in melanoma patients. *J Clin Oncol* 2004;22(22):4463–73.

20 Albertini MR, Hank JA, Gadbaw B, *et al*. Phase II trial of hu14.18-IL2 for patients with metastatic melanoma. *Cancer Immunol Immunother* 2012;61(12):2261–71.

21 Johannsen M, Spitaleri G, Curigliano G, *et al*. The tumour-targeting human L19-IL2 immunocytokine: preclinical safety studies, phase I clinical trial in patients with solid tumours and expansion into patients with advanced renal cell carcinoma. *Eur J Cancer* 2010;46(16):2926–35.

22 Eigentler TK, Weide B, de Braud F, *et al*. A dose-escalation and signal-generating study of the immunocytokine L19-IL2 in combination with dacarbazine for the therapy of patients with metastatic melanoma. *Clin Cancer Res* 2011;17(24):7732–42.

23 Schwager K, Hemmerle T, Aebischer D, Neri D. The immunocytokine L19-IL2 eradicates cancer when used in combination with CTLA-4 blockade or with L19-TNF. *J Invest Dermatol* 2013;133(3):751–8.

24 Platanias LC. Mechanisms of type-I- and type-II-interferon-mediated signalling. *Nat Rev Immunol* 2005;5(5):375–86.

25 Fish EN, Platanias LC. Interferon receptor signaling in malignancy: a network of cellular pathways defining biological outcomes. *Mol Cancer Res* 2014;12(12):1691–703.

26 Kirkwood JM, Strawderman MH, Ernstoff MS, *et al.* Interferon alfa-2b adjuvant therapy of high-risk resected cutaneous melanoma: the Eastern Cooperative Oncology Group Trial EST 1684. *J Clin Oncol* 1996;14:7–17.

27 Kirkwood JM, Ibrahim JG, Sondak VK, *et al.* High- and low-dose interferon alfa-2b in high-risk melanoma: first analysis of intergroup trial E1690/S9111/C9190. *J Clin Oncol* 2000;18(12):2444–58.

28 Kirkwood JM, Ibrahim JG, Sosman JA, *et al.* High-dose interferon alfa-2b significantly prolongs relapse-free and overall survival compared with the GM2-KLH/QS-21 vaccine in patients with resected stage IIB-III melanoma: results of intergroup trial E1694/S9512/C509801. *J Clin Oncol* 2001;19(9):2370–80.

29 Eggermont AM, Suciu S, Testori A, *et al.* Long-term results of the randomized phase III trial EORTC 18991 of adjuvant therapy with pegylated interferon alfa-2b versus observation in resected stage III melanoma. *J Clin Oncol* 2012;30(31):3810–8.

30 Escudier B, Bellmunt J, Négrier S, *et al.* Phase III trial of bevacizumab plus interferon alfa-2a in patients with metastatic renal cell carcinoma (AVOREN): final analysis of overall survival. *J Clin Oncol* 2010;28(13):2144–50.

31 Rini BI, Halabi S, Rosenberg JE, *et al.* Phase III trial of bevacizumab plus interferon alfa versus interferon alfa monotherapy in patients with metastatic renal cell carcinoma: final results of CALGB 90206. *J Clin Oncol* 2010;28(13):2137–43.

32 Chen L, Flies DB. Molecular mechanisms of T cell co-stimulation and co-inhibition. *Nat Rev Immunol* 2013;13(4):227–42.

33 Schneider H, da Rocha Dias S, Hu H, Rudd CE. A regulatory role for cytoplasmic YVKM motif in CTLA-4 inhibition of TCR signaling. *Eur J Immunol* 2001;31(7):2042–50.

34 Hodi FS, O'Day SJ, McDermott DF, *et al.* Improved survival with ipilimumab in patients with metastatic melanoma. *N Engl J Med* 2010;363(8):711–23.

35 Robert C, Thomas L, Bondarenko I, *et al.* Ipilimumab plus dacarbazine for previously untreated metastatic melanoma. *N Engl J Med* 2011;364(26):2517–26.

36 Schadendorf D, Hodi FS, Robert C, *et al.* Pooled analysis of long-term survival data from phase II and phase III trials of ipilimumab in unresectable or metastatic melanoma. *J Clin Oncol* 2015;33(17):1889–94.

37 Eggermont AM, Chiarion-Sileni V, Grob JJ, *et al.* Adjuvant ipilimumab versus placebo after complete resection of high-risk stage III melanoma (EORTC 18071): a randomised, double-blind, phase 3 trial. *Lancet Oncol* 2015;16(5):522–30.

38 Eggermont AM, Chiarion-Sileni V, Grob JJ, *et al.* Prolonged survival in stage III melanoma with ipilimumab adjuvant therapy. *N Engl J Med* 2016;375(19):1845–55.

39 Ribas A, Camacho LH, Lopez-Berestein G, *et al.* Antitumor activity in melanoma and anti-self responses in a phase I trial with the anti-cytotoxic T lymphocyte-associated antigen 4 monoclonal antibody CP-675,206. *J Clin Oncol* 2005;23(35):8968–77.

40 Kirkwood JM, Lorigan P, Hersey P, *et al.* Phase II trial of tremelimumab (CP-675,206) in patients with advanced refractory or relapsed melanoma. *Clin Cancer Res* 2010;16(3):1042–8.

41 Ribas A, Kefford R, Marshall MA, *et al.* Phase III randomized clinical trial comparing tremelimumab with standard-of-care chemotherapy in patients with advanced melanoma. *J Clin Oncol* 2013;31(5):616–22.

42 Zarour HM. Reversing T-cell dysfunction and exhaustion in cancer. *Clin Cancer Res* 2016;22(8):1856–64.

43 Topalian SL, Hodi FS, Brahmer JR, *et al.* Safety, activity, and immune correlates of anti-PD-1 antibody in cancer. *N Engl J Med* 2012;366(26):2443–54.

44 Hamid O, Robert C, Daud A, *et al.* Safety and tumor responses with lambrolizumab (anti-PD-1) in melanoma. *N Engl J Med* 2013;369(2):134–44.

45 Brahmer JR, Tykodi SS, Chow LQ, *et al.* Safety and activity of anti-PD-L1 antibody in patients with advanced cancer. *N Engl J Med* 2012;366(26):2455–65.

46 Wolchok JD, Hoos A, O'Day S, *et al.* Guidelines for the evaluation of immune therapy activity in solid tumors: immune-related response criteria. *Clin Cancer Res* 2009;15(23):7412–20.

47 Robert C, Schachter J, Long GV, *et al.* Pembrolizumab versus ipilimumab in advanced melanoma. *N Engl J Med* 2015;372(26):2521–32.

48 Ribas A, Puzanov I, Dummer R, *et al.* Pembrolizumab versus investigator-choice chemotherapy for ipilimumab-refractory melanoma (KEYNOTE-002): a randomised, controlled, phase 2 trial. *Lancet Oncol* 2015;16(8):908–18.

49 Robert C, Long GV, Brady B, *et al.* Nivolumab in previously untreated melanoma without BRAF mutation. *N Engl J Med* 2015;372(4):320–30.

50 Weber JS, D'Angelo SP, Minor D, *et al.* Nivolumab versus chemotherapy in patients with advanced melanoma who progressed after anti-CTLA-4 treatment (CheckMate 037): a randomised, controlled, open-label, phase 3 trial. *Lancet Oncol* 2015;16(4):375–84.

51 Larkin J, Chiarion-Sileni V, Gonzalez R, *et al.* Combined nivolumab and ipilimumab or monotherapy in untreated melanoma. *N Engl J Med* 2015;373(1):23–34.

52 Reck M, Rodríguez-Abreu D, Robinson AG, *et al.* Pembrolizumab versus chemotherapy for PD-L1-positive non-small-cell lung cancer. *N Engl J Med* 2016;375(19):1823–33.

53 Herbst RS, Baas P, Kim DW, *et al.* Pembrolizumab versus docetaxel for previously treated, PD-L1-positive, advanced non-small-cell lung cancer (KEYNOTE-010): a randomised controlled trial. *Lancet* 2016;387(10027):1540–50.

54 Borghaei H, Paz-Ares L, Horn L, *et al.* Nivolumab versus docetaxel in advanced nonsquamous non-small-cell lung cancer. *N Engl J Med* 2015;373(17):1627–39.

55 Barlesi F, Park K, Ciardiello F, *et al.* Primary analysis from OAK, a randomized phase III study comparing atezolizumab

with docetaxel in 2L/3L NSCLC. Presented at: 2016 ESMO Congress; October 7–11, 2016; Copenhagen, Denmark.

56 Fehrenbacher L, Spira A, Ballinger M, *et al*. Atezolizumab versus docetaxel for patients with previously treated non-small-cell lung cancer (POPLAR): a multicentre, open-label, phase 2 randomised controlled trial. *Lancet* 2016;387(10030):1837–46.

57 Motzer RJ, Escudier B, McDermott DF, *et al*. Nivolumab versus everolimus in advanced renal-cell carcinoma. *N Engl J Med* 2015;373(19):1803–13.

58 Rosenberg JE, Hoffman-Censits J, Powles T, *et al*. Atezolizumab in patients with locally advanced and metastatic urothelial carcinoma who have progressed following treatment with platinum-based chemotherapy: a single-arm, multicentre, phase 2 trial. *Lancet* 2016;387(10031):1909–20.

59 Ansell SM, Lesokhin AM, Borrello I, *et al*. PD-1 blockade with nivolumab in relapsed or refractory Hodgkin's lymphoma. *N Engl J Med* 2015;372(4):311–9.

60 Younes A, Santoro A, Zinzani PL, *et al*. Checkmate 205: nivolumab (nivo) in classical Hodgkin lymphoma (cHL) after autologous stem cell transplant (ASCT) and brentuximab vedotin (BV) – phase 2 study. *J Clin Oncol* 34, 2016 (suppl; abstr 7535).

61 Chow LQ, Haddad R, Gupta S, *et al*. Antitumor activity of pembrolizumab in biomarker-unselected patients with recurrent and/or metastatic head and neck squamous cell carcinoma: results from the Phase Ib KEYNOTE-012 Expansion Cohort. J Clin Oncol 2016 Sep 19. pii: JCO681478.

62 Seiwert TY, Burtness B, Mehra R, *et al*. Safety and clinical activity of pembrolizumab for treatment of recurrent or metastatic squamous cell carcinoma of the head and neck (KEYNOTE-012): an open-label, multicentre, phase 1b trial. *Lancet Oncol* 2016;17(7):956–65.

63 Ferris RL, Blumenschein G Jr, Fayette J, *et al*. Nivolumab for recurrent squamous-cell carcinoma of the head and neck. *N Engl J Med* 2016;375(19):1856–67.

64 Das R, Verma R, Sznol M, *et al*. Combination therapy with anti-CTLA-4 and anti-PD-1 leads to distinct immunologic changes in vivo. *J Immunol* 2015;194(3):950–9.

65 Wolchok JD, Kluger H, Callahan MK, *et al*. Nivolumab plus ipilimumab in advanced melanoma. *N Engl J Med* 2013;369(2):122–33.

66 Postow MA, Chesney J, Pavlick AC, *et al*. Nivolumab and ipilimumab versus ipilimumab in untreated melanoma. *N Engl J Med* 2015;372(21):2006–17.

67 Medina PJ, Adams VR. PD-1 Pathway inhibitors: immuno-oncology agents for restoring antitumor immune responses. *Pharmacotherapy* 2016;36(3):317–34.

68 Hamanishi J, Mandai M, Matsumura N, *et al*. PD-1/PD-L1 blockade in cancer treatment: perspectives and issues. *Int J Clin Oncol* 2016;21(3):462–73.

69 Klebanoff CA, Khong HT, Antony PA, *et al*. Sinks, suppressors and antigen presenters: how lymphodepletion enhances T cell-mediated tumor immunotherapy. *Trends Immunol* 2005;26(2):111–7.

70 Gattinoni L, Finkelstein SE, Klebanoff CA, *et al*. Removal of homeostatic cytokine sinks by lymphodepletion enhances the efficacy of adoptively transferred tumor-specific CD8+ T cells. *J Exp Med* 2005;202(7):907–12.

71 Overwijk WW, Theoret MR, Finkelstein SE, *et al*. Tumor regression and autoimmunity after reversal of a functionally tolerant state of self-reactive CD8+ T cells. *J Exp Med* 2003;198(4):569–80.

72 Rosenberg SA. Raising the bar: the curative potential of human cancer immunotherapy. *Sci Transl Med* 2012;4(127):127–8.

73 Dai H, Wang Y, Lu X, Han W. Chimeric antigen receptors modified T-cells for cancer therapy. *J Natl Cancer Inst* 2016;108(7). pii: djv439.

74 Louis CU, Savoldo B, Dotti G, *et al*. Antitumor activity and long-term fate of chimeric antigen receptor-positive T cells in patients with neuroblastoma. *Blood* 2011;118(23):6050–6.

75 Ahmed N, Brawley VS, Hegde M, *et al*. Human epidermal growth factor receptor 2 (HER2)-specific chimeric antigen receptor-modified T Cells for the immunotherapy of HER2-positive sarcoma. *J Clin Oncol* 2015;33(15):1688–96.

76 Rosenberg SA, Yang JC, Restifo NP. Cancer immunotherapy: moving beyond current vaccines. *Nat Med* 2004;10(9):909–15.

77 Klebanoff CA, Acquavella N, Yu Z, Restifo NP. Therapeutic cancer vaccines: are we there yet? *Immunol Rev* 2011;239(1):27–44.

78 Kantoff PW, Higano CS, Shore ND, *et al*. Sipuleucel-T immunotherapy for castration-resistant prostate cancer. *N Engl J Med* 2010;363(5):411–22.

79 Higano CS, Schellhammer PF, Small EJ, *et al*. Integrated data from 2 randomized, double-blind, placebo-controlled, phase 3 trials of active cellular immunotherapy with sipuleucel-T in advanced prostate cancer. *Cancer* 2009;115(16):3670–9.

80 Sheikh NA, Petrylak D, Kantoff PW, *et al*. Sipuleucel-T immune parameters correlate with survival: an analysis of the randomized phase 3 clinical trials in men with castration-resistant prostate cancer. *Cancer Immunol Immunother* 2013;62(1):137–47.

81 Higano C, Saad F, Somer B, *et al*. A Phase III trial of GVAX immunotherapy for prostate cancer versus docetaxel plus prednisone in asymptomatic, castration-resistant prostate cancer (CRPC) ASCO GU Symposium 2009 (Suppl):Abstr LBA150.

82 Small E, Demkow T, Gerritsen WR, *et al*. A phase III trial of GVAX immunotherapy for prostate cancer in combination with docetaxel versus docetaxel plus prednisone in symptomatic, castration-resistant prostate cancer (CRPC) ASCO GU Symposium. 2009:Abstr 7.

83 Lipson EJ, Sharfman WH, Chen S, *et al*. Safety and immunologic correlates of melanoma GVAX, a GM-CSF secreting allogeneic melanoma cell vaccine administered in the adjuvant setting. *J Transl Med* 2015;13:214.

84 Kruit W, Suciu S, Dreno B, *et al*. Immunization with recombinant MAGE-A3 protein combined with adjuvant systems AS15 or AS02B in patients with unresectable and progressive metastatic cutaneous melanoma: a randomized open-label phase II study of the EORTC Melanoma Group. *J Clin Oncol* 26:2008 (May 20 suppl; abstr 9065).

85 Vansteenkiste J, Zielinski M, Linder A, *et al*. Final results of a multi-center, double-blind, randomized, placebo controlled Phase II study to assess the efficacy of MAGE-A3 immunotherapeutic as adjuvant therapy in stage IB/II Non-Small Cell Lung Cancer (NSCLC). *J Clin Oncol* 2007;25:(June 20 suppl; abstr 7554).

86 Louahed J, Gruselle O, Gaulis S, *et al*. Expression of defined genes by identified by pre-treatment tumor profiling: association with clinical responses to the GSK MAGE-A3 immunotherapeutic in metastatic melanoma patients. *J Clin Oncol* 2008;26:(May 20 suppl; abstr 9045).

87 Vansteenkiste J, Zielinski M, Linder A, *et al*. Association of gene expression signature and clinical efficacy of MAGE-A3 antigen-specific cancer immunotherapeutic (ASCI) as adjuvant therapy in resected stage IB/II non-small cell lung cancer (NSCLC). *J Clin Oncol* 2008;26:(May 20 suppl; abstr 7501).

88 Vansteenkiste JF, Cho BC, Vanakesa T, *et al*. Efficacy of the MAGE-A3 cancer immunotherapeutic as adjuvant therapy in patients with resected MAGE-A3-positive non-small-cell lung cancer (MAGRIT): a randomised, double-blind, placebo-controlled, phase 3 trial. *Lancet Oncol* 2016;17(6):822–35.

89 Shelley MD, Court JB, Kynaston H, *et al*. Intravesical Bacillus Calmette-Guerin in Ta and T1 Bladder Cancer. *Cochrane Database Syst Rev* 2000;(4):CD001986.

90 Pawinski A, Sylvester R, Kurth KH, *et al*. A combined analysis of European Organization for Research and Treatment of Cancer, and Medical Research Council randomized clinical trials for the prophylactic treatment of stage TaT1 bladder cancer. European Organization for Research and Treatment of Cancer Genitourinary Tract Cancer Cooperative Group and the Medical Research Council Working Party on Superficial Bladder Cancer. *J Urol* 1996;156(6):1934–40, discussion 1940–1.

91 Sullivan RJ, Hoshida Y, Brunet J, *et al*. A single center experience with high-dose (HD) IL-2 treatment for patients with advanced melanoma and pilot investigation of a novel gene expression signature as a predictor of response. *J Clin Oncol* 2009;27:15s (suppl; abstr 9003).

92 Andtbacka RH, Kaufman HL, Collichio F, *et al*. Talimogene laherparepvec improves durable response rate in patients with advanced melanoma. *J Clin Oncol* 2015;33(25):2780–8.

93 Callahan MK, Wolchok JD. At the bedside: CTLA-4- and PD-1-blocking antibodies in cancer immunotherapy. *J Leukoc Biol* 2013;94(1):41–53.

94 Intlekofer AM, Thompson CB. At the bench: preclinical rationale for CTLA-4 and PD-1 blockade as cancer immunotherapy. *J Leukoc Biol* 2013;94(1):25–39.

95 Michot JM, Bigenwald C, Champiat S, *et al*. Immune-related adverse events with immune checkpoint blockade: a comprehensive review. *Eur J Cancer* 2016;54:139–48.

96 Chen DS, Mellman I. Oncology meets immunology: the cancer-immunity cycle. *Immunity* 2013;39(1):1–10.

97 Giaccone G, Bazhenova LA, Nemunaitis J, *et al*. A phase III study of belagenpumatucel-L, an allogeneic tumour cell vaccine, as maintenance therapy for non-small cell lung cancer. *Eur J Cancer* 2015;51(16):2321–9.

98 Schuster SJ, Neelapu SS, Gause BL, *et al*. Vaccination with patient-specific tumor-derived antigen in first remission improves disease-free survival in follicular lymphoma. *J Clin Oncol* 2011;29(20):2787–94.

99 Rini B, Stenzl A, Zdrojowy R, *et al*. Results from an open-label, randomized, controlled phase 3 study investigating IMA901 multipeptide cancer vaccine in patients receiving sunitinib as first-line therapy for advanced/metastatic RCC. 2015 European Cancer Congress. Abstract 17LBA. Presented September 27, 2015.

21

Targeted Therapies

Elizabeth Kessler, Paul Brittain, S. Lindsey Davis, Stephen Leong, S. Gail Eckhardt, and Christopher H. Lieu

University of Colorado Anschutz Medical Campus, Aurora, Colorado, USA

Introduction

As the understanding of molecular, genetic, and biochemical changes during carcinogenesis grows, drug development has shifted towards therapies that act on specific molecular targets that drive tumor growth and metastasis. Cell proliferation and differentiation are regulated by numerous hormones, cytokines, and growth factors, and in cancer cells, key components of these pathways may be altered through gene amplification resulting in overexpression or mutation. These abnormal signaling pathways specific to cancer cells represent potential targets for cancer treatments. Targeted therapies are drugs that block the growth and spread of cancer by interfering with specific molecules involved with tumor growth and progression. The development of targeted agents in oncology has rapidly expanded over the past two decades and has led to significant improvements in the treatment of numerous cancers. This chapter will review the basic types of targeted agents as well as the major pathways targeted in cancer that highlight several of the successes and challenges in the development of targeted therapies. Though this chapter is not meant to include all known targets and targeted therapies, various cellular processes regulating oncogenesis targeted by current drugs will be discussed.

Types of Targeted Agents

The advent of technologies to mass produce compounds has made it feasible to target extracellular proteins, cell surface receptors, and cellular processes to inhibit cancer growth and metastasis. Understanding the mechanism of action of these drugs, and how they compare to other cancer therapies, requires basic knowledge about their structure and function. Table 21.1 lists several representative approved therapies mentioned in this chapter. Though there are other categories of targeted agents currently available and under development (e.g., fusion proteins, HDAC inhibitors, proteasome inhibitors, etc.), this

section will focus primarily on antibodies and tyrosine kinase inhibitors (TKIs) as they represent the majority of the current FDA-approved therapies in oncology. Immunotherapies and adoptive cellular therapies are also currently in clinical development, with several agents recently FDA-approved. These will be presented separately in another chapter on immunotherapy.

Antibodies

Nomenclature

- *Monoclonal antibody*: an antibody with a unique specificity for a single antigen.
- *Antigen*: the target molecule for which an antibody has specificity.
- *Fab region (fragment antigen binding)*: the variable end of antibodies unique to a particular antibody that determines the antigenic specificity.
- *Fc region (fragment constant)*: the constant end of an antibody opposite the Fab region. The homogeneous nature of this region allows it to be recognized by the body's immune system regardless of the sequence of the Fab region.
- *Antibody-drug conjugates*: monoclonal antibodies whose Fc region has been linked to or replaced with a secondary molecule (e.g., a drug, toxin, or radioisotope). Drug conjugates take advantage of the specificity of the Fab region of monoclonal antibodies to enable delivery of a secondary molecule to the site of a specific antigen.
- *Antibody-dependent cell-mediated cytotoxicity (ADCC)*: ADCC describes the process through which cells of the innate immune system destroy targets that have been marked by antibodies.
- *Complement-dependent cytotoxicity (CDC)*: the process of cellular destruction by the complement portion of the body's innate immune system, directed at antibody-bound antigens and/or the cells containing specified antigens.
- *Murine Abs*: mouse antibodies, denoted by the suffix -omab. The first antibodies tested for therapy were mouse antibodies, but they generally exhibited poor results due to inefficiency

The American Cancer Society's Principles of Oncology: Prevention to Survivorship, First Edition. Edited by The American Cancer Society.
© 2018 The American Cancer Society. Published 2018 by John Wiley & Sons, Inc.

Table 21.1 Targeted therapies.

Drug	Target	Primary disease site(s)	Known biomarker
Monoclonal antibodies			
Cetuximab	EGFR	Colon, Head and neck	KRAS wild-type
Trastuzumab	HER2/neu	Breast	Her2/neu amplification
Bevacizumab	VEGF	Colon, NSCLC, renal cell, and glioblastoma	
Necitumumab	EGFR	NSCLC	
Ramucirumab	VEGF	Colon, gastric, lung	
Drug conjugates			
Ibritumomab	CD20	Non-Hodgkin lymphoma	
Trastuzumab emtansine	HER2/neu	Breast	HER2/neu amplification
Small molecule inhibitors			
Romidepsin	HDACi	Cutaneous T-cell lymphoma	
Panobinostat	HDACi	Myeloma	
Belinostat	HDACi	Myeloma	
Bortezomib	Proteasome inhibitor	Multiple myeloma	
Ixazomib	Proteasome inhibitor	Multiple myeloma	
Carfilzomib	Proteosome inhibitor	Multiple myeloma	
Vismodegib	Hedgehog	Basal cell carcinoma	
Imatinib	bcr-abl, c-kit, PDGFR	CML, GIST,	
Everolimus	mTOR	renal cell, pancreatic/gastrointestinal/lung Neuroendocrine carcinoma	
Trametinib	MEK	Melanoma	
Sorafenib	VEGFR, PDGFR, RAF	Renal cell and hepatocellular carcinoma	
Vemurafenib	BRAF	Melanoma	BRAF V600E mutation
Dabrafenib	BRAF	Melanoma	BRAF V600E mutation
Cobimetinib	MAPK/MEK1/MEK2	Melanoma	Combination with vemurafenib for V600E/V600K mutations
Crizotinib	ALK/ROS1	Lung adenocarcinoma	ALK/ROS gene rearrangement
Alectinib	ALK	NSCLC	ALK gene rearrangement
Ceritinib	ALK	NSCLC	ALK gene rearrangement
Vandetanib	RET	Medullary thyroid cancer	
Erlotinib	EGFR	Lung adenocarcinoma	EGFR mutation (T790M confers resistance)
Lapatinib	HER1/HER2	Breast	HER2/neu amplification
Osimertinib	EGFR	Non-small cell lung cancer	T790M mutation positive
Lenvatinib	VEGF	Thyroid and renal cell carcinoma	
Idelalisb	PI3Kdelta	Follicular and small lymphocytic lymphomas	

of human immune system stimulation and frequent initiation of anaphylactic reactions.

- *Chimeric Abs*: combination antibodies composed of a murine Fab region, and a human Fc region, denoted by the suffix –ximab. These were the first antibodies developed to avoid the anaphylactic reactions triggered by murine antibodies and to increase antibody half-life.

- *Humanized Abs*: antibodies produced from fully human genes, denoted by the suffix –umab. These antibodies may be produced in cell culture or by transgenic mice.

Mechanism of Action

Monoclonal antibodies exert their antitumor effects through both direct and indirect means. Direct effects result from an

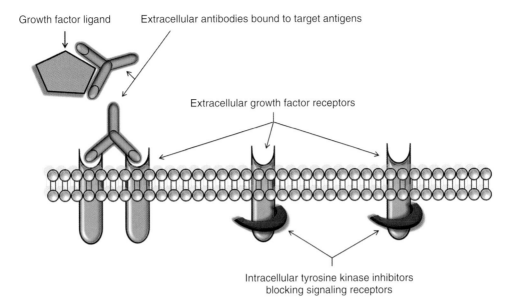

Growth factor ligand   Extracellular antibodies bound to target antigens

Extracellular growth factor receptors

Intracellular tyrosine kinase inhibitors
blocking signaling receptors

Figure 21.1 Sites of action of antibodies and tyrosine kinase inhibitors.

antibody binding to its target molecule through the Fab site and include blockade of ligands or receptors, stimulation of receptors as an agonist, or use as targeting devices (Figure 21.1) [1]. Indirect actions of antibodies take place through the Fc region and require an intact immune system. The immune system recognizes the Fc region of antibodies bound to antigen and eliminates the antigenic targets though mechanisms including CDC and ADCC. In cancer, the antigens may be cancer cells, receptors, or extracellular molecules that promote tumor growth and progression.

Antibody–Drug Conjugates

An antibody–drug conjugate can be thought of as a two-part molecule made up of the Fab portion of an antibody and the Fc portion of an antibody attached to, or replaced by, an antitumor therapy. The concept of drug conjugates takes advantage of the "homing missile" function of the Fab portion of antibodies to selectively deliver toxic moieties such as cytotoxic compounds or radioisotopes directly to a tumor [2]. This delivery method essentially increases the therapeutic index and selectivity of highly toxic agents. For example, brentuximab vedotin a conjugate of a CD30 antibody and auristatin E, is an effective therapy approved for the treatment of lymphoma [3]. The antibody attaches to the CD30 molecule on the surface of the lymphoma cell, and delivers a conjugated toxin directly to the malignant cell.

Tyrosine Kinase Inhibitors

The human genome encodes approximately 90 tyrosine kinases and 43 tyrosine kinase-like genes [4]. Tyrosine kinases serve as activating receptors for complex signaling cascades with diverse effects on normal cellular function and tumorigenesis [4]. Imatinib, a TKI used in chronic myeloid leukemia, was the first success in antineoplastic targeting of tyrosine kinases [5]. Since its development, this mechanism of targeting cancer cells has continued to grow.

Nomenclature

- *Tyrosine kinase*: an enzyme that phosphorylates tyrosine residues, often initiating a signaling transduction cascade. Tyrosine kinases can often function in cell proliferation, differentiation, migration, angiogenesis, and/or cell-cycle regulation [6].
- *Tyrosine kinase inhibitor (TKI)*: a molecule that restrains the action(s) of a tyrosine kinase thus blocking the downstream signaling cascade(s) that would otherwise be activated by the kinase.

Mechanism of Action

Receptor tyrosine kinases function by transferring a phosphate from adenosine triphosphate (ATP) to a protein, thus activating a signaling cascade. Conversely, TKIs block signal transduction through receptors by direct blockade and by competition with the ATP required for activation. Many inhibitors work by binding to the highly conserved ATP binding pocket on the tyrosine kinase receptor, such that an inhibitor of one receptor may also inhibit other receptors within the same family [4]. One TKI may thus exhibit broad effects against multiple tumor targets; however, blockade of several targets on normal tissues may increase toxicity.

Advantages/Disadvantages of Antibodies Versus TKIs

Antibodies are approximately 300 times larger than small molecule inhibitors [7]. Because of their smaller size, oral small molecule TKIs are more readily able to cross the blood–brain barrier and thus may potentially be used to treat CNS disease while antibodies must be given intrathecally to reach the CNS [8]. Antibodies may be too large to traverse the cell membrane and typically act on molecules that are expressed on the cell surface or secreted [9]. Small molecule inhibitors can traverse the cell membrane and inhibit multiple targets and signaling pathways, but at the cost of potentially more toxicity [10].

Antibodies typically have a significantly longer half-life, allowing for weekly to every 3 week dosing, whereas small molecule TKIs typically have a shorter half-life requiring more frequent dosing. Small molecules may be absorbed though the gastrointestinal tract for oral dosing, while antibodies as proteins, are degraded when taken orally and thus require intravenous administration. The differences in administration lead to distinct pharmacokinetic profiles, as oral administration of TKIs may be impacted by variability in gastrointestinal absorption, degradation, metabolism, and excretion while the handling of large proteins by the body, such as antibodies, may be more predictable [11, 12].

The greater specificity of antibodies against targets allows them to serve as targeting devices in antibody–drug conjugates. The Fc regions of antibodies provide indirect effects on ADCC and CDC [13]. While these host-dependent mechanisms may increase the efficacy of antibodies, they likely increase the variability of responses among patients and also complicate preclinical testing *in vitro* and *in vivo*. TKI effects can be measured in cell culture, but antibody responses require more complex *in vivo* models to be measured effectively [14]. For example, cetuximab is a monoclonal antibody that targets a receptor with tyrosine kinase activity but has been shown to exert approximately one-half of its native antitumor activity through the immune system [15]. Thus, the efficacy of antibodies can be significantly reduced in an immunocompromised patient. Conversely, the complexity of immune reliance may be advantageous through modification of the Fc portion of an antibody in order to increase its immunogenicity [16].

Targeted therapy is potentially less toxic than traditional cytotoxic chemotherapies, but the general adverse effects vary based on the drug and the target. Aside from off-target effects, the major dose limiting toxicities of either antibodies or TKIs are often due to effects of target blockade of normal tissue, known as "mechanism-based" toxicity. Examples include the skin rash and diarrhea observed with epidermal growth factor receptor (EGFR) blockade and hypertension and proteinuria with vascular endothelial growth factor (VEGF) blockade [17, 18]. Another concern with monoclonal antibodies is the possibility of an infusion reaction during administration, but with the vast majority of new antibodies being fully humanized, immunogenicity and anaphylactoid reactions are decreasing in incidence and allergic responses can be treated with supportive therapies.

Signal Transduction Pathways Targeted in Cancer

EGFR

The EGFR family, also known as the human epidermal receptor (HER) and Erb family, includes four receptor tyrosine kinases (RTKs) that are ubiquitously expressed and essential for normal development [19]. They exist in their inactivated state as cell surface monomers; however, when bound by their appropriate ligand, they undergo homo- or heterodimerization, leading to transautophosphorylation of the cytoplasmic domain and subsequent downstream signaling via a number of pathways ultimately resulting in cellular proliferation and survival.

The EGFR binds epidermal growth factor (EGF), transforming growth factor-alpha, amphiregulin, betacellulin, heparin-binding EGF (HB-EGF), epiregulin, and neuregulins. Different EGF receptors preferentially modulate particular pathways, with some overlap. The MAPK and PI3K-AKT pathways are important effectors of EGFR activation. EGFR activates Ras through the Grb2 adaptor protein, which is bound to SOS, serving as the first step in induction of the Ras-MAPK pathways [20]. The Src family of kinases has also been implicated in signal transduction from EGFR as either a contributor to activation or a signal transducer, and its overexpression has been shown to enhance EGF-mediated proliferation [21]. Additionally, EGFR activates the JAK/signal transducer and activator of transcription protein (STAT) pathway and the mTOR pathway.

The EGFR may be overexpressed as a result of gene amplification [22], may be constitutively activated by growth factors produced by tumors themselves [23], or may possess somatic mutations in the tyrosine-kinase domain leading to constitutive activation. These kinase domain mutations may preferentially activate the PI3K-Akt or STAT pathways [24]. Occasional mutations in the extracellular dimerization arm also occur allowing for constitutive activation [25]. The receptors may be transactivated by ectodomain shedding of other activators; or by interactions with WNT-FZD, the estrogen receptor, and protein kinase C [26].

Therapeutic targeting of EGFR has been explored both through antibodies and ATP-competitive small-molecule TKIs. EGFR expression is detectable in at least half of non-small cell lung cancers (NSCLC) and point mutations of the ATP binding site, most commonly in exon 19, have been shown to drive a particular subset of these cancers [24, 27]. Gefitinib and erlotinib are reversible TKIs used to treat patients with EGFR mutated NSCLC. However, as often occurs when driver mutations are targeted, a resistance mutation develops at the TKI binding site. Several irreversible inhibitors of EGFR have been developed to overcome this mutation by binding more specifically to the ATP domain. Osimertinib binds irreversibly to the EGFR receptor mutant forms – T790M, L858R and exon 19 deletion and as such is indicated for the treatment of patients with metastatic T790M mutation-positive NSCLC [28]. Additionally, necitumumab is an EGF receptor IgG1 monoclonal antibody used in combination with gemcitabine and cisplatin for first-line treatment of metastatic squamous NSCLC based on an open label phase III trial demonstrating improvement in overall survival [29]. In other cancers, EGFR functions more as a promoter of cellular growth and less as a true driver of the disease. For example, erlotinib is approved in combination with gemcitabine for the treatment of advanced pancreatic adenocarcinoma [30].

Cetuximab and panitumumab are monoclonal antibodies targeting EGFR that are approved for treating patients with KRAS wild-type metastatic colon cancer [31, 32]. Cetuximab is also approved for the treatment of platinum-resistant recurrent or metastatic squamous-cell carcinoma of the head and neck or in first line treatment when combined with chemotherapy [33–35]. Antibodies directed at EGFR family receptors can block receptor function through blockade of ligand binding, increased internalization of receptors [36], and reducing the proteolytic cleavage of receptors [37]. Newer, fully humanized antibodies are under development and additional tumor types are being explored.

HER2

HER2 is a member of the EGFR family of receptors that acts as an important driver of cancer. This transmembrane tyrosine kinase receptor has no known natural ligand but instead functions through dimerization with other members of the HER, or EGFR, family to activate multiple cell survival pathways [38].

Amplification (not receptor mutation) of HER2 is partially responsible for mammary and gastric carcinogenesis, and may play a role in additional tumor types. This receptor is a target of many small molecule inhibitors, both approved and in development. Approximately one third of breast cancers overexpress HER2 and when treated with the monoclonal antibody, trastuzumab, patients have an improved overall survival compared to standard therapy [39, 40]. Trastuzumab is used in both the adjuvant and metastatic setting. It is also approved for the treatment of advanced HER2 overexpressing gastric cancer based on an overall survival benefit when given in combination with chemotherapy [41]. Trastuzumab's mechanism is not fully understood, but it contributes to increased internalization and proteosomic degradation of HER2 resulting in G1 cell cycle arrest and angiogenesis inhibition [42]. Trastuzumab also dissociates the Src adaptor protein, subsequently increasing PTEN translocation to the plasma membrane, thereby negatively influencing Akt and the overall PI3K/Akt/mTOR cell survival pathway [43]. Pertuzumab is another monoclonal antibody directed at HER2, which sterically interferes with the dimerization of the receptor [44]. This agent has been shown to improve survival in patients with HER2 overexpressing breast cancer when used in combination with trastuzumab in either the first- or second-line setting [45]. Lapatanib is a small molecule inhibitor of the HER2 receptor and EGFR, which improved survival when used in combination with chemotherapy for the treatment of metastatic HER2 overexpressing breast cancer and in combination with trastuzumab [46]. Trastuzumab emantasine (T-DM1) is an antibody drug conjugate targeting the HER2 receptor in which trastuzumab tracks to the receptor and a derivative of maytansine, a cytotoxic agent, is then released from a thioether linker. This agent is approved for patients with HER2-positive breast cancer after progression on trastuzumab and a taxane [47].

Insulin-Like Growth Factor-1 Receptor

The insulin-like growth factor-1 receptor (IGF-1R), found mainly in liver, muscle, kidney and adipose tissue, is essential for fetal and postnatal growth and development [48]. This transmembrane tyrosine kinase receptor is important in neoplastic growth through its involvement in the PI3K/Akt and MAPK pathways. The IGF-1R exists in two splice variant isoforms, the first form being more commonly expressed in neoplastic cells and recognizing multiple ligands whereas the second isoform recognizes only insulin; both receptors are very similar to the insulin receptor. Unlike IGF-2R which lacks the ability to signal intracellularly, IGF-1R undergoes autophosphorylation upon ligand binding, recruits a scaffolding protein, and activates downstream signaling through the PI3K/Akt/mTOR and RAS/MAPK pathways respectively. This ultimately results in decreased apoptosis, increased cell growth and increased cell mobility, leading to tumor growth and metastasis [49].

IGF1 signaling is necessary for oncogenic transformation [50]. IGFI, IGFII, and insulin are all ligands of IGF-1R. IGFI is produced in response to growth hormone stimulation predominantly in the liver, whereas IGFII is important in fetal growth but circulates in adults and may be overexpressed in cancer [51]. These factors are regulated by insulin-like growth factor binding proteins (IGF-BP) which alter the levels of circulating ligand. IGFI and insulin have been shown to stimulate the proliferation of tumor cells *in vitro* [52] and decreasing their signaling can decrease *in vivo* tumor growth [49]. Increased circulating levels of IGFI have been associated with an increased risk of breast, prostate and colon cancer and loss of imprinting of IGFII is associated with ovarian and colon cancer [53]. Additionally, levels of circulating insulin may increase one's risk of cancer.

The IGF-1R is highly expressed in breast, colon, lung and prostate cancers as well as sarcomas [54–56]. However, IGF-1R gene amplification is rare and it is thought that the ligands may be more important in the oncogenic role of IGF-1R. The receptor has been targeted using mABs and TKIs in over 100 clinical trials without clearly positive results thus far [57, 58]. Hyperglycemia is a notable side effect reflecting the receptor's homology with the insulin receptor. The small molecule inhibitors are less specific, binding to both the IGF-1R and the insulin receptor but with a shorter half-life that may avoid many of the toxicities associated with antibody treatment. Analogues of the IGFI ligand have been tested in preclinical studies, and antiligand antibodies have also been tested in the clinical arena [59].

c-KIT

c-KIT (CD117) is a receptor tyrosine kinase that is expressed on the surface of hematopoietic stem cells, as well as other cell types. Upon stimulation of the extracellular domain by a ligand known as stem cell factor, the receptor dimerizes and activates the intracellular kinase domain [60]. Multiple adaptor proteins are activated at this site, including Grb2, which in turn stimulates the MAP kinase pathway, and the p85 regulatory subunit of PI3K, which leads to activation of that signaling cascade [61].

Activating mutations of the c-kit gene as well as increased binding of stem cell factor and other ligands to the extracellular receptor have been associated with malignant transformation. Mutations of c-kit are most commonly seen in mastocytoma, gastrointestinal stromal tumor (GIST), and to a lesser degree, sinonasal T-cell lymphoma, seminoma/dysgerminoma, and acute myeloid leukemia. Ligand-associated means of c-KIT activation have been documented in additional tumor types, including thyroid cancers, small cell lung cancer, melanoma, and ovarian cancer [62]. In addition, activating mutations of PDGFRA have been associated with c-KIT pathway activation and GIST formation [63].

Many TKIs designed for other purposes have been subsequently found to inactivate c-KIT in addition to PDGFR, FGFR, and most notably, BCR-ABL [62]. Imatinib mesylate was originally developed and approved as a selective inhibitor of the ABL ATP binding site for treatment of BCR-ABL positive chronic myelogenous leukemia [64]. However, further preclinical evaluation demonstrated potent inhibition of c-KIT and associated signaling pathways [65, 66], and imatinib was approved for use in unresectable and metastatic GIST based on results of a phase

II study showing a response rate of 38% in c-KIT+ patients [67]. The drug was later approved for patients with KIT+ GIST following surgical resection based on a phase III placebo-controlled trial showing improved recurrence-free survival in the treatment group [68].

Despite selecting patients with KIT+ tumors, response to imatinib for treatment of GIST is not universal. Furthermore, resistance to the agent has been demonstrated following initial response to therapy [69]. Specific activating c-kit mutations have been associated with treatment response, most notably the exon 11 mutation, while mutation in exon 9 and PDGFRA D842V mutations have been commonly demonstrated in patients with primary resistance to imatinib. These and others have been demonstrated as secondary mutations in patients with delayed imatinib resistance. Interestingly, regardless of the mechanism of resistance, the c-KIT pathway is found to remain activated [70].

Additional c-KIT targeted agents have been studied in GIST, though thus far only the multikinase inhibitor sunitinib has been approved for such [69]. This drug is known to target FLT3, VEGFR, and PDGFR in addition to c-KIT [71]. Sunitinib was approved for treatment of GIST after progression on imatinib based on a phase III study of the agent versus placebo, which showed significant improvement in time to tumor progression in the sunitinib group [70]. Interestingly, a phase II study demonstrated greatest clinical benefit in those patients with an exon 9 c-kit mutation, with less response in those with exon 11 mutation [72]. The TKI, regorafenib, has also recently been approved for GIST [73]. Studies of other multikinase inhibitors are ongoing, including agents thought to target areas potentially important in imatinib resistance [69].

Mitogen-Activated Protein Kinase Pathway

Normal function of the mitogen-activated protein kinase (MAPK) pathway begins with activation and dimerization of a cell surface receptor tyrosine kinase (RTK), such as EGFR, with resultant stimulation of intracellular kinase domain activity (Figure 21.2) [74]. Adaptor proteins with associated binding domains can then be phosphorylated at this site [75]. Growth factor receptor-bound protein 2 (Grb2) is an example of one such adaptor protein, which is simultaneously bound to son of sevenless (SOS), a guanine-nucleotide exchange factor [76]. This phosphorylation event brings SOS adjacent to RAS proteins located near the plasma membrane, ultimately resulting in GTP binding of GDP-bound RAS [77]. This activity recruits the protein kinase RAF to the membrane and initiates a cascade of phosphorylation. After RAF has been phosphorylated by RAS, it then phosphorylates MAP kinase-kinases MEK1 and MEK2, which subsequently phosphorylate MAP kinases ERK1 and ERK2 [78]. ERK then phosphorylates various intracellular signaling proteins and transcription factors that affect cellular function, including MAPK-interacting serine/threonine kinase (MNK), p90 ribosomal S6 kinase (RSK), erythroblastosis virus E26 oncogene homolog 1-like gene 1 (Elk-1), camp response element binding protein (CREB), c-Fos and c-Jun [76].

Constitutive activation of the MAPK pathway has been associated with malignant transformation [79]. In addition to mutations in RAS, BRAF, or MEK, amplification of these or other pathway activators and altered activity of an associated RTK can also contribute to an overactive pathway [80]. RAS gene mutations, generally somatic mutations of codons 12, 13, or 61, have been identified in 30% of human cancers [81]. Most of these mutations are associated with KRAS and less

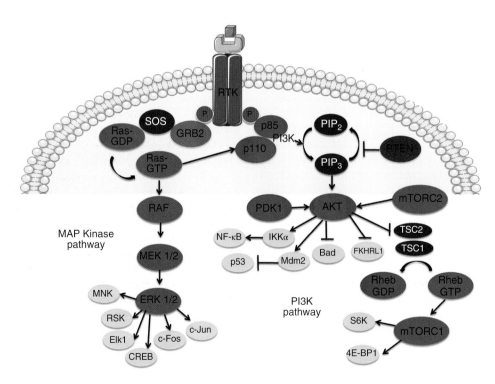

Figure 21.2 Mitogen-activated protein kinase (MAPK) pathway and PI3K pathway with downstream effectors.

commonly with NRAS and HRAS. KRAS mutations have been found to occur with greater frequency in pancreatic, colon, and lung cancers, while NRAS mutations are seen with greater frequency in melanoma [76]. Various BRAF mutations have been recognized in human cancers, with most resulting in disruption of the inactive BRAF protein conformation, leading to chronic activation of the MAPK pathway [82]. The most common BRAF mutation, accounting for approximately 90% of mutations, is the substitution of valine for glutamic acid at position 600 (V600E). Most BRAF mutations are found in melanoma and thyroid cancers, and to a lesser degree, colorectal and ovarian cancers [83]. Mutations of MEK and ERK are rare [84]. Importantly, multiple activating mutations of the same pathway are rarely identified in cancers, as has been demonstrated with BRAF and RAS mutations [82, 85, 86]. This finding suggests that such mutations separately achieve a common outcome of pathway disturbance, and that additive mutations provide no further advantage to the cell [81].

Targeting the MAPK Signaling Pathway

Various effectors within the MAPK signaling cascade have been studied as potential targets for cancer therapy [87]. Targeting the proximal part of the cascade with RAS inhibitors has thus far been unsuccessful. Most efforts at RAS blockade have focused on the use of farnesyltransferase inhibitors (FTI), which interrupt the activity of the enzyme responsible for lipid modification and transportation of RAS to the plasma membrane, a key step in its activation. Clinical trials of multiple agents in RAS dependent cancers have not shown efficacy [88–91]; a possible explanation lies in the resultant activation of geranylgeranyl transferase-1, but preclinical studies targeting this enzyme or both enzymes (FT and GGT) have exhibited unacceptable toxicity thus far [92, 93]. Another effort to inhibit RAS has been made through direct targeting of HRAS through synthetic antisense oligonucleotides that inhibit protein production [94]. Though data in preclinical studies were promising, efficacy in early clinical trials has been less so [76].

Targeting the next effector in the MAPK signaling pathway, RAF, has been more successful. One of the first RAF inhibitors, sorafenib, targets the ATP-binding site of Raf-1 kinase, though it was later discovered to also inhibit BRAF and various RTKs including VEGFR-2, PDGFR-β, Flt-3, c-KIT, and FGFR-1 [95]. Despite negative results in melanoma [96], sorafenib is FDA approved for the treatment of advanced renal cell and unresectable hepatocellular carcinoma, primarily due to its anti-VEGFR and PDGFR properties [10, 97].

A more selective small molecule inhibitor, vemurafenib, was subsequently developed to target the V600E mutated BRAF kinase frequently associated with melanoma. A phase III clinical trial comparing vemurafenib to dacarbazine demonstrated significant improvement in overall survival in the vemurafenib group versus the dacarbazine group, even after crossover at interim analysis [98]. Dabrafenib has also been approved in the treatment of unresectable or metastatic V600E BRAF mutated melanoma [99]. Unfortunately, resistance to vemurafenib therapy was frequently noted, generally after a period of months of disease control [100]. The cause of resistance has been extensively studied, with multiple potential mechanisms identified. NRAS mutations leading to reactivation of the MAPK pathway

has been demonstrated, as has up-regulation of alternative growth pathways through stimulation of RTKs such as PDGFR-β and the PI3K pathway [101]. A subset of V600E mutants have also been identified which lack the RAS-binding domain and are able to dimerize independently of RAS, ultimately leading to pathway reactivation [102]. Other potential acquired resistance mechanisms to BRAF inhibition include transactivation of CRAF, diminution of RAF autoinhibition resulting in MAPK activation in the presence of RAS mutations, and inhibitor-induced drug dependence. Inhibition of alternative effectors in the MAPK pathway to overcome resistance mechanisms to BRAF inhibition have proven successful. Cobimetinib is a reversible inhibitor of MAPK/MEK1 and MEK2 [103]. The BRAF V600E mutation results in constitutive activation of the BRAF pathway inclusive of MEK1 and MEK2, thus use of this inhibitor prevents this alternative growth pathway. This kinase inhibitor is indicated for the treatment of patients with a V600E or V600K mutation in combination with vemurafenib.

Early phase clinical trials of first and second generation MEK inhibitors were disappointing due to lack of clinical efficacy and concerning toxicity, respectively [87]. Toxicity noted in these early phase clinical trials included rash, fatigue, diarrhea, and vision changes. Trametinib is a small molecule that has been shown to specifically and potently inhibit MEK1 and MEK2 kinase activity through binding adjacent to the active site, ultimately preventing RAF phosphorylation as well as downstream activation of ERK1 and ERK2. In additional preclinical experiments, cell lines with activating mutations of up-stream effectors such as BRAF and KRAS were more sensitive to activity of the drug [104]. A phase III trial randomized patients with V600E and V600K mutated melanoma to receive trametinib, dacarbazine, or paclitaxel, with significantly improved progression-free survival (PFS) and 6-month overall survival (OS) in the trametinib group compared to either chemotherapy agent. These outcomes are similar to those with vemurafenib in BRAF-mutated melanoma patients, with no head-to-head study currently underway [105]. The concept of delaying treatment resistance in BRAF-mutated melanoma through combined BRAF and MEK inhibition has been evaluated in early clinical trials with further evaluation planned [106]. Numerous MEK inhibitors are currently in various stages of development.

Phosphoinositide 3-Kinase Pathway

The three classes of lipid kinases that act by phosphorylating phosphoinositides are known as the phosphoinositide 3-kinase (PI3K) family. Of these classes, IA PI3Ks have been linked to carcinogenesis in humans [107]. There are three genes, PIK3CA, PIK3CB, and PIK3CD, encoding highly homologous p110 catalytic isoforms, p110α, p110β, and p110δ respectively. While the expression p110δ is largely restricted to the immune system, p110α and p110β are ubiquitously expressed. At the cellular membrane, PI3K phosphorylates phosphatidylinositol (4,5)-bisphosphate (PIP_2) to phosphatydilinositol-3, 4, 5-triphosphate (PIP_3), leading to activation of cell signaling proteins (Figure 21.2) [108]. This step is negatively regulated by phosphatase and tensin homolog deleted from chromosome 10 (PTEN), which dephosphorylates PIP_3. Activation of the PI3K pathway leads to phosphorylation of downstream effectors, including AKT, which in turn is linked to the mTORC1 complex, comprised of mTOR, the regulatory associated protein of mTOR (RAPTOR), mammalian lethal with secretory 13 protein 8 (mLST8), and proline-rich AKT substrate 40 (PRAS40) [109].

Upregulation of the PI3K pathway has been associated with malignancy and the aberrant activation of various steps in the pathway, including increased RTK activity and mutation or amplification of various downstream effector genes such as including PTEN, PI3K catalytic alpha polypeptide (PIK3CA) gene, and AKT [110]. Mutation of the PTEN tumor suppressor gene was initially thought to prevent the ability of PTEN to dephosphorylate PIP_3, thus precluding its negative regulation of the PI3K pathway [111]. However, additional study has revealed that mutations of PTEN are highly variable, and have been shown to exhibit diverse effects on the signaling pathway [112]. More common sporadic mutations have been identified with high frequency in gliomas, as well as breast, prostate, colon, lung and endometrial cancers [112].

Targeting the PI3K Pathway

There are multiple sites at which the PI3K pathway may be impacted, although most agents are in still in early development. Whereas early agents, such as wortmannin, were less selective and targeted the entire class IA heterodimer, wortmannin derivatives have been shown to be significantly more stable *in vivo*, with cytostatic effects when used as monotherapy [113]. Idelalisib is a PI3 Delta inhibitor which is approved for the treatment of follicular and small lymphocytic lymphomas. Several PI3K-directed inhibitors are in early phase clinical trials with evidence of safety and tolerability thus far [114–116].

Due to the important role of mTOR in the PI3K pathway, agents that target both the p110 catalytic subunit of PI3K and mTOR are currently under investigation and appear promising in preclinical and phase I trials [115]. AKT was initially thought to be an intractable target, but in preclinical studies an AKT1/AKT2 non-catalytic site inhibitor demonstrating activity against breast cancer cell lines with known PIK3CA mutation and HER2 amplification, and a phase I study of a pan-AKT inhibitor has shown promising activity in patients with ovarian cancer [115, 117, 118].

The most developed class of drugs targeting the PI3K pathway has been mTOR inhibitors. Rapamycin and its analogs selectively target the mTORC1 complex and inhibit its kinase function [119]. Temsirolimus is an analog approved for use in patients with advanced recurrent renal cell carcinoma, based on results of a clinical trial which demonstrated improvement in both PFS and OS when compared to interferon [120].

Everolimus was the second rapamycin analog introduced into clinical oncology practice. Due to PFS improvement in a phase III clinical trial of patients with metastatic renal cell carcinoma who had progressed on sunitinib and/or sorafenib [121], the drug was approved by the FDA for use in this patient population. Everolimus has since been approved for use in additional settings. The combination of everolimus and exemestane is approved for hormone receptor-positive, HER2-negative advanced breast cancer, with progression on letrozole or anastrozole based on phase III trial data [122]. An additional indication for everolimus is for use in the setting of unresectable, locally advanced, or metastatic pancreatic, lung and gastrointestinal neuroendocrine tumors [123].

Everolimus has also been approved for treatment of renal angiomyolipoma and subependymal giant cell astrocytoma associated with tuberous sclerosis [124, 125]. Additional rapamycin analogs are under development, including ridaforolimus, which has shown promise in the treatment of sarcoma in a phase II clinical trial [126].

Though mTOR inhibitors have shown promising activity in several studies, only a subset of treated patients has had evidence of disease response. Potential mechanisms contributing to the primary resistance of some cancers to therapy with rapamycin analogs include activation of AKT, and thus the PI3K pathway, upon inhibition of mTORC1 and increased signaling of the MAPK pathway [127]. Preclinical studies with mTOR kinase domain inhibitors have demonstrated greater antiproliferative effects than inhibition from rapamycin alone [128], and the development of combination strategies with MAPK and PI3K inhibitors is currently being tested in preclinical and clinical trials [129, 130].

Anaplastic Lymphoma Kinase

Anaplastic lymphoma kinase (ALK) is a receptor tyrosine kinase that plays an important role in the development of the brain. ALK encodes a receptor tyrosine kinase belonging to the insulin receptor superfamily. The ALK gene often gains oncogenic potential through forming fusion genes. To date, more than 20 different genes have been described as being translocated with ALK [131]. ALK fusion with echinoderm microtubule associated protein-like 4 (EML4) causes ALK to be constitutively active without the need for ligand binding. In 2007 it was described that 2–7% of NSCLCs harbored the ALK/EML4 fusion protein [132]. ALK can activate multiple downstream signaling pathways including PIK/mTOR and the MAP kinase pathways [133]. ALK rearrangements in lung cancer are typically mutually exclusive with EGFR or K-RAS mutations [134]. In lung cancer they tend to be found in younger patients with no or light smoking history [135].

Crizotinib, a multitargeted TKI is effective in treating ALK rearranged lung cancers. Unfortunately, the majority of patients relapse in <12 months on crizotinib [131]. Resistance to ALK inhibition is often secondary to point mutations in the kinase domain of ALK, or through activation of an alternative pathway (EGFR, KIT, or IGF-1) [136, 137]. ALK amplification also results in crizotinib resistance [137]. Second generation ALK inhibitors such as ceritinib and alectinib have been developed and can overcome some of the resistance to crizotinib in the setting of some point mutations given their increased potency [135]. Crizotinib resistance has also been diminished with the use of combination therapy with EGFR, KIT, and IGF-R inhibitors [138]. Ongoing studies are looking at SPTBN1 and other ALK fusion partners in nonlung cancers to help identify other possible ALK driven tumors and possibly expand the role of ALK inhibitors [131].

ROS Proto-Oncogene

The ROS proto-oncogene (ROS1) encodes another insulin-receptor family tyrosine kinase. It was initially discovered as a homolog of the oncogene product from the avian sarcoma RNA virus. There is no known ligand for the ROS1 receptor, but oncogenic gene rearrangements with it have been found in multiple tumor types. These cancers include sarcomas, cholangiocarcinoma, ovarian carcinomas, gastric cancer, glioblastoma, and 1–2% of NSCLCs [139]. The rearrangements lead to fusion of the tyrosine kinase domain of ROS1 with one of 12 different partner proteins. These fusion proteins have constitutive activity and help lead to cellular transformation. In lung cancer, ROS1 gene rearrangements, similar to ALK mutations, are more commonly found in never/light smokers and adenocarcinomas [140]. Inhibition of tumors with ROS1 rearrangements using crizotinib has been shown to have some clinical response and as such it is approved in the treatment of ROS1 rearranged non-small-cell lung cancer [139]. This is likely driven in part by the fact that ALK and ROS1 share 77% amino acid identity within their ATP binding sites. In the phase I study with crizotinib in ALK positive NSCLC patients an objective response was seen in 72% of patients. Unfortunately, response duration to anti-ROS therapy is also limited with most responses stopping by 2–3 years [140]. ROS mutations as well as EGFR and RAS activation have all been identified as sources of resistance to therapy [141–143].

Hedgehog Pathway

Mutation in the Hedgehog (Hh) pathway in adults has been found to affect tissue proliferation and differentiation, and have been associated with tumors of the brain and skin, among others [144]. The association of the Hedgehog pathway with malignancy was first identified through the link of a germline inactivating PTCH mutation to nevoid basal cell carcinoma syndrome (Gorlin syndrome) in which affected patients are predisposed to basal cell carcinomas and medulloblastoma [145]. It was subsequently realized that any cause of pathway upregulation leading to increased expression of the Gil1 gene could lead to the formation of sporadic cancers [146], including activating mutations of SMO [147]. In addition to mutation of the genes in the Hh pathway, autocrine and paracrine Hedgehog signaling has been identified. Autocrine signaling involving tumor production of the Hh ligand which subsequently activates its own Hh pathway has been documented in a broad range of solid tumor types. Less commonly documented is paracrine production of Hh ligand produced by the tumor, stimulating the Hh pathway in surrounding stromal cells [148].

The first drug targeting the Hh pathway was a natural product known as cyclopamine, which blocks the Hh pathway through direct binding and inhibition of SMO; unfortunately, its pharmacokinetic profile limited its clinical use. Synthetic SMO inhibitors have since been developed, with vismodegib the most successful thus far. A phase II study of patients with locally advanced and metastatic basal cell carcinoma showed objective response rates of 30% and 43%, respectively; this agent has now been approved for use in these settings and use in other tumor types is being explored [149]. Another Hh pathway inhibitor, sonidegib, binds to and inhibits Smoothened. This agent was approved based on phase II data revealing an improvement in overall survival of patients with locally advanced basal cell carcinoma recurrent after surgery or radiation – or not amendable to local therapy [150].

Agents in development targeting the Hh pathway include antibodies and small molecules designed to block the Hh ligand and prevent PTCH stimulation, as well as decoy PTCH receptors [148]. GLI1 antagonists are also being studied in the preclinical setting [151].

Basic Cellular Processes Targeted in Cancer

Proteasome Inhibitors

The proteasome is a cellular structure that degrades short-lived proteins which have been marked for degradation. Through a highly regulated system a "marker protein", ubiquitin, is attached to ubiquitin-activating enzyme (E1) and then transferred to ubiquitin-conjugating enzymes (E2) that serve to recognize particular proteins for degradation. The transference of ubiquitin to these proteins marks them for degradation, but the ubiquitin ligase enzyme (E3) completes the conjugation. After ubiquitination, proteins bind to the 19S regulatory subunit of the proteasome that unfolds proteins prior to feeding them into the catalytic inner chamber. This process of breaking the proteins into peptides is important to apoptosis. The caspase family of proteasomes plays a role in the execution of the programmed cell death of apoptosis. Additionally, alteration of proteasome function affects multiple other pathways important in apoptosis such as nuclear factor kB, p53, p21, p27.

The Von Hippel-Lindau (VHL) gene is implicated in many genetic and sporadic renal cell carcinomas. The VHL protein functions as part of an E3 in order to recognize substrates for degradation, so that as the VHL gene is mutated, these substrates accumulate and contribute to the transcription of various pro-angiogenic factors that feed tumor growth.

Given the role of deregulated apoptosis in cancer, proteasome inhibitors are rational therapeutic agents. Most proteasome inhibitors bind to the active site threonine on the 20S core and are further divided based on their structure. Bortezomib, a reversible proteasome inhibitor was approved in the treatment of multiple myeloma in the first line and relapsed setting, as well as for patients with mantle cell lymphoma [152–154]. Carfilzomib, an irreversible inhibitor, is also approved in the treatment of multiple myeloma with other agents also in development [155]. Ixazomib is a proteasome inhibitor that has been approved for the treatment of patients with multiple myeloma having progressed on at least one previous therapy [156, 157].

Histone Deacetylase

Histone deacetylase inhibitors (HDACi) are another way to disrupt basic cellular processes in order to decrease the proliferation of cancer cells. The packaging of chromatin includes DNA which is wrapped around a histone octomer and linker portions of DNA. The nucleosome of the cell determines how chromatin will be packaged, and thus gene activity, as open areas of chromatin are often areas of transcriptionally active genes [158]. This arrangement is not static and the nucleosomal DNA will transiently change and wrap different portions around the histone octomer in order to activate transcription of various genes. The histones also have a charged tail that may be modified by deacetylation, demethylation, and dephosphorylation, all of which influence gene expression without disruption of the genes themselves, and thus are termed epigenetic processes.

Histone modification has long been implicated in the process of cancer [159]. Histones are acetylated by acetyl transferases and these acetyl groups are removed by the histone deacetylases (HDAC). The HDACs function by deacytelating lysine residues on histone tails, thus condensing the chromatin, and inhibiting transcription. HDACs are classified into two classes. Class 1 HDACs are expressed solely in the nucleus and repress transcription while class 2 can be found in the cytoplasm and nucleus. These HDACs target additional proteins beyond just the histone tail [160]. HDACs play a role in regulating the transcription of various factors such as p53, c-Myc, NFkB, HIF1alpha, p21, and the estrogen and androgen receptors [160]. Additionally, HDACs play a role in regulation of proapoptotic and antiapoptotic proteins.

Genetic abnormalities that influence the targets of HDACs or cause differential expression of HDACs may cause functional changes that allow for neoplastic transformation [161]. The best example of the importance of HDAC in cancer is acute promyelocytic leukemia. The retinoic acid receptor (RAR) plays an important role in myeloid differentiation. If no retinoids are available to bind, the RARα and its partner receptor repress transcription by recruiting an HDAC. If ligand is available, the HDAC is released allowing for transcription [162]. In the case of acute promyelocytic leukemia, the RARα and PML portions of chromosome 15 and 17 are fused through translocation. This changes the ability of RARα to bind retinoids and recruit HDACs so that the target genes of RAR are constantly repressed. Thus, HDAC inhibitors restore the sensitivity of the leukemic cells to the retinoids. Many lymphomas have gene fusions that influence the HDAC balance. In 2004, romidepsin received Fast Track designation from the FDA for the treatment of cutaneous T-cell lymphoma, and trials are ongoing in peripheral T-cell lymphoma and multiple myeloma [163, 164]. Panobinostat has also been approved for the treatment of multiple myeloma when used in combination with bortezomib and dexamethasone for patients having received at least two prior lines of therapy. This approval was granted based on PFS data only [165]. Another HDAC inhibitor, vorinostat, is currently approved for the treatment of refractory cutaneous T-cell lymphoma, and promising activity of vorinostat was seen in a phase II study in both follicular and mantle cell lymphoma [166, 167]. Belinostat is an HDAC inhibitor indicated for the treatment of relapsed or refractory peripheral T-cell lymphoma based on tumor response rate; this accelerated approval has not yet established improvement in survival [168]. Solid tumor oncology also relies on HDACs as the MAPK signaling pathway causes HDAC4, a class 2 HDAC, to constitutively localize to the nucleus.

Angiogenesis

Angiogenesis, the growth of new blood vessels, is a central step in the growth and metastatic spread of cancer [169]. Antiangiogenic therapies have been approved in multiple tumor types [170–173]. Though significant progress has been made, the clinical benefits of angiogenic therapy have been relatively modest, and there are many unknown questions regarding the optimal chemotherapy regimens to combine with antiangiogenic therapy, utility in the adjuvant setting, and predictive biomarkers of efficacy.

Angiogenesis is a Critical Step in Tumor Progression

Expansion of a tumor mass beyond the initial microscopic size of a nonangiogenic tumor is dependent on recruitment of endothelial cells that form new blood vessels [174]. This angiogenic phenotype is driven by multiple changes including increased expression of angiogenic factors such as VEGF, placental growth factor (PlGF), and basic fibroblast growth factor (bFGF) [175]. Other changes include decreased expression of endogenous angiogenesis inhibitors, increased expression of angiogenic factors from tumor stromal cells, and recruitment of bone marrow-derived endothelial cell precursors [176].

Preclinical Studies Targeting Angiogenesis

A significant problem in angiogenesis research has been the difficulty of finding suitable methods for assessing the angiogenic response. While *in vitro* assays can be useful in screening specific functions, these assays frequently do not translate into effects on angiogenesis *in vivo* [177]. And, even *in vivo* studies in mice also have a significant limitation in predicting efficacy of angiogenesis inhibitors in humans. Mouse studies using murine or even chimeric antibodies do not predict the impact of an antiglobulin response in humans, an issue that complicated early research with the antihuman VEGF antibody, A4.6.1, subsequently approved for clinical use as bevacizumab, for treatment of patients with multiple tumor types [170–173]. An additional challenge in preclinical angiogenesis research is the rapid vascular growth in preclinical models that leads them to be more responsive to antiangiogenic therapy [178]. Extensive reviews have described the transitory nature of the clinical benefit from angiogenesis inhibitors due to evasive resistance and adaptation to circumvent angiogenic blockade [175, 178]. Investigation is ongoing to target known resistance mechanisms, identify predictive markers of response, and develop combination regimens that synergize with VEGF. Recently, evaluation of the role of PlGF has led to a small improvement in angiogenic therapy in colorectal cancer. PlGF has been shown to be associated with resistance to anti-VEGF therapy in both preclinical models and prospective evaluation in patients treated with anti-VEGF therapy [179, 180]. Results from a recent phase III trial of a dual-inhibitor of PlGF and VEGF-A in patients with metastatic colorectal cancer that have progressed on prior chemotherapy demonstrate that continued blockade of VEGF family members has a modest clinical benefit for patients with acquired resistance to anti-VEGF therapy [181].

Clinical Experience with Angiogenesis Inhibitors

To date, objective tumor responses have been modest for antiangiogenic agents used as monotherapy with the exception of renal cell carcinoma. In 2004, a phase III randomized, placebo-controlled trial reported a significant clinical benefit in patients with advanced colorectal cancer receiving irinotecan-based chemotherapy and bevacizumab versus chemotherapy alone with a 4.4 month improvement in PFS and a 4.7 month improvement in OS [170]. Subsequent studies have confirmed this original finding with a phase III trial investigating oxaliplatin-based chemotherapy (FOLFOX4) with bevacizumab showing a 2.1 month OS benefit compared to FOLFOX4 alone [182]. Unfortunately, addition of bevacizumab to adjuvant chemotherapy did not result in a statistically significant benefit in early stage colorectal cancer [183]. Furthermore, the combination of EGFR inhibition and VEGF inhibition with chemotherapy in advanced colorectal cancer also failed to improve PFS or OS [184, 185]. Although bevacizumab is one of the best-studied antiangiogenic agents in colorectal cancer, further investigation is ongoing to overcome resistance mechanisms and to define predictive biomarkers.

Renal cell carcinoma are often marked by inactivation of the von Hippel-Lindau gene leading to VEGF overexpression [186]. Improved PFS has been seen in randomized clinical trials with bevacizumab, sunitinib, and sorafenib [30, 187, 188]. The benefit of angiogenesis inhibitors in renal cell carcinoma has changed the standard of care dramatically over the last decade but unfortunately, antiangiogenic therapy is not a curative therapy. Recent trials have also investigated the role of mTOR inhibition in patients with metastatic renal cell carcinoma, as mTOR is a downstream effector of VEGF signaling. A phase III study of everolimus versus best supportive care revealed a significant increase in median PFS in patients receiving everolimus [189]. Overall survival was not significantly different, most likely owing to the high rate of crossover (80%) in the trial.

A randomized phase II/III trial of carboplatin and paclitaxel with or without bevacizumab was studied in 878 untreated, advanced (stage IIIB or IB) nonsquamous NSCLC [172, 190]. Patients receiving chemotherapy with bevacizumab had a significantly improved OS of 12.3 months compared to 10.3 months in the chemotherapy-alone group. Clinically significant bleeding (4.4% vs 0.7%) was the most notable difference in side-effects between the bevacizumab group and the chemotherapy only group. A similar randomized phase III trial investigated bevacizumab with another chemotherapy regimen of cisplatin and gemcitabine (AVAIL trial) [191]. PFS was significantly prolonged (6.7 vs 6.1 months) but duration of follow-up was not sufficient for OS analysis. Based on these results, bevacizumab in combination with carboplatin and paclitaxel improves OS, but the results of the AVAIL trial bring into question whether a similar degree of benefit can be expected with any platinum-containing doublet for patients with NSCLC. Studies in NSCLC with VEGFR TKI/chemotherapy combinations are also being evaluated. To date, results have been somewhat mixed due to dose-related adverse events and limited efficacy.

Bevacizumab has also been studied extensively in advanced breast cancer. Prior preclinical studies demonstrated synergistic activity for the combination of the antiangiogenic agent 2-methoxyestradiol and docetaxel chemotherapy against endothelial cells [192], and a phase III study of paclitaxel with or without bevacizumab revealed a significant prolongation of PFS (11.8 vs 5.9 months) but no improvement in OS. Similarly, another phase III study of docetaxel with or without bevacizumab in previously untreated patients with metastatic breast cancer demonstrated an improvement in median PFS but no overall survival advantage was observed. Although the results have been promising for antiangiogenic therapy in front-line, advanced metastatic breast cancer, the lack of overall survival benefit, in addition to the toxicity and cost of bevacizumab, have limited the use of these agents in the metastatic setting.

Antiangiogenic therapy has also shown activity in other solid tumors, including hepatocellular carcinoma. The multitargeted VEGFR TKI, sorafenib, has been evaluated in a phase III randomized, placebo-controlled clinical trial with those patients receiving sorafenib showing a survival benefit (5.5 vs 2.5 months) compared to placebo. In addition, gastric cancer previously treated with fluoropyrimidine- or platinum-containing chemotherapy has shown response to a recombinant human IgG1 monoclonal antibody against VEGF2, ramucirumab [193]. This agent has been approved for the treatment of metastatic colorectal cancer and metastatic NSCLC [194, 195]. Colorectal cancer is also potentially treated with aflibercept, a VEGF-trap which is a high affinity ligand trap blocking the activity of VEGFA and VEGFB, which has been shown to improve survival for patients previously treated with an oxaliplatin-based regimen [196]. Given the promising results of this study, other antiangiogenic agents are currently under investigation. In addition to the above disease types, thyroid cancers seem to be responsive to VEGF inhibition. Lenvatinib is a receptor TKI of VEGFR 1, 2, and 3, fibroblast growth factor receptors 1 through 4, platelet-derived growth factor receptor α, RET, and KIT approved the treatment of locally recurrent, metastatic, or progressive differentiated thyroid carcinoma [197].

Future Directions

Antiangiogenic therapy has improved life expectancy in multiple tumor types, highlighting the proof-of-principle in targeting this critical pathway. Unfortunately, antiangiogenic therapies have not been a curative treatment and benefits have been extremely modest with significant adverse events and cost. As mechanisms of resistance to VEGF pathway inhibitors continue to be elucidated, rational combination therapies will be developed and the timing of administration of various antiangiogenic agents will be refined. More importantly, potential biomarkers for VEGF pathway inhibitors need to be defined to select the patient population most likely to benefit from antiangiogenic therapy.

Conclusion

As we enter the era of targeted therapies, we will be faced with increasing questions and challenges: the vast number of potential targets to evaluate, prioritizing development of competing similar drugs and targets, the development of companion diagnostics for mutations or targets, and obtaining tissue for diagnostic tests and biomarker development. Future clinical trials involving new therapeutics will require novel adaptive designs in order to test drugs with greater efficiency and to potentially decrease the number of patients exposed to drugs unlikely to effectively treat their cancer. The future of targeted therapy will also require the rational use of combination therapy to overcome known acquired resistance mechanisms to improve efficacy and to prevent tumor escape mechanisms. Therefore, understanding the complex mechanisms of resistance to targeted therapies will be a critical component of combination therapies for not only biologic targeted therapy, but for cytotoxic and immunotherapies as well.

References

1 Ciardiello F, Bianco R, Damiano V, *et al.* Antiangiogenic and antitumor activity of anti-epidermal growth factor receptor C225 monoclonal antibody in combination with vascular endothelial growth factor antisense oligonucleotide in human GEO colon cancer cells. *Clin Cancer Res* 2000;6(9):3739–47.

2 Brekke OH, Sandlie I. Therapeutic antibodies for human diseases at the dawn of the twenty-first century. *Nat Rev Drug Discov* 2003;2(1):52–62.

3 Younes A, Bartlett NL, Leonard JP, *et al.* Brentuximab vedotin (SGN-35) for relapsed CD30-positive lymphomas. *N Engl J Med* 2010;363(19):1812–21.

4 Krause DS, Van Etten RA. Tyrosine kinases as targets for cancer therapy. *N Engl J Med* 2005;353(2):172–87.

5 Kantarjian H, Sawyers C, Hochhaus A, *et al.* Hematologic and cytogenetic responses to imatinib mesylate in chronic myelogenous leukemia. *N Engl J Med* 2002;346(9):645–52.

6 Baselga J. Targeting tyrosine kinases in cancer: the second wave. *Science* 2006;312(5777):1175–8.

7 Imai K, Takaoka A. Comparing antibody and small-molecule therapies for cancer. *Nat Rev Cancer* 2006;6(9):714–27.

8 Butowski N, Chang S. Small molecule and monoclonal antibody therapies in neurooncology. *Cancer Control* 2005;12(2):116–24.

9 Carter PJ. Potent antibody therapeutics by design. *Nat Rev Immunol* 2006;6(5):343–57.

10 Llovet JM, Ricci S, Mazzaferro V, *et al.* Sorafenib in advanced hepatocellular carcinoma. *N Engl J Med* 2008;359(4):378–90.

11 Keizer R, Huitema A, Schellens H, Beijnen J. Clinical pharmacokinetics of theapeutic monoclonal antibodies. *Clin Pharmacokinet* 2010;49(8):493–507.

12 Dikshit HK, Sharma TR, Chandra N, Singh BB, Kumari J. Molecular and morphological characterization of advanced breeding lines from diverse cross in mung bean (Vigna radiata (L.) Wilczek). *J Genet* 2009;88(3):341–4.

13 Weiner LM, Dhodapkar MV, Ferrone S. Monoclonal antibodies for cancer immunotherapy. *Lancet* 2009;373(9668):1033–40.

14 Huang S, Armstrong EA, Benavente S, Chinnaiyan P, Harari PM. Dual-agent molecular targeting of the epidermal growth factor receptor (EGFR): combining anti-egfr antibody with tyrosine kinase inhibitor. *Cancer Res* 2004;64(15):5355–62.

15 Murphy K, Travers P, Wolport M (eds) *Immunobiology*, 7th edn. New York: Garland Science, 2007.

16 Idusogie EE, Wong PY, Presta LG, *et al.* Engineered antibodies with increased activity to recruit complement. *J Immunol* 2001;166(4):2571–5.

17 Shih T, Lindly C. Bevacizumab: an angiogenesis inhibitor for the treatment of solid malignancies. *Clinical Therapeutics.* 2006;28(11):1779–802.

18 Cunningham D, Humblet Y, Siena S, *et al.* Cetuximab monotherapy and cetuximab plus irinotecan in irinotecan-refractory metastatic colorectal cancer. *N Engl J Med* 2004;351:337–45.

19 Bogdan S, Klambt C. Epidermal growth factor receptor signaling. *Curr Biol* 2001;11(8):R292–5.

20 Sakaguchi K, Okabayashi Y, Kido Y, *et al.* Shc phosphotyrosine-binding domain dominantly interacts with epidermal growth factor receptors and mediates Ras activation in intact cells. *Mol Endocrinol* 1998;12(4):536–43.

21 Maa MC, Leu TH, McCarley DJ, Schatzman RC, Parsons SJ. Potentiation of epidermal growth factor receptor-mediated oncogenesis by c-Src: implications for the etiology of multiple human cancers. *Proc Natl Acad Sci USA* 1995;92(15):6981–5.

22 Sunpaweravong P, Sunpaweravong S, Puttawibul P, *et al.* Epidermal growth factor receptor and cyclin D1 are independently amplified and overexpressed in esophageal squamous cell carcinoma. *J Cancer Res Clin Oncol* 2005;131(2):111–9.

23 Salomon DS, Brandt R, Ciardiello F, Normanno N. Epidermal growth factor-related peptides and their receptors in human malignancies. *Crit Rev Oncol Hematol* 1995;19(3):183–232.

24 Sordella R, Bell DW, Haber DA, Settleman J. Gefitinib-sensitizing EGFR mutations in lung cancer activate anti-apoptotic pathways. *Science* 2004;305(5687):1163–7.

25 Batra SK, Castelino-Prabhu S, Wikstrand CJ, *et al.* Epidermal growth factor ligand-independent, unregulated, cell-transforming potential of a naturally occurring human mutant EGFRvIII gene. *Cell Growth Differ* 1995;6(10):1251–9.

26 Luttrell DK, Luttrell LM. Not so strange bedfellows: G-protein-coupled receptors and Src family kinases. *Oncogene* 2004;23(48):7969–78.

27 Paez JG, Janne PA, Lee JC, *et al.* EGFR mutations in lung cancer: correlation with clinical response to gefitinib therapy. *Science* 2004;304(5676):1497–500.

28 Janne PA, Yang JC, Kim DW, *et al.* AZD9291 in EGFR inhibitor-resistant non-small-cell lung cancer. *N Engl J Med* 2015;372(18):1689–99.

29 Thatcher N, Hirsch FR, Luft AV, *et al.* Necitumumab plus gemcitabine and cisplatin versus gemcitabine and cisplatin alone as first-line therapy in patients with stage IV squamous non-small-cell lung cancer (SQUIRE): an open-label, randomised, controlled phase 3 trial. *Lancet Oncol* 2015;16(7):763–74.

30 Escudier B, Pluzanska A, Koralewski P, *et al.* Bevacizumab plus interferon alfa-2a for treatment of metastatic renal cell carcinoma: a randomised, double-blind phase III trial. *Lancet* 2007;370(9605):2103–11.

31 Van Cutsem E, Kohne CH, Hitre E, *et al.* Cetuximab and chemotherapy as initial treatment for metastatic colorectal cancer. *N Engl J Med* 2009;360(14):1408–17.

32 Van Cutsem E, Peeters M, Siena S, *et al.* Open-label phase III trial of panitumumab plus best supportive care compared with best supportive care alone in patients with chemotherapy-refractory metastatic colorectal cancer. *J Clin Oncol* 2007;25(13):1658–64.

33 Baselga J, Trigo JM, Bourhis J, *et al.* Phase II multicenter study of the antiepidermal growth factor receptor monoclonal antibody cetuximab in combination with platinum-based chemotherapy in patients with platinum-refractory metastatic and/or recurrent squamous cell carcinoma of the head and neck. *J Clin Oncol* 2005;23(24):5568–77.

34 Bourhis J, Rivera F, Mesia R, *et al.* Phase I/II study of cetuximab in combination with cisplatin or carboplatin and fluorouracil in patients with recurrent or metastatic squamous

cell carcinoma of the head and neck. *J Clin Oncol* 2006;24(18):2866–72.

35 Burtness B, Goldwasser MA, Flood W, Mattar B, Forastiere AA. Phase III randomized trial of cisplatin plus placebo compared with cisplatin plus cetuximab in metastatic/recurrent head and neck cancer: an Eastern Cooperative Oncology Group study. *J Clin Oncol* 2005;23(34):8646–54.

36 Harding J, Burtness B. Cetuximab: an epidermal growth factor receptor chemeric human-murine monoclonal antibody. *Drugs Today (Barc)* 2005;41(2):107–27.

37 Molina MA, Codony-Servat J, Albanell J, Rojo F, Arribas J, Baselga J. Trastuzumab (herceptin), a humanized anti-Her2 receptor monoclonal antibody, inhibits basal and activated Her2 ectodomain cleavage in breast cancer cells. *Cancer Res* 2001;61(12):4744–9.

38 Rubin I, Yarden Y. The basic biology of HER2. *Ann Oncol* 2001;12 Suppl 1:S3–8.

39 Piccart-Gebhart MJ, Procter M, Leyland-Jones B, *et al*. Trastuzumab after adjuvant chemotherapy in HER2-positive breast cancer. *N Engl J Med* 2005;353(16):1659–72.

40 Slamon DJ, Leyland-Jones B, Shak S, *et al*. Use of chemotherapy plus a monoclonal antibody against HER2 for metastatic breast cancer that overexpresses HER2. *N Engl J Med* 2001;344(11):783–92.

41 Bang YJ, Van Cutsem E, Feyereislova A, *et al*. Trastuzumab in combination with chemotherapy versus chemotherapy alone for treatment of HER2-positive advanced gastric or gastro-oesophageal junction cancer (ToGA): a phase 3, open-label, randomised controlled trial. *Lancet* 2010;376(9742):687–97.

42 Holbro T, Beerli RR, Maurer F, *et al*. The ErbB2/ErbB3 heterodimer functions as an oncogenic unit: ErbB2 requires ErbB3 to drive breast tumor cell proliferation. *Proc Natl Acad Sci USA* 2003;100(15):8933–8.

43 Le XF, Lammayot A, Gold D, *et al*. Genes affecting the cell cycle, growth, maintenance, and drug sensitivity are preferentially regulated by anti-HER2 antibody through phosphatidylinositol 3-kinase-AKT signaling. *J Biol Chem* 2005;280(3):2092–104.

44 Franklin MC, Carey KD, Vajdos FF, *et al*. Insights into ErbB signaling from the structure of the ErbB2-pertuzumab complex. *Cancer Cell* 2004;5(4):317–28.

45 Baselga J, Gelmon KA, Verma S, *et al*. Phase II trial of pertuzumab and trastuzumab in patients with human epidermal growth factor receptor 2–positive metastatic breast cancer that progressed during prior trastuzumab therapy. *J Clin Oncol* 2010;28(7):1138–44.

46 Blackwell KL, Burstein HJ, Storniolo AM, *et al*. Overall survival benefit with lapatinib in combination with trastuzumab for patients with human epidermal growth factor receptor 2–positive metastatic breast cancer: final results from the EGF104900 Study. *J Clin Oncol* 2012;30(21):2585–92.

47 Burris HA, 3rd, Rugo HS, Vukelja SJ, *et al*. Phase II study of the antibody drug conjugate trastuzumab-DM1 for the treatment of human epidermal growth factor receptor 2 (HER2)-positive breast cancer after prior HER2-directed therapy. *J Clin Oncol* 2011;29(4):398–405.

48 Yuen JS, Macaulay VM. Targeting the type 1 insulin-like growth factor receptor as a treatment for cancer. *Expert Opin Ther Targets* 2008;12(5):589–603.

49 Pollak M. Insulin and insulin-like growth factor signalling in neoplasia. *Nat Rev Cancer* 2008;8(12):915–28.

50 Baserga R. The insulin-like growth factor I receptor: a key to tumor growth? *Cancer Res* 1995;55(2):249–52.

51 Furstenberger G, Senn HJ. Insulin-like growth factors and cancer. *Lancet Oncol* 2002;3(5):298–302.

52 Osborne CK, Bolan G, Monaco ME, Lippman ME. Hormone responsive human breast cancer in long-term tissue culture: effect of insulin. *Proc Natl Acad Sci USA* 1976;73(12):4536–40.

53 Cui H, Cruz-Correa M, Giardiello FM, *et al*. Loss of IGF2 imprinting: a potential marker of colorectal cancer risk. *Science* 2003;299(5613):1753–5.

54 Riedemann J, Macaulay VM. IGF1R signalling and its inhibition. *Endocr Relat Cancer* 2006;13 Suppl 1:S33–43.

55 Steigen SE, Schaeffer DF, West RB, Nielsen TO. Expression of insulin-like growth factor 2 in mesenchymal neoplasms. *Mod Pathol* 2009;22(7):914–21.

56 Sachdev D. Targeting the type I insulin-like growth factor system for breast cancer therapy. *Curr Drug Targets* 2010;11(9):1121–32.

57 Gualberto A, Pollak M. Clinical development of inhibitors of the insulin-like growth factor receptor in oncology. *Curr Drug Targets* 2009;10(10):923–36.

58 Olmos D, Basu B, de Bono JS. Targeting insulin-like growth factor signaling: rational combination strategies. *Mol Cancer Ther* 2010;9(9):2447–9.

59 Pietrzkowski Z, Wernicke D, Porcu P, Jameson BA, Baserga R. Inhibition of cellular proliferation by peptide analogues of insulin-like growth factor 1. *Cancer Res* 1992;52(23):6447–51.

60 Blume-Jensen P, Claesson-Welsh L, Siegbahn A, *et al*. Activation of the human c-kit product by ligand-induced dimerization mediates circular actin reorganization and chemotaxis. *The EMBO journal*. 1991;10(13):4121–8.

61 Roskoski R, Jr. Signaling by Kit protein-tyrosine kinase–the stem cell factor receptor. *Biochemical and biophysical research communications*. 2005;337(1):1–13.

62 Heinrich MC, Blanke CD, Druker BJ, Corless CL. Inhibition of KIT tyrosine kinase activity: a novel molecular approach to the treatment of KIT-positive malignancies. *J Clin Oncol* 2002;20(6):1692–703.

63 Heinrich MC, Corless CL, Duensing A, *et al*. PDGFRA activating mutations in gastrointestinal stromal tumors. *Science* 2003;299(5607):708–10.

64 Druker BJ, Tamura S, Buchdunger E, *et al*. Effects of a selective inhibitor of the Abl tyrosine kinase on the growth of Bcr-Abl positive cells. *Nature Med* 1996;2(5):561–6.

65 Heinrich MC, Griffith DJ, Druker BJ, *et al*. Inhibition of c-kit receptor tyrosine kinase activity by STI 571, a selective tyrosine kinase inhibitor. *Blood* 2000;96(3):925–32.

66 Mol CD, Dougan DR, Schneider TR, *et al*. Structural basis for the autoinhibition and STI-571 inhibition of c-Kit tyrosine kinase. *J Biol Chem* 2004;279(30):31655–63.

67 Dagher R, Cohen M, Williams G, *et al*. Approval summary: imatinib mesylate in the treatment of metastatic and/or unresectable malignant gastrointestinal stromal tumors. *Clin Cancer Res* 2002;8(10):3034–8.

68 Dematteo RP, Ballman KV, Antonescu CR, *et al*. Adjuvant imatinib mesylate after resection of localised, primary

gastrointestinal stromal tumour: a randomised, double-blind, placebo-controlled trial. *Lancet* 2009;373(9669):1097–104.

69 Giuliani F, Colucci G. Is there something other than imatinib mesilate in therapeutic options for GIST? *Expert Opin Ther Targets* 2012;16 Suppl 2:S35–43.

70 Heinrich MC, Corless CL, Blanke CD, *et al*. Molecular correlates of imatinib resistance in gastrointestinal stromal tumors. *J Clin Oncol* 2006;24(29):4764–74.

71 Mendel DB, Laird AD, Xin X, *et al*. In vivo antitumor activity of SU11248, a novel tyrosine kinase inhibitor targeting vascular endothelial growth factor and platelet-derived growth factor receptors: determination of a pharmacokinetic/ pharmacodynamic relationship. *Clin Cancer Res* 2003;9(1):327–37.

72 Heinrich MC, Maki RG, Corless CL, *et al*. Primary and secondary kinase genotypes correlate with the biological and clinical activity of sunitinib in imatinib-resistant gastrointestinal stromal tumor. *J Clin Oncol* 2008;26(33): 5352–9.

73 Demetri GD, Reichardt P, Kang Y-K, *et al*. Efficacy and safety of regorafenib for advanced gastrointestinal stromal tumours after failure of imatinib and sunitinib (GRID): an international, multicentre, randomised, placebo-controlled, phase 3 trial. *Lancet* 2012;381(9863):295–302.

74 Heldin CH, Ostman A. Ligand-induced dimerization of growth factor receptors: variations on the theme. *Cytokine Growth Factor Rev* 1996;7(1):3–10.

75 Pawson T. Specificity in signal transduction: from phosphotyrosine-SH2 domain interactions to complex cellular systems. *Cell* 2004;116(2):191–203.

76 Downward J. Targeting RAS signalling pathways in cancer therapy. *Nat Rev Cancer* 2003;3(1):11–22.

77 Byrne JL, Paterson HF, Marshall CJ. p21Ras activation by the guanine nucleotide exchange factor Sos, requires the Sos/Grb2 interaction and a second ligand-dependent signal involving the Sos N-terminus. *Oncogene* 1996;13(10): 2055–65.

78 Kyriakis JM, App H, Zhang XF, *et al*. Raf-1 activates MAP kinase-kinase. *Nature* 1992;358(6385):417–21.

79 Mansour SJ, Matten WT, Hermann AS, *et al*. Transformation of mammalian cells by constitutively active MAP kinase kinase. *Science* 1994;265(5174):966–70.

80 Katz M, Amit I, Yarden Y. Regulation of MAPKs by growth factors and receptor tyrosine kinases. *Biochim Biophy Acta* 2007;1773(8):1161–76.

81 De Luca A, Maiello MR, D'Alessio A, Pergameno M, Normanno N. The RAS/RAF/MEK/ERK and the PI3K/AKT signalling pathways: role in cancer pathogenesis and implications for therapeutic approaches. *Expert Opin Ther Targets* 2012;16 Suppl 2:S17–27.

82 Davies H, Bignell GR, Cox C, *et al*. Mutations of the BRAF gene in human cancer. *Nature* 2002;417(6892):949–54.

83 Wellbrock C, Karasarides M, Marais R. The RAF proteins take centre stage. *Nature Rev Mol Cell Biol* 2004;5(11):875–85.

84 Murugan AK, Dong J, Xie J, Xing M. MEK1 mutations, but not ERK2 mutations, occur in melanomas and colon carcinomas, but none in thyroid carcinomas. *Cell Cycle* 2009;8(13):2122–4.

85 Brose MS, Volpe P, Feldman M, *et al*. BRAF and RAS mutations in human lung cancer and melanoma. *Cancer Res* 2002;62(23):6997–7000.

86 Gorden A, Osman I, Gai W, *et al*. Analysis of BRAF and N–RAS mutations in metastatic melanoma tissues. *Cancer Res* 2003;63(14):3955–7.

87 Pratilas CA, Solit DB. Targeting the mitogen-activated protein kinase pathway: physiological feedback and drug response. *Clin Cancer Res* 2010;16(13):3329–34.

88 Tsimberidou AM, Chandhasin C, Kurzrock R. Farnesyltransferase inhibitors: where are we now? *Exp Opin Invest Drugs* 2010;19(12):1569–80.

89 Harousseau JL, Martinelli G, Jedrzejczak WW, *et al*. A randomized phase 3 study of tipifarnib compared with best supportive care, including hydroxyurea, in the treatment of newly diagnosed acute myeloid leukemia in patients 70 years or older. *Blood* 2009;114(6):1166–73.

90 Rao S, Cunningham D, de Gramont A, *et al*. Phase III double-blind placebo-controlled study of farnesyl transferase inhibitor R115777 in patients with refractory advanced colorectal cancer. *J Clin Oncol* 2004;22(19):3950–7.

91 Van Cutsem E, van de Velde H, Karasek P, *et al*. Phase III trial of gemcitabine plus tipifarnib compared with gemcitabine plus placebo in advanced pancreatic cancer. *J Clin Oncol* 2004;22(8):1430–8.

92 Whyte DB, Kirschmeier P, Hockenberry TN, *et al*. K- and N-Ras are geranylgeranylated in cells treated with farnesyl protein transferase inhibitors. *J Biol Chem* 1997;272(22):14459–64.

93 Lobell RB, Omer CA, Abrams MT, *et al*. Evaluation of farnesyl:protein transferase and geranylgeranyl:protein transferase inhibitor combinations in preclinical models. *Cancer Res* 2001;61(24):8758–68.

94 Mukhopadhyay T, Tainsky M, Cavender AC, Roth JA. Specific inhibition of K-ras expression and tumorigenicity of lung cancer cells by antisense RNA. *Cancer Res* 1991;51(6):1744–8.

95 Wilhelm SM, Carter C, Tang L, *et al*. BAY 43-9006 exhibits broad spectrum oral antitumor activity and targets the RAF/ MEK/ERK pathway and receptor tyrosine kinases involved in tumor progression and angiogenesis. *Cancer Res* 2004;64(19):7099–109.

96 Hauschild A, Agarwala SS, Trefzer U, *et al*. Results of a phase III, randomized, placebo-controlled study of sorafenib in combination with carboplatin and paclitaxel as second-line treatment in patients with unresectable stage III or stage IV melanoma. *J Clin Oncol* 2009;27(17):2823–30.

97 Escudier B, Eisen T, Stadler WM, *et al*. Sorafenib for treatment of renal cell carcinoma: Final efficacy and safety results of the phase III treatment approaches in renal cancer global evaluation trial. *J Clin Oncol* 2009;27(20):3312–8.

98 Chapman PB, Hauschild A, Robert C, *et al*. Improved survival with vemurafenib in melanoma with BRAF V600E Mutation. *N Engl J Med* 2011;364(26):2507–16.

99 Hauschild A, Grob JJ, Demidov LV, *et al*. Dabrafenib in BRAF-mutated metastatic melanoma: a multicentre, open-label, phase 3 randomised controlled trial. *Lancet* 2012;380(9839):358–65.

100 Flaherty KT, Puzanov I, Kim KB, *et al.* Inhibition of mutated, activated BRAF in metastatic melanoma. *N Engl J Med* 2010;363(9):809–19.

101 Nazarian R, Shi H, Wang Q, *et al.* Melanomas acquire resistance to B-RAF(V600E) inhibition by RTK or N-RAS upregulation. *Nature* 2010;468(7326):973–7.

102 Poulikakos PI, Persaud Y, Janakiraman M, *et al.* RAF inhibitor resistance is mediated by dimerization of aberrantly spliced BRAF(V600E). *Nature* 2011;480(7377):387–90.

103 Larkin J, Ascierto PA, Dreno B, *et al.* Combined vemurafenib and cobimetinib in BRAF-mutated melanoma. *N Engl J Med* 2014;371(20):1867–76.

104 Gilmartin AG, Bleam MR, Groy A, *et al.* GSK1120212 (JTP-74057) is an inhibitor of MEK activity and activation with favorable pharmacokinetic properties for sustained in vivo pathway inhibition. *Clin Cancer Res* 2011;17(5):989–1000.

105 Flaherty KT, Infante JR, Daud A, *et al.* Combined BRAF and MEK Inhibition in Melanoma with BRAF V600 Mutations. *N Engl J Med* 2012;367(18):1694–703.

106 Flaherty KT, Robert C, Hersey P, *et al.* Improved survival with MEK inhibition in BRAF-mutated melanoma. *N Engl J Med* 2012;367(2):107–14.

107 Samuels Y, Wang Z, Bardelli A, *et al.* High frequency of mutations of the PIK3CA gene in human cancers. *Science* 2004;304(5670):554.

108 Stephens LR, Jackson TR, Hawkins PT. Agonist-stimulated synthesis of phosphatidylinositol(3,4,5)-trisphosphate: a new intracellular signalling system? *Biochim Biophys Acta* 1993;1179(1):27–75.

109 Guertin DA, Sabatini DM. Defining the role of mTOR in cancer. *Cancer Cell* 2007;12(1):9–22.

110 Engleman J LJ, Cantley LC. The evolution of phosphatidylinositol 3-kinases as regulators of growth and metabolism. *Nat Rev Genet* 2006;7:606–19.

111 Myers MP, Pass I, Batty IH, *et al.* The lipid phosphatase activity of PTEN is critical for its tumor supressor function. *Proc Natl Acad Sci USA* 1998;95(23):13513–8.

112 Keniry M, Parsons R. The role of PTEN signaling perturbations in cancer and in targeted therapy. *Oncogene* 2008;27(41):5477–85.

113 Howes AL, Chiang GG, Lang ES, *et al.* The phosphatidylinositol 3-kinase inhibitor, PX-866, is a potent inhibitor of cancer cell motility and growth in three-dimensional cultures. *Mol Cancer Ther* 2007;6(9):2505–14.

114 Ihle NT, Lemos R, Jr., Wipf P, *et al.* Mutations in the phosphatidylinositol-3-kinase pathway predict for antitumor activity of the inhibitor PX-866 whereas oncogenic Ras is a dominant predictor for resistance. *Cancer Res* 2009;69(1):143–50.

115 Courtney KD, Corcoran RB, Engleman JA. The PI3K pathway as drug target in human cancer. *J Clin Oncol* 2010;28(6):1075–83.

116 Gopal AK, Kahl BS, de Vos S, *et al.* PI3Kdelta inhibition by idelalisib in patients with relapsed indolent lymphoma. *N Engl J Med* 2014;370(11):1008–18.

117 Serra V, Markman B, Scaltriti M, *et al.* NVP-BEZ235, a dual PI3K/mTOR inhibitor, prevents PI3K signaling and inhibits the growth of cancer cells with activating PI3K mutations. *Cancer Res* 2008;68(19):8022–30.

118 Tolcher A, Yap T, Fearen I, *et al.* A phase I study of MK-2206, an oral potent allosteric Akt inhibitor (Akti), in patients (pts) with advanced solid tumor (ST). *J Clin Oncol* 2009;27 (suppl) (146s):abstr 3503.

119 Harding MW. Immunophilins, mTOR, and pharmacodynamic strategies for a targeted cancer therapy. *Clin Cancer Res* 2003;9(8):2882–6.

120 Hudes G, Carducci M, Tomczak P, *et al.* Temsirolimus, interferon alfa, or both for advanced renal-cell carcinoma. *N Engl J Med* 2007;356(22):2271–81.

121 Motzer RJ, Escudier B, Oudard S, *et al.* Efficacy of everolimus in advanced renal cell carcinoma: a double-blind, randomised, placebo-controlled phase III trial. *Lancet* 2008;372(9637):449–56.

122 Baselga J, Campone M, Piccart M, *et al.* Everolimus in postmenopausal hormone-receptor-positive advanced breast cancer. *N Engl J Med* 2012;366(6):520–9.

123 Yao JC, Shah MH, Ito T, *et al.* Everolimus for advanced pancreatic neuroendocrine tumors. *N Engl J Med* 2011;364(6):514–23.

124 Lewandoski M, Sun X, Martin GR. Fgf8 signalling from the AER is essential for normal limb development. *Nat Genet* 2000;26:460–3.

125 Reifers F, Bohli H, Walsh EC, *et al.* Fgf8 is mutated in zebrafish acerebellar (ace) mutants and is required for maintenance of midbrain-hindbrain boundary development and somitogenesis. *Development* 1998;125:2381–95.

126 Chawla SP, Staddon AP, Baker LH, *et al.* Phase II study of the mammalian target of rapamycin inhibitor ridaforolimus in patients with advanced bone and soft tissue sarcomas. *J Clin Oncol* 2012;30(1):78–84.

127 Carew JS, Kelly KR, Nawrocki ST. Mechanisms of mTOR inhibitor resistance in cancer therapy. *Target Oncol* 2011;6(1):17–27.

128 Feldman ME, Apsel B, Uotila A, *et al.* Active-site inhibitors of mTOR target rapamycin-resistant outputs of mTORC1 and mTORC2. *PLoS Biol* 2009;7(2):e38.

129 Engleman JA Chen L, Tan X, *et al.* Effective use of PI3K and MEK inhibitors to treat mutant Kras G12D and PIK3CA H1047R murine lung cancers. *Nat Med* 2008;14:1351–6.

130 Kurzrock R, Rosenstein L, *et al.* Phase I dose-escalation of the oral MEK 1/2 inhibitor GSK 1120212 (GSK212) dosed in combination with the oral AKT inhibitor GSK2141795 (GSK795). *J Clin Oncol* 2011;29:abstr 3085.

131 Ying J, Lin C, Wu J, *et al.* Anaplastic lymphoma kinase rearrangement in digestive tract cancer: implication for targeted therapy in Chinese population. *PLoS One* 2015;10(12):e0144731.

132 Soda M, Choi YL, Enomoto M, *et al.* Identification of the transforming EML4-ALK fusion gene in non-small-cell lung cancer. *Nature* 2007;448(7153):561–6.

133 El-Osta H, Shackelford R. Personalized treatment options for ALK-positive metastatic non-small-cell lung cancer: potential role for Ceritinib. *Pharmgenomics Pers Med* 2015;8:145–54.

134 Inamura K, Takeuchi K, Togashi Y, *et al.* EML4-ALK fusion is linked to histological characteristics in a subset of lung cancers. *J Thorac Oncol* 2008;3(1):13–7.

135 Awad MM, Shaw AT. ALK inhibitors in non-small cell lung cancer: crizotinib and beyond. *Clin Adv Hematol Oncol* 2014;12(7):429–39.

136 Choi YL, Soda M, Yamashita Y, *et al*. EML4-ALK mutations in lung cancer that confer resistance to ALK inhibitors. *N Engl J Med* 2010;363(18):1734–9.

137 Katayama R, Shaw AT, Khan TM, *et al*. Mechanisms of acquired crizotinib resistance in ALK-rearranged lung Cancers. *Sci Transl Med* 2012;4(120):120ra17.

138 Liao BC, Lin CC, Shih JY, Yang JC. Treating patients with ALK-positive non-small cell lung cancer: latest evidence and management strategy. *Ther Adv Med Oncol* 2015;7(5):274–90.

139 Matsushime H, Wang LH, Shibuya M. Human c-ros-1 gene homologous to the v-ros sequence of UR2 sarcoma virus encodes for a transmembrane receptorlike molecule. *Mol Cell Biol* 1986;6(8):3000–4.

140 Davies KD, Le AT, Theodoro MF, *et al*. Identifying and targeting ROS1 gene fusions in non-small cell lung cancer. *Clin Cancer Res* 2012;18(17):4570–9.

141 Awad MM, Engelman JA, Shaw AT. Acquired resistance to crizotinib from a mutation in CD74-ROS1. *N Engl J Med* 2013;369(12):1173.

142 Davies KD, Mahale S, Astling DP, *et al*. Resistance to ROS1 inhibition mediated by EGFR pathway activation in non-small cell lung cancer. *PLoS One* 2013;8(12):e82236.

143 Shaw AT, Ou SH, Bang YJ, *et al*. Crizotinib in ROS1-rearranged non-small-cell lung cancer. *N Engl J Med* 2014;371(21):1963–71.

144 Taipale J, Beachy PA. The Hedgehog and Wnt signalling pathways in cancer. *Nature* 2001;411(6835):349–54.

145 Gorlin RJ. Nevoid basal cell carcinoma syndrome. *Dermatol Clin* 1995;13(1):113–25.

146 Dahmane N, Lee J, Robins P, *et al*. Activation of the transcription factor Gli1 and the Sonic hedgehog signalling pathway in skin tumours. *Nature* 1997;389(6653):876–81.

147 Xie J, Murone M, Luoh SM, *et al*. Activating Smoothened mutations in sporadic basal-cell carcinoma. *Nature* 1998;391(6662):90–2.

148 Scales SJ, de Sauvage FJ. Mechanisms of Hedgehog pathway activation in cancer and implications for therapy. *Trends Pharmacol Sci* 2009;30(6):303–12.

149 Sekulic A, Migden MR, Oro AE, *et al*. Efficacy and safety of vismodegib in advanced basal-cell carcinoma. *N Engl J Med* 2012;366(23):2171–9.

150 Migden MR, Guminski A, Gutzmer R, *et al*. Treatment with two different doses of sonidegib in patients with locally advanced or metastatic basal cell carcinoma (BOLT): a multicentre, randomised, double-blind phase 2 trial. *Lancet Oncol* 2015;16(6):716–28.

151 Lauth M, Bergstrom A, Shimokawa T, Toftgard R. Inhibition of GLI-mediated transcription and tumor cell growth by small-molecule antagonists. *Proc Natl Acad Sci USA* 2007;104(20):8455–60.

152 Goy A, Younes A, McLaughlin P, *et al*. Phase II study of proteasome inhibitor bortezomib in relapsed or refractory B-cell non-Hodgkin's lymphoma. *J Clin Oncol* 2005;23(4):667–75.

153 Richardson PG, Sonneveld P, Schuster MW, *et al*. Bortezomib or high-dose dexamethasone for relapsed multiple myeloma. *N Engl J Med* 2005;352(24):2487–98.

154 San Miguel JF, Schlag R, Khuageva NK, *et al*. Bortezomib plus melphalan and prednisone for initial treatment of multiple myeloma. *N Engl J Med* 2008;359(9):906–17.

155 Siegel DS, Martin T, Wang M, *et al*. A phase 2 study of single-agent carfilzomib (PX-171-003-A1) in patients with relapsed and refractory multiple myeloma. *Blood* 2012;120(14):2817–25.

156 Kumar SK, Berdeja JG, Niesvizky R, *et al*. Safety and tolerability of ixazomib, an oral proteasome inhibitor, in combination with lenalidomide and dexamethasone in patients with previously untreated multiple myeloma: an open-label phase 1/2 study. *Lancet Oncol* 2014;15(13):1503–12.

157 Kumar SK, LaPlant B, Roy V, *et al*. Phase 2 trial of ixazomib in patients with relapsed multiple myeloma not refractory to bortezomib. *Blood Cancer J* 2015;5:e338.

158 Jenuwein T, Allis CD. Translating the histone code. *Science* 2001;293(5532):1074–80.

159 Esteller M. Cancer epigenomics: DNA methylomes and histone-modification maps. *Nat Rev Genet* 2007;8(4):286–98.

160 Lane AA, Chabner BA. Histone deacetylase inhibitors in cancer therapy. *J Clin Oncol* 2009;27(32):5459–68.

161 Esteller M, Herman JG. Cancer as an epigenetic disease: DNA methylation and chromatin alterations in human tumours. *J Pathol* 2002;196(1):1–7.

162 Lin RJ, Sternsdorf T, Tini M, Evans RM. Transcriptional regulation in acute promyelocytic leukemia. *Oncogene* 2001;20(49):7204–15.

163 Prince HM, Dickinson M. Romidepsin for cutaneous T-cell lymphoma. *Clin Cancer Res* 2012;18(13):3509–15.

164 Piekarz RL, Frye R, Turner M, *et al*. Phase II multi-institutional trial of the histone deacetylase inhibitor romidepsin as monotherapy for patients with cutaneous T-cell lymphoma. *J Clin Oncol* 2009;27(32):5410–7.

165 San-Miguel JF, Hungria VT, Yoon SS, *et al*. Panobinostat plus bortezomib and dexamethasone versus placebo plus bortezomib and dexamethasone in patients with relapsed or relapsed and refractory multiple myeloma: a multicentre, randomised, double-blind phase 3 trial. *Lancet Oncol* 2014;15(11):1195–206.

166 Mann BS, Johnson JR, Cohen MH, Justice R, Pazdur R. FDA Approval summary: vorinostat for treatment of advanced primary cutaneous T-cell lymphoma. *Oncologist* 2007;12(10):1247–52.

167 Kirschbaum M, Frankel P, Popplewell L, *et al*. Phase II study of vorinostat for treatment of relapsed or refractory indolent non-hodgkin's lymphoma and mantle cell lymphoma. *J Clin Oncol* 2011;29(9):1198–203.

168 O'Connor OA, Horwitz S, Masszi T, *et al*. Belinostat in patients with relapsed or refractory peripheral t-cell lymphoma: results of the pivotal Phase II BELIEF (CLN-19) Study. *J Clin Oncol* 2015;33(23):2492–9.

169 Folkman J, Klagsbrun M, Sasse J, *et al*. A heparin-binding angiogenic protein-–basic fibroblast growth factor-–is stored within basement membrane. *Am J Pathol* 1988;130(2):393–400.

170 Hurwitz H, Fehrenbacher L, Novotny W, *et al*. Bevacizumab plus irinotecan, fluorouracil, and leucovorin for metastatic colorectal cancer. *N Engl J Med* 2004;350(23):2335–42.

171 Yang JC, Haworth L, Sherry RM, *et al*. A randomized trial of bevacizumab, an anti–vascular endothelial growth factor antibody, for metastatic renal cancer. *N Engl J Med* 2003;349(5):427–34.

172 Sandler A, Gray R, Perry MC, *et al*. Paclitaxel-carboplatin alone or with bevacizumab for non-small-cell lung cancer. *N Engl J Med* 2006;355(24):2542–50.

173 Friedman HS, Prados MD, Wen PY, *et al*. Bevacizumab alone and in combination with irinotecan in recurrent glioblastoma. *J Clin Oncol* 2009;27(28):4733–40.

174 Folkman J. What is the evidence that tumors are angiogenesis dependent? *J Natl Cancer Inst* 1990;82(1):4–7.

175 Bergers G, Hanahan D. Modes of resistance to anti-angiogenic therapy. *Nat Rev Cancer* 2008;8(8):592–603.

176 Hicklin DJ, Ellis LM. Role of the vascular endothelial growth factor pathway in tumor growth and angiogenesis. *J Clin Oncol* 2005;23(5):1011–27.

177 Auerbach R, Akhtar N, Lewis RL, Shinners BL. Angiogenesis assays: problems and pitfalls. *Cancer Metastasis Rev* 2000;19(1):167–72.

178 Ellis LM, Hicklin DJ. Pathways mediating resistance to vascular endothelial growth factor-targeted therapy. *Clin Cancer Res* 2008;14(20):6371–5.

179 Carmeliet P, Moons L, Luttun A, *et al*. Synergism between vascular endothelial growth factor and placental growth factor contributes to angiogenesis and plasma extravasation in pathological conditions. *Nat Med* 2001;7(5):575–83.

180 Kopetz S, Hoff PM, Morris JS, *et al*. Phase II Trial of infusional fluorouracil, irinotecan, and bevacizumab for metastatic colorectal cancer: efficacy and circulating angiogenic biomarkers associated with therapeutic resistance. *J Clin Oncol* 2010;28(3):453–9.

181 Van Cutsem E, Tabernero J, Lakomy R, *et al*. Addition of aflibercept to fluorouracil, leucovorin, and irinotecan improves survival in a phase III randomized trial in patients with metastatic colorectal cancer previously treated with an oxaliplatin-based regimen. *J Clin Oncol* 2012;30(28):3499–506.

182 Saltz LB, Clarke S, Diaz-Rubio E, *et al*. Bevacizumab in combination with oxaliplatin-based chemotherapy as first-line therapy in metastatic colorectal cancer: a randomized phase III study. *J Clin Oncol* 2008;26(12):2013–9.

183 Allegra CJ, Yothers G, O'Connell MJ, *et al*. Bevacizumab in stage II-III colon cancer: 5-year update of the National Surgical Adjuvant Breast and Bowel Project C-08 Trial. *J Clin Oncol* 2013;31(3):359–64.

184 Hecht JR, Mitchell E, Chidiac T, *et al*. A randomized phase IIIB trial of chemotherapy, bevacizumab, and panitumumab compared with chemotherapy and bevacizumab alone for metastatic colorectal cancer. *J Clin Oncol* 2009;27(5):672–80.

185 Tol J, Koopman M, Cats A, *et al*. Chemotherapy, bevacizumab, and cetuximab in metastatic colorectal cancer. *N Engl J Med* 2009;360(6):563–72.

186 Motzer RJ, Bander NH, Nanus DM. Renal-cell carcinoma. *N Engl J Med* 1996;335(12):865–75.

187 Motzer RJ, Hutson TE, Tomczak P, *et al*. Overall survival and updated results for sunitinib compared with interferon alfa in patients with metastatic renal cell carcinoma. *J Clin Oncol* 2009;27(22):3584–90.

188 Escudier B, Szczylik C, Eisen T, *et al*. Randomized phase III trial of the Raf kinase and VEGFR inhibitor sorafenib (BAY 43-9006) in patients with advanced renal cell carcinoma (RCC). *J Clin Oncol* 2005;23(16s):LBA4510.

189 Motzer RJ, Escudier B, Oudard S, *et al*. Phase 3 trial of everolimus for metastatic renal cell carcinoma. *Cancer* 2010;116(18):4256–65.

190 Johnson DH, Fehrenbacher L, Novotny WF, *et al*. Randomized phase II trial comparing bevacizumab plus carboplatin and paclitaxel with carboplatin and paclitaxel alone in previously untreated locally advanced or metastatic non-small-cell lung cancer. *J Clin Oncol* 2004;22(11): 2184–91.

191 Reck M, von Pawel J, Zatloukal P, *et al*. Phase III trial of cisplatin plus gemcitabine with either placebo or bevacizumab as first-line therapy for nonsquamous non-small-cell lung cancer: AVAiL. *J Clin Oncol* 2009;27(8):1227–34.

192 Sweeney CJ, Miller KD, Sissons SE, *et al*. The antiangiogenic property of docetaxel is synergistic with a recombinant humanized monoclonal antibody against vascular endothelial growth factor or 2-methoxyestradiol but antagonized by endothelial growth factors. *Cancer Res* 2001;61(8):3369–72.

193 Fuchs CS, Tomasek J, Yong CJ, *et al*. Ramucirumab monotherapy for previously treated advanced gastric or gastro-oesophageal junction adenocarcinoma (REGARD): an international, randomised, multicentre, placebo-controlled, phase 3 trial. *Lancet* 2014;383(9911):31–9.

194 Garon EB, Ciuleanu TE, Arrieta O, *et al*. Ramucirumab plus docetaxel versus placebo plus docetaxel for second-line treatment of stage IV non-small-cell lung cancer after disease progression on platinum-based therapy (REVEL): a multicentre, double-blind, randomised phase 3 trial. *Lancet* 2014;384(9944):665–73.

195 Tabernero J, Yoshino T, Cohn AL, *et al*. Ramucirumab versus placebo in combination with second-line FOLFIRI in patients with metastatic colorectal carcinoma that progressed during or after first-line therapy with bevacizumab, oxaliplatin, and a fluoropyrimidine (RAISE): a randomised, double-blind, multicentre, phase 3 study. *Lancet Oncol* 2015;16(5):499–508.

196 Van Cutsem E, Tabernero J, Lakomy R, *et al*. Addition of aflibercept to fluorouracil, leucovorin, and irinotecan improves survival in a phase III randomized trial in patients with metastatic colorectal cancer previously treated with an oxaliplatin-based regimen. *J Clin Oncol* 2012;30(28):3499–506.

197 Schlumberger M, Tahara M, Wirth LJ, *et al*. Lenvatinib versus placebo in radioiodine-refractory thyroid cancer. *N Engl J Med* 2015;372(7):621–30.

22

Hematopoietic Stem Cell Transplantation for Cancer

Joshua F. Zeidner[1], Christopher G. Kanakry[2], and Leo Luznik[3]

[1] *University of North Carolina, Lineberger Comprehensive Cancer Center, Chapel Hill, North Carolina, USA*
[2] *National Cancer Institute, Experimental Transplantation and Immunology Branch, Bethesda, Maryland, USA*
[3] *Johns Hopkins Hospital, Sidney Kimmel Comprehensive Cancer Center, Bethesda, Maryland, USA*

Introduction

Hematopoietic stem cell transplantation (HSCT) is a procedure that involves the infusion of hematopoietic stem cells after cytotoxic and/or immunosuppressive therapy in order to reconstitute donor hematopoiesis in the host. HSCT can be broadly divided into two groups depending upon the stem cell donor: autologous hematopoietic stem cell transplantation (autoHSCT) and allogeneic stem cell transplantation (alloHSCT). The most common indications for HSCT are in treating malignant and nonmalignant hematological disorders that cannot be cured with conventional therapies [1]. HSCT has undergone dramatic advances and changes over the past two decades, which have made HSCT a safer and more widely available treatment modality for patients who previously would not have been candidates for this approach.

Autologous Hematopoietic Stem Cell Transplantation

Autologous HSCT (autoHSCT) refers to the readministration of the patient's own hematopoietic stem cells as a rescue after interval treatment of the patient with doses of cytotoxic therapy that would normally irreversibly ablate host hematopoiesis [2]. AutoHSCT relies on high doses of chemotherapy and/or radiotherapy to cure malignant disorders. As the patient's pretreatment hematopoietic cells are reinfused, this approach is best utilized in patients with minimal or no disease in the bone marrow (BM). There are recent reports, however, that autologous immune effector cells can lead to an antitumor effect and may also contribute to the therapeutic potential of an autoHSCT [3]. Furthermore, the rapidity of immune reconstitution and the subsets of recovering cells may predict for improved outcomes [4].

The process of autoHSCT begins with the collection of hematopoietic progenitor/stem cells. Peripheral blood stem cells (PBSCs) are preferable to BM cells due to more rapid engraftment [5]. When PBSCs are used, several agents can be used to mobilize hematopoietic stem cells from the BM compartment into the peripheral blood. While the primary means of stem cell mobilization is through the administration of chemotherapy and/or granulocyte colony-stimulating factor (G-CSF), there is emerging evidence on the efficacy of CXCR4 antagonists (e.g. plerixafor) in this setting as well [6]. Following stem cell mobilization, PBSC-enriched peripheral blood is collected via an apheresis catheter and the PBSCs are separated by apheresis. After collection of PBSCs, myeloablative doses of chemotherapy and/or radiotherapy are given to eliminate all hematopoietic cells, including residual hematopoietic stem cells. The harvested PBSCs are then reinfused into the patient to allow for prompt autologous hematologic recovery.

Indications

The most common indications for autoHSCT are multiple myeloma (MM), non-Hodgkin lymphoma (NHL) and Hodgkin lymphoma (HL) (Table 22.1) [1, 7]. Since MM typically cannot be cured with chemotherapy alone, almost all patients with MM will eventually relapse after autoHSCT. AutoHSCT prolongs progression-free survival in MM and earlier studies showed an overall survival (OS) advantage [8, 9]. However, the therapeutic benefit of autoHSCT may be minimized by advances in chemotherapeutic strategies, including the development of proteosome inhibitors and immunomodulatory drugs, and these agents also can be used for maintenance treatment after autoSCT to improve progression-free survival for patients with MM [9–11].

Aggressive NHL and HL are potentially curable by chemotherapy alone. Very high doses of cytotoxic therapy, followed by autoHSCT can produce cures in a significant subset of patients with NHL or HL who relapse after front-line therapy. The utility of autoHSCT for aggressive NHL has been demonstrated by results of a multicenter randomized study, the PARMA trial, which compared chemo-radiotherapy versus chemo-radiotherapy followed

Table 22.1 Indications for an autologous hematopoietic stem cell transplantation.

Disease	When to autoHSCT?
Multiple myeloma	High dose therapy followed by autoHSCT (early) After first relapse (delayed)
Diffuse large B-cell lymphoma	Chemosensitive relapse
Mantle cell lymphoma	Consolidation in CR1 Chemosensitive relapse
Hodgkin's lymphoma	Refractory disease Chemosensitive relapse
Acute myeloid leukemia	Consolidation in CR1 (patients without poor-risk features)[1]
Acute promyelocytic leukemia	Molecular CR2

[1] Although consolidation with autologous hematopoietic stem cell transplantation (autoHSCT) is an option for patients with acute myeloid leukemia without poor-risk features, this is a category 2B indication. Consolidation chemotherapy is strongly recommended for patients with favorable risk features, and an allogeneic hematopoietic stem cell transplantation (alloHSCT) is recommended in patients with intermediate or poor-risk features. AutoHSCT an option for patients with intermediate-risk without an allogeneic donor or if alloHSCT is not an option [93].

by autoHSCT for relapsed chemotherapy sensitive diffuse large B-cell lymphoma. AutoHSCT led to increased rates of event-free survival and OS compared with the chemo-radiotherapy arm, thus becoming a standard treatment for patients with relapsed chemotherapy-sensitive disease [12]. However, the advent of immunotherapy such as rituximab has altered the role of autoHSCT for these patients. The CORAL study, a more recent landmark work, was intended to compare different chemotherapeutic salvage regimens as a bridge to autoHSCT in patients with aggressive NHL [13]. This study showed that while the chemotherapy salvage arms were equivalent, patients who relapsed less than 12 months after first-line therapy R-CHOP (rituximab, cyclophosphamide, doxorubicin, vincristine, and prednisone) had dismal long-term OS despite autoHSCT salvage. Thus, the benefits of autoHSCT previously seen in the pre-rituximab era appear largely restricted to patients who relapse more than 12 months post first-line therapy with R-CHOP. AutoHSCT is also increasingly being studied as a potential salvage option for patients with diffuse large B-cell lymphoma who have a positive interim positron emission tomography scan after initial therapy [14].

The utility of autoHSCT for relapsed chemotherapy sensitive HL has been documented for more than two decades [15]. While response rates and progression-free survival rates are improved compared to other therapies, it is not clear if autoHSCT improves OS. Nonetheless, autoHSCT is considered standard of care for patients with HL as consolidation for relapsed chemosensitive disease [16, 17].

Complications

In general, the complications of autoHSCT are much less severe than those of alloHSCT. AutoHSCT is only rarely associated with graft-versus-host disease (GVHD) or graft failure, both major contributors of morbidity and mortality in alloHSCT.

However, autoHSCT can still lead to severe regimen-related organ toxicities and infectious complications during the peri-transplant period. AutoHSCT leads to infertility in women, and appropriate discussions and planning should be made with women of childbearing age prior to undergoing an autoHSCT when clinically feasible.

Relapse post-autoHSCT

Unfortunately, the rate of relapse following an autoHSCT is high, due to the contamination of the transplanted hematopoietic cells with tumor cells and/or resistance of the tumor cells to the pretransplant cytotoxic therapy (conditioning) [2]. Management of relapse post-autoHSCT depends upon the specific disease state and clinical status of the patient. If a response is obtained after salvage treatment for relapse, there is a growing trend of proceeding to alloHSCT [18].

Allogeneic Hematopoietic Stem Cell Transplantation (alloHSCT)

AlloHSCT refers to the administration of hematopoietic stem cells from one individual (donor) to another (recipient). AlloHSCT is mainly reserved for nonmalignant and malignant hematologic diseases in which conventional therapeutics are ineffective [1]. The efficacy of alloHSCT is due to the replacement of an impaired or defective hematopoietic system for nonmalignant diseases or due to a graft-versus-tumor immune effect in malignant conditions, in which the donor immune system recognizes the malignant condition as foreign and eliminates host tumor cells. Stem cells can come from related or unrelated living donors or umbilical cord blood (UCB) units. Donor availability, traditionally, had been one of the limitations of alloHSCT. However, with recent advances that have allowed the safe utilization of alternative donor options such as partially HLA-mismatched donors or UCB, donor availability is now near universal, with almost all patients having at least one potential donor. Additionally, the development of reduced-intensity conditioning (RIC) regimens has allowed older patients and those with significant comorbidities to safely undergo alloHSCT. There has been substantial improvement in outcomes of patients undergoing alloHSCT over the past two decades, manifested by reductions in overall mortality, relapse, severe GVHD, infection, and organ toxicity [19].

Donor Selection

Human leukocyte antigens (HLA) are widely expressed molecules that present peptides to T cells, prevent the recognition of "self" as foreign, and enable our immune system to recognize foreign antigens. HLA molecules are compared between the diseased patient (recipient) and potential donors in order to find the best "match." There are six major HLA types, although some are more immunogenic and thus important for typing than others. The most common HLA types assessed for a potential match are HLA-A, HLA-B, HLA-C, and HLA-DRB1, with complete typing also including HLA-DQB1 and HLA-DPB1 [20]. The HLA molecules are termed "major determinants", as these antigens are primarily responsible for complications post-alloHSCT, such as GVHD. There is extensive polymorphism among the HLA molecules with extreme diversity between and within different ethnicities and cultures. Currently, the preferred donor is an HLA-matched related sibling (MRD); however, less than 30% of patients will have an MRD [2]. The use of alternative donor sources is thus crucial to allow wider accessibility. The National Marrow Donor Program (NMDP) was established in 1986, creating a database of unrelated donors that can be matched with potential recipients [21]. There are several international registries that have formed as well. It is currently estimated that there are more than 20 million potential donors in the NMDP [22]. However, there are certain ethnic groups that are widely underrepresented in donor registries [23]. Moreover, there is usually a 3-month delay from the time of starting a search for an unrelated donor to the time of collection of stem cells for alloHSCT, and many patients cannot afford this lag time due to high risk for disease relapse. The best outcomes for MUD alloHSCT are seen with donors who are fully HLA matched with the recipient. Several studies have shown that outcomes are similar for recipients of fully HLA matched MUD alloHSCT and MRD alloHSCT [21]. Mismatches at even one of these HLA loci, however, have been associated with increased rates of GVHD and graft rejection, and lower OS rates [24, 25]. There is a growing trend of using other alternative donors such as UCB or partially mismatched living donors. Use of antithymocyte globulin (ATG) and post-transplantation cyclophosphamide (PTCy) show promise in reducing GVHD incidence and improving outcomes in alloHSCT utilizing alternative donor sources [26, 27].

UCB is rich in hematopoietic stem cells, can be cryopreserved for extended periods of time, and leads to a lower risk of GVHD compared with other stem cell sources [2, 28]. However, UCB alloHSCT is associated with delayed immune reconstitution and can thus lead to an increased risk of infectious complications and nonrelapse mortality [28]. Recent data suggests that UCB transplantation may be equivalent to MUD and perhaps even MRD alloHSCT [29].

Haploidentical (haplo) donors are a specific type of partially mismatched donor in which any parent or child, and approximately half of siblings, can be potential haplo donors for a recipient. Early attempts to perform haplo alloHSCTs were unsuccessful due to high rates of graft rejection, GVHD, and nonrelapse mortality [30]. However, newer approaches and novel GVHD prevention methods have allowed haplo alloHSCTs to be successfully performed in the context of either myeloablative conditioning or RIC regimens, with encouraging early results similar to MRD and MUD alloHSCTs [31–33].

For patients without a suitable HLA-identical match (MRD or MUD), the decision between UCB or haplo alloHSCT is largely based on the institution and physician preferences.

Sources of Hematopoietic Stem Cells

BM has traditionally been the primary source of donor cells cells for alloHSCT. BM is harvested in a surgical operating room by repeated BM aspirations from the pelvis under anesthesia. Serious complications are exceedingly rare and are largely related to the complications of anesthesia. The most common complication involves discomfort and pain from the site of the harvest [34]. Hematopoietic stem cells circulate in the blood and can be readily mobilized from the BM with G-CSF or granulocyte macrophage colony- stimulating factor (GM-CSF). PBSCs are then collected by apheresis. Because of the relative ease and convenience of collecting PBSCs as opposed to BM, PBSCs have largely replaced BM collection [2]. However, PBSCs contain more T cells than BM, thereby increasing the rates of chronic GVHD [35–37]. Several studies have compared the results of PBSCs versus BM in MRD alloHSCTs, with similar overall outcomes, but faster engraftment in the PBSC group [38, 39]. A recent phase III multicenter randomized trial comparing PBSC versus BM allografts in MUD alloHSCTs demonstrated similar OS rates but increased rates of graft failure in the BM group, and increased rates of chronic GVHD in the PBSC group [40]. Given these data, PBSC and BM sources are considered roughly equivalent, and decisions regarding which source to use should be guided by physician and donor preferences, as well as disease subtype and conditioning regimens used.

Conditioning Regimens (Myeloablative versus RIC versus Nonmyeloablative)

The treatment given to an individual before the infusion of hematopoietic stem cells is termed the conditioning or preparative regimen. There are three broad classes of conditioning regimens: myeloablative, nonmyeloablative (NMA) and RIC [41]. Myeloablative conditioning regimens utilize intense cytotoxicity against host hematopoietic cells. Without the administration of donor hematopoietic cells, hematopoiesis is irrevocably lost in the host and patients can remain pancytopenic indefinitely [41]. There are a variety of types of myeloablative conditioning regimens used with the most common being a combination of total body irradiation (TBI), delivered in fractions, and cyclophosphamide or a chemotherapy-only regimen comprised of busulfan and cyclophosphamide [42, 43]. Recent data suggest that busulfan may be superior to TBI in patients with acute myeloid leukemia (AML) [44–46]. Myeloablative regimens were originally thought to be necessary to achieve a cure. However, the curative effect of alloSCT was elucidated to be due primarily to an immunologic graft-versus-tumor effect, and not specifically reliant on the conditioning regimen [47, 48]. The concept of NMA and RIC regimens was developed to incorporate the advantage of a donor T cell mediated graft-versus-tumor effect but to decrease transplant-related mortality (TRM) associated with myeloablative conditioning. NMA regimens are primarily immunosuppressive rather than cytotoxic and do not require stem cell infusions for hematologic recovery. RIC regimens, on the other hand, are thought to be of intermediate-intensity, and can cause prolonged aplasia without hematologic recovery [41]. The decision regarding which conditioning regimen to use for an individual patient is determined by multiple factors, including disease type, disease state, age, performance status, comorbidities, organ function, total cumulative prior chemotherapy regimens, and patient/physician preference. In general, NMA and RIC approaches have demonstrated decreased TRM, transplant-related complications and rates of infection, but increased relapse rates when compared with myeloablative regimens [49, 50]. NMA and RIC regimens have permitted patients older than 60–65 years to undergo alloHSCT safely, and is the recommended conditioning approach for patients with significant comorbidities.

Indications for AlloHSCT

Most frequently, alloHSCT is utilized for adults with malignant hematologic disorders that are incurable with conventional chemotherapy agents (Table 22.2). In adults, the most common indication for an alloHSCT is AML (approximately 50% of alloHSCT) [2]. The timing of alloHSCT in AML is critical as the most favorable outcomes are in patients undergoing alloHSCT in first CR (CR1). Meta-analyses have demonstrated increased OS and disease-free survival rates when younger adult patients with AML with intermediate or poor risk cytogenetics undergo an alloHSCT in CR1 [51, 52]. If alloHSCT is deferred until CR2 or higher, OS and event-free survival rates decrease significantly [53]. Therefore, patients with AML without favorable risk features, such as core-binding factor AML, acute promyelocytic leukemia, NPM1 mutation without FLT3-ITD mutation, and CEBPA double mutations, should undergo HLA typing as soon as possible with plans for an alloHSCT during CR1 [54, 55]. Any patient with AML who achieves a CR and subsequently relapses (regardless of risk characteristics) should attempt to undergo an alloHSCT in CR2 unless there are specific contraindications to alloHSCT [55]. Other common indications for alloHSCT include myelodysplasia (MDS), myeloproliferative neoplasms, chronic myelogenous leukemia (CML), acute lymphoblastic leukemia (ALL), NHL, and non-malignant disorders. CML used to be the most common indication for an alloHSCT before the advent of tyrosine kinase inhibitors (TKIs). Now, an alloHSCT is recommended in patients with CML who have failed two or more TKIs, patients with advanced phase disease (accelerated phase or blast crisis) and/or patients with T315I mutations [56, 57]. The most common nonmalignant disorders that are referred for an

alloHSCT include immunodeficiency states, such as Wiskott-Aldrich syndrome, aplastic anemia, thalassemia, and sickle cell anemia, with cure rates as high as 90% [58].

Complications of AlloHSCT (Table 22.3)

Immediate Toxicities

The high doses of chemotherapy and radiation therapy given during conditioning regimens can lead to a variety of early toxicities and complications. Immediate toxicities can vary by the conditioning regimen but include nausea, vomiting, fever, and an erythematous rash. Oral mucositis is common and typically occurs within 5–7 days after alloHSCT, is more commonly seen with myeloablative conditioning, and often requires narcotic medications and pain-controlled analgesia.

Hepatic Sinusoidal Obstruction Syndrome

Hepatic sinusoidal obstruction syndrome (SOS), previously termed veno-occlusive disease of the liver, can be defined by the Baltimore Criteria (bilirubin ≥2 mg/dL with at least two of the three following symptoms: hepatomegaly, ascites and ≥5% weight gain occurring within the first 21 days post-alloHSCT) or McDonald criteria (two of the following: bilirubin ≥2 mg/dL, hepatomegaly or right upper quadrant pain of liver origin, and weight gain >2% of baseline body weight within the first 20 days post-transplant) [59]. The etiology and pathophysiology of SOS is unknown but is thought to be secondary to chemotherapy and radiation toxicity, leading to obstruction of hepatic small venules and consequently sinusoidal obstruction [60]. The incidence of SOS is approximately 5%, and is increased in patients with pre-existing abnormal liver function tests prior to alloSCT [61]. Diagnosis of SOS is usually made clinically. Most patients with mild or moderate SOS recover with normal liver function with supportive care or diuretic therapy. However, the prognosis of severe SOS is extremely poor, and is typically manifested by fulminant liver failure, coagulopathy and multiorgan failure [62]. Defibrotide was recently approved for the management of VOD based on a phase III trial comparing defibrotide 25 mg/kg daily to historical controls receiving best supportive care. Defibrotide led to improved survival at day 100 post-alloHSCT and complete remission rates compared with controls (38.2% vs 25%; $P = 0.011$ and 25.5% vs 12.5%; $P = 0.016$, respectively). The most common serious adverse events include hemorrhage and hypotension [63].

Table 22.2 Neoplastic indications for an allogeneic hematopoietic stem cell transplantation.

Disease	When to alloHSCT?
Acute myeloid leukemia	Consolidation in CR1 (intermediate and poor-risk) CR2
Acute lymphoblastic leukemia	Consolidation in CR1 (Poor-risk) CR2
Myelodysplastic syndrome	High-risk disease (Intermediate-2 and High IPSS score)
Chronic myelogenous leukemia	Advanced phase disease (accelerated phase and blast crisis) Failure to tolerate or resistant to two or more TKIs T315I mutations
Myelofibrosis	Young patients (<60 years) with high-risk disease
Chronic lymphocytic leukemia	High-risk disease Chemosensitive relapse Richter transformation with chemosensitive disease

Table 22.3 Common toxicities post allogeneic hematopoietic stem cell transplantation.

Toxicity	Expected Time of Onset
Oral mucositis	Day 0 – neutrophil recovery
Idiopathic pneumonia syndrome	Day 20–90
Acute GVHD	Day 20–100
Chronic GVHD	> Day 100
Hepatic sinusoidal obstruction syndrome	< Day 30
Infections – early Infections – late	Pre-alloSCT – Day 100 >Day 100

Idiopathic Pneumonia Syndrome

Idiopathic pneumonia syndrome (IPS) typically occurs between 21 and 90 days after alloHSCT and is characterized by fever, cough, tachypnea and hypoxemia, with diffuse infiltrates on radiologic imaging. IPS is more commonly seen after myeloablative conditioning regimens including high-doses of TBI. Pre-existing lung disease, increased age, and prior radiation therapy increase the risk of IPS. Treatment for IPS is unfortunately experimental as there is no universally accepted effective treatment [64].

Graft Failure

Graft failure can occur after any type of alloHSCT and results from host-versus-donor rejection of the donor marrow. Graft failure occurs most commonly when HLA matching is disparate, and when patients have received multiple transfusions prior to alloHSCT [65]. The presence of donor-specific antibodies also increases the risk of graft failure; however, desensitization can effectively reduce the risk of graft failure [66]. Occasionally, patients with graft failure may respond to growth factor support, but the majority of patients will require a second alloHSCT following an immunosuppressive conditioning regimen.

Infections

All patients undergoing alloHSCT will be aplastic for a period of time, and therefore are susceptible to a variety of infections. Patients undergoing alloHSCT also have a high risk of infection due to organ damage and mucositis. Early infections are defined by the initial period of aplasia, occurring within the first 60–90 days after alloHSCT. Antibiotic prophylaxis is recommended during the neutropenic phase to prevent life-threatening bacterial infections. Antifungal prophylaxis has significantly reduced the morbidity and mortality of invasive fungal infections post-alloHSCT [67]. Multiple viral infections can occur in alloHSCT patients. Primary prophylaxis against herpes simplex virus and varicella zoster virus with acyclovir or valacyclovir has markedly reduced the incidence of herpetic infections in patients undergoing alloHSCT [68]. For patients who are serologically CMV-negative and receive allografts from CMV-negative donors, CMV infection can be substantially reduced by using blood products from CMV-negative donors or by leukoreduction of blood products [69]. Pre-emptive ganciclovir or valganciclovir therapy is undertaken in patients with evidence of asymptomatic CMV reactivation and has significantly delayed the onset and reduced the incidence of CMV infection post-alloHSCT [70]. Other viral infections that can occur post-alloSCT include Epstein-Barr virus, adenovirus, human-herpes virus-6 and -7, and respiratory viruses (influenza, respiratory-syncytial virus, parainfluenza, rhinovirus). Late infections are usually defined as infections occurring more than 3 months post-alloHSCT. Patients at highest risk for late infections include patients with chronic GVHD and patients who continue on immunosuppression for either treatment or prevention of GVHD.

GVHD

GVHD occurs when transfused donor T cells recognize the recipient as "foreign", thereby leading to an immune reaction against the host. There are two types of GVHD: acute and chronic. Acute GVHD (aGVHD) typically presents within the first 100 days of alloHSCT, and involves the skin, gut, and/or liver. In most patients, the symptoms of aGVHD begin with an erythematous or maculopapular rash which can affect any part of the body, including the palms and soles. Acute GVHD of the skin is staged into four categories depending upon the amount of body surface area involvement. Skin biopsies are often done but are not specific for aGVHD, and it can be difficult to histologically distinguish aGVHD from other causes of rash, including drug reactions. Acute GVHD of the gut is characterized by diffuse abdominal pain and profuse diarrhea, which can be very severe and life threatening. The severity of aGVHD of the gut is classified by the volume of stool, which can occasionally exceed 10 L/day. It is crucial to monitor patients with aGVHD of the gut closely, as these patients may require several liters of hydration daily [71]. Histologic diagnosis is imperative as other causes of profound diarrhea post-transplant include infectious agents such as CMV, which ideally should be ruled out before empiric therapy for aGVHD is started. Finally, hepatic aGVHD usually presents with a cholestatic picture with elevated bilirubin and alkaline phosphatase and relatively preserved liver function enzymes. However, it is important to note that aGVHD of the liver can occasionally result in high elevations of liver function enzymes with preserved bilirubin and alkaline phosphatase levels. A biopsy may be necessary to differentiate aGVHD of the liver from biliary infections, drug toxicity, and hepatic SOS. Each organ system involved is individually graded and a final aGVHD grade (I–IV) is assigned [72, 73]. The grade of aGVHD is used as a guide for management and prognosis.

Chronic GVHD (cGVHD) typically affects 30–70% of patients undergoing alloHSCTs and is a leading cause of late morbidity and mortality post-transplant. cGVHD resembles a collagen vascular disease that can involve any organ, including the skin, mouth, eyes, liver, lung, joints, gut, and/or genitalia [74]. Skin findings are seen in the majority of patients with cGVHD, and include sclerotic features, lichen planus-like features, poikiloderma, morphea-like features, and lichen sclerosis-like features [75]. Typically, cGVHD occurs more than 100 days after alloHSCT without evidence of aGVHD, but can occur at any time and can occasionally develop as part of an overlap syndrome in which patients simultaneously have features of both aGVHD and cGVHD. Chronic GVHD is more common when patients undergo alloHSCT using PBSCs rather than BM allografts. Incidences of both aGVHD and cGVHD increase with unrelated donors or increasing HLA-mismatching [40].

There are a variety of methods used after alloHSCT to prevent aGVHD. The most widely used regimen is methotrexate and a calcineurin inhibitor (cyclosporine or tacrolimus) [76]. These drugs are usually given for approximately 3 months after alloHSCT and then gradually tapered and eventually discontinued at 6 months post-alloHSCT. Approximately 30% of patients undergoing an alloHSCT with a MRD will develop aGVHD despite GVHD prophylaxis [77]. T-cell depletion of the donor graft is also effective in preventing GVHD, but has been shown to increase both infectious and relapse risks in patients with CML and therefore is less commonly used than pharmacologic approaches at preventing GVHD [78–80]. Unfortunately, most common GVHD preventive strategies are ineffective at preventing cGVHD, though newer approaches, such as ATG and PTCy, show promise in reducing cGVHD rates [81–83].

Treatment of aGVHD is dependent upon the grade and the specific organ(s) involved. In general, mild cases of aGVHD of the skin (grade 1) can be managed with supportive care or with topical steroids alone. Systemic steroids are recommended as the first-line agent in patients with more severe aGVHD of the skin, and for any patient with gut or liver involvement. Second-line agents, such as calcineurin inhibitors, methotrexate, and mycophenolate mofetil, should be initiated promptly if the patient does not respond to steroids within the first 3–5 days or if the presenting symptoms are severe [84].

Treatment of cGVHD also depends on the stage and extent of the disease, and can often be managed with local therapies. More severe cases are often managed with systemic steroids with or without a calcineurin inhibitor but can also include a number of other pharmacologic treatments or dermatologic approaches including ultraviolet light or extracorporeal photopheresis [76]. All patients being treated for aGVHD or cGVHD should be carefully monitored for infectious symptoms and treated with prophylactic antibiotics.

Relapse Post-AlloHSCT

Although alloHSCT can lead to a cure in a significant proportion of patients with otherwise incurable hematologic malignancies, approximately 40–50% of patients will relapse post-alloHSCT [85]. The risk of relapse depends mainly on the disease type, disease characteristics, and the status and burden of disease prior to alloHSCT. The best overall outcomes occur when patients have no detectable disease prior to alloHSCT [86]. Additionally, the use of RIC may lead to increased rates of relapse, which may be counterbalanced by decreased treatment-related morbidity and mortality of the alloHSCT [50].

There is a dearth of options for patients who relapse with their disease post-alloHSCT. Patients on immunosuppression at the time of relapse can occasionally achieve a second remission upon discontinuation of their immunosuppressive medications [87]. The majority of relapsed patients, however, will require more intensive therapy in order to achieve a response. Escalating doses of donor lymphocyte infusions (DLI) were shown to be extremely effective in CML, leading to a graft-versus-tumor effect and consequent GVHD in approximately 70% of chronic phase relapses. Unfortunately, DLI is not very effective in treating AML, MDS, ALL or advanced phase CML relapses post-alloHSCT [88]. Given the lack of alternative options, DLI is often used either as a single agent or combined with chemotherapy in patients that relapse post-alloHSCT. DLI typically takes months to work in order to develop a T-cell mediated graft-versus-tumor effect, so patients with AML and ALL who relapse with a high degree of tumor burden may require cytoreductive therapy prior to initiation of DLI [89]. Recent data suggests that the combination of azacitidine and DLI may be synergistic and is a reasonable consideration for patients with AML who relapse post-alloHSCT, particularly if they are not candidates for intensive chemotherapy [90]. DLI can lead to significant morbidity and mortality, including GVHD in approximately 50% of patients, infections, and myelosuppression, and should therefore be used with caution. TKI therapy has been increasingly used with or without DLI in patients with CML and Philadelphia-chromosome positive ALL who relapse post-alloHSCT. It appears that TKIs may reduce the morbidity and mortality associated with DLI post-alloHSCT [91]. Occasionally, a second alloHSCT can be performed in relapsed patients who achieve a significant response to salvage therapy. NMA conditioning and an alloHSCT from a different donor can lead to long-term responses and overall cures in a subset of patients [92].

References

1 Majhail NS, Farnia SH, Carpenter PA, *et al*. Indications for autologous and allogeneic hematopoietic cell transplantation: guidelines from the American Society for Blood and Marrow Transplantation. *Biol Blood Marrow Transplant* 2015; 21(11):1863–9.

2 Copelan EA. Hematopoietic stem-cell transplantation. *N Engl J Med* 2006;354(17):1813–26.

3 Porrata LF. Autologous graft-versus-tumor effect: reality or fiction? Adv Hematol 2016. doi: 10.1155/2016/5385972. Epub 2016 Aug 22.

4 Porrata LF, Inwards DJ, Ansell SM, *et al*. Day 100 peripheral blood absolute lymphocyte/monocyte ratio and survival in classical Hodgkin's lymphoma postautologous peripheral blood hematopoietic stem cell transplantation. *Bone Marrow Res* 2013;2013:658371.

5 Rancea M, Skoetz N, Monsef I, *et al*. Fourteenth biannual report of the Cochrane Haematological Malignancies Group – focus on autologous stem cell transplantation in hematological malignancies. *J Natl Cancer Inst* 2012;104(14):NP.

6 Vishnu P, Roy V, Paulsen A, Zubair AC. Efficacy and cost-benefit analysis of risk-adaptive use of plerixafor for autologous hematopoietic progenitor cell mobilization. *Transfusion* 2012;52(1):55–62.

7 Baldomero H, Gratwohl M, Gratwohl A, *et al*. The EBMT activity survey 2009: trends over the past 5 years. *Bone Marrow Transplant* 2011;46(4):485–501.

8 Attal M, Harousseau JL, Stoppa AM, *et al*. A prospective, randomized trial of autologous bone marrow transplantation and chemotherapy in multiple myeloma. Intergroupe Francais du Myelome. *N Engl J Med* 1996;335(2):91–7.

9 Child JA, Morgan GJ, Davies FE, *et al*. High-dose chemotherapy with hematopoietic stem-cell rescue for multiple myeloma. *N Engl J Med* 2003;348(19):1875–83.

10 Abidi MH, Gul Z, Abrams J, *et al*. Phase I trial of bortezomib during maintenance phase after high dose melphalan and autologous stem cell transplantation in patients with multiple myeloma. *J Chemother* 2012;24(3):167–72.

11 Attal M, Lauwers-Cances V, Marit G, *et al*. Lenalidomide maintenance after stem-cell transplantation for multiple myeloma. *N Engl J Med* 2012;366(19):1782–91.

12 Philip T, Guglielmi C, Hagenbeek A, *et al*. Autologous bone marrow transplantation as compared with salvage chemotherapy in relapses of chemotherapy-sensitive non-Hodgkin's lymphoma. *N Engl J Med* 1995;333(23):1540–5.

13 Gisselbrecht C, Glass B, Mounier N, *et al*. Salvage regimens with autologous transplantation for relapsed large B-cell

lymphoma in the rituximab era. *J Clin Oncol* 2010;28(27):4184–90.

14 Roland V, Bodet-Milin C, Moreau A, *et al*. Impact of high-dose chemotherapy followed by auto-SCT for positive interim [18F] FDG-PET diffuse large B-cell lymphoma patients. *Bone Marrow Transplant* 2011;46(3):393–9.

15 Linch DC, Winfield D, Goldstone AH, *et al*. Dose intensification with autologous bone-marrow transplantation in relapsed and resistant Hodgkin's disease: results of a BNLI randomised trial. *Lancet* 1993;341(8852):1051–4.

16 Moskowitz CH, Kewalramani T, Nimer SD, *et al*. Effectiveness of high dose chemoradiotherapy and autologous stem cell transplantation for patients with biopsy-proven primary refractory Hodgkin's disease. *Br J Haematol* 2004; 124(5):645–52.

17 Gutierrez-Delgado F, Holmberg L, Hooper H, *et al*. Autologous stem cell transplantation for Hodgkin's disease: busulfan, melphalan and thiotepa compared to a radiation-based regimen. *Bone Marrow Transplant* 2003; 32(3):279–85.

18 Auner HW, Szydlo R, van Biezen A, *et al*. Reduced intensity-conditioned allogeneic stem cell transplantation for multiple myeloma relapsing or progressing after autologous transplantation: a study by the European Group for Blood and Marrow Transplantation. *Bone Marrow Transplant* 2013;48(11):1395–400.

19 Gooley TA, Chien JW, Pergam SA, *et al*. Reduced mortality after allogeneic hematopoietic-cell transplantation. *N Engl J Med* 2010;363(22):2091–101.

20 Ballen KK, Koreth J, Chen YB, Dey BR, Spitzer TR. Selection of optimal alternative graft source: mismatched unrelated donor, umbilical cord blood, or haploidentical transplant. *Blood* 2012;119(9):1972–80.

21 Stroncek D, Bartsch G, Perkins HA, *et al*. The National Marrow Donor Program. *Transfusion* 1993;33(7):567–77.

22 Appelbaum FR. Hematopoietic cell transplantation. In: CL Loprinzi (ed.) *ASCO-SEP Medical Oncology Self-Evaluation Program*. Alexandria, VA: American Society of Clinical Oncology, 2007–2013:451–62.

23 Beatty PG, Mori M, Milford E. Impact of racial genetic polymorphism on the probability of finding an HLA-matched donor. *Transplantation* 1995;60(8):778–83.

24 Lee SJ, Klein J, Haagenson M, *et al*. High-resolution donor-recipient HLA matching contributes to the success of unrelated donor marrow transplantation. *Blood* 2007; 110(13):4576–83.

25 Confer DL, Abress LK, Navarro W, Madrigal A. Selection of adult unrelated hematopoietic stem cell donors: beyond HLA. *Biol Blood Marrow Transplant* 2010;16(1 Suppl):S8–S11.

26 Finke J, Bethge WA, Schmoor C, *et al*. Standard graft-versus-host disease prophylaxis with or without anti-T-cell globulin in haematopoietic cell transplantation from matched unrelated donors: a randomised, open-label, multicentre phase 3 trial. *Lancet Oncol* 2009;10(9):855–64.

27 Brunstein CG, Fuchs EJ, Carter SL, *et al*. Alternative donor transplantation after reduced intensity conditioning: results of parallel phase 2 trials using partially HLA-mismatched related bone marrow or unrelated double umbilical cord blood grafts. *Blood* 2011;118(2):282–8.

28 Ballen KK, Gluckman E, Broxmeyer HE. Umbilical cord blood transplantation: the first 25 years and beyond. *Blood* 2013; 122(4):491–8.

29 Brunstein CG, Gutman JA, Weisdorf DJ, *et al*. Allogeneic hematopoietic cell transplantation for hematologic malignancy: relative risks and benefits of double umbilical cord blood. *Blood* 2010;116(22):4693–9.

30 Powles RL, Morgenstern GR, Kay HE, *et al*. Mismatched family donors for bone-marrow transplantation as treatment for acute leukaemia. *Lancet* 1983;1(8325):612–5.

31 Luznik L, O'Donnell PV, Fuchs EJ. Post-transplantation cyclophosphamide for tolerance induction in HLA-haploidentical bone marrow transplantation. *Semin Oncol* 2012;39(6):683–93.

32 Bashey A, Zhang X, Sizemore CA, *et al*. T-cell-replete HLA-haploidentical hematopoietic transplantation for hematologic malignancies using post-transplantation cyclophosphamide results in outcomes equivalent to those of contemporaneous HLA-matched related and unrelated donor transplantation. *J Clin Oncol* 2013;31(10):1310–6.

33 Robinson TM, O'Donnell PV, Fuchs EJ, Luznik L. Haploidentical bone marrow and stem cell transplantation: experience with post-transplantation cyclophosphamide. *Semin Hematol* 2016;53(2):90–7.

34 Anderlini P, Rizzo JD, Nugent ML, *et al*. Peripheral blood stem cell donation: an analysis from the International Bone Marrow Transplant Registry (IBMTR) and European Group for Blood and Marrow Transplant (EBMT) databases. *Bone Marrow Transplant* 2001;27(7):689–92.

35 Cutler C, Giri S, Jeyapalan S, *et al*. Acute and chronic graft-versus-host disease after allogeneic peripheral-blood stem-cell and bone marrow transplantation: a meta-analysis. *J Clin Oncol* 2001;19(16):3685–91.

36 Stewart BL, Storer B, Storek J, *et al*. Duration of immunosuppressive treatment for chronic graft-versus-host disease. *Blood* 2004;104(12):3501–6.

37 Bensinger WI, Weaver CH, Appelbaum FR, *et al*. Transplantation of allogeneic peripheral blood stem cells mobilized by recombinant human granulocyte colony-stimulating factor. *Blood* 1995;85(6):1655–8.

38 Bensinger WI, Martin PJ, Storer B, *et al*. Transplantation of bone marrow as compared with peripheral-blood cells from HLA-identical relatives in patients with hematologic cancers. *N Engl J Med* 2001;344(3):175–81.

39 Mielcarek M, Storer B, Martin PJ, *et al*. Long-term outcomes after transplantation of HLA-identical related G-CSF-mobilized peripheral blood mononuclear cells versus bone marrow. *Blood* 2012;119(11):2675–8.

40 Anasetti C, Logan BR, Lee SJ, *et al*. Peripheral-blood stem cells versus bone marrow from unrelated donors. *N Engl J Med* 2012;367(16):1487–96.

41 Bacigalupo A, Ballen K, Rizzo D, *et al*. Defining the intensity of conditioning regimens: working definitions. *Biol Blood Marrow Transplant* 2009;15(12):1628–33.

42 Santos GW. The development of busulfan/cyclophosphamide preparative regimens. *Semin Oncol* 1993;20(4 Suppl 4):12–6.

43 Clift RA, Buckner CD, Appelbaum FR, *et al*. Allogeneic marrow transplantation in patients with acute myeloid

leukemia in first remission: a randomized trial of two irradiation regimens. *Blood* 1990;76(9):1867–71.

44 Blaise D, Maraninchi D, Archimbaud E, *et al*. Allogeneic bone marrow transplantation for acute myeloid leukemia in first remission: a randomized trial of a busulfan-Cytoxan versus Cytoxan-total body irradiation as preparative regimen: a report from the Group d'Etudes de la Greffe de Moelle Osseuse. *Blood* 1992;79(10):2578–82.

45 Bredeson C, Lerademacher J, Kato K, *et al*. Prospective cohort study comparing intravenous busulfan to total body irradiation in hematopoietic cell transplantation. *Blood* 2013;122(24):3871–8.

46 Copelan EA, Hamilton BK, Avalos B, *et al*. Better leukemia-free and overall survival in AML in first remission following cyclophosphamide in combination with busulfan compared with TBI. *Blood* 2013;122(24):3863–70.

47 Horowitz MM, Gale RP, Sondel PM, *et al*. Graft-versus-leukemia reactions after bone marrow transplantation. *Blood* 1990;75(3):555–62.

48 Gale RP, Horowitz MM, Ash RC, *et al*. Identical-twin bone marrow transplants for leukemia. *Ann Intern Med* 1994;120(8):646–52.

49 McSweeney PA, Niederwieser D, Shizuru JA, *et al*. Hematopoietic cell transplantation in older patients with hematologic malignancies: replacing high-dose cytotoxic therapy with graft-versus-tumor effects. *Blood* 2001;97(11):3390–400.

50 Giralt S, Thall PF, Khouri I, *et al*. Melphalan and purine analog-containing preparative regimens: reduced-intensity conditioning for patients with hematologic malignancies undergoing allogeneic progenitor cell transplantation. *Blood* 2001;97(3):631–7.

51 Yanada M, Matsuo K, Emi N, Naoe T. Efficacy of allogeneic hematopoietic stem cell transplantation depends on cytogenetic risk for acute myeloid leukemia in first disease remission: a metaanalysis. *Cancer* 2005;103(8):1652–8.

52 Koreth J, Schlenk R, Kopecky KJ, *et al*. Allogeneic stem cell transplantation for acute myeloid leukemia in first complete remission: systematic review and meta-analysis of prospective clinical trials. *JAMA* 2009;301(22):2349–61.

53 Forman SJ, Rowe JM. The myth of the second remission of acute leukemia in the adult. *Blood* 2013;121(7):1077–82.

54 Schlenk RF, Dohner K, Krauter J, *et al*. Mutations and treatment outcome in cytogenetically normal acute myeloid leukemia. *N Engl J Med* 2008;358(18):1909–18.

55 NCCN Clinical Practice Guidelines in Oncology, Acute Myeloid leukemia, version 2.2016. Available at: http://wwwnccn.org (accessed 12 June 2017).

56 Grigg A, Hughes T. Role of allogeneic stem cell transplantation for adult chronic myeloid leukemia in the imatinib era. *Biol Blood Marrow Transplant* 2006;12(8):795–807.

57 NCCN Clinical Practice Guidelines in Oncology, Chronic Myeloid leukemia, version 1.2017. Available at http://wwwnccn.org (accessed 12 June 2017).

58 Buckley RH, Schiff SE, Schiff RI, *et al*. Hematopoietic stem-cell transplantation for the treatment of severe combined immunodeficiency. *N Engl J Med* 1999;340(7):508–16.

59 Blostein MD, Paltiel OB, Thibault A, Rybka WB. A comparison of clinical criteria for the diagnosis of veno-occlusive disease of the liver after bone marrow transplantation. *Bone Marrow Transplant* 1992;10(5):439–43.

60 Wadleigh M, Ho V, Momtaz P, Richardson P. Hepatic veno-occlusive disease: pathogenesis, diagnosis and treatment. *Curr Opin Hematol* 2003;10(6):451–62.

61 DeLeve LD, Shulman HM, McDonald GB. Toxic injury to hepatic sinusoids: sinusoidal obstruction syndrome (veno-occlusive disease). *Semin Liver Dis* 2002;22(1):27–42.

62 McDonald GB, Hinds MS, Fisher LD, *et al*. Veno-occlusive disease of the liver and multiorgan failure after bone marrow transplantation: a cohort study of 355 patients. *Ann Intern Med* 1993;118(4):255–67.

63 Richardson PG, Riches ML, Kernan NA, *et al*. Phase 3 trial of defibrotide for the treatment of severe veno-occlusive disease and multi-organ failure. *Blood* 2016;127(13):1656–65.

64 Panoskaltsis-Mortari A, Griese M, Madtes DK, *et al*. An official American Thoracic Society research statement: noninfectious lung injury after hematopoietic stem cell transplantation: idiopathic pneumonia syndrome. *Am J Respir Crit Care Med* 2011;183(9):1262–79.

65 Anasetti C, Amos D, Beatty PG, *et al*. Effect of HLA compatibility on engraftment of bone marrow transplants in patients with leukemia or lymphoma. *N Engl J Med* 1989;320(4):197–204.

66 Gladstone DE, Zachary AA, Fuchs EJ, *et al*. Partially mismatched transplantation and human leukocyte antigen donor-specific antibodies. *Biol Blood Marrow Transplant* 2013; 19(4):647–52.

67 Marr KA, Seidel K, Slavin MA, *et al*. Prolonged fluconazole prophylaxis is associated with persistent protection against candidiasis-related death in allogeneic marrow transplant recipients: long-term follow-up of a randomized, placebo-controlled trial. *Blood* 2000;96(6):2055–61.

68 Wade JC, Newton B, Flournoy N, Meyers JD. Oral acyclovir for prevention of herpes simplex virus reactivation after marrow transplantation. *Ann Intern Med* 1984;100(6):823–8.

69 Thiele T, Kruger W, Zimmermann K, *et al*. Transmission of cytomegalovirus (CMV) infection by leukoreduced blood products not tested for CMV antibodies: a single-center prospective study in high-risk patients undergoing allogeneic hematopoietic stem cell transplantation (CME). *Transfusion* 2011;51(12):2620–6.

70 Einsele H, Hebart H, Kauffmann-Schneider C, *et al*. Risk factors for treatment failures in patients receiving PCR-based preemptive therapy for CMV infection. *Bone Marrow Transplant* 2000;25(7):757–63.

71 Woodruff JM, Hansen JA, Good RA, Santos GW, Slavin RE. The pathology of the graft-versus-host reaction (GVHR) in adults receiving bone marrow transplants. *Transplant Proc* 1976;8(4):675–84.

72 Przepiorka D, Weisdorf D, Martin P, *et al*. 1994 Consensus Conference on Acute GVHD Grading. *Bone Marrow Transplant* 1995;15(6):825–8.

73 Cahn JY, Klein JP, Lee SJ, *et al*. Prospective evaluation of 2 acute graft-versus-host (GVHD) grading systems: a joint Societe Francaise de Greffe de Moelle et Therapie Cellulaire (SFGM-TC), Dana Farber Cancer Institute (DFCI), and International Bone Marrow Transplant Registry (IBMTR) prospective study. *Blood* 2005;106(4):1495–500.

74 Jacobsohn DA, Kurland BF, Pidala J, *et al*. Correlation between NIH composite skin score, patient-reported skin score, and outcome: results from the Chronic GVHD Consortium. *Blood* 2012;120(13):2545–52.

75 Filipovich AH, Weisdorf D, Pavletic S, *et al*. National Institutes of Health consensus development project on criteria for clinical trials in chronic graft-versus-host disease: I. Diagnosis and staging working group report. *Biol Blood Marrow Transplant* 2005;11(12):945–56.

76 Pavletic SZ, Fowler DH. Are we making progress in GVHD prophylaxis and treatment? *Am Soc Hematol Educ Program* 2012;2012:251–64.

77 Ringden O, Klaesson S, Sundberg B, *et al*. Decreased incidence of graft-versus-host disease and improved survival with methotrexate combined with cyclosporin compared with monotherapy in recipients of bone marrow from donors other than HLA identical siblings. *Bone Marrow Transplant* 1992;9(1):19–25.

78 Ringden O, Remberger M, Aschan J, *et al*. Long-term follow-up of a randomized trial comparing T cell depletion with a combination of methotrexate and cyclosporine in adult leukemic marrow transplant recipients. *Transplantation* 1994;58(8):887–91.

79 Wagner JE, Thompson JS, Carter SL, Kernan NA. Effect of graft-versus-host disease prophylaxis on 3-year disease-free survival in recipients of unrelated donor bone marrow (T-cell Depletion Trial): a multi-centre, randomised phase II-III trial. *Lancet* 2005;366(9487):733–41.

80 Pavletic SZ, Carter SL, Kernan NA, *et al*. Influence of T-cell depletion on chronic graft-versus-host disease: results of a multicenter randomized trial in unrelated marrow donor transplantation. *Blood* 2005;106(9):3308–13.

81 Luznik L, O'Donnell PV, Symons HJ, *et al*. HLA-haploidentical bone marrow transplantation for hematologic malignancies using nonmyeloablative conditioning and high-dose, posttransplantation cyclophosphamide. *Biol Blood Marrow Transplant* 2008;14(6):641–50.

82 Luznik L, Bolanos-Meade J, Zahurak M, *et al*. High-dose cyclophosphamide as single-agent, short-course prophylaxis of graft-versus-host disease. *Blood* 2010;115(16):3224–30.

83 Socie G, Schmoor C, Bethge WA, *et al*. Chronic graft-versus-host disease: long-term results from a randomized trial on graft-versus-host disease prophylaxis with or without anti-T-cell globulin ATG-Fresenius. *Blood* 2011;117(23):6375–82.

84 Bacigalupo A. Management of acute graft-versus-host disease. *Br J Haematol* 2007;137(2):87–98.

85 Pollyea DA, Artz AS, Stock W, *et al*. Outcomes of patients with AML and MDS who relapse or progress after reduced intensity allogeneic hematopoietic cell transplantation. *Bone Marrow Transplant* 2007;40(11):1027–32.

86 Walter RB, Buckley SA, Pagel JM, *et al*. Significance of minimal residual disease before myeloablative allogeneic hematopoietic cell transplantation for AML in first and second complete remission. *Blood* 2013;122(10):1813–21.

87 Collins RH, Jr, Rogers ZR, Bennett M, *et al*. Hematologic relapse of chronic myelogenous leukemia following allogeneic bone marrow transplantation: apparent graft-versus-leukemia effect following abrupt discontinuation of immunosuppression. *Bone Marrow Transplant* 1992;10(4):391–5.

88 Kolb HJ, Schattenberg A, Goldman JM, *et al*. Graft-versus-leukemia effect of donor lymphocyte transfusions in marrow grafted patients. *Blood* 1995;86(5):2041–50.

89 Levine JE, Braun T, Penza SL, *et al*. Prospective trial of chemotherapy and donor leukocyte infusions for relapse of advanced myeloid malignancies after allogeneic stem-cell transplantation. *J Clin Oncol* 2002;20(2):405–12.

90 Schroeder T, Rautenberg C, Haas R, Kobbe G. Hypomethylating agents after allogeneic blood stem cell transplantation. *Stem Cell Invest* 2016;3:84.

91 Hess G, Bunjes D, Siegert W, *et al*. Sustained complete molecular remissions after treatment with imatinib-mesylate in patients with failure after allogeneic stem cell transplantation for chronic myelogenous leukemia: results of a prospective phase II open-label multicenter study. *J Clin Oncol* 2005;23(30):7583–93.

92 Baron F, Storb R, Storer BE, *et al*. Factors associated with outcomes in allogeneic hematopoietic cell transplantation with nonmyeloablative conditioning after failed myeloablative hematopoietic cell transplantation. *J Clin Oncol* 2006;24(25):4150–7.

93 O'Donnell MR, Abboud CN, Altman J, *et al*. Acute myeloid leukemia. *J Natl Compr Canc Netw* 2012;10(8):984–1021.

23

Diet, Physical Activity, and Weight Control for Cancer Patients and Survivors

Wendy Demark-Wahnefried[1], Laura Q. Rogers[1], Catherine M. Alfano[2], Cynthia A. Thomson[3], Kerry S. Courneya[4], Jeffrey A. Meyerhardt[5], Nicole L. Stout[6], Elizabeth Kvale[1], Heidi Ganzer[7], Ted Gansler[8], and Jennifer A. Ligibel[5]

[1] University of Alabama at Birmingham, Birmingham, Alabama, USA

[2] Cancer Control, American Cancer Society, Atlanta, GA

[3] University of Arizona Cancer Center, Tucson, Arizona, USA

[4] University of Alberta, Edmonton, Alberta, Canada

[5] Dana-Farber Cancer Institute, Boston, Massachusetts, USA

[6] National Institutes of Health Clinical Center, Bethesda, Maryland, USA

[7] Minnesota Oncology, St. Paul, Minnesota, USA

[8] American Cancer Society, Atlanta, Georgia, USA

Introduction

It is becoming increasingly clear that good nutrition and a physically active lifestyle should be routinely integrated into cancer care. This chapter serves as a practical guide for healthcare providers who care for cancer patients and survivors and who seek a basic understanding of the relevant diet and exercise literature.

Current ACS Guidelines

The 2012 ACS Guidelines on Nutrition and Physical Activity for Cancer Survivors are summarized in Table 23.1 [1]. These recommendations are based on randomized controlled trials (RCTs) of various lifestyle interventions for improving disease-free and overall survival (most of which involve relatively few subjects), as well as observational studies that examined associations of relevant health behaviors and health-related quality of life, cancer-related symptoms, survival, and other health outcomes.

Weight Management

ACS guideline recommendation: achieve and maintain a healthy weight

If overweight or obese, limit consumption of high-calorie (energy dense) foods and beverages and increase physical activity to promote weight loss.

Until recently, this recommendation has been based largely on the associations between increased body mass index (BMI)

and incidence of several types of cancer. Research supports the conclusion that overweight or obesity after diagnosis seems likely to place patients at risk for second malignant neoplasms [2–5]. Also, it seems reasonable to hypothesize that the mechanisms responsible for associations with incidence might increase risk of cancer progression or recurrence. Evidence indicates that obesity contributes to recurrence and cancer-related mortality [6]. A meta-analysis of 82 observational breast cancer studies found that for each $5\,kg/m^2$ increment in BMI above a normal range, there was a 14–29% increased risk of disease-specific mortality and an 8–17% increased risk of total mortality (women who are underweight also face an unfavorable prognosis) [7]. Likewise, a meta-analysis in prostate cancer demonstrated that each $5 < kg/m^2$ increase in BMI was associated with a 21% increased risk of biochemical recurrence ($P < 0.01$) and a 20% higher risk of disease-specific mortality ($P = 0.06$) [8]. A meta-analysis of 29 colorectal cancer studies demonstrated a summary hazard ratio (HR) of 1.10 (95% CI, 1.06–1.15) for overall survival among individuals with obesity versus normal-weight individuals. Somewhat surprisingly, being overweight (but not obese) was associated with good prognosis. As with breast cancer, being underweight was prognostically unfavorable, although it is difficult to discern whether underweight is the result of unintentional weight loss caused by underlying progressive cancer [9]. Fewer studies have been conducted and to the best of our knowledge meta-analyses have not been reported for other cancers; systematic reviews suggest that obesity is directly associated with shorter disease-free survival and overall survival, although the evidence is less consistent [10, 11].

Obesity increases risk of short-term complications and late adverse effects of cancer treatment such as for poor wound

Table 23.1 American Cancer Society Guidelines on Nutrition and Physical Activity for Cancer Survivors.

Achieve and maintain a healthy weight
- If overweight or obese, limit consumption of high-calorie foods and beverages and increase physical activity to promote weight loss

Engage in regular physical activity
- Avoid inactivity and return to normal daily activities as soon as possible after diagnosis
- Aim to exercise at least 150 min/week
- Include strength training exercises at least 2 days/week

Achieve a dietary pattern that is high in vegetables, fruits, and whole grains
- Follow the American Cancer Society Guidelines on Nutrition and Physical Activity for Cancer Prevention: limit consumption of processed meat and red meat; eat at least 2.5 cups of vegetables and fruits daily; choose whole grains instead of refined grain products; and, if you drink alcoholic beverages, limit consumption to no more than one drink daily for women or two drinks daily for men

Source: Demark-Wahnefried W *et al.* Practical clinical interventions for diet, physical activity, and weight control in cancer survivors. CA: a cancer journal for clinicians 2015;65(3):167–89. Reproduced with permission of John Wiley & Sons.

healing, postoperative infections, and lymphedema. Several common comorbid illnesses (e.g., cardiovascular disease, cerebrovascular disease, and diabetes) and poor functional status are associated with obesity [6, 12]. Obesity also places survivors at greater risk for developing second primary malignancies [13]. These comorbidities are particularly relevant to survivors of certain types of early-stage cancer with a favorable prognosis, who may be more likely to die of comorbid conditions than from recurrent cancer. Furthermore, weight-dependent comorbidities such as diabetes may double the risk of recurrence and death from breast cancer among women initially diagnosed with early stage breast cancer [14].

Most studies of interventions for weight loss among cancer survivors have been single-institution studies with fewer than 100 subjects, and with a few exceptions [15, 16], tend to be limited to breast cancer survivors. These studies have generally focused on the intervention's feasibility and on quality of life and other patient-reported outcomes.

Available evidence supports the feasibility, safety, and benefits of weight loss interventions in cancer populations [16–22]. Reeves *et al.* conducted a systematic review of 14 weight loss trials among breast cancer survivors and observed no adverse events [23]. The vast majority of reported weight loss intervention studies found that cancer patients/survivors can lose at least 5% of initial body weight within a reasonable time frame (<12 months). This amount of weight loss exceeds the 3% threshold associated with a clinically meaningful reduction in cardiovascular risk factors [24], and within the 5–10% range in which greater clinical benefits are observed [25]. In the Exercise and Nutrition to Enhance Recovery and Good health for You (ENERGY) trial among 692 breast cancer survivors, Rock *et al.* found that a group-based weight loss intervention that promoted a weight loss of 6.0% of body weight, as compared to an attention control that resulted in a weight loss of 1.5%, produced significant decreases in both diastolic and systolic blood pressure [26]. Improvements in quality of life and other patient-reported outcomes have been reported, especially with

combined diet plus physical activity interventions. Weight loss interventions for oncology populations can also improve biomarkers linked to cancer risk and outcomes [18, 27, 28].

Interventions have examined a variety of dietary patterns, individually or together with a physical activity component. Results from studies in healthy populations indicate that although caloric restriction is essential for weight loss, exercise and counseling to promote and support behavior change also are required to maintain weight loss long term [25]. Far fewer studies have been conducted in cancer populations, but their results [20, 29] support an important role for exercise and other physical activity in helping survivors achieve and maintain a healthy body weight [30, 31]. In addition, exercise (especially resistance training) can help cancer survivors avoid loss of lean mass that otherwise could accompany weight loss, and is of particular concern for cancer survivors who already may be at risk for chemotherapy-induced or hormonal therapy-induced sarcopenia [32–35].

Guidelines of the American College of Cardiology, the American Heart Association, and The Obesity Society for managing overweight and obesity in the general population of adults do not endorse specific dietary patterns, and emphasize the combination of energy restriction, regular exercise, and behavior modification [25]. In the absence of evidence indicating otherwise, this approach can be reasonably generalized to include most cancer survivors.

Most weight loss studies of cancer survivors to date have enrolled participants after the completion of adjuvant therapy, and most have used short-term interventions. Two notable exceptions are the Reach-out to Enhance Wellness in Older Cancer Survivors (RENEW) and the Lifestyle Intervention in Adjuvant Treatment of Early Breast Cancer (LISA, women with breast cancer receiving letrozole) RCTs, both of which tested distance-based weight loss interventions and demonstrated long-term durability of weight loss [20, 31]. More evidence is needed to optimize effectiveness and cost-effectiveness of weight loss interventions for cancer survivors, with regard to optimal timing (beginning during active treatment or at specific time points thereafter), as well as delivery channel and method (in-person [via individual or group based counseling], telephone counseling, mailed tailored print, or web-based approaches).

Physical Activity

ACS guideline recommendation: engage in regular physical activity

Avoid inactivity and return to normal daily activities as soon as possible following diagnosis; aim to exercise at least 150 min per week; and include strength training exercises at least 2 days per week.

Numerous observational studies support an inverse association between physical activity after a cancer diagnosis and mortality, especially for breast and colon cancer [36, 37]. Increased physical activity also provides many other benefits. The combination of aerobic exercise and resistance training is associated with lower risk and/or better control of cardiovascular disease, osteoporosis, and diabetes, all three of which are common comorbidities of cancer survivors [1, 38]. In addition, some (but not all) studies suggest that the survival benefit of physical activity may interact synergistically with dietary factors, such as the consumption of fruits and vegetables [39–41].

Exercise interventions have resulted in multiple health benefits in several cancer survivor groups [42–48]. Small-to-moderate benefits have been noted in cardiorespiratory fitness [49], muscular strength [50], physical functioning [46], fatigue [51], depression [52], self-esteem [48], and quality of life [53]. There is limited evidence of benefit regarding bone health, muscle mass, peripheral neuropathy, pain, sexual functioning, menopausal symptoms, cognitive function, and sleep [36, 54–62]. Studies of physical activity in cancer patients and survivors demonstrate improvements in levels of various metabolic and immunological biomarkers [63–66] that are reasonable surrogate endpoints for cancer growth and recurrence [36].

Evidence for these benefits is strongest for survivors of breast cancer and prostate cancer [45, 67] whereas other cancer survivor groups remain understudied [35, 55–61, 68–82]. Although exercise during active treatment can be beneficial [46], therapeutic effects may be greater (or adherence improved) after primary treatment [46, 48, 49, 62].

To date, there are no data from adequately powered RCTs testing the effect of increased physical activity after cancer diagnosis on the risk of cancer recurrence or mortality. Although some RCTs in progress are expected to provide relevant evidence [83, 84], additional research is needed. However, at this time, evidence that physical activity can have a beneficial effect on some symptoms of cancer and some side effects of cancer treatment, and that it decreases risk and severity of several common comorbid conditions, seems sufficient to recommend that regular physical activity should be routinely prescribed in cancer populations [1]. An important caveat is that some survivors with ongoing issues such as peripheral neuropathy and resulting balance problems may not safely exercise alone and should be prescribed physical therapy or other cancer rehabilitation interventions prior to initiating lifestyle change.

Additional research is needed to determine the most effective interventions for increasing physical activity among cancer survivors. Reviews of available evidence indicate that the more effective interventions included clearly-stated physical activity goals, generalization of supervised exercise into unsupervised settings, and regular prompting to self-monitor and practice [42]. A simple recommendation by an oncologist can motivate cancer survivors to increase their physical activity [72], as can the provision of print materials [68, 69, 85], particularly if combined with the distribution of a pedometer [68, 69].

Diet Quality

ACS guideline recommendation: achieve a dietary pattern that is high in vegetables, fruits, and whole grains
Follow the American Cancer Society Guidelines on Nutrition and Physical Activity for Cancer Prevention [86]: limit consumption of processed meat and red meat; eat at least 2.5 cups of vegetables and fruits each day; choose whole grains instead of refined grain products; and, if you drink alcoholic beverages, limit consumption to no more than one drink per day for women or two drinks per day for men.

A 2012 meta-analysis evaluating 11 prospective cohort studies indicated that cancer-specific mortality was 22% lower in adults who reported good adherence to dietary guidelines, relative to those who reported poor adherence [87]. Guidelines-based diets, also called prudent diets, that are high in fruits, vegetables, and unrefined grains, and low in red and processed meats, refined grains, and sugars are recommended over "Western" diets that have the opposite pattern and are high in meats, sweets, other processed foods, and dietary fat. To date, four observational studies have compared overall and disease-free survival among cancer survivors who report the consumption of guidelines-based diets versus Western diets. In all three studies of breast cancer cohorts, prudent diets were associated with significantly reduced risk for overall and/or noncancer-related mortality, with reductions that ranged from 15 to 43% [88–90]. In the fourth study, conducted in a sample of patients with stage III colorectal cancer, the prudent diet did not extend overall survival or cancer-specific survival; however, the Western diet was associated with higher cancer-specific and overall mortality rates that were two or three times higher than the rates among patients who did not consume Western diets [91]. These studies suggest that Western diets increase the risk for overall mortality and deaths from causes other than cancer for a broad spectrum of cancer survivors and may increase disease-specific mortality from some cancer types [92].

Two large RCTs have studied whether dietary pattern interventions in women after a breast cancer diagnosis influence their risk of cancer recurrence and mortality. In the Women's Intervention Nutrition Study (WINS), 2437 women with early stage breast cancer who were within 1 year of surgery and had completed primary cancer therapy were randomized to receive counseling and support either on a nutritionally adequate diet or on a nutritionally adequate low-fat diet [93]. Participants who were randomized to the low-fat diet lost an average of 2.7 kg over the 5-year study period. Breast cancer recurrence was reduced by 24% (HR, 0.76; 95% CI, 0.60–0.98) compared with controls. The Women's Healthy Eating and Living (WHEL) study randomized 3088 women who were within 4 years of their diagnosis of early stage breast cancer to a 4-year intervention that promoted five servings of fruits and vegetables daily through mailed print educational materials versus an intervention that promoted 10 servings of fruits and vegetables per day (30 g/day of fiber) combined with a low-fat diet through mailed print materials, group classes, and telephone counseling [94]. The intervention was successful in promoting dietary change, but without weight loss, and without any impact on rates of cancer recurrence after a mean follow-up of 7.3 years. It has been hypothesized that the differences in outcomes of these two trials resulted from: the lack of weight loss among WHEL study participants; the timing of intervention (i.e., within 4 years of diagnosis vs within a year of surgery); ceiling effects due to the high-quality diet and reported consumption of 7.4 servings per day of fruits and vegetables of WHEL participants at baseline; and/or changes in breast cancer therapy, including the widespread use of selective estrogen receptor modulators over the long course of these two trials.

Dietary interventions have been studied in several smaller groups of prostate cancer survivors [95]. For example, a phase 2 study of 161 men who were scheduled for prostatectomy compared the effects of a low-fat diet and/or flaxseed supplementation on the proliferation rate (based on Ki-67 expression) of the resected tumors. Tumors from men in the flaxseed-supplementation arms manifested significantly lower proportions of proliferating cells [96]. Several dietary intervention studies in men electing active surveillance for low-grade localized disease have been completed; none slowed the rates of prostate cancer progression, as measured by prostate-specific antigen levels. Additional studies are currently examining the impact of dietary change on cancer outcomes in prostate cancer. One such study is enrolling patients with clinically localized prostate cancer undergoing active surveillance, and testing the impact of a telephone-based dietary intervention designed to increase vegetable intake on clinical progression (defined by prostate-specific antigen levels or prostate biopsy) [97].

Healthy Lifestyle

Recommendation: concomitant or sequential weight reduction, improvements in dietary quality, and increased physical activity

There is evidence for synergy among weight control, physical activity, high diet quality, and other healthy lifestyle behaviors. Several studies have found that composite scores based on adherence to health behavior guidelines set by the ACS [1, 86] or the World Cancer Research Fund/American Institute for Cancer Research [92] are associated with significant reductions in incidence ranging from 16 to 60% for individuals with the highest as compared to the lowest adherence to these guidelines [95–100]. Healthy lifestyles also have favorable effects on cancer-specific and/or all-cause mortality [96, 101–103]. McCullough *et al.* observed that men and women who adhered to more of the ACS recommendations (scores of 7–8), in comparison with those who adhered to fewer recommendations (scores of 0–2) had significantly lower rates of cancer-related mortality (range, 24–30%), lower all-cause mortality (42%), and lower cardiovascular disease mortality (range, 48–58%) [104]. To date, only one research team has investigated associations between broad patterns of health behaviors and health outcomes of cancer survivors. In a study of postmenopausal breast cancer survivors, Inoue-Choi *et al.* [105] observed a 33% lower mortality rate in women who were most adherent, as compared with those who were least adherent, to the American Institute for Cancer Research/World Cancer Research Fund guidelines [106].

Because of the importance placed on both diet and exercise in managing obesity, diabetes, and cardiovascular disease [107–110] (all three of which are common comorbidities among cancer survivors), several clinical trials of cancer survivors have included both elements. Weight loss is not the only goal of dietary or physical activity interventions; a healthy diet and a physically active lifestyle are still beneficial even in individuals of a healthy weight or in those who are overweight or have obesity if weight loss does not occur. Of the five largest studies of diet and physical activity interventions for cancer survivors [85, 111–113], all but one [114] produced significant improvements in either or both behaviors, as well as in other important outcomes, such as physical functioning [113] and obesity [85].

Lifestyle Behaviors Among Cancer Survivors

Obesity, inactivity, and the ingestion of poor-quality diets are common in cancer survivors [115–117]. Among the 9105 survivors of breast, prostate, colorectal, uterine, bladder, and melanoma skin cancers participating in the ACS Study of Cancer Survivors-II [115], only 14.8–19.1% of survivors consumed at least five daily servings of fruits and vegetables and only 29.6–47.3% of survivors engaged in at least 150 min of moderate-intensity physical activity or 60 min of vigorous physical activity per week. Similar results were found in studies using the National Health Interview Survey [117] and the Canadian Community Health Survey [116]. Among participants in the Nurses' Health Study who developed either breast or colon cancer, only 39% of breast cancer survivors [118] and 42% of colon cancer survivors [119] engaged in at least 150 min of moderate-intensity physical activity or 60 min of strenuous physical activity.

Because most prospective cohort studies collect information regarding lifestyle factors at several time points, these studies can identify changes in these behaviors that occur after cancer diagnosis. For example, among the cohort of 1183 women with early stage breast cancer participating in the Health, Eating, Activity, and Lifestyle (HEAL) study, it was observed that women decreased their total physical activity by approximately 2 h per week (11% of total activity) after diagnosis [120]. Although a decrease in activity, especially among women who received chemotherapy and radiation therapy is not surprising, that study also demonstrated that half of study participants did not return to baseline levels of physical activity even 3 years after diagnosis. The HEAL study also found that 68% of participants gained weight (an average weight gain of 1.7 kg) over the 3 years following diagnosis [121]. Participants in the Nurses' Health Study also tended to gain weight after their breast cancer diagnosis, with 45% of survivors reporting gaining weight [122]. Given evidence that normal-weight patients who remain so after diagnosis are at lowest risk for recurrence and all-cause mortality, there is a need for healthcare providers to emphasize the importance of weight control [122, 123].

Implementing Healthy Lifestyle Change in Cancer Survivors

The Role of the Oncologist

A cancer diagnosis may serve as a "teachable moment", that is, a time when patients are motivated to changes health behaviors that they recognize as being associated with the development of their cancer and with increased risk of its progression [124]. For example, in the ACS Study of Cancer Survivors-II, 40% of survivors reported an attempt to undertake positive dietary changes, 35% reported trying to lose weight, and 29% reported exercising more since their cancer diagnosis [125]. However, despite good intentions, survivors may encounter barriers to achieving and sustaining healthy lifestyles, including limited self-efficacy, knowledge, support, and reinforcement.

Research shows that the clear majority of patients with non-small cell lung cancer desired advice regarding physical activity, with 80% identifying a preference for a face-to-face recommendation by a physician, and 92% stating that they preferred this interaction under the auspices of a cancer center [126]. There is little debate that one of the most powerful influences over patients' health-related behavior is the recommendation of their physician, although most of the supporting evidence is from studies of tobacco cessation and cancer screening [72, 127–136]. A national survey of oncologists found that although 62% agreed that exercise was beneficial and safe for their patients, only 42% ever recommended exercise to their patients, and only 26% reported that they recommended exercise to any of their patients within the past month [137]. In addition to time constraints, the oncologists reported a perceived lack of expertise as a major barrier [137]. In response, some resources or "tool kits" have been developed by organizations like the American Society of Clinical Oncology to enhance oncologists' self-efficacy for delivering health-promotion guidance in areas such as weight control (available at: http://www.asco.org/practice-guidelines/cancer-care-initiatives/prevention-survivorship/obesity-cancer, accessed 24 August 2017) [138]. Also, the oncologist and oncology care team can provide appropriate recommendations and referrals as part of comprehensive survivorship care planning [139, 140].

Although simple approaches and one-time "touches" are unlikely to promote large and durable changes in health behavior or body weight [141], some simple interventions and messaging can offer significant benefit. For example, a clinical trial [72] of 450 patients with newly diagnosed breast cancer found that an oncologist's recommendation to exercise increased physical activity by 3.4 metabolic equivalent hours per week (roughly equivalent to an hour of brisk walking). These data indicate that improvements in health behavior of cancer survivors can be achieved by simple and low-cost interventions. Table 23.2 summarizes some common elements of successful interventions (e.g., incremental goal setting, situational and environmental control, and self-monitoring) [35, 142–145] and organizes these concepts into a "5As" framework that has been used successfully in tobacco cessation. Among these five steps, Asking, Advising, and Arranging appear to be most important for the oncologist's role in catalyzing and reinforcing the behavior change (rather than personally overseeing and supporting the process).

Integration of Weight Management Between Oncology and Primary Care Providers

The incorporation of weight management into oncology care will require a partnership between oncology professionals, who often provide the bulk of medical care to cancer patients in the months to years after cancer diagnosis, and nononcology health providers with experience in treatment of obesity as well as specific expertise in nutrition, physical activity, and behavior change. As with many aspects of survivorship care, coordination and collaboration between oncology and primary care providers are essential to effective weight management in cancer survivor populations. Although primary care physicians typically provide weight management counseling and referrals as a

routine part of their practice, many patients do not seek regular medical care from a primary care physician in the years after cancer diagnosis. Thus, attention to weight management may provide an opportunity to facilitate the transition to effective comanagement of survivorship care.

Specialized Care to Improve Diet and Exercise Behaviors

Long-lasting behavior change often requires a level of ongoing support that can be difficult to provide through a physician's office. Unfortunately, reimbursement for longitudinal weight management services for cancer survivors is limited. However, in some settings, consultation or ongoing support may be available to support dietary and physical activity changes by cancer survivors, especially those with obesity-related comorbidities such as diabetes or cardiovascular disease. Because obesity is now considered a "disease", Medicare coverage is available for weight loss counseling by a primary care physician or other qualified practitioner, for patients whose BMIs are $30\,\mathrm{kg/m^2}$ and above (available at: medicare.gov/coverage/obesity-screening-and-counseling.html, accessed 17 August 2017). Survivors who have ongoing issues such as neuropathy and may not be able to exercise safely on their own may benefit from physical therapy interventions prior to initiating lifestyle change. Cancer rehabilitation interventions are usually covered by insurance.

The American College of Surgeons Commission on Cancer standards and the Association of Community Cancer Centers guidelines both recognize nutrition services as an important element of comprehensive cancer care and call for nutrition screening and assessment, care plans, and early nutrition intervention by a nutrition professional [146, 147]. Both of these organizations recognize that the nutrition professional best able to deliver oncologic nutritional care is the registered dietitian or registered dietitian nutritionist and recommend that registered dietitians/registered dietitian nutritionists working within the oncology setting obtain intensive training and certification in oncology nutrition as Certified Specialists in Oncology Nutrition (CSOs) [148]. A directory of CSOs by state can be found online (available at: http://www.eatright.org/find-an-expert, accessed 17 August 2017). Oncologists are encouraged to refer their patients who require guidance on weight management and nutritional issues to CSOs, although reimbursement for this outpatient care (compared with inpatient care, which is covered) varies from state to state and payer to payer, and also depends on the patient's age, weight status, and comorbidities, as well as the practice setting of the professional delivering this care [148, 149].

Physical activity is beneficial to cancer survivors at any point in their disease trajectory, and should therefore be encouraged for all cancer survivors. An expert roundtable convened by the American College of Sports Medicine concluded that although it is always advisable for a patient to check with their physician before initiating an exercise program, moderate-intensity aerobic exercise could be initiated by most cancer survivors (who do not have other serious comorbidities or toxicities such as neuropathy – see below) without stress testing or other extensive evaluation [150].

Some cancer survivors are at higher risk of adverse events from exercise, either as a result of adverse effects from cancer treatment (e.g., peripheral neuropathy, lymphedema) or

Table 23.2 Sample strategies to promote healthy lifestyles.[1]

Step[2]	Weight Control	Diet Quality	Physical Activity
Ask	Have you tried to lose weight recently (ask only if overweight or obese)?	(a) How many servings of vegetables and fruit do you eat each day? (b) How many servings of red and processed meats do you each week? (c) Do you eat white or whole-grain breads and cereals? (d) What dietary supplements do you use?	On average, how many minutes per week do you do aerobic (or cardio) exercise? How many times a week do you do strengthening exercises? How many hours per day do you spend sitting or watching TV?
Advise	This chart (show Body Mass Index chart) is used to graph people's height and weight to determine whether people are at a healthy weight. That is of concern to me, since I am providing you with cancer treatment that is aimed at prolonging your life. But, if your weight is too high you may be at greater risk for complications that occur later on (lymphedema, heart disease, diabetes, etc.). Therefore, it is important that you lose weight.	Positively reinforce patients if their answers are (a) five or more servings; (b) two or more servings; (c) whole grain; and (d) dietary supplement use is minimal or used to treat a deficiency condition, such as osteoporosis or anemia (not an excessive dose, i.e., within 100% of daily values); if the answers differ, advise that they should be consuming a plant-based diet in which they eat at least five servings of vegetables and fruit per day and no more than two servings of red or processed meat per week and that they should eat whole grain products instead of refined products; moreover, they are to rely on their diets, rather than supplements, to provide needed nutrients.	Positively reinforce patients if they do aerobic exercise for at least 150 min a week or strength training exercises at least twice a week; if not, advise that they should strive to do so; refer to a trained exercise professional for help in initiating strength training if they have lymphedema, colostomy, or other relevant condition; encourage patients to reduce sitting time.
Assess	Losing weight can be hard, but it is important and I am sure that you could do it if you tried – are you ready to lose weight?	Eating a healthy diet is important – are you willing to make a few changes?	Regular exercise is important – are you willing to start?
Assist	If yes... "Great, let me give you this brochure (see resource list), which will help get you on your way"; use tips from Assist and Arrange (below) If no... "OK, but the next time we meet, I will ask again; in the meantime, I want you to read this brochure and just try to do (choose one strategy from Assist items 2 through 5 below)." (1) Set a start date: "Although it would be good to start right away, it is more important to get a good solid start than a fast start; think about any special events in the next week or two, and give yourself time to buy foods that make it easier to diet...lots of raw vegetables and other low calorie foods; look at the calendar—when can you start?" (2) Incremental change: the journey to weight loss goes one step at a time, and even small changes in your diet can make a big difference on the scale over time, for example substituting diet soft drinks or water for regular soft drinks, the use of milk and sweetener in coffee or tea instead of cream (creamer) and sugar.	If yes... "Great, let me give you this brochure (see resource list), which will help get you on your way"; use tips from Assist and Arrange (below) If no... "OK, but the next time we meet, I will ask again; in the meantime, I want you to read this brochure and just try to do (choose one strategy from Assist items 2 through 5 below)." (1) Over the next week, and at every time you eat, ask the question, "Am I making food choices that are healthy?" (2) Incremental change: small changes over time can make a big difference in diet quality, for example, substituting whole grain bread, like whole wheat, rye, or pumpernickel, for white bread; eating brown rice or whole grain pasta instead of white rice or pasta; or snacking on baby carrots, celery sticks, radishes, or cherry tomatoes instead of other things.	If yes... "Great, let me give you this brochure (see resource list), which will help get you on your way"; use tips from Assist and Arrange (below) If no... "OK, but the next time we meet, I will ask again; in the meantime, I want you to read this brochure and just try to do (choose one strategy from Assist items 2 through 5 below)." (1) Set a start date: "It's important to get more physical activity, and walking works for most people. What sort of exercise works best for you—when can you start?" (if interested in strength training, consider referral to trained exercise professional for assistance in proper form and correct choice of exercises) (2) Incremental change: start slowly and then build up, for example, start with 10 min of < walking or other exercise > every day, then add 5 min a day the following week, and so on.

(3) Environmental control examples: taking the stairs instead of the elevator; parking in more distant spaces and walking in; and walking or bicycling to places that are less than a mile away.

(4) Situational control examples: making a point to stand up during TV commercials and move around; and having an exercise buddy (social support) who will accompany you on walks.

(5) Self-monitoring: (a) track the number of minutes you exercise each day and record it on a calendar; (b) wear a pedometer and track the number of steps you take each day, record it on a calendar, and gradually work toward a goal of 10,000 steps per day.

(3) Environmental control examples: making a point to read the label and purchasing fresh and dried fruit for dessert instead of cookies and cakes.

(4) Situational control examples: ordering vegetables or salads instead of potatoes when dining-out; bringing healthy foods to potlucks and parties instead of chips and baked goods; and making a point to always include a vegetable, fruit, nuts, or whole grains when eating a meal or snack.

(5) Self-monitoring: track the number of servings of fruits and vegetables you eat on a daily basis; record it on a calendar.

(3) Environmental control examples: refraining from bringing tempting foods into the home or workplace, storing all food in the pantry or refrigerator (rid the home or office of candy dishes), and limiting eating out to at most once a week.

(4) Situational control examples: plating food at the stove (no serving dishes at the table); and putting down your fork or spoon between bites and savoring the flavors.

(5) Self-monitoring: (a) weigh once a day – record it on a calendar; (b) BEFORE eating anything, record it on paper or use a web-based program (see resource list).

Arrange   Refer to primary care provider
Refer to registered dietitian
Refer to certified exercise professional, for example physiatrist, physical therapist, exercise physiologist

Source: Demark-Wahnefried W *et al.* Practical clinical interventions for diet, physical activity, and weight control in cancer survivors. CA: a cancer journal for clinicians 2015;65(3):167–89. Reproduced with permission of John Wiley & Sons.

[1] Adapted from: Five Major Steps to Intervention (The "5 A's"). Rockville, MD: Agency for Healthcare Research and Quality: 2012. Available at: http://www.ahrq.gov/professionals/clinicians-providers/guidelines-recommendations/tobacco/5steps.html (accessed 17 August 2017).

[2] Steps set in bold text (Ask, Advise, and Arrange) are key points of action for the oncologist.

comorbidities, and some patients will desire to initiate programs that involve more vigorous exercise or carry a higher risk of injury. In these settings, evaluation is ideally undertaken by a healthcare provider with specialized knowledge in exercise physiology and advanced knowledge and skills in cancer rehabilitation [139, 150, 151], with referral to specialized medical or physical therapy interventions. These survivors also may benefit from working with exercise trainers who have cancer expertise. The American College of Sports Medicine allows a wide array of healthcare professionals, as well as athletic trainers and other certified American College of Sports Medicine fitness providers, to participate in their Certified Cancer Exercise Trainer program [152]. This program provides exercise professionals with a better understanding of the impact of cancer treatment side effects on an exercise program. More advanced rehabilitative services can be provided by a physiatrist (a physician who specializes in rehabilitation medicine) or by an occupational or physical therapist. The Oncology Section of the American Physical Therapy Association grants certification to licensed physical therapists who demonstrate specialized knowledge and skills in oncology by offering a Certificate of Achievement in Oncology Physical Therapy. A board certification exam in Oncology rehabilitation which emphasizes exercise physiology, exercise education, and promotion of healthy lifestyles will be available for physical therapists by 2017 [149].

Resources for the Oncology Care Community and the Cancer Survivor

Resources aimed at providing support for both the nutritional and exercise needs of cancer survivors include private agencies and healthcare institutions. However, there is substantial variation in access to and quality of these programs. For this reason, consideration of credentialing as covered in the previous sections can help the oncologist and the patient to select safe and effective resources. Of note, many cancer survivors, especially those who are no longer undergoing active treatment or experiencing significant late effects, can benefit from more broadly administered weight loss programs [153, 154].

Conclusion

The number of cancer survivors is growing rapidly. The Institute of Medicine endorses the importance of weight management, physical activity, and a healthy diet as important components of delivering quality cancer care and as important components of a plan for survivorship care [140, 142]. More research is needed to further define the benefits of lifestyle changes in cancer survivors and to evaluate the most efficacious interventions, and the populations most likely to benefit as well as those who need specialized interventions. However, these gaps in evidence should not distract clinicians from recognizing the importance of routine assessment of lifestyle behavior in cancer patients/survivors, reassessment at regular intervals, and advice and arrangement to optimize the likelihood that all cancer patients will engage in efforts to improve their diet and physical activity.

Disclosures: Dr Demark-Wahnefried was supported by grant CRP-14-111-01-CPPB, and Dr Kvale was supported by grant 121093-CCCDA-11-191-01-CCCDA from the American Cancer Society.

References

1 Rock CL, Doyle C, Demark-Wahnefried W, *et al.* Nutrition and physical activity guidelines for cancer survivors. *CA Cancer J Clin* 2012;62:243–74.

2 Li CI, Daling JR, Porter PL, Tang MT, Malone KE. Relationship between potentially modifiable lifestyle factors and risk of second primary contralateral breast cancer among women diagnosed with estrogen receptor-positive invasive breast cancer. *J Clin Oncol* 2009;27:5312–18.

3 Efstathiou JA, Bae K, Shipley WU, *et al.* Obesity and mortality in men with locally advanced prostate cancer: analysis of RTOG 85–31. *Cancer* 2007;110:2691–9.

4 Majed B, Dozol A, Ribassin-Majed L, Senouci K, Asselain B. Increased risk of contralateral breast cancers among overweight and obese women: a time-dependent association. *Breast Cancer Res Treat* 2011;126:729–38.

5 Druesne-Pecollo N, Touvier M, Barrandon E, *et al.* Excess body weight and second primary cancer risk after breast cancer: a systematic review and meta-analysis of prospective studies. *Breast Cancer Res Treat* 2012;135:647–54.

6 Ligibel JA, Alfano CM, Courneya KS, *et al.* American Society of Clinical Oncology Position Statement on Obesity and Cancer. *J Clin Oncol* 2014;32:3568–74.

7 Chan DS, Vieira AR, Aune D, *et al.* Body mass index and survival in women with breast cancer-systematic literature review and meta-analysis of 82 follow-up studies. *Ann Oncol* 2014;25:1901–14.

8 Cao Y, Ma J. Body mass index, prostate cancer-specific mortality, and biochemical recurrence: a systematic review and meta-analysis. *Cancer Prev Res (Phila)* 2011; 4:486–501.

9 Wu S, Liu J, Wang X, Li M, Gan Y, Tang Y. Association of obesity and overweight with overall survival in colorectal cancer patients: a meta-analysis of 29 studies. *Cancer Causes Control* 2014;25:1489–502.

10 Parekh N, Chandran U, Bandera EV. Obesity in cancer survival. *Annu Rev Nutr* 2012;32:311–42.

11 Arem H, Irwin ML. Obesity and endometrial cancer survival: a systematic review. *Int J Obes (Lond)* 2013;37:634–39.

12 Bennett JA, Winters-Stone KM, Dobek J, Nail LM. Frailty in older breast cancer survivors: age, prevalence, and associated factors. *Oncol Nurs Forum* 2013;40:E126–34.

13 Travis LB, Demark Wahnefried W, Allan JM, Wood ME, Ng AK. Aetiology, genetics and prevention of secondary neoplasms in adult cancer survivors. *Nat Rev Clin Oncol* 2013;10:289–301.

14 Patterson RE, Flatt SW, Saquib N, *et al.* Medical comorbidities predict mortality in women with a history of early stage breast cancer. *Breast Cancer Res Treat* 2010;122:859–65.

15 von Gruenigen V, Frasure H, Kavanagh MB, *et al*. Survivors of uterine cancer empowered by exercise and healthy diet (SUCCEED): a randomized controlled trial. *Gynecol Oncol* 2012;125:699–704.

16 Morey MC, Snyder DC, Sloane R, *et al*. Effects of home-based diet and exercise on functional outcomes among older, overweight long-term cancer survivors: RENEW: a randomized controlled trial. *JAMA* 2009;301:1883–91.

17 Sedlacek SM, Playdon MC, Wolfe P, *et al*. Effect of a low fat versus a low carbohydrate weight loss dietary intervention on biomarkers of long term survival in breast cancer patients ('CHOICE'): study protocol. *BMC Cancer* 2011;11:287.

18 Thompson HJ, Sedlacek SM, Paul D, *et al*. Effect of dietary patterns differing in carbohydrate and fat content on blood lipid and glucose profiles based on weight-loss success of breast-cancer survivors. *Breast Cancer Res* 2012;14:R1.

19 de Waard F, Ramlau R, Mulders Y, de Vries T, van Waveren S. A feasibility study on weight reduction in obese postmenopausal breast cancer patients. *Eur J Cancer Prev* 1993;2:233–8.

20 Goodwin PJ, Segal RJ, Vallis M, *et al*. Randomized trial of a telephone-based weight loss intervention in postmenopausal women with breast cancer receiving letrozole: the LISA trial. *J Clin Oncol* 2014;32:2231–9.

21 Snyder DC, Morey MC, Sloane R, *et al*. Reach out to ENhancE Wellness in Older Cancer Survivors (RENEW): design, methods and recruitment challenges of a home-based exercise and diet intervention to improve physical function among long-term survivors of breast, prostate, and colorectal cancer. *Psychooncology* 2009;18:429–39.

22 Demark-Wahnefried W, Morey MC, Sloane R, *et al*. Reach out to enhance wellness home-based diet-exercise intervention promotes reproducible and sustainable long-term improvements in health behaviors, body weight, and physical functioning in older, overweight/obese cancer survivors. *J Clin Oncol* 2012;30:2354–61.

23 Reeves MM, Terranova CO, Eakin EG, Demark-Wahnefried W. Weight loss intervention trials in women with breast cancer: a systematic review. *Obes Rev* 2014;15:749–68.

24 Jensen MD, Ryan DH, Apovian CM, *et al* 2013 AHA/ACC/TOS guideline for the management of overweight and obesity in adults: a report of the American College of Cardiology/American Heart Association Task Force on Practice Guidelines and The Obesity Society. *J Am Coll Cardiol* 2014;63:2985–3023.

25 Jensen MD RD, Donato KA, Apovian CM, *et al*. Guidelines (2013) for managing overweight and obesity in adults. *Obesity* 2014;22:S1–S410.

26 Rock CL, Flatt SW, Byers TE, *et al*. Results of the Exercise and Nutrition to Enhance Recovery and Good Health for You (ENERGY) trial: a behavioral weight loss intervention in overweight or obese breast cancer survivors. *J Clin Oncol* 2015;33:3169–76.

27 Jen KL, Djuric Z, DiLaura NM, *et al*. Improvement of metabolism among obese breast cancer survivors in differing weight loss regimens. *Obes Res* 2004;12:306–12.

28 Thomson CA, Stopeck AT, Bea JW, *et al*. Changes in body weight and metabolic indexes in overweight breast cancer survivors enrolled in a randomized trial of low-fat vs. reduced carbohydrate diets. *Nutr Cancer* 2010;62:1142–52.

29 Goodwin P, Esplen MJ, Butler K, *et al*. Multidisciplinary weight management in locoregional breast cancer: results of a phase II study. *Breast Cancer Res Treat* 1998;48:53–64.

30 Knobf MT, Winters-Stone K. Exercise and cancer. *Annu Rev Nurs Res* 2013;31:327–65.

31 Demark-Wahnefried W, Platz EA, Ligibel JA, *et al*. The role of obesity in cancer survival and recurrence. *Cancer Epidemiol Biomarkers Prev* 2012;21:1244–59.

32 Weinheimer EM, Sands LP, Campbell WW. A systematic review of the separate and combined effects of energy restriction and exercise on fat-free mass in middle-aged and older adults: implications for sarcopenic obesity. *Nutr Rev* 2010;68:375–88.

33 Demark-Wahnefried W, Campbell KL, Hayes SC. Weight management and its role in breast cancer rehabilitation. *Cancer* 2012;118:2277–87.

34 Demark-Wahnefried W, Peterson BL, Winer EP, *et al*. Changes in weight, body composition, and factors influencing energy balance among premenopausal breast cancer patients receiving adjuvant chemotherapy. *J Clin Oncol* 2001;19:2381–9.

35 Vallance JK, Courneya KS, Plotnikoff RC, Mackey JR. Analyzing theoretical mechanisms of physical activity behavior change in breast cancer survivors: results from the activity promotion (ACTION) trial. *Ann Behav Med* 2008;35:150–8.

36 Ballard-Barbash R, Friedenreich CM, *et al*. Physical activity, biomarkers, and disease outcomes in cancer survivors:a systematic review. *J Natl Cancer Inst* 2012;104:815–40.

37 Schmid D, Leitzmann MF. Association between physical activity and mortality among breast cancer and colorectal cancer survivors: a systematic review and meta-analysis. *Ann Oncol* 2014;25:1293–311.

38 Sturgeon KM, Ky B, Libonati JR, Schmitz KH. The effects of exercise on cardiovascular outcomes before, during, and after treatment for breast cancer. *Breast Cancer Res Treat* 2014;143:219–26.

39 George SM, Irwin ML, Smith AW, *et al*. Postdiagnosis diet quality, the combination of diet quality and recreational physical activity, and prognosis after early-stage breast cancer. *Cancer Causes Control* 2011;22:589–98.

40 Pierce JP, Stefanick ML, Flatt SW, *et al*. Greater survival after breast cancer in physically active women with high vegetable-fruit intake regardless of obesity. *J Clin Oncol* 2007;25:2345–51.

41 Kim EH, Willett WC, Fung T, Rosner B, Holmes MD. Diet quality indices and postmenopausal breast cancer survival. *Nutr Cancer* 2011;63:381–8.

42 Bourke L, Homer KE, Thaha MA, *et al*. Interventions for promoting habitual exercise in people living with and beyond cancer. *Cochrane Database Syst Rev* 2013;9:Cd010192.

43 Braam KI, van der Torre P, Takken T, *et al*. Physical exercise training interventions for children and young adults during and after treatment for childhood cancer. *Cochrane Database Syst Rev* 2013;4:CD008796.

44 Khan F, Amatya B, Ng L, *et al*. Multidisciplinary rehabilitation for follow-up of women treated for breast cancer. *Cochrane Database Syst Rev* 2012;12:CD009553.

45 McNeely ML, Campbell KL, Rowe BH, *et al*. Effects of exercise on breast cancer patients and survivors: a systematic review and meta-analysis. *CMAJ* 2006;175:34–41.

46 Mishra SI, Scherer RW, Geigle PM, *et al.* Exercise interventions on health-related quality of life for cancer survivors. *Cochrane Database Syst Rev* 2012;8:CD007566.

47 Schmitz KH, Holtzman J, Courneya KS, *et al.* Controlled physical activity trials in cancer survivors: a systematic review and meta-analysis. *Cancer Epidemiol Biomarkers Prev* 2005;14:1588–95.

48 Speck RM, Courneya KS, Masse LC, Duval S, Schmitz KH. An update of controlled physical activity trials in cancer survivors: a systematic review and meta-analysis. *J Cancer Surviv* 2010;4:87–100.

49 Jones LW, Liang Y, Pituskin EN, *et al.* Effect of exercise training on peak oxygen consumption in patients with cancer: a meta-analysis. *Oncologist* 2011;16:112–20.

50 Stene GB, Helbostad JL, Balstad TR, Riphagen, II, Kaasa S, Oldervoll LM. Effect of physical exercise on muscle mass and strength in cancer patients during treatment – a systematic review. *Crit Rev Oncol Hematol* 2013;88:573–93.

51 Puetz TW, Herring MP. Differential effects of exercise on cancer-related fatigue during and following treatment: a meta-analysis. *Am J Prev Med* 2012;43:e1–24.

52 Brown JC, Huedo-Medina TB, Pescatello LS, *et al.* The efficacy of exercise in reducing depressive symptoms among cancer survivors: a meta-analysis. *PLoS One* 2012;7:e30955.

53 Ferrer RA, Huedo-Medina TB, Johnson BT, Ryan S, Pescatello LS. Exercise interventions for cancer survivors: a meta-analysis of quality of life outcomes. *Ann Behav Med* 2011;41:32–47.

54 Courneya KS, Segal RJ, Mackey JR, *et al.* Effects of exercise dose and type on sleep quality in breast cancer patients receiving chemotherapy: a multicenter randomized trial. *Breast Cancer Res Treat* 2014;144:361–9.

55 Jacobsen PB, Le-Rademacher J, Jim H, *et al.* Exercise and Stress Management Training Prior to Hematopoietic Cell Transplantation: Blood and Marrow Transplant Clinical Trials Network (BMT CTN) 0902. *Biol Blood Marrow Transplant* 2014;20:1530–6.

56 Midtgaard J, Christensen JF, Tolver A, *et al.* Efficacy of multimodal exercise-based rehabilitation on physical activity, cardiorespiratory fitness, and patient-reported outcomes in cancer survivors: a randomized, controlled trial. *Ann Oncol* 2013;24:2267–73.

57 Mutrie N, Campbell AM, Whyte F, *et al.* Benefits of supervised group exercise programme for women being treated for early stage breast cancer: pragmatic randomised controlled trial. *BMJ* 2007;334:517.

58 Winters-Stone KM, Laudermilk M, Woo K, Brown JC, Schmitz KH. Influence of weight training on skeletal health of breast cancer survivors with or at risk for breast cancer-related lymphedema. *J Cancer Surviv* 2014;8:260–8.

59 Saarto T, Sievanen H, Kellokumpu-Lehtinen P, *et al.* Effect of supervised and home exercise training on bone mineral density among breast cancer patients. A 12-month randomised controlled trial. *Osteoporos Int* 2012;23:1601–12.

60 Hayes SC, Rye S, Disipio T, *et al.* Exercise for health: a randomized, controlled trial evaluating the impact of a pragmatic, translational exercise intervention on the quality of life, function and treatment-related side effects following breast cancer. *Breast Cancer Res Treat* 2013;137:175–86.

61 Speck RM, Gross CR, Hormes JM, *et al.* Changes in the Body Image and Relationship Scale following a one-year strength training trial for breast cancer survivors with or at risk for lymphedema. *Breast Cancer Res Treat* 2010;121:421–30.

62 Demark-Wahnefried W, Case LD, Blackwell K, *et al.* Results of a diet/exercise feasibility trial to prevent adverse body composition change in breast cancer patients on adjuvant chemotherapy. *Clin Breast Cancer* 2008;8:70–9.

63 Irwin ML, Varma K, Alvarez-Reeves M, *et al.* Randomized controlled trial of aerobic exercise on insulin and insulin-like growth factors in breast cancer survivors: the Yale Exercise and Survivorship study. *Cancer Epidemiol Biomarkers Prev* 2009;18:306–13.

64 Lee DH, Kim JY, Lee MK, *et al.* Effects of a 12-week home-based exercise program on the level of physical activity, insulin, and cytokines in colorectal cancer survivors: a pilot study. *Support Care Cancer* 2013;21:2537–45.

65 Ligibel JA, Campbell N, Partridge A, *et al.* Impact of a mixed strength and endurance exercise intervention on insulin levels in breast cancer survivors. *J Clin Oncol* 2008;26:907–12.

66 Lof M, Bergstrom K, Weiderpass E. Physical activity and biomarkers in breast cancer survivors: a systematic review. *Maturitas* 2012;73:134–42.

67 Baumann FT, Zopf EM, Bloch W. Clinical exercise interventions in prostate cancer patients – a systematic review of randomized controlled trials. *Support Care Cancer* 2012;20:221–33.

68 Vallance JK, Courneya KS, Plotnikoff RC, Dinu I, Mackey JR. Maintenance of physical activity in breast cancer survivors after a randomized trial. *Med Sci Sports Exerc* 2008;40:173–80.

69 Vallance JK, Courneya KS, Plotnikoff RC, Yasui Y, Mackey JR. Randomized controlled trial of the effects of print materials and step pedometers on physical activity and quality of life in breast cancer survivors. *J Clin Oncol* 2007;25:2352–9.

70 Courneya KS, McKenzie DC, Gelmon K, *et al.* A multicenter randomized trial of the effects of exercise dose and type on psychosocial distress in breast cancer patients undergoing chemotherapy. *Cancer Epidemiol Biomarkers Prev* 2014;23:857–64.

71 Duijts SF, van Beurden M, Oldenburg HS, *et al.* Efficacy of cognitive behavioral therapy and physical exercise in alleviating treatment-induced menopausal symptoms in patients with breast cancer: results of a randomized, controlled, multicenter trial. *J Clin Oncol* 2012;30:4124–33.

72 Jones LW, Courneya KS, Fairey AS, Mackey JR. Effects of an oncologist's recommendation to exercise on self-reported exercise behavior in newly diagnosed breast cancer survivors: a single-blind, randomized controlled trial. *Ann Behav Med* 2004;28:105–13.

73 Jones LW, Courneya KS, Fairey AS, Mackey JR. Does the theory of planned behavior mediate the effects of an oncologist's recommendation to exercise in newly diagnosed breast cancer survivors? Results from a randomized controlled trial. *Health Psychol* 2005;24:189–97.

74 Courneya KS, Segal RJ, Gelmon K, *et al.* Six-month follow-up of patient-rated outcomes in a randomized controlled trial of exercise training during breast cancer chemotherapy. *Cancer Epidemiol Biomarkers Prev* 2007;16:2572–8.

75 Dolan LB, Gelmon K, Courneya KS, *et al*. Hemoglobin and aerobic fitness changes with supervised exercise training in breast cancer patients receiving chemotherapy. *Cancer Epidemiol Biomarkers Prev* 2010;19:2826–32.

76 Eakin EG, Lawler SP, Winkler EA, Hayes SC. A randomized trial of a telephone-delivered exercise intervention for non-urban dwelling women newly diagnosed with breast cancer: exercise for health. *Ann Behav Med* 2012;43:229–38.

77 Hayes S, Rye S, Battistutta D, *et al*. Design and implementation of the Exercise for Health trial – a pragmatic exercise intervention for women with breast cancer. *Contemp Clin Trials* 2011;32:577–85.

78 Ligibel JA, Meyerhardt J, Pierce JP, *et al*. Impact of a telephone-based physical activity intervention upon exercise behaviors and fitness in cancer survivors enrolled in a cooperative group setting. *Breast Cancer Res Treat* 2012;132:205–13.

79 Carmack Taylor CL, de Moor C, Basen-Engquist K, *et al*. Moderator analyses of participants in the Active for Life after cancer trial: implications for physical activity group intervention studies. *Ann Behav Med* 2007;33:99–104.

80 Carmack Taylor CL, Demoor C, Smith MA, *et al*. Active for Life After Cancer: a randomized trial examining a lifestyle physical activity program for prostate cancer patients. *Psychooncology* 2006;15:847–62.

81 Carmack Taylor CL, Smith MA, de Moor C, *et al*. Quality of life intervention for prostate cancer patients: design and baseline characteristics of the active for life after cancer trial. *Control Clin Trials* 2004;25:265–85.

82 Pinto BM, Papandonatos GD, Goldstein MG. A randomized trial to promote physical activity among breast cancer patients. *Health Psychol* 2013;32:616–26.

83 Courneya KS, Booth CM, Gill S, *et al*. The Colon Health and Life-Long Exercise Change trial: a randomized trial of the National Cancer Institute of Canada Clinical Trials Group. *Curr Oncol* 2008;15:279–85.

84 Courneya KS, Vardy J, Gill S, *et al*. Update on the colon health and life-long exercise change trial: A phase III study of the impact of an exercise program on disease-free survival in colon cancer survivors. *Current Colorectal Cancer Reports* 2014;10:321–8.

85 Demark-Wahnefried W, Clipp EC, Lipkus IM, *et al*. Main outcomes of the FRESH START trial: a sequentially tailored, diet and exercise mailed print intervention among breast and prostate cancer survivors. *J Clin Oncol* 2007;25:2709–18.

86 Kushi LH, Doyle C, McCullough M, *et al*. American Cancer Society Guidelines on nutrition and physical activity for cancer prevention: reducing the risk of cancer with healthy food choices and physical activity. *CA Cancer J Clin* 2012; 62:30–67.

87 Balter K, Moller E, Fondell E. The effect of dietary guidelines on cancer risk and mortality. *Curr Opin Oncol* 2012;24:90–102.

88 Kroenke CH, Fung TT, Hu FB, Holmes MD. Dietary patterns and survival after breast cancer diagnosis. *J Clin Oncol* 2005;23:9295–303.

89 Kwan ML, Weltzien E, Kushi LH, *et al*. Dietary patterns and breast cancer recurrence and survival among women with early-stage breast cancer. *J Clin Oncol* 2009;27:919–26.

90 Vrieling A, Buck K, Seibold P, *et al*. Dietary patterns and survival in German postmenopausal breast cancer survivors. *Br J Cancer* 2013;108:188–92.

91 Meyerhardt JA, Niedzwiecki D, Hollis D, *et al*. Association of dietary patterns with cancer recurrence and survival in patients with stage III colon cancer. *JAMA* 2007;298:754–64.

92 World Cancer Research Fund/American Institute of Cancer Research. Food, Nutrition, Physical Activity, and the Prevention of Cancer: a Global Perspective, second expert report, 2007.

93 Chlebowski RT, Blackburn GL, Thomson CA, *et al*. Dietary fat reduction and breast cancer outcome: interim efficacy results from the Women's Intervention Nutrition Study. *J Natl Cancer Inst* 2006;98:1767–76.

94 Pierce JP, Natarajan L, Caan BJ, *et al*. Influence of a diet very high in vegetables, fruit, and fiber and low in fat on prognosis following treatment for breast cancer: the Women's Healthy Eating and Living (WHEL) randomized trial. *JAMA* 2007;298:289–98.

95 Cerhan JR, Potter JD, Gilmore JM, *et al*. Adherence to the AICR cancer prevention recommendations and subsequent morbidity and mortality in the Iowa Women's Health Study cohort. *Cancer Epidemiol Biomarkers Prev* 2004;13:1114–20.

96 Thomson CA, McCullough ML, Wertheim BC, *et al*. Nutrition and physical activity cancer prevention guidelines, cancer risk, and mortality in the women's health initiative. *Cancer Prev Res (Phila)* 2014;7:42–53.

97 Hastert TA, Beresford SA, Patterson RE, Kristal AR, White E. Adherence to WCRF/AICR cancer prevention recommendations and risk of postmenopausal breast cancer. *Cancer Epidemiol Biomarkers Prev* 2013;22:1498–508.

98 Catsburg C, Miller AB, Rohan TE. Adherence to cancer prevention guidelines and risk of breast cancer. *Int J Cancer* 2014;135:2444–52.

99 Romaguera D, Vergnaud AC, Peeters PH, *et al*. Is concordance with World Cancer Research Fund/American Institute for Cancer Research guidelines for cancer prevention related to subsequent risk of cancer? Results from the EPIC study. *Am J Clin Nutr* 2012;96:150–63.

100 Arab L, Su J, Steck SE, *et al*. Adherence to World Cancer Research Fund/American Institute for Cancer Research lifestyle recommendations reduces prostate cancer aggressiveness among African and Caucasian Americans. *Nutr Cancer* 2013;65:633–643.

101 Hastert TA, Beresford SA, Sheppard L, White E. Adherence to the WCRF/AICR cancer prevention recommendations and cancer-specific mortality: results from the Vitamins and Lifestyle (VITAL) Study. *Cancer Causes Control* 2014;25:541–52.

102 Khaw KT, Wareham N, Bingham S, *et al*. Combined impact of health behaviours and mortality in men and women: the EPIC-Norfolk prospective population study. *PLoS Med* 2008;5:e12.

103 Vergnaud AC, Romaguera D, Peeters PH, *et al*. Adherence to the World Cancer Research Fund/American Institute for Cancer Research guidelines and risk of death in Europe: results from the European Prospective Investigation into Nutrition and Cancer cohort study1,4. *Am J Clin Nutr* 2013;97:1107–20.

104 McCullough ML, Patel AV, Kushi LH, *et al.* Following cancer prevention guidelines reduces risk of cancer, cardiovascular disease, and all-cause mortality. *Cancer Epidemiol Biomarkers Prev* 2011;20:1089–97.

105 Inoue-Choi M, Robien K, Lazovich D. Adherence to the WCRF/AICR guidelines for cancer prevention is associated with lower mortality among older female cancer survivors. *Cancer Epidemiol Biomarkers Prev* 2013;22:792–802.

106 Inoue-Choi M, Lazovich D, Prizment AE, Robien K. Adherence to the World Cancer Research Fund/American Institute for Cancer Research recommendations for cancer prevention is associated with better health-related quality of life among elderly female cancer survivors. *J Clin Oncol* 2013;31:1758–66.

107 Jensen MD, Ryan DH, Apovian CM, *et al.* 2013 AHA/ACC/ TOS guideline for the management of overweight and obesity in adults: a report of the American College of Cardiology/ American Heart Association Task Force on Practice Guidelines and The Obesity Society. *Circulation* 2014;129:S102–38.

108 Liao EP. Management of type 2 diabetes: new and future developments in treatment. *Am J Med* 2012;125:S2–3.

109 Goldstein LB, Adams R, Alberts MJ, *et al.* Primary prevention of ischemic stroke: a guideline from the American Heart Association/American Stroke Association Stroke Council: cosponsored by the Atherosclerotic Peripheral Vascular Disease Interdisciplinary Working Group; Cardiovascular Nursing Council; Clinical Cardiology Council; Nutrition, Physical Activity, and Metabolism Council; and the Quality of Care and Outcomes Research Interdisciplinary Working Group: the American Academy of Neurology affirms the value of this guideline. *Stroke* 2006;37:1583–633.

110 Lloyd-Jones DM, Hong Y, Labarthe D, *et al.* Defining and setting national goals for cardiovascular health promotion and disease reduction: the American Heart Association's strategic Impact Goal through 2020 and beyond. *Circulation* 2010;121:586–613.

111 Bloom JR, Stewart SL, D'Onofrio CN, Luce J, Banks PJ. Addressing the needs of young breast cancer survivors at the 5 year milestone: can a short-term, low intensity intervention produce change? *J Cancer Surviv* 2008;2:190–204.

112 Hawkes AL, Chambers SK, Pakenham KI, *et al.* Effects of a telephone-delivered multiple health behavior change intervention (CanChange) on health and behavioral outcomes in survivors of colorectal cancer: a randomized controlled trial. *J Clin Oncol* 2013;31:2313–21.

113 Demark-Wahnefried W, Clipp EC, Morey MC, *et al.* Lifestyle intervention development study to improve physical function in older adults with cancer: outcomes from Project LEAD. *J Clin Oncol* 2006;24:3465–73.

114 Campbell MK, Carr C, Devellis B, *et al.* A randomized trial of tailoring and motivational interviewing to promote fruit and vegetable consumption for cancer prevention and control. *Ann Behav Med* 2009;38:71–85.

115 Blanchard CM, Courneya KS, Stein K, American Cancer Society's SCS, II. Cancer survivors' adherence to lifestyle behavior recommendations and associations with health-related quality of life: results from the American Cancer Society's SCS-II. *J Clin Oncol* 2008;26:2198–204.

116 Courneya KS, Katzmarzyk PT, Bacon E. Physical activity and obesity in Canadian cancer survivors: population-based estimates from the 2005 Canadian Community Health Survey. *Cancer* 2008;112:2475–82.

117 Bellizzi KM, Rowland JH, Jeffery DD, McNeel T. Health behaviors of cancer survivors: examining opportunities for cancer control intervention. *J Clin Oncol* 2005;23:8884–93.

118 Holmes MD, Chen WY, Feskanich D, Kroenke CH, Colditz GA. Physical activity and survival after breast cancer diagnosis. *JAMA* 2005;293:2479–86.

119 Meyerhardt JA, Giovannucci EL, Holmes MD, *et al.* Physical activity and survival after colorectal cancer diagnosis. *J Clin Oncol* 2006;24:3527–34.

120 Irwin ML, Crumley D, McTiernan A, *et al.* Physical activity levels before and after a diagnosis of breast carcinoma: the Health, Eating, Activity, and Lifestyle (HEAL) study. *Cancer* 2003;97:1746–57.

121 Irwin ML, McTiernan A, Baumgartner RN, *et al.* Changes in body fat and weight after a breast cancer diagnosis: influence of demographic, prognostic, and lifestyle factors. *J Clin Oncol* 2005;23:774–82.

122 Kroenke CH, Chen WY, Rosner B, Holmes MD. Weight, weight gain, and survival after breast cancer diagnosis. *J Clin Oncol* 2005;23:1370–8.

123 Caan BJ, Kwan ML, Shu XO, *et al.* Weight change and survival after breast cancer in the after breast cancer pooling project. *Cancer Epidemiol Biomarkers Prev* 2012;21:1260–71.

124 Demark-Wahnefried W, Aziz NM, Rowland JH, Pinto BM. Riding the crest of the teachable moment: promoting long-term health after the diagnosis of cancer. *J Clin Oncol* 2005;23:5814–30.

125 Hawkins NA, Smith T, Zhao L, *et al.* Health-related behavior change after cancer: results of the American cancer society's studies of cancer survivors (SCS). *J Cancer Surviv* 2010;4:20–32.

126 Philip EJ, Coups EJ, Feinstein MB, *et al.* Physical activity preferences of early-stage lung cancer survivors. *Support Care Cancer* 2014;22:495–502.

127 Bao Y, Duan N, Fox SA. Is some provider advice on smoking cessation better than no advice? An instrumental variable analysis of the 2001 National Health Interview Survey. *Health Serv Res* 2006;41:2114–35.

128 Gritz ER, Fingeret MC, Vidrine DJ, *et al.* Successes and failures of the teachable moment: smoking cessation in cancer patients. *Cancer* 2006;106:17–27.

129 Kreuter MW, Chheda SG, Bull FC. How does physician advice influence patient behavior? Evidence for a priming effect. *Arch Fam Med* 2000;9:426–33.

130 Krupski WC, Nguyen HT, Jones DN, *et al.* Smoking cessation counseling: a missed opportunity for general surgery trainees. *J Vasc Surg* 2002;36:257–62; discussion 262.

131 McRobbie H, Hajek P. Nicotine replacement therapy in patients with cardiovascular disease: guidelines for health professionals. *Addiction* 2001;96:1547–51.

132 Stead LF, Bergson G, Lancaster T. Physician advice for smoking cessation. Cochrane Database Syst Rev 2008:Cd000165.

133 Coups EJ, Dhingra LK, Heckman CJ, Manne SL. Receipt of provider advice for smoking cessation and use of smoking cessation treatments among cancer survivors. *J Gen Intern Med* 2009;24 Suppl 2:S480–6.

134 DuBard CA, Schmid D, Yow A, Rogers AB, Lawrence WW. Recommendation for and receipt of cancer screenings among medicaid recipients 50 years and older. *Arch Intern Med* 2008;168:2014–21.

135 Hay JL, Ford JS, Klein D, *et al*. Adherence to colorectal cancer screening in mammography-adherent older women. *J Behav Med* 2003;26:553–76.

136 Meissner HI, Breen N, Taubman ML, Vernon SW, Graubard BI. Which women aren't getting mammograms and why? (United States). *Cancer Causes Control* 2007;18:61–70.

137 Jones LW, Courneya KS, Peddle C, Mackey JR. Oncologists' opinions towards recommending exercise to patients with cancer: a Canadian national survey. *Support Care Cancer* 2005;13:929–37.

138 Ligibel JA, Alfano CM, Courneya KS, *et al*. American Society of Clinical Oncology position statement on obesity and cancer. *J Clin Oncol* 2014;32:3568–74.

139 Ligibel JA, Denlinger CS. New NCCN guidelines for survivorship care. *J Natl Compr Canc Netw* 2013;11:640–4.

140 Institute of Medicine. *Implementing Cancer Survivorship Care Planning*. Washington, DC: National Academies Press, 2007.

141 Fjeldsoe B, Neuhaus M, Winkler E, Eakin E. Systematic review of maintenance of behavior change following physical activity and dietary interventions. *Health Psychol* 2011;30:99–109.

142 Burke LE, Wang J, Sevick MA. Self-monitoring in weight loss: a systematic review of the literature. *J Am Diet Assoc* 2011;111:92–102.

143 Greaves CJ, Sheppard KE, Abraham C, *et al*. Systematic review of reviews of intervention components associated with increased effectiveness in dietary and physical activity interventions. *BMC Public Health* 2011;11:119.

144 Wing RR, Phelan S. Long-term weight loss maintenance. *Am J Clin Nutr* 2005;82:222s–5s.

145 Pearson ES. Goal setting as a health behavior change strategy in overweight and obese adults: a systematic literature review examining intervention components. *Patient Educ Couns* 2012;87:32–42.

146 American College of Surgeons Commission on Cancer. *Cancer Program Standards 2012*: Ensuring Patient-Centered Care. Chicago, 2012.

147 Association of Community Cancer Centers. Cancer Nutrition Services: A Practical Guide for Cancer Programs, 2012.

148 Kren K, Michael P, Johnson EQ, Thiessen C, Busey JC. Referral systems in ambulatory care–providing access to the nutrition care process. *J Am Diet Assoc* 2008;108:1375–9.

149 Commission on Accreditation of Rehabilitation Facilities. Integrating rehabilitation into cancer care. Available from URL: http://www.carf.org/Programs/Medical/ (acccessed 17 August 2017).

150 Schmitz KH, Courneya KS, Matthews C, *et al*. American College of Sports Medicine roundtable on exercise guidelines for cancer survivors. *Med Sci Sports Exerc* 2010;42:1409–26.

151 Stout NL. Exercise for the cancer survivor: all for one but not one for all. *J Support Oncol* 2012;10:178–9.

152 American College of Sports Medicine. Certified Cancer Exercise Trainer (CET). Available from http://certification. acsm.org/acsm-cancer-exercise-trainer (accessed 17 August 2017).

153 Djuric Z, DiLaura NM, Jenkins I, *et al*. Combining weight-loss counseling with the weight watchers plan for obese breast cancer survivors. *Obes Res* 2002;10:657–65.

154 Greenlee HA, Crew KD, Mata JM, *et al*. A pilot randomized controlled trial of a commercial diet and exercise weight loss program in minority breast cancer survivors. *Obesity (Silver Spring)* 2013;21:65–76.

24

Clinical Trials

Olwen M. Hahn[1] and Richard L. Schilsky[2]

[1] *The University of Chicago, Chicago, Illinois, USA*
[2] *American Society of Clinical Oncology, Alexandria, Virginia, USA*

Introduction: Definition and Importance of Clinical Trials

A clinical trial is a research study designed to answer specific questions about the safety and/or efficacy of new therapies – drugs, devices, or behavioral interventions for primary or secondary prevention of disease, treatment of established disease or mitigation of disease symptoms. Oncology has a rich history of improving patient outcomes and advancing research through clinical trials, in particular randomized controlled trials. These trials have led to the development of new drugs that can potentially cure or improve survival of cancer patients, refined the methods of delivery and scheduling of oncology drugs, identified subpopulations of patients that are most likely to benefit (or be harmed) from a specific therapy, and established the utility of combining different treatment modalities. A trial provides a structured way to select patients, standardizes the delivery of the interventions being studied, and prespecifies the study endpoints and hypotheses as well as the data collection methods and analysis plans. Results from a well-designed and conducted study can provide assurance to physicians and patients that the interventions they employ for cancer treatment, prevention, and screening are based on the highest level of evidence available.

Recent technological innovations and scientific advances in understanding the molecular mechanisms of cancer have accelerated the discovery and development of cancer therapies and diagnostics. In this era, the landscape of clinical trials has evolved. Large randomized controlled trials are often complex and include many correlative science and quality of life objectives. In addition, biomarkers, surrogate endpoints, novel imaging techniques, pharmacokinetics, pharmacodynamics, and genetics have now been incorporated into studies to expedite the development of new therapies and better understand the observed clinical outcomes.

Although clinical trials are the primary means by which scientific advances are translated into improved patient outcomes, they have several limitations and barriers to their development and conduct. The trajectory of a clinical study can be a long and time consuming process from concept, design, implementation, and conduct, to analysis and publication of results. In addition, there are many regulatory and financial hurdles that must be overcome to successfully launch and monitor clinical trials.

Clinical Trial Types and Designs

While the primary focus of this chapter is therapeutic clinical trials, there are many types of clinical trials that are conducted in oncology, including [1]:

1) *Prevention trials*: evaluate interventions that prevent or lower the risk of cancer in individuals with a high risk of developing cancer.
2) *Screening or early detection trials*: assess methods to detect cancer early in its development in asymptomatic individuals.
3) *Therapeutic or treatment trials*: evaluate new cancer therapies, new ways of using current treatments or compare existing cancer treatments.
4) *Quality of life trials*: examine strategies to improve the physical, emotional, and social well-being of cancer patients during or after cancer therapy.
5) *Symptom management trials*: assess interventions that alleviate symptoms of cancer and/or cancer treatment.
6) *Diagnostic trials*: study new tests or procedures that may help diagnose cancer more accurately, monitor outcomes of cancer therapy, or provide predictive or prognostic information.

All clinical trials require careful planning, execution, and analysis. The planning steps culminate in a written protocol document. Table 24.1 summarizes the usual components of a protocol. The protocol document will define the specific question being investigated and objectives of the clinical trial, as well as the scientific rationale for conducting the trial. Additionally, the protocol specifies standardized criteria for the selection of study participants, the therapeutic or diagnostic intervention, required clinical tests and measurements to be performed at

Table 24.1 Major components of a clinical trial protocol.

Introduction and scientific rationale
Objective
Eligibility/selection of patients
Design of study (schema)
Registration, randomization, and stratification information
Treatment plan
Drug information: formulation and preparation
Dose modification and toxicity management
Study calendar: required clinical assessments, including laboratory and radiologic studies
Endpoint definition and criteria for evaluating response/progression/relapse
Statistical plan
Informed consent
Regulatory information, including adverse event reporting
Data forms and data submission

specified intervals, and the statistical analysis plan. Eligibility criteria describe the characteristics of individuals to be enrolled, including the cancer type and stage, prior cancer therapies, medical history, and current health status. These criteria are necessary to define the study population, minimize bias in participant selection, protect the study participants from risk, enable cross study comparisons, and ensure that the trial results are accurate and due to the tested intervention rather than other variables [1]. The statistical analysis plan defines the study endpoints, methods of analysis, and justifies the trial design and sample size of the study.

Ethical Considerations for Clinical Trials

A cornerstone of ethical clinical research is the process of informed consent. While the legal and regulatory system has shaped current requirements for informed consent, the underlying principle is deeply embedded in our culture and is based on the ethical principle of respect for persons [2]. This principle recognizes an individual's right to determine his or her goals and make autonomous choices to achieve those goals.

The present day regulations for research involving human subjects are outlined in the Federal Policy for the Protection of Human Subjects (often referred to as the "Common Rule"), which require several protections to be in place in order to conduct federally funded research on human subjects. As part of these regulations, all research must be approved by an institutional review board whose membership includes community members, and trial participants must be provided with informed consent, which includes a written document as well as discussion with a member of the healthcare team about the risks, benefits, and alternatives of the research project [3].

The process of informed consent includes disclosing to patients the information about the research study, assessing their understanding of the information, and obtaining a patient's voluntary (and written) agreement to participate in the clinical trial. Disclosure of information about the proposed clinical trial must cover a number of specific topics, including: the type and design of the proposed research, the purpose of the research, the unproven nature of research, alternatives to participation in the clinical trial, the potential risks and benefits of participating

in the clinical trial, the voluntary nature of participation in clinical research, and the process of maintaining patient confidentiality [4]. While all of these elements are included in the written informed consent document, the process of informed consent also includes a discussion with the healthcare team; additional written or audiovisual tools may be used to enhance a patient's understanding of the proposed research.

There are ethical issues present in all types of clinical research; however, randomized, phase III trials have been subject to the greatest scrutiny. Much of the attention has focused on the issue of equipoise, which is defined as a state of uncertainty on the part of the clinical investigator and medical community towards the comparative merits of different treatments [5]. For physicians to recommend treatment by randomization ethically, they must have genuine uncertainty about the relative merits of the treatment possibilities, and this uncertainty must be conveyed to patients in an easily understandable way.

Phases of Clinical trials

Although the complexity of clinical trials has increased in recent years in an attempt to address multiple endpoints and objectives, they are still broadly categorized into phases that aim to progressively develop information about the safety, efficacy and effectiveness of the intervention being tested (Table 24.2). Phase 0 trials are small, exploratory studies used as a drug discovery tool to ensure that the novel drug is modulating its intended target. Phase I trials test a new drug, drug combination, or treatment in a small number of patients to evaluate its toxicities, determine the recommended dose for further study, and assess the pharmacokinetic characteristics of the drug being tested. Phase II trials are designed to determine if an intervention has antitumor activity in a specific cancer type as well as to gain additional safety data and, in some cases, to refine dosing. Phase III studies typically enroll several hundred to thousands of patients to compare a novel therapy to the standard therapy or to compare two different therapies to establish their relative efficacy.

Table 24.2 Clinical trial phases.

Phase	Main objective(s)	Notes
0	Modulation of intended target Discovery tool	Small sample size Limited duration
I	Safety, tolerability, identify dose range, Pharmacodynamics, pharmacokinetics	Small sample size Often multiple cancer types
II	Tolerability, preliminary efficacy Proof of concept	Specific cancer type
III	Long term safety, efficacy, Comparison vs standard therapy, Comparative efficacy of several regimens	
IV	Drug effect in various populations Long-term side effects	Performed after drug is marketed/approved

Phase 0 Trials

In recent years, phase 0 studies have been employed to establish, very early during clinical development, whether the agent under investigation is modulating its intended target and to assess the pharmacokinetic (PK) and pharmacodynamic (PD) effects of the drug in humans. Phase 0 studies enroll a very small number of patients (typically fewer than 10), have limited duration (typically less than one week), and administer subtherapeutic doses of the investigational drug; they have no therapeutic or diagnostic intent [6].

The primary purpose of the phase 0 study is to assist in the decision to continue clinical drug development (i.e., go or no-go decision), using human patients instead of animals to confirm the drug's mechanism of action, PK and PD. They are conducted before the traditional phase I dose escalation and toxicity studies. While still not widely conducted, the use of phase 0 studies has increased since 2006, following publication by the FDA of "A Guidance for Industry, Investigators, and Reviewers for Exploratory IND Studies." [7]. Phase 0 studies, while not required, may result in more efficient drug development by improving investigators' understanding of a drug's mechanism of action in humans much earlier than previously. However, phase 0 studies may not be appropriate for some novel agents, for example drugs with multiple targets, those without a well-defined biomarker, or those whose precise mechanism of action is not well defined [8].

Phase I Trials

Phase I trials allow investigators to determine the recommended dose of the drug for further testing, its tolerability and safety profile, its pharmacokinetics (effect of the body on the drug), and pharmacodynamics (effect of the drug on the body). Phase I trials are often the first time the intervention is evaluated in humans. Traditionally, phase I trials of cytotoxic agents have enrolled patients with multiple different cancer types in the same cohort, as the primary objective is to assess safety. Notably, in the era of molecularly targeted agents, phase I trials may limit enrollment to patients with a predefined molecular aberration or specific cancer type that has a high incidence of a particular molecular aberration in order to study the agent in the patients most likely to benefit from the targeted agent. Such studies might also provide a glimpse of the drug's activity in the intended use population. Determining the maximum tolerated dose level (MTD), defined as the dose level at which few patients experience dose limiting toxicities (DLT), is a standard endpoint of phase I trials. Toxicities and adverse events are graded by the National Cancer Institute's (NCI) Common Terminology Criteria for Adverse Events (CTCAE); laboratory abnormalities and symptoms of adverse events are graded on a scale of 1 (mild) to 5 (fatal) and the relationship of the adverse event to exposure to the investigational agent is recorded.

A traditional phase I cancer drug trial is designed to enroll a limited number of patients. The initial cohort enrolls patients at a starting dose level not expected to produce serious toxicity; commonly, 3–6 patients are enrolled per cohort. Enrolled patients will typically receive a predefined number of 'cycles' of the study drug unless severe toxicity or rapid disease progression occurs. The dose is escalated for patients enrolled in subsequent cohorts after observing patients in earlier cohorts to determine if a DLT has occurred. Patients who experience a DLT may be withdrawn from the study. If a DLT is not observed at a given dose level, the dose is escalated for the next cohort of patients. If a DLT is observed at a particular dose level, three more patients are usually enrolled in that cohort to evaluate better the tolerability of that dose; if no further dose-limiting toxicities are seen, then the dose is increased for the next cohort. If the incidence of DLT is greater than 33% in the expanded cohort, then dose escalation will usually stop. The dose recommended for further study in a phase II trial is typically the highest dose that has less than a 33% incidence of DLT.

Several limitations to traditional phase I trials have been described: they may expose many patients to subtherapeutic doses of the new drug; they can take a long time to determine MTD; and they provide limited knowledge about long-term toxicity and interpatient variability [9]. The traditional MTD endpoint may not be relevant for molecularly target agents, which can have a wide therapeutic window due to their mechanism of action on targets differentially expressed on cancer cells versus normal cells [10]. For targeted agents, a primary endpoint of biologically active dose sufficient to inhibit the relevant target may be more appropriate. However, this endpoint requires knowledge of the drug target, as well as a reliable and validated assay to determine target inhibition. A number of novel designs for phase I trials have been proposed to overcome these limitations.

Phase II Trials

Phase II trials are designed to assess the activity of a new agent or therapeutic regimen and to determine if it has sufficient activity to warrant further testing in a phase III setting. Phase II studies must be thoughtfully designed to identify drugs or regimens that are most likely to demonstrate clinical benefit in confirmatory trials. Single agents and/or novel combinations are usually tested in a phase II study in patients with a specific tumor type, although there is increasing interest in evaluating targeted agents against a range of histologies that all harbor the molecular aberration targeted by the drug, so called "basket trials" [11]. This type of enrichment design, in addition to other novel trial designs, has increased in recent years as more widely applied genomic technologies identify molecular subsets of tumors that can be inhibited by targeted agents.

Historically, phase II trials have typically been single arm trials with objective tumor response as the primary endpoint, and without a contemporaneous comparison group; thus the results must be compared against a historical group that is prognostically similar. A traditional design for a phase II study is a two-staged design in which a predefined number of evaluable patients are entered into the first stage of the study. If fewer than a prespecified number of responses is seen, the study is terminated as the tested regimen is determined to have insufficient activity. Otherwise, the study is continued to the next stage in order to reach the total sample size.

In recent years, this traditional phase II study design has been criticized for its limitations as single arm, phase II studies often overestimate the treatment effect of the study drug or drug combination. An analysis of 363 published, phase II combination therapy trials that enrolled over 16,000 patients, of which 94% were single arm studies, revealed that the likelihood that a positive phase II trial will result in a subsequent phase III study that will improve the standard of care is less than 4% [12]. Another limitation of a single arm phase II trial is the inability to assess reliably time to event endpoints such as progression-free survival that might be more relevant for some molecularly-targeted therapies. For these reasons, there is a great deal of interest in alternative phase II trial designs that might be more informative. An example is the increasing use of randomized, phase II trials, which allow for better assessment of time to event endpoints; this design provides the necessary control arm for the natural history of tumor progression in the absence of a therapeutic effect and may result in a more reliable signal of drug activity and better assessment of drug toxicity [13]. Other novel designs for phase II trials include dynamic and adaptive randomization, and the use of biomarkers to enrich the study population for tumors most likely to respond to targeted therapies. There is interest in developing and using more efficient designs that allow trials to change or 'adapt' to new information acquired during the trial; for example, Bayesian and adaptive designs that may reduce the sample size, time, and cost of randomized, phase II trials. Another consideration is the incorporation of interim statistical analyses and early stopping rules for larger, phase II studies. Early stopping rules may limit the number of patients who receive ineffective therapies, which can conserve patient and clinical trial resources. While planned interim analyses are commonplace for phase III studies, they have been incorporated in a minority of randomized, phase II studies. An analysis of 1266 phase II studies revealed that only 27% had a planned interim analysis, but of those studies, 56% stopped early and most of these where stopped due to lack of efficacy [13]. It was estimated that if planned interim analyses had been incorporated into the other randomized, phase II studies, an additional 28% of the studies would have been closed early.

Phase III Trials

Phase III studies are randomized, prospectively controlled trials that are designed to compare the efficacy of two or more treatment regimens. Phase III trials should be designed to answer a clinically meaningful question that can change the standard of care for a particular disease or patient population. Properly designed phase III studies provide the best available scientific evidence of the efficacy of the interventions being studied and form the basis for evidence-based medicine.

Most phase III trials are designed to demonstrate the superiority of a novel therapy over the standard of care. Some studies have a noninferiority design to determine if the new therapy is no worse than the standard of care by a prespecified margin. This design can be useful if the new therapy is less toxic, less invasive, or less expensive than the present standard of care although not necessarily more efficacious. The primary endpoint of a phase III clinical trial should be an outcome that is meaningful for a patient's well-being, such as overall survival, disease-free survival for adjuvant trials, or progression-free survival for certain advanced cancers. Recently, improvement in tumor-related symptoms has been accepted for regulatory approval of new drugs as well. Response rate or tumor shrinkage is not an appropriate endpoint for phase III trials because it often has little correlation with patient benefit.

In a study with multiple treatment arms, patients are randomly assigned to a treatment. The purpose of randomization is to distribute both known and unknown potential biases to ensure that the outcomes observed are due to the treatment intervention rather than confounding factors. When there are known prognostic factors that can affect patient outcome, these factors can be used to stratify the randomization process to ensure equal distribution of patients into the arms of the study. These 'stratification factors' should be specified in the study protocol and built into the randomization process. The stratification factors should be limited to those characteristics that are known to have independent effects on prognosis and outcome.

When patients are randomized to different arms, it may be appropriate to 'blind' or "mask" them, the treating physician, and the study team to the treatment assignment. Blinding is a way to minimize or decrease bias in assessing study outcomes, particularly those that may be subjective in their interpretation such as tumor progression or quality of life. A double-blinded study is when neither the patient nor the study team, including the treating physician, knows the treatment assignment. The treatment is administered in packaging or formulation that does not reveal the treatment assignment and an identical placebo may be used if medically feasible and ethically appropriate. The reporting of side effects and treatment efficacy by patient and study team is thus not biased by knowledge of the treatment received. In unblinded studies, both patient and clinician may be aware of the treatment assignment. A disadvantage of unblinded studies is that patients may be disappointed that they have been randomized to standard treatment and have decreased motivation to continue on the study, thus affecting data collection and endpoint assessment. In unblinded studies, assessments of participants are subject to bias, especially if the physician is enthusiastic about the new treatment, which can affect the reporting of outcomes or side effects. In both blinded and unblinded studies, both arms need to be balanced in terms of required clinical assessments, laboratory studies, radiologic tests and frequency of evaluation.

It may be challenging to enroll patients in placebo-controlled or 'blinded' trials, due to concerns about assignment to the placebo arm. Yet the use of placebos in cancer clinical trials can be medically and ethically appropriate, especially when there is no effective standard of care or when the present standard of care has minimal efficacy or excessive toxicity. In these situations, the patients randomized to the placebo arm, as well as the treatment arm, should also receive the best supportive care, including pain management; ideally, the protocol document will delineate the appropriate components of best supportive care [14].

As phase III trials are typically large studies, enrolling hundreds or even thousands of patients, and are designed to establish a new standard of care, they require detailed planning by investigators and statisticians. The essential elements of the protocol (Table 24.1) require careful execution. One key aspect is the execution of the statistical plan and analysis. In phase III studies, statisticians often plan for a prespecified number of interim analyses while the study is ongoing. In multicenter trials, a data and safety monitoring committee, composed of individuals who are independent from the study team, will review these analyses. This monitoring committee will determine when the trial results are mature and should be released or if the trial should be stopped due to the data crossing a predefined safety or efficacy boundary. Once the committee has determined that the data are sufficiently mature and reliable, it will authorize the study team to release the study results to the public; a publication in a peer reviewed scientific journal should follow shortly afterwards.

Clinical Trials involving Radiation Therapy, Surgery, and Multidisciplinary Therapy

Technology in surgery and radiation oncology has advanced steadily with the development of laparoscopic and robotic operative techniques as well as new radiation therapy approaches such as three-dimensional conformal radiation therapy, intensity-modulated radiation therapy, and stereotactic radiotherapy. As introducing these innovations into clinical practice generally does not require regulatory approval, newer techniques are often adopted in clinical practice without comparative research or randomized controlled trials. Thus, the evidence base to support their widespread use is often lacking. Ideally, trials should be conducted objectively to evaluate a technology to establish its benefit and risks, instead of simply adopting it in clinical practice. Clinical studies can determine if the novel technology or innovation not only decreases therapy-related morbidity, but also provides at least an equivalent, if not superior, oncologic outcome [15, 16].

Cancer Prevention Trials

Cancer prevention research offers the possibility of identifying interventions to prevent cancer in high-risk individuals. Prevention studies pose unique considerations for their design, participant selection, and execution that differ from therapeutic trials. For example, prevention studies are typically sponsored by publicly funded agencies, as these studies require large sample sizes and a long time to reach the primary endpoint, typically reduction in cancer incidence but preferably reduction in cancer mortality. The NCI Division of Cancer Prevention has organized and supported many large trials in cancer prevention. While there have been many successes in cancer prevention, such as the development of tamoxifen, raloxifene and exemestane for breast cancer prevention and the development of the human papilloma virus vaccine to prevent cervical cancer, there have been many high-profile trials, enrolling thousands of patients, that failed to demonstrate a reduction in cancer incidence for the studied intervention. For example, the Alpha-Tocopherol, Beta-Carotene Cancer Prevention Study and the Beta-Carotene and Retinol Efficacy Trial enrolled thousands of high-risk smokers but failed to show a decreased incidence of lung cancer [17, 18]. A large phase III, randomized, double-blind, placebo-controlled trial was conducted to test the efficacy of selenium and vitamin E alone and in combination for preventing prostate cancer. Neither supplement decreased the risk of developing prostate cancer [19], and vitamin E supplementation significantly increased the risk of prostate cancer in healthy men [20]. Thus, despite a sound scientific rationale and supportive preclinical data, these large studies failed to demonstrate a reduction in cancer incidence in the at risk population. Moving forward, investigators hope to be able to identify valid, intermediate-effect biomarkers that could serve as surrogate end points, which could lead to smaller and shorter prevention trials.

Limitations and Challenges of Clinical Trials

While clinical trials have clearly advanced the care of cancer patients, they are not without limitations. The process of developing and activating clinical trials is slow and plagued by a burdensome infrastructure and substantial regulatory oversight. Phase III, randomized trials often require large numbers of patients to identify modest differences between treatments and can take years to accrue and reach the primary endpoint being studied. The conduct of large, phase III trials often requires complex protocols and collection of substantial amounts of patient data which increases the work load and costs for participating sites. Recent studies suggest that a substantial proportion of phase III oncology trials are never completed, wasting both financial and patient resources [21]. As the treatment of cancer advances and new findings are discovered, the delays in start-up and completion of randomized trials may lead to results that are no longer relevant by the time they are reported.

Eligibility criteria, by their very nature, limit the applicability of the trial results. Critics argue that the patient population studied often does not reflect the 'real world' practice of medicine as the inclusion criteria may lead to the selection of only the healthiest patients and may exclude patients with medical comorbidities or borderline organ function. Thus, while a phase III trial may adequately assess the efficacy of an intervention (i.e., what can work); the 'real world' effectiveness that is seen once the intervention is deployed in community practice (i.e., what does work) may be substantially different. The disparity between efficacy and effectiveness is often most apparent in trials designed to obtain regulatory approval for a drug or device, where the selection criteria may be particularly strict and the comparison arm may not reflect current standard practice. In addition, clinical trials often evaluate therapies under idealized clinical conditions including protocol-specified dose modifications and toxicity management; thus the results generated from a study may not be replicated when the therapy is translated to general practice settings and to real world patients.

In addition to the limitations imposed by clinical trial design, logistical, and regulatory hurdles, a major hurdle to conducting clinical trials is the low accrual rate. It is estimated that only 3–5% of adult cancer patients enroll on clinical trials [22]. There are many reasons for the low accrual rates, both on the part of the enrolling physician and the potential study participant, including concerns about randomization, discomfort with research, inadequate knowledge of clinical trials, use of a placebo or no intervention group, health insurance barriers, concern about potential adverse effects of the study treatment, stringent eligibility criteria, and cumbersome requirements of the study protocol [23]. One major barrier to clinical trial enrollment is the failure of physicians to offer enrollment to patients who are eligible to participate in a clinical trial. These enrollment challenges are greater in under-represented minority groups, as well as older adults (age 65 years or older), patients residing in rural areas, and patients of low socioeconomic status.

Public versus Commercial Sponsors of Clinical Trials

There are two main categories of cancer therapeutic trials in the United States (US): (1) publicly sponsored trials, conducted primarily by the NCI through its network of cooperative groups and cancer centers, and (2) commercially sponsored trials. Despite a common mission to improve outcomes of cancer patients, the goals of public and commercial sponsors ultimately diverge (Tables 24.3 and 24.4). Commercial sponsors launch clinical trials that will result in marketing approval, label extension, expansion of market share, and, ultimately, an increase in shareholder value. Publicly sponsored trials seek to optimize therapy for a particular disease, create new knowledge, and improve public health; these trials can also result in label extension of a drug and even in initial drug approval. In general, commercial sponsors have little interest in studying questions that are often of high interest to patients such as the integration of combined modality therapies into treatment paradigms, or comparing the effectiveness of established therapies; such studies are often left to publicly funded research entities. Publicly sponsored trials are also more likely to focus on therapies for rare diseases and to study survivorship and quality of life. By collecting and banking biospecimens, these trials may be able to

Table 24.3 Goals of therapeutic clinical trials.

Commercial sponsor	Public sponsor
Drug registration	Optimize treatment
Label extension	Label extension
Epand market share	Create new knowledge
Create shareholder value	Improve public health

Table 24.4 Role of publicly funded trials.

- Compare the effectiveness of various treatment options
- Combine/compare drugs developed by different sponsors
- Develop therapies for rare diseases
- Address optimal dosing
- Test multi-modality therapies such as radiation therapy in combination with drugs
- Identify patient and tumor subsets most likely to benefit from interventions
- Study screening and prevention strategies
- Focus on survivorship and quality of life
- Publish negative results
- Assess cost and cost-effectiveness
- Provide "gold standard" databases for registry studies

identify patient and tumor subsets that are most likely to benefit from the intervention being studied, or to experience severe toxicities or poor outcomes. Given the public nature of the funding, clinical investigators are expected to publish their results, even if the outcome is unfavorable for the investigational therapy.

National Clinical Trials Network

The national cooperative group program was established in 1955 with the goals of conducting clinical trials of new cancer treatments, studying cancer prevention and detection, and assessing quality of life during and after cancer treatment. The cooperative groups have an established infrastructure with administrative and data management centers that are organized to develop and conduct trials; and quality assurance programs to ensure proper study conduct and accurate data. With the inclusion of the Community Clinical Oncology program (CCOP) program, many trials have been conducted in community settings that are similar to those in which the intervention will be employed in practice [24]. The cooperative group program includes more than 14,000 oncology professionals working at more than 3100 unique sites and enrolls patients that are representative of the US population as a whole [25]. With its biorepositories, image archives, and references laboratories, the Cooperative Group Program is able to collect high quality biospecimens and images for research that will allow investigators to develop personalized cancer care further.

Despite its robust infrastructure and past achievements, the national cooperative group program has been criticized for its operational inefficiencies and slow adaptation to new scientific opportunities. In 2009, the Institute of Medicine (IOM) issued a report that lauded the accomplishments of the NCI Cooperative Group Program but also delineated important deficiencies in the system [21]. The report noted system inefficiencies such as prolonged start up times for trials and a 50% rate of successful trial accrual. It was noted that the program has been hampered by funding reductions and a cumbersome oversight structure that impedes efficiency. The IOM report called for strengthening the publicly funded cancer clinical trials system in the US, as well as for modifying the system so that it is scientifically nimble, more efficient, and accessible to all members of the US population. The panel developed an extensive list of recommendations to achieve the goals of: (1) improving the speed and efficiency of design and conduct of trials; (2) incorporating innovative science and trial design into clinical trials; (3) improving trial prioritization, selection and support; and (4) incentivizing physician and patient participation. In addition, the NCI established an operational efficiency working group with a goal of reducing study activation time by 50% by placing strict timelines on the clinical trial development process [26].

In response to the IOM report the NCI reorganized and restructured the cooperative group program to form the National Clinical Trials Network (NCTN). The goals of the NCTN are: to provide an essential national infrastructure for publicly funded trials in cancer prevention, screening, diagnosis, and treatment; to provide a unified national platform for translational research; and to efficiently answer important clinical questions that are not well supported in a commercial environment. The nine adult cooperative groups consolidated into four groups, joining the existing single pediatric cooperative group, and the CCOPs and NCI's Community Cancer Center Programs merged to form the NCI Community Oncology Research Program (NCORP). NCORP now supports cancer control, prevention, treatment, and screening clinical trials and is expanding its research scope to include cancer care delivery research.

It is anticipated that the NCORP sites will provide 30–40% of enrollment to treatment trials in the NCTN [27]. The NCORP structure will provide an opportunity for community oncologists and their research teams to provide scientific and feasibility input to academic investigators developing clinical trials. Community organizations participating in NCORP include practices, health systems, and public institutions with a track record of clinical trial accrual and ability to maintain the minimum requirements to support cancer care delivery and research that have been defined by the American Society of Clinical Oncology [28]. By becoming members of NCORP, community sites and investigators are able to participate in a large menu of cancer clinical trials and benefit from the operational standards set by the NCTN.

Clinical Trials in the Era of Genomic Medicine and Personalized Medicine

Our growing knowledge of the human genome and the molecular basis of cancer will shape the design of clinical trials in the future. Many new anticancer therapies target specific protein products of genes identified as key driver mutations; this 'precision oncology' approach may lead to cancer patients experiencing a long-lasting remission or improved survival as cancer therapies that target specific mutations present in an individual's cancer are identified and developed. The selection of patients whose tumors contain the intended target adds complexity to designing clinical trials. With the declining cost of genome sequencing, many future clinical trials may rely on tumor genome sequencing to direct patients to optimal treatment and/or to determine trial eligibility.

In years past, a particular cancer was treated as a homogenous disease; for example, breast cancer treatment trials enrolled patients regardless of tumor hormone receptor or HER2-neu status. Breast cancer patients are now selected for clinical trials based not only on hormone receptor and HER2-neu status, but also on gene expression signatures, such as the 21 gene recurrence score (Oncotype Dx®) and the 70 gene profile (MammaPrint). The era of genomic and personalized medicine depends not only on developing targeted therapies, but also on developing and validating reliable and reproducible biomarker tests that will identify patients who will benefit from a particular therapy.

The oncology community has begun to make great strides to study rigorously the potential of precision medicine. Since 2014, NCI and the NCTN, in a partnership with pharmaceutical partners and the private sector, have launched a series of precision medicine clinical trials. One notable example, NCI-Molecular Analysis for Therapy Choice (NCI-MATCH), enrolls patients with refractory solid tumors and lymphoma and analyzes their tumors to determine if there is an actionable mutation; based on the genomic analysis, patients are assigned to a treatment arm with a matched targeted therapy. NCI-MATCH will help determine whether treating cancers according to their molecular alterations can efficiently identify signals of drug activity; this study opened in August 2015, and has a total of 24 treatment arms, with each arm anticipating the enrollment of a maximum of 35 patients. The NCTN's Lung Master Protocol (Lung-MAP) is another precision oncology study that enrolls patients with squamous cell lung cancer, analyzes their tumor for genomic alterations in >200 cancer-related genes, and assigns them a substudy with a matched, targeted therapy based on the genomic analysis. Both NCI-MATCH and LUNG-MAP employ a single genomic assay to assign patients to a parent protocol with multiple substudies [29].

The precision oncology strategy is also being tested in the adjuvant setting. The Adjuvant Lung Cancer Enrichment Marker Identification and Sequencing Trials (ALCHEMIST) are a group of randomized clinical trials, sponsored by NCI and NCTN, studying adjuvant therapies for patients with early-stage NSCLC, where better curative therapies are urgently needed. Approximately 6,000–8,000 patients will have their tumor tissue tested for the ALCHEMIST trials. The ALCHEMIST trials are testing therapies that target two types of rare genetic changes that are thought to drive lung cancer growth: mutations in the *EGFR* gene (approximately 20% of NSCLC) and a rearrangement of the *ALK* gene (5–6% of NSCLC). Therapies that inhibit these two targets are approved for patients with advanced NSCLC. Patients whose tumors do not have the *EGFR* or *ALK* gene change may be able to enroll in a third ALCHEMIST treatment trial that is comparing the immune checkpoint inhibitor nivolumab to observation.

Despite the excitement and promise of precision oncology, much work remains before the majority of cancer patients benefit. At the interim analysis of NCI-MATCH in May 2016, despite enrolling 795 patients, only 2% of patients were paired with a targeted therapy [30]. While there is great promise in precision oncology, the field is still evolving and much progress is needed. Fortunately, the public and private sectors are dedicating significant resources to advancing cancer research, by developing information platforms that integrate tumor genomic information and treatment outcomes. The National Cancer Moonshot, with its $1 billion investment in cancer research and its goal of accelerating cancer research in the next 5 years, will hopefully further these efforts by enhancing data access, and facilitating collaborations among researchers, physicians, patients, and industry.

As our knowledge of the genetics of cancer increases, the way we conduct clinical trials to study new therapies will also need to evolve. To transition into the era of personalized medicine, cancer clinical trials will need to improve in a number of ways including: Involvement, Informativeness, Innovation, and Interconnectedness [31]. Increased involvement from oncology patients and physicians, particularly community physicians, is critical. Informativeness and innovation will require the development and adoption of novel approaches for study design, data collection and analysis, as well as maximizing learning from early stage trials to better identify the optimal dose, schedule, and patient selection tools for late phase trials. The development of next generation sequencing techniques has enabled investigators to simultaneously study hundreds or even thousands of genes in a small sample of tumor. This amount of data requires advances and innovation in the area of bioinformatics to analyze genomic information in concert with clinical data. Improved interconnectedness, by increasing the collaboration among industry, public sponsors, academic centers, and organizations with an interest in cancer research, has the potential to efficiently generate new knowledge that will rapidly improve the outcomes of cancer patients.

References

1 National Cancer Institute. NCI's Clinical Trials Programs and Initiatives. Updated: June 24, 2016. https://www.cancer.gov/research/areas/clinical-trials (accessed 18 August 2017).

2 The National Commission for the Protection of Human Subjects of Biomedical and Behavioral Research. The Belmont Report: Ethical Principles and Guidelines for the Protection of Human Subjects of Research. 1979.

3 Office for Human Research Protections. Federal Policy for the Protection of Human Subjects ('Common Rule'). In: U.S. Department of Health & Human Services 1991. http://www.hhs.gov/ohrp/humansubjects/commonrule (accessed 18 August 2017).

4 Daugherty CK. Impact of therapeutic research on informed consent and the ethics of clinical trials: a medical oncology perspective. *J Clin Oncol* 1999;17(5):1601–17.

5 Fried C. *Medical Experimentation: Personal Integrity and Social Policy*. Amsterdam: North Holland Publishing, 1974.

6 Kinders R, Parchment RE, Ji J, *et al*. Phase 0 clinical trials in cancer drug development: from FDA guidance to clinical practice. *Mol Interv* 2007;7(6):325–34.

7 U.S. Department of Health and Human Services; Food and Drug Administration. Guidance for Industry, Investigators, and Reviewers: Exploratory IND Studies. http://www.fda.gov/downloads/Drugs/GuidanceComplianceRegulatoryInformation/Guidances/ucm078933.pdf. 2006 (accessed 18 August 2017).

8 LoRusso PM. Phase 0 clinical trials: an answer to drug development stagnation? *J Clin Oncol* 2009;27(16):2586–8.

9 Von Hoff DD. There are no bad anticancer agents, only bad clinical trial designs: Twenty-first Richard and Hinda Rosenthal Foundation Award Lecture. *Clin Cancer Res* 1998;4:1079–86.

10 Kummar S, Gutierrez M, Doroshow JH, Murgo AJ. Drug development in oncology: classical cytotoxics and molecularly targeted agents. *Br J Clin Pharmacol* 2006;62(1):15–26.

11 Sleijfer S, Bogaerts J, Siu LL. Designing transformative clinical trials in the cancer genome era. *J Clin Oncol* 2013;31(15):1834–41.

12 Maitland ML, Hudoba C, Snider KL, Ratain MJ. Analysis of the yield of phase II combination therapy trials in medical oncology. *Clin Cancer Res* 2010;16(21):5296–302.

13 Lee JJ, Feng L. Randomized phase II designs in cancer clinical trials: current status and future directions. *J Clin Oncol* 2005;23(19):4450–7.

14 Daugherty CK, Ratain MJ, Emanuel EJ, Farrell AT, Schilsky RL. Ethical, scientific, and regulatory perspectives regarding the use of placebos in cancer clinical trials. *J Clin Oncol* 2008;26(8):1371–8.

15 Giuliano AE, Hunt KK, Ballman KV, *et al*. Axillary dissection vs no axillary dissection in women with invasive breast cancer and sentinel node metastasis: a randomized clinical trial. *JAMA* 2011;305(6):569–75.

16 Clinical Outcomes of Surgical Therapy Study Group. A comparison of laparoscopically assisted and open colectomy for colon cancer. *N Engl J Med* 2004;350(20):2050–9.

17 Virtamo J, Pietinen P, Huttunen JK, *et al*. Incidence of cancer and mortality following alpha-tocopherol and beta-carotene supplementation: a postintervention follow-up. *JAMA* 2003;290(4):476–85.

18 Hennekens CH, Buring JE, Manson JE, *et al*. Lack of effect of long-term supplementation with beta carotene on the incidence of malignant neoplasms and cardiovascular disease. *N Engl J Med* 1996;334(18):1145–9.

19 Lippman SM, Klein EA, Goodman PJ, *et al*. Effect of selenium and vitamin E on risk of prostate cancer and other cancers: the Selenium and Vitamin E Cancer Prevention Trial (SELECT). *JAMA* 2009;301(1):39–51.

20 Klein EA, Thompson IM, Jr., Tangen CM, *et al*. Vitamin E and the risk of prostate cancer: the Selenium and Vitamin E Cancer Prevention Trial (SELECT). *JAMA* 2011;306(14):1549–56.

21 Institute of Medicine. A National Cancer Clinical Trials System for the 21st Century: Reinvigorating the NCI Cooperative Group Program, 2010.

22 Cassileth BR. Clinical trials: time for action. *J Clin Oncol* 2003;21(5):765–6.

23 Mills EJ, Seely D, Rachlis B, *et al*. Barriers to participation in clinical trials of cancer: a meta-analysis and systematic review of patient-reported factors. *Lancet Oncol* 2006;7(2):141–8.

24 Minasian LM, Carpenter WR, Weiner BJ, *et al*. Translating research into evidence-based practice: the National Cancer Institute Community Clinical Oncology Program. *Cancer* 2010;116(19):4440–9.

25 National Cancer Institute. NCI's Clinical Trials Cooperative Group Program. https://www.cancer.gov/research/areas/clinical-trials (accessed 22 August 2017).

26 Compressing Timelines for CTEP-Supported Cancer Treatment Trials – A Response to the OEWG Report. http://ctep.cancer.gov/SpotlightOn/OEWG.htm (accessed 18 August 2017).

27 McCaskill-Stevens W, Lyss AP, Good M, Marsland T, Lilenbaum R. The NCI Community Oncology Research Program: what every clinician needs to know. *Am J Soc Clin Oncol Educ Book* 2013. doi: 10.1200/EdBook_AM.2013.33.e84.

28 Zon R, Meropol NJ, Catalano RB, Schilsky RL. American Society of Clinical Oncology Statement on minimum standards and exemplary attributes of clinical trial sites. *J Clin Oncol* 2008;26(15):2562–7.

29 McNeil C. NCI-MATCH launch highlights new trial design in precision–medicine era. *J Natl Cancer Inst* 2015;107(7): djv193 doi: 10.1093/jnci/djv193.

30 ECOG-ACRIN. Executive Summary: Interim Analysis of the NCI-MATCH Trial May 6, 2016. http:// ecog-acrin.org/nci-match-eay131/interim-analysis (accessed 18 August 2017).

31 Maitland ML, Schilsky RL. Clinical trials in the era of personalized oncology. *CA Cancer J Clin* 2011;61(6): 365–81.

25

Complementary and Alternative (Integrative) Oncology

Gabriel Lopez[1], Richard Lee[2], M. Kay Garcia[1], Alejandro Chaoul[1], and Lorenzo Cohen[1]

[1] *University of Texas MD Anderson Cancer Center, Houston, Texas, USA*
[2] *Case Western Reserve University, Cleveland, Ohio, USA*

Introduction

Complementary and alternative medicine (CAM) approaches have gained increasing acceptance in western medicine. With an increasing number of CAM offerings, patients need guidance in navigating the available information to make informed decisions about their use. Integrative medicine practitioners can include physicians, midlevel providers, and nurses with an integrative medicine focus, and other practitioners already part of most interdisciplinary integrative teams including psychologists, acupuncturists, massage, art, and music therapists. Developing an integrative care plan requires a thoughtful, evidence-based, and safe approach to incorporating nonconventional CAM therapies with conventional disease-directed therapeutics.

Definitions: Alternative, Complementary, Integrative

In the United States (US), CAM is defined by the National Center for Complementary and Integrative Health (NCCIH) as "a group of diverse medical and healthcare systems, practices, and products that are not normally considered to be part of conventional medicine" [1]. NCCIH is part of the National Institutes of Health and classifies CAM therapies into three broad categories: natural products, mind and body medicine, and other complementary medicine approaches (see Table 25.1) [2].

It is important to recognize the distinction between alternative, complementary, and integrative medicine [3]. Alternative medicine is defined as use of a nonconventional modality for which there is no scientific evidence of efficacy in place of conventional medicine. Although alternative medicine is not discussed in this chapter, that topic (including consequences of foregoing evidence-based treatment) has been reviewed elsewhere [4–6]. Complementary medicine is an approach combining conventional treatment with CAM or nonconventional therapies for which there may or may not exist scientific evidence of safety and effectiveness. Integrative medicine, on the other hand, seeks to merge conventional medicine and complementary therapies in a manner that is comprehensive, personalized, evidence based, and safe in order to achieve optimal health and healing. The Academic Consortium for Integrative Medicine and Health has defined this term as the practice of medicine that "reaffirms the importance of the relationship between practitioner and patient, focuses on the whole person, is informed by evidence, and makes use of all appropriate therapeutic and lifestyle approaches, healthcare professionals and disciplines to achieve optimal health and healing" [7]. To more accurately reflect the goals of integrative medicine, the term CIM, or complementary and integrative medicine, has seen increasing use in the literature, replacing CAM. Although applying the concept of integrative medicine to cancer care is still in its formative years, a number of comprehensive cancer centers in the US are putting this concept into practice under the term *Integrative Oncology*.

Prevalence of CIM

CIM use is common worldwide, with increasing availability to the general population as well as cancer patients in the US. The World Health Organization (WHO) estimates that up to 80% of people in developing countries rely on nonconventional traditional medicines for primary healthcare [8]. People in more developed countries also seek out these medicines and practices assuming that they are effective and may be safer than allopathic medicine because they are natural. Data from a 2012 survey shows 33.2% of the US adult population using CIM therapies excluding prayer in the previous 12 months [9]. CIM therapies are used by up to 69% of cancer patients, with increased use in those with advanced cancers [10–12]. The greatest concern is when these therapies, especially biological products like herbs and supplements, have the potential to adversely impact conventional treatment outcomes, either decreasing treatment

Table 25.1 National Institutes of Health – National Center for Complementary and Integrative Health.

Complementary health approaches	Examples
Natural products	Dietary supplements: • Herbal medicines (botanicals) • Vitamins • Minerals • Probiotics
Mind and body practices	Meditation Yoga Acupuncture Tai chi and Qigong Massage therapy Relaxation techniques: • Breathing exercises • Guided imagery • Progressive muscle relaxation Movement therapies: • Feldenkrais • Pilates Spinal manipulation: • Chiropractic • Osteopathic • Physical therapy Energy therapies: • Healing touch • Reiki • Magnet therapy Hypnotherapy
Other complementary health approaches	Whole medical systems: • Traditional healers • Ayurvedic medicine • Traditional Chinese medicine • Homeopathy • Naturopathy

Source: adapted from NCCIH Pub No. D347; https://nccih.nih.gov/health/integrative-health (accessed 21 August 2017).

efficacy by speeding up drug metabolism or possibly increasing toxicity by enhancing bioavailability of the drugs.

In the general population, individuals who use CIM are not disappointed or dissatisfied with conventional medicine [13]. Cancer patients and survivors report using CIM because they seek to reduce side effects such as organ toxicity, to improve quality of life, to protect and stimulate immunity, or to prevent further cancers or recurrences [11, 14, 15]. Whether or not patients living with cancer use CIM therapies to treat cancer or its effects, they may also use them to treat other chronic conditions such as arthritis, heart disease, diabetes, and chronic pain.

CIM and Symptom Management

Routine assessment for interest in and prior use of CIM approaches alongside symptom assessment is critical to the ongoing care of patients, ensuring the highest quality care

[16, 17]. A collaborative approach involving the patient's main hematology-oncology team and colleagues in integrative medicine, palliative care, pain management, psychiatry, and rehabilitation can more effectively meet patient needs. For those seeking integrative medicine approaches for the management of their symptoms, initial and follow-up symptom assessment is critical. CIM approaches can be incorporated into the healthcare plan from diagnosis, through active treatment, survivorship, and end-of-life. A personalized symptom management strategy utilizing an evidence-based application of conventional and nonconventional therapies can help improve quality of life and optimize treatment outcomes.

Communicating about CIM

Using a receptive, nonjudgmental approach to ask patients about CIM use is an important first step to developing an integrative care plan. Research indicates that neither adult nor pediatric cancer patients receive sufficient information or discuss CIM therapies with physicians, pharmacists, nurses, or CIM practitioners [18]. Most patients do not bring up the topic of CIM because no one asks; thus, patients may believe it is unimportant. It is estimated that 38–60% of patients with cancer used complementary approaches without informing their healthcare team [10, 11]. This lack of discussion is of concern because biologically based therapies (such as herbs) may interact unfavorably with cancer treatments. Patients are commonly unaware of differences between the US Food and Drug Administration (FDA) approval process for medications and the limited extent of regulation for dietary supplements under the Dietary Supplement Health and Education Act (DSHEA) of 1994 [19]. Supplements under this legislation are exempt from the same scrutiny the FDA imposes on medications; these supplements are not intended to treat, prevent, or cure diseases and such products should be labeled with this statement.

The common belief by patients that "natural" means safe is misplaced and appropriate education in this area is necessary. Some herbs and supplements have been associated with drug interactions [20], increased cancer risk [21], and organ toxicity [22]. Existing research suggests that the majority of cancer patients desire communication with their doctors about CIM [23]. If the topic of CIM arises, clinicians need to develop an empathic communication strategy [24]. The strategy needs to balance clinical objectivity and creation of a therapeutic alliance, benefitting both patient and healthcare provider [25, 26]. Patients need reliable information on CIM from reliable resources, with adequate time to discuss this information with their oncologists [27] (see Table 25.2).

CIM Modalities

Patients may have a variety of motivations for seeking nonconventional therapies, including a desire to improve quality of life and prolong life, boost the immune system, and aid conventional medical treatments [11, 28]. An evidence-based approach to the integration of these nonconventional therapies can help patients develop realistic expectations, optimize safety, and improve outcomes. Natural products, mind–body approaches, massage, acupuncture, and music therapy are commonly used nonconventional therapies encountered in a variety of healthcare settings.

Natural Products

Natural products include a variety of substances such as herbs, vitamins, minerals, probiotics, and extracts. Biologically based CIM therapies such as natural products have the potential to cause harm. There is also great interest in investigating how these substances can be used safely along with conventional treatment approaches to improve cancer treatment outcomes. Issues to consider when discussing natural products include quality control, metabolic interactions, treatment interactions, organ toxicity, and cancer growth.

Quality Control

Concerns regarding herbs and supplements are also related to the quality of the manufactured product being sold. Herbs and other supplements available to patients over the counter are often manufactured with no strict regulation to ensure the quality of the product. With no standardized administration of the manufacturing process, concerns arise regarding the potential introduction of contaminants and lack of reliability with regard to the labeled dose or ingredients [29–32]. Herbs and supplements should be considered biological substances, similar to prescription medications, and, therefore, may be useful but could also lead to harm.

Metabolic Interactions

Drug–herb interactions have the potential to increase treatment-related toxicity and/or decrease treatment efficacy [33–35]. The clinical efficacy of chemotherapy or chemopreventive agents metabolized through the hepatic cytochrome P450 (CYP) system may be compromised by herbs or supplements acting as inducers or inhibitors [36, 37]. As an example, St John's wort (*Hypericum perforatum*), a herbal product popularly used to treat depression, is an inducer of CYP 3A4 and 2C9 [38]. As such, it may reduce clinical efficacy of irinotecan or imatinib [37]. A thorough review of herbs, vitamins, and supplements patients are using is critical to maximize patient safety during and after the completion of cancer-directed therapies.

Treatment Interactions

The use of antioxidants has been proposed for cancer prevention and treatment. Examples include vitamins A, C, E, selenium, and green tea extract. However, antioxidant supplementation may interfere with radiation and chemotherapy agents that depend on oxidative damage to exert their cytotoxic effects (i.e., alkylating agents, anthracyclines, or platinums) [39, 40]. Antioxidant supplements require further study of their safety and efficacy when used during active therapy or as chemoprevention [41]. Current recommendations are to obtain antioxidants through whole food sources until more evidence becomes available regarding the safe use of antioxidant supplements.

Organ Toxicity

Prolonged use of concentrated natural products may lead to organ toxicity. Green tea preparations have been associated with liver toxicity, most commonly leading to an elevation in liver enzymes [22]. While short-term exposure to hepatotoxins or nephrotoxins present in natural products may lead to transient and reversible organ injury, prolonged exposure can lead to organ failure. Certain herbs and supplements, such as *Ginkgo biloba*, saw palmetto, fish oil, and garlic, have been associated with increased risk of bleeding [20]. These agents should be discontinued before surgical procedures, and should be used cautiously with other agents that increase bleeding risk.

Cancer Growth

A common concern is the potential for herbs and supplements to stimulate cancer growth, leading to the development of new primary cancers or recurrences. As an example, phytoestrogens are plant-based compounds structurally similar to estradiol, able to bind estrogen receptors. Black cohosh, red clover, dong quai and flax contain phytoestrogens [42]. Randomized clinical trials are needed before a definitive recommendation can be made regarding their safe use in patients with hormone positive cancers. However, phytoestrogens in soy consumed as part of a healthy diet and as a whole food (not supplements, powders, or processed soy products) have been documented in multiple observational studies in the US and China to pose no risk for breast cancer patients and may have benefits [43–47].

Table 25.2 Recommended websites for evidence-based resources (all accessed 21 August 2017).

Organization/website (alphabetical order)	Address/URL
American Cancer Society	www.cancer.org/treatment/treatmentsandsideeffects/complementaryandalternativemedicine/index
Cochrane Review Organization	www.cochrane.org
Memorial Sloan-Kettering Cancer Center Integrative Medicine Service	www.mskcc.org/cancer-care/treatments/symptom-management/integrative-medicine/herbs
National Center for Complementary and Integrative Health (NCCIH)	nccih.nih.gov/
Natural Medicines	naturalmedicines.therapeuticresearch.com/
NCI Office of Cancer Complementary and Alternative Medicine (OCCAM)	cam.cancer.gov/
University of Texas MD Anderson Cancer Center, Integrative Medicine Center	www.mdanderson.org/integrativemedcenter

Mind–Body

Mind–body practices can be used by patients at any point throughout their cancer journey. Mind–body practices are defined by NCCIH as "a large and diverse group of techniques that are administered or taught to others by a trained practitioner or teacher" [2]. Mind–body techniques include relaxation, hypnosis, visual imagery, meditation, biofeedback, cognitive-behavioral therapies, group support, autogenic training, and spirituality as well as expressive arts therapies such as art, music, or dance. They also include practices such as yoga, tai chi, and qigong where focused attention on movement, breath, or sound can increase self-awareness and relieve stress and anxiety.

Newell *et al.* [48] reviewed psychological therapies for cancer patients and concluded that interventions involving self-practice and hypnosis for managing nausea and vomiting could be recommended, but further research was suggested to examine the benefits of relaxation training and guided imagery. Further research was also warranted to examine the benefits of relaxation and guided imagery for managing general nausea, anxiety, quality of life, and overall physical symptoms. Ernst *et al.* examined changes in the state of the evidence for mind–body therapies for various medical conditions between 2000 and 2005 and found that, over that period, maximal evidence had appeared for the use of relaxation techniques for anxiety, hypertension, insomnia, and nausea due to chemotherapy [49].

Research examining yoga, tai chi/qigong, and meditation incorporated into cancer care suggests that these mind–body practices help improve quality of life through improved mood, sleep quality, physical functioning, and overall well-being [50–54]. Mind–body practices have an excellent safety profile, with some practices requiring more physical activity than others. Mind–body practitioners with experience in cancer patient populations can provide guidance to help patients engage safely in practices such as meditation, yoga, and tai chi. As research continues, those treatments found beneficial will continue to be integrated into conventional medical care.

Managing aspects of mental health in oncology is critically important, as mood disorders can adversely affect mortality [55–57]. Mind–body approaches should be considered as well as more conventional therapies such as psychotherapy, cognitive behavioral therapy, and psychotropic medications (see Chapter 27 for more information on management of psychiatric complications of cancer care).

Massage

As a manipulative touch-based therapy, massage can benefit cancer patients when it is performed by individuals who have an awareness of their special needs [58]. A massage therapist with special training in oncology massage is the best equipped to safely deliver the massage. Risk of bruising, bleeding, or injury can be minimized by careful application of pressure, avoiding massage into the deep tissue or bone in selected patients. Areas that have recently had surgery or radiation should be avoided. In patients with extremities subject to lymphedema, therapists will need to adjust their technique to maximize safety. Patients may benefit from formal lymphedema therapy as part of a physical therapy program [59].

Research to date suggests that massage is helpful at relieving pain, anxiety, fatigue, distress and increasing relaxation [60, 61]. Benefit on mood and pain relief is limited to the more immediate effect of massage, with no current studies demonstrating long-term relief [62–64]. Anecdotal and case report evidence has suggested benefit of massage for relief of chemotherapy induced peripheral neuropathy [65]. A massage to the feet, hands, and head can provide therapeutic benefit as these areas are especially sensitive to tactile stimulation and can result in relaxation and increased well-being [66]. Massage provided by caregivers may offer a unique opportunity for interaction between patient and caregiver that can help enhance the well-being of both [67]. In addition to symptomatic relief, studies have also demonstrated systemic effects of massage, with decreases in cortisol levels resulting from a massage intervention [68, 69]. More research is needed to understand better the role of massage therapy in cancer symptom management.

Acupuncture

The traditional theory behind the benefits of acupuncture is that the placement of needles, heat, or pressure at specific places on the body can help to regulate the flow of qi (vital energy). The most common form of acupuncture involves the practice of inserting needles into the skin at specific points throughout the body to achieve a desired effect. Depending on the condition being treated, heat may be applied to the needles after insertion. Small stainless steel or gold studs or tacks are sometimes placed or taped at specific points on the ears and left in place for several days, which can be stimulated by pressure. For some patients, acupressure may be used, which involves applying pressure to acupoints instead of puncturing the skin.

In 1997, an NIH consensus statement supported the use of acupuncture for postoperative and chemotherapy-related nausea and vomiting and some types of pain. Previous studies have found acupuncture may help treat nausea caused by chemotherapy drugs and surgical anesthesia [70, 71] and although further scientifically rigorous research is needed, it is often used for other symptom management such as pain, chemotherapy-induced peripheral neuropathy, dry mouth, hot flashes, fatigue, and mood or sleep disturbances [72]. The mechanisms involved are believed to include enhanced conduction of bioelectromagnetic signals, activation of opioid systems, and activation of the autonomic and central nervous systems causing the release of various neurotransmitters and neurohormones [73].

A systematic review of studies involving cancer patients evaluated 42 randomized-controlled trials involving the use of acupuncture to help manage eight symptoms (nausea, pain, hot flashes, fatigue, radiation-induced xerostomia, prolonged postoperative ileus, anxiety/mood disorders, and sleep disturbance) [74]. This review also found the strongest evidence to date is in support of its use for pain, nausea, and vomiting. Although nausea and vomiting are among the top three most commonly reported side effects of cancer treatment, pain is the most common reason cancer patients use acupuncture.

When performed correctly, acupuncture has been shown to be a safe, minimally invasive procedure with few side effects [75, 76]. The most commonly reported complications are fainting, bruising, and mild pain. Infection is also a potential risk, although very uncommon. Acupuncture should only be performed by a healthcare professional with an appropriate license and preferably one who has had experience in treating patients with malignant diseases.

Music Therapy

Music therapy uses music (music making, songwriting, singing, listening) in a prescriptive manner for nonmusical goals, including improving quality of life [77]. Trained music therapists choose a music approach most appropriate to help patients achieve a desired result. Evidence suggests music therapy can help with management of mood disturbances, including anxiety [78, 79]. One technique, the ISO-Vectoring principle, calls for the music therapist to match the patient's mood with the music tempo; a subsequent increase or decrease in tempo can result in a change in the patient's mood [80]. Patients taught the ISO principle can learn to develop an individualized musical playlist to change their mood, for relaxation or stimulation. An integrative medicine practitioner can help identify those patients most likely to benefit from consultation with a music therapist.

Nutrition and Exercise

Growing evidence supports the important role of physical activity and nutrition in the health of cancer patients, and these factors have been correlated with improved clinical outcomes [81–87]. An integrative care plan is not complete without a personalized discussion regarding a patient's individual dietary needs and physical activity goals.

Nutrition

Patients are flooded with a number of dietary approaches and need guidance. Diets labeled as "anti-cancer" composed strictly of raw foods, juiced fruits and vegetables, animal protein sources or alkaline foods have no evidence to support their use and may be harmful during active treatment, lacking important nutrients necessary for proper healing and recovery. Some choices are offered to patients as an alternative to conventional treatment which can lead to delays in therapy and poor outcomes. As a general approach, a diet rich in fruits, vegetables, whole grains, and lean meats with an avoidance of processed foods can be part of a healthy lifestyle. Referral to a dietician can help patients and survivors identify how to best meet their nutritional needs during their cancer journey (see Chapter 23).

Exercise

Exercise can be important to patients receiving active treatment as well as survivors, helping to improve physical function and quality of life [88–90]. Regular exercise during cancer therapies such as chemotherapy or radiation has the potential to decrease treatment-related fatigue [91]. ACS guidelines for cancer prevention recommend avoidance of sedentary behavior, encouraging 150 min of moderate physical activity spread throughout the week [86]. Specialists in Cancer Rehabilitation can help develop an individualized, safe, and structured program of exercise for patients and survivors, taking into account

pre-existing comorbidities in the context of cancer- and cancer treatment-related impairments [92] (see Chapter 9).

CIM and Survivorship

Cancer survivors look to CIM therapies for a number of reasons, including a desire to decrease risk of recurrence, decrease risk of developing new cancers, manage residual cancer- or cancer treatment-related symptoms, and prevent other diseases [15]. Survivors also report using CIM therapies to treat chronic conditions such as arthritis, heart disease, diabetes, and chronic pain. It is important for survivors to discuss use of CIM therapies with their healthcare team to develop a plan for their safe and appropriate use.

CIM Research

CIM approaches are a challenge to investigate as they do not always lend themselves well to clinical trial approaches used for conventional drug therapies. Challenges in massage research include decisions regarding dosage (frequency and duration of massage) and design of a believable control group [93]. In acupuncture research, challenges include comparison of sham acupuncture versus true acupuncture [94]. For both acupuncture and massage research, it is important to account for the impact of therapeutic presence (patient–practitioner interaction) versus the therapeutic intervention (massage, acupuncture, etc.) on study outcomes.

Proper design of research trials, including control groups when appropriate, is crucial to be able to increase the amount of quality data available to support use of CIM therapies. To serve the public's best interests, it is important to be able to predict which patients might benefit most from a specific treatment approach versus those who may not benefit at all. Optimizing CIM treatment methods and understanding putative mechanisms can only be achieved through rigorous scientific endeavor and are the moral and ethical responsibility of CIM investigators. For evidence-based reviews of CIM modalities refer to the resources listed in Table 25.2.

Summary

Integrative oncology is an expanding discipline holding tremendous promise for additional treatment and symptom control options. An integrative approach provides patients, from diagnosis through survivorship, with a comprehensive system of care to help meet their needs. The majority of cancer patients are either using complementary medicines or want to know more about them, so it is incumbent on the conventional medical system to provide appropriate education and evidenced-based clinical services. The clinical model for integrative care requires a patient-centered approach with attention to patient concerns and enhanced communication skills. In addition, it is essential that conventional and nonconventional practitioners work together in developing a comprehensive, integrative care plan. In this way, cancer patients will receive the best medical care making use of all appropriate treatment modalities in a safe evidence-based manner to achieve optimal clinical outcomes.

References

1 National Center for Complementary/Integrative Health (NCCIH) of the National Institutes of Health. Are You Considering Complementary Medicine? Created December 2006; last updated September 2016. NCCAM Pub No. D339. Available from https://nccih.nih.gov/health/decisions/consideringcam.htm (accessed 21 August 2017).

2 National Center for Complementary/Integrative Health (NCCIH) of the National Institutes of Health. What is complementary and alternative medicine? Created October 2008; last updated June 2016. NCCAM Pub No. D347. Available from http://nccih.nih.gov/health/whatiscam/ (accessed 21 August 2017).

3 Deng G, Cassileth B. Complementary or alternative medicine in cancer care – myths and realities. *Nat Rev Clin Oncol* 2013;10:656–64.

4 Cassileth BR, Yarett IR. Cancer quackery: the persistent popularity of useless, irrational 'alternative' treatments. *Oncology* 2012;26:754.

5 Vickers A. Alternative cancer cures: "unproven" or "disproven"? *CA Cancer J Clin* 2004;54:110–8.

6 Johnson SB, Park HS, Gross CP, Yu JB. Use of alternative medicine for cancer and its impact on survival. *JNCI* 2018;110(1). djx145, https://doi.org/10.1093/jnci/djx145

7 Consortium of Academic Health Centers for Integrative Medicine (CAHCIM). Definition of Integrative Medicine. Developed and Adopted by The Consortium, May 2004. http://www.imconsortium.org/about/home.html.

8 World Health Organization. Traditional medicine. Fact Sheet No. 134. Geneva: WHO, 2003.

9 Clarke TC, Black LI, Stussman BJ, Barnes PM, Nahin RL. *Trends in the use of complementary health approaches among adults: United States, 2002–2012*. National health statistics reports; no 79. Hyattsville, MD: National Center for Health Statistics, 2015. https://www.cdc.gov/nchs/data/nhsr/nhsr079.pdf (accessed 21 August 2017).

10 Navo MA, Phan J, Vaughan C, *et al*. An assessment of the utilization of complementary and alternative medication in women with gynecologic or breast malignancies. *J Clin Oncol* 2004;22:671–7.

11 Richardson MA, Sanders T, Palmer JL, Greisinger A, Singletary SE. Complementary/alternative medicine use in a comprehensive cancer center and the implications for oncology. *J Clin Oncol* 2000;18:2505–14.

12 Dy GK, Bekele L, Hanson LJ, *et al*. Complementary and alternative medicine use by patients enrolled onto phase I clinical trials. *J Clin Oncol* 2004;22:4810–5.

13 Eisenberg DM, Kessler RC, Van Rompay MI, *et al*. Perceptions about complementary therapies relative to conventional therapies among adults who use both: results from a national survey. *Ann Intern Med* 2001;135:344–51.

14 Molassiotis A, Fernandez-Ortega P, Pud D, *et al*. Use of complementary and alternative medicine in cancer patients: a European survey. *Ann Oncol* 2005;1:65–3.

15 Mao JJ, Palmer CS, Healy KE, *et al*. Complementary and alternative medicine use among cancer survivors: a population-based study. *J Cancer Surviv* 2011;5:8–17.

16 Paterson C, Thomas K, Manasse A, Cooke H, Peace G. Measure Yourself Concerns and Wellbeing (MYCaW): an individualised questionnaire for evaluating outcome in cancer support care that includes complementary therapies. *Complement Ther Med* 2007;15:38–45.

17 Frenkel M, Cohen L, Peterson N, *et al*. Integrative medicine consultation service in a comprehensive cancer center: findings and outcomes. *Integr Cancer Ther* 2010;9:276–83.

18 Oneschuk D, Fennell L, Hanson J, Bruera E. The use of complementary medications by cancer patients attending an outpatient pain and symptom clinic. *J Palliat Care* 1998;14:21–6.

19 103rd Congress. Dietary Supplement Health and Education Act of 1994 (DSHEA). Public Law 1994;103–417.

20 Ulbricht C, Chao W, Costa D, *et al*. Clinical evidence of herb-drug interactions: a systematic review by the natural standard research collaboration. *Curr Drug Metab* 2008;9:1063–120.

21 Klein EA, Thompson IM Jr, Tangen CM, *et al*. Vitamin E and the risk of prostate cancer: the Selenium and Vitamin E Cancer Prevention Trial (SELECT). *JAMA* 2011 306:1549–56.

22 Mazzanti G, Menniti-Ippolito F, Moro PA, *et al*. Hepatotoxicity from green tea: a review of the literature and two unpublished cases. *Eur J Clin Pharmacol* 2009;65:331–41.

23 Verhoef MJ, White MA, Doll R. Cancer patients' expectations of the role of family physicians in communication about complementary therapies. *Cancer Prev Control* 1999;3:181–7.

24 Berk LB. Primer on integrative oncology. *Hematol Oncol Clin North Am* 2006;20:213–31.

25 Sugarman J, Burk L. Physicians' ethical obligations regarding alternative medicine. *JAMA* 1998;280:1623–5.

26 Robotin MC, Penman AG. Integrating complementary therapies into mainstream cancer care: which way forward? *Med J Aust* 2006;185:377–9.

27 Weiger WA, Smith M, Boon H, *et al*. Advising patients who seek complementary and alternative medical therapies for cancer. *Ann Intern Med* 2002;137:889–903.

28 Nahleh Z, Tabbara IA. Complementary and alternative medicine in breast cancer patients. *Palliat Support Care* 2003;1:267–73.

29 Gilroy CM, Steiner JF, Byers T, Shapiro H, Georgian W. *Echinacea* and truth in labeling. *Arch Intern Med* 2003;163:699–704.

30 Saper RB, Philips RS, Sehgal A, *et al*. Lead, mercury, and arsenic in US- and Indian-manufactured Ayurvedic medicines sold via the Internet. *JAMA* 2008;300:915–23.

31 Posadzki P, Watson L, Ernst E. Contamination and adulteration of herbal medicinal products (HMPs): an overview of systematic reviews. *Eur J Clin Pharmacol* 2013;69:295–307.

32 Newmaster SG, Grguric M, Shanmughanandhan D, Ramalingam S, Ragupathy S. DNA barcoding detects contamination and substitution in North American herbal products. *BMC Med* 2013;11:222.

33 Palmer ME, Haller C, McKinney PE, *et al*. Adverse events associated with dietary supplements: an observational study. *Lancet* 2003;361(9352):101–6.

34 Izzo AA. Interactions between herbs and conventional drugs: overview of the clinical data. *Med Princ Pract* 2012;21:404–28.

35 Hardy ML. Herb-drug interactions: an evidence-based table. *Alt Med Alert* 2000;3:1.

36 Mathijssen RHJ, Verweij J, DeBruijn P. Modulation of irinotecan (CPT-11) metabolism by St John's wort in cancer patients. American Association for Cancer Research, 93rd Annual Meeting, San Francisco, April 6–10, 2002.

37 Smith P, Bullock JM, Booker BM, *et al*. The influence of St John's wort on the pharmacokinetics and protein binding of imatinib mesylate. *Pharmacotherapy* 2004;24:1508–14.

38 Markowitz JS, Donovan JL, DeVane CL, *et al*. Effect of St John's wort on drug metabolism by induction of cytochrome P450 3A4 enzyme. *JAMA* 2003;290:1500–4.

39 Lawenda BD, Kelly KM, Ladas EJ, *et al*. Should supplemental antioxidant administration be avoided during chemotherapy and radiation therapy? *J Natl Cancer Inst* 2008;100:773–83.

40 Bairati I, Meyer F, Gélinas M, *et al*. Randomized trial of antioxidant vitamins to prevent acute adverse effects of radiation therapy in head and neck cancer patients. *J Clin Oncol* 2005;23:5805–13.

41 Martinez ME, Jacobs ET, Baron JA, *et al*. Dietary supplements and cancer prevention: balancing potential benefits agains proven harms. *J Natl Cancer Inst* 2012;104:732–9.

42 Ososki, AL, Kennelly EJ. Phytoestrogens: a review of the present state of research. *Phytother Res* 2003;17:845–869.

43 Boyapati SM, Shu XO, Ruan ZX, *et al*. Soyfood intake and breast cancer survival: a follow up of the Shanghai Breast Cancer Study. *Breast Cancer Res Treat* 2005; 92:11–17.

44 Fink BN, Steck SE, Wolff MS, *et al*. Dietary flavonoid intake and breast cancer survival among women on Long Island. *Cancer Epidemiol Biomarkers Prev* 2007; 6:2285–92.

45 Guha N, Kwan ML, Quesenberry CP Jr, *et al*. Soy isoflavones and risk of cancer recurrence in a cohort of breast cancer survivors: the Life After Cancer Epidemiology study. *Breast Cancer Res Treat* 2009;118:395–405.

46 Shu XO, Zheng Y, Cai H, *et al*. Soy food intake and breast cancer survival. *JAMA* 2009; 302:2437–43.

47 Dong J-Y, and Qin L-Q. Soy isoflavones consumption and risk of breast cancer incidence or recurrence: a meta-analysis of prospective studies. *Breast Cancer Res Treat* 2011;125:315–23.

48 Newell SA, Sanson-Fisher W, Savolainen NJ. Systematic review of psychological therapies for cancer patients: overview and recommendations for future research. *J Natl Cancer Inst* 2002;94:558–84.

49 Ernst E, Pittler MH, Wider B, *et al*. Mind-body therapies: are the trial data getting stronger? *Altern Ther Health Med* 2007;13:62–64.

50 Syrjala, KL, Chapko ME. Evidence for a biopsychosocial model of cancer treatment-related pain. *Pain* 1995;61:69–79.

51 Cohen L, Warneke C, Fouladi RT, Rodriguez MA, Chaoul-Reich A. Psychological adjustment and sleep quality in a randomized trial of the effects of a Tibetan yoga intervention in patients with lymphoma. *Cancer* 2004;100:2253–60.

52 Bower JE, Woolery A, Sternlieb B, *et al*. Yoga for cancer patients and survivors. *Cancer Control* 2005;12:165–71.

53 Chandwani KD, Thornton B, Perkins GH, *et al*. Yoga improves quality of life and benefit finding in women undergoing radiotherapy for breast cancer. *J Soc Integr Oncol* 2010;8:43–55.

54 Oh B, Butow PN, Mullan BA, *et al*. Effect of medical Qigong on cognitive function, quality of life, and a biomarker of inflammation in cancer patients: a randomized controlled trial. *Supp Care Cancer* 2012;20:1235–42.

55 Satin JR, Linden W, Phillips MJ. Depression as a predictor of disease progression and mortality in cancer patients: a meta-analysis. *Cancer* 2009;115:5349–61.

56 Giese-Davis J, Collie K, Rancourt KM, *et al*. Decrease in depression symptoms is associated with longer survival in patients with metastatic breast cancer: a secondary analysis. *J Clin Oncol* 2011;29:413–20.

57 Cohen L, Cole SW, Sood AK, *et al*. Depressive symptoms and cortisol rhythmicity predict survival in patients with renal cell carcinoma: role of inflammatory signaling. *PLoS One* 2012;7:e42324.

58 Collinge W, MacDonald G, Walton T. Massage in supportive cancer care. *Semin Oncol Nurs* 2012;28:45–54.

59 Torres Lacomba M, Yuste Sanchez MJ, Zapico Goni A, *et al*. Effectiveness of early physiotherapy to prevent lymphoedema after surgery for breast cancer: randomised single blinded, clinical trial. *BMJ* 2010; 340:b5396.

60 Cassileth, BR, Vickers, AJ. Massage therapy for symptom control: outcome study at a major cancer center. *J Pain Symptom Manage* 2004; 28:244–9.

61 Russell NC, Sumler SS, Beinhorn CM, Frenkel MA. Role of massage therapy in cancer care. *J Altern Complement Med* 2008;14:209–14.

62 Kutner JS[1], Smith MC, Corbin L, Hemphill L, *et al*. Massage thcrapy versus simple touch to impove pain and mood in patient with advanced cancer: a randomized trial. *Ann Intern Med* 2008;149:369–79.

63 Wilkinson SM[1], Love SB, Westcombe AM, *et al*. Effectiveness of aromatherapy massage in the management of anxiety and depression in patients with cancer: a multicenter randomized controlled trial. *J Clin Oncol* 2007;25:532–9.

64 Campeau MP, Gaboriault R, Drapeau M, *et al*. impact of massage therapy on anxiety levels in patients undergoing radiation therapy: randomized controlled trial. *J Soc Integr Oncol* 2007;5:133–8.

65 Cunningham JE, Kelechi T, Sterba K, *et al*. Case report of a patient with chemotherapy-induced peripheral neuropathy treated with manual therapy (massage). *Support Care Cancer* 2011;19:1473–6.

66 Grealish L, Lomasney A, Whiteman B. Foot massage. A nursing intervention to modify the distressing symptoms of pain and nausea in patients hospitalized with cancer. *Cancer Nursing* 2000;23:237–43.

67 Collinge W, Kahn J, Walton T, *et al*. Touch, caring, and cancer: randomized controlled trial of a multimedia caregiver education program. *Support Care Cancer* 2013;21:1405–14.

68 Stringer J, Swindell R, Dennis M. Massage in patients undergoing intensive chemotherapy reduces serum cortisol and prolactin. *Psychooncology* 2008;17:1024–31.

69 Listing M, Krohn M, Liezmann C, *et al*. The efficacy of classical massage on stress perception and cortisol following primary treatment of breast cancer. *Arch Womens Ment Health* 2010;13:165–73.

70   Lee A, Done ML. The use of nonpharmacologic techniques to prevent postoperative nausea and vomiting: a meta-analysis. *Anesth Analg* 1999;88:1362–9.

71   Ezzo J, Vickers A, Richardson MA, *et al.* Acupuncture-point stimulation for chemotherapy-induced nausea and vomiting. *J Clin Oncol* 2005;23:7188–98.

72   Acupuncture (PDQ) – Health Professional Version. National Cancer Institute. https://www.cancer.gov/about-cancer/treatment/cam/hp/acupuncture-pdq (accessed 21 August 2017).

73   Helms JM. *Acupuncture Energetics: A Clinical Approach for Physicians.* Berkeley: Medical Acupuncture Publishers, 1997:20–42.

74   Garcia MK, McQuade J, Haddad R, *et al.* Systematic review of acupuncture in cancer care: a synthesis of the evidence. JCO 2012 (review pending). *J Clin Oncol* 2013;31:952–60.

75   Ernst, E, White AR. Prospective studies of the safety of acupuncture: a systematic review. *Am J Med* 2001;110:481–5.

76   Filshie J. Safety aspects of acupuncture in palliative care. *Acupunct Med* 2001;19:117–22.

77   Hilliard RE. the effects of music therapy on the quality and length of life of people diagnosed with terminal cancer. *J Music Ther* 2003;40:113–37.

78   Cassileth, BR, Vickers AJ, Magill LA. Music therapy for mood disturbance during hospitalization for autologous stem cell transplantation: a randomized controlled trial. *Cancer* 2003;15:98:223–9.

79   Bradt J, Dileo C, Grocke D, *et al.* Music interventions for improving psychological and physical outcomes in cancer patients. Cochrane Database Syst Rev 2011; :CD006911.

80   Richardson M, Babiak-Vazquez AE, Frenkel MA. Music therapy in a comprehensive cancer center. *J Soc Integrat Oncol* 2008;6:76–81.

81   Chlebowski RT, Blackburn GL, Thomson CA, *et al.* Dietary fat reduction and breast cancer outcome: interim efficacy results from the Women's Intervention Nutrition Study. *J Natl Cancer Inst* 2006;98:1767–76.

82   Meyerhardt JA, Heseltine D, Niedzwiecki D, *et al.* Impact of physical activity on cancer recurrence and survival in patients with stage III colon cancer: findings from CALGB 89803. *J Clin Oncol* 2006;24:3535–41.

83   Meyerhardt JA, Niedzwiecki D, Hollis D, *et al.* Association of dietary patterns with cancer recurrence and survival in patients with stage III colon cancer. *JAMA* 2007;298:754–64.

84   Pierce JP, Natarajan L, Caan BJ, *et al.* Influence of a diet very high in vegetables, fruit, and fiber and low in fat on prognosis following treatment for breast cancer: the Women's Healthy Eating and Living (WHEL) randomized trial. *JAMA* 2007;298:289–98.

85   Pierce JP, Stefanick ML, Flatt SW, *et al.* Greater survival after breast cancer in physically active women with high vegetable-fruit intake regardless of obesity. *J Clin Oncol* 2007;25:2345–51.

86   Kushi LH, Doyle C, McCullough M, *et al.* American Cancer Society Guidelines on Nutrition and Physical Activity for Cancer Prevention: Reducing the Risk of Cancer With Healthy Food Choices and Physical Activity. *CA Cancer J Clin* 2012;62:30–67.

87   Rock CL, Doyle C, Demark-Wahnefried W, *et al.* Nutrition and Physical Activity Guidelines for Cancer Survivors. *CA Cancer J Clin* 2012;62:242–74.

88   Courneya KS, Segal RJ, Mackey JR, *et al.* Effects of aerobic and resistance exercise in breast cancer patients receiving adjuvant chemotherapy: a multicenter randomized controlled trial. *J Clin Oncol* 2007;25:4396–404.

89   Courneya KS, Sellar CM, Stevinson C, *et al.* Randomized controlled trial of the effects of aerobic exercise on physical functioning and quality of life in lymphoma patients. *J Clin Oncol* 2009;27:4605–12.

90   Vallance JK, Courneya KS, Plotnikoff RC, *et al.* Randomized controlled trial of the effects of print materials and step pedometers on physical activity and quality of life in breast cancer survivors. *J Clin Oncol* 2007;25:2352–9.

91   Cramp F, Byron Daniel J. Exercise for the management of cancer-related fatigue in adults. *Cochrane Database Syst Rev* 2012;11:CD006145.

92   Silver JK, Baima J, MayerRS. Impairment-driven cancer rehabilitation: an essential component of quality care and survivorship. *CA Cancer J Clin* 2013;63:295–317.

93   Smith M, Kutner J, Hemphill L, *et al.* Developing treatment and control conditions in a clinical trial of massage therapy for advanced cancer. *J Soc Integr Oncol* 2007;5:139–46.

94   Witt CM, Schützler L. The gap between results from sham-controlled trials and trials using other controls in acupuncture research-the influence of context. *Complement Ther Med* 2013;21:112–4.

Section 5

Geriatric Oncology

26

Geriatric Oncology
Arvind M. Shinde[1], Sumanta K. Pal[2], and Arti Hurria[2]

[1] *Samuel Oschin Comprehensive Cancer Institute, Cedars-Sinai, Los Angeles, California, USA*
[2] *City of Hope Comprehensive Cancer Center, Duarte, California, USA*

Introduction

The United States (US) is undergoing a demographic change resulting in an older population [1]. In 1980, adults age 65 or older numbered 25 million, and this increased to 35 million in the year 2000. As the baby boomer generation ages, the US Census Bureau projects that by the year 2030, the number of individuals over the ages of 65 and 85 will more than double to nearly 62 million and 10 million, respectively [2, 3]. Furthermore, the centenarians are predicted to be the fastest growing segment of this population. Cancer occurs with greater frequency in older adults [1]. As the population of the US ages, it is expected that the number of cases of cancer will also increase. From 2010 to 2030, the total projected cancer incidence will increase by approximately 45% from 1.6 to 2.3 million. Based upon this demographic shift, a 67% increase in cancer incidence is predicted in older adults (age $\geq$ 65), as compared to an 11% increase in younger adults. Furthermore, from 2010 to 2030, the percentage of all cancers diagnosed in older adults will increase from 61 to 70% [3].

Caring for older patients with cancer creates a number of unique challenges. Aging is associated with decreased physiological reserve, functional dependence, increased comorbidities, and changes in cognitive functioning. These changes may have a direct impact on an individual's life expectancy, risk of further functional decline, risk of hospitalization, and other morbidities. [4–7]. However, chronological age may not accurately predict this decline, which is highly variable from individual to individual [8]. Furthermore, aging is associated with changes in social support structure and psychosocial well-being which can modulate these outcomes and add additional complexity to predicting an individual's physical tolerance and aging trajectory [9–11]. Many of these changes associated with aging can affect a patient's ability to tolerate cancer therapy.

Furthermore, changes in an individual's goals of therapy can influence the discussion regarding the appropriate therapeutic options.

The challenge in treating the older patient with cancer lies in an understanding of their individual vulnerability to the cancer-directed therapies, and the development of a good understanding of the balance between the risk and benefit associated with that therapy. To date, only a few oncologic studies have specifically incorporated baseline functional metrics in the elderly population to assess its impact on outcome. The most utilized indicators of functional status as predictors of risk for adverse outcomes of cancer therapy have been the Eastern Cooperative Oncology Group (ECOG) and Karnofsky Performance Status (KPS). Unfortunately, these indicators do not capture the variability and nuance in functional status in the geriatric population, nor do they incorporate external factors which can affect outcomes [12, 13]. Furthermore, older adults have been under-represented in oncologic clinical trials to date, and only a few published studies have focused on older patients who have been considered physically unable to tolerate standard cancer therapies [14, 15]. Because of the paucity of data in the oncologic literature, it can be helpful to apply principles from the geriatric literature to the treatment of older patients with cancer. Specifically, these principles coalesce around the utilization of a comprehensive geriatric assessment (CGA) to aid the clinician in assessing an older individual's risk of morbidity and mortality. More recently, studies are underway to incorporate a CGA tool into prospective oncologic clinical trials to expand our evidence-based knowledge of the impact of treatment in this patient population.

In this chapter, we will attempt to provide a brief overview of the important aspects of assessing the geriatric patient with cancer, with the goal of providing practical guidance on how to approach the management of the geriatric patient who is diagnosed with a malignancy.

The American Cancer Society's Principles of Oncology: Prevention to Survivorship, First Edition. Edited by The American Cancer Society.
© 2018 The American Cancer Society. Published 2018 by John Wiley & Sons, Inc.

"Geriatric"

The *Oxford Dictionary* defines geriatric as or "relating to old people, especially with regard to their health care", or "an old person, especially one receiving special care" [16]. Geriatric adults are often classified into three broad groups based upon their age: patients aged 65–75 years, patients aged 75–85 years, and patients who are older than 85 years of age [17]. As a generality, older patients have diminished physical reserves, increased comorbidities, and a greater risk of mortality. However, chronological age alone is not a reliable indicator of an individual's functional reserve, their psychosocial well-being, life expectancy, or tolerance to oncological therapies [8]. The treatment decisions for an older adult should be based upon an understanding of the potential risks and benefits of treatment in the context of an understanding of the individual's life expectancy. If an individual is expected to die from something other than their malignancy even if untreated, oncologic care should focus on supportive therapies. Patients who would be expected to live long enough to face the possibility of death from their malignancy should be evaluated for cancer therapy. While it is not possible for a physician to predict the life expectancy of an individual with precision, it is within the realm of their expertise to provide an estimation of whether the individual is expected to live longer, shorter, or on par with others of the same age. This determination can then be applied to life table data to estimate the life expectancy of an individual at any age [18]. Alternatively, validated tools such as the one developed by Lee *et al.* can be used to prognosticate the risk of 4-year mortality utilizing demographic variables, comorbid conditions, and functional variables [7, 19]. Web-based prognostic tools can also be used to estimate an individual's life expectancy without the diagnosis of cancer [20].

Assessing the Older Patient with Cancer

While estimation of life expectancy can assist in estimating which patients would not be expected to live long enough to achieve benefit from cancer-directed therapies, it does not provide enough information to determine which patients would be able to tolerate therapy well and those who would be expected to experience increased morbidity as a result of the therapy. In the field of geriatric medicine, the CGA has been utilized to predict the risk of morbidity and mortality in older adults. The CGA consists of multiple domains of assessment, each with independent predictive capabilities of morbidity and mortality. Components of the CGA have been associated with survival in older patients with specific cancer types [21–24]. The domains of the CGA include functional status, comorbidities, nutritional status, psychological state, cognitive function, and social support. In addition, a medication review is performed to identify if there is evidence of polypharmacy. These domains of a CGA and key questions to consider in daily practice are summarized below.

Functional Status

"Does my patient need help with basic activities needed to maintain independence at home or in the community?"

Table 26.1 ADLs and IADLs [27, 28].

Activities of Daily Living (ADLs)	Instrumental ADL (IADLs)
• Bathing	• Ability to use telephone
• Dressing	• Shopping
• Toileting	• Food preparation
• Transferring	• Housekeeping
• Continence	• Laundry
• Feeding	• Mode of transportation
	• Ability to take own medications
	• Ability to handle finances

The need for functional assistance has been demonstrated prospectively to be associated with morbidity and mortality in the geriatric population [25]. A number of tools have been developed and validated to describe the functional status of an older patient [26]. A commonly utilized tool evaluates an individual's ability to complete activities of daily living (ADLs) and instrumental activities of daily living (IADLs) (Table 26.1). ADLs encompass those basic skills of self-care required to maintain independence in the home [27]. IADLs encompass those more complex skills necessary to maintain independence in the community [28]. The need for assistance with ADLs and IADLs has been demonstrated to be predictive of severity of treatment-related toxicity, psychological distress, morbidity, and mortality in older patients with cancer [8, 21, 23, 29–32].

Comorbidities

"How will my patient's other medical problems impact their ability to tolerate cancer treatments and affect their life expectancy?"

Older adults have an increased prevalence and severity of comorbidities. Comorbidities can substantially impact treatment tolerance, morbidity, and mortality in adults with cancer [33, 34]. The US Preventive Services Task Force and the American Cancer Society recommend evaluating comorbid conditions and the implications for prognosis when developing an individualized screening plan for breast and colorectal cancer [35–37].

Common comorbidities present in the elderly population can impact treatment tolerance and morbidity. For example, cardiovascular disease, manifest as decreased left ventricular ejection fraction, may preclude a patient from receiving specific cancer therapies associated with an increased risk of heart failure, such as anthracyclines and trastuzumab. Impaired renal function, in the form of diminished glomerular filtration rate, may result in increased toxicity of administered drugs which are excreted by the kidney, or metabolized to toxic or active forms by the kidney.

Comorbid conditions such as diabetes, may impact cancer outcomes. For example, patients with diabetes, diagnosed with breast or colon cancer, experience a higher all-cause mortality rate, as well as an increased risk of chemotherapy associated toxicity and recurrence, respectively [38, 39]. Furthermore, poorly controlled diabetes may preclude a patient from receiving steroid therapies which are utilized as premedication for chemotherapeutic agents. Neuropathy, as a consequence of long-standing diabetes, may result in poor tolerance to chemotherapeutic agents that can cause neuropathy, such as taxanes and platinums. Furthermore, cardiovascular disease, renal dysfunction, and diabetes, when poorly controlled can increase the morbidity associated with oncologic surgery.

Indices for evaluating comorbidities have been developed and validated. The Charlson Comorbidity Index [40], the Adult Comorbidity Evaluation-27 Index [33], the Cumulative Illness Rating Scale [41] and the OARS Multidimensional Functional Assessment Questionnaire [42] are commonly used to capture and quantify comorbidity in the research setting. These comorbidity tools have been utilized to demonstrate a relationship between comorbidities and certain chemotherapy-associated toxicities, treatment discontinuation, infectious complications and reduction in overall survival.

Polypharmacy

"What medications is my patient taking? Is my patient at increased risk for drug interactions or side effects? What will be the effect of these medications on their cancer-directed treatment and outcomes?"

Older individuals are more susceptible to polypharmacy [43]. "Polypharmacy" can be defined as taking a large number of medications or taking clinically inappropriate medications, which includes unnecessary medications and duplicate medications [44, 45]. Older adults are at risk for polypharmacy given the increase in comorbidities with age, and an associated increase in the number of prescribed medications. Alterations in drug metabolism observed with aging can contribute to adverse drug reactions (ADRs) and interactions [45, 46]. ADRs can in turn facilitate functional decline and lead to geriatric syndromes. Furthermore, the use of multiple medications as is observed in older patients with cancer can increase the likelihood of non-adherence, as well as the potential for drug–drug interactions [44, 45, 47–49]. Certain classes of drugs have been implicated with a higher frequency of ADRs [50]. These include anticoagulants (specifically warfarin), benzodiazepines, anticholinergics, and corticosteroids, which are notable for their frequent use in patients with malignancies, for cancer-related thrombosis, management of anxiety, nausea, and edema [51, 52]. Given the strong association between polypharmacy and potential for poor outcomes in elderly patients, a medication review for inappropriate and duplicative medications is recommended at each clinical visit. This requires collaboration between patients, caregivers, and clinicians to keep and update a medication list and share the information amongst one another. Furthermore, asking patients to bring all medications to each visit can aid in the assessment.

Nutritional Status

"Has my patient experienced unintentional weight loss? Do they have a low or high body mass index? Is my patient able to meet their nutritional needs while undergoing therapy?"

Malnutrition among older adults is both a prevalent and serious condition. A number of studies in older adults have demonstrated that the prevalence of malnutrition rises with increasing comorbidity and functional dependence, with a relatively low rate in independent, community-dwelling older adults (2–16%), and a significantly higher rate in hospitalized or institutionalized older adults (20–65%) [53]. Several studies have also identified an association between a low body mass index and an increased risk of mortality [54–57]. This relationship highlights the importance of adequate nutrition. In patients with cancer, an association has also been observed across multiple malignancies between weight loss and poorer outcomes, including lower response rates to chemotherapy and decreased survival [58–60]. While some of the malnutrition can be attributed to the severity of the underlying illness, it is an independent predictor for morbidity [61]. Furthermore, cancer-related treatments can contribute to malnutrition in older adults. Chemotherapy-induced nausea, vomiting, diarrhea and mucositis can decrease an individual's oral intake. Treatment-related diarrhea can impair adequate caloric absorption. Furthermore, cancer and treatment-related fatigue can impair an individual's functional status, making it more difficult for them to obtain and prepare foods to meet their nutritional needs.

Cognitive Function

"Can my patient make treatment-related decisions, follow a treatment plan, and know what to do if they need help?"

A decline in cognitive function is associated with rising age and an increased risk for all-cause mortality [62, 63]. Older patients who are cognitively impaired have an elevated risk of functional dependence, depression, and mortality [64, 65]. The level of cognitive functioning is also predictive of medication adherence regardless of medical diagnosis or medication regimen [66]. Impairment in a patient's cognitive functioning may affect their capacity to assess the risks and benefits associated with cancer treatments. It may also affect their ability to adhere to a treatment plan, and to bring to medical attention the potentially dangerous adverse side effects of the cancer therapy. Therefore, it is important to evaluate cognitive function as well as the capacity to make treatment-related decisions prior to and during cancer therapy. Validated instruments are available to screen for impairment in cognitive function, and assess for decision-making capacity. Importantly, the determination of decision-making capacity focuses on the patient's ability to understand relevant information about the proposed treatments, to understand their current situation, to reason about the risks and benefits of specific actions or inaction, and to communicate their choice [67]. Delirium and depression are common causes of cognitive impairment that may improve when appropriately diagnosed and treated. Similarly, medications such as anticholinergics, antipsychotics, benzodiazapines, corticosteroids, and opioids can cause cognitive impairment in the older adult, and their use should be evaluated carefully, and discontinued when suspected of impacting cognitive function [65].

Social Support

"Does my patient have people in their lives to help to care for them?"

Numerous studies have demonstrated an association between social isolation and mortality across many disease states [9–11, 64]. This association has been confirmed in elderly patients with cancer [68]. In part, it is believed that the survival disadvantage is due to a lack of access to medical care and/or caregiving from friends, relatives, and adult children. Therefore, a patient's social support and presence of a caregiver should be assessed and taken into consideration when developing a care plan for an older patient with cancer.

Geriatric Syndromes

"Have my patient's age-associated medical conditions been optimized prior to treatment?"

Geriatric syndromes are "clinical conditions which are highly prevalent in older adults, especially in those who are vulnerable or frail, and cannot be attributed to a specific disease category" [69]. The geriatric syndromes of dementia, delirium, depression, distress, frailty, falls, and osteoporosis, are common in elderly patients with cancer and appear to increase in prevalence with age [22, 51]. Geriatric syndromes are more prevalent in older patients with cancer [69, 70]. Furthermore, these syndromes have been associated with increased risk of multiple adverse clinical outcomes [71]. Data from randomized studies indicate that interventions to mitigate the progression or effects of geriatric syndromes can result in improved functional status and mental well-being in older adults [72]. These data highlight the importance of early diagnosis and interventions to improve health outcomes in older patients with geriatric syndromes. Collaboration with rehabilitation services before, during, and after treatment can help to optimize and preserve a patient's functional status [73].

Coordination of Care: Role of the Multidisciplinary Team

The assessment of the above domains can be performed in collaboration with a multidisciplinary team, which is the cornerstone of geriatric medicine. The responsibility of the treating physician lies in recognizing if impairments exist, and if so, either treating them (depending on their level of comfort and expertise) or referring to the appropriate specialist who can address the impairment. Rapid screening for impairment can be achieved by systematically asking the questions associated with each of the above domains during the office visit. When an impairment is identified, referral to specialists within the local healthcare system can be made. Alternatively, community and governmental resources can be queried. An example of a government-funded resource which can assist with identifying local resources is the National Association of Area Agencies on Aging.

Diminished Physiological Capacity and Reserve

As an individual ages, there is a progressive decline in organ reserve [17, 74]. This impacts, for example, nerve conduction velocities, the cardiac output and resilience of the cardiovascular system, the maximum breathing capacity of the pulmonary system, the glomerular filtration rate of the kidneys, the risk of infection, and the regenerative capacity of the hematopoietic system. Furthermore, at a cellular level, the ability to maintain homeostasis is impaired. This decline can diminish an individual's ability to tolerate treatments directed towards their malignancy. Special attention must be given when utilizing chemotherapeutic drugs that can affect these systems in older patients. Furthermore, physiological mechanisms which are designed to restore homeostasis can also be impaired, resulting in a more rapid decline of function. For example, elderly patients may have a diminished thirst response when experiencing dehydration from poor oral intake resulting from mucositis. This can, in turn, further impair renal function, resulting in further loss of fluid homeostasis and oral intake. Therefore, a solid understanding of an individual's physiological reserve is important prior to initiating therapy. During treatment, close monitoring with attention to small changes in function are critical to prevent a rapid decline in overall functioning.

Predicting Chemotherapy-Associated Toxicity

Identifying which older patients are at high risk of developing chemotherapy-associated toxicities informs treatment decisions, including choice of cancer-directed treatments and intensity of supportive care. Recently, Extermann *et al.* published data on the capacity of the Chemotherapy Risk Assessment Scale for High-Age Patients (CRASH) score to predict the risk of severe chemotherapy toxicity (grade 4 hematologic, or grade 3/4 nonhematologic) in patients aged ≥ 70 years who were starting chemotherapy. The score was validated in its ability to stratify patients into four risk categories (low, medium-low, medium-high, and high) utilizing the individual's clinical, laboratory, and functional variables, with chemotherapy regimen specific toxicity criteria. It is noteworthy that even patients in the low risk category experienced significant grade 4 hematologic and grade 3/4 nonhematologic toxicities, emphasizing the importance of close monitoring of these patients [75].

Hurria *et al.* have developed a brief, but comprehensive geriatric assessment for older patients with cancer, which is largely patient administered and which assesses the functional age of the patient by evaluating the domains of functional status, comorbidity, cognition, psychological status, social functioning and support, and nutrition [76, 77]. A prospective evaluation of this tool in older patients (mean age of 73) found that it could be completed by the majority of older patients without assistance and that it identified important deficits and problems that may impact morbidity and mortality. A subsequent prospective study by the Cancer and Aging Research Group investigated pretreatment factors, including geriatric assessment questions, in order to formulate a predictive model for grade 3–5 toxicity from chemotherapy treatments in 500 patients with a mean age of 73 years undergoing treatment for a solid malignancy. In addition to the variables obtained as part of standard clinical oncologic practice (i.e., age, tumor, treatment, and laboratory values), geriatric assessment questions were independent predictors of chemotherapy toxicity. Specifically, functional status as assessed by the ability to walk one block, decreased social activities because of physical or emotional problems, falls in the last 6 months, need for assistance with taking medications, and poor hearing were predictors of chemotherapy toxicity. Interestingly, KPS did not identify patients at risk of chemotherapy toxicity, while the predictive model including geriatric assessment questions could identify those at risk [78]. This predictive model was subsequently validated in an independent cohort ($n = 250$) of older adults starting a new chemotherapy regimen [79].

Approach to the Older Patient with Cancer

It is important to recognize that no treatment plan is appropriate for all individuals. However, all patients should receive adequate supportive care and symptom management. The variability in the care plan arises from the question of who should receive additional cancer therapies. There is great heterogeneity in both physiologic age as well as the goals and values of each older adult. An individually tailored plan takes into consideration this diversity. The National Comprehensive Cancer Network guidelines for older adult oncology provide a useful algorithm for the management of the older patient diagnosed with a malignancy [80]. If a patient is expected to have a life expectancy that is short, such that they are likely to die from a cause other than the malignancy, the treatments should focus on symptom management and supportive care. If the patient is expected to live long enough that they are at a moderate to high risk of dying from the cancer without cancer-directed therapy, then the next step is to assess whether they have decision-making capacity. If not, the patient's proxy should be involved in the management decisions. If the patient does have capacity, are the goals and values of the patients consistent with wanting cancer-directed therapies? If no, care should focus on symptom management and supportive care. If yes, risk factors such as comorbidities, functional status, and nutritional issues should be assessed as described above.

If risk factors are found, they should be modified, if possible, prior to assessing the patient for therapy. If the risk factors are not modifiable, then these risk factors need to be considered in formulating the treatment plan. A regimen with a different toxicity profile and/or specific supportive therapies to decrease the risk of side effects should be considered depending on the specific risk factors identified. If a patient has no risk factors and is functionally independent, they should be considered a good candidate for most forms of cancer treatment, regardless of age. For patients who are expected to undergo standard cancer-directed therapies, treatment should be based upon the same treatment guidelines indicated for younger patients [81].

While in general it is expected that older adults with cancer derive the same benefit from chemotherapy treatment as do younger patients, the physiological changes associated with aging can result in an increased risk of toxicities from therapy. The most common complications observed in older patients receiving chemotherapy include prolonged myelosuppression (anemia, thrombocytopenia, neutropenia), mucositis, diarrhea, renal toxicity, neurotoxicity, and cardiac toxicity. Furthermore, these toxicities in conjunction with the tumor and the underlying physiological changes associated with aging, can lead to increased risk of infection, diarrhea, dehydration, malnutrition, electrolyte abnormalities, delirium, and functional dependence. Therefore, close monitoring and intervention, as necessary, is essential to successful completion of therapy and avoidance of severe complications. There should be a low threshold for inpatient hospitalization as these patients may have limited reserve capacity and may decline rapidly.

Older patients can benefit from treatments directed towards their cancers. However, more research needs to be done to evaluate which therapies provide the greatest benefit and the least associated morbidity. A comprehensive approach to evaluating older patients can be helpful in determining which patients would benefit from cancer-directed therapies, and optimizing those patients with modifiable risk factors. Predictive models of chemotherapy toxicity have been developed and validated in the geriatric population.

References

1 He W, Sengupta M, Velkoff VA, DeBarros KA, US Census Bureau. Current Population Reports P23–209. 65+ in the United States: 2005. Washington DC: US Government Printing Office, 2005.

2 Federal Interagency Forum on Aging-Related Studies. Older Americans 2008: *Key Indicators of Well Being.* Wasington DC: US Government Printing Office, March 2008.

3 Smith BD, Smith GL, Hurria A, Hortobagyi GN, Buchholz TA. Future of cancer incidence in the United States: burdens upon an aging, changing nation. *J Clin Oncol* 2009;27:2758–65.

4 Klein BE, Klein R, Knudtson MD, Lee KE. Frailty, morbidity and survival. *Arch Gerontol Geriatr* 2005;41:141–9.

5 Inouye SK, Peduzzi PN, Robison JT, *et al.* Importance of functional measures in predicting mortality among older hospitalized patients. *JAMA* 1998;279:1187–93.

6 Walter LC, Brand RJ, Counsell SR, *et al.* Development and validation of a prognostic index for 1-year mortality in older adults after hospitalization. *JAMA* 2001;285:2987–94.

7 Lee SJ, Lindquist K, Segal MR, Covinsky KE. Development and validation of a prognostic index for 4-year mortality in older adults. *JAMA* 2006;295:801–8.

8 Wedding U, Rohrig B, Klippstein A, Pientka L, Hoffken K. Age, severe comorbidity and functional impairment independently contribute to poor survival in cancer patients. *J Cancer Res Clin Oncol* 2007;133:945–50.

9 Iwasaki M, Otani T, Sunaga R, *et al.* Social networks and mortality based on the Komo-Ise cohort study in Japan. *Int J Epidemiol* 2002;31:1208–18.

10 Seeman TE, Kaplan GA, Knudsen L, Cohen R, Guralnik J. Social network ties and mortality among the elderly in the Alameda County Study. *Am J Epidemiol* 1987;126:714–23.

11 Tomaka J, Thompson S, Palacios R. The relation of social isolation, loneliness, and social support to disease outcomes among the elderly. *J Aging Health* 2006;18:359–84.

12 Repetto L, Fratino L, Audisio RA, *et al.* Comprehensive geriatric assessment adds information to Eastern Cooperative Oncology Group performance status in elderly cancer patients: an Italian Group for Geriatric Oncology Study. *J Clin Oncol* 2002;20:494–502.

13 Extermann M, Overcash J, Lyman GH, Parr J, Balducci L. Comorbidity and functional status are independent in older cancer patients. *J Clin Oncol* 1998;16:1582–7.

14 Hutchins LF, Unger JM, Crowley JJ, Coltman CA, Jr., Albain KS. Underrepresentation of patients 65 years of age or older in cancer-treatment trials. *N Engl J Med* 1999;341:2061–7.

15 Extermann M. *Conducting clinical trials for patients who are frail or elderly*. Alexandria, Virginia: American Society of Clinical Oncology, 2009.

16 Oxford Dictionaries Online - American English (US). Geriatric.

17 Balducci L, Extermann M. Management of cancer in the older person: a practical approach. *Oncologist* 2000;5:224–37.

18 Walter LC, Covinsky KE. Cancer screening in elderly patients: a framework for individualized decision making. *JAMA* 2001;285:2750–6.

19 Carey EC, Walter LC, Lindquist K, Covinsky KE. Development and validation of a functional morbidity index to predict mortality in community-dwelling elders. *J Gen Intern Med* 2004;19:1027–33.

20 ePrognosis – Estimating Prognosis for Elders. http://eprognosis.ucsf.edu (accessed 23 August 2017).

21 Maione P, Perrone F, Gallo C, *et al.* Pretreatment quality of life and functional status assessment significantly predict survival of elderly patients with advanced non-small-cell lung cancer receiving chemotherapy: a prognostic analysis of the multicenter Italian lung cancer in the elderly study. *J Clin Oncol* 2005;23:6865–72.

22 Koroukian SM, Murray P, Madigan E. Comorbidity, disability, and geriatric syndromes in elderly cancer patients receiving home health care. *J Clin Oncol* 2006;24:2304–10.

23 Winkelmann N, Petersen I, Kiehntopf M, *et al.* Results of comprehensive geriatric assessment effect survival in patients with malignant lymphoma. *J Cancer Res Clin Oncol* 2011;137:733–8.

24 Clough-Gorr KM, Thwin SS, Stuck AE, Silliman RA. Examining five- and ten-year survival in older women with breast cancer using cancer-specific geriatric assessment. *Eur J Cancer* 2012;48:805–12.

25 Reuben DB, Rubenstein LV, Hirsch SH, Hays RD. Value of functional status as a predictor of mortality: results of a prospective study. *Am J Med* 1992;93:663–9.

26 Applegate WB, Blass JP, Williams TF. Instruments for the functional assessment of older patients. *N Engl J Med* 1990;322:1207–14.

27 Katz S, Ford AB, Moskowitz RW, Jackson BA, Jaffe MW. Studies of illness in the aged. The index of ADL: a standardized measure of biological and psychosocial function. *JAMA* 1963;185:914–9.

28 Lawton MP, Brody EM. Assessment of older people: self-maintaining and instrumental activities of daily living. *Gerontologist* 1969;9:179–86.

29 Koroukian SM, Xu F, Bakaki PM, *et al.* Comorbidities, functional limitations, and geriatric syndromes in relation to treatment and survival patterns among elders with colorectal cancer. *J Gerontol A Biol Sci Med Sci* 2010;65:322–9.

30 Freyer G, Geay JF, Touzet S, *et al.* Comprehensive geriatric assessment predicts tolerance to chemotherapy and survival in elderly patients with advanced ovarian carcinoma: a GINECO study. *Ann Oncol* 2005;16:1795–800.

31 Garman KS, Pieper CF, Seo P, Cohen HJ. Function in elderly cancer survivors depends on comorbidities. *J Gerontol A Biol Sci Med Sci* 2003;58:M1119–24.

32 Hurria A, Li D, Hansen K, *et al.* Distress in older patients with cancer. *J Clin Oncol* 2009;27:4346–51.

33 Piccirillo JF, Tierney RM, Costas I, Grove L, Spitznagel EL, Jr. Prognostic importance of comorbidity in a hospital-based cancer registry. *JAMA* 2004;291:2441–7.

34 Yancik R. Cancer burden in the aged: an epidemiologic and demographic overview. *Cancer* 1997;80:1273–83.

35 Walter LC, Lewis CL, Barton MB. Screening for colorectal, breast, and cervical cancer in the elderly: a review of the evidence. *Am J Med* 2005;118:1078–86.

36 U.S. Preventive Task Force Guidelines for Screening Mammography, 2009. http://www.ahrq.gov/clinic/USpstf/uspsbrca.htm (accessed 23 August 2017).

37 Levin B, Lieberman DA, McFarland B, *et al.* Screening and surveillance for the early detection of colorectal cancer and adenomatous polyps, 2008: a joint guideline from the American Cancer Society, the US Multi-Society Task Force on Colorectal Cancer, and the American College of Radiology. *CA Cancer J Clin* 2008;58:130–60.

38 Srokowski TP, Fang S, Hortobagyi GN, Giordano SH. Impact of diabetes mellitus on complications and outcomes of adjuvant chemotherapy in older patients with breast cancer. *J Clin Oncol* 2009;27:2170–6.

39 Meyerhardt JA, Catalano PJ, Haller DG, *et al.* Impact of diabetes mellitus on outcomes in patients with colon cancer. *J Clin Oncol* 2003;21:433–40.

40 Charlson ME, Pompei P, Ales KL, MacKenzie CR. A new method of classifying prognostic comorbidity in longitudinal studies: development and validation. *J Chron Dis* 1987;40:373–83.

41 Linn BS, Linn MW, Gurel L. Cumulative illness rating scale. *J Am Geriatr Soc* 1968;16:622–6.

42 Fillenbaum GG, Smyer MA. The development, validity, and reliability of the OARS multidimensional functional assessment questionnaire. *J Gerontol* 1981;36:428–34.

43 Yancik R, Ershler W, Satariano W, *et al.* Report of the national institute on aging task force on comorbidity. *J Gerontol A Biol Sci Med Sci* 2007;62:275–80.

44 Maggiore RJ, Gross CP, Hurria A. Polypharmacy in older adults with cancer. *Oncologist* 2010;15:507–22.

45 Tam-McDevitt J. Polypharmacy, aging, and cancer. *Oncology* 2008;22:1052–5, discussion 5, 8, 60.

46 Popa MWK, Brunello A, Extermann M. The impact of polypharmacy on toxicity from chemotherapy in elderly patients: focus on cytochrome P-450 inhibition and protein binding effects [abstract]. *J Clin Oncol* 2008; 26(Suppl 15).

47 O'Mahony D, Gallagher PF. Inappropriate prescribing in the older population: need for new criteria. *Age Ageing* 2008;37:138–41.

48 Riechelmann RP, Saad ED. A systematic review on drug interactions in oncology. *Cancer Inv* 2006;24:704–12.

49 Riechelmann RP, Tannock IF, Wang L, *et al.* Potential drug interactions and duplicate prescriptions among cancer patients. *J Natl Cancer Inst* 2007;99:592–600.

50 Hanlon JT, Pieper CF, Hajjar ER, *et al.* Incidence and predictors of all and preventable adverse drug reactions in frail elderly persons after hospital stay. *J Gerontol A Biol Sci Med Sci* 2006;61:511–5.

51 Flood KL, Carroll MB, Le CV, *et al.* Geriatric syndromes in elderly patients admitted to an oncology-acute care for elders unit. *J Clin Oncol* 2006;24:2298–303.

52 Flood KL, Carroll MB, Le CV, Brown CJ. Polypharmacy in hospitalized older adult cancer patients: experience from a prospective, observational study of an oncology-acute care for elders unit. *Am J Geriatr Pharmacother* 2009;7:151–8.

53 Wells JL, Dumbrell AC. Nutrition and aging: assessment and treatment of compromised nutritional status in frail elderly patients. *Clinical Intervent Aging* 2006;1:67–79.

54 Reynolds MW, Fredman L, Langenberg P, Magaziner J. Weight, weight change, mortality in a random sample of older community-dwelling women. *J Am Geriatr Soc* 1999;47:1409–14.

55 Wallace JI, Schwartz RS, LaCroix AZ, Uhlmann RF, Pearlman RA. Involuntary weight loss in older outpatients: incidence and clinical significance. *J Am Geriatr Soc* 1995;43:329–37.

56 Wallace JI, Schwartz RS. Involuntary weight loss in elderly outpatients: recognition, etiologies, and treatment. *Clin Geriatr Med* 1997;13:717–35.

57 Kane RL, Shamliyan T, Talley K, Pacala J. The association between geriatric syndromes and survival. *J Am Geriatr Soc* 2012;60:896–904.

58 Dewys WD, Begg C, Lavin PT, *et al.* Prognostic effect of weight loss prior to chemotherapy in cancer patients. Eastern Cooperative Oncology Group. *Am J Med* 1980;69:491–7.

59 Buccheri G, Ferrigno D. Importance of weight loss definition in the prognostic evaluation of non-small-cell lung cancer. *Lung Cancer* 2001;34:433–40.

60 Aaldriks AA, Maartense E, le Cessie S, *et al.* Predictive value of geriatric assessment for patients older than 70 years, treated with chemotherapy. *Crit Rev Oncol Hematol* 2011;79:205–12.

61 Bozzetti F. Nutritional aspects of the cancer/aging interface. *J Geriatr Oncol* 2011;2:177–86.

62 Eagles JM, Beattie JA, Restall DB, *et al.* Relation between cognitive impairment and early death in the elderly. *BMJ* 1990;300:239–40.

63 Wolfson C, Wolfson DB, Asgharian M, *et al.* A reevaluation of the duration of survival after the onset of dementia. *N Engl J Med* 2001;344:1111–6.

64 Sampson EL, Bulpitt CJ, Fletcher AE. Survival of community-dwelling older people: the effect of cognitive impairment and social engagement. *J Am Geriatr Soc* 2009;57:985–91.

65 Extermann M. Older patients, cognitive impairment, and cancer: an increasingly frequent triad. *J Natl Compr Canc Netw* 2005;3:593–6.

66 Stilley CS, Bender CM, Dunbar-Jacob J, Sereika S, Ryan CM. The impact of cognitive function on medication management: three studies. *Health Psychol* 2010;29:50–5.

67 Sessums LL, Zembrzuska H, Jackson JL. Does this patient have medical decision-making capacity? *JAMA* 2011;306:420–7.

68 Ellis J, Lin J, Walsh A, *et al.* Predictors of referral for specialized psychosocial oncology care in patients with metastatic cancer: the contributions of age, distress, and marital status. *J Clin Oncol* 2009;27:699–705.

69 Mohile SG, Fan L, Reeve E, *et al.* Association of cancer with geriatric syndromes in older Medicare beneficiaries. *J Clin Oncol* 2011;29:1458–64.

70 Mohile SG, Xian Y, Dale W, *et al.* Association of a cancer diagnosis with vulnerability and frailty in older Medicare beneficiaries. *J Natl Cancer Inst* 2009;101:1206–15.

71 Inouye SK, Studenski S, Tinetti ME, Kuchel GA. Geriatric syndromes: clinical, research, and policy implications of a core geriatric concept. *J Am Geriatr Soc* 2007;55:780–91.

72 Phelan EA, Balderson B, Levine M, *et al.* Delivering effective primary care to older adults: a randomized, controlled trial of the senior resource team at group health cooperative. *J Am Geriatr Soc* 2007;55:1748–56.

73 Silver JK, Baima J, Mayer RS. Impairment-driven cancer rehabilitation: an essential component of quality care and survivorship. *CA Cancer J Clin* 2013;63:295–317.

74 Balducci L, Extermann M. Cancer and aging. An evolving panorama. *Hematol/Oncol Clin North Am* 2000;14:1–16.

75 Extermann M, Boler I, Reich RR, *et al.* Predicting the risk of chemotherapy toxicity in older patients: the Chemotherapy Risk Assessment Scale for High-Age Patients (CRASH) score. *Cancer* 2012;118:3377–86.

76 Hurria A, Gupta S, Zauderer M, *et al.* Developing a cancer-specific geriatric assessment: a feasibility study. *Cancer* 2005;104:1998–2005.

77 Hurria A, Cirrincione CT, Muss HB, *et al.* Implementing a geriatric assessment in cooperative group clinical cancer trials: CALGB 360401. *J Clin Oncol* 2011;29:1290–6.

78 Hurria A, Togawa K, Mohile SG, *et al.* Predicting chemotherapy toxicity in older adults with cancer: a prospective multicenter study. *J Clin Oncol* 2011;29:3457–65.

79 Hurria A, Mohile SG, Gajra A, *et al.* Validation of a prediction tool for chemotherapy toxicity in older adults with cancer. *J Clin Oncol* 2016;34:2366–71.

80 VanderWalde N, Jagsi R, Dotan E, *et al.* NCCN Guidelines Insights: older adult oncology, version 2.2016. *J Natl Compr Canc Netw* 2016;14:1357–70.

81 Hurria A, Browner IS, Cohen HJ, *et al.* Senior adult oncology. *J Natl Compr Canc Netw* 2012;10:162–209.

Section 6

Symptom Management, Palliative Care, Complications and Toxicities of Treatment, Patient-Reported Outcomes, etc.

27

Palliative and Supportive Care

Rony Dev and Eduardo Bruera

The University of Texas MD Anderson Cancer Center, Houston, Texas, USA

Introduction

Despite advances in cancer therapy, the prognosis of many cancer patients remains poor [1, 2]. Cancer patients and their family face physical, psychosocial, and financial distress [3, 4] at the time of diagnoses as well as at the end of life.

Palliative medicine is an interdisciplinary medical specialty which focuses on preventing and relieving unnecessary suffering of cancer patients and their family. The essential principles of palliative care consist of a thorough assessment and treatment of symptoms, eliciting patient's goals of care and implementing a patient-centered treatment plan, facilitating open and honest communication, and providing psychosocial, spiritual and practical support for both patients and their family.

In the past, a palliative medicine consultation for cancer patients often has been initiated when patients were not candidates for cancer treatment or as they were being transitioned to end-of-life care (Figure 27.1) [5–7]. Recently, integration of palliative care earlier in the disease trajectory has been advocated to improve symptom management, provide greater psychosocial support, and ease the transition to end-of-life care for cancer patients.

Palliative care was developed in the United Kingdom in the late 1960s in conjunction with development of hospice services [8]. In the early years, programs addressing end-of-life care were community based and referrals to a hospice were late in the disease trajectory. Often, the most distressed patients died in acute care hospitals without access to hospice care [9, 10]. In the 1980s, academic acute care hospitals and cancer centers in Canada developed inpatient consultation services and later acute palliative care units to manage hospitalized cancer patients with the highest symptom burden prior to discharge back into the community [11].

Recently, hospice and palliative medicine has been recognized as a medical subspecialty by the American Board of Medical Specialties in the United States (US), as well as other countries including the United Kingdom, Australia, Canada, and many European nations [12]. Other countries are developing pathways for certification in palliative medicine which is a

rapidly growing field. Clinicians trained in palliative medicine have expertise in pain and symptom management, communication with both patients and their family regarding goals of care and end-of-life discussions, assessing and treating psychosocial and spiritual distress, and coordinating the care of frail patients across various settings from the hospital to the home [13].

This chapter will describe the components of a palliative medicine service and the necessary members of an interdisciplinary palliative care team, outline models for the integration of palliative care in cancer centers as well as barriers to implementation, and describe the management of common symptoms for cancer patients.

Definitions of Palliative Medicine

Various nationally and internationally recognized organizations have reflected on and, over the years, refined the definition of palliative care:

- The Centers for Medicare and Medicaid Services define palliative care as "patient and family-centered care that optimizes quality of life by anticipating, preventing, and treating suffering. Palliative care throughout the continuum of illness involves addressing physical, intellectual, emotional, social, and spiritual needs and facilitating patient autonomy, access to information, and choice" [14].
- The Center to Advance Palliative Care definition is: "Palliative care, and the medical sub-specialty of palliative medicine, is specialized medical care for people living with serious illness. It focuses on providing relief from the symptoms and stress of a serious illness. The goal is to improve quality of life for both the patient and the family. Palliative care is provided by a team of palliative care doctors, nurses, social workers and others who work together with a patient's other doctors to provide an extra layer of support. It is appropriate at any age and at any stage in a serious illness and can be provided along with curative treatment" [15].
- The World Health Organization definition is "... an approach that improves the quality of life of patients and their families

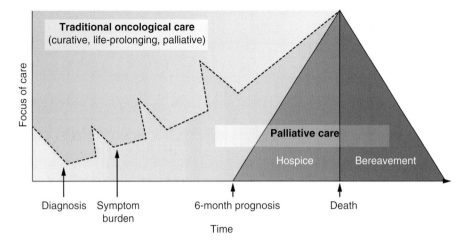

Figure 27.1 Model of palliative care for patients with cancer. *Source:* Campbell TC, Roenn JH. Semin Intervent Radiol 2007;24:375–81. Reproduced with permission of Thieme Publishers. Originally adapted from Emanuel LL, Ferris FD, von Gunten CF, Von Roenn, JH. EPEC-O: Education in Palliative and End-of-Life Care—Oncology (The EPEC Project, Chicago, 2005).

facing the problems associated with life-threatening illness, through the prevention and relief of suffering by means of early identification and impeccable assessment and treatment of pain and other problems, physical, psychosocial, and spiritual" [16].

Components for a Palliative Care Program

As outlined by the American Academy of Hospice and Palliative Medicine [17], palliative care programs would include the following components.

An Interdisciplinary Palliative Care Team

Palliative care teams consist of a palliative care physician, preferably board certified in hospice and palliative care, a nurse, social worker, psychologist/psychiatrist, chaplain, and a pharmacist. Other members of an interdisciplinary team may include art, music, and massage therapists, a dietician, a holistic health or integrative medicine expert, a bereavement counselor, volunteers, a physiotherapist, and respiratory and recreational therapists [18]. Some evidence exists supporting the management of cancer patients by an interdisciplinary palliative care team [19–23]; however, more research is needed on how best to deliver palliative care in a cost-effective manner, essential disciplines to include in the interdisciplinary team, and overall organizational structure for a viable palliative care program.

A Mobile Consultation Service

This is a consultation service which is available to provide palliative care recommendations for patients in all inpatient floors of a cancer center including the Intensive Care Unit and Emergency Room. A consultative team often requires less resources in cases where the primary team retains the primary responsibility for the care of the patient and is able to deliver palliative care to more cancer patients distributed throughout the hospital.

An Inpatient Acute Palliative Care Unit

A Palliative Care Unit (PCU) is a designated section of the hospital staffed by a board certified palliative care physician, nurses with training in palliative care, and an interdisciplinary team consisting of a chaplain, counselors, child life experts, a social worker, and case manager. All members of the team should be trained in palliative care and be able to interact and communicate with each other as an interdisciplinary team. Patients admitted to a PCU should ideally be managed primarily by the palliative care team.

Cancer patients admitted to a PCU are often the most distressed [24] and reasons to transfer to an inpatient PCU include difficult-to-control symptoms, poor communication or coordination of care secondary to multiple healthcare providers, difficult patient or family characteristics such as patients who are coping poorly with their illness or have personality disorders and dysfunctional family members which makes the medical management more complicated, or patients with high psychosocial or existential distress which is not manageable by the mobile consultation team. PCUs have been shown to reduce hospital costs [25, 26] while maintaining a high quality of care for cancer patients with a poor prognosis with studies reporting an increased satisfaction with end-of-life care among family caregivers of patients who died [27].

The Outpatient Supportive Care Center

This is an outpatient center which is staffed by board certified palliative care physicians, nurses, counselors, and social workers with a background and training in palliative care. It should ideally operate from 8 a.m. to 5 p.m., 5 days a week and have the capabilities to communicate with patients and their distressed family caregivers via a phone service during working hours and afterhours [28].

The Outpatient Supportive Care Center best serves patients with complex or advanced illnesses and a high symptom burden, often in conjunction with curative treatment. Ambulatory outpatient centers have shown to improve the quality of life of patients and may improve survival when introduced early in the disease trajectory of cancer patients [29, 30].

Hospice Service – Home and Inpatient Care

The interdisciplinary palliative care team should be able to provide palliative care consultations and follow-up visits across multiple settings outside the hospital or outpatient supportive care ambulatory clinics, including long-term acute care facilities, skilled nursing care, and the home setting. Medicare and Medicaid, as well as other insurances, cover the benefits of hospice care which delivers end-of-life symptom management for patients with a terminal illness, that is, a prognosis of less than 6 months [31]. Treatment is directed at controlling symptoms and psychosocial support for patient and their family caregivers as opposed to "curative" treatment [31]. Hospice services can be provided in the home or inpatient setting for patients with a terminal disease. Patients who are cognitively impaired or who have a poor functional status resulting in a higher burden for their family caregivers are often referred to inpatient hospices rather than the home service [32].

Palliative Care in the Intensive Care Unit

In the US, roughly one in five deaths occurs in the intensive care unit (ICU) setting [33] which would argue for a need to integrate palliative care with critical care in cancer centers. Among individuals aged 65 years or older who die of cancer, approximately 22.2% of deaths occur in an acute care hospital and 27.2% have at least one intensive care admission during their last 30 days of life [34]. Often, distinguishing critical illness and terminal illness is difficult. The goal of relieving unnecessary suffering can coexist with the curative treatment offered in the ICU [35]. When critically ill cancer patients are not responsive to medical therapy, the goal of palliation can take precedence and be seamlessly continued if palliative care has been integrated in the ICU setting.

In the ICU, effective communication with patients and family is essential. Mixed messages by the ICU staff including clinicians, nurses, respiratory therapists, pharmacists, social workers and chaplains, primary oncologist, and other consulting services have been associated with increased anxiety and depression in family members [36]

An observational study conducted in the ICU setting reported that increased collaboration by an interdisciplinary team resulted in decreased mortality, shorter length of stay, lower rates of admission, and decreased workplace stress, for nurses in particular [37]. More research is needed to determine how best to integrate palliative care into ICU settings in cancer centers.

Growth of a Palliative Care Program

The number of hospital-based palliative care programs has increased rapidly [38]. In 2011, the Center for Advancement of Palliative Care (CAPC) reported that roughly 63% of hospitals in the US with 50 beds or more had some type of palliative care program [39]. Despite the rapid growth of palliative care programs across the nation, a survey of 71 National Cancer Institute-designated cancer centers and a random sample of 71 non-National Cancer Institute cancer centers reported the scope of services and degree of integration of palliative care in the institutions varied widely [40]. In the cancer centers surveyed, 80% had a mobile consultation team, but less than half had outpatient clinics or institution sponsored hospice services and only 30% had acute inpatient palliative care beds.

As outlined by the CAPC, factors which influence the number of consultations requested by palliative care healthcare providers include: the type and size of the hospital; degree of acceptance and awareness of palliative medicine, and the availability of palliative care consultation; and the degree of internal support and funding from the hospital administration [41].

The Supportive Care and Palliative Care Program at the University of Texas MD Anderson Cancer Center is one of the most comprehensive palliative care programs among cancer centers in the US [40]. Over a 10-year period, clinical activity consistently grew from year to year in the institution (Figure 27.2) [42]. A review of referral patterns at MD Anderson Cancer Center reveals increased clinical activity across all tumor types; however, patients with solid tumors were referred earlier than patients with hematological malignancies [43]. Growth of palliative care was engineered, following the theory of adoption of innovation [44], which emphasizes initially winning over a small core of early adopters and advocates who eventually were enlisted to persuade detractors to consider the integration of palliative care within our tertiary care cancer center [45].

Barriers to Access Palliative Care

Barriers to palliative care access include the limited resources and staffing at the majority of cancer centers in the US to accommodate increased or early referral [40]. Currently, rates of consultation with palliative care are unpredictable, often delayed and vary among institutions depending on the degree of integration. Clinical care pathways have been proposed for triggering palliative care consultation at the appropriate time. For example, patients may be systematically screened for various sentinel events including poor performance status, severe symptom distress, or cachexia which would trigger a palliative care consultation [46].

In addition, the terminology of end-of-life care influences its integration into cancer centers (Figure 27.3). In a recent survey, the term "supportive care" resulted in less distress than "palliative care" among oncologists and nurse practitioners [47] and a name change from "palliative care" to "supportive care" resulted in a 41% increase in the number of consultations, mainly inpatient, and earlier consultations with a median survival time increased to 6.2 months from 4.7 months in the outpatient clinic [48].

Despite having a supportive administrative team, experienced leaders and palliative care team, and commitment to the hard work required to establish a viable palliative care program, the institutional medical culture – defined as "the customary beliefs, social forms, and material traits of a racial, religious, or social group" [49] – has a strong influence on the success of integration [50].

In the earliest stage, an institution's medical culture may lack awareness of the importance of palliative care and its benefits for patients and their family. Monica Mueller coined

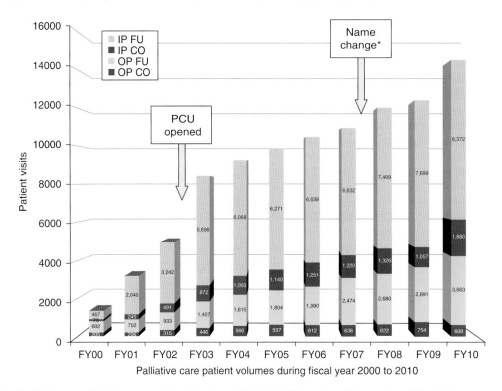

Figure 27.2 Growth of palliative care clinical encounters from fiscal years 2000–2010. IP, inpatient; OP, outpatient; CO, palliative care consultation; FU, follow-up clinical visit; PCU, palliative care unit. *Name change (supportive care from palliative care). *Source:* Dev R, Del Fabbro E, Miles M, *et al.* [42]. Reproduced with permission of Elsevier.

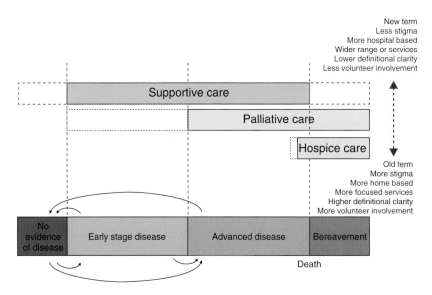

Figure 27.3 Conceptual framework for "Supportive Care", "Palliative Care", and "Hospice Care". "Hospice Care" is part of "Palliative Care", which in turn is under the umbrella of "Supportive Care". "Palliative Care" predominantly addresses the care needs for patients with advanced cancer in both acute care facilities and the community, whereas "Supportive Care" provides an even broader range of services for patients throughout various stages of the disease, including diagnosis, active treatment, end of life, and survivorship. *Source:* Hui D, De La Cruz M, Mori M, *et al.* Concepts and definitions for "palliative care", "supportive care", "best supportive care", and "hospice care" in the published literature, dictionaries, and textbooks. Supp Care Cancer 2013;21:659–85. Reproduced with permission of Springer.

the following terms to describe the cultural evolution of hospitals: the stages of institutional transformation to adopt palliative care consist of an initial period of palliphobia, followed by pallilalia, and finally a palliactive stage [50]. Palliaphobic institutions have a culture which acknowledges the need for palliative care, but exhibits a fear of adoption secondary to the belief that palliative care undermines their own professional competencies involving symptom management, empathetic communication and end-of-life discussions, and overall treatment strategy for cancer patients. The next stage, pallilalia is characterized by institutions which are vocal about the importance of integrating palliative care but the hospital administration fails to financially support or foster success. In the final palliative stage, hospitals provide the appropriate financial, administrative, and logistical support to develop a viable palliative care team.

From a clinician perspective, a survey conducted in the US revealed that physicians recognized that quality of life for seriously ill patients was more important than prolonging life with every possible medical intervention. However, they also acknowledged concerns regarding integrating palliative care alongside curative treatment secondary to a belief that palliative care would interfere with treatment directed at prolonging life, inadequate patient resources and reimbursement, and a shortage of well-trained palliative care physicians and healthcare providers [51]. In the same survey, physicians acknowledged significant gaps in education regarding palliative medicine with a lack of exposure to palliative care for the majority of physicians during their clinical training. In the current healthcare climate where resources are constrained, establishing a viable palliative care program may be viewed with apprehension since resources may have to be diverted away from other departments and goals such as developing curative treatments for cancer.

In addition to the medical culture, the perceptions of patients and family may influence the acceptance of palliative care interventions. A public opinion poll conducted in 2011 reported that over 90% of those polled agreed that it is important for palliative care services to be available for hospitalized patients with a critical illness [52]. However, in the same study, lack of awareness of palliative care services and healthcare providers equating palliative care to "end-of-life" care was noted to be a barrier to timely access.

Medicare hospice benefits are designed for palliative care services to be provided at home with a sole emphasis on comfort. Numerous studies suggest that the majority of individuals want to die at home. Between 49 and 70% of the general public have been reported to prefer a home death [53]. In a recent study, 51–52% of cancer patients die in hospitals compared with just 34–35% home deaths [54]. However, not all patients and their family caregivers want a home death, and as many as 48% of patients have been reported to want access to all available treatments at the end of life [55]. Currently, restrictive enrollment policies of hospice programs present a barrier to the integration of palliative care [56]. Secondary to inadequate reimbursement, enrollment barriers for cancer patients encountered when enrolling in hospice care include the following: the need to receive palliative radiation therapy, blood or platelet transfusions, parenteral nutrition/fluids or tube feeding, antibiotics for serious infections, and anticoagulation therapy for pulmonary embolism or deep venous thrombosis.

In addition to the culture of the hospital, racial factors may influence the integration of palliative care with cancer treatment. African Americans and other minority patients have a higher cancer-related mortality rate than other racial groups in the US [57–60]. Delays in diagnosis of cancer and less than optimal treatment has been reported for patients belonging to minority groups [61–63]. Researchers have argued that the association between race/ethnicity and poor health outcomes is largely due to poor socioeconomic conditions [64], which also may play a role in access for minority groups to high quality end-of-life care. In addition, media coverage in the African American community is significantly less likely to publicize adverse events or treatment failures of chemotherapy, issues regarding death and dying, and options for end-of-life care including palliative medicine and hospice care [65, 66], which results in a lack of awareness and misunderstandings about the benefits of palliative medicine and hospice care.

Very few studies have examined the role of racial and ethnic discrepancies to access to palliative care for cancer patients [67, 68]. A recent retrospective study reported no significant difference in timing of referral to a palliative medicine consultation based on race, but did confirm that Hispanics and non-Hispanic blacks had a higher symptom burden [68].

Benefits of Palliative Care

Consultation with an interdisciplinary palliative care team for cancer patients has been shown to provide improved symptom control and reduce suffering in the ICU, inpatient and outpatient settings [69–72]. In addition to symptom improvement, financial burden for both patient and family [73, 74] and survival outcomes [75] have been shown to improve with earlier palliative care consultation. Temel *et al.* [75] performed a pivotal randomized controlled trial of early palliative care consultation for patients with metastatic non-small cell lung cancer within 8 weeks of their diagnosis, and reported a better quality of life and improved survival rates.

The benefits of cost avoidance as a result of implementing palliative care has been emphasized to persuade hospital administrators to invest in palliative care programs since revenue generated by clinical encounters is insufficient to support a palliative medicine program [76]. Some palliative care organizations have reported their own experience resulting in cost avoidance [77, 78]; however, cost avoidance without improvements in the quality of patient care will likely discourage patients, their family caregivers, and healthcare providers from seeking access to palliative care or enrolling in hospice services.

Access and Integration of Palliative Care with Cancer Therapy

The American Society of Clinical Oncology has recently published an updated clinical opinion advocating for routine palliative care consultation for all patients with incurable cancer [79]. Limited studies exist examining the proportion of cancer patients who had access to palliative care prior to death. In a large retrospective study, 45% of cancer patients who died had access to palliative care. Patients with gynecologic malignancies had the highest rate at 66% and those with hematologic malignancies were less likely to have palliative care consultation at the end of life, having a rate of only 33% and consultation occurring with a median time of 0.4 months before death (Figure 27.4). [80]. The study also reported that younger or married patients were more likely to have access to palliative care consultation prior to death.

Other studies have reported similar findings, with patients with hematologic disorders more likely to receive aggressive therapy at the end of life [81], to have late palliative care

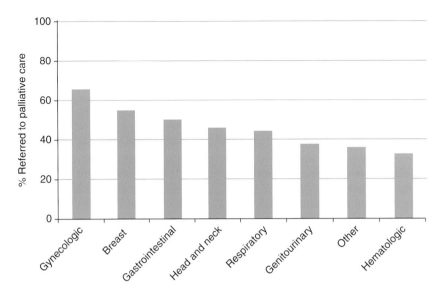

Figure 27.4 Percentage of patients with access to palliative care according to tumor type. *Source:* Hui *et al.* [80]. Reproduced with permission of AlphaMed Press.

consultation [80], and die in the ICU [71]. A study examining the characteristics of patients referred earlier versus late reported similar symptom burden between the two groups but patients referred earlier were younger, less likely to be married, and were more likely to be receiving active chemotherapy [82]. In addition, patients with head and neck cancers were noted to be referred earlier mainly for symptoms of pain secondary to mucositis [83].

Late referral to palliative care was reported to be a common occurrence in a survey of palliative care services at designated cancer centers [40, 84–86]. In 2014, 35.5% of patients were referred to a hospice in the last week of life with a median length of stay of 17.4 days [87]. Referral to palliative or hospice care late in the disease trajectory may limit the benefits of physical and psychosocial interventions for patients and their family and links palliative medicine and hospice services with the treatment of "actively" dying patients when treatment is directed at solely controlling symptoms associated with impending death. Recently published research shows that although there is increased use of hospice [87] and palliative care services [88] resulting in increased deaths at home over the years, ICU hospitalizations prior to death and transition to "comfort care" only in the last 3 days of life or less have also increased [89], which arguably results in no cost savings and poor end-of-life care.

Models of Delivery of Palliative Medicine

Three models have been proposed on how palliative care can be integrated into oncology practice: the Solo Practice Model, the Congress Practice Model, and the Integrated Care Model (Figure 27.5) [90].

In the Solo Practice Model, oncologists provide all aspects of cancer therapy and supportive/palliative care. The lack of time to assess and diagnose cancer patients, formulate a treatment plan, and simultaneously assess and treat both physical and psychosocial distress limits the effectiveness of this model [91].

In addition, the limited educational training in the field of palliative medicine does not prepare oncologists to treat pain [92] and other symptoms adequately.

The Congress Practice Model, where oncologists refer to multiple services and disciplines, may address the deficits encountered in the Solo Practice Model but is hindered by the lack of coordination of care and potential to undergo treatments prescribed by multiple healthcare providers that, at times, are counter effective. In addition, critically ill, frail patients have difficulty with the need to have multiple assessments and the financial burden of multiple visits and lost time at work for the patient and/or their family caregivers.

The Integrated Care Model addresses the limitations of the other practice patterns and by active collaboration delivers efficient cancer therapy in conjunction with supportive care and assists with a seamless transition to end-of-life care managed by the palliative care team when patients are not candidates for curative treatment.

Communication

Timely, open, and honest communication is essential in order to provide effective palliation of symptoms for cancer patients and their family. Information regarding medical findings, disease severity and complications, risks and benefits of medications and other cancer treatments, may have to be repeated to ensure understanding. Research has shown that the use of visual graphs or written material [93], question prompt lists [94], or audiocassette recordings of consultations can increase recall and satisfaction [95].

For patients with advanced cancer, decisions to pursue aggressive treatment versus pursuit of "comfort care" often depend on the disclosure of a poor prognosis provided by their physicians and their own goals of care [96]. Clinicians often overestimate survival for patients at the end of life [97], which often influences a patient's desire for further diagnostic testing,

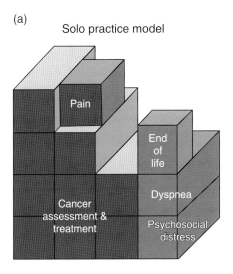

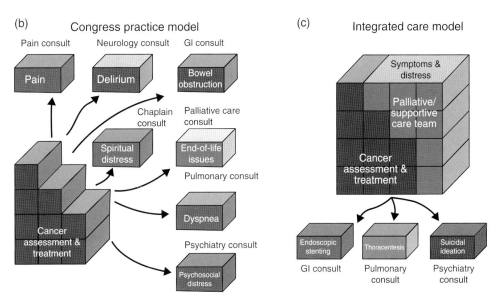

Figure 27.5 The cancer care package. (a) In the Solo Practice Model, the oncologist provides both cancer assessment and treatment, and addresses a variety of supportive care issues such as pain and dyspnea. However, the lack of time and expertise means that these issues may not be managed adequately. (b) In the Congress Practice Model, the oncologist refers the patient to various specialities for all the supportive care issues. This could result in fragmented and expensive care. (c) In the Integrated Care Model, the oncologist routinely refers patients to palliative care for their supportive care needs. This helps to ensure patients receive comprehensive and integrated care, and it streamlines the provision of care. *Source:* Bruera E, Hui D. Conceptual models for integrating palliative care at cancer centers. J Palliat Med 2012;15:1261–9.

pursuit of cancer therapy, and enrollment in clinical trials versus hospice care.

Unrealistic expectations of patients can be secondary to the poor communication by healthcare professionals, inability of patients to understand the information provided by their clinicians, or patients being in a stage of denial, which helps them cope with the thoughts of impending death. In addition, poor communication can be exacerbated by the terminology used to communicate the effects of treatment, such as "response" or "tumor shrinkage", which may be easily misinterpreted by patients and family caregivers.

Breaking bad news is difficult for clinicians and is an important skill not only for the palliative care professional but also for oncologists and other healthcare providers taking care of cancer patients. Guidelines have been developed to assist clinicians

with this important task (Table 27.1) [98–102]. Initial disclosure of a poor prognosis often results in brief periods of hopelessness and emotional distress for patients and their family. With time and proper psychosocial support, the loss of hope for a cure or treatment is often transformed to a more realistic hope such as a good quality of life or a peaceful death.

A recent study reported that clinicians who communicated an optimistic view of the benefits of treatment were perceived as having better communications skills [103]. In the same study, more than two-thirds of the patients in the study had expectations that chemotherapy would provide a cure for their cancer. Oncologists have raised concerns that a move to palliative medicine with no options to receive chemotherapy including clinical trials is accepting a state of hopelessness [104]; however, unrealistic hope for patients and families can be quite detrimental.

Table 27.1 Recommendation for patient-centered communication when discussing bad news [100–102].

Recommendation	Comments
Prioritize: prioritize what you want to accomplish during the discussion	Ask yourself: what are two to four key points that the patient should retain? What decisions should be made during this encounter? What is reasonable to expect from the patient during this encounter?
Practice and prepare: practice giving bad news; arrange for an environment conducive to delivering the news	Rehearse the discussion; arrange for a private location without interruptions; set cell phones and pagers to vibrate or turn them off; ask the patient if he or she wants to invite family members
Assess patient understanding: start with opening questions, rather than medical statements, to determine the patient's level of understanding about the situation	Ask the patient: "What do you already know about your condition?" "What does it mean to you?" "What do you think will happen?"
Determine patient preferences: ask what and how much information the patients wants to know	Assess how the patient wants the information presented; ask the patient, "Some of my patients prefer hearing only the big picture, whereas others want a lot of details. Which do you prefer?"
Present information: deliver information to the patient using language that is easy to understand (do not use medical jargon); provide a small amount of information at a time; check periodically for patient comprehension	Provide a few pieces of information, and then ask the patient to repeat it back to you
Provide emotional support: allow the patient to express his or her emotions; respond with empathy	Assess the patient's emotional state directly and often (ask the patient: "How are you doing?" "Is this hard for you?" "Let me know when we should continue"); use nonverbal cues such as eye contact; listen to what the patients says and validate his or her reactions with empathic statements such as "I understand that is very difficult news"
Discuss options for the future: devise a plan for subsequent visits and care	Help the patient understand the expected disease course and how the disease may or may not respond to treatment; schedule follow-up visits (ask the patient: "Can we meet next week to discuss treatment options and any questions you may have?"
Offer additional support: provide information about support services	Bring handouts and pamphlets to the visit; refer the patient to support groups, psychologists, social workers, or chaplains
Consider individual preferences: assess patient preferences, and tailor the discussion appropriately	Consider the patient's sex, age, health literacy, health status, previous healthcare experiences, social status, culture, and race/ethnicity; avoid assumptions about what the patient is likely to want; ask the patient directly about values and preferences

Source: Ngo-Metzger Q, August KJ, Srinivasan M, Liao S, Meyskens. End-of-Life Care: Guidelines for Patient-Centered Communication. Am Fam Physician 2008;77(2):167–74. Reproduced with permission of American Academy of Family Physicians.

In addition, a growing body of research suggests that having end-of-life discussions does not result in higher rates of depression [105], loss of hope [106], or decreased survival [107].

Family conferences have been advocated by some healthcare providers to improve communication regarding end-of-life discussions for cancer patients and their family. In the ICU setting, prospective cohort trials have shown that end-of-life discussions conducted in a family meeting were associated with improvements in overall family satisfaction with care provided, reduced length of stay in the ICU, and increased access to palliative care and hospice enrollment without an increase in mortality [108, 109].

Similar studies of family conferences that occur in cancer centers are lacking. A recent prospective study examining 140 family conferences revealed that they facilitated end-of-life discussions regarding the patient's and family's understanding of the disease burden and treatment options, prognosis, symptom management, need for transition to non-curative treatment, and hospice education [110]. In the same study, patient participation in the family meetings resulted in discussions regarding prognosis and what patients may experience during the dying phase to occur less often. Qualitative studies have shown that information needs of critically ill patients and their family caregivers often differ [111]. As the cancer progresses, patients often ask fewer questions about their diagnosis and are less involved in the decision making of their cancer treatment, relying more on their family caregivers [112].

Symptoms Assessment and Management

A thorough assessment of symptoms is critical to providing palliative care. Evidence exists that relying on a patient's response or on responses to open-ended questions is inferior to assessing with a standardized screening tool [113–116].

A number of assessment tools have been validated and are useful for repeated measurements of the intensity of symptoms for patients with cancer [117]. These assessment tools can be visually displayed which communicates the symptom burden of cancer patients to other healthcare providers. Often, the assessment tools display the severity of symptoms as either numbers, words, colors, circles of gradually increasing sizes, or graphs. An example of an assessment tool which has been validated and integrated into clinical practice in a cancer center is the Edmonton symptom assessment scale (ESAS) (Figure 27.6) [118]. The ESAS is used by clinicians to systematically assess 10

Participant's Initials:_____   Acc#:_____   Date:___/___/___

Edmonton Symptom Assessment System (ESAS)

Please circle the number that best describes your symptoms in the last 24 hours:

| No pain | 0 1 2 3 4 5 6 7 8 9 10 | Worst pain imaginable |

| No fatigue | 0 1 2 3 4 5 6 7 8 9 10 | Worst fatigue imaginable |

| No nausea | 0 1 2 3 4 5 6 7 8 9 10 | Worst nausea imaginable |

| No depression | 0 1 2 3 4 5 6 7 8 9 10 | Worst depression imaginable |

| No anxiety | 0 1 2 3 4 5 6 7 8 9 10 | Worst anxiety |

| No drowsiness | 0 1 2 3 4 5 6 7 8 9 10 | Worst drowsiness imaginable |

| No shortness of breath | 0 1 2 3 4 5 6 7 8 9 10 | Worst shortness of breath imaginable |

| Best appetite | 0 1 2 3 4 5 6 7 8 9 10 | Worst appetite imaginable |

| Best feeling of well-being | 0 1 2 3 4 5 6 7 8 9 10 | Worst feeling of well-being |

| Other problem | 0 1 2 3 4 5 6 7 8 9 10 | Worst imaginable |

Signature: _____

Figure 27.6 Edmonton Symptom Assessment System. *Source:* Bruera E, Kim HN. Cancer pain. JAMA 2003;290:2476–9. Reproduced with permission of American Medical Association.

common symptoms (pain, fatigue, nausea, depression, anxiety, drowsiness, shortness of breath, appetite, feeling of well-being) experienced by cancer patients over the past 24 h [118].

Pain

Pain is one of the most feared symptoms that cancer patients may experience. Unfortunately, inadequate treatment of cancer pain is not uncommon [90] and is due to the clinician's lack of knowledge, limited availability and governmental regulation of opioid medications, and the physician's fear of litigation for prescribing opioids to patients who may abuse or divert medications for illegal use [119].

Surveys have found that 30–50% of cancer patients receiving active therapy and 60–90% of advanced cancer patients have pain [120, 121]. Cancer pain may arise from the growth and destruction of surrounding tissue by the tumor or indirectly by inflammatory mediators secreted by the cancer, or as a result of cancer treatments. Nociceptive pain is associated with ongoing tissue damage and can be divided into somatic or visceral origin, while neuropathic pain results from the dysfunction of the nervous system. Somatic pain is reported to be well localized and often described as aching, throbbing and gnawing discomfort. Visceral pain is poorly localized aching, cramping, or pressure-like sensation. Neuropathic pain is often characterized by patients as burning, tingling, shooting, stabbing, itching, and numbing discomfort.

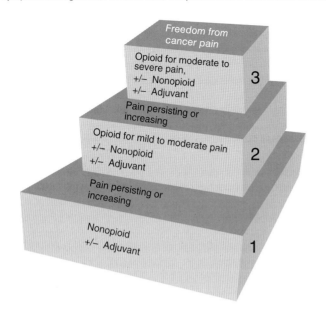

Figure 27.7 WHO's Pain Relief Ladder. *Source:* http://www.who.int/cancer/palliative/painladder/en/ (accessed 24 August 2017). Reproduced with permission of WHO.

Pain is subjective and the expression of pain varies from patient to patient as a result of multiple factors including a patient's cognitive state, mood, cultural beliefs and attitudes toward pain, and past experiences. It is critical for physicians to assess pain intensity in cancer patients. Intensity of pain can be easily measured by numerical, verbal, or visual scales or more complex pain questionnaires [118]. In addition to the assessment of pain intensity, psychosocial, cognitive, cultural beliefs, and practical concerns, such as financial burden, must be thoroughly reviewed to determine "total pain" better prior to initiating treatment, which should be directed at not only physical pain but also the other underlying factors.

The World Health Organization has proposed a step-wise ladder for the pharmacologic management of cancer-related pain (Figure 27.7) [122]. Low-potency opioids commonly prescribed include codeine, tramadol, and hydrocodone which are indicated for mild to moderate pain. Often, these medications are combined with acetaminophen which limits the maximum dose. High-potency opioids include morphine, oxycodone, hydromorphone, fentanyl, and methadone.

The first step in the treatment of cancer pain is to assess the intensity, which will determine if a low potency opioid or a high-potency drug, like morphine, is needed. Most cancer patients will require strong, high-potency analgesics. Pain expression should be assessed in conjunction with a patient's psychosocial symptoms.

The second step is to assess for past history of opioid use and abuse, side effects, and review existing medications, such as benzodiazepines, which may potentially interact with the opioid prescribed. Patient-to-patient variability in analgesic response to opioids has been acknowledged [123] and the past experience will often dictate which opioid is dispensed.

The third step after selecting the type of opioid is to determine the dosing and frequency. Cancer patients without a history of exposure to opioid therapy often require lower doses initially, and as they develop a degree of tolerance, the dose may

be titrated upwards to control their cancer pain. Patients who have previously developed a tolerance to opioid therapy often require higher doses or a stronger opioid regimen. For patients with continuous or frequent episodes of pain, around the clock or a long-acting preparation of a strong opioid is required. In addition to scheduled opioids, rescue doses should be prescribed as often as once every hour as needed for breakthrough pain. Rescue doses are typically 10–20% of the total 24-h opioid requirements for cancer patients.

The final step is to monitor for side effects and efficacy. If cancer patients continue to have uncontrolled pain over time, dosage titration upward is warranted if patients are not experiencing side effects. Prior to escalation, assessment for the presence of side effects and factors which modify pain expression such as anxiety, delirium, and depression must be addressed and treated accordingly. Side effects of opioids include sedation, nausea and vomiting, constipation, urinary retention, myoclonus, pruritis, delirium, and respiratory depression. Some side effects can be managed, such as sedation, with either a decrease in dosage or treatment with a central nervous stimulant such as methylphenidate [124], nausea and vomiting can often be managed with metoclopramide, and constipation is prevented with coadministration of opioids with a bowel stimulant (e.g., senna) and preparations such as polyethylenene glycol. More serious side effects such as urinary retention, pruritis with evidence of an allergic reaction, persistent myoclonus, and delirium secondary to opioids should be managed with either a decrease in dosage or an opioid rotation.

Respiratory depression is a rare side effect in patients who are on chronic opioids and is often preceded by other side effects such as myoclonus or delirium. In patients with rapid escalation, accidental overdose, or who have been prescribed another sedative agent that results in respiratory depression, such as a benzodiazepine, opioids can be temporarily discontinued or the dosage lowered when the respiratory function is intact. When respiratory function is compromised, the opioid antagonist naloxone can be administered to restore respiratory function. Naloxone is administered in 40 µg increments rather than as a bolus to avoid opioid withdrawal.

Opioid rotation, the switch from one opioid to another, is the treatment of choice for cancer patients experiencing serious side effects from opioid therapy such as myoclonus and delirium or when pain is refractory to treatment [125]. Opioid rotation, based on the concept of incomplete cross-tolerance between opioids, requires a working knowledge of an equianalgesic dosing and requires the substitution of one opioid with an alternative analgesic resulting in better pain control and permits the body to clear neurotoxic metabolites which can accumulate due to chronic use.

Of the high-potency opioids, morphine is the gold-standard drug and has the advantage of low cost, ease of use, analgesic potency, and availability in most countries around the world. It is converted to morphine-3-glucuronide and morphine-6-glucuronide by the liver. Morphine-6-glucuronide has noted opioid activity and is thought to be responsible for sedation, based on animal studies. Morphine-3-glucuronide has been implicated in the development of neuroexcitatory toxicities [126]. Morphine should be used with caution in cancer patients with renal dysfunction.

Oxycodone is equal to or slightly greater in potency than morphine. It is available as a time-released long-acting form and immediate release short-acting oral medication.

Hydromorphone is a short-acting opioid which is five to seven times stronger than morphine and can be administered as an oral pill or intravenous medication. Recently, a long-acting, time-released oral capsule administered daily has been introduced, but its use is limited by high cost.

Fentanyl, a semisynthetic opioid, is available in parenteral, transdermal, and oral preparations. Fentanyl has a rapid onset and short duration which is ideal for patient-controlled analgesic pumps. For cancer patients with stable pain, fentanyl can be administered as a patch which is changed every 72 h and takes up to 18 h to reach its peak [127]. Recently, an oral transmucosal fentanyl has been approved as a rescue dose for breakthrough pain.

Methadone is an inexpensive opioid and is accepted as a second-line opioid for the treatment of cancer-related pain. The two main indications for methadone in palliative care are the treatment of cancer patients who have a high tolerance for opioids and as a second-line agent in an opioid rotation. Interindividual variation in the pharmacokinetics of methadone has been attributed to the differences in metabolism via the cytochrome P450 hepatic enzymes. Caution should be practiced by physicians when prescribing methadone with P450 inhibitors such as antifungals, antiviral, antidepressants, and certain antibiotics. In addition, P450 inducers such as anticonvulsants, rifampin, and corticosteroids may alter the analgesic potency of methadone. Methadone should be also used cautiously for patients with QTc prolongation (>450 cm) which can result in torsades de points [128].

Adjuvant therapies for pain have analgesic properties but are nonopioid medications. They are used for specific pain syndromes, often in conjunction with opioid therapy in patients with cancer.

Acetaminophen is an antipyretic analgesic which may inhibit cyclo-oxygenase in the central nervous system and has inhibitory effects on the serotonergic system [129]. Liver function abnormalities and increased risk of serious liver toxicity are noted when exceeding 4 g of acetaminophen per day [130], especially in patients with comorbid liver disease. It may be used for mild pain and in conjunction with stronger opioids for moderate to severe pain.

NSAIDs, including the nonspecific COX inhibitors and selective COX-2 inhibitors, block the synthesis of prostaglandins resulting in less pain and inflammation. They are useful in treating bone pain and as adjuvant therapy with opioid medications for a variety of pain syndromes. Limitations in the management of cancer pain are the potential for long-term side effects including gastric and duodenal ulceration, cardiovascular and renal toxicity, and bleeding risk associated with their use in thrombocytopenic patients.

Patients are often unaware of their own daily use of acetaminophen and NSAIDs in over-the-counter medications which are often combined with other analgesics. Patient education about toxicities of acetaminophen and NSAIDs is critical and attention focused on educating patients on the content of their over-the-counter medications is recommended.

Both tricyclic antidepressants (amitriptyline and nortriptyline) and anticonvulsants (gabapentin, pregabalin, and lamotrigine) are useful for the treatment of neuropathic pain.

For neuropathic pain, gabapentin is the gold-standard and sedation is the notable side effect. Typically, gabapentin is started at low doses and titrated to control symptoms.

Anorexia–Cachexia Syndrome

Anorexia is characterized by the loss of appetite or decreased caloric intake, whereas cachexia is defined as a complex metabolic syndrome associated with an underlying illness, such as cancer, and is associated with a loss of muscle mass with or without a loss of fat [131]. A recent international group of researchers defined cancer cachexia as weight loss greater than 5%, or weight loss greater than 2% in patients with the depletion of skeletal muscle mass, or a body mass index (BMI) of $< 20\,kg/m^2$ [132]. Others have hypothesized that cachexia progresses through distinct stages – precachexia to cachexia to refractory cachexia [133], and interventions directed at reversing or stabilizing weight loss may be more effective in the early, precachectic stage versus the refractory stage. In advanced cancer patients with refractory cachexia, psychosocial support and education about the therapeutic limitations may be more important than pharmaceutical interventions.

In cancer cachexia, the supplementation of nutrition by parenteral feeding results in minimal weight gain [134, 135]. Unlike starvation which is correctable by refeeding and associated with decreased metabolic rate and increased efficiency of energy utilization, cachexia is characterized by increased activity of catabolic pathways and increased metabolism [136].

Nutritional status in cancer patients can be assessed by evaluating the following: caloric intake, degree of weight loss, laboratory indicators of malnourishment, and evaluation of risk factors which compromise nutritional intake. Risk factors, such as uncontrolled pain, nausea, and clinical depression, can result in decreased caloric intake and the anorexia–cachexia syndrome. In cancer patients, inadequate caloric intake is common, occurring in roughly 40% of cancer patients, and often is inadequate to support a patient's basal metabolic demands [136]. Wide variations in nutritional intake exist in cancer patients, with cachexia being strongly associated with decreased frequency of eating and with oral intake which consists predominantly of liquids [137].

Measurement of weight can be represented by the BMI – calculated by an individual's body mass divided by the square of his or her height (kg/m^2). Unfortunately, BMI can be misleading since cachectic patients who often loose predominantly muscle mass may continue to have BMI values in the normal range. In the research setting, dual-energy X-ray absorptiometry is highly accurate and can measure weight as well as differentiate fat, lean body mass, and bone.

Nutritional counseling has shown to increase the caloric intake of cachectic patients with cancer but results in no weight gain. In advanced cancer patients with cachexia, psycho-social support and counseling is critical. Anorexia and cachexia resulting in alterations of a patient's appearance can be distressing. Counseling with an emphasis on the social benefits of eating at the dinner table and the pleasure of tasting food should be emphasized over the amount of caloric intake. Patients and family should be educated that increasing caloric intake does not reverse the metabolic derangements which result in cachexia and that weight loss is a common symptom and a natural often irreversible process at the end of life.

Pharmacologic treatments of cancer cachexia include megestrol acetate, a progesterone derivative with progestational and antigonadotropic effects [138]. In several systematic reviews [139–141], researchers have concluded that megestrol acetate does improve appetite. However, there is no overall benefit on lean body mass or global quality of life scales. Side effects of megestrol acetate include edema, adrenal insufficiency, thromboembolism, and hypogonadism in male patients [142].

Corticosteroids, including prednisolone, dexamethasone, and methylprednisolone, have been shown to stimulate appetite in cancer patients, but the beneficial effects diminish over time [143]. More research is needed on the optimal dosing and duration of corticosteroids in the treatment of cancer cachexia. Side effects of steroid administration include insulin resistance, suppression of the immune system, myopathy, and risk of adrenal insufficiency if abruptly discontinued.

Investigational treatments include omega-3 fatty acids (eicosapentaenoic acid and docosahexaenoic acid), amino acids supplementation with glutamine or L-carnitine, NSAIDs, and mirtazapine.

Fatigue

Fatigue, also known as weakness or asthenia – is the most common symptom experienced by cancer patients and increases in intensity at the end of life. It is often misdiagnosed and undertreated [144] and systematic assessment and treatment should be offered to all cancer patients. The National Comprehensive Cancer Network defines cancer-related fatigue as "a distressing, persistent, subjective sense of physical, emotional, and/or cognitive tiredness or exhaustion related to cancer or cancer treatment that is not proportional to recent activity and interferes with usual functioning" [145]. Cancer-related fatigue is not relieved by rest and is felt to be mediated by pro-inflammatory cytokines as a result of the cancer or its treatment.

As the cancer progresses, the etiology of fatigue becomes more complex and multidimensional. For example, the contribution of anemia to the symptom of fatigue is significant during the early stages of cancer when patients are undergoing treatment; however, as cancer patients approach the end of life, the significance of anemia as the underling etiology of fatigue becomes less important [146]. It is only one factor which can contribute to the symptom of fatigue in advanced cancer patients, along with other factors including sleep disturbances, psychological symptoms such as anxiety and depression, deconditioning, cachexia, side effects of medications, autonomic dysfunction, hypogonadism in men, delirium, and infections.

A comprehensive history and physical examination is indicated with attention to reversible factors. Identification of drug–drug interactions or polypharmacy resulting in the side effects of fatigue is important to review. Medications including antihistamines, beta-blockers, diuretics, muscle relaxants, and benzodiazepines can often be modified resulting in improvements in the level of fatigue in cancer patients. The initial management of fatigue is to treat underlying factors which may be reversible such as complications of delirium or clinical depression.

If no reversible factors are discovered, symptomatic treatment is indicated. Non-pharmacologic treatment may be advisable to attempt initially and include exercise, yoga, and cognitive behavioral therapy. Exercise has been extensively researched and has been demonstrated to improve symptoms of fatigue in cancer patients. Even in patients with advanced cancer, a twice-a-week group exercise program showed improvements in mood and physical fatigue [147].

If cancer-related fatigue persists, which is debilitating despite conservative treatment, established pharmacological interventions for the treatment of fatigue are corticosteroids and megestrol acetate. For cancer patients with fatigue and anorexia, a trial of megestrol acetate may be attempted which can potentially improve both symptoms. For advanced cancer patients with a high symptom burden, a trial of glucocorticoids is reasonable.

Psychostimulants, such as methylphenidate, dextroamphetamine, and modafanil, have also been found to be useful for some cancer patients but should be used with caution in patients with cognitive disturbances and cardiac disease. Studies have reported that methylphenidate is effective for symptoms of opioid-induced sedation, depression, and in pilot studies, cancer-related fatigue. However, a recent randomized controlled trial reported that methylphenidate and/or a nursing telephone intervention were not superior to placebo for the treatment of cancer-related fatigue [148]. Because of rapid onset and short half-life, a brief trial of methylphenidate can be attempted for fatigue in cancer patients. If after a few doses, it is found to be ineffective, it can be discontinued.

Nausea

Patients with cancer often experience chronic nausea with and without vomiting. Initial assessment of cancer patients with nausea includes a detailed history and physical examination which may indicate the underlying mechanism and help tailor the therapy to each individual patient. Often, more than one etiology may contribute to the symptom of nausea in patients with cancer.

History should be thorough with attention to symptoms which may contribute to nausea. Symptoms of early satiety may indicate autonomic dysfunction resulting in gastroparesis which is not uncommon in patients with advanced cancer and those who are on opioid medications [149]. Symptoms of nausea and vomiting in the early hours of the day associated with head discomfort suggest increased intracranial pressure. Nausea relieved by a large volume emesis suggests a possible bowel obstruction. Cancer patients with disease in the liver, peritoneum, or brain often have high rates of nausea and vomiting. Also, a history of anxiety, constipation, infections, or metabolic abnormalities, as well as radiation therapy to the abdomen or pelvis can increase the risk of having nausea with or without vomiting.

A review of a patient's medication regimen is also critical to treat symptoms of nausea. Commonly prescribed medications which may result in symptoms of nausea and vomiting include opioids, certain chemotherapies, or antibiotics. During the physical examination, attention should be directed at assessing the heart rate for loss of variability or orthostatic hypotension

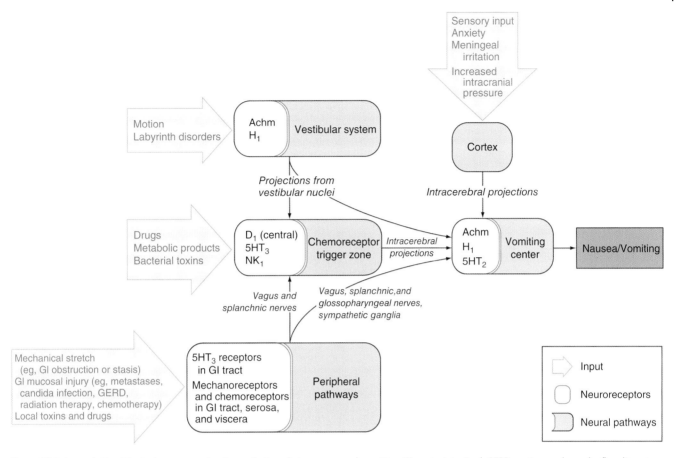

Figure 27.8 Interrelationships between neural pathway that mediate nausea and vomiting. GI, gastrointestinal. GERD, gastroesophageal reflux disease. *Source:* Wood GJ, Shega JW, Lynch B, Von Roenn JH. Management of intractable nausea and vomiting in patients at the end of life "I was feeling nauseous all of the time…nothing was working". JAMA 2007;298:1196–207. Reproduced with permission of American Medical Association.

which indicates autonomic dysfunction and gastroparesis. The oral mucosa should be examined for signs of mucositis or thrush, which may result in nausea as a result of oropharyngeal and esophageal irritation. Evidence of abdominal distention or masses on the physical examination may indicate ascites or possible bowel obstruction. Rectal examination is recommended to look for signs of hard stool or impaction suggesting constipation which needs to be treated.

Symptoms of nausea and vomiting are the result of stimulation of one or more of the following pathways: the chemoreceptor trigger zone, cortex with input from the senses, mechanoreceptors from the gastrointestinal tract, vagus and splanchnic nerves, glossopharyngeal nerves, and sympathetic ganglia, and the vestibular system (Figure 27.8).

In clinical practice, advanced cancer patients have multiple underlying factors which trigger symptoms of nausea and vomiting. Reversible underlying etiologies such as constipation must be treated aggressively. Two symptomatic approaches to managing chronic nausea in cancer patients have been proposed. One approach is to treat with an empirical antiemetic regimen, usually a D2 antagonist such as haloperidol or metoclopramide, irrespective of the underlying etiology [150]. Another approach which has been advocated involves treatment based on the underlying mechanism of nausea and

vomiting and was reported to be effective in 90% of patients with advanced disease (Table 27.2) [151].

Depression and Anxiety

Clinical depression in cancer patients is often underdiagnosed and undertreated. Depression is the most common mood abnormality faced by cancer patients and can increase the risk of suicide for this vulnerable patient population.

In cancer patients, the challenge for healthcare providers is to distinguish clinical or major depression from symptoms of depressed mood, sadness, anticipatory grief, or an adjustment reaction which are all common responses. Across the spectrum of depressive symptoms, cancer patients with the most severe feelings of depression benefit the most from antidepressants [152]. Cancer patients with an adjustment reaction often have changes in mood and anxiety temporarily associated with an acute stressor such as when they are given a diagnosis of cancer or other setbacks, including recurrences and relapses. An anticipatory grief reaction is not uncommon when cancer patients are informed of a poor prognosis or approaching end of life. The majority of cancer patients will cope and adapt reasonably well to their illness, often with brief episodes of anxiety and depressed mood which fluctuates and improves over a period of

Table 27.2 Selected studies supporting use of common antiemetics[1].

Source	Intervention	Design	No. of participants	Setting	Outcomes	Length of follow-up	Results	Adverse events
Robbins and Nagel,[60] 1975	Haloperidol 1 mg IM × 1 vs placebo	RCT	28	Nursing home residents with nausea and vomiting due to GI tract disorders	Failure: vomiting after antiemetic	12 h	86% Haloperidol group completed study vs 43% placebo[2] Less nausea and vomiting observed in haloperidol group[2]	None
Barton,[61] 1975	Haloperidol 1 mg IM × 1 vs placebo	RCT	62	Postoperative patients who developed nausea	Vomiting and report of nausea	3 h	Haloperidol more effective (83% vs 29% with no vomiting at 1 h, 71% vs 20% with no nausea)[2]	No serious adverse effects
Bruera et al.,[62] 2000	Controlled-release metoclopramide 40 mg orally every 12 h vs placebo	RCT	26	>1 month of cancer-associated dyspepsia syndrome	Nausea and vomiting self-report on 100 mm VAS in daily journal	4 day in each arm of cross-over design	5-Point lower nausea score in cohort receiving controlled-release metoclopramide[2]	No difference from placebo
Gralla et al.,[63] 1981	Metoclopramide 10 mg/kg vs prochlorperazine 50 mg vs placebo over study period	RCT	41	Patients with advanced cancer receiving cisplatin	Episodes of emesis, volume of emesis, duration of nausea	9 h	Fewer vomiting episodes with metoclopramide (10.5) vs placebo (1)[2] and metoclopramide (12) vs prochlorperazine (1)[2] Reduced emesis volume and nausea duration with metoclopramide[2]	Mild sedation with metoclopramide; 1 patient in the metoclopramide group had brief extrapyramidal reaction
Ernst et al.,[64] 2000	Prochlorperazine 10 mg IV vs promethazine 25 mg IV	RCT	84	Adults treated at emergency department for gastritis or gastroenteritis	Patient report of nausea on 100 mm VAS, time to complete relief	60 min	Scores: Prochlorperazine baseline, 65; 30 min, 29; and 60 min, 4.5; Promethazine baseline, 73; 30 min, 46; and 60 min, 26[2] Prochlorperazine was also superior in time to complete relief[2]	14% Akathisia or extrapyramidal reactions in both groups Less sedation in prochlorperazine (38% vs 71%)
Bardfeld,[65] 1966	Trimethobenzamide 200 mg IM vs prochlorperazine 10 mg IM vs placebo	RCT	126	Mostly ambulatory patients with nausea and vomiting	Patient self-report	24 h	Prochlorperazine superior: no relief in 21% of placebo, 18% of trimethobenzamide, and 7% of prochlorperazine (*P* value range, 0.07–0.08)	Drowsiness and pain at injection site in 12 of 41 patients receiving prochlorperazine
Pykko et al.,[66] 1985	Transdermal scopolamine (1 patch delivering 5 µg/h vs 2 patches delivering 10 µg/h) vs dimenhydrinate 100 mg with 50 mg of caffeine vs placebo	RCT	16	Experimentally induced motion sickness in healthy volunteers	Self-report of nausea on 0–100 numerical scale	Duration of experimental induction of nausea	Mean score for scopolamine 1 patch (40), 2 patches (23), and dimenhydrinate (18), all superior to placebo (61)[2]	Dry mouth more often than placebo with all 3 treatments; vertigo and gait disturbances in 3 participants treated with 2 scopolamine patches

Study	N	Design	Intervention	Population	Outcome measure	Duration	Results	Adverse effects
Marty et al.,[67] 1990	76	RCT	Ondansetron 8 mg IV before cisplatin then 1 mg/h for 24 h vs metoclopramide 3 mg/kg before cisplatin then 0.5 mg/kg for 8 h then placebo for 16 h	Cancer patients receiving cisplatin	Observed emesis, self-report of nausea by graded scale, VAS, and patient preference	24 h	2 or fewer episodes of vomiting in 75% of patients treated with ondansetron vs 42% treated with metoclopramide[2] Ondansetron also superior for nausea control[2]	Dystonic reactions in 3 patients treated with metoclopramide, more sedation with metoclopramide (12 vs 5 patients)
Theobald et al.,[68] 2002	20	Open-label crossover trial	Mirtazapine 15 and 30 mg orally as needed	Cancer patients taking opioids for pain	Self-report of nausea on 1-10 scale	6 week	Nausea decreased from 2.4 to 0.9 ($P = 0.10$)	Not reported
Mystakidou et al.,[57] 1998	160	RCT	Chlorpromazine 25 mg 2/day + dexamethasone 2 mg daily vs chlorpromazine 25 mg 2/day + tropisetron 5 mg/day vs chlorpromazine 25 mg 2/day + dexamethasone 2 mg/day vs tropisetron 5 mg/day	Terminally ill patients with cancer with no readily identifiable cause of nausea and vomiting	Patient report of nausea and vomiting with total control defined as no nausea and vomiting	15 day	Total control nausea/vomiting in 18 (33.9%) of chlorpromazine + dexamethasone, 74.4 (84.6%) of chlorpromazine + tropisetron, 85 (92.5%) of chlorpromazine + tropisetron + dexamethasone, 65.8 (78.9%) of tropisetron All tropisetron-containing regimens superior to chlorpromazine + dexamethasone[2]	No difference in adverse effects and none that forced discontinuation of therapy
Braude, et al.,[69] 2006	97	RCT	Droperidol 1.25 mg vs metoclopramide 10 mg vs prochlorperazine 10 mg vs placebo All received IV fluids	Adults in emergency department with nausea	100 mm VAS	60 min	Droperidol (−54.5 mm), metoclopramide (−40.2 mm), prochlorperazine (−40.5 mm), and placebo (−38.7 mm)[2]	Droperidol (71.4%) caused more self-reported anxiety or restlessness than all others (23.5%)

Source: Wood GJ, Shega JW, Lynch B, Von Roenn JH. Management of intractable nausea and vomiting in patients at the end of life "I was feeling nauseous all of the time…nothing was working." JAMA 2007;298(10):1196–207. Reproduced with permission of American Medical Association.

Abbreviations: IM, intramuscular; IV, intravenous; RCT, randomized controlled trial; VAS, visual analog scale.

[1] Study selection based primarily on quality of evidence and secondarily on how well the study population approximates patients near the end of life.

[2] Statistically significant at $P < 0.05$.

a few weeks. Healthcare providers can decrease the psychological burden faced by cancer patients with empathetic care and attention to the treatment of both physical and psychological distress.

Rates of depression vary depending on criteria used to diagnose clinical depression; the best estimate is a range of 10–25% in cancer patients. Risk factors for clinical depression in cancer patients include a family or past history of depression, female gender, poor social support and family dysfunction, uncontrolled pain, and external stressors. Malignancies which are associated with a higher rate of depression include retroperitoneal tumors including pancreatic cancers, brain malignancies, and head and neck cancers. In addition, medical comorbidities such as hypothyroidism, poorly controlled pain, and hypogonadism must be addressed prior to diagnosing clinical depression. Medications which may exacerbate symptoms of depression, such as corticosteroids, anticonvulsants, alpha interferon and interleukin-2, sedatives, and beta-blockers, should also be minimized.

A single screening question – "Are you depressed most of the time?" – has been found to be a brief, reliable screen for depression in advanced cancer patients [153]. However, a thorough diagnostic interview is the gold standard workup needed to determine in difficult cases if a cancer patient is clinically depressed and in need of pharmacologic interventions. To distinguish clinical depression, assessing patients for symptoms of pervasive hopelessness, helplessness, worthlessness, excess guilt, anhedonia, or suicidal ideation are the best, most specific diagnostic indicators. In addition, vegetative signs not explained by the underlying medical condition such as insomnia, poor concentration, loss of appetite, and psychomotor retardation may also indicate clinical depression.

Advanced cancer patients, who are appropriately adjusting to their illness, may lose hope for a cure but will be able to transfer hope for a more realistic goal, such as a good quality of life. Anhedonia, the inability to experience pleasure in life activities, may be difficult to assess in cancer patients who have a functional decline, but loss of joy in long-standing relationships with family and friends is an important history to obtain and a marker for clinical depression.

In cases of doubt, judicious use of antidepressant medications in conjunction with supportive psychotherapy is required to treat depression in patients with cancer. Selective serotonin reuptake inhibitors (SSRIs) are antidepressants which are useful in treating clinical depression but take time for the full therapeutic effect to be felt. Side effects of SSRIs including nausea, insomnia, and sexual dysfunction should be monitored. Tricyclic antidepressants (TCAs) are sedating and may be useful for cancer patients with insomnia. However, side effects of TCAs may be serious and include hypotension, arrhythmias, and constipation. When a rapid response is required, psychostimulants, such as methylphenidate, may be initiated while the benefits of selective SSRIs take effect (which may take a few weeks).

Cancer patients may experience symptoms of anxiety which often is associated with receiving bad news regarding the diagnosis or treatment of their illness. For most cancer patients, the emotional reaction is brief and resolves over time with no impact on a patient's ability to function with the support of family, friends, and empathetic healthcare providers.

Common medical conditions often associated with anxiety include pulmonary emboli, hypoxia with symptoms of dyspnea, bleeding, or complications of delirium and must be ruled out. If present, appropriate treatment of the medical complication will result in a reduction in the level of anxiety in patients with cancer. Medication side effects and withdrawal states are often overlooked as possibly underlying factors which result in symptoms of anxiety. Antiemetic medications including metoclopramide, prochlorperazine, promethazine, and haloperidol can result in akathisia which can resemble an anxious state and can be easily treated by discontinuation of the medication. Withdrawal from excessive alcohol consumption, benzodiazepine use, or abuse of sedative barbiturates can also be misdiagnosed as anxiety and must be treated appropriately.

Prior to treatment, underlying medical problems should be corrected and symptoms such as pain should be managed. Behavioral or pharmacologic treatments for anxiety may be useful if a patient's level of distress is debilitating. Non-pharmacologic treatments including relaxation exercises, slow, deep breathing, and distraction techniques may be helpful for some patients. Supportive counseling is an important intervention for patients with advanced cancer who are facing death. Cancer patients may be unable to disclose their fears regarding death to friends and family, and a trained counselor may be able to facilitate open and frank discussions with the goal of normalizing and demystifying the process in order to reach a state of acceptance and peace of mind.

Anxiety medications can be used safely to treat acute and chronic symptoms of debilitating anxiety in patients with cancer. For situational anxiety, when symptoms are associated with procedures or tests, a short-acting benzodiazepine such as alprazolam or lorazepam may be indicated. For patients with chronic anxiety, a longer acting benzodiazepine, like clonazepam, may be indicated. For cancer patients on opioids, healthcare providers should prescribe benzodiazepines cautiously and educate patients on potential interactions of opioids with sedatives which may result in serious side effects such as delirium or respiratory depression. In addition, the lowest effective dose should be administered and supportive psychotherapy should complement any pharmacologic treatment of anxiety.

End-of-Life Care

Dyspnea

Dyspnea is a common symptom in patients with advanced cancer [154]. Air hunger or the uncomfortable awareness of breathing is more common in primary lung cancer or intrathoracic metastatic disease but can also be present in cancer patients without cardiopulmonary involvement. Dyspnea may be a result of increased ventilatory demand, impairment in the mechanical process of breathing, or a combination of both mechanisms.

Dyspnea is a subjective symptom which patients self-report and may or may not be associated with objective measures of ventilation such as oxygen saturation, respiratory rate, or arterial blood gas measurements. The first step in the management of dyspnea is the correction of underlying factors such as the treatment of pneumonia with antibiotics, anticoagulation therapy for patients with pulmonary embolism, or transfusions of red blood cells for anemic patients.

Conservation interventions for the treatment of dyspnea include breathing training and relaxation exercises, alterations of activity level with the use of bathroom aids, portable oxygen and wheelchairs, and chest wall vibration therapy. Cool air directed on the face may benefit some cancer patients with symptoms of dyspnea [155]. When dyspnea is refractory to medical therapy and conservative treatments have failed to alleviate feelings of dyspnea, systemic opioid therapy carefully titrated to control air hunger is the treatment of choice [156]. Hypoxemic patients may benefit from oxygen supplementation [157]. Anxiety often accompanies symptom of dyspnea, and with appropriate control of air hunger can often be managed without anxiolytics. Benzodiazepines can precipitate symptoms of delirium or result in respiratory depression and should be used cautiously for cancer patients with anxiety associated with dyspnea.

Delirium

For patients with advanced cancer, irreversible global cerebral dysfunction results in delirium which is the most common neuropsychiatric complication at the end of life [107]. Delirium precedes death and often is associated with agitation which can be distressing for patients, family members, and healthcare providers [158],

For cancer patients, a number of factors may contribute to the presentation of delirium and include the following:

- Opioid-induced neurotoxicity
- Cancer metastases to the brain
- Treatment with chemotherapy or radiation
- Metabolic factors including hypercalcemia and hyponatremia
- Dehydration
- Organ failure
- Infections
- Medications including benzodiazepines, glucocorticoids, psychotropic medications.

Screening tools for delirium have been developed and validated in patients with cancer including the Memorial Delirium Assessment Scale (Figure 27.9) [159] and the Confusion Assessment Method [160].

In cancer patients with delirium, every attempt should be made to investigate and treat underlying reversible causes – change the type of opioid therapy, treat infections with antibiotics, discontinue benzodiazepines if not being used on a chronic basis, or fluid resuscitate dehydrated patients. For symptoms of agitation, delusions, or hallucinations, haloperidol is the treatment of choice [161]. In cancer patients, preliminary studies show that inadequate doses of neuroleptics, which are often too low, are used by clinicians to treat agitation due to delirium [162] resulting in poor control. More research is needed in order to develop the best approach.

For cancer patients with delirium who are refractory to haloperidol (daily doses exceeding 10–20 mg), other more sedating medications could be considered including olanzapine or chlorpromazine. Patients who fail to respond to neuroleptics may benefit from palliative sedation [163].

Palliative Sedation

Palliative sedation is the treatment of last resort for uncontrolled, refractory symptoms in patients with advanced cancer who have a poor prognosis. Uncontrolled symptoms are refractory after all attempts, ideally by an interdisciplinary team with either a specialist in pain management or a palliative care professional, have been exhausted. Consensus is lacking for the indications for palliative sedation, which varies widely between different groups and settings. Palliative sedation may be indicated emergently in cancer patients with intractable convulsions, massive hemorrhage, asphyxiation, terminal dyspnea or agitated delirium refractory to medical therapy [164]. For advanced cancer patients with refractory depression, anxiety, or existential distress, no clear consensus exists among specialists who practice palliative care regarding the role of sedation [165].

A few of the problems with the use of palliative sedation identified by the European Association of Palliative Care include: the practice of initiating palliative sedation to hasten death, healthcare providers inadequately trained to treat symptoms resorting to sedation out of frustration or burnout, and substandard implementation of palliative sedation with inadequate monitoring of the level of sedation, unwarranted escalation, or use of inappropriate medications (e.g., opioids) [166].

Benzodiazepines are the most commonly used sedatives with parentally administered midazolam being the most frequently used medication [167]. Midazolam, which has anxiolytic and anticonvulsant properties, has a short half-life and is easily titrated to control symptoms. Barbiturates, such as propofol and phenobarbital, have also been administered to provide palliative sedation for cancer patients. Opioids are not useful agents for palliative sedation since they provide only transient sedation and when escalated result in severe side effects including agitated delirium, myoclonus, and respiratory depression, which can be fatal. Cancer patients on chronic opioids, however, should be maintained on their opioid regimen and palliative sedation, if indicated, be provided by another alternative sedative.

Conclusion

Cancer patients and their family face a host of stressors during the diagnosis and treatment of their cancer. Palliative care professionals can assist oncologists and other colleagues with the physical pain, psychosocial distress, spiritual conflict, and practical concerns of cancer patients at any point in the trajectory of their disease. Although the field of palliative care is expanding, integration of palliative care services, including the availability of inpatient consultation palliative care teams,

PCUs, outpatient ambulatory clinics, and home care/hospice services, has been variable within cancer centers. Barriers to access and availability of palliative care services must be addressed and more research is needed on how to judiciously spend limited resources to integrate and maintain viable palliative care programs in institutions dedicated to treating cancer.

Evidence suggests improvements in symptom control, psychosocial and spiritual well-being, and possible survival with the integration of palliative care with cancer treatment. Therefore, it is critical that palliative care services along with surgical, radiation, and medical oncology services work in tandem to care for cancer patients.

Appendix 1
Memorial Delirium Assessment Scale (MDAS)

INSTRUCTIONS: Rate the severity of the following symptoms of delirium based on current interaction with subject or assessment of his/her behavior or experience over past several hours (as indicated in each time.)

ITEM 1-REDUCED LEVEL OF CONSCIOUSNESS (AWARENESS): Rate the patient's current awareness of and interaction with the environment (interviewer, other people/objects in the room; for example; ask patients to describe their surroundings).
☐ 0: none   (patient spontaneously fully aware of environment and interacts appropriately)
☐ 1: mild   (patient is unaware of some elements in the environment, or not spontaneously interacting appropriately with the interviewer; becomes fully aware and appropriately interactive when prodded strongly; interview is prolonged but no seriously disrupted)
☐ 2: moderate (patient is unaware of some or all elements in the environment, or not spontaneously interacting with the interviewer; becomes in completely aware and inappropriately interactive when prodded strongly: interview is prolonged but not seriously disrupted)
☐ 3: severe   (patient is unaware of all elements in the environment with no spontaneous interaction of awareness of the interviewer, so that the interview is difficulty-to-impossible even with maximal prodding

ITEM 2-DISORENTATION: Rate current state by asking the following 10 orientation items: date, month day, year, season, floor, name of hospital, city, state, and country.
☐ 0: none   (patient knows 9-10 items)
☐ 1: mild   (patient knows 7-8 items)
☐ 2: moderate (patient knows 5-6 items)
☐ 3: severe   (patient know no more than 1 item)

ITEM 3-SHORT-TERM MEMORY IMPAIRMENT: Rate current state by using repetition and delayed recall of 3 words [patient must immediately repeat and recall words 5 min later after an intervening task. Use alternate sets of 3 words for successive evaluations (for example, apple, table, tomorrow, sky, cigar, justice)].
☐ 0: none   (all 3 words repeated and recalled)
☐ 1: mild   (all 3 repeated, patient fails to recall 1)
☐ 2: moderate (all 3 repeated, patient fails to recall 23)
☐ 3: severe   (patient fails to repeat 1 or more words)

ITEM 4-IMPAIRED DIGIT SPAN: Rate current performance by asking subjects to repeat first 3, 4, then 5 digits forward and then 3, then 4 backwards; continue to the next step only if patient succeeds at the previous one.
☐ 0: none   (patient can do at least 5 numbers forward and 4 backward)
☐ 1: mild   (patient can do at least 5 numbers forward and 3 backward)
☐ 2: moderate (patient can do 4-5 numbers forward, cannot do 3 backward)
☐ 3: severe   (patient can no more than 3 numbers forward)

ITEM 5-REDUCED ABILITY TO MAINTAIN AND SHIFT ATTENTION: As indicated during the interview by questions needing to be rephrased and/or repeated because patient's attention wanders, patient loses track, patient is distracted by outside stimuli or over-absorbed in a task.
☐ 0: none   (none of the above, patient maintains and shifts attention normally)
☐ 1: mild   (above attentional problems occur once or twice without prolonging the interviews)
☐ 2: moderate (above attentional problems occur often, prolonging the interview without seriously disrupting it)
☐ 3: severe   (above attentional problems occur constantly, disrupting and making the interview difficult-to-impossible

ITEM 6-DISORGANIZED THINKING: As indicated during the interview by rambling irrelevant, or incoherent speech, or by tangential, circumstantial, or faculty reasoning. Ask patient a some a somewhat complex question (for example, "Describe your current medical condition").
☐ 0: none   (patient's speech is coherent and goal-directed)
☐ 1: mild   (patient's speech is slightly difficult to follow: responses to questions are slightly off target but not so much as to prolong the interview)
☐ 2: moderate (disorganized thoughts or speech are clearly present, such that interview is prolonged but not disrupted)
☐ 3: severe   (examination is very difficult or impossible due to disorganized thinking or speech)

Figure 27.9 Memorial Delirium Assessment Scale (MDAS). *Source:* Breitbart W, Rosenfeld B, Roth A, *et al.* [159]. Reproduced with permission of Elsevier.

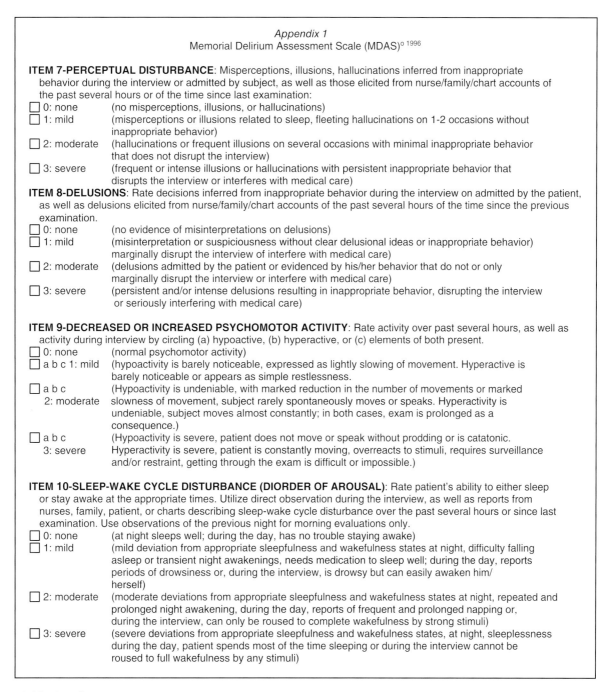

Figure 27.9 (Continued)

References

1 Walling A, Lorenz KA, Dy SM, *et al.* Evidence-based recommendations for information and care planning in cancer care. *J Clin Oncol* 2008;26:3896–902.

2 Siegel RL, Miller KD, Jemal A. Cancer statistics, 2017. *CA Cancer J Clin* 2017;67:7–30.

3 Whelan TJ, Mohide EA, Willan AR, *et al.* The supportive care needs of newly diagnosed cancer patients attending a reginal cancer center. *Cancer* 1997;80:1518–24.

4 Alifrangis C, Koizia L, Rozario A, *et al* The experiences of cancer patients. *QJM* 2011;104:1075–81.

5 Field MJ, Cassel CK (eds). *Approaching Death: Improving Care at the End of Life.* Washington, DC: National Academy Press, 1997.

6 Fadul N, Elsayem A, Palmer JL, *et al.* Supportive versus palliative care: what's in a name? A survey of medical oncologist and midlevel providers at a comprehensive cancer center. *Cancer* 2009;115:2013–21.

7 Hillier R. Palliative medicine. *BMJ* 1988;297:874–5.

8 Clark D. The development of palliative medicine in the UK and Ireland. In: Bruera E, Higginson IJ, Ripamonti R, von Gunten

(eds) *Textbook of Palliative Medicine*. London: Hodder Arnold, 2006:3–11.

9 Fukui S, Fujita J, Tsujimura M, *et al*. Late referrals to home palliative cares service affecting death at home in advanced cancer patients in Japan: a nationwide survey. *Ann Oncol* 2011;22:2113–20.

10 Teno JM, Shu JE, Casarett D, *et al*. Timing of referral to hospice and quality of care: length of stay and bereaved family members' perceptions of the timing of hospice referral. *J Pain Symptom Manage* 2007;34:120–5.

11 MacDonald N. The development of palliative care in Canada. In: Bruera E, Higginson IJ, Ripamonti R, von Gunten C (eds) *Textbook of Palliative Medicine*. London: Hodder Arnold, 2006:22–8.

12 Centeno C, Noguera A, Lynch T, Clark D. Official certification of doctors working in palliative medicine in Europe: data from and EAPC study in 52 European countries. *Palliat Med* 2007;21:683–7.

13 Morrison RS, Meier DE. Clinical practice. *Palliative care. N Engl J Med* 2004;350:2582–90.

14 Federal Register 2008 – 73 FR 32204, June 5, 2008.

15 Center to Advance Palliative Care (CAPC). About Palliative Care. https://www.capc.org/about/palliative-care/ (accessed 24 August 2017).

16 World Health Organization (WHO) definition of palliative care, available online at http://www.who.int/cancer/palliative/definition/en (accessed 24 August 2017)

17 Bruera E, Billings JA, Lupu D, Ritchie CS. AAHPM position paper: requirements for the successful development of academic palliative care programs. *J Pain Symptom Manage* 2010;39:743–55.

18 Cummings I. The interdisciplinary team. In: Doyle D, Hanks G, MacDonald N (eds) *Oxford Textbook of Palliative Medicine*. Oxford: Oxford University Press, 1998.

19 Strasser F, Sweeney C, Willey J, *et al*. Impact of a half-day multidisciplinary symptom control and palliative care outpatient clinic in a comprehensive cancer center on recommendations, symptom intensity, and patient satisfaction. A retrospective descriptive study. *J Pain Symptom Manage* 2004;27:481–91.

20 Bruera E, Michaud M, Vigano A. Multidisciplinary symptom control clinic in a cancer center: a retrospective study. *Support Care Cancer* 2001;9:162–8.

21 Higginson IJ, Wade AM, McCarthy M. Effectiveness of two palliative support teams. *J Public Health Med* 1992;14:50–6.

22 Addington-Hall JM, MacDonald LD, Anderson HR, *et al*. Randomized controlled trial of effects of coordinating care for terminally ill cancer patients. *BMJ* 1992:305:1317–22.

23 Pituskin E, Fairchil A, Dutka J, *et al*. Multidisciplinary team contributions within a dedicated outpatient palliative radiotherapy clinic: a prospective descriptive study. *Int J Radiat Oncol Biol Phys* 2010;78:527–32.

24 Bruera E, Hui D. Palliative care units: the best option for the most distressed. *Arch Intern Med* 2011;171:1601.

25 Elsayem A, Swint K, Fisch MJ, *et al*. A high-volume specialist palliative care unit and team may reduce in-hospital end-of-life care costs. *J Palliat Med* 2003;6:699.

26 Smith TJ, Coyne P, Cassel B, *et al*. Do hospital-based palliative teams improve care for patients or families at the end of life? *J Pain Symptom Manage* 2002;23:96.

27 Casarett D, Johnson M, Smith D, Richardson D. The optimal delivery of palliative care: a national comparison of the outcomes of consultation teams vs inpatient units. *Arch Intern Med* 2011;171:649–55.

28 Bradford N, Irving H, Smith AC, Pedersen LA, Herbert A. Palliative care afterhours: a review of a phone support service. *J Pediatr Oncol Nurs* 2012;29:141–50.

29 Temel JS, Greer JA, Muzikansky A, *et al*. Early palliative care for patients with metastatic non-small-cell lung cancer. *N Engl J Med* 2010;363:733.

30 Rabow MW, Dibble SL, Pantilat SZ, McPhee SJ. The comprehensive care team: a controlled trial of outpatient palliative medicine consultation. *Arch Intern Med* 2004;164:83.

31 Medicare Hospice Benefits. Centers for Medicare and Medicaid Services 2016. https://www.medicare.gov/Pubs/pdf/02154-Medicare-Hospice-Benefits.PDF (accessed 24 August 2017).

32 Fainsinger RL, Demoissac D, Cole J, *et al*. Home versus hospice inpatient care: discharge characteristics of palliative care patients in an acute care hospital. *J Palliat Care* 2000;16:29.

33 Angus DC, Barnato AE, Linde-Zwirble WT, *et al*. Use of intensive care at the end of life in the United States: an epidemiologic study. *Crit Care Med* 2004;32:638–43.

34 Bekelman JE, Halpern SD, Blankart CR, *et al*. Comparison of site of death, health care utilization, and hospital expenditures for patients dying with cancer in 7 developed countries. *JAMA* 2016;315:272–83.

35 Shimabukuro-Vornhagen A, Böll B, Kochanek M, *et al*. Critical care of patients with cancer. *CA: Cancer J Clin* 2016;66:496–517.

36 Pochard F, Azoulay E, Chevret S, *et al*. Symptoms of anxiety and depression in family members of intensive care unit patients: ethical hypothesis regarding decision-making capacity. *Crit Care Med* 2001;29:1893–7.

37 Curtis JR, Shannon SE. Transcending the silos: toward an interdisciplinary approach to end-of-life care in the ICU. *Intensive Care Med* 2006;32:15–17.

38 Morrison RS, Maroney-Galin C, Kralovec PD, Meier DE. The growth of palliative care programs in United States hospitals. *J Palliat Med* 2005;8:1127.

39 www.CAPC.org (accessed 24 August 2017).

40 Hui D, Elsayem A, De La Cruz, *et al*. Availability and integration of palliative care at US cancer centers. *JAMA* 2010;303:1054–61.

41 Center to Advance Palliative Care. Tools for palliative care programs. Estimating consult volume. Available from https://www.capc.org/topics/metrics-and-measurement-palliative-care (accessed 24 August 2017).

42 Dev R, Del Fabbro E, Miles M, *et al*. Growth of an academic palliative medicine program: patient encounters and clinical burden. *J Pain Symptom Manage* 2013;45:261–71.

43 Fadul NA, El Osta B, Dalal S, Poulter VA, Bruera E. Comparison of symptom burden among patients referred to palliative care with hematologic malignancies versus those with solid tumors. *J Palliat Med* 2008;11:422–6.

44 Rogers E, Shoemaker FF. *Communication of Innovations; A Cross-Cultural Approach*, 2nd edn. New York: New York Free Press, 1971.

45 Holland WE. The adoption of palliative care. The engineering of organizational change. In: Bruera E, Higginson IJ, Ripamonti C, Gunten CV (eds) *Textbook of Palliative Medicine*. London: Hodder Arnold, 2006: 231–7.

46 Dudgeon D, King S, Howell D, *et al*. Cancer Care Ontario's experience with implementation of routine physical and psychological symptom distress screening. *Psychooncology* 2012;21:357–64.

47 Fadul N, Elsayem A, Palmer JL, *et al*. Supportive versus palliative care: what's in a name? A survey of medical oncologists and midlevel providers at a comprehensive cancer center. *Cancer* 2009;115:2013–21.

48 Dalal S, Palla S, Hui D, *et al*. Association between a name change from palliative to supportive care and the timing of patient referrals at a comprehensive cancer center. *The Oncologist* 2011;16:105–11.

49 Merriam Webster. Online Dictionary, Available at www.merriam-webster.com/cgi-bin/dictionary?book=Dictionary&va=culture (accessed 24 August 2017).

50 Bruera E. The development of a palliative care culture. *J Palliat Care* 2004;20:316–19.

51 The Regence Foundation Living Well at the End of Life Poll Results. http://syndication.nationaljournal.com/communications/NationalJournalRegenceDoctorsToplines.pdf (accessed 24 August 2017).

52 Center to Advance Palliative Care 2011 Public Opinion Research on palliative care. https://media.capc.org/filer_public/18/ab/18ab708c-f835-4380-921d-fbf729702e36/2011-public-opinion-research-on-palliative-care.pdf (accessed 24 August 2017).

53 Gomes B, Calanzani N, Gysels M, Hall S, Higginson IJ. Heterogeneity and changes in preferences for dying at home: a systematic review. *BMC Palliat Care* 2013;12:7.

54 Bruera E, Sweeney C, Russell N, Willey JS, Palmer JL. Place of death of Houston area residents with cancer over a two year period. *J Pain Symptom Manage* 2003;26:637–43.

55 Steinhauser KE, Christakis NA, Clipp EC, *et al*. Factors considered important at the end of life by patients, family, physicians, and other care providers. *JAMA* 2000;284:2476–82.

56 Carlson MDA, Barry CL, Cherlin EJ, McCorkle R, Bradley. Hospices' enrollment policies may contribute to underuse of hospice care in the United States. *Health Aff* 2012;31:2690–8.

57 American Cancer Society. *Cancer Facts and Figures*, 2009. Atlanta: American Cancer Society, 2009.

58 Gadgeel SM, Kalemkerian GP. Racial differences in lung cancer. *Cancer Metastasis Rev* 2003;22:39–46.

59 Newman LA, Griffith KA, Jatoi I, *et al*. Meta-analysis of survival in African American and white American patients with breast cancer: ethnicity compared with socioeconomic status. *J Clin Oncol* 2006;24:1342–9.

60 Platz EA, Rimm EB, Willett WC, Kantoff PW, Giovannucci E. Racial variation in prostate cancer incidence and in hormonal system markers among male health professionals. *J Natl Cancer Inst* 2000;92:2009–17.

61 Elmore JG, Nakano CY, Linden HM, *et al*. Racial inequities in the timing of breast cancer detection, diagnosis, and initiation of treatment. *Med Care* 2005;43:141–8.

62 Kerner JF, Yedidia M, Padgett D, *et al*. Realizing the promise of breast cancer screeing: clinical follow-up after abnormal screening among Black women. *Prev Med* 2003;37:92–101.

63 Shavers VL, Brown ML. Racial and ethnic disparities in the receipt of cancer treatment. *J Natl Cancer Inst* 2002;94:334–57.

64 Aday LA. Equity, accessibility, and ethical issues: is the U.S. health care reform debate asking the right questions? *Am Behav Sci* 1993;36:724–40.

65 Fishman JM, Have TT, Casarett DC. Is public communication about end-of-life care helping to inform all? Cancer news coverage in African American versus mainstream media. *Cancer* 2012;118:2157–62.

66 Payne R, Medina E, Hamptom JW. Quality of life concerns in patients with breast cancer: evidence for disparity of outcomes and experiences in pain management and palliative care among African-American women. *Cancer* 2003;97:311–17.

67 Francoeur RB, Payne R, Raveis VH, Shim H. Palliative care in the inner city. Patient religious affiliation, underinsurance, and symptom attitude. *Cancer* 2007;109:425–34.

68 Reyes-Gibby CC, Anderson KO, Shete S, Burea E, Yennurajalingam S. Early referral to supportive care specialist for symptom burden in lung cancer patients. a comparison of Non-Hispanic Whites, Hispanics, and Non-Hispanic Blacks. *Cancer* 2012;118:856–63.

69 Strasser F, Sweeney C, Willey J, *et al*. Impact of half-day multidisciplinary symptom control and palliative care outpatient clinic in a comprehensive cancer center on recommendations, symptom intensity, and patient satisfaction. A retrospective descriptive study. *J Pain Symptom Manage* 2004;27:481–91.

70 Modonesi C, Scarpi E, Maltoni M, *et al*. Impact of palliative care unit admission on symptom control evaluated by the Edmonton Symptom Assessment System. *J Pain Symptom Manage* 2005;30:367–73.

71 Delgado-Guay MO, Parsons HA, Li Z, *et al*. Symptom distress, interventions, and outcomes of intensive care unit cancer patients referred to a palliative care consult team. *Cancer* 2009;115:437–45.

72 Goodwin DM, Higginson IJ, Myers K, *et al*. Effectiveness of palliative day care in improving pain, symptom control, and quality of life. *J Pain Symptom Manage* 2003;25:201–12.

73 Elsayem A, Swint K, Fisch MJ, *et al*. Palliative care inpatient service in a comprehensive cancer center: clinical and financial outcomes. *J Clin Oncol* 2004;22:2008–14.

74 Morrison RS, Penrod JD, Cassel JB, *et al*. Cost savings associated with US hospital palliative care consultation programs. *Arch Intern Med* 2008;168:1783–90.

75 Temel JS, Greer JA, Muzikansky A, *et al*. Early palliative care for patients with metastatic non-small-cell lung cancer. *N Engl J Med* 2010;363:733–42.

76 von Gunten CF. Financing palliative care. *Clin Geriatr Med* 2004;20:767–81.

77 Smith TJ, Coyne P, Cassel JB, *et al*. a high volume specialist palliative care unit and team may reduce in-hospital end of life care cost. *J Palliat Med* 2003; 6:699–705.

78 Naik G. Unlikely way to cut costs: comfort the dying. *Wall Street J* 2004:A1.

79 Ferrell BR, Temel JS, Temin S, *et al*. Integration of Palliative Care Into Standard Oncology Care: American Society of Clinical Oncology Clinical Practice Guideline Update. *J Clin Oncol* 2017;35:96–112.

80 Hui D, Kim SH, Kwon JH, *et al*. Access to palliative care among patients treated at a comprehensive cancer center. *Oncologist* 2012;17:1574–80.

81 Hui D, Elsayem A, Li Z, *et al*. Antineoplastic therapy use in patients with advanced cancer admitted to an acute palliative care unit at a comprehensive cancer center: a simultaneous care model. *Cancer* 2010;116:2036–43.

82 Fadul N, Elsayem A, Palmer JL, *et al*. Predictors of access to palliative care services among patients who died at a comprehensive cancer center. *J Palliat Med* 2007;10: 1146–52.

83 Kwon JH, Hui D, Chisholm G, *et al*. Clinical characteristics of cancer patients referred early to supportive and palliative care. *J Pall Med* 2012;16:148–55.

84 Ferrel BR. Late referrals to palliative care. *J Clin Oncol* 2005;23:2588–9.

85 Morita T, Akechi T, Ikenaga M, *et al*. Late referrals to specialized palliative care service in Japan. *J Clin Oncol* 2005;23:2637–44.

86 Morita T, Miyashita M, Tsuneto S, *et al*. Late referrals to palliative care units in Japan: nationwide follow-up survey and effects of palliative care team involvement after the Cancer Control Act. *J Pain Symptom Manage* 2009;38:191–6.

87 National Hospice and Palliative Care Organization (NHPCO). Facts and Figures on Hospice. NHPCO. 2015. p. 1–17. https://www.nhpco.org/sites/default/files/public/Statistics_Research/2015_Facts_Figures.pdf (accessed 24 August 2017).

88 Morrison RS, Maroney-Galin C, Kralovec PD, Meier DE. The growth of palliative care programs in United States hospital. *J Palliat Med* 2005;8:1127–34.

89 Teno JM, Gozalo PL, Bynum JPW, *et al*. Change in end-of-life care for Medicare beneficiaries. site of death, place of care, and health care transitions in 2000, 2005, and 2009. *JAMA* 2013;309:470–7.

90 Bruera E, Hui D. Integrating supportive and palliative care in the trajectory of cancer: establishing goals and models of care. *J Clin Oncol* 2010;28:4013–17.

91 Erikson C, Salsberg E, Forte G, Bruinooge S, Goldstein M. Future supply and demand for oncologists: challenges to assuring access to oncology services. *J Oncol Pract* 2007;3:79–86.

92 Fisch MJ, Lee JW, Weiss M, *et al*. Prospective, observational study of pain and analgesic prescribing in medical oncology outpatients with breast, colorectal, lung, or prostate cancer. *J Clin Oncol* 2012;30:1980–8.

93 Azoulay E, Pochard F, Chevret S, *et al*. Impact of a family information leaflet on effectiveness of information provided to family members of intensive care unit patients: a multicenter, prospective, randomized, controlled trial. *Am J Respir Crit Care Med* 2002;165:438.

94 Clayton JM, Butow PN, Tattersall MH, *et al*. Randomized controlled trial of a prompt list to help advanced cancer patients and their caregivers to ask questions about prognosis and end-of-life care. *J Clin Oncol* 2007;25:715.

95 Tattersall MH, Butow PN, Griffin AM, Dunn SM. The take-home message: patients prefer consultation audiotapes to summary letters. *J Clin Oncol* 1994;12:1305.

96 Hui D, Con A, Christie G, Hwaley PH. Goals of care and end-of-life decision making for hospitalized patients at a Canadian tertiary care cancer center. *J Pain Symptom Manage* 2009;38:871–81.

97 Lamont EB, Christakis NA. Prognostic disclosure to patients with cancer near the end of life. *Ann Intern Med* 2001;38:871–81.

98 Back AL, Arnold RM. Discussing prognosis: "how much do you want to know?" Talking to patients who do not want information or who are ambivalent. *J Clin Oncol* 2006;24:4214.

99 Back AL, Arnold RM. Discussion prognosis: "how much do you want to know?" Talking to patients who are prepared for explicit information. *J Clin Oncol* 2006;24:4209.

100 Baile WF, Buckman R, Lenzi R, *et al*. SPIKES – a six-step protocol for delivering bad news: application to the patient with cancer. *Oncologist* 2000;5:302.

101 Ambuel B, Mazzone MF. Breaking bad news and discussing death. *Prim Care*. 2001;28(2):249–267.

102 Schofield PE, Butow PN, Thompson JF, *et al*. Psychological responses of patients receiving a diagnosis of cancer. *Ann Oncol* 2003;14(1):48–56.

103 Weeks JC, Catalano PJ, Cronin A, *et al*. Patients' expectation about effects of chemotherapy for advanced cancer. *N Engl J Med* 2012;367:1616–25.

104 Freireich EJ, Kurzrock. The role of investigational therapy in management of patients with advanced metastatic malignancy. *J Clin Oncol* 2009;27:304–6.

105 Wright AA, Zhang B, Ray A, *et al*. Associations between end-of-life discussions, patient mental health, medical care near death, and caregiver bereavement adjustment. *JAMA* 2008;300:1665.

106 Smith TJ, Dow LA, Virago EA, *et al*. A pilot trial of decision aids to give truthful prognostic and treatment information to chemotherapy patients with advanced cancer. *J Support Oncol* 2011;9:79–86.

107 Connor SR, Pyenson B, Fitch K, Spence C, Iwasaki K. Comparing hospice and nonhospice patient survival among patients who die with a three-year window. *J Pain Symptom Manage* 2007;33:238–46.

108 Lilly CM, Sonna LA, Haley KJ, Massaro AF. Intensive communication: four-year follow-up from a clinical practice study. *Crit Care Med* 2003;31(5 Suppl):S394.

109 Lautrette A, Darmon M, Megarbane B, *et al*. A communication strategy and brochure for relatives of patients dying in the ICU. *N Engl J Med* 2007;356:469.

110 Dev R, Coulson L, Del Fabbro E, *et al*. A prospective study of family conferences: effects of patient presence on emotional expression and end-of-life discussions. *J Pain Sympt Manage* 2013;46:536–45.

111 Clayton JM, Butow PN, Tatersall MH. The needs of terminally ill cancer patients versus those of caregivers for information regarding prognosis and end-of-life issues. *Cancer* 2005;103:1957.

112 Butow PN, Maclean M, Dunn SM, Tattersall MH, Boyer MJ. The dynamics of change: cancer patient's preferences for

information, involvement and support. *Ann Oncol* 1997;8:857.

113 Homsi J, Walsh D, Rivera N, *et al.* Symptom evaluation in palliative medicine: patient report vs systematic assessment. *Support Care Cancer* 2006;4:444–53.

114 Stromgren AS, Groenvold M, Sorensen A, *et al.* Symptom recognition in advanced cancer. A comparison of nursing records against patient self-rating. *Acta Anaesthesiol Scand* 2001;45:1080–5.

115 Stromgren AS, Groenvold M, Pedersen L, Andersen L. Does the medical record cover the symptoms experienced by cancer patients receiving palliative care? A comparison of the record and patient self-rating. *J Pain Symptom Manage* 2001;21:189–96.

116 Sneeuw KCA, Sprangers MAG, Aaronson NK. The role of health care providers and significant others in evaluating the quality of life of patients with chronic disease. *J Clin Epidemiol* 2012;55:1130–43.

117 Bruera E. Patient assessment in palliative cancer care. *Cancer Treat Rev* 1996;22(Suppl A):3.

118 Bruera E, Kuehn N, Miller MJ, Selmser P, Macmillan K. The Edmonton Symptom Assessment System (ESAS): a simple method for the assessment of palliative care patients. *J Palliat Care* 1991;7:6–9.

119 Koshy RC, Rhodes D, Devi S, Grossman SA. Cancer pain management in developing countries: a mosaic of complex issues resulting in inadequate analgesia. *Support Care Cancer* 1998;6:430–7.

120 Foley KM. Pain syndromes in patients with cancer. In Bonica JJ, Ventafridda V (Eds), *Advances in Pain Research and Therapy*. New York: Raven Press, 1979:59–75.

121 Twycross RG, Fairfield S. Pain in far-advanced cancer. *Pain* 1982;14:303–10.

122 World Health Organization. Cancer pain relief and palliative care: report of a WHO Expert Committee. *World Health Organ Tech Rep Ser* 1990;804:11–12.

123 Galer BS, Coyle N, Pasternak GW, Portenoy RK. Individual variation in the response to different opioids-report of five cases. *Pain* 1992;49:87–91.

124 Bruera E, Chadwick S, Brenneis C, Hanson J, MacDonald RN. Methylphenidate associated with narcotics for the treatment of cancer pain. *Cancer Treat Rep* 1987;71:67–70.

125 Indelicato RA, Portenoy RK. Opioid rotation in the management of refractory cancer pain. *J Clin Oncol* 2002;20:348–52.

126 Andersen G, Christrup L, Sjogren P. Relationships among morphine metabolism, pain and side effects during long-term treatment: an update. *J Pain Symptom Manage* 2003;25:74–91.

127 Skaer TL. Transdermal opioids for cancer pain. *Health Qual Life Outcomes* 2006;4:24.

128 Krants M, Martin J, Stimmel B, *et al.* QTc interval screening in methadone treatment. *Ann Intern Med* 2009;150:387–95.

129 Pickering G, Loriot MA, Libert F, *et al.* Analgesic effect of acetaminophen in humans: first evidence of a central serotonergic mechanism. *Clin Pharmacol Ther* 2006;79:371–8.

130 Watkins PB, Kaplowitz N, Slattery JT, *et al.* Aminotransferase elevation in healthy adults receiving 4 grams of acetaminophen daily: a randomized controlled trial. *JAMA* 2006:296:87–93.

131 Evans WJ, Morley JE, Argiles J, *et al.* Cachexia: a new definition. *Clin Nutr* 2008;27:793–9.

132 Fearon K, Strasser F, Anker SD, *et al.* Definition and classification of cancer cachexia: an international consensus. *Lancet Oncol* 2011;12:489–95.

133 Bozzetti F, Mariani L. Defining and classifying cancer cachexia: a proposal by the SCRINIO Working Group. *J Parenter Enteral Nutr* 2009;33:489–95.

134 Grosvenor M, Bulcavage L, Chlebowski RT. Symptoms potentially influencing weight loss in a cancer population. Correlations with primary site, nutritional status, and chemotherapy administration. *Cancer* 1989;63:330–4.

135 Evan WK, Makuch R, Clamon GH, *et al.* Limited impact of total parenteral nutrition on nutritional status during treatment for small cell lung cancer. *Cancer Res* 1985;45:3347–53.

136 Bosaeus I, Daneryd P, Svanberg E, Lundholm K. Dietary intake and resting energy expenditure in relation to weight loss in unselected cancer patients. *Int J Cancer* 2001;93:380–3.

137 Hutton JL, Martin L, Field CJ, *et al.* Dietary patterns in patients with advanced cancer: implications for anorexia-cachexia therapy. *Am J Clin Nutr* 2006;22:376–82.

138 Neruman F. The physiological action of progesterone and the pharmacological effects of progestogens – a short review. *Postgrad Med J* 1978;54:11–24.

139 Berenstein EG, Ortiz Z. Megestrol acetate for the treatment of anorexia-cachexia syndrome. *Cochrane Database Syst Rev* 2005;18(2).

140 Ruiz-Garcia V, Joan O, Perez Hoyos S, *et al.* Megestrol acetate: a systematic review usefulness about the weight gain in neoplastic patients with cancer. *Med Clinica* 2002;119:166–70.

141 Maltoni M, Nanni O, Scarpi E, *et al.* High-dose progestins for the treatment of cancer anorexia-cachexia syndrome: a systematic review of randomized clinical trials. *Ann Oncol* 2001;12:289–300.

142 Dev R, Del Fabbro E, Burera E. Association between megestrol acetate treatment and symptomatic adrenal insufficiency and hypogonadism in male patients with cancer. *Cancer* 2007;110:1173.

143 Yavuzsen T, Davis MP, Walsh D, LeGrand S, Lagman R. Systematic review of the treatment of cancer-associated anorexia and weight loss. *J Clin Oncol* 2005;23:8500–11.

144 Curt GA, Breitbart W, Cella D. Impact of cancer-related fatigue on the lives of patients new findings from the Fatigue Coalition. *Oncologist* 2000;5:353–60.

145 Berger AM, Mooney K, Banerjee C, *et al.* NCCN Clinical Practice Guidelines in Oncology: Cancer-Related Fatigue. Version 1.2017, December 19, 2016. Nccn.org. Accessed 14 January 2017

146 Munch TN, Zhang T, Willey J, Palmer JL, Bruera E. The association between anemia and fatigue in patients with advanced cancer receiving palliative care. *J Palliat Med* 2005;8:1144.

147 Oldervoll LM, Loge JH, Paltiel H, *et al.* The effect of a physical exercise program in palliative care. *J Pain Symptom Manage* 2006;31:421–30.

148 Bruera E, Yennurajalingam S, Palmer JL, *et al.* Methylphenidate and/or a nursing telephone intervention for fatigue in patients with advanced cancer: a randomized, placebo-controlled, Phase II trial. *J Clin Oncol* 2013;31:2421–7.

149 Fadul N, Strasser F, Palmer JL, *et al.* The association between autonomic dysfunction and survival in male patients with advanced cancer: a preliminary report. *J Pain Symptom Manage* 2010;39:283–90.

150 Bruera E, Seifert L, Watanabe S, *et al.* Chronic nausea in advanced cancer patients: a retrospective assessment of a metoclopramide-based antiemetic regimen. *J Pain Symptom Manage* 1996;11:147–53.

151 Stephenson J, Davies A. An assessment of etiology-based guidelines for the management of nausea and vomiting in patients with advanced cancer. *Support Care Cancer* 2006;14:348–53.

152 Fisch M. Use of antidepressants for depression in patients with advanced cancer. *Lancet Oncol* 2007;8:567–8.

153 Chochinov H, Wilson K, Enns M, Lander S. 'Are you depressed?' *Screening for depression in the terminally ill. Am J Psychiatry* 1997;12:439–45.

154 Ripamonti C, Fulfaro F, Burera E. Dyspnoea in patients with advanced cancer: incidence, causes and treatments. *Cancer Treat Rev* 1998;24:69.

155 Bausewein C, Booth S, Gysels M, Kuhback R, Higginson IJ. Effectiveness of a hand-held fan for breathlessness: a randomized phase II trial. *BMC Palliat Care* 2010;9:22.

156 Del Fabbro E, Dalal S, Bruera E. Symptom control in palliative care. Part III. Dyspnea and delirium. *J Palliat Med* 2006;9:422–36.

157 Abernethy AP, McDonald CF, Frith PA, *et al.* Effect of palliative oxygen versus room air in relief of breathlessness in patients with refractory dyspnoea: a double-blind, randomized controlled trial. *Lancet* 2010;376:784–93.

158 Bruera E, Bush SH, Willey J, *et al.* Impact of delirium and recall on the level of distress in patients with advanced cancer and their family caregivers. *Cancer* 2009;115:2004.

159 Breitbart W, Rosenfeld B, Roth A, *et al.* The Memorial Delirium Assessment Scale. *J Pain Symptom Manage* 1997;13:128.

160 Inouye SK, van Dyck CH, Alessi CA, *et al.* Clarifying confusion: the confusion assessment method. *A new method for detection of delirium. Ann Intern Med* 1990;113:941.

161 Breitbart W, Marotta R, Platt MM, *et al.* A double-blind trial of haloperidol, chlorpromazine, and lorazepam in the treatment of delirium in hospitalized AIDS patients. *Am J Psychiatr* 1996;153:231–7.

162 Hui D, Bush SH, Gallo LE, *et al.* Neuroleptic dose in the management of delirium in patients with advanced cancer. *J Pain Symptom Manage* 2010;39:186–96.

163 Bottomley DM, Hanks GW. Subcutaneous midazolam infusion in palliative care. *J Pain Symptom Manage* 1990;5:259.

164 Nauck F, Alt-Epping B. Crises in palliative care – a comprehensive approach. *Lancet Oncol* 2008;9:1086–91.

165 de Graeff A, Dean M. Palliative sedation therapy in the last weeks of life: a literature review and recommendations for standards. *J Palliat Med* 2007;10:67–85.

166 Cherny NI, Radbruch L. European Association for Palliative Care (EAPC) recommended framework for the use of sedation in palliative care. *Palliat Med* 2009;23:581–93.

167 Chater S, Viola R, Paterson J, Jarvis V. Sedation for intractable distress in the dying: a survey of experts. *Palliat Med* 1998;12:255–69.

28

Sexuality and Fertility

Jeanne Carter, Shari B. Goldfarb, Yukio Sonoda, Christian J. Nelson, Maura N. Dickler, and John P. Mulhall

Memorial Sloan Kettering Cancer Center, New York, New York, USA

Introduction

With the United States (US) population of cancer survivors expected to grow to 20 million by 2026 [1, 2], the need to address survivorship and quality of life (QOL) issues, including sexual function and fertility needs [3, 4], has become increasingly important. The normal aging process prompts physical changes that influence reproductive organs and sexual function, and cancer and its treatment can compound these issues or induce symptoms earlier [3–6]. In this chapter we summarize the major sexual health issues associated with cancer and treatment; discuss fertility preservation, reproductive concerns, and the impact of cancer-related infertility; and provide suggestions for enhanced patient–physician communication in addressing these issues.

Cancer and Sexuality

The epidemiology of sexual dysfunction in cancer populations has not been extensively studied across all disease sites [7]. However, cancer and its treatments (surgery, chemotherapy, and radiation therapy [RT]), can contribute to a decrease in sexual activity. Particular cancer diagnoses and demographic factors (i.e., age, relationship status) can present unique challenges. Body image concerns, cultural factors, medical comorbidities, and the natural aging process can all impact intimacy and sexual health. For women, dyspareunia and loss of desire are the most common sexual problems after cancer treatment [8–14], and persistent menopausal symptoms have been associated with greater distress [15]. For men, pelvic floor weakness (incontinence and prolapse) and erectile dysfunction (ED) can influence sexual health and functioning by reducing desire and arousal [11]. In the effort to focus on "fighting the disease", these sexual health issues are often overlooked.

Distinctions by Disease Site

Breast Cancer

Breast cancer is the most common cancer in women in the US, with approximately 252,700 cases annually, accounting for 30% of all cancers diagnosed among females. There are approximately 3,561,000 female breast cancer survivors (44% of female cancer survivors) [1, 2]. Endocrine therapies such as tamoxifen and aromatase inhibitors (AIs) are used in the treatment of early-stage and metastatic hormone receptor-positive breast cancer (approximately 80% of breast cancers are hormone receptor-positive) and for chemoprevention for high-risk unaffected women. Endocrine therapies antagonize the action of estrogen in breast tissue (tamoxifen) or inhibit estrogen synthesis (AIs), improving disease-free and overall survival, but can also negatively impact sexual function [16–19].

Tamoxifen users have reported increased hot flashes, which can lead to poorer sleep and subsequent loss of energy and libido. They may also experience vaginal discharge, which can make a woman believe she does not need vaginal moisturizers, leading to pain if vaginal atrophy is present [16]. Breast cancer patients treated with AIs have been shown to experience significantly lower desire than tamoxifen-treated patients and controls ($P = 0.05$) [17], but their distress about decreased desire has been reported to be dramatically less (tamoxifen, 10.3% vs AIs, 21.2%) than their loss of libido (28.6% and 50%, respectively) [20]. Recent research suggests that libido levels may never return to pretreatment levels even after treatment cessation [13]. Some women treated with endocrine therapy, especially AIs, for an extended period develop vaginal dryness, gross architectural changes to the vulva, vaginal and clitoral atrophy, adhesions and/or phimosis, and severe narrowing or stenosis of the vaginal introitus [20–24].

Gynecologic Cancers

Gynecologic cancers account for approximately 13% of newly diagnosed cancers in women in the US and more than 16% worldwide [1, 25]. *Ovarian cancer* treatment generally involves bilateral oophorectomy, resulting in hormonal deprivation and adverse sexual and vaginal health (i.e., vaginal atrophy) [12], even for postmenopausal women, in whom the ovaries produce androgens that aromatize to estrogens [26, 27]. Ovarian cancer is at times a chronic condition requiring long-term chemotherapy, which is associated with toxicities (such as fatigue and neuropathy) that can negatively impact intimacy [28–30].

Endometrial cancer treatment generally includes surgical staging with the removal of the uterus, fallopian tubes, ovaries, and lymph node sampling [31, 32]. Recently, minimally invasive and nerve-sparing surgical techniques have been applied during hysterectomy procedures to decrease rates of sexual dysfunction and bladder and bowel difficulties that may arise from damage to the autonomic nerves in the pelvis [33, 34]. RT is recommended for patients with high-risk features or advanced disease [35], but can adversely impact a woman's sexual and vaginal health. Irradiation of the vagina can create agglutination, ulceration, stenosis, and/or scar tissue [36, 37], reduce vaginal depth and elasticity [38, 39], and diminish sexual function [36, 40–42].

Vaginal and vulvar cancers are less common and occur mostly in older women. Treatment of invasive vulvar cancer or vulvar intraepithelial neoplasia (VIN) may require local vulvar excision or radical vulvectomy. In some cases, resection of the clitoral area, which could inhibit a woman from experiencing pleasurable sensation and clitoral orgasm, is warranted [43, 44]. Radical vulvar excisions are significantly associated with lower sexual function and QOL, particularly in older women [43].

Conservative surgical approaches for *cervical cancer* have been established to allow for the preservation of the uterus for those desiring future fertility [45–47]. The median age at which women are diagnosed with cervical cancer is 49 years; 13.8% are between ages 20 and 34 years, and another 24.9% are between ages 35 and 44 years [48]; however, approximately 20% of new cervical cancer cases and greater than 36% of all cervical cancer deaths involve women over the age of 65 [49–51]. Regardless of age, nerve-sparing techniques may produce better QOL while minimizing bladder, intestinal, and sexual abnormalities [52]. For more advanced cervical cancer, chemoradiotherapy can result in significant vaginal toxicity and sexual dysfunction (i.e., vaginal stenosis, dryness, atrophy, and dyspareunia) [44, 53, 54].

Prostate Cancer

Prostate cancer is the most common malignancy in US men, with approximately 160,000 new cases per year, and it is the second leading cause of cancer death among US men [1]. There are more than 3.3 million prostate cancer survivors in the US [2]. Treatment options for localized prostate cancer include radical prostatectomy (RP), a variety of pelvic RT delivery modalities, and androgen deprivation therapy (ADT) [55, 56]. RP, through cavernous nerve trauma, arterial injury (accessory pudendal arteries), and cavernosal smooth muscle structural changes, leads to transient ED in many patients and permanent ED in some. A recent meta-analysis demonstrated that approximately 50% of men are left with permanent ED 2 years postsurgery. Although reported rates of erectile function preservation vary widely (14–97%) [57], predictors of ED after RP include patient age, baseline erectile function, nerve-sparing status, comorbidity profile, and surgeon experience [58]. RT, in all of its modalities, is associated with ED risk.

The rates of ED development are quite disparate, ranging from 30 to 50% 12–24 months after RT [59]. The poorest erectile function occurs sometime between 3 and 5 years after treatment. Predictors of ED after RT include patient age, baseline erectile function, comorbidities, RT dose, and use of neoadjuvant ADT [60]. Testosterone is a crucial hormone needed for libido, orgasmic function, and erectile function in men. Many patients with prostate cancer will be required to undergo ADT if high-risk features or metastatic disease is present. ADT induces the complete absence of testosterone, resulting in the loss of libido in up to 90% of men. Unfortunately, treatment longer than 6 months in duration can lead to permanent structural changes in the erectile tissue, resulting in ED in nearly all men [61].

Lung Cancer

Lung cancer is a leading cause of cancer death in men and women in the US [1]. Treatment for lung cancer may include surgical resection [62], chemotherapy [63], and RT, which have consequences on health-related QOL (HRQOL) and function [64]. There are limited data examining the sexual concerns of lung cancer patients, although they appear common [65, 66] and associated with physical and emotional factors. In particular, shortness of breath and emotional distress impact sexual enjoyment, interest, and performance [65]. A prospective study showed that patients experienced poor HRQOL and decreased breathing, sleeping, activities, and sexual function after lobectomy or bilobectomy for lung cancer [62]. In-depth interviews with couples impacted by lung cancer revealed that although there were negative effects of cancer and its treatment, there were also positive effects on intimacy, with increased noncoital physical closeness and partner appreciation [67].

Colorectal and Anal Cancers

Although colorectal cancer is the fourth most common cancer in the US [1], anal cancer is a rare malignancy. Regardless, effective treatments tend to be multimodal therapy (chemotherapy, RT) and can include surgery, which places individuals at risk of sexual problems [68–70]. Older women and those with poor global QOL have been shown to be at greater risk for sexual difficulties [69]. The presence of a stoma also potentially has a negative physical and psychological impact on QOL [71]. Long-term bowel issues [71] and fear of urinary and fecal incontinence post-treatment are significant concerns [70, 72] that can interfere with sexual activity. Pelvic floor exercises can help reduce incontinence by strengthening the pelvic floor muscles while simultaneously improving circulation for arousal [73, 74]. Erection (cavernous) nerve injury can occur with low radical rectal surgery, although it is more likely with RP. Total mesorectal excision of rectal cancer has been associated with permanent ED in 11–25% of patients and permanent ejaculatory dysfunction (failure to ejaculate) in 19–54% [75]. Depending on the chemotherapy regimen (agents, dose, duration), patients may experience hypogonadism or ovarian failure and associated sequelae, and as mentioned previously, RT to the pelvis is associated with vascular damage, potentially impairing erections and engorgement [39, 76] as well as dyspareunia [77].

Bladder Cancer

Bladder cancer is newly diagnosed in approximately 60,000 men and 19,000 women in the US annually, with estimates of 766,000 survivors [1]. Muscle invasive bladder cancer is treated by radical cystectomy and urinary diversion with or without neo-adjuvant chemotherapy (typically, gemcitabine, cisplatin) [78]. In men, the surgical treatment is radical cystoprostatectomy, which is associated with cavernous nerve injury, leading to similar sexual problems as those experienced by RP patients [79]. While there are no data on bladder cancer chemotherapy-associated hypogonadism, clinical experience suggests there may be a link between the two.

Postradical cystoprostatectomy ED appears to be associated with factors such as age, baseline function, nerve-sparing status, and type of urinary diversion [79]. Although postoperative sexual function data are sparse, it is reasonable to expect that the erectile function recovery rates will be lower, as these patients tend to be older in comparison to prostate cancer patients.

In women, treatment for bladder cancer involves radical cystectomy and the removal of the urethra, anterior vaginal wall, uterus, and ovaries. Parasympathetic and sympathetic nerves essential to the sexual response may also be removed [80] or damaged [81]. Fortunately, with the advances in minimally invasive surgery, robotic approaches can minimize sexual sequelae [82]. For patients who are eligible, sexuality-preserving cystectomy with construction of a neobladder results in tissue preservation and normal sexual function and reasonable urinary tract reconstruction [80]. When the bladder is removed, continent diversions can be associated with a higher likelihood of sexual recovery following cystectomy, although there may be confounding factors related to the management of diversions and age factors [80].

Hematologic Cancer

Treatment for hematologic cancers may encompass multiagent chemotherapy, RT, and possible hematopoietic stem cell transplantation (HCT) [81–86]. Alkylating chemotherapy agents, used particularly with HCT, are widely associated with sexual difficulties [85,[86]. Surveys with leukemia/lymphoma survivors have identified sexual issues as an unmet need [87]. Long-term survivors of Hodgkin lymphoma commonly report decreased sexual activity (54%) and decreased interest (41.4%) [84]. More than half of non-Hodgkin lymphoma survivors report dissatisfaction with their sex life, despite being sexually active [83]. Predictors of decreased sexual activity include older age, lack of a partner, and below-average physical function [83].

HCT patients/survivors may develop graft versus host disease (GVHD). Vaginal scarring and stenosis have been reported in nearly half of women with GVHD [85]. Severe vaginal pain [12] caused by GVHD can be treated with topical estrogen plus systemic and topical immunosuppressant drugs. Early identification is ideal for effective treatment [86,[88].

Sexual Rehabilitation and Solutions

The current treatments for sexual dysfunction are most effective when medical treatment is paired with psychoeducation and counseling for both men (e.g., PDE5 inhibitor [PDE5i] targeting ED) and women (vaginal moisturizers targeting dryness and pain).

Specific Issues for Women

Estrogen Deprivation Symptoms

Chemotherapy, a moderate dose of radiation to the ovaries, or bilateral oophorectomy can trigger premature ovarian failure with more abrupt, intense, and/or prolonged estrogen deprivation symptoms than natural menopause [12, 89–91]. Estrogen deprivation effects include vulvovaginal atrophy (VVA), with the loss of genital tissue elasticity, lubrication and symptoms of dryness, irritation, itching, discharge, and dyspareunia [92–95]. VVA symptoms can be more challenging for the female cancer patient/survivor due to an abrupt onset of estrogen deprivation resulting from treatment. Estrogen-deprivation-associated VVA can lead to loss of sexual desire and arousal, as well as orgasm difficulties stemming from vaginal dryness, pain, and stenosis [92, 93, 96, 97]. For female cancer patients treated with pelvic radiation, AIs, or allogeneic HCT with graft versus host disease, vaginal pain can be even more severe with these treatments [12]. Vaginal health is not only important to sexual function but comfort with gynecologic examinations – a crucial component of cancer surveillance. Indirectly, hormonal deprivation can impair sleep, causing fatigue and overall poor QOL, which in turn can negatively influence sexual function and interest [98, 99].

Nonhormonal Strategies

Vaginal lubricants and moisturizers are simple solutions, but many patients and healthcare providers are unclear about their potential benefits, respective uses, and/or ideal administration in this population [73]. Vaginal lubricants are used to supplement women's lubrication response, aiding in vaginal insertion and/or manual stimulation by decreasing dryness and friction, thereby reducing irritation and discomfort [73]. Water-based lubricants break down easily after washing with warm water and soap and are therefore recommended. Silicone-based lubricants are another option, but are not as easily washed off. Petroleum-based lubricants (i.e., Vaseline) are not usually recommended, as they may increase the risk of vaginal infections and render latex condoms ineffective [73]. Vaginal moisturizers (creams, gels, suppositories, or ovules) differ from lubricants; these products are meant to hydrate the vaginal tissues and improve vaginal pH [73, 100] and are not generally used for direct sexual activity. Natural products containing vitamin E and/or hyaluronic acid may be beneficial in the treatment of vaginal atrophy [101, 102]. Moisturizers should be applied before bedtime for optimal absorption and should be used on a regular basis, at least three to five times per week to address acute symptoms experienced in the cancer setting [73] and externally to treat vulvar discomfort/atrophy.

Hormonal Strategies

Topical or systemic estrogen therapy is effective in treating vaginal atrophy in the general menopausal population [103]; however, postmenopausal hormone therapy can be a complex issue in the cancer setting [104]. The Women's Health Initiative (WHI) Estrogen plus Progestin study presented concerns about risks of systemic hormone replacement, which appeared to outweigh the benefits [105]. This study highlighted the potential increased risk of breast cancer, but other studies have suggested that unopposed estrogen may not increase breast cancer risk [106, 107]. A meta-analysis found a significant association of increased risk of breast cancer with the use of estrogen plus progestin versus estrogen therapy, and risk increased with more than 5 years of use [108]. However, very low doses of vaginal estrogen can alleviate vaginal atrophy, with little elevation of systemic serum estrogen levels; yet in some women, even these products may generate an elevation in serum estradiol levels [109]. Currently, we do not know if a transient elevation impacts treatment with AIs. A small study (*n* = 6) raised concern about the safety of low-dose estrogen (Vagifem®, 25 µg) in breast cancer survivors taking AIs [110] followed by a second study noting postinsertion estradiol levels were significantly higher in women on AIs than controls [111]. Vagifem is now available at a lower dose (10 µg), which has been shown to be effective in the treatment of vaginal atrophy in women without a breast cancer history. Recently, no statistically significant change in estradiol was found in postmenopausal breast cancer patients on AIs who were given Vagifem® 10 µg for 12 weeks [112].

Cancer survivors, particularly breast cancer survivors, often refuse hormones because of fear of cancer recurrence risk [113, 114]. Hormone therapy should be accompanied with a discussion of treatment risks, benefits, and alternatives. A conservative approach would be to start with non-hormonal strategies, re-evaluating often, and advance to vaginal estrogens if symptoms persist [73, 115]. Cancer survivors, particularly those with nonhormone-dependent cancer, are ideal candidates for vaginal estrogens in combination with nonhormonal strategies. In regard to systemic estrogen treatment, it is not recommended for women with a history of endometrial cancer and has not been proven safe in breast cancer survivors [116].

Dehydroepiandrosterone (DHEA), a precursor to estrogens and androgen, has been investigated for the treatment of menopausal sexual dysfunction. A recent review questioned the value of oral DHEA therapy [117], but a small randomized trial of intravaginal DHEA was found to lessen vaginal atrophy and increase sexual functioning [104, 118–120], with serum steroid levels remaining in the postmenopausal range [104]. The FDA also recently approved Ospemifene, an oral selective estrogen receptor modulator, for the treatment of VVA in postmenopausal women [108]. This product was shown to improve vaginal health without any negative effects on the endometrium. Physiologic changes of improvement in vaginal pH scores and percentages of superficial and parabasal cells, in addition to relief of VVA symptoms, were noted [121]. However, these products need to be studied in cancer populations.

Vaginal laser therapy for treatment of VVA: this novel and experimental treatment (not covered by insurance) is performed in the outpatient setting. The aim of the procedure is to promote collagen production and restoration of vaginal epithelium. A recent 12-week evaluation in postmenopausal women showed improvement in VVA symptoms [122]. In a small study (*n* = 50) with breast cancer patients at 11 months posttreatment, 52% reported satisfaction [123]. These results are promising, but further research is needed to examine duration of efficacy and placebo effect with randomized controlled trials comparing treatment versus a

Strategies to Address Vaginal Pain/Dyspareunia

Dilators are an important tool for addressing vaginal pain, stenosis, and agglutination, while also allowing women the opportunity to gain confidence and a greater understanding of their own anatomy. Although dilators are most commonly used after RT to treat and/or prevent stenosis, they can be extremely useful for any woman experiencing vaginal pain or having difficulty tolerating pelvic examinations [73]. Dilators are available in sets of increasing size for a gradual stretching process, while reducing a woman's anxiety and enhancing confidence about vaginal comfort [73]. If one lacks a partner or chooses not to be sexually active, dilators can be a rehabilitative resource. Adherence with the use of dilators can be a challenge for some, but women will be more motivated if they are provided with information and believe that pelvic examinations can be more comfortable [124]. Dilator therapy may be most helpful when including pelvic floor exercises. By practicing contraction and relaxation of pelvic and vaginal muscles, women gain awareness and control over their muscles, thereby decreasing pain associated with reflexively tightening [125, 126]. A recent study investigated the use of liquid topical lidocaine applied to the vulvar vestibular tissues before vaginal penetration in breast cancer survivors. Reduced distress and improved comfort were noted [127]. However, only 28% had ever tried a moisturizer, which may also have been helpful.

Specific Issues for Male Cancer Patients/Survivors

Erectile Difficulties

Erectile difficulty is the most common male sexual dysfunction, affecting 50% of all men older than 40 years of age [128]. Causes of ED in cancer patients, besides the diagnosis itself, include radical pelvic surgery, pelvic RT, and testosterone deficiency (secondary to treatment). After RP, nearly all men have at least temporary ED, with optimal recovery 18–24 months after surgery. Younger patient age, better baseline function, and greater degree of nerve sparing during RP are the major predictors of erectile function recovery after RP [129]. RT causes erectile problems due to a direct injurious effect to smooth muscle (the crus of the penis lies 1–2 cm below the prostate) and endarteritis obliterans [59], a progressive structural change in endothelium associated with diminished endothelial function. After RT, most men experience a minimal negative effect on erectile function for the first 12 months, but nearly all men will experience some decrement in erectile function over the ensuing 2–3 years. While there are no data demonstrating that any specific means of RT delivery is better at erectile function preservation, it is well accepted that the dose of radiation delivered is a critical predictor of erectile function preservation [59].

The management of ED includes modifiable risk factors (diabetes, hypertension, dyslipidemia), lifestyle alterations (alcohol, cigarette consumption), addressing psychosocial issues, and from a drug therapy standpoint, PDE5is, such as sildenafil, vardenafil, and tadalafil. PDE5is have been available for 15 years and are safe and effective but require a functioning cavernous nerve to donate nitric oxide for them to work. Two populations responding most poorly to these agents are those with diabetes and those with a history of radical pelvic surgery [130]. Recent evidence suggests that these medications work best in a eugonadal environment [131] and when a patient has hypogonadism and therapy with a PDE5i fails, supplementation of testosterone may be indicated, when medically appropriate, to improve PDE5i response. Most common side effects with PDE5i agents include: headache, facial flushing, nasal congestion, heartburn, and visual disturbances (diplopia, blurred vision, temporary loss of color vision), but there is no robust evidence demonstrating a causal link between PDE5i and sudden blindness or hearing loss. Most men fail to respond to PDE5i in the first year after RP due to the neuropraxia that the operation induces. As nerve recovery occurs, PDE5i response rates increase and optimize sometime between 18 and 24 months postoperatively [130]. Sildenafil and vardenafil are short-acting PDE5is with erectogenic windows of opportunity of 8–12 h [132]. Both should be taken on an empty stomach, and all PDE5is require sexual stimulation for maximal effect. Tadalafil is a long-acting PDE5i with an erectogenic window of opportunity of at least 36 h for most men. This agent is not affected by food [132].

Second-line therapy consists of penile injection therapy, intraurethral prostaglandin suppository, and/or vacuum devices. Injection therapy is a safe and effective treatment, although it does involve the use of a diabetic-type syringe and needle for injection of vasoactive medications directly into the corpus cavernosum, 5–10 min prior to anticipated sexual relations [133]. There are numerous vasoactive agents used for this therapy, with success rates of greater than 90% in certain ED populations [133]. Priapism is the most concerning side effect of injection therapy, although rates are less than 1% with proper patient education and monitoring.

Third-line therapy involves penile implant surgery, which is typically reserved for men who have tried and failed to respond to penile injection therapy or find injections unpalatable [134].

Hypogonadism

Testosterone replacement therapy has advanced significantly, providing multiple options, with four transdermal agents, intramuscular agents, and subcutaneous pellets currently available [131]. Transdermal testosterone agents have been approved in the US for almost two decades. There are currently four that are applied to the upper arm/chest area (androgen, Testim), inner thigh (Fortesta), and axilla (Axiron). The gels combine testosterone with a permeating agent to enhance absorption across the skin. More than 80% of men will achieve eugonadal serum testosterone levels with such agents. The concerns with such agents include cost and the fear of transference to women and children. Digital rectal examination to assess prostate size and consistency as well as serum hematocrit levels (below 50%) are important for baseline assessment [135, 136]. Hematocrit levels can be elevated to the point of polycythemia with testosterone supplementation; however, this is less than 2%, but may be as high as 20% with intramuscular therapy. Direct testosterone supplementation suppresses pituitary gonadotropin production, which is an important consideration for men concerned about fertility. In such cases, clomiphene citrate or intramuscular/subcutaneous human chorionic gonadotropin injection are excellent choices [137]. The latter therapies work best in men with reasonable testis function (low to normal luteinizing hormone levels).

Sexual Response

Sexual Desire Disorder

Sexual desire disorder, defined as the persistent or recurrent deficiency (or absence) of sexual fantasies and interest in sexual activity, has been associated with hormonal deprivation in women due to surgical menopause or ovarian failure post-treatment [138, 139] and endocrine therapies both in women [16, 20, 138–140] and men [61].

Testosterone is required for sexual function in men, including erectile function, orgasm, and libido [141]. Testosterone therapy may be helpful in addressing decreased libido, although decreased libido is a nonspecific sign with many causes, including medications (psychotropics, antiandrogens, estrogenic agents, 5-alpha reductase inhibitors), endocrinopathies (hypogonadism, hyperprolactinemia, thyroid dysfunction), and psychological causes (relationship conflict, orientation conflict, the presence of a sexual dysfunction in a patient or partner). Improvement in libido, felt to be the result of hypogonadism, should resolve within a few weeks of normalization of eugonadal testosterone levels. However, for men that require ADT as part of their prostate cancer treatment, complete absence of testosterone will result in loss of libido in up to 90% of men [61]. Such patients also experience significant ED and routine failure to achieve orgasm [61].

Loss of desire can also result from pain due to atrophic vaginitis, which occurs from estrogen deprivation [142]. For the female cancer patient/survivor, this issue can be more prominent due to the nature of many cancer therapies (i.e., RT, oophorectomy), and in many cases, the abrupt onset of symptoms. Improvement of vaginal dryness and comfort often leads to more interest in sexual activity, subjective arousal, and capacity to reach orgasm. Randomized controlled trials targeting menopausal symptoms have shown improvement in sexual function of cancer survivors [143, 144].

In August 2015, the FDA approved Flibanserin for the treatment of decreased libido in premenopausal women. Flibanserin is a 5-hydroxytryptamine (5-HT1A) agonist and 5-HT2A antagonist. A recent report of four randomized, placebo-controlled trials of 3414 premenopausal women found improvement in satisfying sexual events ($P < 0.000001$) and scores on the Female Sexual Function Index (FSFI) desire domain ($P < 0.00001$) in the Flibanserin group compared to the placebo group ($P < 0.000001$) [145]. A novel agent (non-FDA approved) being studied is Bremelanotide, an agonist to the melanocortin-receptor-4 agonist to modulate sexual response pathways [146]. A recent randomized, placebo-controlled, dose-ranging study in premenopausal women found that Bremelanotide effectively increased satisfying sexual events and scores on the FSFI [146]. These promising results offer hope for treating desire disorders, but it is unclear how they will perform in postmenopausal women and cancer survivors.

Sexual Arousal Disorders

Arousal disorders can occur when circulation and blood flow to the genitals is diminished, preventing adequate engorgement (vasocongestion). A sexual arousal disorder is defined as persistent or recurrent inability to attain sexual arousal until completion [147, 148]. Pelvic floor exercises, self-stimulation, vibrators, and vacuum devices can be helpful for facilitating arousal response by drawing blood flow and promoting circulation in the pelvic area [73, 74].

A clitoral vacuum device was approved by the FDA for the treatment of female arousal disorders. The vacuum device is applied over the clitoral area to pull blood flow to the pelvis, thereby promoting engorgement [132]. Improvements in arousal were noted in the general population and in a cohort of cancer patients post-RT [149, 150] with possible rehabilitative effects to the tissues [150].

Of note, the definition of arousal disorders is debatable, since the Diagnostic and Statistical Manual of Mental Disorders, fourth edition (DSM-IV) focuses on physical factors and excludes subjective perception of arousal [147]. Arousal is in fact a multifaceted process, and some recent studies demonstrated the disconnect that can exist. Sildenafil citrate was tested in women with female arousal disorder. The goal was to increase blood flow to the clitoris and vagina, a concept hypothesized from research on ED in men. The study findings noted an increase in vasocongestion and vaginal engorgement in the presence of stimuli; however, subjective arousal did not significantly increase [151–154]. In contrast, emotional and cognitive strategies have been found to promote subjective arousal, despite physical limitations. A recent mindfulness intervention demonstrated improved perception of arousal, despite no physical improvements in engorgement, demonstrating the power of the mind–body connection to adapt and overcome in the face of physical impairments [155].

Male sexual arousal has historically been classified as physiological and assessed as a man's ability to have an erection [156]. Emerging evidence suggests the subjective aspect of arousal may play an important role for men [157, 158]. Based on this concept, Althof *et al.* recently developed a scale that measures the multidimensional aspects of subjective sexual arousal in men and provided important validation data on this scale [159]. The Subjective Sexual Arousal Scale for Men (SSASM) highlights five areas important to subjective arousal: sexual performance, mental satisfaction, sexual assertiveness, partner communication, and partner relationship. These researchers hope that by highlighting the subjective component of arousal in men, pharmacological and psychological therapies can be developed.

Psychosocial Implications

Performance anxiety or despondence that the sexual attempt will ultimately end in failure can be experienced by both genders. Men who experience ED tend to avoid sexual contact because of this [160], and it can also be the case for women experiencing pain and vulvovaginal dryness [161, 162]. Avoidance can lead to a reduction in the couple's sense of intimacy, sexual frequency [163, 164], and sexual satisfaction, as shown in men [164] and women with cancers [165, 166]. This avoidance of sexual contact has also been linked to an increase in sexual dysfunction in the other partner [167]. The depression and distress associated with sexual dysfunction can lead to a loss of sexual satisfaction and intimacy in one's relationships, potentially leading to relationship conflict [168, 169]. Greater fear of sex (due to pain) and poorer quality relationships can contribute to sexual dysfunction in female survivors [162], and if bothersome

estrogen deprivation symptoms (i.e., vaginal dryness and pain) persist, distress and depression may increase [170].

The prevalence of depression in men with ED has been reported to be as high as 56%, and the relationship between ED and depression has been demonstrated in three large, well-designed, population-based studies of aging men in the US, Finland, Brazil, Japan, and Malaysia [171–173]. Depressive symptoms and sexual bother are related to poor erectile function following prostate cancer treatments [172]. Longitudinal data following RP indicated that sexual bother significantly increased post-treatment and remained consistently high throughout the follow-up period of 24 months post-treatment [174]. Of note, the sexual bother scale queries "general happiness in life", indicating that ED in men (as seen in prostate cancer) can impact a man's general outlook on life.

In a study examining the characteristics of colorectal and anal cancer survivors seeking sexual intervention, self-reported body image was a significant predictor of sexual function. Sexual and relationship satisfaction was also positively associated with QOL, emotional functioning, and body image [175]. It is important to recognize that sexual QOL is multifaceted and includes not only activity, but satisfaction, and perception. Depression and distress can also influence sexual function and negatively impact one's perception of themselves as a sexual being [176, 177].

Strategies to improve sexual function by reducing anxiety/distress and enhance attention to pleasurable bodily sensations are important for sexual rehabilitation after cancer treatment. Sensate Focus is a classical technique to help couples focus on physical and sexual touch to enhance pleasure without intercourse, thus reducing sexual (performance) anxiety. Initially, touch or massage occurs without including the breast or genital area; the second phase allows for sensual touch but without intercourse; and the third phase continues sensual touch with the option of intercourse. Sensate Focus in combination with PDE5i agents is often successful in treating anxiety-mediated ED. Once confidence has been achieved with combined therapy, transitioning off PDE5is can occur with natural erections. This strategy can also reduce anxiety associated with sexual touch for women experiencing dyspareunia. Recent mindfulness interventions have also demonstrated improvement in sexual response and satisfaction, with decreased sexual distress in female cancer patients [178]. This study also noted an improvement in the perception of arousal, even when no physical improvements in engorgement were noted [155].

The fields of sexual medicine and psycho-oncology provide us with insight into effective modalities. Crisis interventions can accelerate the return to sexual activity [179]. Long-term (12-week) interventions show improved sexual function and mood [180]. Brief consultations with mental health professionals demonstrate a positive effect on coping and QOL of newly diagnosed patients [181]. Psychoeducational interventions can decrease fear about sexual activity, increase knowledge, and promote compliance with dilators post-RT [182]. Mindfulness training can positively affect the sexual response, particularly perception of arousal, and decrease sexual distress, while promoting overall wellbeing [178]. Psychoeducational interventions have been successfully in helping cancer patients struggling with sexual health and QOL issues [143, 144, 182–187]. Online modalities have also been recently tested to reach patients more broadly and conveniently [188, 189]. However, more research is needed, particularly in cancer populations and with control-group designs [190].

Reproductive Issues

In 2004, a report by the President's Cancer Panel recommended informing all patients of reproductive age who are diagnosed with cancer about the possibility of treatment-related infertility and the options for preserving fertility [191]. These sentiments were echoed by the American Society of Clinical Oncology (ASCO), which issued guidelines and recommendations for addressing the fertility risks and preservation options for men and women coping with cancer [192] to encourage oncology providers to discuss and provide this information as early as medically possible and to provide referrals [193]. The lack of infrastructure and resources at many cancer centers has made this challenging [194].

Among individuals diagnosed with cancer in their reproductive years, 40–80% of women and 30–75% of men are at risk of cancer-related infertility [195]. Any surgical cancer treatment that removes all or part of a reproductive organ can impair reproductive function. Chemotherapy can cause: loss or damage of germ cells and developing sperm [196, 197]; Leydig cell dysfunction, causing lower testosterone production in men; and depletion of primordial follicles and oocytes, lowering ovarian reserve and function (premature menopause) [198]. Alkylating agents pose the highest risk of cancer-related infertility [192, 199, 200]. Spermatogonia and stem cells are sensitive to chemotherapy [196]. The extent of damage depends on the type of drug involved and the cumulative dose. Importantly, synergism between individual agents when administered concurrently may lower the threshold doses needed to impact fertility [197, 199–202].

RT causes the same impairments stated above but also reduces vascularity to the uterus and can cause fibrosis interfering with conception and gestation [203]. The testis is one of the most radiosensitive organs in the body [204]. As the dose increases, injury to different types of germ cells results, leading to more profound oligo/azoospermia and more delayed recovery and higher rates of failure to have sperm return to the ejaculate. Fractionated doses of more than 1.2 Gy are associated with permanent sterility [205, 206]. The most common cause of gonadal impairment post-RT is scatter from radiation directed at adjacent tissues. Notably, the testicles may receive up to 1–2% of abdominopelvic-directed RT during treatment for malignancies of the prostate, bladder, and rectum [207].

Briefly summarized below are the available options that can be explored between the patient and provider, ideally prior to initiation of treatment.

Female Fertility Preservation Strategies

Embryo Cryopreservation

Embryo cryopreservation is probably the most reliable method of fertility preservation. The woman's ovaries are stimulated, and then oocyte (egg) retrieval is performed using ultrasound guidance. The oocytes can then be fertilized, and the resulting embryos are frozen for future use. This process typically requires a 2–4 week delay in cancer treatment. If there is concern that ovarian stimulation will cause high serum concentrations of estrogen, alternative protocols to stimulate follicle growth using tamoxifen and letrozole to reduce the potential risk of estrogen exposure can be used [208]. Tamoxifen is a selective estrogen receptor modulator that is often used in breast cancer treatment. It has been used to stimulate follicle growth during IVF treatment, producing more oocytes and embryos [209]. Letrozole is an AI that blocks the conversion of androgenic substances to estrogens. It has been used as an ovulation induction agent and is associated with a lower estradiol level [210]. Fertilized follicles can be cryopreserved. Reported survival rates per thawed embryo range from 35 to 90%, implantation rates range from 8 to 30%, and cumulative pregnancy rates can be greater than 60% [208, 211]. Despite these encouraging numbers, embryo cryopreservation does require a partner's or donor's sperm, which may not be possible or acceptable to some patients.

Oocyte Cryopreservation

Oocyte cryopreservation is an option for women who may not have a partner or desire to maintain future options. The delicate nature of the oocyte makes it sensitive to ice crystals during freezing and thawing. Vitrification is a newer method of cryopreservation that employs a highly concentrated cryoprotectant and ultrarapid freezing process that avoids ice crystal formation. As experience has grown with these methods, rates of fertility have approached those seen with fresh oocytes [212, 213].

Ovarian Tissue Cryopreservation

Ovarian tissue cryopreservation is an experimental technique that does not require a delay for ovarian stimulation or a sperm donor. The ovarian cortex, which contains the primordial follicles, is harvested surgically, followed by subsequent cyropreservation. After cancer treatment, the ovarian tissue is thawed and reimplanted into the ovarian fossa (orthotopic) or into the forearm or abdominal wall (heretotopic). Some issues with this include the ischemic-reperfusion injury that occurs between transplantation and revascularization of the ovarian tissue [214]. Although most primordial follicles can survive the freeze–thaw cycles, two-thirds are lost after transplantation [215]. *In vitro* maturation of these primordial follicles is being investigated as a way of alleviating this problem.

Ovarian Transposition

Ovarian transposition is used in women who need pelvic RT. The ovaries are detached from the uterus and physically moved out of the pelvis while maintaining the integrity of the ovarian vessels. The ovaries are usually transposed to the lateral paracolic gutters, but location may vary depending on the radiation field to be prescribed. The procedure can typically be performed using a minimally invasive approach. Although the chance of success in preserving ovarian function is 63.6–88.6%, there are concerns regarding altered blood flow and scatter of RT [216, 217]. The location of the transposed ovary predicts whether patients retain normal ovarian function, thereby preventing menopause and allowing for reproductive options [218]. Patients should be informed that due to the distorted anatomy, assisted reproductive techniques such as IVF are usually required to achieve pregnancy.

Conservative Surgical Approaches

For patients diagnosed with early-stage *cervical cancer*, radical trachelectomy, which spares the uterus while resecting the cervix, is a safe surgical alternative. Cervical cancer is the most common cancer in women under 40 years of age. Approximately 48% of women diagnosed with early-stage cervical cancer meet criteria for radical trachelectomy [219]. Radical trachelectomy has demonstrated similar recurrence rates to those of radical hysterectomy, with excellent obstetrical outcomes [220–227]. This procedure has been performed predominantly with a vaginal approach, but radical abdominal trachelectomy is showing encouraging results as well [222]. Traditionally, women with lesions larger than 2 cm or with extensive stromal involvement were excluded from trachelectomy [225]; however, the use of abdominal radical trachelectomy and neoadjuvant chemotherapy may allow for the expansion of the eligibility criteria [225, 226]. Two prospective studies of women undergoing radical trachelectomy versus radical hysterectomy found no differences in mood, distress, sexual function, and QOL [227, 228]. The short-term recovery period was identified as another time point of vulnerability, implying that preoperative consults and/or additional support during the immediate postoperative setting could be beneficial. Patients should be informed that radical trachelectomy can lead to dysmenorrhea (24%), neocervical stenosis (10–40%), and dyspareunia (10–30%) [161, 229].

For patients with *endometrial cancer*, hysterectomy, bilateral salpingo-oophorectomy, and lymph node sampling are the standard of care. Twenty-five percent of endometrial cancer patients are premenopausal [230, 231]. In women with a precancerous condition of complex atypical hyperplasia or with low-risk endometrial cancer, hormonal treatment may be considered. Complex atypical hyperplasia of the endometrium is often treated with hysterectomy due to the high risk (29%) of progression to endometrial cancer [232], as well as the 25–42% risk of having unidentified endometrial cancer within the specimen [233, 234]. Prognosis of endometrial cancer is based on several factors, including stage, histologic grade, depth of myometrial invasion, cervical involvement, vascular space involvement, and nodal involvement [235, 236]. Therefore, women should only be considered for conservative management after careful evaluation, including a dilatation and curettage and radiologic imaging [237, 238]. Data on conservative therapy with hormonal treatment are limited, but one study demonstrated a 76% response rate to hormonal treatment, with no evidence of disease in 81 women [239]. Another study reported 56 children born in 101 patients treated with nonsurgical hormonal treatment [240]. Patients should be extensively counseled as to the limited data on conservative therapy, risk of disease progression both during and after progestin therapy, duration of treatment, and follow-up procedures. Discussions should also address the 5% risk of metastases to ovary [235, 241] and the 10–29% risk of

synchronous ovarian malignancy [241, 242]. Patients considered for fertility-preserving management with hormones should have low-grade tumors limited to the endometrium [230, 231, 235] and should be highly motivated and compliant because surveillance is essential, with endometrial sampling recommended every 3–6 months [235]. Some experts advocate definitive surgical treatment upon completion of childbearing or tumor recurrence [241, 243–245]. The increased risk of ovarian cancer has also led to the recommendation of bilateral salpingo-oophorectomy, but others have questioned its necessity [240, 241]. Because of limited data, patients undergoing conservative management should be encouraged to enroll in tumor registries or clinical trials, when possible.

Among women with *ovarian cancer*, fertility-sparing approaches many be considered for those with malignant germ cell tumors, sex cord tumors, tumors of low-malignant potential, or stage IA invasive ovarian cancers [237, 238, 246–249]. Malignant germ cell tumors have an excellent prognosis and tend to be confined to one ovary, with the exception of dysgerminoma, which can be bilateral in 15% [237]. One of the largest series on the experience of treating young women with fertility-sparing surgery for the treatment of malignant germ cell tumors showed 81% of the women undergoing unilateral salpingo-oophorectomy with staging and demonstrated a 90–100% survival rate [247]. Adult granulosa cell tumors have a favorable prognosis, but some variation has been shown based on stage of disease, with higher survival rates with less-advanced disease [250, 251]. A conservative fertility-sparing approach can be considered in young women with stage IA disease, but an endometrial biopsy should be performed to rule out concomitant uterine cancer. Overall, adult granulosa cell tumors of the ovary exhibit disease unilaterally, yet 2–8% present bilaterally [252, 253]. It is reasonable (but controversial) to consider removal of the other ovary and completion hysterectomy in women treated conservatively after childbearing has been completed.

In a series of 339 women diagnosed with borderline (low malignant potential) tumors, there was a 12% recurrence rate in the 164 stage I patients who underwent fertility-sparing surgery. Despite conservative surgery being associated with a higher incidence of recurrence than radical surgery, due to the indolent nature of borderline tumors, most of the recurrences were salvaged by surgery without negatively impacting survival rates [247]. Stage I epithelial ovarian cancer confined to the ovary can be managed conservatively in some cases. However, preservation of the uterus and contralateral ovary needs to be conducted in the setting of a comprehensive surgical staging procedure with extensive discussions about the risk of recurrence and possible adjuvant therapy. Patients treated conservatively for stage I ovarian cancer should also be closely followed with CA-125 monitoring every 3 months and transvaginal ultrasounds for a minimum of 2 years. A large multisite series demonstrated that successful reproduction is possible with fertility-preserving surgery (71%), with 5- and 10-year survival rates of 98% and 93%, respectively [249]. Fertility-sparing surgery should be considered in women with early-stage disease who desire further fertility [248, 254]. However, after completion of family building, definitive surgery may be advised.

Male Fertility Preservation Strategies

Sperm Cryopreservation (Banking)

Sperm cryopreservation (banking) is the most reliable method of preserving male fertility prior to cancer therapy. With advances in IVF, even patients with very few spermatozoa present in the ejaculate are candidates for sperm cryopreservation. Sperm can be stored for several decades. Overall, IVF success rates for cryopreserved sperm in cancer patients are similar to those of patients who have cryopreserved sperm for other male-factor reasons [255]. Sperm banking should be performed prior to the commencement of cancer therapy, as sperm analysis has shown that the integrity of sperm DNA may be affected after even one treatment session [256]. However, if a patient decides to attempt sperm cryopreservation after cancer treatment, experts recommend waiting at least 12 months after the last treatment session (chemotherapy or RT) [257]. The most commonly used method for semen collection for sperm cryopreservation is ejaculation through masturbation. We suggest separating the sample into multiple vials for freezing. More than one third of viable sperm may be lost upon thawing of a cryopreserved specimen [258].

In a survey of 200 young male cancer survivors, most of whom were treated at a dedicated cancer center, only 51% recalled being offered sperm banking prior to their cancer treatment [259]. The optimal time for fertility preservation is before the initiation of oncological therapy, so it is essential that fertility management is discussed before treatment commences. In a study of more than 6,000 men diagnosed with cancer before the age of 21 and who had survived more than 5 years, cancer survivors were 44% less likely to have a family compared with their siblings [260].

Electroejaculation

Electroejaculation is an option for some patients who are unable to ejaculate on demand for a variety of reasons, including sickness, age (being prepubertal), pain, or due to psychological, cultural, or religious barriers [261]. Although a semen specimen can be obtained rapidly via electroejaculation, this method requires general anesthesia. This technique involves the placement of a narrow (1 inch) probe into the rectum. Low-energy electrical current is transmitted through the probe giving patients an erection, and nearly all ejaculate. As patients have urinary catheterization during the procedure, the only adverse effect is the potential for a urinary infection.

Testicular Sperm Extraction

Testicular sperm extraction (TESE) is a method to extract sperm from the testes or occasionally from the epididymis (MESA, microsurgical epididymal sperm aspiration; PESA, percutaneous epididymal sperm aspiration) when electroejaculation is unsuccessful. In the patient who has a high likelihood of good spermatogenesis, this can be achieved by a percutaneous sample or aspiration. For most cancer patients with azoospermia, a surgical incision in the scrotum is required [262]. In the postchemotherapy patient with azoospermia, TESE yields good results [263]. In the prechemotherapy setting, one study found that approximately 45% of adult cancer patients with pretreatment azoospermia had successful sperm retrieval on open biopsy prior to initiation of chemotherapy [264]. In the postchemotherapy patient with azoospermia, TESE yields good results, with sperm retrieval rates of approximately 40% reported from large centers [263].

Gonadal Shielding

Gonadal shielding during abdominopelvic radiation is a well-established method for minimizing scatter radiation to the testicles [265]. In children and adolescents, it has been shown to protect testicular growth and function from inadvertent scatter radiation [266].

Cancer-Related Infertility

Loss of fertility is faced by a significant number of cancer patients/survivors whose reproductive organs have been impacted either directly or indirectly by cancer treatment [192]. Multiple organizations have published position statements and recommendations for fertility preservation in cancer patients to enhance awareness and communication [192, 267]. Nonetheless, time constraints, lack of resources, concerns about treatment delays, and patient distress have impeded this process [268], despite data showing that reproductive concerns are significantly linked to QOL [6]. Infertility has been identified as an emotionally devastating experience, marked by grief and loss [269,270]. For women, this is usually accompanied by premature menopause, with greater acuity and duration of symptoms [89, 90] and a negative impact to sexual function [10, 11,91, 271–274]. Therefore, it is imperative that cancer survivors who are unable to use fertility-sparing approaches or are unsuccessful in achieving fertility preservation receive information about alternative ways to build a family [259, 270].

Alternative Family Building Options

Third-party parenting has been successful and is gaining recognition, although there are a lack of data on the awareness and use of these techniques in cancer survivors [192]. Third-party parenting involves the use of a third person to build a family by the donation of gametes (i.e., oocyte, embryo, or sperm donation) and/or surrogacy [275]. Unfortunately, there is limited research on how survivors are addressing their impaired fertility and the psychosocial impact of utilizing fertility preservation [192, 270, 276].

Adoption is another alternative. The literature shows that among cancer survivors, adoption is viewed as more acceptable than third-party parenting [15, 270, 277, 278], although there are potential concerns about discrimination during the adoption process [275]. Table 28.1 lists patient education resources regarding family building after cancer.

Communication

Patients show interest in communicating about intimacy, sexuality, and fertility after cancer treatment, yet many medical professionals prefer to focus exclusively on "combating the disease" [203, 268, 279]. Doctor–patient communication is imperative, as many patients have misconceptions and unrealistic expectations

Table 28.1 Resources for oncology providers and patients.

Cancer (general)	National Cancer Institute (NCI) Office of Cancer Survivorship	http://dccps.nci.nih.gov
	American Cancer Society (ACS)	http://www.cancer.org
	LIVESTRONG	http://www.livestrong.org
	NCCN	http://nccn.org
Sexuality/ menopause	American Association of Sex Education Counselors and Therapists (AASECT)	http://www.aasect.org
	North American Menopause Society (NAMS)	http://www.menopause.org
	American Cancer Society "Cancer and Sexuality"	https://www.cancer.org/treatment/treatments-and-side-effects/physical-side-effects/fertility-and-sexual-side-effects/sexuality-for-women-with-cancer/problems.html
	National Cancer Institute "Sexuality and Cancer"	https://www.cancer.gov/about-cancer/treatment/side-effects/sexuality-fertility-women
Fertility	The Oncofertility Consortium	www.oncofertility.northwestern.edu
	American Society for Reproductive Medicine	www.ASRM.org
	Fertile Hope	fertilehopes.org
	My OncoFertility	www.myoncofertility.org
	SaveMyFertility	www.savemyfertility.org
	LIVESTRONG's Fertile Hope – Fertility Resource Guide	https://www.livestrong.org/tags/fertile-hope
Family-building options		
Specific for adolescents	NCCN Clinical Practice Guidelines in Oncology for Adolescent and Young Adult Oncology	https://www.nccn.org/patients/guidelines/aya/files/assets/common/.../aya.pdf
	Cancer.Net	www.cancer.net (Search cancer in teens/cancer and your body/fertility and reproductive)
	KidsHealth	www.kidshealth.org (Search under Teens/Disease and Tumors/Can I Have Children After Cancer Treatments?)
	CureSearch	www.curesearch.org (Search male or female reproductive health)

regarding their treatment, recovery, and function in cancer survivorship. Table 28.2 lists and summarizes communication models for addressing sexual health. The PLISSIT model has been widely published to enhance discussions on sexuality in the medical setting [280, 281]. Bober *et al.* adapted a behavioral health counseling model [282] called the '5 As' for sexual health communication targeting the oncology team and a multidisciplinary approach [283, 284]. We propose one model to integrate, explore, and act on the sexual and reproductive concerns of men and women facing cancer – the STAT model for sexual and reproductive health communication: S, screen about knowledge and concern about issues; T, target important issues or symptoms; A, act by providing information re: target area, offer strategies or referrals; and T, teamwork, which needs investment and follow-up by both the medical provider and patient. Our goal is to consolidate both issues into one model to enable all practitioners to routinely query both important issues (sexuality/reproductive concerns) with their patients throughout the continuum of care.

Appropriate support, services, and information are vital throughout the continuum of care [155, 285, 286]. Recent patient interviews highlighted the importance and need for discussions between survivors and their medical team [287]. Surveys have revealed unmet service and informational needs [91, 287, 288]. Most recently, in 476 survivors surveyed, 41%

($n = 297$) reported an unmet need regarding sexual issues, in addition to emotional, financial, and insurance concerns [287]. In fact, a recent survey demonstrated that 40–68% of gynecologic and breast cancer patients felt it would be helpful to speak with a sexual health expert, but only 7–10% had done so [289]. There has been a strong movement to improve fertility preservation survivorship care. Facilities, such as the Survivorship Centers of Excellence throughout the US, have been created to support patients post-treatment [290]. The goal of this movement is to provide access or referral for survivors and includes: treatment summaries and care plans for survivorship, screening guidelines, symptom management, health promotion education, resources (sexual and reproductive health), and strategies for coordination of care between primary care and oncology [290].

Conclusions

Cancer diagnosis and treatment can negatively impact sexual functioning and fertility in a variety of ways. These complex issues encompass both physical and emotional components that can remain long after cancer treatment ends. Regardless of whether one is sexually active, an assessment of potential difficulties should be a standard part of clinical care. Reproductive

Table 28.2 Communication models for addressing sexual health.

Model	Components	Description	Application
PLISSIT	P – Permission	Normalize the topic with patients	"It is common for patients to have sexual/vaginal changes after cancer. Is it ok if we discuss this issue?"
	LI – Limited Information	Offer limited information to identify the effect of cancer/treatment on sexuality	"Treatment side-effects can have a big impact on sexual activity. You mentioned that intercourse has been painful for you. How is this pain affecting your sex life?"
	SS – Specific Suggestions	Provide specific suggestions to manage sexual side effects	"There are many ways couples can adjust to the effect of cancer treatment. Consider which activities you can still enjoy. How would you and your partner feel about focusing on other types of sexual activity?"
	IT – Intensive Treatment	Identify further support for the identified issues and refer when appropriate	"Would you like to see a counselor who's experienced in this area?"
5 A's	A – Ask	Bring up the topic	"How has your treatment affected your sex life?"
	A – Advise	Take time to normalize symptoms for patients	"Many patients struggle with changes in sexual function."
	A – Assess	Take a history of sexual functioning, assess symptoms and develop treatment plan	"Are you experiencing any symptoms from or after cancer treatment that are affecting your sexual functioning?"
	A – Assist	Inform patients about available resources	Provide patient education materials about: Symptoms (i.e., vaginal moisturizers and lubricants) Sexuality (ACS – Sexuality after Cancer Booklet) Referrals (see resource list)
	A – Arrange Follow-Up	Check in with patients regularly	"Did you find the materials helpful" "Are you still having sexual/ vaginal health concerns"
STAT Model for Sexual and Reproductive Health Communication	S – Screen	Screening about knowledge and concern about issues	Screening tools: use formal ACOG, checklists, information from the medical chart Empirical measures: PCI/EPIC, IEEF, FSFI, PROMIS
	T – Target Symptoms	Target important issues/symptoms (VVA, erectile dysfunction, etc.)	See Sexual Rehabilitation and Solutions section
	A – Act	Provide patient info, education, and referrals regarding target area	Suggest developing patient education materials (See Sexual Rehabilitation and Solutions section) Identify experts or practitioners in your local area for a referral list See Table 28.1 (national resource list)
	T – Teamwork	This process needs investment and follow-up by both patient and medical provider	Suggest making a note in the patient chart so topic can be readdressed at follow ups

concerns need to be addressed, ideally prior to cancer treatment but also post-treatment in cancer survivorship. Research indicates patients are not receiving information about how cancer treatment can impact their sexual function and reproductive health despite a desire for information on the topic [291]. It is recommended that members of the oncology team prepare patients pretreatment about potential challenges, as well as screening post-treatment for symptoms or concerns [69, 267]. Furthermore, future prospective clinical trials need to incorporate these issues as study endpoints using validated measures [291–293] in order to advance sexual and reproductive medicine research in the oncology field.

References

1 Siegel RL, Miller KD, Jemal A. Cancer statistics, 2017. *CA Cancer J Clin* 2017;67:7–30.
2 Miller KD, Siegel RL, Lin CC, *et al.* Cancer treatment and survivor statistics. *CA Cancer J Clin* 2016;66:271–89.
3 Kent EE, Arora NK, Rowland JH, *et al.* Health information needs and health-related quality of life in a diverse population of long-term cancer survivors. *Patient Educ Couns* 2012;89:345–52.

4 Beckjord EB, Arora NK, McLaughlin W, *et al.* Health-related informational needs in a large and diverse sample of adult cancer survivors: implications for care. *J Cancer Survivors* 2008;2:179–89.
5 Husson O, Mols F, van de Poll-Franse LV. The relation between informational provision and health-related quality of life, anxiety and depression among cancer survivors: a systematic review. *Ann Oncol* 2010;22:761–72.

6 Wenzel L, Dogan-Ates A, Habbal R, *et al.* Defining and measuring reproductive concerns of female cancer survivors. *J Natl Cancer Inst Monogr* 2005;34:94–8.

7 Palacios SCR, Grazziotin A. Epidemiology of female sexual dysfunction. *Maturitas* 2009;63:119–23.

8 Carter J, Rowland K, Chi D, *et al.* Gynecologic cancer treatment and the impact of cancer-related infertility. *Gynecol Oncol* 2005;97:90–5.

9 Cella D, Fallowfield LJ: Recognition and management of treatment-related side effects for breast cancer patients receiving adjuvant endocrine therapy. *Breast Cancer Res Treat* 2008;107:167–80.

10 Ganz PA, Rowland JH, Desmond K, *et al.* Life after breast cancer: understanding women's health-related quality of life and sexual functioning. *J Clin Oncol* 1998;16:501–14.

11 Rutledge TL, Heckman SR, Qualls C, *et al.* Pelvic floor disorders and sexual function in gynecologic cancer survivors: a cohort study. *Am J Obstet Gynecol* 2010;203:514 e1–7.

12 Schover LR. Premature ovarian failure and its consequences: vasomotor symptoms, sexuality, and fertility. *J Clin Oncol* 2008;26:753–8.

13 Carter J, Stabile C, Seidel B, *et al.* Baseline characteristics and concerns of female cancer patients/survivors seeking treatment at a Female Sexual Medicine and Women's Health Program. Support Care Cancer 2015: Jan 8.

14 Huffman LB, Hartenbach EM, Carter J, Rash JK, Kushner DM. Maintaining sexual health throughout gynecologic cancer survivorship: a comprehensive review and clinical guide. *Gynecologic Oncol* 2016;140:359–68.

15 Carter J, Raviv L, Applegarth L, *et al.* A cross-sectional study of the psychosexual impact of cancer-related infertility in women: third-party reproductive assistance. *J Cancer Surviv* 2010;4:236–46.

16 Fallowfield LJ, Kilburn LS, Langridge C, *et al.* Long-term assessment of quality of life in the Intergroup Exemestane Study: 5 years post-randomisation. *Br J Cancer* 2012;106:1062–7.

17 Early Breast Cancer Trialists' Collaborative Group (EBCTCG). Effects of chemotherapy and hormonal therapy for early breast cancer on recurrence and 15-year survival: an overview of the randomised trials. *Lancet* 2005;365:1687–717.

18 Baum M, Budzar AU, Cuzick J, *et al.* Anastrozole alone or in combination with tamoxifen versus tamoxifen alone for adjuvant treatment of postmenopausal women with early breast cancer: first results of the ATAC randomised trial. *Lancet* 2002;359:2131–9.

19 Howell A, Cuzick J, Baum M, *et al.* Results of the ATAC (Arimidex, Tamoxifen, Alone or in Combination) trial after completion of 5 years' adjuvant treatment for breast cancer. *Lancet* 2005;365:60–2.

20 Baumgart J, Nilsson K, Evers AS, *et al.* Sexual dysfunction in women on adjuvant endocrine therapy after breast cancer. *Menopause* 2013;20:162–8.

21 Mok K, Juraskova I, Friedlander M. The impact of aromatase inhibitors on sexual functioning: current knowledge and future research directions. *Breast* 2008;17:436–40.

22 Lester J, Pahouja G, Anderson B, Lustberg M. Atrophic vaginitis in breast cancer survivors: a difficult survivorship issue. *J Personal Med* 2015;5:50–66.

23 Bernhard J, Luo W, Ribi K Colleoni M, *et al.* Patient-reported outcomes with adjuvant exemestane versus tamoxifen in premenopausal women with early breast cancer undergoing ovarian suppression (TEXT and SOFT): a combined analysis of two phase 3 randomised trials. *Lancet Oncol* 2015;16:848–58.

24 Burstein HJ, Lacchetti C, Anderson H, *et al.* Adjuvant endocrine therapy for women with hormone receptor positive breast cancer: American Society of Clinical Oncology Clinical Practice Guideline Update on ovarian suppression. *J Clin Oncol* 2016;34:1689–701.

25 Torre LA, Bray F, Siegel RL, *et al.* Global cancer statistics, 2012. *CA Cancer J Clin* 2015;65:87–108.

26 Finch A, Narod SA. Quality of life and health status after prophylactic salpingo-oophorectomy in women who carry a BRCA mutation: a review. *Maturitas* 2011;70:261–5.

27 Hughes CL, Jr., Wall LL, Creasman WT. Reproductive hormone levels in gynecologic oncology patients undergoing surgical castration after spontaneous menopause. *Gynecol Oncol* 1991;40:42–5.

28 Krychman ML, Pereira L, Carter J, *et al.* Sexual oncology: sexual health issues in women with cancer. *Oncology* 2006;71:18–25.

29 Domenici L, Innocenza P, Giorgini M, *et al.* Sexual health and quality of life assessment among ovarian cancer patients during chemotherapy. *Oncology* 2016;4:205–10.

30 Westin S, Sun C, Tung C, *et al.* Survivors of gynecologic malignancies: impact of treatment on health and well-being. *J Cancer Surviv* 2016;10:261–70.

31 Benedetti Panici P, Basile S, Maneschi F, *et al.* Systematic pelvic lymphadenectomy vs no lymphadenectomy in early-stage endometrial carcinoma: randomized clinical trial. *J Natl Cancer Inst* 2008;100:1707–16.

32 Kitchener H, Swart AM, Qian Q, *et al.* Efficacy of systematic pelvic lymphadenectomy in endometrial cancer (MRC ASTEC trial): a randomised study. *Lancet* 2009;373:125–36.

33 de Kroon CD, Gaarenstroom KN, van Poelgeest MI, *et al.* Nerve sparing in radical surgery for early-stage cervical cancer: yes we should! *Int J Gynecol Cancer* 2010;20:S39–41.

34 Walker JL, Piedmonte MR, Spirtos NM, *et al.* Laparoscopy compared with laparotomy for comprehensive surgical staging of uterine cancer: Gynecologic Oncology Group Study LAP2. *J Clin Oncol* 2009;27:5331–6.

35 Alektiar KM, Venkatraman E, Chi DS, *et al.* Intravaginal brachytherapy alone for intermediate-risk endometrial cancer. *Int J Radiat Oncol Biol Phys* 2005;62:111–7.

36 Bergmark K, Avall-Lundqvist E, Dickman PW, *et al.* Vaginal changes and sexuality in women with a history of cervical cancer. *N Engl J Med* 1999;340:1383–9.

37 Saibishkumar EP, Patel FD, Sharma SC. Evaluation of late toxicities of patients with carcinoma of the cervix treated with radical radiotherapy: an audit from India. *Clin Oncol (R Coll Radiol)* 2006;18:30–7.

38 Bruner DW, Lanciano R, Keegan M, *et al.* Vaginal stenosis and sexual function following intracavitary radiation for the treatment of cervical and endometrial carcinoma. *Int J Radiat Oncol Biol Phys* 1993;27:825–30.

39 Flay LD, Matthews JH. The effects of radiotherapy and surgery on the sexual function of women treated for cervical cancer. *Int J Radiat Oncol Biol Phys* 1995;31:399–404.

40 Jensen PT, Groenvold M, Klee MC, *et al.* Longitudinal study of sexual function and vaginal changes after radiotherapy for cervical cancer. *Int J Radiat Oncol Biol Phys* 2003;56:937–49.

41 Onujiogu N, Johnson T, Seo S, *et al.* Survivors of endometrial cancer: who is at risk for sexual dysfunction. *Gynecol Oncol* 2011;123:356–9.

42 Damast S, Alektiar K, Eaton A, *et al.* Comparative patient-centered outcomes (health state and adverse sexual symptoms) between adjuvant brachytherapy versus no adjuvant brachytherapy in early stage endometrial cancer. *Ann Surg Oncol* 2014;21:2740–50.

43 Likes WM, Stegbauer C, Tillmanns T, *et al.* Correlates of sexual function following vulvar excision. *Gynecol Oncol* 2007;105:600–3.

44 Katz A. *Breaking the Silence on Cancer and Sexuality.* Pittsburgh, PA: Oncology Nursing Society, 2007.

45 Abu-Rustum NR, Neubauer N, Sonoda Y, *et al.* Surgical and pathologic outcomes of fertility-sparing radical abdominal trachelectomy for FIGO stage IB1 cervical cancer. *Gynecol Oncol* 2008;111:261–4.

46 Lanowska M, Mangler M, Spek A, *et al.* Radical vaginal trachelectomy (RVT) combined with laparoscopic lymphadenectomy: prospective study of 225 patients with early-stage cervical cancer. *Int J Gynecol Cancer* 2011;21:1458–64.

47 Plante M. Vaginal radical trachelectomy: an update. *Gynecol Oncol* 2008;111:S105–10.

48 *SEER Cancer Statistics Factsheets: Cervix Uteri Cancer.* Bethesda: National Cancer Institute. http://seer.cancer.gov/statfacts/html/cervix.html (accessed 28 August 2017).

49 Montgomery K, Bloch JR, Bhattacharya A, *et al.* Human papillomavirus and cervical cancer knowledge, health beliefs, and preventative practices in older women. *J Obstet Gynecol Neonatal Nurs* 2010;39:238–49.

50 Centers for Disease Control and Prevention: Human Papillomavirus. www.cdc.gov/aging (accessed 28 August 2017).

51 Ries LAG, Krapcho M. *SEER Cancer Statistics Review, 1975–2004.* Bethesda: National Cancer Institute, 2007.

52 Ditto A, Martinelli F, Borreani C, *et al.* Quality of life and sexual, bladder, and intestinal dysfunctions after class III nerve-sparing and class II radical hysterectomies: a questionnaire-based study. *Int J Gynecol Cancer* 2009;19:953–7.

53 Roth AJ, Nelson CJ. Sexuality after cancer. In: JC Holland, WS Breitbart, PB Jacobsen, *et al.* (eds) *Psycho-oncology*, 2nd edn. New York: Oxford University Press, 2010:245–50.

54 Schover LR, Fife M, Gershenson DM. Sexual dysfunction and treatment for early stage cervical cancer. *Cancer* 1989;63:204–12.

55 Anastasiadis AG, Salomon L, Katz R, *et al.* Radical retropubic versus laparoscopic prostatectomy: a prospective comparison of functional outcome. *Urology* 2003;62:292–7.

56 Han M, Partin AW, Pound CR, *et al.* Long-term biochemical disease-free and cancer-specific survival following anatomic radical retropubic prostatectomy. The 15-year Johns Hopkins experience. *Urol Clin North Am* 2001;28:555–65.

57 Tal R, Alphs HH, Krebs P, *et al.* Erectile function recovery rate after radical prostatectomy: a meta-analysis. *J Sex Med* 2009;6:2538–46.

58 Mulhall JP. Exploring the potential role of neuromodulatory drugs in radical prostatectomy patients. *J Androl* 2009;30:377–83.

59 van der Wielen GJ, Mulhall JP, Incrocci L. Erectile dysfunction after radiotherapy for prostate cancer and radiation dose to the penile structures: a critical review. *Radiother Oncol* 2007;84:107–13.

60 Incrocci L, Slob AK, Levendag PC. Sexual (dys)function after radiotherapy for prostate cancer: a review. *Int J Radiat Oncol Biol Phys* 2002;52:681–93.

61 Mazzola CR, Deveci S, Heck M, Mulhall JP. Androgen deprivation therapy before radical prostatectomy is associated with poorer postoperative erectile function outcomes. *BJU Int* 2012;110:112–6.

62 Ilonen IK, Rasanen JV, Knuuttila A, *et al.* Quality of life following lobectomy or bilobectomy for non-small cell lung cancer, a two-year prospective follow-up study. *Lung Cancer* 2010;70:347–51.

63 Schwartz S, Plawecki HM. Consequences of chemotherapy on the sexuality of patients with lung cancer. *Clin J Oncol Nurs* 2002;6:212–6.

64 Schag CA, Ganz PA, Wing DS, *et al.* Quality of life in adult survivors of lung, colon and prostate cancer. *Qual Life Res* 1994;3:127–141.

65 Reese JB, Shelby RA, Abernethy AP. Sexual concerns in lung cancer patients: an examination of predictors and moderating effects of age and gender. *Support Care Cancer* 2011;19:161–5.

66 Shell JA, Carolan M, Zhang Y, *et al.* The longitudinal effects of cancer treatment on sexuality in individuals with lung cancer. *Oncol Nurs Forum* 2008;35:73–9.

67 Lindau ST, Surawska H, Paice J, *et al.* Communication about sexuality and intimacy in couples affected by lung cancer and their clinical-care providers. *Psychooncology* 2011;20:179–85.

68 Den Oudsten BL, Traa MJ, Thong MS, *et al.* Higher prevalence of sexual dysfunction in colon and rectal cancer survivors compared with the normative population: a population-based study. *Eur J Cancer* 2012;48:3161–70.

69 Milbury K, Cohen L, Jenkins R, *et al.* The association between psychosocial and medical factors with long-term sexual dysfunction after treatment for colorectal cancer. *Support Care Cancer* 2013;21:793–802.

70 Bentzen AG, Balteskard L, Wanderas EH, *et al.* Impaired health-related quality of life after chemoradiotherapy for anal cancer: late effects in a national cohort of 128 survivors. *Acta Oncol* 2013;52:736–44.

71 Jansen L, Koch L, Brenner H, *et al.* Quality of life among long-term (>/=5 years) colorectal cancer survivors–systematic review. *Eur J Cancer* 2010;46:2879–88.

72 Panjari M, Bell RJ, Burney S, *et al.* Sexual function, incontinence, and wellbeing in women after rectal cancer – a review of the evidence. *J Sex Med* 2012;9:2749–58.

73 Carter J, Goldfrank D, Schover LR. Simple strategies for vaginal health promotion in cancer survivors. *J Sex Med* 2011;8:549–59.

74 Lowenstein L, Gruenwald I, Gartman I, *et al.* Can stronger pelvic muscle floor improve sexual function? *Int Urogynecol J* 2010;21:553–6.

75 Havenga K, Enker WE, McDermott K, *et al.* Male and female sexual and urinary function after total mesorectal excision

with autonomic nerve preservation for carcinoma of the rectum. *J Am Coll Surg* 1996;182:495–502.

76 Mulhall JP, Hall M, Broderick GA, Incrocci L. Radiation therapy in Peyronie's disease. *J Sex Med* 2012;9:1435–41.

77 Traa M, De Vries J, Roukema J, Rutten H, Den Oudsten B. The sexual health care needs after colorectal cancer: the view of patients, partners, and health care professionals. *Support Care Cancer* 2014;22:763–71.

78 Gallagher DJ, Milowsky MI. Bladder cancer. *Curr Treat Options Oncol* 2009;10:205–15.

79 Porter MP, Penson DF. Health related quality of life after radical cystectomy and urinary diversion for bladder cancer: a systematic review and critical analysis of the literature. *J Urol* 2005;173:1318–22.

80 Horenblas S, Meinhardt W, Ijzerman W, *et al.* Sexuality preserving cystectomy and neobladder: initial results. *J Urol* 2001;166:837–40.

81 Zippe CD, Raina R, Shah AD *et al.* Female sexual dysfunction after radical cystectomy: a new outcome measure. *Urology* 2004;63:1153–57.

82 Menon M, Hemal AK, Tewari A, *et al.* Robot-assisted radical cystectomy and urinary diversion in female patients: technique with preservation of the uterus and vagina. *J Am Coll Surg* 2004;198:386–93.

83 Beckjord EB, Arora NK, Bellizzi K, *et al.* Sexual well-being among survivors of non-Hodgkin lymphoma. *Oncol Nurs Forum* 2011;38:E351–9.

84 Recklitis CJ, Sanchez Varela V, Ng A, *et al.* Sexual functioning in long-term survivors of Hodgkin's lymphoma. *Psychooncology* 2010;19:1229–33.

85 Stratton P, Turner ML, Childs R, *et al.* Vulvovaginal chronic graft-versus-host disease with allogeneic hematopoietic stem cell transplantation. *Obstet Gynecol* 2007;110:1041–9.

86 Nakayama K, Liu P, Detry M, *et al.* Receiving information on fertility and menopause related treatment effects among women who undergo hematopoietic stem cell transplantation: changes in perceived importance over time. *Biol Blood Marrow Transplant* 2009;15:1465–74.

87 Parry C, Lomax JB, Morningstar EA, *et al.* Identification and correlates of unmet service needs in adult leukemia and lymphoma survivors after treatment. *J Oncol Pract* 2012;8:e135–41.

88 Olsson C, Sandin-Bojo A, Bjuresater K, Larsson M. *Patients treated for hematologic malignancies: affected sexuality and health-related quality of life: Cancer Nurs* 2015;38:99–110.

89 Crandall C, Petersen L, Ganz PA, *et al.* Association of breast cancer and its therapy with menopause-related symptoms. *Menopause* 2004;11:519–30.

90 Gupta P, Sturdee DW, Palin SL, *et al.* Menopausal symptoms in women treated for breast cancer: the prevalence and severity of symptoms and their perceived effects on quality of life. *Climacteric* 2006;9:49–58.

91 Harris PF, Remington PL, Trentham-Dietz A, *et al.* Prevalence and treatment of menopausal symptoms among breast cancer survivors. *J Pain Symptom Manage* 2002;23:501–9.

92 Schover LR. Sexuality and fertility after cancer. Hematology Am Soc Hematol Educ Program 2005;523–7.

93 Levine KB, Williams RE, Hartmann KE. Vulvovaginal atrophy is strongly associated with female sexual dysfunction among

sexually active postmenopausal women. *Menopause* 2008;15:661–6.

94 Sturdee DW, Panay N. Recommendations for the management of postmenopausal vaginal atrophy. *Climacteric* 2010;13:509–22.

95 Nappi RE, Kokot-Kierepa M. Vaginal Health: Insights, Views & Attitudes (VIVA) – results from an international survey. *Climacteric* 2012;15:36–44.

96 Avis NE, Brockwell S, Randolph JF, Jr., *et al.* Longitudinal changes in sexual functioning as women transition through menopause: results from the Study of Women's Health Across the Nation. *Menopause* 2009;16:442–52.

97 Lindau ST, Schumm LP, Laumann EO, *et al.* A study of sexuality and health among older adults in the United States. *N Engl J Med* 2007;357:762–74.

98 Joffe H, Soares CN, Thurston RC, *et al.* Depression is associated with worse objectively and subjectively measured sleep, but not more frequent awakenings, in women with vasomotor symptoms. *Menopause* 2009;16:671–9.

99 Williams RE, Levine KB, Kalilani L, *et al.* Menopause-specific questionnaire assessment in US population-based study shows negative impact on health-related quality of life. *Maturitas* 2009;62:153–9.

100 van der Laak JA, de Bie LM, de Leeuw H, *et al.* The effect of Replens on vaginal cytology in the treatment of postmenopausal atrophy: cytomorphology versus computerised cytometry. *J Clin Pathol* 2002;55:446–51.

101 Costantino D, Guaraldi C. Effectiveness and safety of vaginal suppositories for the treatment of the vaginal atrophy in postmenopausal women: an open, non-controlled clinical trial. *Eur Rev Med Pharmacol Sci* 2008;12:411–6.

102 Ekin M, Yasar L, Savan K, *et al.* The comparison of hyaluronic acid vaginal tablets with estradiol vaginal tablets in the treatment of atrophic vaginitis: a randomized controlled trial. *Arch Gynecol Obstet* 2011;283:539–43.

103 Suckling J, Lethaby A, Kennedy R. Local oestrogen for vaginal atrophy in postmenopausal women. Cochrane Database Syst Rev: CD001500, 2006.

104 Labrie F, Cusan L, Gomez JL, *et al.* Effect of one-week treatment with vaginal estrogen preparations on serum estrogen levels in postmenopausal women. *Menopause* 2009;16:30–6.

105 Rossouw JE, Anderson GL, Prentice RL, *et al.* Risks and benefits of estrogen plus progestin in healthy postmenopausal women: principal results From the Women's Health Initiative randomized controlled trial. *JAMA* 2002;288:321–33.

106 Anderson GL, Limacher M, Assaf AR, *et al.* Effects of conjugated equine estrogen in postmenopausal women with hysterectomy: the Women's Health Initiative randomized controlled trial. *JAMA* 2004;291:1701–12.

107 Jick SS, Hagberg KW, Kaye JA, *et al.* Postmenopausal estrogen-containing hormone therapy and the risk of breast cancer. *Obstet Gynecol* 2009;113:74–80.

108 Shah NR, Borenstein J, Dubois RW. Postmenopausal hormone therapy and breast cancer: a systematic review and meta-analysis. *Menopause* 2005;12:668–78.

109 Simon J, Nachtigall L, Gut R, *et al.* Effective treatment of vaginal atrophy with an ultra-low-dose estradiol vaginal tablet. *Obstet Gynecol* 2008;112:1053–60.

110 Kendall A, Dowsett M, Folkerd E, Smith I. Caution: vaginal estradiol appears to be contraindicated in postmenopausal women on adjuvant aromatase inhibitors. *Ann Oncol* 2006;17:584–7.

111 Wills S, Ravipati A, Venuturumilli M, *et al.* The efects of vaginal estrogens (VE) on serum estradiol levels in postmenopausal breast cancer survivors receiving an aromatase inhibitor (AI) or a selective estrogen receptor modulator (SERM). *Cancer Research Suppl* 2009;69:24(suppl; abstr 806).

112 Goldfarb S, Dickler M, Dnistrian A, *et al.* Absorption of low dose 10 μg intravaginal 17-β Estradiol (Vagifem®) in postmenopausal women with breast cancer on aromatase inhibitors. Poster presentation at San Antonio Breast Cancer Symposium, San Antonio, Texas, December 2012.

113 Biglia N, Cozzarella M, Cacciari F, *et al.* Menopause after breast cancer: a survey on breast cancer survivors. *Maturitas* 2003;45:29–38.

114 Ganz PA, Greendale GA, Kahn B, *et al.* Are older breast carcinoma survivors willing to take hormone replacement therapy? *Cancer* 1999;86:814–20.

115 The North American Menopause Society. The role of local vaginal estrogen for treatment of vaginal atrophy in postmenopausal women: 2007 position statement of The North American Menopause Society. *Menopause* 2007;14:355–69; quiz 370–1.

116 The North American Menopause Society. Estrogen and progestogen use in postmenopausal women: 2010 position statement of The North American Menopause Society. *Menopause* 2010;17:242–55.

117 Panjari M, Davis SR. DHEA for postmenopausal women: a review of the evidence. *Maturitas* 2010;66:172–9.

118 Labrie F, Archer D, Bouchard C, *et al.* Serum steroid levels during 12-week intravaginal dehydroepiandrosterone administration. *Menopause* 2009;16:897–906.

119 Labrie F, Archer DF, Bouchard C, *et al.* Intravaginal dehydroepiandrosterone (prasterone), a highly efficient treatment of dyspareunia. *Climacteric* 2011;14:282–8.

120 Labrie F, Martel C, Pelletier G. Is vulvovaginal atrophy due to a lack of both estrogens and androgens? Menopause 2016:452–61.

121 Portman D. *Outcome of the visual evaluation of the vagina in phase 3 studies of oral ospemifene for vulvar/vaginal atrophy.* International Society for the Study of Women's Sexual Health. New Orleans, 2013.

122 Salvatore S, Maggiore U, Origoni M, *et al.* Microablative fractional CO_2 laser improves dyspareunia related to vulvovaginal atrophy: a pilot study. *J Endometr Pelvic Pain Dis* 2014;6:150–6.

123 Pieralli A, Fallani MG, Becorpi A, *et al.* Fractional CO_2 laser for vulvovaginal atrophy (VVA) dyspareunia relief in breast cancer survivors. *Arch Gynecol Obstet* 2016;294:841–6.

124 Friedman LC, Abdallah R, Schluchter M, *et al.* Adherence to vaginal dilation following high dose rate brachytherapy for endometrial cancer. *Int J Radiat Oncol Biol Phys* 2011;80:751–7.

125 Goldfinger C, Pukall CF, Gentilcore-Saulnier E, *et al.* A prospective study of pelvic floor physical therapy: pain and psychosexual outcomes in provoked vestibulodynia. *J Sex Med* 2009;6:1955–68.

126 Rosenbaum TY. Pelvic floor involvement in male and female sexual dysfunction and the role of pelvic floor rehabilitation in treatment: a literature review. *J Sex Med* 2007;4:4–13.

127 Goetsch MF, Lim JY, Caughey AB. A practical solution for dyspareunia in breast cancer survivors: a randomized control trial. *J Clin Oncol* 2015;33:3394–400.

128 Feldman HA, Goldstein I, Hatzichristou DG, *et al.* Impotence and its medical and psychological correlates: results of Massachusetts male aging study. *J Urol* 1994;151:54–61.

129 Rabbani F, Stapleton, Kattan MW, *et al.* Factors predicting recovery of erections after radical prostatectomy. *J Urol* 2000;164:1929–34.

130 Montorsi F, McCullough A. Efficacy of sildenafil citrate in men with erectile dysfunction following radical prostatectomy: a systematic review of clinical data. *J Sex Med* 2005;2:658–67.

131 Buvat J, Montorsi F, Maggi M, *et al.* Hypogonadal men nonresponders to the PDE5 inhibitor tadalafil benefit from normalization of testosterone levels with a 1% hydroalcoholic testosterone gel in the treatment of erectile dysfunction (TADTEST study). *J Sex Med* 2011;8:284–93.

132 Uckert S, Kuczyk MA, Oelke M. Phosphodiesterase inhibitors in clinical urology. *Exp Rev Clin Pharmacol* 2013;6:323–32.

133 Tal R, Mulhall JP. Intracavernosal injections and fibrosis: myth or reality? *BJU Int* 2008;102:525–6.

134 Tal R, Jacks LM, Elkin E, Mulhall JP. Penile implant utilization following treatment for prostate cancer: analysis of the SEER-Medicare database. *J Sex Med* 2011;8(6):1797–804.

135 Coviello AD, Kaplan B, Lakshman KM, *et al.* Effects of graded doses of testosterone on erythropoiesis in healthy young and older men. *J Clin Endocrinol Metab* 2008;93:914–9.

136 Fernández-Balsells MM, Murad MH, Lane M, *et al.* Clinical review 1: adverse effects of testosterone therapy in adult men: a systematic review and meta-analysis. *J Clin Endocrinol Metab* 2010;95:2560–75.

137 Katz DJ, Nabulsi O, Tal R, Mulhall JP. Outcomes of clomiphene citrate treatment in young hypogonadal men. *BJU Int* 2012;110:573–8.

138 Shifren JL, Schiff I. Role of hormone therapy in the management of menopause. *Obstet Gynecol* 2010;115:839–55.

139 West SL, D'Aloisio AA, Agans RP, *et al.* Prevalence of low sexual desire and hypoactive sexual desire disorder in a nationally representative sample of US women. *Arch Intern Med* 2008;168:1441–9.

140 Segraves R, Woodard T. Female hypoactive sexual desire disorder: history and current status. *J Sex Med* 2006;3:408–18.

141 Morley JE. Testosterone and behavior. *Clin Geriatr Med* 2003;19:605–16.

142 Basson R. Sexuality and sexual disorders. Clin Update Womens Health Care II 2003:1–94.

143 Ganz PA, Greendale GA, Petersen L, *et al.* Managing menopausal symptoms in breast cancer survivors: results of a randomized controlled trial. *J Natl Cancer Inst* 2000;92:1054–64.

144 Schover LR, Jenkins R, Sui D, *et al.* Randomized trial of peer counseling on reproductive health in African American breast cancer survivors. *J Clin Oncol* 2006;24:1620–6.

145 Gao Z, Yang D, Yu L, Cui Y. Efficacy and safety of Flibanserin in women with hypoactive sexual desire disorder: a systematic review and meta-analysis. *J Sex Med* 2015;12(11):2095–104.

146 *Jordan R, Edelson J, Greenberg S, et al. Efficacy of subcutaneous bremelanotide self-administered at home by premenopausal women with female sexual dysfunction: a placebo-controlled dose-ranging study.* International Society for the Study of Women's Sexual Health. New Orleans, 2013.

147 Clayton AH, DeRogatis LR, Rosen RC, Pyke R. Intended or unintended consequences? The likely implications of raisng the bar for sexual dysfunction diagnosis in the proposed DSM-V Revisions: 2. For women with loss of subjective sexual arousal. *J Sex Med* 2012;9:2040–6.

148 *American Psychiatric Association: Diagnostic and Statistical Manual of Mental Disorders*, 4th edn. Washington, DC, 2000.

149 Billups KL, Berman L, Berman J, *et al.* A new non-pharmacological vacuum therapy for female sexual dysfunction. *J Sex Marital Ther* 2001;27:435–41.

150 Schroder M, Mell LK, Hurteau JA, *et al.* Clitoral therapy device for treatment of sexual dysfunction in irradiated cervical cancer patients. *Int J Radiat Oncol Biol Phys* 2005;61:1078–86.

151 Basson R, Brotto LA. Sexual psychophysiology and effects of sildenafil citrate in oestrogenised women with acquired genital arousal disorder and impaired orgasm: a randomised controlled trial. *BJOG* 2003;110:1014–24.

152 Basson R, McInnes R, Smith MD, *et al.* Efficacy and safety of sildenafil citrate in women with sexual dysfunction associated with female sexual arousal disorder. *J Womens Health Gend Based Med* 2002;11:367–77.

153 Berman JR, Berman LA, Toler SM, *et al.* Safety and efficacy of sildenafil citrate for the treatment of female sexual arousal disorder: a double-blind, placebo controlled study. *J Urol* 2003;170:2333–8.

154 Caruso S, Intelisano G, Lupo L, *et al.* Premenopausal women affected by sexual arousal disorder treated with sildenafil: a double-blind, cross-over, placebo-controlled study. *BJOG* 2001;108:623–8.

155 Brotto LA, Erskine Y, Carey M, *et al.* A brief mindfulness-based cognitive behavioral intervention improves sexual functioning versus wait-list control in women treated for gynecologic cancer. *Gynecol Oncol* 2012;125:320–5.

156 Sachs BD. A contextual definition of male sexual arousal. *Horm Behav* 2007;51:569–78.

157 Basson R. Human sex-response cycles. *J Sex Marital Ther* 2001;27:33–43.

158 Ferretti A, Caulo M, Del Gratta C, *et al.* Dynamics of male sexual arousal: distinct components of brain activation revealed by fMRI. *Neuroimage* 2005;26:1086–96.

159 Althof SE, Perelman MA, Rosen RC. The Subjective Sexual Arousal Scale for Men (SSASM): preliminary development and psychometric validation of a multidimensional measure of subjective male sexual arousal. *J Sex Med* 2011;8:2255–68.

160 Hedon F. Anxiety and erectile dysfunction: a global approach to ED enhances results and quality of life. *Int J Impot Res* 2003;15 Suppl 2:S16–9.

161 Carter J, Sonoda Y, Chi DS, *et al.* Radical trachelectomy for cervical cancer: postoperative physical and emotional concerns. *Gynecol Oncol* 2008;111:151–7.

162 Carter J, Huang H, Chase DM, *et al.* Sexual function of endometrial cancer patients enrolled on the Gynecologic Oncology Group LAP2 study. *Int J Gynecol Cancer* 2012;22:1624–33.

163 Carroll JL, Bagley DH. Evaluation of sexual satisfaction in partners of men experiencing erectile failure. *J Sex Marital Ther* 1990;16:70–8.

164 Müller MJ, Ruof J, Graf-Morgenstern M, *et al.* Quality of partnership in patients with erectile dysfunction after sildenafil treatment. *Pharmacopsychiatry* 2001;34:91–5.

165 Stafford L, Judd F. Partners of long-term gynaecologic cancer survivors: psychiatric morbidity, psychosexual outcomes and supportive care needs. *Gynecol Oncol* 2001;118: 268–73.

166 Carmack Taylor CL, Basen-Engquist K, Shinn EH, Bodurka DC. Predictors of sexual functioning in ovarian cancer patients. *J Clin Oncol* 2004;22:881–9.

167 Nelson CJ. The impact of male sexual dysfunction on the female partner. *Curr Sex Health Rep* 2006;3:37–41.

168 Bokhour BG, Clark JA, Inui TS, *et al.* Sexuality after treatment for early prostate cancer: exploring the meanings of "erectile dysfunction". *J Gen Intern Med* 2001;16:649–55.

169 Moore TM, Strauss JL, Herman S, Donatucci CF. Erectile dysfunction in early, middle, and late adulthood: symptom patterns and psychosocial correlates. *J Sex Marital Ther* 2003;29:381–99.

170 Carter J, Chi DS, Brown CL, *et al.* Cancer-related infertility in survivorship. *Int J Gynecol Cancer* 2010;20:2–8.

171 Araujo AB, Durante R, Feldman HA, *et al.* The relationship between depressive symptoms and male erectile dysfunction: cross-sectional results from the Massachusetts Male Aging Study. *Psychosom Med* 1998;60:458–65.

172 Nelson CJ, Mulhall JP, Roth AJ. The association between erectile dysfunction and depressive symptoms in men treated for prostate cancer. *J Sex Med* 2011;8:560–6.

173 Shiri R, Koskimaki J, Tammela TL, *et al.* Bidirectional relationship between depression and erectile dysfunction. *J Urol* 2007;177:669–73.

174 Nelson CJ, Deveci S, Stasi J, *et al.* Sexual bother following radical prostatectomy. *J Sex Med* 2010;7:129–35.

175 Philip EJ, Nelson C, Temple L, *et al.* Psychological correlates of sexual dysfunction in female rectal and anal cancer survivors: analysis of baseline intervention data. *J Sex Med*, 2013;10:2539–48.

176 Andersen BL, Woods XA, Copeland LJ. Sexual self-schema and sexual morbidity among gynecologic cancer survivors. *J Consult Clin Psychol* 1997;65:221–9.

177 Carpenter KM, Andersen BL, Fowler JM, *et al.* Sexual self schema as a moderator of sexual and psychological outcomes for gynecologic cancer survivors. *Arch Sex Behav* 2009;38:828–41.

178 Brotto LA, Heiman JR, Goff B, *et al.* A psychoeducational intervention for sexual dysfunction in women with gynecologic cancer. *Arch Sex Behav* 2008;37:317–29.

179 Capone MA, Westie KS, Chitwood JS, *et al.* Crisis intervention: a functional model for hospitalized cancer patients. *Am J Orthopsychiatry* 1979;49:598–607.

180 Caldwell R, Classen C, Lagana L, *et al.* Changes in sexual functioning and mood among women treated for gynecological cancer who receive group therapy: a pilot study. *J Clin Psychol Med Settings* 2003;10:149–56.

181 Powell CB, Kneier A, Chen LM, *et al.* A randomized study of the effectiveness of a brief psychosocial intervention for women attending a gynecologic cancer clinic. *Gynecol Oncol* 2008;111:137–43.

182 Robinson JW, Faris PD, Scott CB. Psychoeducational group increases vaginal dilation for younger women and reduces sexual fears for women of all ages with gynecological carcinoma treated with radiotherapy. *Int J Radiat Oncol Biol Phys* 1999;44:497–506.

183 Mishel MH, Belvea M, Germino BB, *et al.* Helping patients with localized prostate carcinoma manage uncertainty and treatment side effects. *Nurse-delivered psychoeducational intervention over the telephone Cancer* 2002;94:1854–66.

184 Canada AL, Neese LE, Sui D, Schover LR. Pilot intervention to enhance sexual rehabilitation for couples after treatment for localized prostate carcinoma. *Cancer* 2005;104: 2689–700.

185 Canada AL, Schover LR, Li Y. A pilot intervention to enhance psychosexual development in adolescents and young adults with cancer. *Pediatr Blood Cancer* 2007;49:824–8.

186 Molton IR, Siegel SD, Penedo FJ, *et al.* Promoting recovery of sexual functioning after radical prostatectomy with group-based stress management: the role of interpersonal sensitivity. *J Psychosom Res* 2008;64:527–36.

187 Wiljer D, Urowitz S, Barbaera L, *et al.* A Qualitative study of an internet-based support group for women with sexual distress due to gyecologic cancer. *J Canc Educ* 2011;26: 451–8.

188 Classen C, Chivers M, Urowitz S, *et al.* Psychosexual distress in women with gynecologic cancer: a feasibility study of an online support group. *Psycho-Oncology* 2013;22:930–5.

189 Brotto L, Atallah S, Johnson-Agbakwu C, *et al.* Psychological and interpersonal dimensions of sexual function and dysfunction. *J Sex Med* 2016;13:538–71.

190 Brotto LA, Yule M, Breckon E. Psychological interventions for the sexual sequelae of cancer: a review of the literature. *J Cancer Surviv* 2010;4:346–60.

191 National Cancer Institute: President's Cancer Panel 2003–2004 Annual Report Supplement: Living Beyond Cancer: A European Dialogue, 2004. http://deainfo.nci.nih.gov/advisory/pcp/annualReports/pcp03-04rpt/Supplement.pdf (accessed 28 August 2017).

192 Lee SJ, Schover LR, Partridge AH, *et al.* American Society of Clinical Oncology recommendations on fertility preservation in cancer patients. *J Clin Oncol* 2006;24:2917–31.

193 Reinecke JD, Kelvin JF, Arvey SR, *et al.* Implementing a systematic approach to meeting patients' cancer and fertility needs: a review of the Fertile Hope Centers of Excellence Program. *J Oncol Pract* 2012;8:303–8.

194 Clayman M, Harper M, Quinn GP *et al.* The status of oncofertility resources at NCI designated comprehensive cancer centers. *J Clin Oncol* 2011;29:580s (suppl; abstr 9123).

195 King L, Quinn GP, Vadaparampil ST, *et al.* Oncology nurses' perceptions of barriers to discussion of fertility preservation with patients with cancer. *Clin J Oncol Nurs* 2008;12:467–76.

196 Bucci LR, Meistrich ML. Effects of busulfan on murine spermatogenesis: cytotoxicity, sterility, sperm abnormalities, and dominant lethal mutations. *Mutat Res* 1987;176:259–68.

197 Ginsberg JP. Educational paper: the effect of cancer therapy on fertility, the assessment of fertility and fertility preservation options for pediatric patients. *Eur J Pediatr* 2011;170:703–8.

198 Levine J, Canada A, Stern CJ. Fertility preservation in adolescents and young adults with cancer. *J Clin Oncol* 2010;28:4831–41.

199 van der Kaaij MA, van Echten-Arends J, Simons AH, Kluin-Nelemans HC. Fertility preservation after chemotherapy for Hodgkin lymphoma. *Hematol Oncol* 2010;28:168–79.

200 Colpi GM, Contalbi GF, Nerva F, *et al.* Testicular function following chemo-radiotherapy. *Eur J Obstet Gynecol Reprod Biol* 2004;113 Suppl 1:S2–6.

201 Mackie EJ, Radford M, Shalet SM. Gonadal function following chemotherapy for childhood Hodgkin's disease. *Med Pediatr Oncol* 1996;27:74–8.

202 DeSantis M, Albrecht W, Höltl W, Pont J. Impact of cytotoxic treatment on long-term fertility in patients with germ-cell cancer. *Int J Cancer* 1999;83:864–5.

203 Duffy C, Allen S. Medical and psychosocial aspects of fertility after cancer. *Cancer J* 2009;15:27–33.

204 Rowley MJ, Leach DR, Warner GA, Heller CG. Effect of graded doses of ionizing radiation on the human testis. *Radiat Res* 1974;59:665–78.

205 Speiser B, Rubin P, Casarett G. Aspermia following lower truncal irradiation in Hodgkin's disease. *Cancer* 1973;32:692–8.

206 Centola GM, Keller JW, Henzler M, Rubin P. Effect of low-dose testicular irradiation on sperm count and fertility in patients with testicular seminoma. *J Androl* 1994;15: 608–13.

207 Budgell GJ, Cowan RA, Hounsell AR. Prediction of scattered dose to the testes in abdominopelvic radiotherapy. *Clin Oncol (R Coll Radiol)* 2001;13:120–5.

208 Sonmezer M, Oktay K. Fertility preservation in female patients. *Hum Reprod Update* 2004;10:251–66.

209 Oktay K, Buyuk E, Davis O, *et al.* Fertility preservation in breast cancer patients: IVF and embryo cryopreservation after ovarian stimulation with tamoxifen. *Hum Reprod* 2003;18:90–5.

210 Mitwally MF, Casper RF. Aromatase inhibitors in ovulation induction. *Semin Reprod Med* 2004;22:61–78.

211 Son WY, Yoon SH, Yoon HJ, *et al.* Pregnancy outcome following transfer of human blastocysts vitrified on electron microscopy grids after induced collapse of the blastocoele. *Hum Reprod* 2003;18:137–9.

212 Rienzi L, Cobo A, Paffoni A, *et al.* Consistent and predictable delivery rates after oocyte vitrification: an observational longitudinal cohort multicentric study. *Hum Reprod* 2012;27:1606–12.

213 Grifo JA, Noyes N. Delivery rate using cryopreserved oocytes is comparable to conventional in vitro fertilization using fresh

oocytes: potential fertility preservation for female cancer patients. *Fertil Steril* 2010;93:391–6.

214 Noyes N, Knopman JM, Long K, *et al.* Fertility considerations in the management of gynecologic malignancies. *Gynecol Oncol* 2011;120:326–33.

215 Lobo RA. Potential options for preservation of fertility in women. *N Engl J Med* 2005;353:64–73.

216 Bisharah M, Tulandi T. Laparoscopic preservation of ovarian function: an underused procedure. *Am J Obstet Gynecol* 2003;188:367–70.

217 Pahisa J, Alonso I, Torne A. Vaginal approaches to fertility-sparing surgery in invasive cervical cancer. *Gynecol Oncol* 2008;110:S29–32.

218 Hwang JH, Yoo HJ, Park SH, *et al.* Association between the location of transposed ovary and ovarian function in patients with uterine cervical cancer treated with (postoperative or primary) pelvic radiotherapy. *Fertil Steril* 2012;97:1387–93.

219 Sonoda Y, Abu-Rustum NR, Gemignani ML, *et al.* A fertility-sparing alternative to radical hysterectomy: how many patients may be eligible? *Gynecol Oncol* 2004;95:534–8.

220 Boss EA, van Golde RJ, Beerendonk CC, Massuger LF. Pregnancy after radical trachelectomy: a real option? *Gynecol Oncol* 2005;99:S152–6.

221 Plante M, Renaud MC, Hoskins IA, Roy M. Vaginal radical trachelectomy: a valuable fertility-preserving option in the management of early-stage cervical cancer. A series of 50 pregnancies and review of the literature. *Gynecol Oncol* 2005;98:3–10.

222 Shepherd JH, Mould T, Oram DH. Radical trachelectomy in early stage carcinoma of the cervix: outcome as judged by recurrence and fertility rates. *BJOG* 2001;108:882–5.

223 Wenzel L, Carter J, Chase D, *et al. Quality of Life Issues in Gynecologic Oncology*, 5th edn. Lippincott Williams & Wilkins: Philadelphia, 2009.

224 Rob L, Pluta M, Strnad P, *et al.* A less radical treatment option to the fertility-sparing radical trachelectomy in patients with stage I cervical cancer. *Gynecol Oncol* 2008;111:S116–20.

225 Wethington SL, Sonoda Y, Park KJ, *et al.* Expanding radical trachelectomy for cervical cancer with tumor >2 centimeters: a report of 29 cases. Annual Meeting of the Society of Gynecologic Oncology, 2013.

226 Robova H, Halaska M, Pluta M, *et al.* The role of neoadjuvant chemotherapy and surgery in cervical cancer. *Int J Gynecol Cancer* 2010;20(11 Suppl 2):S42–6.

227 Carter J, Sonoda Y, Baser RE, *et al.* A 2-year prospective study assessing the emotional, sexual, and quality of life concerns of women undergoing radical trachelectomy versus radical hysterectomy for treatment of early-stage cervical cancer. *Gynecol Oncol* 2010;119:358–65.

228 Song T, Choi CH, Lee YY, *et al.* Sexual function after surgery for early-stage cervical cancer: is there a difference in it according to the extent of surgical radicality? *J Sex Med* 2012;9:1697–704.

229 Alexander-Sefre F, Chee N, Spencer C, *et al.* Surgical morbidity associated with radical trachelectomy and radical hysterectomy. *Gynecol Oncol* 2006;101:450–4.

230 Benshushan A. Endometrial adenocarcinoma in young patients: evaluation and fertility-preserving treatment. *Eur J Obstet Gynecol Reprod Biol* 2004;117:132–7.

231 Crissman JD, Azoury RS, Barnes AE, *et al.* Endometrial carcinoma in women 40 years of age or younger. *Obstet Gynecol* 1981;57:699–704.

232 Kurman RJ, Kaminski PF, Norris HJ. The behavior of endometrial hyperplasia. A long-term study of "untreated" hyperplasia in 170 patients. *Cancer* 1985;6:403–12.

233 Trimble CL, Kauderer J, Zaino R, *et al.* Concurrent endometrial carcinoma in women with a biopsy diagnosis of atypical endometrial hyperplasia: a Gynecologic Oncology Group study. *Cancer* 2006;106:812–9.

234 Kurman RJ, Norris HJ. Evaluation of criteria for distinguishing atypical endometrial hyperplasia from well-differentiated carcinoma. *Cancer* 1982;49:2547–59.

235 Creasman WT, Morrow CP, Bundy BN, *et al.* Surgical pathologic spread patterns of endometrial cancer. *A Gynecologic Oncology Group Study. Cancer* 1987;60:2035–41.

236 Barakat RR. Contemporary issues in the management of endometrial cancer. *CA Cancer J Clin* 1998;48:299–314.

237 Gershenson DM. Fertility-sparing surgery for malignancies in women. *J Natl Cancer Inst Monogr* 2005;34:43–7.

238 Leitao MM, Chi DC. Fertility-sparing options for patients with gynecologic malignancies. *Oncologist* 2005;10:613–22.

239 Ramirez PT, Frumovitz M, Bodurka DC, *et al.* Hormonal therapy for the management of grade 1 endometrial adenocarcinoma: a literature review. *Gynecol Oncol* 2004;95:133–8.

240 Gotlieb WH, Beiner ME, Shalmon B, *et al.* Outcome of fertility-sparing treatment with progestins in young patients with endometrial cancer. *Obstet Gynecol* 2003;102:718–25.

241 Duska LR, Garrett A, Rueda BR, *et al.* Endometrial cancer in women 40 years old or younger. *Gynecol Oncol* 2001;83:388–93.

242 Walsh C, Holschneider C, Hoang Y, *et al.* Coexisting ovarian malignancy in young women with endometrial cancer. *Obstet Gynecol* 2005;106:693–9.

243 Jadoul P, Donnez J. Conservative treatment may be beneficial for young women with atypical endometrial hyperplasia or endometrial adenocarcinoma. *Fertil Steril* 2003;80:1315–24.

244 Lowe MP, Cooper BC, Sood AK, *et al.* Implementation of assisted reproductive technology following conservative management of FIGO grade I endometrial adenocarcinoma and/or complex hyperplasia with atypia. *Gynecol Oncol* 2003;91:569–72.

245 Niwa K, Tagami K, Lian Z, *et al.* Outcome of fertility-preserving treatment in young women with endometrial carcinomas. *BJOG* 2005;112:317–20.

246 Low JJ, Perrin LC, Crandon AJ, *et al.* Conservative surgery to preserve ovarian function in patients with malignant ovarian germ cell tumors. A review of 74 cases. *Cancer* 2000;89:391–8.

247 Zanetta G, Rota S, Chiari S, *et al.* Behavior of borderline tumors with particular interest to persistence, recurrence, and progression to invasive carcinoma: a prospective study. *J Clin Oncol* 2001;19:2658–64.

248 Morice P, Camatte S, El Hassan J, *et al.* Clinical outcomes and fertility after conservative treatment of ovarian borderline tumors. *Fertil Steril* 2001;75:92–6.

249 Schilder JM, Thompson AM, DePriest PD, *et al.* Outcome of reproductive age women with stage IA or IC invasive epithelial ovarian cancer treated with fertility-sparing therapy. *Gynecol Oncol* 2002;87:1–7.

250 Sehouli J, Drescher FS, Mustea A, *et al.* Granulosa cell tumor of the ovary: 10 years follow-up data of 65 patients. *Anticancer Res* 2004;24:1223–9.

251 Kim YM, Jung MH, Kim KR, *et al.* Adult granulosa cell tumor of the ovary: 35 cases in a single Korean Institute. *Acta Obstet Gynecol Scand* 2006;85:112–5.

252 Ohel G, Kaneti H, Schenker JG. Granulosa cell tumors in Israel: a study of 172 cases. *Gynecol Oncol* 1983;15:278–86.

253 Savage P, Constenla D, Fisher C, *et al.* Granulosa cell tumours of the ovary: demographics, survival and the management of advanced disease. *Clin Oncol (R Coll Radiol)* 1998;10:242–5.

254 Brown CL, Dharmendra B, Barakat RR. Preserving fertility in patients (Pts) with epithelial ovarian cancer (EOC): the role of conservative surgery in the treatment of early stage disease. 31st Annual Meeting of the Society of Gynecologic Oncologists. Gynecol Oncol 2000;76:240 [Abstract #36].

255 Hourvitz A, Goldschlag DE, Davis OK, *et al.* Intracytoplasmic sperm injection (ICSI) using cryopreserved sperm from men with malignant neoplasm yields high pregnancy rates. *Fertil Steril* 2008;90:557–63.

256 Chung K, Irani J, Knee G, *et al.* Sperm cryopreservation for male patients with cancer: an epidemiological analysis at the University of Pennsylvania. *Eur J Obstet Gynecol Reprod Biol* 2004;113 Suppl 1:S7–11.

257 Fosså SD, Magelssen H. Fertility and reproduction after chemotherapy of adult cancer patients: malignant lymphoma and testicular cancer. *Ann Oncol* 2004;15 Suppl 4:iv259–65.

258 O'Connell M, McClure N, Lewis SE. The effects of cryopreservation on sperm morphology, motility and mitochondrial function. *Hum Reprod* 2002;17:704–9.

259 Schover LR, Brey K, Lichtin A, *et al.* Knowledge and experience regarding cancer, infertility, and sperm banking in younger male survivors. *J Clin Oncol* 2002;20:1880–9.

260 Green DM, Kawashima T, Stovall M, *et al.* Fertility of male survivors of childhood cancer: a report from the Childhood Cancer Survivor Study. *J Clin Oncol* 2010;28:332–9.

261 Pacey AA. Fertility issues in survivors from adolescent cancers. *Cancer Treat Rev* 2007;33:646–55.

262 Schlegel PN. Testicular sperm extraction: microdissection improves sperm yield with minimal tissue excision. *Hum Reprod* 1999;14:131–5.

263 Hsiao W, Stahl PJ, Osterberg EC, *et al.* Successful treatment of postchemotherapy azoospermia with microsurgical testicular sperm extraction: the Weill Cornell experience. *J Clin Oncol* 2011;29:1607–11.

264 Schrader M, Müller M, Sofikitis N, *et al.* "Onco-tese": testicular sperm extraction in azoospermic cancer patients before chemotherapy-new guidelines? *Urology* 2003;61:421–5.

265 Bieri S, Rouzaud M, Miralbell R. Seminoma of the testis: is scrotal shielding necessary when radiotherapy is limited to the para-aortic nodes? *Radiother Oncol* 1999;50:349–53.

266 Ishiguro H, Yasuda Y, Tomita Y, *et al.* Gonadal shielding to irradiation is effective in protecting testicular growth and function in long-term survivors of bone marrow transplantation during childhood or adolescence. *Bone Marrow Transplant* 2007;39:483–90.

267 Johnson RH, Kroon L. Optimizing fertility preservation practices for adolescent and young adult cancer patients. *JNCCN* 2013;11: 71–7.

268 Quinn GP, Vadaparampil ST, Lee JH, *et al.* Physician referral for fertility preservation in oncology patients: a national study of practice behaviors. *J Clin Oncol* 2009;27:5952–7.

269 Domar AD, Zuttermeister PC, Friedman R. The psychological impact of infertility: a comparison with patients with other medical conditions. *J Psychosom Obstet Gynaecol* 1993;14 Suppl:45–52.

270 Schover LR. Psychosocial aspects of infertility and decisions about reproduction in young cancer survivors: a review. *Med Pediatr Oncol* 1999;33:53–9.

271 Partridge AH, Gelber S, Peppercorn J, *et al.* Web-based survey of fertility issues in young women with breast cancer. *J Clin Oncol* 2004;22:4174–83.

272 Carmack Taylor CL, Basen-Engquist K, Shinn EH, *et al.* Predictors of sexual functioning in ovarian cancer patients. *J Clin Oncol* 2004;22:881–9.

273 Frumovitz M, Sun CC, Schover LR, *et al.* Quality of life and sexual functioning in cervical cancer survivors. *J Clin Oncol* 2005;23:7428–36.

274 Matulonis UA, Kornblith A, Lee H, *et al.* Long-term adjustment of early-stage ovarian cancer survivors. *Int J Gynecol Cancer* 2008;18:1183–93.

275 Rosen A. Third party reproduction and adoption in cancer patients. *JNCI* 2005;34:91–3.

276 Nieman CL, Kazer R, Brannigan RE, *et al.* Cancer survivors and infertility: a review of a new problem and novel answers. *J Support Oncol* 2006;4:171–8.

277 Schover LR, Rybicki LA, Martin BA, Bringelsen KA. Having children after cancer: a pilot survey of survivors' attitudes and experiences. *Cancer* 1999;86:697–709.

278 Schover LR. Patient attitudes toward fertility preservation. *Pediatr Blood Cancer* 2009;53:281–4.

279 Hordern AJ, Street AF. Communicating about patient sexuality and intimacy after cancer: mismatched expectations and unmet needs. *Med J Aust* 2007;186:224–7.

280 Penson RT, Gallagher J, Gioiella ME, *et al.* Sexuality and cancer: conversation comfort zone. *Oncologist* 2000;5:336–44.

281 von Eschenbach AC, Schover LR. The role of sexual rehabilitation in the treatment of patients with cancer. *Cancer* 1984;54:2662–7.

282 Fiore MC, Bailey WC, *et al. Treating tobacco use and dependence, Clinical Practice Guideline.* Rockville: US Department of Health and Human Services, 2000.

283 Bober SL, Carter J, Falk S. Addressing female sexuality after cancer by internist and primary care providers. *J Sex Med* 2013;10(suppl. 1):112–19.

284 Park ER, Norris RL, Bober SL. Sexual health communication during cancer care: barriers and recommendations. *Cancer J* 2009;15:74–7.

285 Carter J, Chi DS, Abu-Rustum N, *et al.* Brief report: total pelvic exenteration – a retrospective clinical needs assessment. *Psychooncology* 2004;13:125–31.

286 Corney RH, Crowther ME, Everett H, *et al.* Psychosexual dysfunction in women with gynaecological cancer following radical pelvic surgery. *Br J Obstet Gynaecol* 1993;100:73–8.

287 Parry C, Lomax JB, Morningstar EA, *et al.* Identification and correlates of unmet service needs in adult leukemia and lymphoma survivors after treatment. *J Oncol Pract* 2012;8:e135–41.

288 Kornblith AB, Anderson J, Cella DF, *et al.* Hodgkin disease survivors at increased risk for problems in psychosocial adaptation. The Cancer and Leukemia Group B. *Cancer* 1992;70:2214–24.

289 Hill EK, Sandbo S, Abramsohn E, *et al.* Assessing gynecologic and breast cancer survivors' sexual health care needs. *Cancer* 2011;117:2643–51.

290 Rechis R, Arvey SR, Beckjord EB. Perspectives of a lifelong cancer survivor – improving survivorship care. *Nat Rev Clin Oncol* 2013;10:117–20.

291 Flynn KE, Reese JB, Jeffery DD, *et al.* Patient experiences with communication about sex during and after treatment for cancer. *Psychooncology* 2012;21:594–601.

292 Baser RE, Li Y, Carter J. Psychometric validation of the Female Sexual Function Index (FSFI) in cancer survivors. *Cancer* 2012;118:4606–18.

293 Jeffery DD, Tzeng JP, Keefe FJ, *et al.* Initial report of the cancer Patient-Reported Outcomes Measurement Information System (PROMIS) sexual function committee: review of sexual function measures and domains used in oncology. *Cancer* 2009;115:1142–53.

29

Psychiatric Issues in Cancer Patients

Andrew J. Roth[1] and Adrienne Jaeger[2]

[1] *Memorial Sloan Kettering Cancer Center; Weill Cornell Medical Center, New York, New York, USA*
[2] *Yale School of Nursing, Yale University, New Haven, Connecticut, USA*

Introduction

Psychological Impact of Cancer

People who receive diagnoses of cancer exhibit characteristic normal responses. An initial period of disbelief, denial, or despair is common [1] and can last from days to weeks. Patients often state "This just can't be happening to me", or "Pathology must have mixed up my slides", or "What's the point of taking any treatment, it won't work; cancer kills". A second phase, characterized by dysphoric mood, anxiety, appetite changes, insomnia, or irritability follows, and can last another few weeks or even months. The ability to concentrate and to carry out usual daily activities is impaired, and intrusive thoughts of the illness and uncertainty about the future are present. Often as treatment gets underway or is completed, adaptation begins and continues for months as patients integrate new information, confront reality issues such as actual rather than feared complications of treatment, find reasons for optimism, resume activities and adjust to a 'new normal' or baseline as a cancer survivor [2].

Patients' perceptions of the disease, its manifestations, and the stigma commonly attached to cancer contribute to these responses. Many adults fear a painful death. Most patients fear potential disability, dependency on family and healthcare providers, altered appearance, and changed body function. The new role of 'patient' involves a change in nearly every aspect of adults' or children's lives, if only temporarily. The fear of being separated from or abandoned by family, friends, and colleagues is common. These concerns in older patients are influenced by previous experiences with cancer in friends and family and the death of loved ones.

The initial level of psychological distress is highly variable and often relates to three factors: (i) *medical* (cancer type and site; stage at diagnosis; critical symptoms such as pain, bleeding or shortness of breath; treatments required; rehabilitation available; clinical course of illness; predicted prognosis and medical caregiver attitudes about treatment and prognosis; and associated medical and psychiatric conditions); (ii) *patient-related* (level of cognitive and psychological development; ability to cope with stressful events; emotional maturity; ability to accept altered life goals; prior experiences with cancer; concurrent life losses and stresses; emotional and economic support by family and others); and (iii) *societal and cultural* (attitudes toward cancer and treatment) [3]. Consideration of these factors enables general physicians and oncology treatment teams to evaluate the patient better and propose more individualized recommendations for support.

Cancer treatment can be lengthy and arduous, often necessitating flexibility in patterns of emotional adaptation. Beyond the initial adjustment, the possibility of cure changes the threat of death to a focus on uncertainty and management of treatment side effects. Simultaneously, patients must meet usual school, work, and family obligations, must negotiate flexibility with various degrees of control and at times wavering confidence in the outcome, and they must manage financial burdens.

Pediatric and Family Issues

Discussing a cancer diagnosis with sick children is as routine in pediatric care as in the care of adult patients. The diagnosis and prognosis, including the issue of death, are discussed in a developmentally appropriate manner on several occasions with participation of the family [4]. Efforts to reduce "keeping secrets" will diminish the possibility of problematic communication patterns in affected families. Compliance is enhanced by a child's sense of involvement in the treatment.

Families as well as patients are affected by a cancer diagnosis. Pre-existing family difficulties may be aggravated. In the pediatric patient, additional attention is placed on potential developmental issues while in treatment and follow-up afterwards. Behavioral, school, and cognitive problems due to chemotherapy and radiation therapy have been documented.

Major Psychiatric Disorders in Oncology

Prevalence of Psychiatric Disorders in Cancer Patients

Myths about psychological reactions in cancer patients vary from the expectation for all patients to be overwhelmed and depressed by cancer to the other extreme that awards heroism to those who engage in battle with a nonwavering positive attitude, and either don't succumb or die trying until their last breath. In the most comprehensive study to date, the Psychosocial Collaborative Oncology Group in 1983 used criteria from the Diagnostic and Statistical Manual of Mental Disorders to determine the prevalence of psychiatric disorders in randomly assessed hospitalized and ambulatory adult patients with cancer [5]. Slightly more than half (53%) adjusted normally to the crisis of illness. The remainder met diagnostic criteria for a psychiatric disorder. Adjustment disorder with depressed and/or anxious mood was by far the most common diagnosis (68%). More recent studies have found adjustment disorder, major depression, delirium, and anxiety occur in between 10 and 34% of cancer patients [6–11].

Many individual factors affect overall coping and risk of psychiatric disorders. Older men with prostate cancer reported less distress and anxiety [12], and better emotional quality of life in one study, but were also more likely to have noteworthy depressive symptoms. Weiss *et al.* [13] looked at similar constructs in older male and female cancer patients and also found patients had less anxiety, but depression levels remained stable with increasing with age.

Integrating Mental Health Care into Cancer Care

The Institute of Medicine (IOM) made specific recommendations in 2008 for the psychological care of cancer patients: "Attending to psychosocial needs should be an integral part of quality cancer care. All components of the health care system involved in cancer care should explicitly incorporate attention to psychosocial needs into their policies, practices, and standards addressing clinical care" [14]. The IOM recommended: facilitating effective communication between patients and care providers; identifying each patient's psychosocial health needs; and designing and implementing a plan that links patients with needed psychosocial services and that coordinates and integrates a patient's biomedical and psychosocial care. The American College of Surgeons' Commission on Cancer is phasing in Psychosocial Screening [15]. All approved cancer programs need to demonstrate that they screen patients diagnosed with cancer for distress, and identify the issues that can negatively impact treatment and outcome. It should be emphasized that routine screening for distress does not eliminate the need for individual assessment by a trained clinician prior to instituting any particular psychosocial intervention.

Psychosocial care for patients may depend on the setting and location of treatment. Although attention has increased on integrated mental health care [16] in subspecialty medical clinics, there have been very few studies on the effectiveness of integrated care for patients with cancer. In recent years, the Symptom Management Research Trials (SMaRT) in the United Kingdom have shown positive results. Patients received screening and management of depressive symptoms in subspecialty oncology clinics by trained cancer nurses and psychiatrists.

In the SMaRT Oncology-1 and 2 trials, treatment was found to improve depression scale scores more than usual care [17, 18]. In addition, this method of delivering care was also found to be cost effective [17]. These studies offer promising insights into addressing the psychosocial needs of people with cancer. The IMPACT trial (Improving Mood-Promoting Access to Collaborative Treatment) program, a stepped care collaborative care management program for depression in primary care patients, was shown to be feasible and effective for older cancer patients [19]. In the oncology setting, screening questionnaires can be helpful in identifying patients who may need additional support or mental health referrals. Clinical screening tools that help clinicians identify psychological distress in cancer patients include the Distress Thermometer [20, 21], Patient Health Questionnaire for Depression [22], and the Hospital Anxiety and Depression Scale [23].

Psychotherapeutic Interventions for Cancer Patients

The types of psychotherapeutic interventions used most commonly by mental health professionals working with cancer patients include education, behavioral training, group interventions, and individual psychotherapy [24]. The cornerstone of psychological interventions in cancer is emotional support [25]. Psychosocial interventions significantly improve distress, anxiety, and depression in cancer patients. However, early claims that psychotherapy improves longevity have not been substantiated [26–28]. Psycho-educational counseling that focuses on advice-giving and information about illness can be helpful to both patients and family members, and can be carried out by different members of the treatment team. Behavioral therapies emphasize self-regulatory interventions. Many learn relaxation exercises, visual imagery for distraction, self-hypnotic suggestions and the importance of health status-appropriate physical exercise. These techniques are effective in reducing anticipatory nausea and vomiting in patients receiving chemotherapy, mobilizing patients complaining of fatigue, and in relieving pain. Recent studies have also demonstrated the efficacy of mindfulness-based therapy, a therapy that stems from eastern meditations and yoga traditions [29]. Religious or spiritual counseling is meaningful for many patients during the existential crisis created by cancer. In the last decade new therapies such as Meaning Centered Psychotherapy [30] and Dignity Conserving Therapy [31] have been developed to help patients and families cope with advanced cancer and end-of-life issues.

Psychotherapy in the cancer setting consists of short-term, crisis-oriented supportive therapy to assist patients to strengthen adaptive defenses and to cope better with the problems of illness. Including a spouse, partner, or family member in some sessions may enhance support at home. Supportive psychotherapy, crisis intervention, family therapy, group therapy, cognitive behaviorally oriented therapy, problem solving therapy, and interpersonal psychotherapy all help a patient manage the stressors at hand [9]. Group therapy may have an educational function, orienting and teaching patients as well as relieving anxiety by allowing individuals to share similar problems and solutions, and to reduce isolation. It is important to account for patient energy level, symptoms, and scheduled trips to the cancer center when considering a format for psychotherapy in terms of length and frequency of sessions, as well as type of psychotherapy—one size does not fit all. Advances in tele/video psychiatry may facilitate mental health treatment for patients living far distances from cancer treatment centers.

Specific Disorders

A number of psychiatric disorders occur frequently enough in cancer to warrant a description of their clinical picture. Some are direct responses to illness, while others are pre-existing conditions that may be exacerbated by illness. Sometimes an overlap is not easily distinguishable.

Adjustment Disorders

Adjustment disorder, sometimes referred to as "reactive" or "situational" anxiety and/or depression, is characterized by severe symptoms of distress in response to a life stressor; the key features are the unusual persistence of symptoms and undue interference with occupational, social, or school functioning. It is sometimes difficult to differentiate an adjustment disorder from major depression or generalized anxiety disorder. Since an initial diagnosis of adjustment disorder may be the beginning stages of a more severe mental disorder [9], regular patient follow up is needed to clarify diagnostic uncertainties.

Interventions are directed at helping the patient adapt to, and cope with, the stresses of cancer. Individual psychotherapy helps clarify the medical situation and treatments, as well as the meaning of illness for a particular person and family while introducing or reinforcing successful coping strategies. The decision to prescribe psychotropic medication is based on a consistent high level of distress or an inability to carry out daily activities. A therapeutic trial of a benzodiazepine such as lorazepam, alprazolam or clonazepam, on an as needed basis may control symptoms such as intermittent worry or insomnia.

Depressive Disorders

The overlap of physical illness and symptoms of depression is widely recognized. A major depressive episode in physically healthy adults is based upon the presence of neurovegetative complaints – insomnia, anorexia, fatigue, and weight loss – in addition to depressed mood, hopelessness, guilt or worthlessness, and suicidal ideation. These physical symptoms, however, are common to cancer, cancer treatment, and depression. Thus in cancer patients, diagnosis often depends on identification of: dysphoric mood, apathy, crying, anhedonia, feelings of helplessness, hopelessness decreased self-esteem, guilt, social withdrawal, and thoughts of "wishing for death" or suicide [32].

Depression in both adult and pediatric cancer patients has been studied using a range of assessment methods [33–35]. Several studies using patient self-report and observer ratings found major depression in approximately 25% of hospitalized adult cancer patients [33, 34]. This prevalence is similar to that seen in patients with other serious medical illnesses, suggesting that the level of illness, not the specific diagnosis, is a primary determinant [36, 37]. Factors associated with a higher prevalence of depression in cancer patients usually include: greater level of physical impairment, advanced stages of illness, inade-

quately controlled pain, prior history of depression, and the presence of other significant life stresses or losses [34]. Patients with specific cancers, including pancreatic, oropharyngeal, gastric and lung cancer also have higher rates of depression [9]. Furthermore, the incidence of depression in men and women with cancer appears to be relatively equal [9].

The clinical evaluation of patients includes a careful assessment of previous depressive episodes, family history of depression or suicide, concurrent life stresses, recent losses, and level of social support. The contribution of pain and other quality-of-life parameters such as fatigue, nausea, and substance use to depressive symptoms, must be considered and addressed [38].

Symptoms of depression can be produced by various medications such as barbiturates, calcium channel blockers, benzodiazepines, hormonal agents such as aromatase inhibitors, gonadotropin releasing hormones (GnRH) analogs, and selective estrogen receptive modulators, amphotericin B, opioids, statins, and varenicline for smoking cessation. Relatively few chemotherapeutic agents produce depressive symptoms: prednisone, dexamethasone, vincristine, vinblastine, procarbazine, asparaginase, tamoxifen, interferon, and interleukin-2. Many metabolic, nutritional, and endocrine disorders such as: abnormal levels of potassium, sodium, or calcium; deficiencies of folate or vitamin B12; hypothyroidism, hyperthyroidism or adrenal insufficiency can produce depressive symptoms [39].

Suicidal ideation requires careful and urgent assessment to determine whether those thoughts of wanting to die reflect an emergency that demands providing immediate safety for a patient or a less action-oriented expression of a wish to have ultimate control over potentially intolerable symptoms. There are many suicidal assessment methods including both short and longer measures [40, 41]. Though absolute numbers are not high, one study recently found that cancer patients were more likely to commit suicide than individuals in the general populations [32] and should therefore be asked about suicidal ideation. Adult cancer patients at higher risk are those with poor prognosis, advanced stage of illness, a psychiatric history or history of substance abuse, previous suicide attempts or a family history of suicide [42–45], or those with lung, stomach, pharyngeal, or laryngeal cancers [32]. A recent death of a friend or partner, few social supports, depression with extreme hopelessness [46], poorly controlled pain, delirium with poor impulse control, or helplessness in the context of depression, or recent information of a grave prognosis are also significant risk factors [42].

If a patient is expressing suicidal thoughts, psychiatric consultation and possible inpatient hospitalization must be weighed against end-of-life and palliative care considerations. Care should focus on developing and maintaining a supportive relationship, good communication, and offering the patient a sense of autonomy by helping him/her focus on that which can be controlled. It is important to convey the attitude that improvement in quality, if not quantity, of life is a realistic goal, by addressing symptoms of pain, nausea, insomnia, anxiety or restlessness, depression, confusion and fatigue, possibly with the help of a palliative care team.

Treatment of Depressive Disorders

Usually, prolonged and severe depression requires treatment that combines psychotherapeutic techniques noted earlier with

Table 29.1 Medications frequently used to treat depression in cancer patients.

Medication	Starting daily dose (mg PO)	Comments
Serotonin Reuptake Inhibitors (SSRIs)		
Fluoxetine	10	All SSRIs can cause sexual dysfunction; they may increase energy but overshoot to anxiety and insomnia; they may be calming but overshoot to daytime sleepiness; they may cause gastric upset. Overall – well tolerated.
Sertraline	25	
Paroxetine	10	
Citalopram	10	
Escitalopram	5	
Serotonin-Norepinephrine (SNRIs)		
Venlafaxine	25	SNRIs have similar side effect profiles as SSRIs. Additionally, they are used to treat neuropathic pain syndromes.
Duloxetine	20	
Others		
Mirtazapine	15–30	Mirtazapine has no gastric side effects and may improve appetite. It can be sedating and help sleep. Bupropion is energizing and can help fatigue. It is contraindicated in people with seizure history or bulimia; it does not cause sexual dysfunction; it is also used as a smoking cessation aide.
Bupropion	100 mg slow release	
Psychostimulants		
Dextroamphetamine	2.5 at 8 a.m. and 1 p.m.	Modafinil is a gentler and more easily tolerated stimulant than the others. It is safer in those with history of seizures or cardiac arrhythmias.
Methylphenidate	2.5 at 8 a.m. and 1 p.m.	
Modafinil	50 in the morning	

Source: adapted from Roth AJ, Massie MJ. Psychiatric complications in cancer patients. In: RE Lenhard Jr, RT Osteen, T Gansler (eds) Clinical Oncology. Atlanta: American Cancer Society, 2001: 842 [113].
PO, per os.

psychotropic medication. Table 29.1 lists pharmacologic treatments used frequently to treat depression in adult cancer patients including the selective serotonin reuptake inhibitors (SSRIs), the serotonin-norepinephrine reuptake inhibitors (SNRIs), and the psychostimulants. All antidepressants are started at low doses and require at least 2–5 weeks at any particular dose to show efficacy. Patients who are not told this when beginning treatment may stop the medicine prematurely. The dose may need to be increased after this initial period.

The SSRIs and SNRIs are safer and more easily tolerated than older antidepressants, with fewer sedating, cardiovascular, and autonomic side effects. The most common side effects of SSRIs and SNRIs are mild nausea and gastrointestinal disturbance, headache, a calming feeling that can exceed into daytime somnolence or an energizing effect that can extend to anxiety or insomnia; hyponatremia and bleeding abnormalities are uncommon but problematic adverse effects. These drugs may cause appetite suppression with some cancer patients experiencing transient weight loss; however, weight usually returns to baseline level. There have been recent concerns about higher doses of citalopram and escitalopram prolonging cardiac QTc intervals. EKG recordings should therefore be monitored regularly while on these drugs. Paroxetine, sertraline, citalopram and escitalopram have shorter half-lives than fluoxetine; this helps avoid accumulation of the drug and allows for more precise titration. Abruptly stopping SSRIs and SNRIs can potentially cause a discontinuation syndrome (DS), or withdrawal. Though not life threatening, DS can be extremely uncomfortable, with significant anxiety, agitation and restlessness, difficulty sleeping, irritability, flu-like symptoms, and dizziness; DS may be avoided by slow taper or by the addition of a longer acting SSRI such as fluoxetine. Antidepressants can potentially cause unacceptable sexual dysfunction in both men, such as delayed ejaculation, and women, such as decreased arousal and anorgasmia, that often leads to stopping the medication [47].

Bupropion, an activating antidepressant that works primarily on the dopaminergic neurotransmitter system, is useful in fatigued or lethargic medically ill patients; it should be used cautiously in those with anxiety, and avoided in patients with a history of seizures and in those who are malnourished. Slow-release bupropion may also be helpful to decrease anxiety bursts and for smoking cessation. It is less likely to cause sexual side effects than other antidepressants. Mirtazapine is a sedating antidepressant that primarily works on the serotonergic system. It has been found to be efficacious for people with anxiety, agitated depressions, and insomnia. It has fewer gastrointestinal side effects than other antidepressants and may therefore be useful for patients who have nausea; it may increase appetite as well. Its soluble tablet formulation may be helpful for people who have difficulty swallowing. Mirtazapine is also less likely to cause sexual dysfunction than the SSRIs and SNRIs.

Low doses of a psychostimulant (i.e., dextroamphetamine, methylphenidate, modafinil, or armodafinil) promote a sense of well-being in cancer patients; they may also improve focus and concentration, decrease fatigue, and in low doses stimulate appetite. The often rapid onset of mood elevation compared to traditional antidepressants makes psychostimulants particularly useful for people at the end of life who cannot wait weeks to see improvement. Psychostimulants can potentiate the analgesic effects of opioid analgesics and counteract opioid-induced sedation. Side effects at low doses include anxiety, insomnia, tachycardia, euphoria, and mood lability. High doses and long-term use may produce nightmares, insomnia, tics and paranoia. Patients should be cardiologically and neurologically stable without a history of arrhythmia or seizures before starting a stimulant such as methylphenidate or dextroamphetamine [48, 49].

Modafinil, a gentler wakefulness agent, usually is an excellent drug for frail, debilitated patients who cannot tolerate the potentially stronger side effects of the more traditional psychostimulants [50–53]. It is not unusual for a patient to be started on a stimulant and antidepressant simultaneously, benefiting from the activating effect of the stimulant within days and the longer acting benefits of the antidepressant effects in 2–5 weeks.

Choosing an antidepressant depends on the nature of the depressive symptoms, the medical problems present, and the secondary effects of the specific drug that may benefit a patient or that should be avoided. For instance, depressed patients who are agitated and have insomnia will benefit from the use of an antidepressant that has sedating effects, such as mirtazapine. Patients with psychomotor and cognitive slowing will benefit from medications with the most energy enhancing and least sedating effects, such as bupropion, fluoxetine, or desipramine, or a psychostimulant. Patients who have stomatitis or dry mouth due to chemotherapy or radiotherapy or who have slowed intestinal motility or urinary retention should receive an antidepressant with the least anticholinergic effects, such as most SSRIs or SNRIs, or bupropion. Low doses of an SNRI such as duloxetine or TCAs can be useful in those with neuropathic pain syndromes. People who are unable to swallow pills may be able to take an elixir form of an antidepressant or a soluble tablet formulation (mirtazapine). Patients who are taking tamoxifen should not be concurrently prescribed strong inhibitors of CYP2D6, including antidepressants such as bupropion, paroxetine, sertraline, and fluoxetine. Though still clinically controversial, the concern is that these medications may interfere with the metabolism of tamoxifen to its active metabolite endoxifen, thereby decreasing the anticancer value of the medication. Venlafaxine, mirtazapine and citalopram should be considered first [54].

Anxiety Disorders

Anxiety syndromes encountered in the oncology setting include acute anxiety related to the stress of cancer diagnosis and its treatment, as well as chronic anxiety disorders that antedate the cancer diagnosis and are exacerbated during treatment [55]. Situational anxiety is common. Many patients are nervous: after biopsies while waiting to hear their diagnosis; before stressful or painful procedures such as bone marrow aspiration, chemotherapy administration, radiotherapy, or wound debridement; prior to surgery; during prolonged imaging procedures in close environments like MRI scanners; and while awaiting laboratory or imaging test results that may indicate the presence or progression of cancer. Anxiety is present with varying intensity, yet most patients manage with the reassurance and support from their physicians and families.

Anxiety often worsens and becomes more prevalent as cancer progresses. Anxiety can also paradoxically increase following the conclusion of cancer treatment because patients feel more vulnerable and fearful without active therapy to fight the cancer, and without the ongoing presence of the oncology team [55]. Extreme fearfulness, inability to cooperate or understand procedures, a prior history of panic attacks, needle phobia, or claustrophobia may require reassurance, education, relaxation and other behaviorally oriented interventions, and possibly a low dose of an anxiolytic medication such as lorazepam, alprazolam, or clonazepam to reduce symptoms to a manageable level. Sleep medications like zolpidem at bedtime are also useful.

The differential diagnosis of anxiety in cancer patients can be complex. Patients who have severe pain may appear anxious or agitated and usually respond to adequate pain control with analgesics. The anxiety that accompanies a reversible cause of respiratory distress, such as hypoxia or a pulmonary embolus, or while weaning from a ventilator, often benefits from the anxiolytic effects of an atypical antipsychotic like olanzapine or quetiapine, which will not depress respiratory function as benzodiazepines can. Many patients on steroids experience insomnia and anxiety; this angst and restlessness is treated with benzodiazepines or atypical antipsychotics. Anxiety symptoms are also features of intoxication or withdrawal from alcohol, narcotics, benzodiazepines, and barbiturates. Physicians should consider substance withdrawal in all patients who develop otherwise unexplained anxiety symptoms during the first week or two of hospitalization. Other medical conditions causing anxiety include hyperthyroidism, hypoglycemia, hypocalcemia, and hormone-secreting tumors. Antiemetics such as prochlorperazine and metoclopramide can cause akathisia, a feeling of inner restlessness or severe anxiety that can be relieved by benzodiazepines or beta blockers.

Phobias of blood, needles, doctors, and hospitals and panic disorders can worsen in medical settings [56] and compromise medical treatment. Occasionally, patients have their first episode of panic while being treated for a medical problem. People with advanced stages of cancer who have dependent children are at greater risk for experiencing panic [8]. Those with claustrophobia may have extreme anxiety in the confined spaces of diagnostic scanning devices, radiotherapy treatment rooms, or very small examining rooms.

Careful attention to preparation of children (e.g., role playing) in advance of painful procedures may limit the incidence of anxiety. Specific behavioral interventions, including relaxation training, self-hypnosis and distraction, may be indicated for specific symptoms [57].

Post-traumatic stress disorder (PTSD) is a specific type of anxiety disorder caused by the effects of traumatic experiences, including military combat, natural catastrophes, assault, rape, accidents, and life-threatening illness, such as cancer. The prevalence of PTSD in cancer patients ranges from 5 to 19% [58]. Reminders of prior painful or frightening treatments are common stimuli of post-traumatic stress symptoms in cancer patients, especially children. Illness can also exacerbate feelings about earlier traumas, noted particularly in combat veterans and holocaust survivors. In general, younger age, less education, and lower socioeconomic status are correlated with more symptoms of PTSD [56]. The underdeveloped emotional and language state of children prevents them from using various adaptive strategies; the elderly may have fixed coping mechanisms that minimize their flexibility in dealing with trauma.

In adults, the typical presenting symptoms include periods of intrusive repetition of the stressful event (nightmares, flashbacks, re-experiencing old traumas, avoidance of situations, hyperarousal such as restlessness and pacing, startle responses and intrusive thoughts) along with avoidance, emotional numbness, and depression. A syndrome of recurrent nightmares, separation anxiety, and emotional blunting consistent with the diagnosis of PTSD has been reported in children being treated for cancer [59]. Generally, play therapy is indicated for children with PTSD, while adults benefit from relaxation and distraction techniques, and psychopharmacological treatments to prevent and alleviate symptoms [8]. Relaxation and behavioral interventions described earlier can improve anxiety and panic symptoms significantly. When not successful, pharmacologic interventions are appropriate, often in combination with psychotherapeutic techniques.

Benzodiazepines are the drugs of choice for acute anxiety states. The most common side effects – sedation and confusion – occur more frequently in older people and in those with impaired liver or brain function. Short-acting benzodiazepines, such as alprazolam, lorazepam, and oxazepam often are prescribed. However, their short-acting nature may lead to rebound anxiety. Oxazepam and lorazepam are metabolized by conjugation and are excreted by the kidney and, hence, are better tolerated by patients with impaired hepatic function. Lorazepam helps reduce vomiting in cancer patients receiving emetogenic chemotherapeutic agents. Clonazepam, a longer-acting benzodiazepine, is useful for individuals who have end-of-dose failure or rebound anxiety from short-acting benzodiazepines.

Table 29.2 lists the approximate dose equivalents, the initial doses, the half-lives and some specific comments about benzodiazepines often used in the oncology setting. The dose schedule depends on patients' tolerance and the anxiolytics duration of action. Increasing the dose is preferred to switching to another agent in patients with persistent symptoms. Since many patients are worried about becoming "addicted" to medications, it is important to have a discussion at the beginning of benzodiazepine therapy regarding the distinctions between: (i) physical dependence, which is likely in most, if not all, patients within a month of daily use, and can lead to withdrawal symptoms if the medicine is abruptly stopped; (ii) physical tolerance, which after a few months or longer of daily therapy may lead to some patients requiring a higher dose to obtain the same amount of relief they got with lower doses earlier on; and (iii) addiction, understood as the use of an agent despite harm. Addiction means that the substance is often taken in larger amounts than is indicated, there is a persistent desire or unsuccessful efforts to cut down or control substance use, a great deal of time is spent in activities necessary to obtain or use the substance, such as visiting multiple doctors, or recovering from its effects, and important social, occupational, or recreational activities are given up or impeded because of substance use.

Patients who experience severe anticipatory anxiety before chemotherapy administration or a medical procedure may be given an anxiolytic (e.g., lorazepam) the night before and immediately prior to the treatment. Patients with chronic anxiety states may require anxiolytics daily or intermittently for months or years. People requiring chronic medication may do better with buspirone or an antidepressant for chronic anxiety, which usually do not cause tolerance, addiction, or abuse, although they must be taken daily.

The most common side effects of benzodiazepines are dose dependent and include drowsiness and potential falls, confusion, and motor incoordination. Sedation is most common and most severe in patients with impaired liver or renal function. Medications that have CNS-depressant properties, such as opioids, may have synergistic effects with benzodiazepines. It is important to be cognizant of the potential signs of benzodiazepine withdrawal, which include: anxiety, restlessness and rarely, seizures, regardless of whether the medication was used to treat anxiety or nausea. Vital signs should be monitored regularly;

Table 29.2 Commonly prescribed benzodiazepines in cancer patients.

Drug name (by class)	Approximate dose equivalent (mg PO)	Initial dosage (mg PO)	Elimination half-life drug metabolites (h)/active metabolite	Comments
Shorter acting				
Alprazolam	0.5	0.25–0.5	10–15/Yes	Best for as-needed panic symptoms. Possible rebound anxiety. Difficult to taper. Higher addictive risk. Oxazepam is good for those with liver dysfunction.
Oxazepam	10.0	10–15	5–15/No	
Intermediate acting				
Lorazepam	1.0	0.5–2.0	10–20/Yes	May also help with nausea and appetite problems.
Longer acting				
Diazepam	5.0	5–10	20–100/Yes	Good for preventing panic symptoms and more generalized anxiety. Valium has higher addictive risk.
Clonazepam	0.5	0.25–1	18–50/No	

Source: adapted from Roth AJ, Massie MJ. Psychiatric complications in cancer patients. In: RE Lenhard Jr, RT Osteen, T Gansler (eds) Clinical Oncology. Atlanta: American Cancer Society, 2001:846 [113].
PO, per os.

as with alcohol withdrawal, suspicion must be maintained if the patient is on a beta blocker for cardiovascular illness, as it may mask some of the autonomic dysregulation of withdrawal.

Low-dose sedating antipsychotic medications such as olanzapine and quetiapine are effective in patients with severe anxiety that is not controlled with maximal therapeutic doses of benzodiazepines or for those patients who cannot tolerate side effects of benzodiazepines, such as sedation or respiratory depression. Patients who are not depressed but who have difficulty falling asleep may also benefit from sedating medications in the antidepressant family such as mirtazapine, amitriptyline, trazodone, or doxepin.

Treatment of Acute Agitation, Mania and Bipolar Disorder

In the cancer setting, stabilization of mood lability and acute agitation is attained with atypical antipsychotic medications such as olanzapine or quetiapine, or with a combination of haloperidol and a benzodiazepine. These medications can bring rapid relief to agitation and high-energy states caused by manic exacerbations of bipolar disorder, or by medications such as corticosteroids. Patients who have been receiving lithium carbonate for bipolar affective disorder prior to developing cancer should be maintained as best as possible on the agent throughout cancer treatment. Close monitoring is necessary when the intake of fluids and electrolytes is restricted, such as during preoperative, postoperative, or bone marrow or stem cell transplant settings. The maintenance dose of lithium may have to be reduced in seriously ill patients. Lithium should be prescribed with caution in patients receiving cisplatin or other potentially nephrotoxic drugs. Use of carbamazepine as a mood stabilizer can be problematic in cancer patients because of its bone marrow-suppressing properties. Valproic acid, gabapentin, and lamotrigine use in this population appears to be well tolerated for longer-term use and mood stabilization.

Occasionally, electroconvulsive therapy (ECT) is considered for adult cancer patients whose depression is resistant to less invasive interventions and in whom it represents a life-threatening complication during cancer treatment, such as for catatonia. In addition, ECT should be considered in patients who are unable to tolerate medications due to unacceptable side effects. Referral to an ECT program or psychiatric consultation may be useful in determining whether ECT is appropriate. Apart from various case reports, literature is sparse about the benefits and complications of using ECT in cancer patients.

Delirium

Delirium, the most common neuropsychiatric diagnosis among cancer patients [10], is due either to the direct effects of cancer on the central nervous system (CNS) or the indirect CNS complications of the disease and/or cancer treatment. Delirium is experienced as distressing by patients, family and hospital staff [60]. The prevalence of delirium increases as cancer progresses, with up to 85% of terminally ill patients diagnosed with this syndrome. Early symptoms of delirium are often misinterpreted as anxiety or depression, and hence, are underdiagnosed and undertreated. Any adult who shows acute onset of agitation, behavioral changes, impaired cognitive function, altered attention span, or fluctuating level of consciousness should be evaluated for the presence of delirium. Children may exhibit

symptoms of agitation, confusion, and fear. Delirium is due to one or more physiological causes: medications such as corticosteroids or the cumulative effects of antihistamines, benzodiazepines, and analgesics; electrolyte imbalance; nutritional deficiencies; metabolic abnormalities; infections; hematologic abnormalities; vascular complications [10]; hormone-producing tumors, or paraneoplastic syndromes [61]. Advanced age and pre-existing neurocognitive dysfunction, such as dementia, also increase patients' risk for developing delirium [62].

Delirium has been associated with cancer-treating medications such as methotrexate (by intrathecal or intravenous administration), 5-fluorouracil, vincristine, vinblastine, bleomycin, carmustine (BCNU), cisplatin, asparaginase, procarbazine, cytosine arabinoside, ifosfamide, and corticosteroids. Other medications prescribed for cancer patients such as interleukin-2, amphotericin, voriconazole and acyclovir, and especially benzodiazepines and opioids, can also cause confusional states.

Steroid compounds (i.e., prednisone, dexamethasone) are frequent causes of delirium. Psychiatric disturbances range from minor mood disturbances to psychosis [63], including paranoia, suspiciousness, delusions, irritability, and hallucinations. More severe symptoms also can develop while patients are on a maintenance dose or on intermittently high doses commonly prescribed for antiemetic therapy. No relationship has been shown between the development of steroid-induced mental status changes and premorbid personality or psychiatric history [64].

Management of delirium requires re-evaluation of the necessity of all sedating drugs and other medications that can cause mental status changes mentioned above. Important nonpharmacologic interventions include: providing a safe and supportive environment for patient, staff, and family; reassurance to family of the medical and likely transient nature of delirium, unless the patient is near end of life; a well-lit room; visible clock, calendar and frequent reorientation; familiar people, objects, photos; early mobilization; and communicating with patient and family about the goals of care and desirable outcomes, that is sedation versus awake but agitated, as well as hallucinations and their management or meaning.

Interim symptomatic treatment with antipsychotics to control psychotic symptoms may be needed. Verbal reassurance by a consistent companion can decrease distress; correction of the underlying medical or physiological causes as well as interim symptomatic treatment with antipsychotic medications to control psychotic symptoms, given occasionally with benzodiazepines, will help sedate agitated patients. Benzodiazepines should not be given alone to treat delirious patients as they can worsen confusion and cause paradoxical agitation [65].

Haloperidol is the antipsychotic medication prescribed most commonly because of its excellent safety record, producing little effect on heart rate, blood pressure, respiration, or cardiac output. It can be given orally in tablet or concentrate form or can be administered parenterally, initially started at low dosages. There is a black box warning for all antipsychotic medications for potential prolongation of EKG QTc intervals. EKGs should be monitored at baseline and followed regularly. The effects of prolonged QTc are more prominent with intravenous haloperidol, and lower potency antipsychotics. A QTc of 450 msec or higher is concerning and cardiological consultation should be considered. When QTc exceeds 500 msec or increases by 60 msec compared to baseline, providers may want to stop the offending medication and consider alternative treatments [66]. All other medications that a delirious patient is receiving should be reviewed for potential QTc prolonging tendencies including methadone and ondansetron to see what else can be manipulated should the antipsychotic be vital for control of dangerous agitation. Side effects of the traditional high potency antipsychotics like haloperidol can include parkinsonism, with extrapyramidal symptoms and gait disturbance.

The newer atypical antipsychotic medications may be useful because of improved though different side effect profiles. Olanzapine and quetiapine, which are sedating, can be useful for agitated patients who have difficulty sleeping. However, they cannot be given intravenously. Olanzapine does come in a wafer formulation that dissolves on the tongue and allows for monitored adherence, but the medication must still be swallowed and absorbed in the gut to be effective. With prolonged use and higher doses, these medications can cause metabolic syndromes and increased glucose levels. There is a black box warning for all atypical antipsychotic medications which can cause stroke in elderly patients with histories of dementia. As with their biochemical predecessors, prochlorperazine and metoclopramide, newer antipsychotics may help relieve nausea. Clinicians should be aware that lower potency antipsychotics like chlorpromazine, whose sedating properties can help with agitated confused patients, can also cause orthostatic hypotension and anticholinergic side effects that could increase the risk of falling and further confusion in an already delirious patient.

Symptoms and Situations not Otherwise Classified in Oncology Settings

Though many mild to moderately severe psychiatric disorders are managed successfully by oncologists and a sensitive support staff, some situations and symptoms require accurate assessment and precise and effective intervention by mental health professionals. Severe psychiatric problems, such as schizophrenia, bipolar disorders, and treatment resistant depression require close collaboration between oncologists and psychiatrists. Additional indications for involvement of psychiatrists and other mental health practitioners, and at times hospital administrative staff discussed in the following sections include coping with physical symptoms of pain, fatigue, sexual dysfunction, and cognitive well-being. A multidisciplinary group of mental health, medical, ethics and administrative staff may use the information in the next section to provide needed comprehensive assessment and consultation of the capacity of patients to participate in treatment decisions or to leave a hospital against medical advice. We also discuss the challenges of transitioning into survivorship, or postacute treatment phases of cancer, and helping patients understand the complexity of increasing data about genetic risks and how that data relates to individual treatment decisions. Finally, we discuss the importance of grief education for patients, families and staff and how to promote oncology staff health.

Psychiatric Issues in Cancer Patients with Pain

People with uncontrolled pain have a higher prevalence of psychiatric diagnosis [67] that may be ameliorated with pain management. Requests by patients with cancer pain for hastened death were decreased as depression improved [68]. Unfortunately, underlying depression is often unrecognized in these people. Acute anxiety, depression with despair, agitation, irritability, lack of cooperation, anger, and insomnia may be the emotional or behavioral concomitants of pain. In physically ill children, chronic pain may present with symptoms of apathy, withdrawal, and clinging behaviors.

Undertreatment of pain is a major problem in both adult and pediatric settings [69]. Aggressive pain management strategies, including opioids, are essential to the emotional care of physically ill children and adults (see Chapter 27). Clinicians should continue to reassess patients' mental state as pain is controlled to determine whether a lingering psychiatric disorder persists. Long-term psychiatric sequelae are less likely in children whose pain is well treated. Little evidence substantiates increased risk of subsequent drug abuse in either children or adults receiving opioid analgesia. In fact, patients associate the opioid effects with the unpleasant aspects of the illness and seek to avoid them during the recovery phase. This is probably also true regarding the benefits of addressing and managing all quality-of-life symptoms such as fatigue and nausea [70–73].

Fatigue

Cancer-related fatigue is extremely common. In evaluating fatigue, overlapping problems should be considered including depression, anxiety, sleep disturbances, and pain. The NCCN practice guidelines for fatigue recommend screening for fatigue using a 0–10 rating scale. It is recommended that underlying causes of fatigue should be identified and treated if possible. Nonpharmacological treatments of fatigue include increasing physical activity, increasing psychosocial support, addressing sleep, and addressing any nutritional deficiencies [74]. Exercise and cognitive behavioral therapy have been found to be effective treatment against cancer-related fatigue [75, 76].

Psychopharmacologic interventions have also been used. In clinical practice, although stimulants are often used to address sedation due to opioid therapy, the evidence for effectiveness to treat cancer-related fatigue is mixed. In a small randomized, double-blind, placebo-controlled design, methylphenidate appeared to be effective for fatigue in prostate cancer patients [77]. In addition, several open-label studies have shown positive results [78, 79] although a placebo-controlled trial suggests a large placebo effect [80] which may mask the effectiveness of these medications. Side effects of psychostimulants may include irritability, insomnia, and agitation. There is limited evidence for the use of modafinil or armodafinil for cancer-related fatigue. One study found clinical benefit for modafinil in patients with severe fatigue, but not for mild or moderate fatigue [52]. Another study investigating the use of modafinil versus placebo for fatigue in patients with non-small cell lung cancer found no significant difference between the two groups [81]. A recent study using armodafinil for cancer-related fatigue in multiple myeloma patients found no significant difference over placebo [82]. In summary, although evidence has not consistently supported the use of stimulants for cancer-related fatigue, we believe practitioners should consider their prudent use in patients whose fatigue is significantly interfering with their quality of life, while monitoring vital signs. Evidence regarding antidepressant medications for cancer-related fatigue has been mixed as well, highlighting the need for good scientific research for pharmacologic treatments in this area.

Sexual Dysfunction

Infertility and sexual dysfunction may be unavoidable consequences of irradiation, surgery, chemotherapy [83], and hormonal therapy for cancer. In men, the opportunity for sperm banking before potential fertility-compromising treatment can both arouse and assuage concerns about having children in the future. Information given to men with newly diagnosed prostate cancer about the likelihood of erectile dysfunction with different treatment options can aid treatment decisions, though it can also begin a trail of worry about sexual functioning, intimacy and sexual and self-identity. In women, education and psychological preparation helps decrease worry for various possible outcomes, such as premature menopause and sterility associated with chemotherapy, altered sexual function that results from gynecologic surgery, and body image complications in women with breast cancer. Survivors who are single or divorced may worry about dating and deciding when to tell a potential partner about their cancer history and subsequent sexual difficulties, if any. Oncology teams and psycho-oncologists should initiate discussions about sexual activity early on during their interactions with patients, in an attempt to establish a baseline of sexual interest, performance, relationships and support status, and to alert the patient that their medical team is interested and capable of participating in potentially embarrassing conversations. Most patients are reassured to learn that the sexual consequences of cancer treatment are important to their treating physicians and will be monitored during and after cancer treatment. Despite the importance of informing patients about what they might expect regarding sexual problems like erectile dysfunction, dry orgasms and dyspareunia, sexual issues are not often adequately screened for or treated in the cancer population [84–86]. Therapists can help affected patients maintain physical intimacy during cancer treatment and in restoring a healthy new baseline for sexuality after treatment. Recent studies indicate that behavioral and pharmacological interventions lead to improvements in sexual functions [87], while couples interventions can also be beneficial [88].

Cancer Therapy-Associated Cognitive Change

Cancer therapy-associated cognitive change, or 'chemobrain', is an entity that has been identified in people with a variety of cancers who have had chemotherapy and/or hormonal therapy, and who have experienced difficulty in executive functions, multitasking, short-term memory recall and attention [89, 90]. Impaired processing speed has also been noted [91]. Up to 75% of patients may experience cognitive impairment [92]. This neurotoxicity adversely impacts patients' and survivors' quality of life, including occupational and social functioning, and results in increased healthcare and societal costs. Cognitive changes in patients with cancer were initially thought to be related to treatment only, thus the term "chemobrain". However, research studies have shown evidence of cognitive deficits in patients even before chemotherapy [93, 94], suggesting additional factors that contribute to cognitive changes in people

with cancer. Pertinent factors may include chemotherapy dose, cognitive reserve, and presence of an APOEε4 allele. Additionally, depression, stress, anxiety, other side effects of chemotherapy, effects of menopause and hormonal treatment, as well as local radiation and surgery in the case of brain lesions must be considered. Cognitive changes associated with chemotherapy seem to be dose dependent, and certain chemotherapeutic agents are associated with worse cognitive effects [91]. Stimulants have been used clinically to counter cognitive slowing in this population, although rigorous evidence of efficacy is still lacking. Similarly, the evidence regarding the use of donepezil for cancer-related cognitive dysfunction remains unclear [91]. Positive results have been found with cognitive rehabilitation techniques in breast cancer patients [95], although these techniques are limited by the frequency of needed sessions or lack of available trained therapists. Cognitive training programs, which focus on the practice of specific skills through the use of computers, have shown some benefit in preliminary studies [91]. Some of these training programs can also be used at home, and are less expensive than in-office cognitive rehabilitation programs.

Capacity to Consent To or Refuse Treatment, or Leave Against Medical Advice

A psychiatric consultation is often requested to assess the capacity of a patient to give informed consent or to refuse a procedure critical to survival. Consultations for refusal of treatment recommendations are more frequent than when a patient is agreeing to recommendations, even when their cognition and degree of understanding may be compromised [96]. Occasionally, legal advice or a judge's decision is necessary for emergency treatment. A court direction may also be needed when elective treatment is planned for a mentally or cognitively impaired inpatient with no family available. A common concern is with patients who refuse a clearly life-sustaining treatment, such as dialysis or first-line chemotherapy. Often, oncologists and nurses are not certain whether such patients are truly capable of assessing all their options. The presence of acute depression, delirium, or dementia, which dulls mental or cognitive processes and strongly biases decisions, poses a difficult and sometimes urgent reason for psychiatric consultation [97]. Assessment of capacity takes into account a patient's understanding of pertinent medical issues and recommended treatment, the pros and cons of accepting or refusing the recommendations, and the ability of a patient to state a preference [98]. Capacity to understand and participate in decision-making usually encompasses a particular situation and decision rather than a person's global and general ability to make decisions [99]. Particular challenges arise in consultation with patients who do not speak English or who cannot speak because of their medical condition, but must communicate by other means such as writing or using writing tablets.

Requests to leave the hospital against medical advice are often due to the presence of a confusional state secondary to illness or medication and, as such, may represent an acute danger to self, permitting brief restraint and treatment until psychiatric evaluation is completed. An acute psychotic state may also result in poor judgment. The cause of the behavior must be determined, and a decision must be made as to whether patients can be managed safely at home, alone or with a relative or companion, or whether they must remain in the hospital. Often, the severity of a patient's medical status prevents safe transfer to a psychiatric unit.

Survivorship

The long-term adjustment of survivors of childhood cancer appears largely unimpaired [100], though there may be cancer and cancer treatment-specific quality-of-life concerns, as well as family and individual issues. Cured cancer patients have special medical and psychiatric concerns, including: preoccupation with disease recurrence; a sense of greater vulnerability to illness; pervasive awareness of mortality; difficulty with reentry into normal life; persistent guilt; difficulty adjusting to physical losses and handicaps; diminished self-esteem or confidence; disclosure of diagnosis or long-term treatment complications to friends and potential partners; perceived loss of job mobility; fear of second malignancies; and fear of insurance discrimination. It is only recently that health insurance companies have been directed not to discriminate against people with pre-existing conditions like cancer when they change jobs or careers. "Survivorship clinics" can be found in increasing numbers to address the concerns of cured patients and those living with chronic illness.

Psychological Challenges in Genetically High-Risk Individuals

The current explosion of information about the genetic contribution to the development of cancer has brought into existence a new population of people whose family history puts them at higher risk for certain cancers. It is useful to differentiate between people who are afraid they *might be* at risk and people who are afraid because they *know* they are at risk. Those in the first group benefit from education about what, if any, are their increased risks. Unfortunately, increased data does not mean complete data that comes with assurances about the future. Some will remain excessively anxious even in the absence of objective reason and may be said to suffer from cancer phobia; they may be considered the 'worried well'. These people may benefit from psychological support and regular checkups with a trusted internist to prevent them from squandering time and resources consulting with numerous physicians and getting multiple tests looking for cancer.

Patients who are at known increased genetic risk need detailed genetic and psychological counseling to help them in making difficult decisions regarding genetic testing, marriage, childbearing, prenatal testing, or risk-reducing surgeries (e.g., prophylactic mastectomy or oophorectomy).

Management of Grief

Grief is frequently encountered in the oncology setting, and is often present even before a patient dies; this is called anticipatory grief. People cope with real losses that arise from a cancer diagnosis and treatment such as the inability to do certain activities, as well as intangible losses such as the sense of health they knew before the cancer or the now uncertain hopes and plans that they imagined for their future. Staff acknowledgement of these losses can positively affect the nature of bereavement and influence the family's long-term adjustment. Once death has occurred, grieving has acute and chronic components [101]. Reminders of the deceased often precipitate waves of an overwhelming sense of loss, crying, fatigue, and agitation. Sometimes, the reminders may be subtle, such as a smell, a photo, or even a television commercial about a health product. The intense distress of the first few months is often characterized by social withdrawal, preoccupation with the deceased, diminished concentration, restlessness, depressed mood, anxiety, insomnia, or anorexia. The bereaved spouse or parent often recalls how the final days were handled, how the painful news of dire prognosis and death were conveyed, and how sensitively the final moments were managed. The surviving relatives may search for fault and tend to blame both themselves and staff members, and sometimes blame the patient for giving up too soon. Sometimes caregivers feel guilt for wishing that death would come soon to relieve everyone's suffering, or for feeling relief after the death. A condolence card or a telephone call from staff can be an important expression of human connection and a healing gesture to a bereaved family member. Over months, grief usually diminishes in intensity. The duration of normal grieving is much more variable than originally assumed and often extends well beyond a year. Often, parents and older spouses from a long union report that they are "never the same again"; some truly never recover [102]. Caregivers under the age of 60 caring for terminally ill cancer patients have demonstrated higher levels of "complicated grief" (characterized by intense yearning, difficulty accepting death, bitterness, and emptiness) than older caregivers [103]. These grieving caregivers are at increased risk for a major depression [104], which can be as high as 40% 6 months post-loss [105]. Complicated grief is treated as a major depression with both psychotherapeutic and psychopharmacologic interventions.

Oncology Staff Stress: Compassion Fatigue and Burnout

In reviewing psychiatric considerations for patients, oncology staff should also be aware of the impact on providers caring for patients with cancer, to identify and potentially intervene early to avoid compassion fatigue and burnout.

"Debilitating weariness brought about by repetitive, empathic responses to the pain and suffering of others" describes compassion fatigue [106, 107]. Burnout has been defined as the presence of emotional exhaustion, depersonalization, and a sense of low personal accomplishment [108, 109], or as the chronic psychological syndrome of perceived demands from work outweighing perceived resources in the work environment [110]. Burnout may affect a large percentage of professionals caring for cancer patients [106]. These practitioners may be at increased risk for substance use, sleep problems, changes in appetite and weight, fatigue, somatic complaints and detachment from patients. In addition, quality of care and professionalism may suffer as a result of physician burnout [111]. Nurses demonstrate higher levels of emotional exhaustion compared to physicians [112]. One recent study on burnout in oncologists found approximately 45% of oncologists had at least one symptom of burnout [111]. Personal stressors outside of the workplace may further exacerbate workplace pressure. Recognizing limitations, developing a compatible perspective on self and work, accepting personal and medical inadequacies, using humor to lighten painful events, working a normal workday, stopping when others do, taking a long weekend off, regular exercise and socializing outside of work are common survival tactics. Personal mental health treatment should be sought when symptoms do not remit. The work environment should emphasize healthy outlets for stress, and support for recognizing and addressing burnout.

Conclusion

Meeting the psychiatric and palliative care needs of oncology patients is an essential component of comprehensive care from initial cancer diagnosis through survivorship. Although the most common psychiatric complications in patients with cancer are depression, anxiety, and delirium, patients may present with other quality-of-life symptoms that set in motion psychiatric, mental health, or palliative care consultations, such as pain, fatigue, sexual or cognitive dysfunction. In addition, certain situations that arise in the oncology context are managed with the help of mental health specialists, such as the assessment of capacity to make medical decisions if cognition is compromised, adjusting to survivorship after acute cancer treatment, individuals and families coping with genetic vulnerabilities and uncertainties of state of the art cancer treatment strategies, as well as grief before and after a loved one has died. Improved identification, evaluation, and treatment of these problems that span the psychiatric–medical and palliative care spectrum are essential to promoting patient comfort, improved cancer treatment and compliance, and better quality of life for both patients and their families.

Research in psycho-oncology over the last decade has added to our understanding and amelioration of the psychiatric and palliative care needs of patients undergoing cancer treatment and survivors. In this chapter, we reviewed strategies for psychotherapeutic and psychopharmacologic interventions to help oncology teams manage cancer patients' psychosocial needs when mental health specialists are not readily available. Additional investigation is warranted to give cancer clinicians more reliable tools to improve patient reported outcomes regarding quality of life further. Finally, we briefly addressed the psychological well-being and potential burnout of oncology staff, an area of increasing concern among practitioners as it may directly impact the care of patients. This work is rewarding yet demanding. Helping ourselves as we help our patients is not just common sense—it is essential in order to continue to reliably and effectively treat cancer.

Acknowledgment

The authors gratefully acknowledge the meticulous and dedicated assistance of Ms. Annie Kong in the preparation of this manuscript. This work was supported in part by The Research and Therapeutics Program in Prostate Cancer of Memorial Sloan-Kettering Cancer Center, The Silbermann Foundation and the Muriel Duenewald Lloyd Fund.

References

1 Massie MJ, Holland JC. Consultation and liaison issues in cancer care. *Psych Med* 1987;5(4):343–59.

2 Wachsman DS. *P.C.:A Layman's Guide to the Prostate Cancer Experience.* Bloomington: iUniverse, 2011.

3 Holland J. Psychological aspects of cancer. In: J Holland, E Frei (eds) *Cancer Medicine*, 2nd edn. Philadelphia: Lea & Febiger, 1982:1175–203, 2325–31.

4 Zadeh S, Wiener L, Pao M. Helping Providers to Help Adolescents and Young Adults be Involved in End-of-Life Care: The Conversation No One Wants to Have. American Psychosocial Oncology Society Annual Meeting, Huntington Beach, CA, 2013.

5 Derogatis LR, Morrow GR, Fetting J, *et al.* The prevalence of psychiatric disorders among cancer patients. *JAMA* 1983;249(6):751–7.

6 Zabora J, BrintzenhofeSzoc K, Curbow B, Hooker C, Piantadosi S. The prevalence of psychological distress by cancer site. *Psycho-oncology* 2001;10(1):19–28.

7 Roth AJ, Kornblith AB, Batel-Copel L, *et al.* Rapid screening for psychologic distress in men with prostate carcinoma: a pilot study. *Cancer* 1998;82(10):1904–8.

8 Traeger L, Greer JA, Fernandez-Robles C, Temel JS, Pirl WF. Evidence-based treatment of anxiety in patients with cancer. *J Clin Oncol* 2012;30(11):1197–205.

9 Li M, Fitzgerald P, Rodin G. Evidence-based treatment of depression in patients with cancer. *J Clin Oncol* 2012;30(11):1187–96.

10 Breitbart W, Alici Y. Evidence-based treatment of delirium in patients with cancer. *J Clin Oncol* 2012;30(11):1206–14.

11 Zabora JR, Macmurray L. The history of psychosocial screening among cancer patients. *J Psychosoc Oncol* 2012;30(6):625–35.

12 Nelson CJ, Weinberger MI, Balk E, *et al.* The chronology of distress, anxiety, and depression in older prostate cancer patients. *Oncologist* 2009;14(9):891–9.

13 Weiss T, Nelson C, Tew W, *et al. The Relationship among Age, Anxiety, and Depression in Older Adults with Cancer.* The American Society of Clinical Oncology (ASCO) Annual Meeting, Chicago, 2012.

14 Adler NE, Page AEK (eds) *Cancer Care for the Whole Patient: Meeting Psychosocial Health Needs.* Washington DC: National Academies Press, 2008.

15 Cancer Program Standards 2012: Ensuring Patient-Centered Care. https://www.facs.org/~/media/files/quality%20programs/cancer/coc/programstandards2012.ashx (accessed 29 August 2017).

16 Archer J, Bower P, Gilbody S, *et al.* Collaborative care for depression and anxiety problems. *Cochrane Database Syst Rev* 2012;10:CD006525.

17 Strong V, Waters R, Hibberd C, *et al.* Management of depression for people with cancer (SMaRT oncology 1): a randomised trial. *Lancet* 2008;372(9632):40–8.

18 Sharpe M, Walker J, Holm Hansen C, *et al.* Integrated collaborative care for comorbid major depression in patients with cancer (SMaRT Oncology-2): a multicentre randomised controlled effectiveness trial. *Lancet* 2014;384(9948):1099–108.

19 Fann JR, Fan MY, Unützer J. Improving primary care for older adults with cancer and depression. *J Gen Intern Med.* 2009;24(Suppl 2):S417–24.

20 Roth AJ, Kornblith AB, Batel-Copel L, *et al.* Rapid screening for psychologic distress in men with prostate carcinoma: a pilot study. *Cancer* 1998;82(10):1904–8.

21 Ransom S, Jacobsen PB, Booth-Jones M. Validation of the Distress Thermometer with bone marrow transplant patients. *Psycho-oncology* 2006;15(7):604–12.

22 Fann JR, Berry DL, Wolpin S, *et al.* Depression screening using the Patient Health Questionnaire-9 administered on a touch screen computer. *Psycho-oncology* 2009;18(1):14–22.

23 Zigmond AS, Snaith RP. The hospital anxiety and depression scale. *Acta Psychiatr Scand* 1983;67(6):361–70.

24 Fawzy FI, Fawzy NW, Arndt LA, Pasnau RO. Critical review of psychosocial interventions in cancer care. *Arch Gen Psych* 1995;52(2):100–13.

25 Sourkes BM, Massie MJ, Holland JC. Psychotherapeutic issues. In: J Holland J (ed.) *Psycho-Oncology.* New York: Oxford University Press, 1998:694–700.

26 Spiegel D, Bloom JR, Kraemer HC, Gottheil E. Effect of psychosocial treatment on survival of patients with metastatic breast cancer. *Lancet* 1989;2(8668):888–91.

27 Daniels J, Kissane DW. Psychosocial interventions for cancer patients. *Curr Opin Oncol* 2008;20(4):367–71.

28 Goodwin PJ, Leszcz M, Ennis M, *et al.* The effect of group psychosocial support on survival in metastatic breast cancer. *N Engl J Med* 2001;345(24):1719–26.

29 Piet J, Wurtzen H, Zachariae R. The effect of mindfulness-based therapy on symptoms of anxiety and depression in adult cancer patients and survivors: a systematic review and meta-analysis. *J Consult Clin Psychol* 2012;80(6):1007–20.

30 Breitbart W, Poppito S, Rosenfeld B, *et al.* Pilot randomized controlled trial of individual meaning-centered psychotherapy for patients with advanced cancer. *J Clin Oncol* 2012;30(12):1304–9.

31 Chochinov HM, Kristjanson LJ, Breitbart W, *et al.* Effect of dignity therapy on distress and end-of-life experience in terminally ill patients: a randomised controlled trial. *Lancet Oncol* 2011;12(8):753–62.

32 Snyderman D, Wynn D. Depression in cancer patients. *Primary Care* 2009;36(4):703–19.

33 Bukberg J, Penman D, Holland JC. Depression in hospitalized cancer patients. *Psychosom Med* 1984;46(3):199–212.

34 DeFlorio ML, Massie MJ. Review of depression in cancer: gender differences. *Depression* 1995;3(1-2):66–80.

35 Massie M, Popkin M. Depressive disorders. In: J Holland J (ed.) *Psycho-Oncology.* New York: Oxford University Press, 1998.

36 Moffic HS, Paykel ES. Depression in medical in-patients. *Br J Psych* 1975;126:346–53.

37 Schwab JJ, Bialow M, Brown JM, Holzer CE. Diagnosing depression in medical inpatients. *Ann Intern Med* 1967;67(4):695–707.

38 Massie MJ, Holland JC. The cancer patient with pain: psychiatric complications and their management. *Med Clin N Am* 1987;71(2):243–58.

39 Hall RC, Popkin MK, Devaul RA, Faillace LA, Stickney SK. Physical illness presenting as psychiatric disease. *Arch Gen Psych* 1978;35(11):1315–20.

40 Horowitz LM, Snyder D, Ludi E, *et al.* Ask suicide-screening questions to everyone in medical settings: the asQ'em Quality Improvement Project. *Psychosomatics* 2013;54(3):239–47.

41 Posner K, Brown GK, Stanley B, *et al.* The Columbia-Suicide Severity Rating Scale: initial validity and internal consistency findings from three multisite studies with adolescents and adults. *Am J Psychiatry* 2011;168(12):1266–77.

42 Breitbart W. Suicide in cancer patients. In: J Holland, J Rowland (eds) *Handbook of Psycho-oncology: Psychological Care of the Patient with Cancer.* New York: Oxford University Press, 1989:291–9.

43 Zweig RA, Hinrichsen GA. Factors associated with suicide attempts by depressed older adults: a prospective study. *Am J Psych* 1993;150(11):1687–92.

44 Dubovsky SL. Averting suicide in terminally ill patients. *Psychosomatics* 1978;19(2):113–5.

45 Murphy GE. Suicide and attempted suicide. *Hosp Pract* 1977;12(11):73–81.

46 Breitbart W, Rosenfeld B, Pessin H, *et al.* Depression, hopelessness, and desire for hastened death in terminally ill patients with cancer. *JAMA* 2000;284(22):2907–11.

47 Kennedy SH, Rizvi S. Sexual dysfunction, depression, and the impact of antidepressants. *J Clin Psychopharm* 2009;29(2):157–64.

48 Lower EE, Fleishman S, Cooper A, *et al.* Efficacy of dexmethylphenidate for the treatment of fatigue after cancer chemotherapy: a randomized clinical trial. *J Pain Symptom Manage* 2009;38(5):650–62.

49 Breitbart W, Alici Y. Psychostimulants for cancer-related fatigue. *J Natl Comp Cancer Net* 2010;8(8):933–42.

50 Gehring K, Patwardhan SY, Collins R, *et al.* A randomized trial on the efficacy of methylphenidate and modafinil for improving cognitive functioning and symptoms in patients with a primary brain tumor. *J Neuro-oncol* 2012;107(1):165–74.

51 Wirz S, Nadstawek J, Kuhn KU, *et al.* [Modafinil for the treatment of cancer-related fatigue: an intervention study]. *Schmerz (Berlin, Germany)* 2010;24(6):587–95.

52 Jean-Pierre P, Morrow GR, Roscoe JA, *et al.* A phase 3 randomized, placebo-controlled, doubleblind, clinical trial of the effect of modafinil on cancer-related fatigue among 631 patients receiving chemotherapy: a University of Rochester Cancer Center Community Clinical Oncology Program Research base study. *Cancer* 2010;116(14):3513–20.

53 Cooper MR, Bird HM, Steinberg M. Efficacy and safety of modafinil in the treatment of cancer-related fatigue. *Ann Pharmacother* 2009;43(4):721–5.

54 Breitbart W. Do antidepressants reduce the effectiveness of tamoxifen? *Psycho-oncology* 2011;20(1):1–4.

55 Noyes R, Holt C, Massie M. Anxiety disorders. In: J Holland J (ed.) *Psycho-Oncology*. New York: Oxford University Press, 1998:548–63.

56 Miller K, Massie MJ. Depression and anxiety. *Cancer J* 2006;12(5):388–97.

57 Redd WH, Jacobsen PB, Die-Trill M, *et al.* Cognitive/attentional distraction in the control of conditioned nausea in pediatric cancer patients receiving chemotherapy. *J Consult Clin Psychol* 1987;55(3):391–5.

58 Rustad JK, David D, Currier MB. Cancer and post-traumatic stress disorder: diagnosis, pathogenesis and treatment considerations. *Palliat Support Care* 2012;10(3):213–23.

59 Nir Y. Post-traumatic stress disorder in children with cancer. In: R Pynoose, S Eth (eds) *Post-Traumatic Stress Disorder in Children*. Washington, DC: American Psychiatric Press, 1985:121–32.

60 Breitbart W, Gibson C, Tremblay A. The delirium experience: delirium recall and delirium-related distress in hospitalized patients with cancer, their spouses/caregivers, and their nurses. *Psychosomatics* 2002;43(3):183–94.

61 Lipowsky Z. *Delirium: Acute Brain Failure in Man.* Springfield: Charles C. Thomas, 1980.

62 Centeno C, Sanz A, Breura E. Delerium in advanced cancer patients. *Palliat Med* 2004;18(3):184–94.

63 Hall RC, Popkin MK, Stickney SK, Gardner ER. Presentation of the steroid psychoses. *J Nerv Mental Dis* 1979;167(4):229–36.

64 Stiefel FC, Breitbart WS, Holland JC. Corticosteroids in cancer: neuropsychiatric complications. *Cancer Invest* 1989;7(5):479–91.

65 Breitbart W, Marotta R, Platt MM, Weisman H, Derevenco M, Grau C, *et al.* A double-blind trial of haloperidol, chlorpromazine, and lorazepam in the treatment of delirium in hospitalized AIDS patients. *Am J Psych* 1996;153(2):23–7.

66 Drew BJ, Ackerman MJ, Funk M, *et al.* Prevention of torsade de pointes in hospital settings: a scientific statement from the American Heart Association and the American College of Cardiology Foundation. *Circulation* 2010;121(8):1047–60.

67 Pao M, Kazak AE (eds) *Anxiety and Depression.* Charlottesville: IPOS Press, 2009.

68 O'Mahony S, Goulet J, Kornblith A, *et al.* Desire for hastened death, cancer pain and depression: report of a longitudinal observational study. *J Pain Symptom Manage* 2005;29(5):446–57.

69 Weisman SJ, Schechter NL. The management of pain in children. *Pediatr Rev* 1991;12(8):237–43.

70 Rosenfeld B, Breitbart W, Galietta M, *et al.* The schedule of attitudes toward hastened death: measuring desire for death in terminally ill cancer patients. *Cancer* 2000;88(12):2868–75.

71 Chochinov HM, Wilson KG, Enns M, *et al.* Desire for death in the terminally ill. *Am J Psych* 1995;152(8):1185–91.

72 Wilson KG, Chochinov HM, McPherson CJ, *et al.* Suffering with advanced cancer. *J Clin Oncol* 2007;25(13):1691–7.

73 Chochinov HM, McClement SE, Hack TF, *et al.* The Patient Dignity Inventory: applications in the oncology setting. *J Palliat Med* 2012;15(9):998–1005.

74 Berger AM, Mooney K, Banerjee C, *et al.* NCCN Guideline. NCCN Clinical Practice Guidelines in Oncology: Cancer-Related Fatigue. Version 1.2017, December 19, 2016. Nccn.org.

75 Campos MP, Hassan BJ, Riechelmann R, Del Giglio A. *Cancer-related fatigue: a review. Rev Assoc Med Brasil (1992)*:2011;57(2):211–9.

76 Ruddy KJ, Barton D, Loprinzi CL. Laying to rest psychostimulants for cancer-related fatigue? *J Clin Oncol* 2014;32(18):1865–7.

77 Roth AJ, Nelson C, Rosenfeld B, *et al.* Methylphenidate for fatigue in ambulatory men with prostate cancer. *Cancer* 2010;116(21):5102–10.

78 Sarhill N, Walsh D, Nelson KA, Homsi J, LeGrand S, Davis MP. Methylphenidate for fatigue in advanced cancer: a prospective open-label pilot study. *Am J Hosp Palliat Care* 2001;18(3):187–92.

79 Bruera E, Driver L, Barnes EA, *et al.* Patient-controlled methylphenidate for the management of fatigue in patients with advanced cancer: a preliminary report. *J Clin Oncol* 2003;21(23):4439–43.

80 Bruera E, Valero V, Driver L, *et al.* Patient-controlled methylphenidate for cancer fatigue: a double-blind, randomized, placebo-controlled trial. *J Clin Oncol* 2006;24(13):2073–8.

81 Spathis A, Fife K, Blackhall F, *et al.* Modafinil for the treatment of fatigue in lung cancer: results of a placebo-controlled, double-blind, randomized trial. *J Clin Oncol* 2014;32(18):1882–8.

82 Berenson JR, Yellin O, Shamasunder HK, *et al.* A phase 3 trial of armodafinil for the treatment of cancer-related fatigue for patients with multiple myeloma. *Support Care Cancer* 2015;23:1503–12.

83 Schover L. *Sexuality and Fertility After Cancer.* New York: Wiley, 1997.

84 Bober SL, Varela VS. Sexuality in adult cancer survivors: challenges and intervention. *J Clin Oncol* 2012;30(30):3712–9.

85 Desimone M, Spriggs E, Gass JS, *et al.* Sexual dysfunction in female cancer survivors. *Am J Clin Oncol* 2012;37:101–6.

86 Wiggins DL, Wood R, Granai CO, Dizon DS. Sex, intimacy, and the gynecologic oncologists: survey results of the New England Association of Gynecologic Oncologists (NEAGO). *J Psychosoc Oncol* 2007;25(4):61–70.

87 Shell JA. Evidence-based practice for symptom management in adults with cancer: sexual dysfunction. *Oncol Nurs Forum* 2002;29(1):53–66;

88 Badr H, Taylor CL. Sexual dysfunction and spousal communication in couples coping with prostate cancer. *Psycho-oncology* 2009;18(7):735–46.

89 Hurria A, Somlo G, Ahles T. Renaming "chemobrain". *Cancer Invest* 2007;25(6):373–7.

90 Nelson CJ, Nandy N, Roth AJ. Chemotherapy and cognitive deficits: mechanisms, findings, and potential interventions. *Palliat Supp Care* 2007;5(3):273–80.

91 Wefel JS, Kesler SR, Noll KR, Schagen SB. Clinical characteristics, pathophysiology, and management of noncentral nervous system cancer-related cognitive impairment in adults. *CA Cancer J Clin* 2015;65(2):123–38.

92 Janelsins MC, Kohli S, Mohile SG, Usuki K, Ahles TA, Morrow GR. An update on cancer- and chemotherapy-related cognitive dysfunction: current status. *Semin Oncol* 2011;38(3):431–8.

93 Wefel JS, Lenzi R, Theriault RL, Davis RN, Meyers CA. The cognitive sequelae of standard-dose adjuvant chemotherapy in women with breast carcinoma: results of a prospective, randomized, longitudinal trial. *Cancer* 2004;100(11):2292–9.

94 Jansen CE, Cooper BA, Dodd MJ, Miaskowski CA. A prospective longitudinal study of chemotherapy-induced cognitive changes in breast cancer patients. *Support Care Cancer* 2011;19(10):1647–56.

95 Ferguson RJ, McDonald BC, Rocque MA, *et al.* Development of CBT for chemotherapy-related cognitive change: results of a waitlist control trial. *Psycho-oncology* 2012;21(2):176–86.

96 Stowell C, Barnhill J, Ferrando S. Characteristics of Patients with Impaired Decision-Making Capacity Academy of Psychosomatic Medicine Annual Meeting November 17, 2007. Amelia Island, Florida 2007.

97 Massie MJ, Spiegel L, Lederberg M, Holland J. Psychiatric complications in cancer patients. In: G Murphy, W Lawrence Jr, R Lenhard Jr |(eds) *American Cancer Society Textbook of Clinical Oncology*, 2nd edn. Atlanta: American Cancer Society, 1995.

98 Lederberg MS. Making a situational diagnosis. Psychiatrists at the interface of psychiatry and ethics in the consultation-liaison setting. *Psychosomatics* 1997;38(4):327–38.

99 Roth AJ, Weiss T. Psychiatric emergencies In: J Holland J (ed.) *Psycho-Oncology*. New York: Oxford University Press, 1998;297–302.

100 Greenberg HS, Kazak AE, Meadows AT. Psychologic functioning in 8- to 16-year-old cancer survivors and their parents. *J Pediatr* 1989;114(3):488–93.

101 Osterweis M, Solomon F, Green M (eds) *Bereavement Reactions, Consequences and Care*. Washington: National Academy Press, 1984.

102 Parkes C, Wess R. *Recovery of Bereavement*. New York: Basic Books, 1983.

103 Tomarken A, Holland J, Schachter S, *et al.* Factors of complicated grief pre-death in caregivers of cancer patients. *Psycho-oncology* 2008;17(2):105–11.

104 Chiu YW, Huang CT, Yin SM, *et al.* Determinants of complicated grief in caregivers who cared for terminal cancer patients. *Support Care Cancer* 2010;18(10):1321–7.

105 Guldin MB, Vedsted P, Zachariae R, Olesen F, Jensen AB. Complicated grief and need for professional support in family caregivers of cancer patients in palliative care: a longitudinal cohort study. *Support Care Cancer* 2012;20(8):1679–85.

106 La Rowe K. *Breath of Relief: Transforming Compassion Fatigue into Flow*. Boston: Acanthus Publishing, 2005.

107 Perry B, Toffner G, Merrick T, Dalton J. An exploration of the experience of compassion fatigue in clinical oncology nurses. *Can Oncol Nurs J* 2011;21(2):91–105.

108 Trufelli DC, Bensi CG, Garcia JB, *et al.* Burnout in cancer professionals: a systematic review and meta-analysis. *Eur J Cancer Care* 2008;17(6):524–31.

109 Demirci S, Yildirim YK, Ozsaran Z, *et al.* Evaluation of burnout syndrome in oncology employees. *Med Oncol* 2010;27(3):968–74.

110 Potter P, Deshields T, Divanbeigi J, *et al.* Compassion fatigue and burnout: prevalence among oncology nurses. *Clin J Oncol Nurs* 2010;14(5):E56–62.

111 Shanafelt TD, Gradishar WJ, Kosty M, *et al.* Burnout and career satisfaction among US oncologists. *J Clin Oncol* 2014;32(7):678–86.

112 Alacacioglu A, Yavuzsen T, Dirioz M, Oztop I, Yilmaz U. Burnout in nurses and physicians working at an oncology department. *Psycho-oncology* 2009;18(5):543–8.

113 Roth AJ, Massie MJ. *Psychiatric complications in cancer patients In: RE Lenhard Jr, RT Osteen, T Gansler (eds) Clinical Oncology*. Atlanta: American Cancer Society, 2001:837–51.

30

Oncologic Emergencies

Mark A. Lewis[1], William J. Hogan[2], and Timothy J. Moynihan[2]

[1] *Intermountain Healthcare, Salt Lake City, Utah, USA*
[2] *Mayo Clinic, Rochester, Minnesota, USA*

Introduction

Oncologic emergencies comprise many different syndromes that can significantly and adversely affect patients with cancer. Prompt recognition and treatment can reduce morbidity, relieve symptoms, and improve quality and quantity of life for these patients.

Infectious Emergencies

Neutropenic Fever

Pathophysiology

Febrile neutropenia is an oncologic emergency that carries a 9.5% inpatient mortality rate with a median hospital stay of 11.5 days at a cost of more than $19,000 per episode based on a report from 2006 [1]. The most common cause is myelotoxic chemotherapy. Other etiologies exist, but usually these can be quickly excluded by a careful history and review of recent treatment. Most of the common outpatient chemotherapy regimens for solid tumors produce a neutrophil nadir between 5 and 10 days after administration; although some regimens have a nadir up to several weeks after administration. The risk corresponds both to the depth as well as the duration of the nadir [2]. Additional risk factors include the prior use of chemotherapy or immunosuppressive medications and other comorbid conditions including hepatic dysfunction, renal insufficiency, pulmonary compromise, and age greater than 65 years [3]. Anthracyclines, taxanes, topoisomerase inhibitors, platinums, gemcitabine, vinorelbine, and alkylators such as cyclophosphamide and ifosfamide are most likely to produce febrile neutropenia [4].

An offending infectious agent is identified in a minority (approximately 10–30%) of cases [5]. When cultures are positive, gram-positive organisms including *Staphylococcus aureus*, *Staphylococcus epidermidis* (especially in patients with indwelling devices), *Streptococcus pneumoniae*, *Streptococcus pyogenes*, the viridians Streptococci, and *Enterococcus faecalis* and *faecium* and *Corynebacterium* are the most frequently identified.

Escherichia coli, *Klebsiella* species, and *Pseudomonas aeruginosa* [6] represent the most common gram-negative species while *Candida* is the most common fungal organism [7]. *Aspergillus* and *Zygomycetes* have a predilection for angioinvasion and a more challenging clinical course, but rarely have positive blood cultures.

Presentation

An infectious etiology is believed to be responsible more that 50% of the time even though only a minority can be microbiologically documented [8]. Other causes for fever should be considered including tumor-induced febrile episodes, drug reactions, and thrombotic complications such as pulmonary embolism. Fever is defined as a single oral temperature $\geq 38.3\,°C$ (101 °F), or temperatures $\geq 38.0\,°C$ (100.4 °F) measured one hour apart [8]. A patient's reduced ability to mount an inflammatory response can limit localizing signs and symptoms, so fever may be the only abnormal finding. Due to the dearth of neutrophils, erythema, induration, abscesses or pulmonary infiltrates may be absent in the presence of infection.

Diagnosis

Neutropenia is defined as an absolute neutrophil count of $< 0.5 \times 10^9$/L (500 cells/mm^3). Infectious risk increases as the absolute neutrophil count falls such that one-fifth of all patients with ANC $< 0.5 \times 10^9$/L are bacteremic [8, 9].

Evaluation begins with a careful history and physical examination with attention to any focal areas of infection; inspection of mucosal barriers, especially the gums, pharynx, perineum, and anus, avoiding digital rectal examination; and inspection of any vascular access or percutaneous drain sites. Patients with hematologic malignancies or more prolonged neutropenia should also undergo funduscopy, as well as palpation of the maxillary and frontal sinuses.

Two sets of blood cultures should be drawn, at least one from each lumen of any indwelling vascular access device. Peripheral blood cultures should also be obtained and the time of each specimen collection carefully recorded. Catheter-related infection should be suspected if the time to a positive culture from the catheter is significantly less than that obtained from the peripheral blood [10]. Absence of pyuria does not exclude urinary tract infection so both urinalysis and urine culture should also be obtained. Laboratory assessment of renal and hepatic function should be performed and chest imaging is recommended to evaluate respiratory symptoms.

Treatment

The presence of comorbidities has a major impact on outcomes from febrile neutropenia, with a large study of over 40,000 patients suggesting that patients without any major comorbidities had a 2.6% risk of mortality, those with one major comorbidity had a mortality of 10.3%, and those with more than one comorbidity incurred a 21.4% mortality. Validated risk stratification tools help gauge the probability of complications, the need for hospitalization, and antibiotic choices in patients with febrile neutropenia. The Multinational Association of Supportive Care in Cancer (MASCC) score [11–13] uses simple clinical criteria to divide patients into high risk < 21 and low risk > 21 with a positive predictive value of 91% and a specificity of 68% and a sensitivity of 71% (Table 30.1).

Immediate empiric antibiotic treatment is recommended for all patients due to the potential for development of sepsis, with subsequent adjustment based on culture results and clinical response. Treatment guidelines have been published by the American Society of Clinical Oncology (ASCO) [14], National Comprehensive Cancer Network (NCCN) [15], and Infectious Diseases Society of America (IDSA) [16]. High-risk patients should be hospitalized for intravenous (IV) therapy with a fourth-generation cephalosporin (e.g. cefepime), a carbapenem, or piperacillin-tazobactam. Routine empiric use of vancomycin is reserved for patients with suspected catheter-related, skin, or soft tissue infection, pneumonia, previous quinolone prophylaxis, or hemodynamic compromise [16]. Growth factors are not routinely recommended. A study in 600 hospitals showed a high level of compliance with initial antibiotic coverage, but poor compliance with recommendations to avoid use of empiric vancomycin and growth factors [17].

Low-risk patients can be treated as outpatients with intravenous antimicrobial therapy or occasionally an oral quinolone and amoxicillin/clavulanic acid, but should receive close follow-up observing for complications or persistent (>48 h) fever, with hospitalization if these occur [16].

Table 30.1 Multinational Association of Supportive Care in Cancer (MASCC) score.

Burden of illness: no or mild symptoms	5
Moderate symptoms	3
No hypotension	5
No chronic obstructive pulmonary disease	4
Solid tumor or no previous invasive fungal infection	4
Outpatient status	3
No dehydration	3
Aged < 60 years	2

Culture-negative patients who are clinically improving should remain on empiric antibiotics until the ANC is $> 0.5 \times 10^9$/L and rising. Patients who remain febrile after 4–7 days of antibiotics with no identifiable source of infection should have antifungal therapy added to their regimen [16].

Staphylococcus aureus, Pseudomonas aeruginosa, fungi, or mycobacteria-infected catheters do require device removal followed by at least 14 days of antimicrobial therapy [16]. Patients with catheter-related infections with coagulase-negative Staphylococcus species or other more sensitive organisms do not always require device removal, but carry a risk for subsequent infection [18].

Colony-stimulating factors are not generally recommended in patients who present with febrile neutropenia but prophylactic use of these agents is recommended for patients receiving chemotherapy that carries a greater than 20% [19] risk of febrile neutropenia or in patients who have had a prior episode of febrile neutropenia [20].

White blood cell transfusions are not routinely recommended and are reserved for special circumstances such as refractory fungal infections in patients with prolonged neutropenia [21]. Prophylactic antiviral therapy is not recommended for most patients being treated for solid tumors.

Neurologic Emergencies

Malignant Spinal Cord Compression

Malignant spinal cord compression (MSCC) occurs in up to 2.5% of all cancer patients in the 5 years prior to death from solid tumors [22]. Preservation of neurologic function and improved overall survival requires early diagnosis and treatment. Breast, prostate, and lung cancer each account for approximately 15–20% of the cases, with non-Hodgkin lymphoma, renal cell carcinoma, and myeloma each causing 5–10% of cases [2, 23]. A minority of cases [22, 24, 25] will have spinal cord compression as the initial manifestation of malignancy.

Pathophysiology

Indentation, displacement, or encasement of the thecal sac that surrounds the spinal cord or cauda equina by cancer is the hallmark of malignant spinal cord compression [26]. Compression most commonly occurs by extension of vertebral body metastases, but can also occur through a paraspinous mass growing in through the vertebral foramen (seen in 15% of cases, most commonly neuroblastomas, lymphomas or paraspinous sarcomas [26, 27]). Metastases directly to the spinal cord or meninges are rare [27–29]. More than half of all patients will have multiple levels of the spine involved, most commonly the thoracic spine (60%) followed by the lumbosacral region (30%) and cervical spine (10%) [23, 28].

Presentation

The single most important prognostic factor for neurologic function after treatment of MSCC is pretreatment neurologic status [30–33]. Presentation will vary depending on severity, location, and duration of the compression. Back pain occurs in approximately 90% of the cases [26]. Back pain often precedes neurologic symptoms by weeks to months and may present as referred pain, depending on the location and nature of the compression [25, 34].

Neurologic progression can be quite rapid, including motor weakness, sensory impairment, and autonomic dysfunction. Lumbar involvement may cause cauda equina syndrome with urinary retention, overflow incontinence, and decreased sensation over the buttocks, posterior-superior thighs, and perineal region [23, 33].

Location of the lesion and the duration/degree of impingement will affect physical examination findings. Hyperreflexia, spasticity, and loss of sensation (position, temperature, pinprick, vibratory) can occur early. Deep tendon reflexes may then become hypoactive or absent. Late signs include weakness, sensory loss, Babinski signs, and decreased anal sphincter tone.

Diagnosis

New-onset back pain in cancer patients should prompt an immediate assessment for possibility of spinal cord compression. While not all patients require imaging of the spine, those with new neurologic deficits need emergent evaluation (Figure 30.1) [28].

Magnetic resonance imaging (MRI) has a sensitivity of 93%, specificity of 97%, and overall accuracy of 95% [28, 35, 36]. Plain radiographs of the spine may demonstrate areas of vertebral body involvement but cannot be used to rule out compression [24, 28]. Imaging must include the entire thecal sac [37]. In a series of 337 patients with MSCC at the Mayo Clinic, 30% had multiple lesions. CT myelography can be used if MRI is unavailable or contraindicated [2, 29].

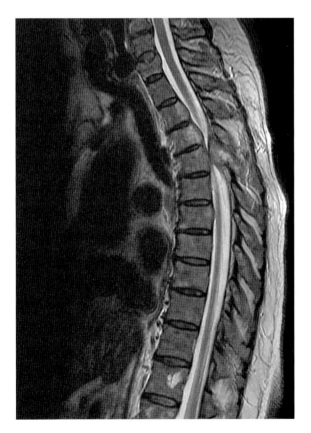

Figure 30.1 Spinal cord compression from metastatic breast cancer.

Treatment

Initial management of MSCC includes glucocorticoids, external beam radiation therapy, and/or surgical decompression with stabilization [25, 26, 38]. Chemosensitive cancers such as malignant germ cell tumors or lymphomas can respond well to systemic therapy.

Unless strongly contraindicated, all patients with MSCC should receive corticosteroids. The ideal dose has not been firmly established based on level one evidence. A randomized trial of 96 mg/day versus 16 mg/day of dexamethasone did not show any difference in clinical benefit for ambulation, survival, or toxicity although the trial did not complete accrual [39]. Three other clinical trials [39–41] and a meta-analysis were unable to show that 96 mg/day dosing offered any superior outcomes, but was associated with a higher incidence of gastrointestinal ulcers, psychosis and infection [39, 40]. It has been our practice to give 10–16 mg IV bolus followed by 4–6 mg every 4 h, with a taper during or immediately after completion of radiation [2, 23, 28]. Some clinicians choose to treat patients having severe neurologic deficits with 96 mg dexamethasone IV, followed by 24 mg four times daily for 3 days, then tapered over 10 days [28].

Definitive treatment depends largely on spinal column stability, degree of compression, and radiosensitivity of the tumor. The only prospective trial [42] randomized 101 patients to resection plus radiation versus radiation therapy only, with all patients receiving high dose steroids. Surgical patients were more likely to regain or retain ambulation for a longer period (84% vs 57%, $P < 0.001$), had better maintenance of urinary continence (74% vs 57%, $P < 0.005$), duration of continence (median 157 days vs 17 days, $P < 0.016$), and improved functional status. Surgical patients had a 26-day improvement in median survival (126 days vs 100 days, $P < 0.033$). A meta-analysis similarly showed a benefit to ambulation in patients treated surgically [43]. Patients over 65 years did not seem to derive the same benefit as younger patients [44]. These findings have led to the development of the Patchell criteria [42] (Table 30.2).

Surgical decompression and stabilization should be considered when spinal instability is present [26, 38]. The Spine

Table 30.2 Patchell Criteria for operative intervention in cord compression.

Inclusion criteria	Exclusion criteria
Age 18 or older	Multiple discrete lesions
Biopsy proven cancer[1]	Radiosensitive tumors
General medical status acceptable for surgery	Compression of only the cauda equina or spinal roots
At least one neurologic sign/symptom (including pain)	Pre-existing neurologic problems not related to cord compression
No paraplegia > 48 h	Prior radiation therapy to region
MSCC restricted to one area[2] MRI evidence of MSCC[3] Expected survival greater than 3 months	

[1] Not of CNS and/or spinal origin.
[2] Can include several contiguous spinal or vertebral segments.
[3] Defined as displacement of the spinal cord by an epidural mass.

Oncology Study Group has established a novel classification system for spinal instability, with patients scoring 7 or higher warranting surgical consultation. Spinal column location of tumor, pain, bone lesion quality (lytic/blastic/mixed), spinal alignment, vertebral body collapse, and posterior involvement of the spinal elements are the key components [45]. Performance status, disease burden, and overall prognosis should also be considered [29, 42].

Radiation plays a crucial role in management of MSCC, but the exact dose and fractionation scheme have not been definitively identified. Regimens include 30 cGy in 20 fractions, 16 cGy in two fractions, or 8 cGy in a single fraction [46]. Radiation doses > 30 Gy have not been shown to improve outcomes [23, 38, 47, 48]. For patients with a poor prognosis and significant pain, a brief course of one or two fractions of 8 Gy can provide palliation [49]. In radioresistant tumors such as renal cell carcinoma and melanoma, SBRT in a single fraction can be utilized for effective pain relief and local control [46, 50, 51].

Increased Intracranial Pressure

Intracranial metastases or primary brain neoplasms can lead to elevated intracranial pressure with significant morbidity and mortality. Prompt recognition and treatment can avoid devastating neurologic injury. The vast majority of adult intracranial tumors arise from metastatic disease, most commonly lung (20%), renal (10%), melanoma (7%), breast (5%), and colorectal cancers (1%) [52–57]. Primary central nervous system (CNS) malignancies are less common, with approximately 23,130 cases estimated in 2013 compared to an estimated 200,000-plus metastatic brain tumors [58]. Prognosis is dependent upon performance status, extent of systemic disease and type of primary tumor [59].

Pathophysiology

Brain metastases occur via hematogenous spread and tend to occur in the watershed areas and gray–white matter junctions. Location of metastases reflects relative blood flow volume, with the cerebrum most commonly affected, followed by the cerebellum and brainstem [54]. Growing tumor mass (either primary or metastatic) as well as peritumoral edema produced by local cytokines, including VEGF, lead to blood–brain barrier dysfunction; both contribute to the mass effect and impact treatment choices [60, 61].

Presentation

The most common clinical presentation for brain metastases is headache, seen in 48% of patients and frequently described as "tension" [62] that tends to worsen with positional changes (such as bending over) or Valsalva maneuvers and may be accompanied by nausea and/or emesis. Early morning predilection only occurred in a minority (36%) of cases [62]. Approximately 10–20% of brain metastases present with seizures and almost exclusively occur in patients with supratentorial lesions. Stroke-like presentations can be seen with tumor emboli or intratumoral hemorrhage. Hemorrhage is more commonly associated with melanoma, choriocarcinoma, thyroid or renal cell cancers [58].

Any patient with cancer with new focal neurologic symptoms or new severe headaches should be evaluated for intracranial metastases. Physical examination helps to delineate focal deficits and papilledema. Cushing response (hypertension with wide pulse pressure, bradycardia, and irregular respiratory rate) is a late sign and raises concerns for impending brainstem herniation.

Diagnosis

Contrast-enhanced MRI is the imaging modality of choice and is more sensitive than CT with contrast [63, 64]. CT scans are useful for intracranial hemorrhage or hydrocephalus [2, 58, 65].

Treatment

Dexamethasone with its lack of mineralocorticoid activity and low infection risk is the initial treatment of choice and can reduce peritumoral edema and local brain compression within hours [66, 67]. The best dose is controversial, with high doses (96–100 mg bolus) not clearly demonstrating any significant advantage over 10–20 mg bolus, with repeated doses of 4–8 mg every 6 h [2, 58]. Downregulation of VEGF, upregulation of angiopoietin-1, and increased clearance of peritumoral edema are the proposed mechanisms of action of dexamethasone [68]. Patients not responding to standard therapy can be given mannitol as an IV bolus or as a continuous infusion. Intubation and hyperventilation will also acutely decrease cerebral edema, but the effects of both mannitol and hyperventilation are transient and some more definitive therapy needs to be planned in these cases [69].

Surgical debulking is the most rapid way to decrease intracranial pressure, but should be reserved for patients with a good performance status, relatively limited CNS disease, and systemic disease that is controlled. Patients unlikely to live more than a few weeks due to systemic disease are less likely to benefit from an aggressive neurosurgical procedure.

Radiation therapy options include whole brain radiation, localized radiation with stereotactic or gamma knife, or a combination of the two. There is no overall survival difference when whole brain radiation is compared to either focal radiation alone or the combination of whole brain and focal radiation [70]. Patients who had whole brain radiation were less likely to suffer a recurrent intracranial event, but had more neurologic sequelae [58, 69].

In cases of highly chemotherapy-sensitive tumors such as germ cell tumors, lymphoma, or small cell carcinomas, chemotherapy can be used, especially if radiation therapy is not an option.

Bevacizumab has been studied as an agent to decrease peritumoral edema and mass effect in primary brain tumors, metastatic lesions, and radiation necrosis. Dramatic responses to edema have been reported and one very small (*n* = 14) randomized trial of bevacizumab 7.5 mg/kg given once every 3 weeks for four doses versus placebo in radiation necrosis did show level one evidence of the effectiveness of this therapy, with decreased edema and decreased use of dexamethasone [71].

Seizures

Approximately 10–20% of patients with brain metastases or primary brain tumors present with seizures. Status epilepticus is an oncologic emergency and requires treatment, typically with

Table 30.3 Treatment of hypercalcemia.

Medication	Usual dose	Points to remember
Normal saline	Rapid infusion 300–500 cm^3/h until euvolemic	Caution in patients with heart failure
Furosemide	20–40 mg IV q 12–24 h	Only after adequate hydration
Pamidronate	60–90 mg IV	Adjust infusion time to creatinine clearance
Zoledronic acid	4 mg IV	Consider alternative treatment in renal failure
Calcitonin	4–8 IU/kg SQ or IM q 12 h	Tachyphylaxis occurs quickly
Steroids	Hydrocortisone 100 mg IV q 6 h; or prednisone 60 mg po daily	Role usually limited to lymphomas; anticipate hyperglycemia
Denosumab	120 mg SQ (dose to be repeated no earlier than 1 week from first administration)	Also approved for prevention of skeletal-related events from bone metastases

IV, intravenous; SQ, subcutaneous; IM, intramuscular; IU, international Units; po, per oral.

lorazepam, phenytoin, valproic acid, or fosphenytoin [2, 38, 58]. Prophylactic antiseizure therapy is not required in patients with brain metastases or primary brain tumors if they have never had a seizure [72].

Metabolic Emergencies

Hypercalcemia

Hypercalcemia will be experienced by up to one-third of cancer patients [73]. It is frequently associated with breast, lung, and renal cell carcinomas, as well as with multiple myeloma [73, 74]. Cancer-related hypercalcemia is humoral in up to 80% of cases, caused by tumor production of parathyroid-related peptide (PTHrP), most often seen in squamous cell carcinomas. Malignant hypercalcemia can also result from tumor destruction of bone, or, rarely, arise from tumor secretion of vitamin D analogues.

Presentation

Skeletal pain, polyuria, polydipsia, nephrolithiasis, abdominal discomfort, constipation, nausea, anorexia, diffuse weakness, and altered mentation are the most common presenting symptoms of hypercalcemia. Bone pain is usually related to discrete metastases. Abdominal pain can arise from dysregulated intestinal motility, pancreatitis, or severe constipation. Changes in sensorium can occur along a spectrum from lethargy to coma.

Diagnosis

Ionized calcium is the most reliable laboratory test to detect hypercalcemia and is considered elevated above 1.29 mmol/L. If measuring total calcium, correct for hypoalbuminemia: corrected calcium, in mg/dL = measured total calcium, in mg/dL + 0.8(4 − measured albumin, in g/dL). There is no absolute level of calcium at which patients will become symptomatic, and the rate of increase is likely more significant than the magnitude of elevation; relatively high levels may be well-tolerated if the rate of rise has been gradual [38].

PTHrP level seldom affects outcome or alters management and should not be routinely measured.

Treatment

The 30-day mortality rate of cancer patients hospitalized with hypercalcemia approaches 50% [75]. Even in advanced malignancies when efforts to lower calcium do not demonstrably prolong life, there can be a palliative benefit to treating hypercalcemia [75]. Urgent intervention is needed to normalize symptomatic hypercalcemia (Table 30.3).

Hydration is the initial management as almost all patients with clinically meaningful hypercalcemia have intravascular volume depletion. Correction of volume depletion should restore brisk urine output. If the patient has intact left ventricular systolic function, normal saline can be safely infused at rates up to 500 mL/h until hypovolemia has resolved. At this time, loop diuretics, such as 40 mg furosemide IV every 12–24 h, can be initiated to promote calciuresis. Thiazide diuretics should be avoided as they promote the retention of calcium. Exogenous sources of calcium and vitamin D should be curtailed. Intravenous phosphates should be avoided due to the potential for calciphylaxis when the calcium-phosphorus product exceeds 70 mg^2/dL^2 [74].

Bisphosphonates block bone resorption by osteoclasts but, even when given intravenously, do not lower calcium rapidly enough to replace aggressive hydration as the first step in management. Calcium usually declines within 48–96 h of infusion and nadirs at 1 week [76]. Adverse effects include acute bone pain, ocular inflammation [77], and electrolyte abnormalities like hypophosphatemia or "overshoot" hypocalcemia [78]. Zoledronic acid 4 mg can be infused more quickly than 60–90 mg of pamidronate (15 min vs 4–6 h), but zoledronic acid is relatively contraindicated in severe renal insufficiency (glomerular filtration rate < 30 mL/min or serum creatinine > 3.0). Pamidronate can be more safely administered in renal insufficiency but still carries the risk of nephrotoxicity [79]. Hemodialysis can quickly correct hypercalcemia in patients with diminished kidney function [80], heart failure, or other conditions that preclude high volumes of IV fluids [81].

Calcitonin administration lowers the calcium more quickly than bisphosphonates, often producing normocalcemia within 12–24 h, but it rapidly loses efficacy through tachyphylaxis [82]. It should not be used as a single agent due to rebound hypercalcemia. Calcitonin can be administered by the intramuscular or subcutaneous routes at 4–8 units/kg every 12 h, but intranasal administration is not effective in this setting. Salmon-derived calcitonin carries a risk of hypersensitivity reaction but anaphylaxis is sufficiently rare that a test dose is no longer routinely recommended [83].

Glucocorticoids (60 mg prednisone orally daily or 100 mg hydrocortisone IV every 6 h) can be helpful when hypercalcemia is driven by vitamin D analogues, typically associated with lymphoma. In addition to their direct lympholytic effect, steroids inhibit calcitriol production and appreciably lower the calcium level within 3–5 days of administration. The duration of use should be limited to minimize steroid toxicities.

Receptor activator of nuclear factor κB (RANK) is found on the surface of osteoclast precursors. Its ligand (RANKL) is found on the surface of osteoblasts and stimulates osteoclast precursors to differentiate and begin bone resorption, liberating calcium [74]. Denosumab is a fully humanized monoclonal antibody with high affinity and specificity for RANKL that is approved for use in the prevention of skeletal events from bone metastases [84] and has additional application in managing hypercalcemia of malignancy [85, 86, 87].

Cinacalcet is a calcimimetic that activates the calcium-sensing receptor, which is present in the parathyroid glands, where it regulates the release of parathyroid hormone, as well as the renal tubules, where it inhibits calcium reabsorption. Approved for the management of secondary hyperparathyroidism, it may have a niche application in severe hypercalcemia associated with parathyroid carcinoma [88].

Hyponatremia

The amount of sodium in the body, not the plasma sodium concentration, determines the volume of fluid outside the cells, and this volume can be readily measured by physical examination. If the total body sodium is high, then the extracellular fluid volume is large and the patient will appear edematous. If the total body sodium is low, then the extracellular space (including the circulatory volume) will contract and the patient will progressively develop tachycardia and hypotension. A low plasma sodium concentration (hyponatremia) can be associated with clinical hypervolemia, hypovolemia, or euvolemia. The physician must correctly evaluate the hyponatremic patient's volume to understand both their sodium and water balance and then select the appropriate treatment [89].

Euvolemic hyponatremic patients have normal extracellular fluid volume, but excessive water in the intravascular space, most commonly mediated through the syndrome of inappropriate antidiuretic hormone (SIADH). Antidiuretic hormone promotes free water uptake in the distal tubules by binding to the vasopressin 2 (V_2) receptor. SIADH should be suspected based upon the site(s) of the primary and metastatic tumors, as SIADH is more commonly encountered in diseases originating in or involving the lungs, pleura, thymus, and brain. Between 10 and 45% of patients with small cell lung cancer will show evidence of SIADH [90]. Iatrogenic causes of hyponatremia include cisplatin [91], cyclophosphamide [92], ifosfamide [93], the vinca alkaloids [94], and imatinib [95]. Drugs with high emetogenic potential can stimulate ADH release through nausea, an appropriate physiologic response that may be confused with SIADH.

Diagnosis

Hyponatremia can be classified as mild (131–135 mmol/L), moderate (126–130 mmol/L), or severe (<125 mmol/L). Hyperglycemia can create spurious hyponatremia and can be adjusted for using the formula: corrected sodium, in mmol/L = measured serum sodium, in mmol/L + 0.016 (measured glucose, in mg/dL – 100).

SIADH is diagnosed when, after exclusion of adrenal insufficiency and hypothyroidism [96], the effective serum osmolality – calculated by subtracting (BUN/2.8) from the measured osmolality – is < 275 mOsm/kg of water, and the urine osmolality exceeds 100 mOsm/kg of water [97]. Urine sodium > 40 mmol/L in the absence of excessive dietary sodium intake supports the diagnosis of SIADH [98].

Treatment

Treatment of hyponatremia in malignancy is dependent upon the underlying cause. Sodium concentrations below 125 mmol/L can create life-threatening cerebral edema. The rate at which hyponatremia develops will primarily determine the patient's symptomatology. Chronic "severe" hyponatremia by laboratory criteria may be better tolerated than "moderate" hyponatremia that develops acutely [90]. The most concerning symptoms of hyponatremia are neurologic, including lethargy, delirium, seizures, and coma, all of which merit urgent treatment.

Hypovolemic hyponatremic patients require sodium-containing fluids. Severe hyponatremia with neurologic symptomatology can merit very careful use of hypertonic (3%) saline. Otherwise normal (0.9%) saline is an appropriate infusate. The serum sodium should not be corrected at a rate > 0.5 mEq/L/h to avoid central pontine myelinolysis [78]. The sodium correction per liter of infusate can be estimated by the following formula: change in serum Na (mEq/L) = [(infusate Na – serum Na) / (total liters of body water +1)] (reference values: infusate Na = 513 mEq in 3% saline, infusate Na = 154 mEq in 0.9% saline, total liters of body water = weight in kilograms × 0.6) [99].

Asymptomatic, euvolemic hyponatremic cancer patients are treated by removing the offending stimulus for their ADH secretion, such as controlling nausea, lessening pain, and treating the underlying malignancy. Restriction of free water intake to 500–1000 mL/day will increase plasma osmolality and normalize the sodium level in many SIADH patients. Demeclocycline, a tetracycline antibiotic with the side effect of inducing nephrogenic diabetes insipidus, can be used at a dosage of 600–1200 mg/day [99], but patients need to be monitored for polyuria and can actually develop hypernatremia if their restriction to free water is continued. The vaptans are non-peptide vasopressin antagonists that bind competitively to the V_2 receptors in the collecting duct where ADH exerts its effect on the kidney. IV conivaptan [100] (20 mg infused over 30 min, then 20 mg infused over 24 h) and oral tolvaptan [101] (starting at 15 mg daily) have been shown in clinical trials to achieve rapid correction of hyponatremia through almost pure aquaresis, and are thus absolutely contraindicated in hypovolemia. The rate of vaptan-induced sodium correction needs to be closely monitored to ensure it is not excessive [102], and then the patient also needs to be monitored for hyponatremic relapse after discontinuation of the vaptan if the agent was used for longer than 5 days [103].

Tumor Lysis Syndrome

Tumor lysis occurs when cancer cells release their intracellular contents into the bloodstream, either spontaneously or following antineoplastic therapy [104, 105]. When large, rapid circulatory shifts of electrolytes and nucleic acids occur, the sudden development of hyperkalemia, hyperuricemia, and hyperphosphatemia can have life-threatening end-organ effects on the myocardium, kidneys, and central nervous system. Hypocalcemia, a consequence of hyperphosphatemia, is included in the constellation of metabolic disturbances known as tumor lysis syndrome (TLS).

Presentation

Clinical TLS is diagnosed when one or more of three conditions arise: acute renal failure (a rise in creatinine to ≥ 1.5 times the upper limit of normal), arrhythmias (including sudden cardiac death), and seizures. Acute renal failure can manifest as a decrease in urine output, uremia-related altered sensorium, or crystalline obstructive uropathy.

Tumor lysis syndrome is more common in rapidly proliferating hematologic malignancies, like acute lymphoblastic leukemia, acute myeloid leukemia, and Burkitt's lymphoma, but has been documented in solid tumors like small cell lung cancer [106] and germ cell tumors [107]. The onset of TLS can be delayed by days to weeks after treatment in a solid malignancy [105].

Diagnosis

The laboratory definition of TLS includes a 25% increase in uric acid, potassium, or phosphorous and/or a 25% decrease in calcium within 3 days before and 7 days after the initiation of treatment (Table 30.4) [108]. Absolute values of uric acid ≥ 8 mg/dL, potassium ≥ 6 mEq/L, phosphorus ≥ 4.5 mg/dL, or calcium ≤ 7 mg/dL are also considered significant [108]. Because of the need to establish a temporal relationship to treatment, the same criteria do not apply to spontaneous TLS. The severity of TLS has a formal grading system (Table 30.5).

Treatment

Prophylaxis is appropriate in high-risk patients, including those with bulky tumors, rapidly proliferating disease, expectations of immediately effective cytotoxic treatment, and baseline renal insufficiency, volume depletion, or hyperuricemia. Complex algorithms can be used to estimate the disease-specific risk for TLS [109].

Allopurinol inhibits xanthine oxidase, thus decreasing uric acid production, and can be given preventively starting up to 48 h before treatment at doses of 100 mg/m^2 every 8 h (maximum daily dose: 800 mg). Allopurinol does not alter uric acid that has already formed and is not recommended for patients with pretreatment hyperuricemia ≥ 7.5 mg/dL. (At the time of this writing, the relative merits of febuxostat, a xanthine oxidase inhibitor like allopurinol, are debatable, but in a large trial of over 300 patients with hematologic malignancies at intermediate to high risk of TLS, the mean area under the concentration–time curve of serum uric acid from days 1 through 8 was significantly lower with febuxostat.) [110].

Rasburicase is recombinant urate oxidase, which converts uric acid into water-soluble allantoin (0.15–0.2 mg/kg/day for up to 7 days) and is used for patients with hyperuricemia [111]. Due to its expense, it should be used judiciously, and patients should be screened for G6PD deficiency.

The electrolyte complications of TLS are not directly remedied by allopurinol or rasburicase (Table 30.6). Hyperkalemia can be treated with loop diuretics. Immediate reduction in serum potassium through intracellular shifting can be achieved by injection

Table 30.4 Laboratory definition of tumor lysis syndrome using Cairo-Bishop classification.

Laboratory tumor lysis syndrome

Uric acid ≥ 8 mg/dL (≥ 476 μmol/L) or 25% increase from baseline

Potassium ≥ 6 mEq/L (≥ 6 mmol/L) or 25% increase from baseline

Phosphorus ≥ 6.5 mg/dL (≥ 2.1 mmol/L) or 25% increase from baseline

Calcium ≤ 7 mg/dL (≤ 1.75 mmol/L) or 25% decrease from baseline

Clinical tumor lysis syndrome

Creatinine ≥ 1.5 times upper limit of normal

Cardiac arrhythmia or sudden death

Seizure

Note: two or more laboratory changes must be observed within 3 days before or 7 days after cytotoxic therapy.

Table 30.5 Grading of tumor lysis syndrome complications.

Complication	Grade					
	0	1	2	3	4	5
Creatinine	$\geq 1.5 \times$ ULN	$1.5 \times$ ULN	>1.5–$3.0 \times$ ULN	>3.0–$6.0 \times$ ULN	$>6.0 \times$ ULN	Death
Cardiac arrhythmia	None	Intervention not indicated	Nonurgent medical intervention indicated	Symptomatic and incompletely controlled medically or controlled with device (e.g., defibrillator)	Life-threatening (e.g., arrhythmia associated with HF, hypotension, syncope, shock)	Death
Seizure	None	-	One brief, generalized seizure; seizure(s) well controlled by anticonvulsants or infrequent focal motor seizures not interfering with ADL	Seizure in which consciousness is altered; poorly controlled seizure disorder; with breakthrough generalized seizures despite medical intervention	Seizure of any kind which are prolonged, repetitive or difficult to control (eg, status epilepticus, intractable epilepsy)	Death

ULN, upper limits of normal.

Table 30.6 Treatment of metabolic alterations in tumor lysis syndrome.

Problem	Treatment	Dose	Comments
Renal failure/ hypovolemia	Intravenous fluids	Normal saline 3 L/m^2/day	Caution in heart disease
	Dialysis		For fluid nonresponsive or heart failure
Hyperuricemia	Allopurinol	100 mg/m^2 per dose q 8 h (daily max 800 mg)	Prophylaxis only. Caution with 6MP, azathioprine
	Rasburicase	0.15–0.2 mg/kg/d IV	Contraindicated pregnancy and G6PD
Hyperphosphatemia	Limit dietary PO4	Limit dairy/bread	
	Aluminum hydroxide or carbonate	30 mL po q 6 h	
	Dialysis if unresponsive		
Hyperkalemia	Regular insulin	10 IU IV	Insulin and dextrose are administered together
	Dextrose	50 mL of 50% IV push, then 50–75 mL 10% over 1 h	
	Albuterol	10 to 20 mg in 4 mL of saline by nebulization over 10 minutes	
	Dialysis if unresponsive		
	Calcium gluconate	1000 mg IV	If EKG changes present
Hypocalcemia	Calcium gluconate	200 mg/min IV up to 1000 mg total	Caution in severe hyperphosphatemia

EKG, electrocardiogram; IU, international units; IV, intravenous; po, per oral.

of 10 units of regular insulin, followed immediately by 50 mL of 50% dextrose and then an hour long infusion of 50–75 mL of 10% dextrose to prevent hypoglycemia [112]. Inhaled beta-agonists, such as 10–20 mg (4–8 times the dose used for asthma) of nebulized albuterol, can lower potassium [113]. Cation exchange resins like sodium polystyrene sulfonate are not routinely recommended. A 1000 mg infusion of calcium gluconate can reverse electrocardiographic changes such as first-degree AV block and a widened QRS [114].Hyperphosphatemia is managed by a phosphorous-restricted diet or by short-term use of oral phosphate binders, e.g. aluminum. Dialysis may ultimately be necessary to treat any refractory, life-threatening electrolyte derangements, especially in the context of volume overload and renal insufficiency.

Cardiovascular Emergencies

Pericardial Effusion and Cardiac Tamponade

Malignant pericardial effusions develop through direct or metastatic involvement of the pericardial sac. The most common tumors are lung cancer, breast cancer, and mediastinal lymphoma [115]. Fluid in the pericardial space accumulates until diastolic pressures equalize throughout the chambers of the heart and adversely affects cardiac output by compromising filling [116], at which point tamponade physiology emerges.

Presentation
Pericardial effusions can be asymptomatic, although their presence portends a poor prognosis. Tamponade classically presents with Beck's triad: hypotension, elevated jugular venous pressure, and a muffled precordium, but a minority of patients

will demonstrate all three signs [117]. Most patients complain of dyspnea and chest discomfort, which may begin abruptly. Tamponade physiology can arise from volumes of as little as 100 mL if effusions develop rapidly [118].

Diagnosis
On physical examination, tachycardia is nearly universal, and an elevated pulsus paradoxus of >10 mmHg is an ominous finding [119].

Chest X-ray may show cardiomegaly and the classic "water bottle" cardiac silhouette. Electrocardiogram can show low voltage and electrical alternans. Echocardiography is the definitive test, demonstrating right ventricular collapse during early diastole.

Treatment
Sonographically-guided pericardiocentesis is the treatment of choice [120, 121]. A catheter can be placed into the sac to drain residual or reaccumulating fluid. Surgical creation of a pericardial window or pericardiectomy is generally reserved for cases refractory to catheter drainage.

Patients often report immediate symptomatic improvement from pericardiocentesis but still require close monitoring. Decompression can produce paradoxical hemodynamic instability requiring ICU admission and pressor support.

Superior Vena Cava Syndrome

The thin-walled superior vena cava (SVC) returns all blood from the cranial, neck, and upper extremity vasculature to the right side of the heart. Primary or metastatic tumors can cause SVC compression. Thrombosis, particularly due to an underlying hypercoagulable state or endothelial damage from an indwelling vascular device, can also obstruct venous return.

Presentation

The extent of SVC obstruction and acuity of development dictate the patient's presentation. Blockage is better tolerated when there has been time for collateral veins to develop over weeks to months. The veins on the patient's chest wall may be visibly distended. Edema in the arms, facial plethora (not necessarily unilateral), chemosis, and periorbital edema may also occur. Stridor is an alarming sign that edema is narrowing the luminal diameter of the pharynx and larynx. Confusion may indicate cerebral edema. These symptoms may be more noticeable when the patient is supine.

Cancers classically associated with SVC syndrome include: lung cancer (particularly right-sided), breast cancer, lymphoblastic lymphoma, thymoma, and mediastinal germ cell tumors.

Diagnosis

Radiographic imaging is crucial to diagnosis and treatment planning, especially if radiation and endovascular stents are potential interventions. While the gold standard for localizing obstruction remains selective venography, CT or MRI are preferable for their non-invasiveness, easier availability, and decreased contrast load [122].

Treatment

SVC syndrome requires prompt recognition and treatment, but the clinical course typically permits completion of appropriate diagnostic studies before definitive therapy begins [123]. Thus, when SVC syndrome heralds malignancy, there is usually still time to perform biopsies or other diagnostic procedures without endangering the patient. Patients with neurologic symptoms or airway compromise merit immediate treatment. Endovascular stenting can provide prompt palliation that should not interfere with further diagnostic maneuvers and generally relieves symptoms more quickly than chemoradiation [122].

Determining the histology of the responsible malignancy can often guide therapy. Chemotherapy may be the only necessary treatment in patients presenting in non-emergent fashion with small cell lung cancer, lymphoma, or germ cell tumors. Radiation remains the mainstay of treatment for most causes of SVC syndrome.

Respiratory Emergencies

Malignant Airway Obstruction

Airway obstruction may result from malignant infiltration of the oropharynx, trachea, and bronchi, or by extrinsic compression of the respiratory tree by tumor or lymphadenopathy. Primary bronchogenic carcinomas are the most common cause; other culprit tumor types include those arising from the tongue, oropharynx, and thyroid.

Presentation

The clinical manifestations of malignant airway obstruction depend on the severity and location of the obstruction. The most common presentation is dyspnea, while the patient is lying supine. Patients often have a productive cough or hemoptysis and wheezing. Stridor may be present if the obstruction is located in the trachea or carina [124].

Diagnosis

Airway obstruction needs to be considered in the differential diagnosis of patients with a history of malignancy presenting with new respiratory symptoms. Crackles or fremitus, along with poor expansion of the lung, may be found on physical examination [125]. Chest X-rays should be rapidly obtained to determine the presence of a tumor, or indirect evidence of obstruction such as tracheal deviation or airway narrowing, although CT scanning is preferred. Pulse oximetry will aid in determining the degree of hypoxemia. Bronchoscopy allows for direct visualization of the obstruction, as well as providing a method for obtaining tissue for diagnosis and immediate treatment [38, 124, 125]. This must be done in a controlled setting as bronchoscopy can further increase the obstruction and the accompanying anesthesia may also decrease the gas exchange.

Treatment

The mainstay of treatment is stenting via bronchoscopy, which also aids in diagnosis. Rigid bronchoscopy is preferred for significant airway obstruction, as it allows for placement of metallic self-expanding stents that are particularly useful for cases of extrinsic airway compression or to tamponade a bleeding lesion. Stents are the treatment of choice in acute airway obstruction due to extrinsic tumor compression [126] or in patients with tracheoesophageal fistulas [127]. Neodymium yttrium (Nd:YAG) or CO_2 lasers can be used to open the airway as well [38, 128] but the effects tend to be transient and some other form of more definitive tumor control should follow, such as radiation or chemotherapy [38, 125, 129–131].

Chemotherapeutic Emergencies

Extravasation of Chemotherapy

Pathophysiology

Extravasation is the unintended leakage of a chemotherapy drug into the extravascular space. Vesicants, including the anthracyclines, vinca alkaloids, and mitomycin C, are chemotherapy agents that have the ability to induce tissue necrosis, resulting in functional impairment and disfigurement. Irritants, such as the platinum compounds, taxanes, and topoisomerase I inhibitors, cause an inflammatory reaction rather than tissue necrosis, although this classification is not absolute because the severity of tissue injury is dependent on drug concentration and volume [132]. Recent reports suggest as many as 3% of patients receiving IV fosaprepitant may have a local injection site reaction [133].

Presentation

Signs and symptoms of pain, blistering, and induration may occur immediately after the incident or develop in days or weeks. Ulceration may be delayed and continue to worsen for months. In severe cases, necrosis of the skin and the underlying tissues may develop, leading to infection, scars, treatment delay, functional deficits, amputation, and, rarely, death [126, 128, 129, 134, 135]. In the case of irritant extravasation, symptoms include erythema, swelling, and tenderness. Phlebitis, hyperpigmentation, and sclerosis can subsequently develop along the vein, but these symptoms usually resolve within weeks and long-term sequelae are extremely rare. Factors that increase the risk of extravasation include small or deep veins, damaged veins secondary to multiple venipunctures, impaired neurologic ability to detect changes in sensation, obesity, and movement during chemotherapy administration [126,129,135].

Diagnosis

A change in the rate of infusion or absence of blood return from the vascular access device may be the initial sign, followed by leakage of fluid around the IV site, pain, erythema, and swelling.

Treatment

Prevention through careful chemotherapy administration is the most effective approach. Once extravasation is suspected, even if asymptomatic, the infusion should be discontinued immediately and the affected limb elevated [126,129,134]. The access device should not be removed, but rather should be used to attempt to aspirate fluid from the area [131]. The next step of treatment is dependent on the specific drug and, in many cases, remains controversial. Application of ice to the affected area is recommended for extravasation of most vesicants and irritant drugs, as the cooling causes vasoconstriction to reduce the extent of local injury and also reduce pain [129]. Cold is contraindicated for vinca alkaloids and epipodophyllotoxins, as this worsens the ulceration in animal models [129,135] and heat is recommended to increase perfusion, theoretically enhancing removal of these drugs [126,135].

Non-surgical treatment modalities have been investigated in vesicant extravasation, mainly in animal studies or in studies without a control arm. Although agents such as topical or injected dimethyl sulfoxide, hyaluronidase, and corticosteroids are used, only dexrazoxane has been FDA approved for the treatment of extravasation resulting from anthracycline therapy [132].

Anaphylactic Reactions to Chemotherapy

Essentially any chemotherapeutic agent has the potential to cause infusion reactions, which can range significantly in severity. Anaphylaxis is rare with most conventional cytotoxic agents, although it is well recognized with the taxanes and the platinums, especially after multiple exposures to the latter [136]. Carboplatin hypersensitivity is seen in up to 16% of the gynecologic oncology population [137,138].

Presentation

Anaphylactic reactions caused by chemotherapeutic agents present with the same variety of signs and symptoms as do anaphylactic reactions secondary to other medications. Urticaria and angioedema are most common (up to 90% of cases), followed by respiratory symptoms such as wheezing and dyspnea (up to 70% of cases). Gastrointestinal complaints of abdominal pain, diarrhea, or emesis, and cardiovascular events like hypotension and syncope occur in up to 35% of cases [136,139,140].

Anaphylaxis may occur in response to the drug vehicle rather than the chemotherapeutic agent itself. Acute reactions

to paclitaxel and docetaxel tend to present shortly after the infusion is initiated, and nearly 95% of cases develop within the first two cycles of therapy [141,142]. Paclitaxel is formulated with Cremophor, a polyethoxylated castor oil that is also used to deliver drugs such as ixabepilone, diazepam, and vitamin K [143]. Paclitaxel should be avoided in patients who had a severe reaction to one of these drugs. Abraxane (nanoparticle albumin-bound paclitaxel) can be used in patients who have reactions to Cremophor [144]. Docetaxel, like IV etoposide, is formulated with polysorbate-80, a vehicle to which reactions can include chest discomfort, bronchospasm, and angioedema [145].

Treatment

In mild infusion reactions, without any features of anaphylaxis, the infusion should be temporarily discontinued until proper evaluation of the patient has occurred. Diphenhydramine (50 mg IV) can help relieve mild symptoms. The infusion can be restarted at a slow rate with close monitoring. In cases of anaphylaxis, the infusion should be discontinued immediately, with subsequent treatment identical to management of other causes of anaphylaxis. Close assessment of airway, breathing, and circulation should occur. Administration of epinephrine (intramuscular; 0.3–0.5 mg, 1:1000) should be given immediately and can be repeated every 3–5 min as necessary. Patients should also be given oxygen and IV fluids. Antihistamines and glucocorticoids can be helpful. Epinephrine infusions, vasopressors, and glucagon may be necessary if the patient is refractory to these initial therapies.

Hematologic Emergencies

Hyperleukocytosis and Leukostasis

Hyperleukocytosis describes a laboratory abnormality of elevated leukocyte count (arbitrarily defined as > 100 ×10⁹/L) that may or may not be associated with a medical emergency (leukostasis/blast crisis). Leukostasis represents end-organ dysfunction as a result of impaired tissue perfusion due to increased viscosity and impaired flow through the microvasculature. Altered tissue perfusion is dependent on multiple factors (e.g. phenotype of leukemia, blast characteristics) and cannot necessarily be predicted based on the leukocyte count alone. Leukostasis is seen more commonly in patients with acute myeloid leukemia or chronic myeloid leukemia (CML) in blast phase. In contrast, patients with chronic lymphocytic leukemia can have extremely elevated leukocyte counts (>400 × 10⁹/L) and remain asymptomatic. It is critical to recognize and rapidly treat leukostasis to prevent devastating complications such as CNS injury, respiratory failure, and visual loss [146].

Pathophysiology

The pathophysiology appears to be a result of interplay between the volume of leukocytes/blasts (leukocrit), characteristics such as expression of adhesion molecules (more common in myeloid leukemias), and endothelial interactions. Leukostasis in the absence of significant leukocytosis has occasionally been described, emphasizing the potential importance of leukocyte–endothelium interactions. The reduced pliability of large myeloid blasts may also contribute to microvascular occlusion. Local tissue hypoxemia can be aggravated by the high metabolic requirement of leukemic blasts combined with cytokine-induced tissue damage.

Presentation/Diagnosis

Hyperleukocytosis occurs in approximately 5–15% of patients presenting with acute myeloid leukemia, more commonly in M4, M5 and the microgranular variant of acute promyelocytic leukemia [147]. Leukostasis is more likely if the leukocyte count and especially if the blast count is $> 100 \times 10^9$/L.

Hyperleukocytosis occurs in approximately 10–30% of patients with acute lymphoblastic leukemia, most commonly in male infants and adolescents and those with T cell phenotype or high-risk cytogenetics such as t(4;11) and t(9;22). Hyperleukocytosis is relatively common in chronic lymphocytic leukemia and CML in chronic phase; however, leukostasis is relatively rare except in the presence of CML with myeloid blast crisis.

Patients presenting with leukostasis are typically acutely ill, due to impaired organ perfusion. Symptoms most commonly result from involvement of the brain, lungs, and eyes and most early deaths result from intracranial bleeding (40%) or respiratory failure (30%). It is imperative to recognize and intervene quickly, as mortality can be up to 40% without appropriate intervention. Patients are often febrile and may have major metabolic derangements and/or coexistent coagulopathy related to thrombocytopenia or disseminated intravascular coagulation (40%), spontaneous tumor lysis (10%), or infection complicating the presentation.

Respiratory involvement can range from mild dyspnea to florid respiratory failure. Common findings include fever (80%) and interstitial or alveolar pulmonary infiltrates, which can coexist with pneumonia. Typically, such patients are treated empirically for infection while awaiting the results of additional investigations such as blood cultures and the response to myelosuppressive therapy and leukapheresis. Neurological signs include headache, visual changes, dizziness, tinnitus, and altered mental status ranging from mild confusion to coma. Other manifestations may include myocardial, bowel, or limb ischemia, or occasionally priapism.

Diagnostic pitfalls can include spuriously low results from direct measurement of arterial pO_2 due to oxygen consumption by metabolically active leukocytes after the specimen is drawn (pulse oximetry may be more accurate) and pseudohyperkalemia due to potassium leakage from leukocytes in transit (plasma potassium will be more accurate than serum potassium). Overestimation of the platelet count can also occur by automated counters due to leukocyte fragments being erroneously counted as platelets. In this setting, manual review of the smear can more accurately assess platelet count.

Treatment

Effective therapy of leukostasis requires a high index of suspicion, rapid and effective initial cytoreduction, and institution of definitive therapy as soon as possible. The choice of initial cytoreduction may depend on the situation. In a patient presenting de novo with leukostasis, initial leukapheresis and hydroxyurea are frequently used while the leukemia is further

characterized [148]. Leukapheresis should reduce the blast count by 30–50% and may help reduce the risk of devastating tumor lysis by physical removal of the blasts. It must be accompanied by myelosuppressive therapy [149,150], initially hydroxyurea (e.g. 1.5–2.5 g every 6 h, maximum dose usually 8–10 g/day for a couple of days) and subsequently definitive lineage-specific chemotherapy once the diagnosis is established. High doses of hydroxyurea may not be well tolerated due to nausea and emesis, which can complicate management.

Patients with leukostasis are also at risk for disseminated intravascular coagulopathy and TLS, which may worsen after chemotherapy. Aggressive hydration, electrolyte monitoring, allopurinol, and possibly rasburicase can be helpful. Platelet transfusions may need to be used liberally given the potential for devastating hemorrhage and worsening thrombocytopenia. In patients with symptomatic leukostasis there is concern that rapid increases in viscosity associated with packed red cell transfusions could potentially exacerbate the situation and this should be administered cautiously, typically during or after leukapheresis. Specific chemotherapy should be instituted as soon as possible, as this is likely to have the greatest impact on survival. The role of cranial and pulmonary radiation in symptomatic patients is controversial and typically not used, but may be a consideration in circumstances where rapid access to leukapheresis is not available in a rapidly decompensating patient.

Hyperviscosity

Hyperviscosity typically results from excessive accumulation of monoclonal proteins in the context of a dysproteinemic disorder.

Pathophysiology

The likelihood of hyperviscosity depends on the amount of the protein in addition to its characteristics; the high molecular weight and pentameric structure of IgM is much more likely to result in clinically relevant increases in viscosity (85–90% of cases of hyperviscosity occur in Waldenström's macroglobulinemia). Rarely, overproduction of other proteins such as IgA or, less likely, IgG or kappa light chains [151] can also be responsible.

Presentation/Diagnosis

Hyperviscosity causes symptoms by compromising the microcirculation of critical organs, frequently the brain and eye, resulting in symptoms such as fatigue, dizziness, visual, or hearing loss, altered mental status and progressing to confusion, seizures, and coma. Altered platelet function can lead to mucosal and retinal hemorrhages. Ultimately, end-organ failure including cardiac and renal failure can result. The diagnosis is confirmed by measuring serum viscosity. A normal value is usually 1.4–1.8 centipoise (cP); values < 3 cP are rarely associated with symptoms, and typically symptoms begin at values > 5 cP, which often correlates with IgM levels > 4 g/dL. Almost all patients with values > 10 cP will be symptomatic.

Treatment

For patients presenting with symptomatic hyperviscosity, especially with neurologic manifestations, emergency plasmapheresis is indicated to rapidly reduce the serum viscosity [152]. IgM is predominantly intravascular and tends to respond better to plasmapheresis compared to other smaller monoclonal proteins such as IgA and IgG which redistribute from the extravascular space. Definitive therapy of the underlying plasma cell disorder should commence promptly as plasmapheresis is only a tempo-

rizing measure. The choice of definitive therapy will depend on contemporary recommendations but for de novo Waldenström's disease presenting with hyperviscosity, plasmapheresis followed by initiation of a rituximab- and/or bendamustine-containing regimen could be considered [153,154].

References

1 Kuderer NM, Dale DC, Crawford J, Cosler LE, Lyman GH. Mortality, morbidity, and cost associated with febrile neutropenia in adult cancer patients. *Cancer* 2006;106(10):2258–66.

2 Halfdanarson TR, Hogan WJ, Moynihan TJ. Oncologic emergencies: diagnosis and treatment. *Mayo Clin Proc* 2006;81(6):835–48.

3 Lugtenburg P, Silvestre AS, Rossi FG, *et al.* Impact of age group on febrile neutropenia risk assessment and management in patients with diffuse large B-cell lymphoma treated with R-CHOP regimens. *Clin Lymphoma Myeloma Leuk* 2012;12(5):297–305.

4 Lyman GH, Kuderer NM, Crawford J, *et al.* Predicting individual risk of neutropenic complications in patients receiving cancer chemotherapy. *Cancer* 2011;117(9):1917–27.

5 Ramphal R. Changes in the etiology of bacteremia in febrile neutropenic patients and the susceptibilities of the currently isolated pathogens. *Clin Infect Dis* 2004;39(Suppl 1):S25–31.

6 Zinner SH. Changing epidemiology of infections in patients with neutropenia and cancer: emphasis on gram-positive and resistant bacteria. *Clin Infect Dis* 1999;29(3):490–4.

7 Kanamaru A, Tatsumi Y. Microbiological data for patients with febrile neutropenia. *Clin Infect Dis* 2004;39 Suppl 1:S7–S10.

8 Hughes WT, Armstrong D, Bodey GP, *et al.* 2002 guidelines for the use of antimicrobial agents in neutropenic patients with cancer. *Clin Infect Dis* 2002;34(6):730–51.

9 Bodey GP, Buckley M, Sathe YS, Freireich EJ. Quantitative relationships between circulating leukocytes and infection in patients with acute leukemia. *Ann Intern Med* 1966;64(2):328–40.

10 Raad I, Hanna HA, Alakech B, *et al.* Differential time to positivity: a useful method for diagnosing catheter-related bloodstream infections. *Ann Intern Med* 2004;140(1):18–25.

11 Talcott JA, Siegel RD, Finberg R, Goldman L. Risk assessment in cancer patients with fever and neutropenia: a prospective, two-center validation of a prediction rule. *J Clin Oncol* 1992;10(2):316–22.

12 Klastersky J, Paesmans M, Rubenstein EB, *et al.* The Multinational Association for Supportive Care in Cancer risk index: a multinational scoring system for identifying low-risk febrile neutropenic cancer patients. *J Clin Oncol* 2000;18(16):3038–51.

13 Klastersky J, Paesmans M, Georgala A, *et al.* Outpatient oral antibiotics for febrile neutropenic cancer patients using a score predictive for complications. *J Clin Oncol* 2006;24(25):4129–34.

14 Flowers CR, Seidenfeld J, Bow EJ, *et al.* Antimicrobial prophylaxis and outpatient management of fever and neutropenia in adults treated for malignancy: American Society of Clinical Oncology clinical practice guideline. *J Clin Oncol* 2013;31(6):794–810.

15 NCCN Clinical Practice Guidelines in Oncology: Prevention and treatment of cancer-related infections, Version 1.2017. December 21, 2016 (cited 4 January 2017).

16 Freifeld AG, Bow EJ, Sepkowitz KA, *et al.* Clinical practice guideline for the use of antimicrobial agents in neutropenic patients with cancer: 2010 update by the Infectious Diseases Society of America. *Clin Infect Dis* 2010;52(4):427–31.

17 Wright JD, Neugut AI, Ananth CV, *et al.* Deviations from guideline-based therapy for febrile neutropenia in cancer patients and their effect on outcomes. *JAMA Inter Med* 2013;173(7):559–68.

18 Raad I, Kassar R, Ghannam D, *et al.* Management of the catheter in documented catheter-related coagulase-negative staphylococcal bacteremia: remove or retain? *Clin Infect Dis* 2009;49(8):1187–94.

19 Smith TJ, Khatcheressian J, Lyman GH, *et al.* 2006 update of recommendations for the use of white blood cell growth factors: an evidence-based clinical practice guideline. *J Clin Oncol* 2006;24(19):3187–205.

20 Aapro MS, Bohlius J, Cameron DA, *et al.* 2010 update of EORTC guidelines for the use of granulocyte-colony stimulating factor to reduce the incidence of chemotherapy-induced febrile neutropenia in adult patients with lymphoproliferative disorders and solid tumours. *Eur J Cancer* 2010;47(1):8–32.

21 Lee JJ, Chung IJ, Park MR, *et al.* Clinical efficacy of granulocyte transfusion therapy in patients with neutropenia-related infections. *Leukemia* 2001;15(2):203–7.

22 Loblaw DA, Laperriere NJ, Mackillop WJ. A population-based study of malignant spinal cord compression in Ontario. *Clin Oncol* 2003;15(4):211–7.

23 Abrahm JL, Banffy MB, Harris MB. Spinal cord compression in patients with advanced metastatic cancer: "all I care about is walking and living my life". *JAMA* 2008;299(8):937–46.

24 Schiff D. Spinal cord compression. *Neurol Clin* 2003;21(1):67–86, viii.

25 Schiff D, O'Neill BP, Suman VJ. Spinal epidural metastasis as the initial manifestation of malignancy: clinical features and diagnostic approach. *Neurology* 1997;49(2):452–6.

26 Prasad D, Schiff D. Malignant spinal-cord compression. *Lancet Oncol* 2005;6(1):15–24.

27 Gilbert RW, Kim JH, Posner JB. Epidural spinal cord compression from metastatic tumor: diagnosis and treatment. *Ann Neurol* 1978;3(1):40–51.

28 Cole JS, Patchell RA. Metastatic epidural spinal cord compression. *Lancet Neurol* 2008;7(5):459–66.

29 Kwok Y, Tibbs PA, Patchell RA. Clinical approach to metastatic epidural spinal cord compression. *Hematol Oncol Clin North Am* 2006;20(6):1297–305.

30 Maranzano E, Latini P. Effectiveness of radiation therapy without surgery in metastatic spinal cord compression: final

results from a prospective trial. *Int J Radiat Oncol Biol Phys* 1995;32(4):959–67.

31 Bach F, Larsen BH, Rohde K, *et al.* Metastatic spinal cord compression. Occurrence, symptoms, clinical presentations and prognosis in 398 patients with spinal cord compression. *Acta Neurochir (Wien)* 1990;107(1–2):37–43.

32 Kim RY, Spencer SA, Meredith RF, *et al.* Extradural spinal cord compression: analysis of factors determining functional prognosis–prospective study. *Radiology* 1990;176(1):279–82.

33 Martenson JA, Jr., Evans RG, Lie MR, *et al.* Treatment outcome and complications in patients treated for malignant epidural spinal cord compression (SCC). *Journal of neuro-oncology.* 1985;3(1):77–84.

34 Deyo RA, Rainville J, Kent DL. What can the history and physical examination tell us about low back pain? *JAMA* 1992;268(6):760–5.

35 Li KC, Poon PY. Sensitivity and specificity of MRI in detecting malignant spinal cord compression and in distinguishing malignant from benign compression fractures of vertebrae. *Magn Reson Imaging* 1988;6(5):547–56.

36 Yuh WT, Zachar CK, Barloon TJ, *et al.* Vertebral compression fractures: distinction between benign and malignant causes with MR imaging. *Radiology* 1989;172(1):215–8.

37 van der Sande JJ, Kroger R, Boogerd W. Multiple spinal epidural metastases; an unexpectedly frequent finding. *J Neurol Neurosurg Psych* 1990;53(11):1001–3.

38 Behl D, Hendrickson AW, Moynihan TJ. Oncologic emergencies. *Crit Care Clin* 2010;26(1):181–205.

39 Graham PH, Capp A, Delaney G, *et al.* A pilot randomised comparison of dexamethasone 96 mg vs 16 mg per day for malignant spinal-cord compression treated by radiotherapy: TROG 01.05 Superdex study. *Clin Oncol* 2006;18(1):70–6.

40 Sorensen S, Helweg-Larsen S, Mouridsen H, Hansen HH. Effect of high-dose dexamethasone in carcinomatous metastatic spinal cord compression treated with radiotherapy: a randomised trial. *Eur J Cancer* 1994;30A(1):22–7.

41 Vecht CJ, Haaxma-Reiche H, van Putten WL, *et al.* Initial bolus of conventional versus high-dose dexamethasone in metastatic spinal cord compression. *Neurology* 1989;39(9):1255–7.

42 Patchell RA, Tibbs PA, Regine WF, *et al.* Direct decompressive surgical resection in the treatment of spinal cord compression caused by metastatic cancer: a randomised trial. *Lancet* 2005;366(9486):643–8.

43 Klimo P, Jr., Thompson CJ, Kestle JR, Schmidt MH. A meta-analysis of surgery versus conventional radiotherapy for the treatment of metastatic spinal epidural disease. *Neuro-oncology* 2005;7(1):64–76.

44 Chi JH, Gokaslan Z, McCormick P, *et al.* Selecting treatment for patients with malignant epidural spinal cord compression-does age matter?: results from a randomized clinical trial. *Spine* 2009;34(5):431–5.

45 Fisher CG, DiPaola CP, Ryken TC, *et al.* A novel classification system for spinal instability in neoplastic disease: an evidence-based approach and expert consensus from the Spine Oncology Study Group. *Spine* 2010;35(22):E1221–9.

46 Gerszten PC, Burton SA, Ozhasoglu C, Welch WC. Radiosurgery for spinal metastases: clinical experience in 500 cases from a single institution. *Spine* 2007;32(2):193–9.

47 Ushio Y, Posner R, Posner JB, Shapiro WR. Experimental spinal cord compression by epidural neoplasm. *Neurology* 1977;27(5):422–9.

48 Rades D, Karstens JH, Hoskin PJ, *et al.* Escalation of radiation dose beyond 30 Gy in 10 fractions for metastatic spinal cord compression. *Int J Radiat Oncol Biol Phys* 2007;67(2):525–31.

49 Rades D, Stalpers LJ, Veninga T, *et al.* Evaluation of five radiation schedules and prognostic factors for metastatic spinal cord compression. *J Clin Oncol* 2005;23(15):3366–75.

50 Yamada Y, Bilsky MH, Lovelock DM, *et al.* High-dose, single-fraction image-guided intensity-modulated radiotherapy for metastatic spinal lesions. *Int J Radiat Oncol Biol Phys* 2008;71(2):484–90.

51 Moulding HD, Elder JB, Lis E, *et al.* Local disease control after decompressive surgery and adjuvant high-dose single-fraction radiosurgery for spine metastases. *J Neurosurg Spine* 2010;13(1):87–93.

52 Posner JB. Management of brain metastases. *Rev Neurol (Paris)* 1992;148(6–7):477–87.

53 Barnholtz-Sloan JS, Sloan AE, Davis FG, *et al.* Incidence proportions of brain metastases in patients diagnosed (1973 to 2001) in the Metropolitan Detroit Cancer Surveillance System. *J Clin Oncol* 2004;22(14):2865–72.

54 Schouten LJ, Rutten J, Huveneers HA, Twijnstra A. Incidence of brain metastases in a cohort of patients with carcinoma of the breast, colon, kidney, and lung and melanoma. *Cancer* 2002;94(10):2698–705.

55 Patchell RA. The management of brain metastases. *Cancer Treat Rev* 2003;29(6):533–40.

56 Posner JB, Chernik NL. Intracranial metastases from systemic cancer. *Adv Neurol* 1978;19:579–92.

57 Wen PY BP, Loeffler JS. Treatment of metastatic cancer. In: VT DeVita Jr, TS Lawrence, SA Rosenberg (eds) *Cancer: Principles and Practice of Oncology*, 6th edn. Philadelphia: Lippincott Williams & Wilkins, 2001:2655–70.

58 Nutt SH, Patchell RA. Intracranial hemorrhage associated with primary and secondary tumors. *Neurosurg Clin N Am* 1992;3(3):591–9.

59 Tosoni A, Ermani M, Brandes AA. The pathogenesis and treatment of brain metastases: a comprehensive review. *Crit Rev Oncol Hematol* 2004;52(3):199–215.

60 Ay I, Francis JW, Brown RH, Jr. VEGF increases blood-brain barrier permeability to Evans blue dye and tetanus toxin fragment C but not adeno-associated virus in ALS mice. *Brain Res* 2008;1234:198–205.

61 Argawa AT, Gurfeina BT, Zhanga Y, Zameera A, Johna GR. VEGF-mediated disruption of endothelial CLN-5 promotes blood-brain barrier breakdown *Proc Natl Acad Sci USA* 2009;106(6):1977–82.

62 Forsyth PA, Posner JB. Headaches in patients with brain tumors: a study of 111 patients. *Neurology* 1993;43(9):1678–83.

63 Davis PC, Hudgins PA, Peterman SB, Hoffman JC, Jr. Diagnosis of cerebral metastases: double-dose delayed CT vs contrast-enhanced MR imaging. *Am J Neuroradiol* 1991;12(2):293–300.

64 Schaefer PW, Budzik RF, Jr., Gonzalez RG. Imaging of cerebral metastases. *Neurosurg Clin N Am* 1996;7(3):393–423.

65 Lee EL, Armstrong TS. Increased intracranial pressure. *Clin J Oncol Nurs* 2008;12(1):37–41.

66 Alberti E, Hartmann A, Schutz HJ, Schreckenberger F. The effect of large doses of dexamethasone on the cerebrospinal fluid pressure in patients with supratentorial tumors. *J Neurol* 1978;217(3):173–81.

67 Jarden JO, Dhawan V, Moeller JR, Strother SC, Rottenberg DA. The time course of steroid action on blood-to-brain and blood-to-tumor transport of 82Rb: a positron emission tomographic study. *Ann Neurol* 1989;25(3):239–45.

68 Kim H, Lee JM, Park JS, *et al.* Dexamethasone coordinately regulates angiopoietin-1 and VEGF: a mechanism of glucocorticoid-induced stabilization of blood-brain barrier. *Biochem Biophys Res Commun* 2008;372(1):243–8.

69 Peacock KH, Lesser GJ. Current therapeutic approaches in patients with brain metastases. *Curr Treat Options Oncol* 2006;7(6):479–89.

70 Tsao MN, Lloyd N, Wong RKS, *et al.* Whole brain radiotherapy for the treatment of newly diagnosed multiple brain metastases. *Cochrane Database Syst Rev* 2012(4):CD003869.

71 Levin VA, Bidaut L, Hou P, *et al.* Randomized double-blind placebo-controlled trial of bevacizumab therapy for radiation necrosis of the central nervous system. *Int J Radiat Oncol Biol Phys* 2011;79(5):1487–95.

72 Sirven JI, Wingerchuk DM, Drazkowski JF, Lyons MK, Zimmerman RS. Seizure prophylaxis in patients with brain tumors: a meta-analysis. *Mayo Clin Proc* 2004;79(12):1489–94.

73 Vassilopoulou-Sellin R, Newman BM, Taylor SH, Guinee VF. Incidence of hypercalcemia in patients with malignancy referred to a comprehensive cancer center. *Cancer* 1993;71(4):1309–12.

74 Sargent JT, Smith OP. Haematological emergencies managing hypercalcaemia in adults and children with haematological disorders. *Br J Haematol* 2010;149(4):465–77.

75 Ralston SH, Gallacher SJ, Patel U, Campbell J, Boyle IT. Cancer-associated hypercalcemia: morbidity and mortality. Clinical experience in 126 treated patients. *Ann Intern Med* 1990;112(7):499–504.

76 Stewart AF. Clinical practice. Hypercalcemia associated with cancer. *N Engl J Med* 2005;352(4):373–9.

77 Tanvetyanon T, Stiff PJ. Management of the adverse effects associated with intravenous bisphosphonates. *Ann Oncol* 2006;17(6):897–907.

78 Kacprowicz RF, Lloyd JD. Electrolyte complications of malignancy. *Emerg Med Clin North Am* 2009;27(2):257–69.

79 Kyle RA, Yee GC, Somerfield MR, *et al.* American Society of Clinical Oncology 2007 clinical practice guideline update on the role of bisphosphonates in multiple myeloma. *J Clin Oncol* 2007;25(17):2464–72.

80 Wang CC, Chen YC, Shiang JC, *et al.* Hypercalcemic crisis successfully treated with prompt calcium-free hemodialysis. *Am J Emerg Med* 2009;27(9):1174 e1–3.

81 Pelosof LC, Gerber DE. Paraneoplastic syndromes: an approach to diagnosis and treatment. *Mayo Clin Proc* 2010;85(9):838–54.

82 Davidson TG. Conventional treatment of hypercalcemia of malignancy. *Am J Health Syst Pharm* 2001;58 Suppl 3:S8–15.

83 Porcel SL, Cumplido JA, de la Hoz B, Cuevas M, Losada E. Anaphylaxis to calcitonin. *Allergol Immunopathol (Madr)* 2000;28(4):243–5.

84 Lee RJ, Saylor PJ, Smith MR. Treatment and prevention of bone complications from prostate cancer. *Bone* 2011;48(1):88–95.

85 Lumachi F, Brunello A, Roma A, Basso U. Cancer-induced hypercalcemia. *Anticancer Res* 2009;29(5):1551–5.

86 Boikos SA, Hammers HJ. Denosumab for the treatment of bisphosphonate-refractory hypercalcemia. *J Clin Oncol* 2012;30(29):e299.

87 Hu MI, Glezerman IG, Leboulleux S, *et al.* Denosumab for treatment of hypercalcemia of malignancy. *J Clin Endocrinol Metab* 2014 Sep;99(9):3144–52. doi: 10.1210/jc.2014-1001. Epub 2014 Jun 10.

88 Sternlicht H, Glezerman IG. Hypercalcemia of malignancy and new treatment options. *Ther Clin Risk Manag* 2015;11:1779–88.

89 Onitilo AA, Kio E, Doi SA. Tumor-related hyponatremia. *Clin Med Res* 2007;5(4):228–37.

90 Raftopoulos H. Diagnosis and management of hyponatremia in cancer patients. *Supp Care Cancer* 2007;15(12):1341–7.

91 Hamdi T, Latta S, Jallad B, *et al.* Cisplatin-induced renal salt wasting syndrome. *South Med J* 2010;103(8):793–9.

92 Jayachandran NV, Chandrasekhara PK, Thomas J, Agrawal S, Narsimulu G. Cyclophosphamide-associated complications: we need to be aware of SIADH and central pontine myelinolysis. *Rheumatology (Oxford)* 2009;48(1):89–90.

93 Kirch C, Gachot B, Germann N, Blot F, Nitenberg G. Recurrent ifosfamide-induced hyponatraemia. *Eur J Cancer* 1997;33(14):2438–9.

94 Ginsberg SJ, Comis RL, Fitzpatrick AV. Vinblastine and inappropriate ADH secretion. *N Engl J Med* 1977; 296(16):941.

95 Liapis K, Apostolidis J, Charitaki E, *et al.* Syndrome of inappropriate secretion of antidiuretic hormone associated with imatinib. *Ann Pharmacother* 2008;42(12):1882–6.

96 Sherlock M, Thompson CJ. The syndrome of inappropriate antidiuretic hormone: current and future management options. *Eur J Endocrinol* 2010;162(Suppl 1):S13–8.

97 Ellison DH, Berl T. Clinical practice. The syndrome of inappropriate antidiuresis. *N Engl J Med* 2007;356(20):2064–72.

98 Reddy P, Mooradian AD. Diagnosis and management of hyponatraemia in hospitalised patients. *Int J Clin Pract* 2009;63(10):1494–508.

99 Adrogue HJ. Consequences of inadequate management of hyponatremia. *Am J Nephrol* 2005;25(3):240–9.

100 Ghali JK. Mechanisms, risks, and new treatment options for hyponatremia. *Cardiology* 2008;111(3):147–57.

101 Ghali JK, Hamad B, Yasothan U, Kirkpatrick P. Tolvaptan. *Nat Rev Drug Discov* 2009;8(8):611–2.

102 Velez JC, Dopson SJ, Sanders DS, Delay TA, Arthur JM. Intravenous conivaptan for the treatment of hyponatraemia caused by the syndrome of inappropriate secretion of antidiuretic hormone in hospitalized patients: a single-centre experience. *Nephrol Dial Transplant* 2010;25(5):1524–31.

103 Gross P. Clinical management of SIADH. *Ther Adv Endocrinol Metab* 2012;3(2):61–73.

104 Tufan A, Unal N, Koca E, *et al.* Spontaneous tumor lysis syndrome in a patient with diffuse large B cell lymphoma and Richter syndrome. *Ann Hematol* 2006;85(3):183–4.

105 Gemici C. Tumour lysis syndrome in solid tumours. *Clin Oncol* 2006;18(10):773–80.

106 Kallab AM, Jillella AP. Tumor lysis syndrome in small cell lung cancer. *Med Oncol* 2001;18(2):149–51.

107 Pentheroudakis G, O'Neill VJ, Vasey P, Kaye SB. Spontaneous acute tumour lysis syndrome in patients with metastatic germ cell tumours. Report of two cases. *Supp Care Cancer* 2001;9(7):554–7.

108 Cairo MS, Bishop M. Tumour lysis syndrome: new therapeutic strategies and classification. *Br J Haematol* 2004;127(1):3–11.

109 Cairo MS, Coiffier B, Reiter A, Younes A. Recommendations for the evaluation of risk and prophylaxis of tumour lysis syndrome (TLS) in adults and children with malignant diseases: an expert TLS panel consensus. *Br J Haematol* 2010;149(4):578–86.

110 Spina M, Nagy Z, Ribera JM, *et al.* FLORENCE: a randomized, double-blind, phase III pivotal study of febuxostat versus allopurinol for the prevention of tumor lysis syndrome (TLS) in patients with hematologic malignancies at intermediate to high TLS risk. *Ann Oncol* 2015;26(10):2155–61.

111 Cortes J, Moore JO, Maziarz RT, *et al.* Control of plasma uric acid in adults at risk for tumor Lysis syndrome: efficacy and safety of rasburicase alone and rasburicase followed by allopurinol compared with allopurinol alone–results of a multicenter phase III study. *J Clin Oncol* 2010;28(27):4207–13.

112 Ngugi NN, McLigeyo SO, Kayima JK. Treatment of hyperkalaemia by altering the transcellular gradient in patients with renal failure: effect of various therapeutic approaches. *East Afr Med J* 1997;74(8):503–9.

113 Allon M, Dunlay R, Copkney C. Nebulized albuterol for acute hyperkalemia in patients on hemodialysis. *Ann Intern Med* 1989;110(6):426–9.

114 Rampello E, Fricia T, Malaguarnera M. The management of tumor lysis syndrome. *Nat Clin Pract Oncol* 2006;3(8):438–47.

115 Maisch B, Ristic A, Pankuweit S. Evaluation and management of pericardial effusion in patients with neoplastic disease. *Prog Cardiovasc Dis* 2010;53(2):157–63.

116 Spodick DH. Acute cardiac tamponade. *N Engl J Med* 2003;349(7):684–90.

117 Sternbach G. Claude Beck: cardiac compression triads. *J Emerg Med* 1988;6(5):417–9.

118 Jacob S, Sebastian JC, Cherian PK, Abraham A, John SK. Pericardial effusion impending tamponade: a look beyond Beck's triad. *Am J Emerg Med* 2009;27(2):216–9.

119 Shabetai R, Fowler NO, Fenton JC, Masangkay M. Pulsus paradoxus. *J Clin Invest* 1965;44(11):1882–98.

120 Tsang TS, Enriquez-Sarano M, Freeman WK, *et al.* Consecutive 1127 therapeutic echocardiographically guided pericardiocenteses: clinical profile, practice patterns, and outcomes spanning 21 years. *Mayo Clin Proc* 2002;77(5):429–36.

121 Cooper JP, Oliver RM, Currie P, Walker JM, Swanton RH. How do the clinical findings in patients with pericardial effusions influence the success of aspiration? *Br Heart J* 1995;73(4):351–4.

122 Ganeshan A, Hon LQ, Warakaulle DR, Morgan R, Uberoi R. Superior vena caval stenting for SVC obstruction: current status. *Eur J Radiol* 2009;71(2):343–9.

123 Schraufnagel DE, Hill R, Leech JA, Pare JA. Superior vena caval obstruction. Is it a medical emergency? *Am J Med* 1981;70(6):1169–74.

124 Lemaire A, Burfeind WR, Toloza E, *et al.* Outcomes of tracheobronchial stents in patients with malignant airway disease. *Ann Thorac Surg* 2005;80(2):434–7; discussion 7–8.

125 Suh JH, Dass KK, Pagliaccio L, *et al.* Endobronchial radiation therapy with or without neodymium yttrium aluminum garnet laser resection for managing malignant airway obstruction. *Cancer* 1994;73(10):2583–8.

126 Langer SW. Extravasation of chemotherapy. *Curr Oncol Rep* 2010;12(4):242–6.

127 Berghammer P, Pohnl R, Baur M, Dittrich C. Docetaxel extravasation. *Supp Care Cancer* 2001;9(2):131–4.

128 Langer SW, Sehested M, Jensen PB. Treatment of anthracycline extravasation with dexrazoxane. *Clin Cancer Res* 2000;6(9):3680–6.

129 Bertelli G. Prevention and management of extravasation of cytotoxic drugs. *Drug Saf* 1995;12(4):245–55.

130 Jacobson JO, Polovich M, McNiff KK, *et al.* American Society of Clinical Oncology/Oncology Nursing Society chemotherapy administration safety standards. *Oncol Nurs Forum* 2009;36(6):651–8.

131 Wengstrom Y, Margulies A. European Oncology Nursing Society extravasation guidelines. *Eur J Oncol Nurs* 2008;12(4):357–61.

132 Mouridsen HT, Langer SW, Buter J, *et al.* Treatment of anthracycline extravasation with Savene (dexrazoxane): results from two prospective clinical multicentre studies. *Ann Oncol* 2007;18(3):546–50.

133 Canada MF. Product monograph: Emend IV (fosaprepitant). 2012 Jan 30.

134 Schulmeister L. Preventing and managing vesicant chemotherapy extravasations. *J Support Oncol* 2010;8(5):212–5.

135 Dorr RT, Alberts DS. Vinca alkaloid skin toxicity: antidote and drug disposition studies in the mouse. *J Natl Cancer Inst* 1985;74(1):113–20.

136 Sampson HA, Munoz-Furlong A, Campbell RL, *et al.* Second symposium on the definition and management of anaphylaxis: summary report – Second National Institute of Allergy and Infectious Disease/Food Allergy and Anaphylaxis Network symposium. *J Allergy Clin Immunol* 2006;117(2):391–7.

137 Polyzos A, Tsavaris N, Kosmas C, *et al.* Hypersensitivity reactions to carboplatin administration are common but not always severe: a 10-year experience. *Oncology* 2001;61(2):129–33.

138 Navo M, Kunthur A, Badell ML, *et al.* Evaluation of the incidence of carboplatin hypersensitivity reactions in cancer patients. *Gynecol Oncol* 2006;103(2):608–13.

139 Sampson HA, Munoz-Furlong A, Bock SA, *et al.* Symposium on the definition and management of anaphylaxis: summary report. *J Allergy Clin Immunol* 2005;115(3):584–91.

140 Brown SG. Clinical features and severity grading of anaphylaxis. *J Allergy Clin Immunol* 2004;114(2):371–6.

141 Robinson JB, Singh D, Bodurka-Bevers DC, *et al.* Hypersensitivity reactions and the utility of oral and intravenous desensitization in patients with gynecologic malignancies. *Gynecol Oncol* 2001;82(3):550–8.

142 Weiss RB. Hypersensitivity reactions. *Semin Oncol* 1992;19(5):458–77.

143 Szebeni J, Muggia FM, Alving CR. Complement activation by Cremophor EL as a possible contributor to hypersensitivity to paclitaxel: an in vitro study. *J Natl Cancer Inst* 1998;90(4):300–6.

144 Gradishar WJ, Tjulandin S, Davidson N, *et al.* Phase III trial of nanoparticle albumin-bound paclitaxel compared with polyethylated castor oil-based paclitaxel in women with breast cancer. *J Clin Oncol* 2005;23(31): 7794–803.

145 Millward MJ, Newell DR, Mummaneni V, *et al.* Phase I and pharmacokinetic study of a water-soluble etoposide prodrug, etoposide phosphate (BMY-40481). *Eur J Cancer* 1995;31A(13–14):2409–11.

146 Dutcher JP, Schiffer CA, Wiernik PH. Hyperleukocytosis in adult acute nonlymphocytic leukemia: impact on remission rate and duration, and survival. *J Clin Oncol* 1987;5(9):1364–72.

147 Cuttner J, Conjalka MS, Reilly M, *et al.* Association of monocytic leukemia in patients with extreme leukocytosis. *Am J Med* 1980;69(4):555–8.

148 Kasner MT, Laury A, Kasner SE, Carroll M, Luger SM. Increased cerebral blood flow after leukapheresis for acute myelogenous leukemia. *Am J Hematol* 2007;82(12):1110–2.

149 Porcu P, Danielson CF, Orazi A, *et al.* Therapeutic leukapheresis in hyperleucocytic leukaemias: lack of correlation between degree of cytoreduction and early mortality rate. *Br J Haematol* 1997;98(2):433–6.

150 Giles FJ, Shen Y, Kantarjian HM, *et al.* Leukapheresis reduces early mortality in patients with acute myeloid leukemia with high white cell counts but does not improve long- term survival. *Leukemia Lymphoma* 2001;42(1–2):67–73.

151 Carter PW, Cohen HJ, Crawford J. Hyperviscosity syndrome in association with kappa light chain myeloma. *Am J Med* 1989;86(5):591–5.

152 Drew MJ. Plasmapheresis in the dysproteinemias. *Ther Apher* 2002;6(1):45–52.

153 Ansell SM, Kyle RA, Reeder CB, *et al.* Diagnosis and management of Waldenstrom macroglobulinemia: Mayo stratification of macroglobulinemia and risk-adapted therapy (mSMART) guidelines. *Mayo Clin Proc* 2010;85(9):824–33.

154 Treon SP. How I treat Waldenstrom macroglobulinemia. *Blood* 2015;126(6):721–32.

31

Patient-Reported Outcomes in Cancer: Application and Utility in Clinical Practice and Research

Kevin D. Stein[1], Tenbroeck Smith[2], Joseph E. Bauer[2], Deborah L. Driscoll[2], and Dexter L. Cooper[3]

[1] Emory University Rollins School of Public Health, Atlanta, Georgia, USA
[2] American Cancer Society, Atlanta, Georgia, USA
[3] Morehouse School of Medicine, Atlanta, Georgia, USA

Introduction

This chapter provides an overview of patient-reported outcomes (PROs) in the context of cancer clinical care and research. It is not meant to make the reader a PRO specialist or expert; rather it is intended to help the reader become an educated consumer of information about PROs and to understand the advantages and challenges of the use of PROs in their respective settings. To that end, the first section of the chapter focuses on the concept of the PRO, delineating what is and what is not considered to be a PRO and why these measures are increasingly being viewed as important outcomes in oncology. The advantages of including PRO measures alongside the biomedical and clinical measures traditionally used to assess the quality of cancer care are also explored in this section. In the second and third sections, we discuss how PROs are used in both clinical and research settings. Specifically, we provide examples of different PROs, address how PROs are used to measure symptoms and functioning in different domains, and discuss strategies for the selection and development of PROs for specific purposes and populations. We conclude the chapter with a discussion of the key challenges and issues oncology professionals should consider in the selection and use of PROs. Throughout the chapter, the reader is referred to resources, including websites and further reading on the topic of PROs, should a greater depth of knowledge on a particular issue or topic be of interest.

What are PROs and What are Their Advantages?

Cancer and the varied treatment options used to combat the disease can lead to a wide range of symptoms and side effects that may affect the patient's functioning and overall quality of life [1]. The biomedical outcomes that have traditionally been used to assess the quality and efficacy of cancer care, such as tumor progression, laboratory values and test results, and objective physiological measures, provide important information regarding the clinical progression and prognosis of the individual's disease. However, such biomedical measures fail to capture the viewpoint of the patient and may not represent outcomes that are important to them. For example, treatment-related symptoms such as pain, fatigue, and impaired bowel function can significantly impact patients' quality of life but are not captured by biomedical measures. To evaluate and compare the effectiveness of different treatment options and models of care and aid in treatment decision making, it is critical to collect data on outcomes that are meaningful and matter most to patients. Without this self-reported data, the comprehensive information needed for important clinical decision-making is not complete. In the past, physicians often made ratings of their patients' functioning (e.g. performance status) in relevant domains. However, ratings of patient's functioning provided by healthcare providers may fail to represent the patient experience accurately. In fact, healthcare providers may be poor estimators of their patients' symptom severity and subjective experience [2]. Only by asking patients directly about their experiences can we fully understand the impact of a disease and its treatments. Such subjectively-collected outcomes are often referred to as PROs.

According to the FDA report entitled "Patient-Reported Outcome Measures: Use in Medical Product Development to Support Labeling Claims", a PRO is defined as "any report of the status of patient's health condition that comes directly from the patient, without interpretation of the patient's response by a clinician or anyone else" [3]. Many types of outcomes are included in this broad definition, including reports of symptoms, functioning, and overall quality of life. A PRO may be preference-based, which includes the patient's own ratings of what outcomes are or are not important. For example, in a PRO instrument assessing functional status, a patient may rate mobility highly important and fatigue less important.

This rating would then be incorporated into a weighted overall utility score for the PRO measure and could lead the healthcare provider to focus more on their patient's mobility, rather than his or her fatigue. PROs also include other important indicators relevant to health and health care. Patient satisfaction with care, adherence to treatment regimens and health behavior recommendations from providers, and assessments of the quality of the communications with healthcare providers and allied health teams are important PROs that must be considered when assessing the quality of care a patient receives.

Assessing PROs in cancer clinical trials has become standard practice as a method to differentiate between treatment modalities in comparative effectiveness research (CER). For example, if two treatments are equally effective in controlling one's disease, the deciding factor in choosing which treatment to use can be to review the impact of each treatment on one's function in domains measured via PROs, such as treatment-related symptoms or overall quality of life. However, outside of the regulatory context, there are no widely accepted standards around the collection and reporting of PROs in oncology and guidelines around their collection are only beginning to emerge [4]. For example, the American College of Surgeon's Commission on Cancer (CoC) has implemented a requirement that all CoC accredited facilities begin to routinely collect PROs, such as screening for psychosocial distress, of patients treated at their facilities. Periodic updates regarding CoC patient-centered care standards can be viewed at https://www.facs.org/publications/newsletters/coc-source/special-source/standard3132 (accessed 6 September 2017). Likewise, the National Comprehensive Care Network (NCCN) has established Clinical Practice Guidelines for assessment and management of PROs such as pain, fatigue, and emotional distress [5–7]. However, despite the establishment of these new standards and guidelines, much confusion remains about the inclusion of PROs in clinical care settings and CER. Using a consensus-building approach, Basch *et al.* attempted to address this issue by developing a set of 11 recommendations for the inclusion of PROs in the design and implementation of CER [4]. These recommendations were intended to help create a framework for more widescale adoption and appropriate use of PROs in the oncology setting. Key recommendations centered around ensuring the inclusion of PROs in CER; selecting PRO tools relevant to the symptom profile of the population being studied; using psychometrically reliable, valid, and sensitive PRO measures; employing methods to minimize burden on respondents and reduce the likelihood of missing data; using standard data reporting conventions (e.g. reporting means and percentages); and publishing PRO results alongside traditional biomedical outcomes (see Basch *et al.* [4] for complete set of recommendations). More recently, investigators have conducted surveys of PRO researchers and clinicians to develop *minimum standards* for the design and selection of PRO measures in patient-centered outcomes and CER paradigms, but acknowledge that efforts are still needed to identify best practices for selecting decision-relevant PROs [8].

Inclusion of PROs and measures of quality of life in clinical care and research and in CER has been advanced by recent federal legislation that led to the creation of the Patient-Centered Outcomes Research Institute (PCORI) via the US Patient Protection and Affordable Care Act [9]. The mission of PCORI is to help people make informed healthcare decisions and improve healthcare delivery and outcomes by funding research that is guided by patients, caregivers, and the broader healthcare community [10]. Thus far, PCORI has committed more than $1 billion to fund patient-centered CER in which PROs are a central and integral component.

PROs use patient feedback to provide measures for monitoring clinical conditions, informing decision-making, and potentially improving the delivery of care. PROs gather information in a standardized way, which give healthcare personnel and researchers insights into the patient's perspectives and experiences. Information collected by these measures allow the outcomes that patients care about to be assessed [11]. A broad array of PRO tools that provide valid, reliable, and accurate measures of the patient's status are available for use in both clinical and research settings, and make it possible to track patient outcomes over time and to compare patients to other patients [12]. PRO measures are typically relatively easy for patients to complete and provide the end user with immediate feedback regarding the patients' subjective experience of functioning in the domain of interest. Selecting an appropriate PRO and putting it into practice may present more of a challenge. Specifically, the collection of PROs also facilitates communication between patients and providers, resulting in improved care provision. Thus, PROs are systematic measures for capturing patient information. The specific domains often include physical, psychological, and social components of outcomes. Table 31.1 describes the constructs that can be assessed using PRO measures and provides examples of commonly used instruments [11].

Use of PROs in Clinical Practice

PRO measures can convey important information to healthcare personnel to supplement traditional biomedical outcome measures in the assessment of the overall burden of cancer and the effectiveness of interventions [13]. As noted previously, these measures are most often defined as the physical, emotional, or social functioning of the patient, but in a more pragmatic sense include the perceptions of patients and thus are not limited to functional status alone. For example, a patient may have significant functional deficits and still perceive that their quality of life is good. PRO measures can be used to obtain data from the patient's perspective to help guide healthcare personnel in making clinical decisions as well as monitoring the outcomes of interventions. They can be used as baseline assessments to identify patient needs, and they can be used to aid patient–doctor communications. PRO measures could even be administered in clinical settings for audit and quality improvement/quality assurance purposes – for example, in assessing the effectiveness of different procedures. Additionally, as health care shifts from the volume of services delivered to the value created for patients, PROs will become increasingly important in reflecting the outcomes that matter to patients.

Table 31.1 Classification of PROs and selected measures*. Ahmed *et al.* 2012 [11]. Reproduced with permission of Wolters Kluwer Health, Inc.[†].

Construct	Description	Example measures
Symptoms	Measures that evaluate the frequency, severity, and impact of symptoms [16,17]	Brief Pain Inventory (BPI)[18] MD Anderson Symptom Inventory (MDASI)[19] Memorial Symptom Assessment Scale Short Form (MSAS-SF)[20] SF-36 Vitality Scale[21] Center for Epidemiologic Studies Depression Scale (CESD)[22]
Functional status	Functional status measures assess a person's ability to carry out daily activities such as walking, working, or attending social events[14]	Distress Thermometer[23] McGill pain questionnaire[24,25] Kidscreen[26] Arthritis impact measurement scales[27] Saint George's respiratory questionnaire[28] Functional Assessment of Cancer Therapy (FACT) core plus symptom modules[29]
HRQoL	The extent to which one's usual or expected physical, emotional, and social well-being is affected by a medical condition and/or treatment	European Organization for Research of Cancer Quality of Life Questionnaire Core-30 (EORTC QLQ-C30) plus symptom modules [29,30] SF-36 [21,29]
Non-preference	These generic measures provide data on functioning relative to both a minimal and maximal level of performance for each health concept and can be used with any group of individuals	World Health Organization Quality of Life Assessment, Brief Form (WHO QOL-BREF)[29,31]
Preference	The relative value or utility weight assigned to each of the levels of health is assessed based on patient preferences	EuroQoL (EQ-5D) Short Form 6D (SF-6D) Health Utility Index (HUI) Quality of Well-Being scale
Health behaviors		
Health-directed behavior	The healthful behaviors individuals engage in aimed at disease prevention and/or health promotion	Health education impact questionnaire (heiQ)
Adherence	The extent to which the patient continues the agreed- upon mode of treatment under limited supervision when faced with conflicting demands, as distinguished from compliance or maintenance[32]	Simplified medication adherence questionnaire (SMAQ)[33] Parent Adherence Report Questionnaire[34]
Satisfaction with care	Patient satisfaction with care received	Consumer Assessment of Health Plans Surveys (CAHPS)[35]

* Selected measures are only select examples and may assess more than one construct.
[†] Note citations refer to the original article (this publication falls under STM opt-out).

How are PROs Different from Traditional Clinical Measures?

Traditional clinical measures include physiologic measures that require professional knowledge to interpret and to utilize in making clinical/medical decisions. In contrast, PROs are self-reported measures of health and quality of life that often have more meaning to the persons who are affected by disease, who are undergoing active treatment(s), or who are trying to maintain or restore their health. Although clinical measurements remain the primary method for assessing patients' physical health, there is an increasing awareness of the importance of using PROs to assess the patient's perspective and experiences. Quite often it is these perceptions and experiences of health and illness that influence what people think about their health, as well as what people do about their health.

Overall, traditional clinical and PRO measures differ from each other in three important ways. First, self-reported measures are increasingly used to help determine whether treatments are doing more harm than good. However, they often correlate poorly with clinical physiologic measures, meaning that one cannot substitute one type of measure for the other; they are both important. Second, two patients with the same clinical status or physiologic state may have dramatically different perceptions of their quality of life. Thus, clinical measures by themselves do not always provide enough information to measure patient differences in response to treatment. Third, and perhaps most importantly, clinicians may assume that physiological clinical measures align well with patient preferences, but this is often not the case, and using PROs in clinical practice can provide a standardized way to collect information on patient preferences [2]. It is increasingly important that clinicians are able to understand and use outcomes measured from both the clinical and patient perspectives to inform their practice. Wu *et al.* provide a 'Clinician's Checklist' to help practicing physicians understand clinical research articles that include PROs so that the information can be used for decision making [14].

Consideration of Variation in Clinical Populations in the Use and Selection of PROs

When considering the use of a PRO in a clinical setting, one should select an instrument that measures constructs that are relevant to the patient's disease or condition, and which is also appropriate for the patient's cultural background, which may require accounting for racial, ethnic, nation of origin, language, literacy, and/or sociodemographic differences. More technically – one must know whether the measurement tool was validated (does it measure what you think it is measuring) and whether this measure is reliable (does it measure things consistently). Further discussion of validity and reliability are found in the section of this chapter focusing on the use of PROs in a research context. There can be major variations/differences in clinical populations; thus the choice of a PRO must be thought about and made with care [15]. The better the 'fit' that the PRO has with these kinds of variations/differences, the more specific the information derived from the PRO will be.

Selecting an Appropriate PRO for Assessment in a Clinical Setting

It can be challenging to select the most appropriate PRO measure(s), because of the sheer number of instruments that have been developed, and because of the varying clinical environments and patient populations that one may encounter. However, some questions about a patient's health can only be answered by the patient themselves, and PROs give healthcare personnel the means to incorporate the patient's perspective into clinical decision making. Including PROs as part of an information capture strategy in clinical settings is part of a patient-centric culture, and may lead to a higher quality of patient care. When the aim is to use PRO data at the bedside (non-research), the measure(s) need to provide clear and interpretable data to healthcare personnel and the patient, but also be easy to administer and interpret. Given the widening array of diagnostic and treatment options, PROs facilitate informed decision-making, taking into account the patient's needs as well as their view of the likely impact of treatment [12]. For additional information on sources for PRO measures, interested readers may wish to visit the website (http://www.nihpromis. org/, accessed 6 September 2017) for the Patient-Reported Outcomes Measurement Information System (PROMIS), a system of highly reliable, precise measures of patient-reported health status for physical, mental, and social well-being, the development of which was funded by the National Institutes of Health (NIH). PROMIS provides item banks – groups of questions measuring the same underlying concept. An item is a single question on a questionnaire or PRO measure. PROMIS uses item response theory and computer adaptive testing to improve measurement precision while limiting respondent burden by

decreasing the number of items required to assess a given concept accurately [16]. Cancer clinicians may be particularly interested in reading about PROMIS for Clinicians (http://www. nihpromis.org/Clinicians/InClinicians, accessed 6 September 2017), which provides an overview of the PROMIS system and its relevance to cancer care.

Additionally, the website of the International Society for Quality of Life Research (http://www.isoqol.org/research/ isoqol-publications, accessed 6 September 2017) includes the "User's Guide to Implementing Patient-Reported Outcomes Assessment in Clinical Practice" [17]. The purpose of this User's Guide is to help clinicians or other healthcare personnel who are interested in using PROs in their clinical practice as a tool in patient management. This online resource is updated periodically, with the most recent update added in 2015 [17]. Snyder *et al.* [18] summarized the key issues from the User's Guide and provide a quick overview. A podcast, in which two physicians who have integrated PROs into their clinical practice recount their experiences, is posted on the ISOQOL website at http:// www.isoqol.org/UserFiles/media/ISOQOL_2_3_2012.mp3 (accessed 6 September 2017). A review paper provides detailed examples of innovative systems used at institutions in the United States and United Kingdom for incorporating PRO assessment into clinical care, in which electronic surveys (web based or phone based) are completed by patients from home or in the clinic, and the results are relayed to providers in individual reports or sent directly to the electronic medical record [19]. These resources should give the reader the opportunity to learn more about PROs and their use in a clinical setting.

How are PROs used in Clinical and Public Health Research?

Incorporation of PROs in observational studies and clinical trials provides the patient perspective on disease and treatment that is essential for gaining a full understanding of cancer care and the impact of cancer on people's lives. For example, a PRO may be a primary outcome in an observational study estimating pain prevalence or in a clinical trial of an intervention designed to decrease pain among cancer patients. PROs can also provide important explanatory variables. For example, PROs are important explanatory variables in studies of adherence to treatment because they are good at assessing treatment-related side effects such as nausea and fatigue known to predict non-adherence [20, 21]. PROs also play an important role in providing information about treatment choices when biomedical outcomes are equivalent. For example, the recommended treatment options for local prostate cancer provide similar survival benefits, so the comparison of the relative treatment side effects, such as incontinence and erectile dysfunction – best assessed with PRO measures – is an important part of decision making. PROs also make important contributions to research in cases where they provide a reliable, cost-effective alternative to standard clinical measures. For example, when conducting a study of adherence to home use of hormone therapy, it may be most efficient to rely on patient-reported data. PRO-based research informs our understanding of the patient side of the cancer experience.

The importance of PROs in clinical and public health research has increased in parallel with the greater focus on patients' perspectives and patient-centered care that is reflected in a number of recent events. First, the Food and Drug Administration (FDA) now accepts PRO data to support medical product labeling, given applicable requirements are met. The FDA requires the use of a "well-defined and reliable PRO instrument in appropriately designed investigations" [22]. Second, the European Agency for the Evaluation of Medicinal Products has similarly acknowledged the essential role of PROs in clinical trials [23]. Third, the National Cancer Institute (NCI) has signaled the importance of PROs through efforts to increase and improve their use as primary and secondary endpoints in clinical trials through the creation of the Symptom Management and Health-Related Quality of Life Steering Committee [13, 24]. Fourth, the previously-mentioned PCORI promotes CER to inform healthcare decisions and improve healthcare outcomes. Finally, recognizing the potential for patient satisfaction data to empower consumers, the Centers for Medicare and Medicaid Services and the National Committee on Quality Assurance require health organizations to report data from the Consumer Assessment of Health Providers and Systems (CAHPS) surveys publicly. All these initiatives reflect the increasing importance of PROs in research.

Research Design, PRO Structure and Psychometric Properties

PRO data are only as good as the methodology of the protocol used to collect it. To be informed consumers, investigators and health professionals need some understanding of the methodological issues relevant to PROs. In addition to the information provided in this chapter, clinicians can inform their understanding of PRO research with the "Clinician's Checklist for Reading and Using an Article About Patient-Reported Outcomes" [14]. The validity and interpretation of research with patient-reported outcomes depend on many of the same factors important to research using other measures. For example, the eligibility criteria and research setting should reflect the target population. The design and execution of protocols lead to varying levels of external and internal validity. For the purposes of this chapter, focus will be on methodological issues unique to PROs. For example, experimental blinding may be especially important in clinical trials with PRO assessments because knowledge of experimental conditions may influence participant response patterns. Steps can be taken to increase the reliability of measurement (e.g., using multiple questions to assess single concepts) and improve the validity of measurement (e.g., avoiding questions that ask participants to summarize benefits of an intervention or changes over time). Assessing participants' current status at multiple points in time (longitudinal design) is recommended. Survey administration methods should also be considered; participants may respond to a sensitive question (e.g., about sexual functioning) more honestly when self-administered via paper or computer questionnaires than when interviewed on the telephone or in person.

Multi-item PRO instrument structure may be unidimensional, measuring one concept, or multidimensional, measuring a group of related concepts. When a PRO instrument uses multiple items to assess a single underlying concept, the resulting measure is referred to as a scale. For example, the SF-36, a commonly used PRO instrument, uses 10 items in a physical functioning subscale. Using multiple items usually improves reliability. On the other hand, single item measures can be reliable and have lower respondent burden. The items in a multidimensional PRO instrument usually contribute to one of several domains or subscales, each of which produces a score. Subscales can also often be combined into a summary score. For example, the SF-36 has four measures of physical health that can be combined into one Physical Component Summary score.

Just as with the biomedical measurement instruments, PRO instruments have properties that indicate the degree to which they reliably measure the intended concept. Many aspects of PRO instrument quality can be evaluated statistically. One of the most important aspects of PRO instrument quality is validity, or the degree to which the instrument is measuring the construct it is intended to measure. There are several forms or types of validity. *Content validity* reflects the degree to which a given PRO covers all aspects of the intended concept. For example, a measure of depression that assessed the emotional but not the behavioral aspects of depression lacks content validity. *Construct validity* refers to the degree to which scores derived from a PRO correlate with other measures as one would expect based upon theory and *a priori* hypotheses. For example, data collected from a PRO measuring dyspnea (difficult or labored breathing) should correlate with results of a six-minute walk test.

Another important indicator of instrument quality is reliability. Reliability statistics estimate the tendency of an instrument to produce stable scores over time. As with validity, there are several methods of measuring reliability. *Test–retest reliability* measures the consistency of a PRO over repeated measures, ideally when little or no change is expected between measurements. *Internal consistency* describes the homogeneity of items within a given domain/subscale. High scores on measures of *internal consistency* (e.g., Cronbach's Alpha) suggest that items are measuring the same underlying construct. Provided are a few common examples of indicators of the psychometric performance of a measure (see Streiner [25] and DeVellis [26] for thorough descriptions of scale structure, reliability, and validity estimates).

Interpretation of group differences or longitudinal changes in PRO scores should be informed by minimal clinically important differences (MCID). The MCID has been defined as the smallest difference in PRO scores "that patients perceive as important, either beneficial or harmful, and which would lead the clinician to consider a change in the patient's management" [27]. While there are a number of methods for determining MCID, *effect size* is a common approach. Effect size is especially helpful when interpreting results from studies with large samples, which can lead to statistical significance between groups that are *not* substantively different. Effect size also plays an important role in summarizing results from multiple studies via meta-analyses. Some criticize effect size because it is data-driven and does not gather patient input on the magnitude of change that is meaningful. MCIDs are an intuitively appealing and practical way of interpreting differences in PRO scores in the clinical and research setting. The topic of MCIDs is complex with a variety of related but separate approaches; the reader is referred to King [28] for additional considerations of MCIDs.

Selecting PRO Concepts and Instruments

When designing a study protocol involving PROs and prior to selecting PRO instruments, considerable care should be taken selecting the concepts to be measured. A good first step is to write well-formulated, concise research questions that include the concepts that will be measured by PRO instruments in the study. These concepts should be precisely defined and more specific than "quality of life" or "satisfaction", which are general and cover many different concepts. For example, a study of a physical rehabilitation intervention might measure physical functioning and the degree to which physical impairments interfere with usual activities rather than or in addition to quality of life or satisfaction.

Research questions and study protocols will benefit from the use or creation of a conceptual model (sometimes referred to as a "logic model"), especially when research includes multidimensional, latent concepts which are not readily observable. A conceptual model is a simplified representation of reality intended to improve understanding and communication among those developing and reading the research proposal, protocol, or manuscript. Unlike biomedical conceptual models that focus on biological/clinical processes and outcomes, PRO conceptual models describe the interrelation of different PRO concepts. Figure 31.1 is an example of a conceptual model showing the interrelation of a variety of health-related quality of life concepts among cancer survivors. Conceptual models may include only PRO concepts or explicate the interface between PROs and biomedical concepts. Concept selection should also be influenced by the particulars of the study. For example, a clinical trial conducted among patients with a specific type and stage of disease (e.g., local breast cancer) will benefit from instruments that capture the symptoms and side effects associated with that disease (e.g., pain, fatigue, lymphedema). Once the research questions are written and the concepts identified, the investigator can select PRO instruments.

Selection of PRO Instruments

The first step in PRO instrument selection is determining whether adequate PRO instruments exist, an existing instrument can be modified, or a new one is required. When appropriate, using existing, valid PRO instruments is preferred because it saves the expense, time and effort required to develop and validate a new instrument. Using existing instruments also increases comparability of study results with previous studies using the same instrument. Noncomparable data stifles meta-analyses and other efforts to summarize studies with PRO endpoints. The NIH and the NCI have created systems to address this issue and help investigators select PRO instruments. The aforementioned PROMIS is available at no charge for use by researchers and clinicians, offering normative data

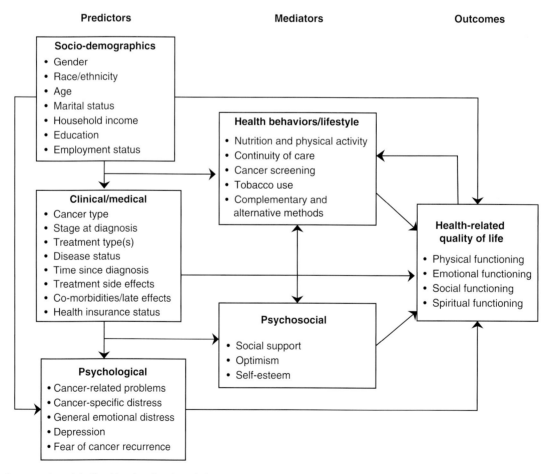

Figure 31.1 Conceptual model of health-related quality of life in cancer survivors.

for healthy individuals as well as individuals with chronic conditions for comparison purposes. Another NIH/NCI product, the grid-enabled measures (GEM), is a dynamic web-based database that catalogues behavioral and social science measures organized by theoretical constructs. Readers are referred to the GEM website (https://cancercontrol.cancer.gov/brp/research/gem.html, accessed 6 September 2017) for additional information. Previously developed instruments can also be identified through reviews of the scientific literature, especially in papers reviewing instruments relevant to the area of investigation. Organizations with a particular research focus, such as palliative care or shared decision making, are increasingly assembling and publicizing lists of relevant PRO measures through their websites.

When previously developed instruments do not exist, the investigator may adapt available validated instruments or develop new ones. Adaptation of existing instruments requires many of the same steps as scale development. The development of a new PRO instrument is labor- and time-intensive. The process starts with creating a list of questions. This usually involves qualitative studies intended to capture all the relevant questions from stakeholders and experts such as patients, health professionals and researchers, thus assuring *content validity*. Instructions must be written and response format selected – Likert scales (e.g., strongly agree, agree, neutral, disagree, strongly disagree) are a commonly used response format. Cognitive testing, involving administration of the instrument with several individuals, followed by one-on-one in-depth interviews, is used to determine if study participants interpret the instructions, questions and response format as intended (see Willis [29] for more on cognitive testing). Cognitive testing is often iterative; for example, early findings in cognitive testing may lead to reworded questions which are then tested again. The next stage is collecting quantitative data from a pilot version of the PRO instrument. Pilot data are used to determine factor structure (i.e., dimensionality) and psychometric characteristics (validity and reliability). All of these steps can be combined into one mixed-methods study protocol (see Creswell [30] for a comparison of qualitative, quantitative and mixed methods research). PRO instrument development may be especially challenging for measures of multidimensional, latent concepts such as depression or fatigue. See Streiner [25], DeVellis [26] and Patrick *et al.* [31] for thorough descriptions of scale development procedures. Guidance documents such as minimum standards for PROs in patient-centered outcomes and CER or for reporting PROs in clinical trials may also be helpful. Those who are involved with clinical research are likely familiar with CONSORT (Consolidated Standards for Reporting Trials). Specifically, the CONSORT statement provides evidence-based recommendations to improve completeness of reporting in RCTs and has been endorsed by a number of major journals and editorial groups [32]. More recently, Calvert *et al.* [33] developed an extension of the CONSORT statement to address the inclusion of PROs in clinical trials. This CONSORT PRO extension describes the methods used to gain consensus on the extension and also provides both rationale for each new recommended item and examples of good reporting. Additional

factors to be considered when selecting or developing PRO measures are found in the Challenges and Considerations section of this chapter.

Challenges and Considerations in the Use of PRO Measures

Several challenges and considerations need to be addressed when measuring PROs. Selecting the correct tool depends on: (i) the purpose of the evaluation, (ii) the key outcomes of interest, (iii) the target population being assessed, and (iv) the cultural, language, literacy, racial and ethnic diversity of those being surveyed. The target population may be narrowly defined, such as those using an individual clinic or being treated for a specific disease, or more broadly defined to a general public health area or population. No single tool can meet every need, so careful consideration must be given to selecting the most appropriate, practical and feasible instrument that will work for the given situation and population [11]. The final choice of the PRO instrument(s) to be used for a particular evaluation will depend on answers to the following questions:

- Are the questions in the instrument acceptable for the individuals(s) being surveyed, or will they make the respondent uncomfortable? This can happen if the questions ask for information the patient considers sensitive or culturally inappropriate.
- Are the questions and response options able to be adequately presented in the native language and style of the respondent? This can be important if the original English questions or response categories do not easily translate. Response options such as *rarely*, *sometimes*, *a little bit* may not invoke the same concept of quantity in all respondents or have equivalent words in another language [2].
- Is there research literature confirming that the instrument can provide an accurate measure of the outcome it was designed to assess and that the results will be applicable to the population being evaluated?
- Are the questions in the instrument appropriate for the particular disease or target population? In some cases, an instrument may be designed for a broad audience and may not be appropriate for the more specific population being targeted; conversely, the instrument may be designed for a specific population and not be appropriate for a broader application.
- Does the instrument ask for information that the respondent considers confidential, which they would not normally provide? A respondent who is not confident that this information will be handled properly may be reluctant to answer these questions [13].

If the answers to these questions are negative, then the choice of a more appropriate PRO instrument for the target population and planned application should be considered. Additional practical issues also need to be addressed when planning the use of any PRO instrument. How long and how much effort it will take to answer all of the questions will be a top concern for the potential respondent. The staff or organization administering the instrument will be concerned with the time and effort needed to collect the information and to analyze the responses. Analysis issues related to the handling of incomplete or missing data also affect the time and effort needed. All issues relating to time and effort affect the costs involved in the use of a selected instrument. Factors such as patient age, fatigue and severity of illness/side effects may affect the respondent's ability or desire to complete the survey. The length of the survey, the method of administration (e.g., online vs paper vs smartphone/tablet), when it is to be completed (previsit or during a visit), and how often it will be given also play a role in getting and keeping respondents. These same issues are generally key factors in determining the time and costs to the staff/organization administering the survey. The burdens to the patient and the healthcare provider must be carefully considered when deciding which particular PRO instrument to use.

Analyzing the data collected using PRO tools can also pose challenges. Frequently PROs are administered multiple times over the course of a person's illness. People may discontinue participation for many reasons: they feel too ill, feel much better, move away, succumb to their illness, or are simply bored or tired and are no longer interested. Questions not answered (skipped) can result in gaps in the data, forcing those cases to be excluded from the analyses or values to be imputed. Either approach can lead to biases that affect analysis results and potentially limit the usefulness of final conclusions and recommendations. For example, if a number of the most ill patients discontinue participation, then disease burden may be underestimated. Similarly, if patients stop participating once they feel better, response to treatment may be underestimated [11]. These analysis issues with PRO data are not different than what is typically seen with other biomedical data [13], although when using a PRO instrument, the amount of missing data may be greater and dealing with this will need to be planned for accordingly.

Collecting and using PRO instrument data requires careful attention to several important ethical issues. For example, if during the course of collecting data, it is noticed that a patient's depression level has increased by a significant amount, the patient should be referred for treatment, have their medications adjusted, and be evaluated frequently. Conversely, a patient can be informed during consent and at the beginning or end of a survey that their clinician will not see the data and if they have medical needs they must contact their provider themselves. When selecting a PRO instrument, each of the issues identified above must be addressed, paying attention to staff and participant burden as well as costs compared to the value of the information being collected. As discussed earlier, PROs can be used in clinical trials and research studies. These instruments may also encourage discussions between patients and healthcare professionals, providing useful information for changes in symptoms, side effects and other health-related issues. Greenhalgh summarizes the evidence for PROs as "having much greater impact on the discussion and detection of patient problems within the consultation than on the ways in which clinicians subsequently manage these problems or on the patient's eventual health outcomes" [34]. Thus, we have much work to do to ensure that PROs are used and appropri-

ately impact clinical cancer care. Greenhalgh recommends the adoption of a theory-driven approach, using both qualitative and quantitative methods and greater scientific rigor to judge and demonstrate the effectiveness and impact of the use of PROs in clinical practice and research [34].

Electronic health record (EHR) use is standard practice and data collected via electronic technologies is increasing [35, 36]. Allowing EHRs to record and include PROs will assist in implementation and usability of PROs in the clinical and research setting. However, using this ability is not without challenges. Lack of industry standards and time to learn new EHR systems, along with multiple updates/upgrades/new versions to these systems, adds additional challenges to those already described [23].

Summary

The use of PROs in cancer clinical practice and research is increasing in importance. PROs provide unique and direct insight into the patient's perspective on their functioning across a number of domains, as well as information about their attitudes regarding the quality and efficacy of their cancer care, including the degree to which they feel that they can communicate effectively with their healthcare providers. In the clinical setting, PROs offer a number of benefits not provided by traditional biomedical measures. While biomedical measures are clearly important to assessing the overall prognosis and health status, they often fail to capture other facets of disease and treatment that are important to patients. Healthcare providers may fail to elicit such information for a number of reasons, including limited time due to competing demands, limited training in speaking with patients about such issues, or simply failure to ask the question(s) that would elicit such data. Patients also bear responsibility in that they may neglect to inform their providers about issues that are of concern to them out of fear that it may distract their provider from focusing on their cancer care or perceptions that their providers are too busy or otherwise unavailable to discuss their concerns.

From a clinical research perspective, PROs are becoming increasingly commonplace, if not standard, as they offer an efficient and economical method of collecting reliable and valid data about the patient's functioning. Through careful selection and use of an appropriate PRO, a researcher can have greater confidence that any given study will provide a comprehensive and representative picture that can be used to guide research priorities and healthcare policy decisions. While PROs offer numerous advantages, their use must be considered in the context of several limitations and challenges. In particular, the efficacy and utility of a PRO depends on the characteristics of the population in which it is being used, the appropriateness of the instrument for the population, setting, and type of information needed, and the time and effort needed from a patient to complete the PRO, which may lead to unwanted patient burden. Missing and biased data are also a concern that may diminish the accuracy of the information collected. For these reasons, it is often wise to consult with an expert prior to implementing PROs in the clinical care or research setting.

References

1 Stein KD, Syrjala KL, Andrykowski MA. Physical and psychological long-term and late effects of cancer. *Cancer* 2008;112(11 Suppl):2577–92.

2 Office of Behavioral and Social Sciences Research. Patient Reported Outcomes 2013. Available from: http://www.esourceresearch.org/ (accessed 7 September 2017).

3 US Food and Drug Administration. *Patient reported outcome measures: use in medical product development to support labeling claims*, 2009. Rockville: Food and Drug Administration: Final guidance document. https://www.fda.gov/ucm/groups/fdagov-public/@fdagov-drugs-gen/documents/document/ucm193282.pdf (accessed 7 September 2017).

4 Basch E, Abernethy AP, Mullins CD, *et al*. Recommendations for incorporating patient-reported outcomes into clinical comparative effectiveness research in adult oncology. *J Clin Oncol* 2012;30(34):4249–55.

5 Swarm RA, Anghelescu DL, Benedetti C, *et al*. NCCN clinical practice guidelines in oncology (NCCN Guidelines®). Adult cancer pain version 2.2016. NCCN.org.

6 Berger AM, Mooney K, Banerjee BC, *et al*. NCCN Clinical Practice Guidelines in Oncology (NCCN Guidelines®) Cancer-Related Fatigue Version 1.2017. NCCN.org.

7 Holland J, Jacobsen PB, Andersen B, *et al*. NCCN Clinical Practice Guidelines in Oncology (NCCN Guidelines) Distress Management Version 2.2016. NCCN. org.

8 Reeve BB, Wyrwich KW, Wu AW, *et al*. ISOQOL recommends minimum standards for patient-reported outcome measures used in patient-centered outcomes and comparative effectiveness research. *Qual Life Res* 2013;22:1889–905.

9 Patient Protection and Affordable Care Act of 2010. Pub. L. No. 114–48 (March 23, 2010), as amended through May 1, 2010. 2012.

10 Patient-Centered Outcomes Research Institute. About Us, 2016 (accessed 7 September 2017).

11 Ahmed S, Berzon RA, Revicki DA, *et al*. The use of patient-reported outcomes (PRO) within comparative effectiveness research: implications for clinical practice and health care policy. *Med Care* 2012;50(12):1060–70.

12 Wu AW, Snyder C, Clancy CM, Steinwachs DM. Adding the patient perspective to comparative effectiveness research. *Health Aff (Millwood)* 2010;29(10):1863–71.

13 Lipscomb J, Gotay CC, Snyder CF. Patient-reported outcomes in cancer: a review of recent research and policy initiatives. *CA Cancer J Clin* 2007;57(5):278–300.

14 Wu AW, Bradford AN, Velanovich V, *et al*. Clinician's checklist for reading and using an article about patient-reported outcomes. *Mayo Clin Proc* 2014;89(5):653–61.

15 Lohr KN, Zebrack BJ. Using patient-reported outcomes in clinical practice: challenges and opportunities. *Qual Life Res* 2009;18(1):99–107.

16 Cella D, Yount S, Rothrock N, *et al*. The Patient-Reported Outcomes Measurement Information System (PROMIS): progress of an NIH Roadmap cooperative group during its first two years. *Med Care* 2007;45(5 Suppl 1):S3–S11.

17 Aaronson N, Elliott T, Greenhalgh J, *et al*. User's Guide to Implementing Patient-Reported Outcomes Assessment in Clinical Practice. *International Society for Quality of Life Research, Version* 2, 2015.

18 Snyder CF, Aaronson NK, Choucair AK, *et al*. Implementing patient-reported outcomes assessment in clinical practice: a review of the options and considerations. *Qual Life Res* 2012;21(8):1305–14.

19 Bennett AV, Jensen RE, Basch E. Electronic patient-reported outcome systems in oncology clinical practice. *CA: Cancer J Clin* 2012;62(5):336–47.

20 Banna GL, Collova E, Gebbia V, *et al*. Anticancer oral therapy: emerging related issues. *Cancer Treat Rev* 2010;36(8):595–605.

21 Cella D, Fallowfield LJ. Recognition and management of treatment-related side effects for breast cancer patients receiving adjuvant endocrine therapy. *Breast Cancer Res Treat* 2008;107(2):167–80.

22 US Food and Drug Administration. Guidance for industry: patient-reported outcome measures: use in medical product development to support labeling claims. *Federal Register* 2009;74(235):65132–3.

23 Gondek K, Sagnier PP, Gilchrist K, Woolley JM. Current status of patient-reported outcomes in industry-sponsored oncology clinical trials and product labels. *J Clin Oncol* 2007;25(32):5087–93.

24 Clauser SB, Ganz PA, Lipscomb J, Reeve BB. Patient-reported outcomes assessment in cancer trials: evaluating and enhancing the payoff to decision making. *J Clin Oncol* 2007;25(32):5049–50.

25 Streiner DL, Norman GR, Cairney J. *Health Measurement Scales: A Practical Guide to Their Development and Use*, 5th edn. Oxford: Oxford University Press, 2014.

26 DeVellis RF. *Scale Development: Theory and Applications*, 4th edn. Los Angeles: Sage Publications, 2016.

27 Guyatt GH, Osoba D, Wu AW, *et al*. Methods to explain the clinical significance of health status measures. *Mayo Clin Proc* 2002;77(4):371–83.

28 King MT. A point of minimal important difference (MID): a critique of terminology and methods. *Expert Rev Pharmacoecon Outcomes Res* 2011;11(2):171–184.

29 Willis GB. *Cognitive Interviewing: A Tool for Improving Questionnaire Design*. Los Angeles: Sage Publications, 2004.

30 Creswell JW. *Research Design: Qualitative, Quantitative, and Mixed Methods Approaches*. Los Angeles: Sage Publications, 2013.

31 Patrick DL, Burke LB, Gwaltney CJ, *et al*. Content validity – establishing and reporting the evidence in newly developed patient-reported outcomes (PRO) instruments for medical product evaluation: ISPOR PRO Good Research Practices Task Force Report: Part 1—Eliciting Concepts for a New PRO instrument. *Value Health* 2011;14(8):967–77.

32 Moher D, Hopewell S, Schulz KR, *et al*. CONSORT 2010 explanation and elaboration: updated guidelines for reporting parallel group randomised trials. *Int J Surg* 2012;10(1):28–55.

33 Calvert M, Blazeby J, Altman DG, *et al*. Reporting of patient-reported outcomes in randomized trials: the CONSORT PRO extension. *JAMA* 2013;309(8):814–22.

34 Greenhalgh J. The applications of PROs in clinical practice: what are they, do they work, and why? *Qual Life Res* 2009;18(1):115–23.

35 Chung AE, Basch EM. Potential and challenges of patient-generated health data for high-quality cancer care. *J Oncol Pract* 2015;11(3):195–7.

36 Howell D, *et al*. Patient-reported outcomes in routine cancer clinical practice: a scoping review of use, impact on health outcomes, and implementation factors. *Ann Oncol* 2015;26(9):1846–58.

32

Survivorship Care

Emily Tonorezos, Shrujal S. Baxi, Victoria Blinder, Darren R. Feldman, Danielle Novetsky Friedman, Matthew Matasar, Talya Salz, Armin Shahrokni, and Kevin C. Oeffinger

Memorial Sloan Kettering Cancer Center, New York, New York, USA

Introduction

There are currently over 15.5 million cancer survivors in the United States (US), a number which is expected to reach 18 million by the year 2020 [1]. The dramatic improvements in cancer prevention, screening, and treatment, as well as the aging of the general population, account for this growing population of cancer survivors. Nonetheless, cancer survivors have an increased incidence of chronic health problems compared with similarly aged individuals in the general population who have not had cancer [2, 3]. These problems may occur during therapy and persist for many years (e.g., vincristine-related neuropathy) or develop many years later as a direct or indirect consequence of the cancer therapy (e.g., anthracycline-related cardiomyopathy). Collectively, when these conditions occur in excess (risk) of what would have been expected if the individual did not have cancer, they are referred to as late effects.

The incidence and severity of many late effects of cancer therapy can be substantially reduced with risk-based healthcare, and thus the life expectancy and the quality of life of a survivor can be maximized [2, 3]. The cornerstone of the risk-based approach is anticipatory, proactive care that includes a systematic plan of prevention and surveillance based on risks associated with the cancer therapy, genetic predispositions, lifestyle behaviors, and comorbid health conditions [4].

This chapter highlights key late effects for different cancer groups that can be prevented or diminished in severity by early intervention. We begin by discussing several topics that are relevant to all cancer survivors, followed by a discussion of several of the major cancer types, a special therapeutic modality (allogeneic hematopoietic cell transplant), and two particularly vulnerable populations (childhood and elderly cancer survivors).

For All Cancer Survivors

Some health issues should be considered when evaluating any cancer survivor. For example, psychosocial difficulties including depression, anxiety, post-traumatic stress and social withdrawal are frequently described [2, 5, 6]. An analysis of the National Health Interview Survey revealed a higher prevalence of poor mental and physical health among cancer survivors than among the general population [7]. Up to a third of survivors complain of debilitating fatigue and/or pain [8].

Healthy lifestyle practices such as tobacco avoidance or cessation, regular exercise, weight loss or maintenance, and maintaining a healthy diet are important for all survivors. Benefits of tobacco cessation after a cancer diagnosis include improving survival and lowering the risk of a second primary malignancy (SPM), metastasis, or recurrence [9, 10]. Obesity at the time of cancer diagnosis and weight gain following diagnosis have been associated with poor outcomes [11–13], while the Women's Intervention Nutrition Study found a significant reduction in the risk of breast cancer recurrence among a subset of women randomized to a low-fat diet [14]. Of note, while other studies have demonstrated that cancer survivors can achieve significant dietary improvement, and that healthy diets can improve adverse metabolic outcomes such as insulin resistance and visceral adiposity [15], the benefit to cancer-related outcomes has been mixed [16–18]. Exercise has been demonstrated to be safe during and after the cancer diagnosis, and potential benefits include [19, 20] improved quality of life, reduced fatigue and depressive symptoms, as well as lower risk of diabetes and cardiovascular disease [21]. Additionally, cancer-specific benefits including reductions in recurrence and mortality have been observed [22, 23]. Initiating an exercise routine can be challenging for both the provider and the survivor; the American College of Sports Medicine advises a gradual progression to 150 min of aerobic exercise per week, with complementary flexibility and resistance training, as is recommended for the nonsurvivor adult population [24].

Many cancer survivors present for follow-up with questions about how their primary treatment may have affected reproductive health [25, 26]. Cancer therapies that may affect reproductive health include: surgery on the reproductive organs, radiation to the brain, testes, pelvis or abdomen; and chemotherapy (e.g., alkylating agents including cyclophosphamide)

[27, 28]. Risk factors such as age at treatment and underlying medical conditions affect risk. Additionally, some female survivors may retain ovarian function early in adulthood but develop premature menopause [29]. Survivors at risk for reduced fertility should undergo an annual physical examination including Tanner stage (if relevant) and periodic assessment of hormone levels such as follicle stimulating hormone, luteinizing hormone, and estradiol or testosterone, and semen analysis among men [27, 30]. Couples who are struggling with conception should be promptly referred to a reproductive endocrinologist, if desired [31].

Since blood transfusions and blood products are often needed as supportive care during marrow suppressing therapy, many cancer survivors treated in the 1960s to the early 1990s are at risk for blood-borne infections. This risk is often forgotten when taking a history and thus there is a reasonable proportion of cancer survivors with undiagnosed latent infections. For cancer survivors treated before 1972, screening for chronic hepatitis B is recommended. Those treated before 1993 should be tested for hepatitis C, while those diagnosed between 1977 and 1985 should also be tested for HIV [30]. These dates, which are based on the screening of the US blood supply, may differ for those survivors treated internationally.

The Role of the Primary Care Provider

The primary care clinicians' long-term relationship with patients and expertise in preventive care and management of chronic conditions place them in an ideal position to manage

TREATMENT SUMMARY AND SURVIVORSHIP CARE PLAN
Date of preparation: 2013

Name: John Doe	Date of Birth: 1/1/1985

Cancer Diagnosis: Acute Myelocytic Leukemia (AML)

Treatment center: Children's Cancer Hospital
Date of diagnosis: 1/1/2004
Age at diagnosis: 19
Date of completion of therapy: 7/5/2004

Surgery

Date	Procedure
6/15/2004	Bone marrow harvest

Radiation Therapy

Date start	Date stop	Field	Dose (cGy)
7/1/2004	7/5/2004	Total body irradiation	1500
7/2/2004	7/4/2004	A/P chest wall boost	600
7/5/2004	7/5/2004	Testes	400

Chemotherapy

Drug Name	Dose (units or mg/m^2)
Daunomycin	320 mg/m^2
Cytarabine	
Etoposide	
Thioguanine	
Dexamethasone	
Cyclophosphamide	3.6 grams/m^2

Autologous bone marrow transplant on 7/5/2004

Cytoreduction with total body irradiation, etoposide, and cyclophosphamide

Potential Late Effects	Screening Recommendations**
• Heart problems • Lung problems • Osteoporosis • Thyroid problems • Fertility problems • Dental problems • Cataracts • Second cancers	• Annual lab to include: CBC, comprehensive metabolic profile, TSH, urinalysis, lipid panel, LH, FSH, testosterone • Echocardiogram/EKG every year • Pulmonary Function Test baseline • Bone density study (DXA) baseline • Regular dental check-ups and cleaning • Eye exam yearly • Semen analysis as indicated

**Screening recommendations adapted from the
CureSearch Children's Oncology Group Long-Term Follow-Up Guidelines
http://www.survivorshipguidelines.org.

Figure 32.1 Sample cancer treatment summary and survivorship care plan.

most cancer survivors. However, to provide such care, the primary care clinician must be informed by the oncologist or cancer team of the patient's cancer therapy, risks for late effects, and recommended screening and surveillance. The Institute of Medicine advocates that a Cancer Treatment Summary and Survivorship Care Plan be prepared for all cancer survivors (Figure 32.1 provides an example of the two documents combined into a single page form) [2, 3]. These documents should be shared with both the patient and the primary care clinician as the patient is transitioned back to a primary care setting. For those interested in reading more about the shared care approach, in which primary care clinicians and cancer specialists work together to optimize outcomes, the reader is referred to two recent papers [4,32].

Breast Cancer Survivors

Breast cancer is the most common malignancy in the US. There are currently approximately 3.56 million female breast cancer survivors living in this country [1].

Potential Late Effects Following Breast Cancer Therapy

A detailed list of late effects associated with specific treatment exposures can be found in Table 32.1. Additional problems reported by survivors include fatigue, cognitive changes, and weight gain. Lymphedema is associated with axillary lymph node surgery or radiation; the risk is higher among patients who undergo an axillary node dissection rather than or in addition to a sentinel lymph node biopsy [33–35]. Lymphedema is associated with a higher risk of cellulitis, so patients are instructed to be vigilant of the arm on the side of their surgery and monitor for signs of infection, such as new swelling, erythema, or warmth. Small cuts and abrasions can sometimes lead to serious infections, so special care should be taken to monitor the arm if these occur.

Cardiomyopathy can be a complication of treatment with both anthracyclines, which are used in some of the most common chemotherapy regimens, and trastuzumab. Patients who develop symptoms of heart failure should be promptly assessed and referred to a cardiologist for management.

Table 32.1 Late and long-term effects among breast cancer survivors.

Late or long-term effect	Exposure	Incidence
Leukemia	• Chemotherapy (especially anthracyclines) • Radiation therapy	• ≤1% [180]
Endometrial cancer	• Tamoxifen	• 2–3% (depending on duration of therapy) [181]
Other second solid tumors (sarcoma, esophageal or lung cancer, contralateral breast cancer)	• Radiation therapy	• 1–3% [180]
Congestive heart failure	• Anthracyclines (irreversible) • Trastuzumab (reversible)	• 1–4% (anthracyclines) [182,183] • 1–12% (trastuzumab) [182,183]
Ischemic heart disease	• Radiation therapy	• Risk depends on fields irradiated (internal mammary chain, left vs right breast), and technology used [184]
Lymphedema	• Axillary surgery (higher risk associated with axillary node dissection compared to sentinel lymph node biopsy; supraclavicular/axillary radiation)	• 17–20% [185] (overall 1-40% depending on risk factors [186])
Osteopenia/osteoporosis	• Aromatase inhibitors[1]	• 8.7% [187]
Impaired fertility and premature ovarian failure[2]	• Chemotherapy	• 15% (age < 35), 39% (age 35–40) [188]
Sexual dysfunction, vaginal dryness	• Hormonal therapy (tamoxifen, aromatase inhibitors)	• 70% [189]
Vasomotor symptoms (hot flashes)	• Hormonal therapy (tamoxifen, aromatase inhibitors)	• 77–81% [189,190]
Peripheral neuropathy (hands and feet)[3]	• Chemotherapy (especially paclitaxel, docetaxel, and carboplatin)	• 15–81% [191,192]

[1] Chemotherapy associated amenorrhea and premature ovarian failure also increase the risk of bone loss.
[2] Data for impaired fertility and premature menopause are limited by differences in the definition and measurement of menopause and impaired fertility. Rates of impaired fertility and premature menopause vary by age group and chemotherapy regimen received.
[3] Most data were reported in clinical trials with relatively short follow-up for late effects. Up to 81% of breast cancer survivors in a small study of long-term neuropathy after treatment with taxanes reported ongoing symptoms.

Second Primary Malignancy in Breast Cancer Survivors

Some treatments for breast cancer are associated with an increased risk of SPMs. For example, anthracyclines are associated with a small risk of leukemia, and radiation therapy is associated with a small risk of sarcoma. Additional details about exposure-related risk of second primary malignancies are included in Table 32.1.

Recommendations for Follow-Up of Breast Cancer Survivors

The 5-year risk of locoregional recurrence (recurrence in the affected breast or skin or in regional lymph nodes in the absence of metastatic disease) after lumpectomy is 7% among patients receiving radiation therapy and 26% among those not treated with radiation therapy [36]. The 5-year risk of locoregional recurrence after mastectomy ranges from 2 to 23% depending on factors such as lymph node involvement and whether or not postmastectomy radiation therapy is administered [36].

The risk of distant recurrence depends on factors including the size of the tumor, number of lymph nodes involved, estrogen/progesterone receptor status, HER2 status, and a variety of other pathologic criteria [37, 38].

The 20-year risk of contralateral breast cancer, which is generally considered to be a new primary breast cancer, is approximately 12% [39]. This risk is reduced by the use of endocrine therapy [40]. Certain patients, such as those with mutations in the *BRCA 1* or *2* genes, are at higher risk of a second breast cancer as well as ovarian and other cancers. Importantly, carriers of *BRCA 1* or *BRCA 2* should be followed by a specialist who is familiar with this population.

The American Cancer Society (ACS)/American Society of Clinical Oncology (ASCO) guideline [41, 42] recommends that breast cancer survivors be followed with a detailed cancer-related history and physical examination every 3–6 months during the first 3 years after completion of primary treatment, every 6–12 months during years 4 and 5, and annually thereafter. Mammograms should be performed on an annual basis for women who have undergone breast-conserving surgery. No imaging of the affected breast is recommended in the setting of a mastectomy, but screening for breast cancer in the contralateral breast should continue. Magnetic resonance imaging (MRI) is not recommended for early detection of a new breast cancer unless a woman meets high-risk criteria for increased breast cancer surveillance. Routine blood tests (including complete blood counts, chemistry panels, and tumor markers) are not recommended for asymptomatic patients [43]. Patients should receive education regarding signs and symptoms of local and regional recurrence; family history should be assessed and, as appropriate, genetic counseling should be offered. They should also receive counseling regarding adherence to adjuvant therapy, and an annual gynecologic assessment for postmenopausal women on selective estrogen receptor modulator therapies. Screening for cancers of other sites should follow guidelines for the general population.

Breast cancer survivors should undergo assessment and management of long-term and late effects including body image concerns, lymphedema, cardiotoxicity, cognitive impairment, distress/depression/anxiety, fatigue, bone health, musculoskeletal health, pain and neuropathy, infertility, sexual health, premature menopause, and hot flashes. Health promotion should include information and physician counseling regarding obesity, nutrition, and smoking cessation (as relevant). Care coordination should include a survivorship care plan, communication between primary care clinicians and the oncology team, and inclusion of family members.

Prostate Cancer Survivors

There are currently nearly 3.31 million men with a diagnosis of prostate cancer living in the US, comprising 45% of male cancer survivors [1]. More than 75% of prostate cancer survivors are 65 years of age or older.

Late Effects Following Prostate Cancer Therapy

Persistent treatment-related morbidity associated with prostate cancer therapy primarily involves sexual dysfunction, urinary incontinence, and bowel toxicity. Sexual dysfunction is a major source of morbidity associated with treatment of prostate cancer. In the acute post-treatment period, radical prostatectomy and brachytherapy are associated with higher rates of acute sexual dysfunction. In contrast, in long-term survivors, external beam radiation (EBRT) has the greatest negative impact on sexual function [44]. About a quarter of patients will be able to maintain erectile function 2 years after radical prostatectomy compared to 50–70% of men treated with radiation [45]. Urinary dysfunction is frequent immediately following radical prostatectomy, but tends to improve somewhat over the first 2 years. Unfortunately, thereafter, further recovery is rarely noted. In a group of long-term survivors (>4 years from treatment), patients who received radiation therapy appeared to have worsening urinary control manifested as urinary dribbling and an increase in pad requirements over time [44]. However, other series found no significant deterioration in urinary function between 4 and 8 years postradiation treatment [46]. Bowel function which includes symptoms of bowel urgency, frequency, fecal control, hematochezia and rectal pain, is seen acutely following radiation treatment with more frequent dysfunction following brachytherapy as compared to EBRT. However, over time, there is more improvement in patients treated with brachytherapy, such that about 6 years post-treatment, relative rates of bowel symptoms are similar for both radiation approaches with 10–15% of men still reporting some problem with overall bowel habits [44].

Even active surveillance can be associated with long-term morbidity. In a randomized study of radical prostatectomy vs active surveillance for the management of men with localized prostate cancer, a weak urinary stream was significantly more common in the active surveillance group (44% vs 28%) at a median of 4 years from the time of randomization. Erectile dysfunction (80% vs 45%) and urinary leakage (49% vs 21%) were more common in the radical prostatectomy group [47].

The late effects of hormone therapy are systemic reflecting the absence of androgens in the body. In a cohort of patients with locally advanced disease or rising prostate specific antigen (PSA), men treated with androgen deprivation therapy reported decreased quality of life, increased fatigue, more sexual problems, and decreased physical functioning compared to patients who did not receive androgen deprivation therapy [48]. Based on the duration of treatment, patients are at risk of decreased bone mineral density, anemia, fatigue, erectile dysfunction, decreased libido, weight gain, cardiovascular disease, diabetes, and emotional lability [49]. Denosumab and bisphosphonate therapy have been shown to prevent bone loss in men receiving androgen-deprivation therapy for prostate cancer [50, 51].

Second Primary Malignancy in Prostate Cancer Survivors

Survivors who received radiation to the prostate have a higher risk of bladder, colon, and rectal cancer compared to men who underwent prostatectomy alone [52]. Nieder *et al.* reported a 42% increase in bladder cancer risk following EBRT and a 10% increase in risk following brachytherapy, as compared to expected rates in the US male population [52]. Only EBRT (and not brachytherapy) was associated with an increased risk of rectal cancer [52]. Thus, the method of radiation delivery and dose delivered to surrounding tissue is an important factor in the development of SPM. It is not yet clear if newer methods of EBRT delivery, such as intensity modulated and conformal beam radiation therapy will have a different risk of SPM.

Recommendations for Follow-Up of Prostate Cancer Survivors

The ACS guideline [53] for prostate cancer survivorship care recommends that prostate cancer survivors be followed with serum PSA levels every 6–12 months for the first 5 years, then annually thereafter, and an annual digital rectal examination (coordinated between the cancer specialist and primary care clinician to avoid duplication).

Screening for cancers of other sites should follow guidelines for the general population.

Prostate cancer survivors should undergo assessment and management of long-term and late effects including urinary dysfunction (slow urinary stream, difficulty emptying the bladder, nocturia, incontinence), anemia (a risk for men receiving ADT), bowel dysfunction (e.g., rectal bleeding, sphincter dysfunction, rectal urgency, and frequency), cardiovascular and metabolic effects (a risk for men receiving ADT), hematuria, osteoporosis and fracture risk (a risk for men receiving ADT), sexual dysfunction, vasomotor symptoms (e.g., hot flushes, a risk for men receiving ADT), and issues with body image or intimacy, distress/depression/PSA anxiety.

Health promotion should include information related to prostate cancer and its treatment, side effects, other health concerns, and available support services and physician counseling regarding overweight and obesity, physical activity, nutrition, alcohol consumption, and tobacco cessation with clinical interventions as appropriate.

Care coordination should include a survivorship care plan, communication between primary care clinicians and the oncology team, and inclusion of caregivers, spouses, or partners.

Colorectal Cancer Survivors

An estimated 1.45 million people in the US had ever been diagnosed with colorectal cancer, making it the third largest population of cancer survivors among both men and women [1].

Late Effects Following Colorectal Cancer Therapy

Colorectal cancer survivors generally have a good quality of life [54]. Late effects from colorectal cancer are predominantly lingering toxicities and complications from treatment as opposed to late-occurring complications. Patients treated with oxaliplatin commonly experience peripheral neuropathy, which may persist years into the post-treatment setting [55]. Four years after treatment with oxaliplatin, 15% of survivors experience neuropathy [56]. Chemotherapy-induced neuropathy most typically includes numbness and tingling in upper and lower extremities [55]. No pharmaceutical agents or other interventions have proven successful in ameliorating chemotherapy-induced neuropathy [57]. Survivors whose treatment included the creation of a permanent ostomy may suffer additional complications, including hernia, urinary dysfunction, hemorrhage, skin conditions at the ostomy site, intestinal obstruction, and fistulas, compared with those who had a temporary ostomy [58].

Second Primary Malignancy in Colorectal Cancer Survivors

Colorectal cancer survivors are at risk for local recurrence and second colorectal cancers [59, 60]. Five years after diagnosis with stage II or III colorectal cancer, 1.5% of survivors will experience a second primary colorectal cancer, with a mean time of 18.4 months to diagnosis of a second cancer [59]. Local recurrences occur in 2–4% of those treated for colon cancer, and the rates are up to ten times higher for rectal cancer [60].

Recommendations for Follow-Up of Colorectal Cancer Survivors

The American Cancer Society Colorectal Cancer Survivorship Care Guideline [61] includes recommendations regarding surveillance for recurrence and screening for early detection of second primary cancers. During the first 2 years after treatment, the guidelines recommend a cancer-related history and physical examination every 3–6 months, serum carcinoembryonic antigen (CEA) levels every 3–6 months for patients who are potential candidates for further intervention, chest/abdominal/pelvic CT every 12 months for patients with stage III disease and those with stages I–II if at high risk for recurrence, and colonoscopy in year 1 (repeated in 1 year if an advanced adenoma is detected). During post-treatment years 3–5, the guidelines recommend a cancer-related history and physical examination every 6 months, CEA levels every 6 months for potential candidates for further intervention, chest/abdominal/pelvic CT every 12 months for patients with stage III disease and those with stages I–II if at high risk for recurrence, and colonoscopy during year 4 (repeated every 5 years if no advanced adenomas are detected). Survivors 5 or more years post-treatment should undergo colonoscopy every 5 years (more often if advanced adenomas are detected). Other blood tests and imaging tests (including positron emission tomography (PET)/computed tomography) (CT)) are not routinely recommended for patients without signs or symptoms of recurrence. In the absence of documented or suspected cancer predisposition syndromes, screening for cancers of other sites should follow guidelines for the general population.

Patients should receive education regarding signs and symptoms of recurrence; family history should be assessed and, as appropriate, genetic counseling should be offered. They should also receive counseling regarding weight management, physical activity, a dietary pattern high in vegetables, fruits and whole grains, limiting or avoiding alcohol consumption, and tobacco cessation (as appropriate).

Colorectal cancer survivors should undergo assessment and management of long-term and late effects including bowel/gastrointestinal dysfunction or bleeding, cognitive function, dental/oral issues, distress/depression/anxiety, fatigue, neuropathy, ostomy-related issues, pain, sexuality and fertility issues, and urinary tract/bladder issues.

Care coordination should include a treatment summary and survivorship care plan, and communication between primary care clinicians and the oncology team.

A recent systematic review of 32 studies of adherence to surveillance guidelines found a general pattern of underuse of colonoscopy and CEA testing [62]. At the same time, some studies found evidence of overly frequent colonoscopies and CT imaging, as well as the use of chest X-rays and other tests for metastatic disease not recommended by any guidelines. While underuse of recommended testing carries the obvious risk of missing possibly treatable disease, overuse and inappropriate use of testing can bring about unnecessary harms and costs. Chest X-rays and other metastatic disease markers are not recommended for colorectal cancer survivors [63].

Lymphoma Survivors

In the US, there are 219,570 survivors of Hodgkin lymphoma (HL) and over 686,370 survivors of non-Hodgkin lymphoma (NHL) [1].

Late Effects Following Lymphoma Therapy

Curative therapy for lymphoma can be associated with acute toxicities that persist long after the completion of therapy, and can also increase the risk for late effects. These are predominantly influenced not by the underlying disease, but by the components of therapy – chemotherapeutic agents and radiotherapy dose and field. Given the differences in treatment regimens between HL and NHL, these will be discussed separately, although the fact that many elements of therapy are common to both diseases, such as anthracycline chemotherapy and the use of radiotherapy, leads to some similar risks of late effects.

Hodgkin Lymphoma (HL) Survivors

Late effects of treatment for HL can be significant; by 22 years post-treatment, risk of death due to causes other than HL surpass that due to HL itself; this is largely driven by increased risks of SPMs and cardiovascular disease associated with HL therapy. Cardiovascular risks are increased in HL survivors; mediastinal radiation can lead to increased risk of coronary artery disease or congestive heart failure [64]. By 30 years after mediastinal radiation, the incidence of coronary artery disease is 20%, and of myocardial infarction, 13%. Doxorubicin increases the risk of congestive heart failure; while risks are dose related, some patients are highly sensitive to anthracy-

cline-induced cardiomyopathy even at low doses [65]. Valvular disease is increased in HL survivors following mediastinal radiation, with an over eightfold increase in odds of having undergone valve surgery by 22 years post-treatment [66]. Pericardial disease and arrhythmias may also occur as consequences of mediastinal radiotherapy.

Bleomycin can lead to pneumonitis that can either be subclinical, presenting with asymptomatic decline in the diffusing capacity for carbon monoxide or overt, with nonspecific interstitial pneumonitis, bronchiolitis obliterans organizing pneumonia, or diffuse alveolar damage. Other common toxicities during treatment include nausea, fatigue, and neuropathy. If radiotherapy is used, acute toxicity depends on the treated field; for mediastinal treatment, skin changes and esophagitis are the most typical side effects, although they are transitory.

Infertility is common with full-course escalated BEACOPP (bleomycin, etoposide, doxorubicin, cyclophosphamide, vincristine, procarbazine, prednisolone), although ABVD and the Stanford V regimen have far less impact on male or female fertility. Hypothyroidism can result in as many as half of patients receiving radiotherapy to the thyroid gland. Neck drop, resulting from nemaline myopathy following radiation therapy to the neck, can have significant cosmetic and functional impact on survivors. Survivors of HL also experience ongoing infectious risks, including *Varicella zoster* reactivation (shingles) and higher rates of influenza infection. Patients who underwent diagnostic splenectomy are also at increased risk of overwhelming sepsis from infection with encapsulated organisms, and require both specific vaccination strategies as well as a heightened awareness of the need for prompt antibiotics at the onset of fever.

NHL Survivors

Late effects among NHL survivors are largely similar to those seen among HL survivors, with a few exceptions.

Treatment-related myelodysplasia or acute myelogenous leukemia (AML) can occur after R-CHOP (rituximab, cyclophosphamide, doxorubicin, vincristine, prednisolone) for NHL, although it is a rare event [67]. Rituximab, an anti-CD20 monoclonal antibody, improves cure rates, but is associated with hypogammaglobulinemia, resulting classically in recurrent sinopulmonary infections. Rarely, rituximab may be associated with progressive multifocal leukoencephalopathy, a devastating and typically fatal neurological syndrome caused by a reactivation of latent JC polyomavirus [68]. Given that radiation therapy is less frequently used in NHL than in HL, fewer patients are at risk for late radiotherapy complications, but risks are similar to those discussed above.

Second Primary Malignancy in Lymphoma Survivors

SPM risk is closely associated with treatment and patient factors. As mentioned, risks of myelodysplasia or AML are associated with cumulative dosages of doxorubicin and etoposide [69].

The majority of SPM risk among lymphoma survivors is associated with radiation therapy. The breast parenchyma is exposed to radiation with mantle or mediastinal field radiotherapy. In women treated under age 35, these fields are associated with a substantially increased risk of breast cancer at a young age. A woman irradiated at age 25 may have a risk of breast cancer by age 55 of 30% [70, 71]. Thoracic radiation with lung tissue in the field increases the risk of nonsmall cell lung carcinoma as a second malignancy; such patients have a sixfold greater risk of lung cancer, an eightfold increased risk if treatment also included alkylating chemotherapy, and a 20-fold increased risk if they were smokers before diagnosis or during treatment [72]. Procarbazine appears to potentiate the risk of gastric cancer and colorectal cancer following abdominal radiotherapy, although the risk of gastrointestinal cancer following procarbazine alone may not be elevated [73, 74]. Thyroid carcinoma may occur when the thyroid receives radiation, particularly in younger patients, with peak odds when the thyroid is exposed to 10–30 Gy of radiation and diminished odds with exposure of either less than 10 Gy or more than 40 Gy of radiation [75, 76]. Soft-tissue sarcoma may occur in the radiation field, but absolute excess risk remains modest given how uncommon they are. Lastly, nonmelanoma skin cancer (basal and squamous cell carcinomata) often occurs within the radiation field [77].

Recommendations for Follow-Up of Lymphoma Survivors

The majority of relapses occur during the first 5 years post-treatment for lymphoma, although late relapses can occur. The optimal surveillance strategy for monitoring for recurrence is unknown. For HL, National Comprehensive Cancer Network (NCCN) guidelines recommend routine physical examination and laboratory analyses (complete blood count, chemistry profile, and erythrocyte sedimentation rate) every 3-6 months for 1–2 years, and then every 6–12 months until year 3, and then annually until 5 years post-treatment. Surveillance CT scans can be performed at 6, 12, and 24 months after completion of treatment, and then as indicated. Routine imaging with PET is not recommended. Survivors should receive a treatment summary and should be counseled regarding reproduction, health habits, psychosocial and cardiovascular late effects, breast self-examination and skin cancer risk. Longer-term follow-up guidelines include recommendations for vaccination (influenced by type of treatment), for detection of endocrine late effects (especially hypothyroidism), and for early detection of second primary cancers using regimens based on increased risk [78].

Follow-up recommendations for survivors of NHL are more variable, depending on the type and location of disease, as well as the treatment modalities and drugs administered. General themes for survivorship care include monitoring for recurrence with history and physical examination, with imaging tests (as indicated by the type, stage, and location of disease), and by blood tests. Likewise, long-term and late effects also depend on similar factors related to the patient, the lymphoma, and the treatment have been developed to aide physicians and patients in reducing morbidity and mortality from an SPM [30, 79]. Patients at higher risk of breast cancer should routinely be screened with annual mammography and breast MRI beginning 8 years post-treatment or age 25, whichever comes last. Adult patients at high risk of lung cancer due to treatment exposure and a smoking history can be screened with annual low-dose chest CT, although the optimal schedule and duration of screening is not known. For patients who received abdominal radiation, colorectal screening with colonoscopy should be performed

at least every 5 years starting 10 years after radiation or age 35, whichever occurs last.

Patients at high risk of cardiovascular disease due to therapy can undergo periodic echocardiography; stress echo can be considered 10 years post-treatment as well, although the optimal approach for cardiac screening is unclear [80]. Optimizing traditional cardiac risk factors, including maintaining a normal blood pressure, optimal lipids, tobacco avoidance or cessation, and maintaining a healthy lifestyle, is of critical importance; primary prophylaxis with aspirin starting 5 years post-treatment is a common consideration as well.

For patients receiving radiation to the thyroid, annual thyroid palpation and serum TSH evaluation is recommended. If a thyroid nodule is detected, it should be further evaluated. Men should undergo repeat semen analysis 1–2 years post-treatment to evaluate spermatogenesis, and women should typically seek the advice of a reproductive endocrinologist. Premature ovarian failure places women at higher risk for osteoporosis, and hormonal repletion (in addition to calcium and vitamin D supplementation as needed) is routine.

Testicular Cancer Survivors

There are currently more than 266,550 testicular cancer survivors living in the US [1].

Potential Late Effects Following Testicular Cancer Therapy

Cardiovascular disease (CVD) is an important cause of morbidity and death among testicular cancer survivors. The relative risk of CVD with cisplatin-based chemotherapy has varied widely in series from 1.4-fold to sevenfold, depending on the definition of CVD, the median length of follow-up and the control group used [81–83]. Nevertheless, the absolute incidence of CVD appears to be very similar across series, occurring in 5–10% of testicular cancer survivors treated with cisplatin-based chemotherapy [81–83]. If heart failure and stroke are also included as cardiac events, the incidence increases further, up to 18% in one series [83]. Gonadal dysfunction and infertility are major sources of morbidity in this population and can arise from radiation, chemotherapy, or surgery. Radiation and chemotherapy are cytotoxic to germ cells and can lead to oligospermia or azoospermia. In addition, radiation and chemotherapy can cause a hypogonadal state, which may be exacerbated in the setting of having only one remaining testis. Testosterone deficiency causes decreased libido and erectile dysfunction, symptoms that can be extremely disconcerting to young men. Fatigue, osteoporosis, weight gain, and the metabolic syndrome are additional potential complications of testosterone deficiency. Paternity rates following chemotherapy or radiation therapy for testicular cancer are approximately 60–80%, with higher chemotherapy doses associated with lower success [84]. Retroperitoneal lymph node dissection (RPLND) can also lead to infertility through transection of the lumbar nerves which control ejaculation, resulting in retrograde ejaculation. Despite the employment of nerve-sparing techniques, retrograde ejaculation still occurs in 1–10% of patients undergoing RPLND in the prechemotherapy setting

[85, 86] and 10–30% of men undergoing RPLND in the postchemotherapy setting [85, 87, 88]. Since many men have not yet started or completed their families at the time of diagnosis, infertility is a major source of morbidity in this population and may have significant psychological ramifications.

The risk of infertility underscores the fact that all men should be encouraged to undergo sperm banking prior to surgery, radiation, or RPLND. Unfortunately, many are not made aware of the risk of infertility and are not offered sperm banking prior to treatment. In addition, financial restrictions, perceived urgency of initiating treatment, and lack of foresight lead many men to forego sperm banking. Some men may be unable to bank for religious reasons.

Peripheral neuropathy and ototoxicity, primarily tinnitus but occasionally loss of high frequency hearing, represent additional potential long-term toxicities of cisplatin-based chemotherapy. These adverse effects develop in 50% of patients acutely during or right after receiving cisplatin-based chemotherapy and can persist chronically in 20–40% [89–92]. Depending on the patient's occupation, this can have serious detrimental effects for musicians and people who rely on fine motor skills, such as tailors and electricians, for example. The severity and frequency of these effects increases with cumulative exposure to neurotoxic agents.

Second Primary Malignancy in Testicular Cancer Survivors

Secondary nongerm cell tumor malignancies represent the primary late effect of radiation therapy but are also increased among patients treated with chemotherapy. In a retrospective study of patients who had survived at least 1 year from their diagnosis of testicular cancer, 5.6% developed a second nongerm cell tumor malignancy with a median follow-up of 11.3 years [93]. There was an approximately twofold increased risk of malignancy among patients who had received radiation therapy with several malignancies within the radiation port (pancreas, bladder, stomach, and connective tissue) demonstrating the greatest relative increase in risk [93]. Additional studies from Europe have demonstrated similar findings. A study from the Netherlands reported a 2.2-fold increased risk of developing a nongerm cell tumor following radiation therapy and 1.7-fold increased risk following chemotherapy [94]. In addition, both series found that patients who received both radiation and chemotherapy had the greatest risk, more than three times higher than that expected in an age-matched control population [93, 94]. The risk appears to continue throughout a patient's lifetime and was estimated as being as high as 37% for a patient with an attained age of 75 who was treated for testicular cancer at the age of 35 [93]. A recent study of testicular cancer survivors found that the relative risk of gastric cancer was nearly 10-fold higher among patients who had received 20 Gy or higher doses of radiation [74].

Recommendations for Follow-Up of Testicular Cancer Survivors

Surveillance for testicular cancer recurrence involves physical examination with special attention to the contralateral testis and serial evaluations of serum tumor markers (alpha-fetoprotein, human chorionic gonadatrophin, and usually lactate dehy-

drogenase), chest X-rays, and CT scans of the abdomen +/- pelvis. Although several groups have put forth guidelines on the frequency with which visits and tests are necessary, their approaches often differ significantly with relatively little data to suggest superiority of any one group's recommendations. All guidelines tend to adjust the frequency of visits, markers, and imaging by stage of disease, histology (seminoma or nonseminoma) and treatment (radiation, chemotherapy, surveillance) received. In recent years, the trend has been toward decreasing the intensity of follow-up, especially the frequency of CT imaging due to the potential for development of an SPM related to radiation exposure associated with this imaging modality. The true nature of this risk remains to be defined in future studies but nevertheless, MRI is currently being evaluated as an alternative to CT. The NCCN guidelines are perhaps the most widely used and offer a reasonable strategy for surveillance [95].

Patients treated with radiation should be made aware of their risk of secondary malignancies and should undergo age-appropriate screening. Most of the cancers with the highest relative risk do not have a screening test available so it is important that they bring symptoms to the attention of their oncologist or primary care physician in a timely fashion. Consideration should be given to initiating colorectal cancer screening at age 40, rather than 50. For patients treated with chemotherapy, cholesterol and blood pressure should be monitored annually, and patients should be counseled on the risks of weight gain and metabolic syndrome. Testosterone levels should be evaluated for symptoms of hypogonadism and/or if the metabolic syndrome develops.

Head and Neck Cancer Survivors

There are approximately 436,060 head and neck squamous cell cancer (HNSCC) survivors living in the US; an additional 61,760 cases are diagnosed annually [96].

Potential Late Effects Following HNSCC Therapy

Patients are at risk for many functional difficulties in the oral cavity including trismus, xerostomia, dental caries, and osteoradionecrosis of the jaw. Survivors can also experience difficulty hearing and tinnitus as a result of radiation and cisplatin chemotherapy. Other chronic effects include dysphagia, speech articulation, dysphonia, and chronic pain [97, 98]. There is also a growing concern about late developing dysphagia associated with high-dose radiation to the head and neck which places survivors at risk for aspiration pneumonia and poor nutritional status [99]. In addition, patients who receive treatment to the neck with either surgery or radiation are at an increased risk for cervical radiculopathy, neck stiffness, lymphedema, shoulder pain and dysfunction [100]. Head and neck cancer patients treated with radiation are also at risk for hypothyroidism [101]. Survivors of HNSCC, often due to their prior tobacco and alcohol history, are at risk of death from multiple competing causes including cardiovascular and pulmonary disease [102]. These patients have a particular risk of cerebrovascular disease given the radiation-induced endothelial changes to the carotid arteries. However, no routine vascular screening is recommended [103].

Second Primary Malignancies in HNSCC Survivors

New cancers represent a major challenge to long-term survival in a subset of HNSCC survivors. The annual incidence of SPM is 3–7%, and the cumulative rate at 10 years from diagnosis is 10–30% due to field carcinogenesis from tobacco or alcohol exposure of the upper aerodigestive tract (head and neck, lung, and esophagus) [104–110]. Approximately one-third of SPM in HNSCC survivors arise in the lung, representing a fourfold higher rate compared to the general population [104, 108]. Screening with low-dose chest CT should be considered in HNSCC survivors with a tobacco history [111]. At this time, screening for esophageal cancer, even in high-risk adults, is controversial [112]. Patients treated with radiation to the head and neck region are at risk for radiation-induced SPMs, such as thyroid cancer. At present, there is no additional recommendation for screening beyond the routine head and neck physical examination, but physicians caring for patients who have received high-doses of radiation should always be cognizant of the possibility.

Recommendations for Follow-Up of HNSCC Survivors

The risk of recurrent HNSCC decreases over time with almost 90% detected within the first three years following treatment [113]. The NCCN recommends a schedule of frequent routine visits immediately following treatment and then less frequently over time [114]. Post-treatment imaging with a PET, CT or MRI is recommended to establish a new baseline, but there is no role for routine imaging in surveillance of HNSCC [114].

The American Cancer Society Head and Neck Cancer Survivorship Care Guideline [96] includes recommendations regarding surveillance for recurrence and screening for early detection of second primary cancers. A detailed cancer-related history and physical examination (including follow-up with an otolaryngologist or head and neck cancer specialist for a focused examination) is recommended every 1–3 months for the first year after primary treatment, every 2–6 months in the second year, every 4–8 months in year 3–5, and annually after 5 years. Screening for cancers of other sites should follow ACS guidelines for the general population, including screening for lung cancer as indicated by smoking history. Because survivors of some types of head and neck cancer are at increased risk for related second primary cancers, these survivors should undergo screening for head and neck cancers and esophageal cancer. Patients should receive education regarding signs and symptoms of local recurrence and referred to a specialist as appropriate.

Potential psychosocial long-term and late effects should be assessed at each follow-up visit and managed appropriately. These long-term and late effects include spinal accessory nerve palsy, cervical dystonia/muscle spasms/neuropathies, shoulder dysfunction, trismus, dysphagia/aspiration/stricture, gastroesophageal reflux disease, lymphedema, fatigue, altered taste or loss of taste, hearing loss, vertigo, vestibular neuropathy, sleep disturbance/sleep apnea, speech/voice issues, hypothyroidism, body and self-image issues, and distress/depression/anxiety. Primary care, oncology specialty, and dental professionals should coordinate care to prevent, recognize, and manage oral complications including caries, periodontitis, xerostomia, osteonecrosis, and oral infections.

Health promotion should include education and counseling information needs, weight management, physical activity, tobacco avoidance/cessation, and personal oral hygiene. Care coordination should include a treatment summary and survivorship care plan, and communication among primary care clinicians, the oncology team, and dental health professionals, with the inclusion of caregivers, spouses, or partners in usual HNSCC survivorship care and support.

Lung Cancer Survivors

There are approximately 224,390 patients in the US diagnosed with lung cancer each year and currently there are more than 526,510 lung cancer survivors living in the US [1].

Late Effects Following Lung Cancer Therapy

The main symptoms reported in long-term survivors of lung cancer are fatigue, dyspnea, hearing loss, neuropathy, pain, anxiety, and depression which are impacted by treatment received, age at diagnosis, and comorbidity [115–117]. In a national survey, survivors of lung cancer reported significantly poorer general health and more psychological problems compared to other cancer survivors [118]. In prior studies of lung cancer survivors who have survived at least 5 years from diagnosis, 70% reported good general health status despite 70% having comorbid medical conditions [119]. About half of long-term survivors have measureable impaired pulmonary function ($FEV_1 < 70\%$ predicted), but two-thirds reported respiratory symptoms. The presence of symptoms, not measurable dysfunction, predicts worse overall quality of life [120]. While exercise is associated with an improved quality of life, most lung cancer survivors do not meet recommended levels of physical activity [121].

Second Primary Malignancy Following Lung Cancer

Patients with a history of lung cancer remain at risk for a subsequent lung cancer. About 85–90% of lung cancers are attributed to a prior smoking history and these patients are at an elevated risk of other tobacco-related malignancies in the head and neck, esophagus, and bladder [122]. These patients are already being screened for subsequent lung cancers as part of their cancer surveillance. There are no other cancer screening recommendations for this cohort aside from age appropriate recommendations.

Recommendations for Follow-Up of Lung Cancer Survivors

The NCCN recommends surveillance after recovery from primary therapy for small cell lung cancer according to the following schedule: every 3–4 months during the first 2 years, every 6 months during years 3–5, and annually thereafter. Each follow-up visit should include a medical history and physical examination, CT of the chest/liver/adrenals, and blood tests as clinically indicated. The NCCN guideline also recommends against use of PET/CT for routine follow-up [123]. Following curative-intent therapy for nonsmall cell lung cancer, the NCCN recommends follow-up history and physical examination and a chest CT with or without contrast every 6–12 months for 2 years, followed by annual history and physical examination and CT without contrast [124]. No other imaging is currently recommended.

Assessment of tobacco use at each follow-up visit (and for smoking cessation counseling or referral) is an extremely important aspect of care for lung cancer survivors, and is recommended by the NCCN. There are growing methods to assist survivors with cessation. Chronic smoking is associated with an increased risk of cancer, osteoporosis, cardiac disease, hypertension, renal insufficiency, and other competing causes of death in this cohort [122]. NCCN guidelines also recommend regular medical care including blood glucose screening, blood pressure measurement, cholesterol monitoring, bone mineral density testing as appropriate, routine dental care, and routine sun protection, as well as assuring that survivors are up-to-date with immunizations for influenza, herpes zoster, and pneumococcus. Health promotion should include counseling regarding weight management, physical activity, nutrition, and avoiding or limiting consumption of alcoholic beverages [124]. Similar recommendations were recently published by the American College of Chest Physicians. This guideline also recommends use of validated health-related quality-of-life instruments for patients who have undergone curative-intent therapy for nonsmall cell lung cancer, and recommends against use of biomarker testing outside of clinical trials [125].

Special Therapeutic Modality: Allogeneic Hematopoietic Stem Cell Transplantation

Allogeneic transplants (alloHCT) are those in which the patient receives blood-forming stem cells from someone other than him/herself or a twin. As of 2009, over 40,000 survivors of alloHCT were living in the US [126].

Contemporary alloHCT

Children and adults with a wide variety of conditions, including high-risk leukemias, certain myeloproliferative and myelodysplastic syndromes, and bone marrow failure syndromes, may be treated with alloHCT. To reduce or avoid long-term sequelae associated with traditional, myeloablative regimens, reduced intensity conditioning regimens have been increasingly used prior to transplantation.

Potential Late Effects Following alloHCT

Survivors of alloHCT are at risk for a wide variety of treatment-related late effects depending on underlying diagnosis and pre-HCT therapy, preparative regimens used for HCT, and post-HCT events. Potential late effects may impact ocular, dermatologic, audiologic, oral, craniofacial, cardiovascular, endocrine, pulmonary, hepatic, gastrointestinal, renal, genitourinary, musculoskeletal, neurologic, psychiatric, and reproductive health. Providers must also consider potential dysfunctional immune reconstitution and concomitant risk of infection, psychosocial development, and the occurrence of SPMs following alloHCT [127].

Endocrine complications are among the most common chronic health conditions to develop after HCT and include thyroid dysfunction, osteoporosis, gonadal dysfunction, growth impairment (with possible growth hormone deficiency), and metabolic syndrome [128, 129]. HCT survivors primarily develop hypothyroidism, although hyperthyroidism, immune-mediated thyroiditis and thyroid nodules can occur as well [130, 131]. Osteopenia and osteoporosis are primarily related to the use of steroids – either for treatment of the primary disease or for treatment of graft-versus-host disease (GvHD) [132]. Other risk factors for endocrine dysfunction include treatment with craniospinal, gonadal, total lymphoid, or total body irradiation (TBI) [133]. Irreversible gonadal damage is known to result from the intensity of preparative regimens in patients undergoing HCT, particularly when TBI is included [134]. HCT survivors have also been found to have an increased risk of metabolic syndrome, a constellation of factors that are associated with cardiovascular disease and type 2 diabetes, and include central obesity, hypertension, high fasting blood glucose, and dyslipidemia [135]. Survivors of alloHCT are two times more likely to report hypertension and four times more likely to report diabetes than their siblings [136]. Exposure of children to TBI is specifically associated with subsequent development of metabolic syndrome [137, 138] with HCT recipients exposed to TBI reported to have a 3.9-fold elevated risk when compared with those treated with conventional therapy without radiation [139].

Related to this increased risk of cardiovascular risk factors, alloHCT survivors also face an increased risk of cardiac disease, including cardiomyopathy, congestive heart failure, valvular dysfunction, arrhythmia, and pericarditis [140] with a 2.3-fold increased risk of cardiac-related premature death compared to the general population [141]. Risk is associated with a combination of pre-HCT therapies, transplant-related conditioning, post-HCT GvHD, and existent comorbidities. Potential risk factors unique to HCT recipients include conditioning with high-dose chemotherapy, TBI, and incidence of chronic GvHD after transplant [127].

In addition to treatment-related late effects, long-term survivors of HCT are at risk for additional late effects related specifically to GvHD [142]. Patients with GvHD may manifest symptoms of a sicca syndrome with xerostomia, vaginitis, dryness of the skin, and ocular manifestations such as reduced tear flow, sterile conjunctivitis, corneal ulceration and clinical signs of keratitis. Ocular GvHD, specifically, occurs in 40–60% of survivors of alloHCT and negatively impacts quality of life [143]. The mouth is also frequently affected in patients with chronic GvHD [144] with patients reporting oral pain, dryness, difficulty and/or painful swallowing, sensitivity, lichenoid changes, and restriction of mouth opening due to skin sclerosis [145]. Chronic GvHD is also associated with secondary malignancies, particularly squamous cell carcinomas of the oral cavity [146]. In addition to sicca syndrome, ocular, and oral complications, chronic GvHD is a major cause of liver dysfunction; myositis or polymyositis, sclerosis of the skin and subcutaneous tissues, and skin complaints with sclerosis, nail dystrophy, and skin depigmentation are frequently reported [147].

Second Primary Malignant Neoplasms in alloHCT Recipients

An increased risk of SPMs, ranging from four- to 11-fold that of the general population, has been reported following alloHCT [148]. Patients treated with alloHCT are specifically at risk for: therapy-related myelodysplasia (t-MDS) and acute myeloid leukemia (t-AML); lymphoma, including post-transplant lymphoproliferative disorders (PTLD); and nonhematopoietic tumors such as cancers of the skin, breast, and thyroid [149]. Generally, t-MDS/AML and lymphoma develop soon after HCT while secondary solid tumors have a longer latency. A PTLD, such as a lymphoma, is the most common second cancer in the first year following T-cell depleted alloHCT and is associated with Epstein-Barr virus infection as well as T-cell depletion of the donor graft, anti-thymocyte globulin use, presence of acute or chronic GvHD, older age at HCT, and multiple transplants [150]. Late-occurring lymphomas are associated with extensive chronic GvHD and tend to have longer latency (>2.5 years). Solid tumors have an even longer latency with breast cancer occurring a median of 12.5 years after HCT and thyroid cancer occurring at a median of 8.5 years [127].

Recommendations for Follow-Up of alloHCT Survivors

In 2012, the Center for International Blood and Marrow Transplant Research, the European Group for Blood and Marrow Transplantation, and the American Society of Blood and Marrow Transplantation provided updated consensus recommendations for risk-based screening and preventive practices for alloHCT recipients [147]. The guidelines, based on treatment exposures and organized by organ system, offer suggested screening recommendations and preventive measures for patients who have survived more than 6 months after transplantation. Comprehensive guidelines for long-term follow-up of pediatric cancer survivors (including recipients of alloHCT) have also been developed by the Children's Oncology Group (COG) to provide a framework for monitoring late effects among long-term survivors of childhood and young adult cancer [30].

Screening recommendations are tailored to individual exposures received. Patients at risk for t-AML and t-MDS are screened with an annual complete blood count for 10 years after treatment. Patients at risk for radiation-related second cancers are screened annually through routine examinations of the skin and underlying tissues within the radiation field. Those at risk for radiation-related colorectal cancer (radiation doses ≥ 30 Gy to the abdomen, pelvis, or spine) are advised to receive a colonoscopy every 5 years beginning at age 35 or 10 years following radiation (whichever occurs later). Screening for thyroid cancer consists of annual thyroid palpation; no routine imaging is recommended, given the indolent natural history of the disease.

Special Population: The Childhood Cancer Survivor

As of January 2011, there were 388,501 survivors of childhood cancer living in the US [151].

Potential Late Effects Following Childhood Cancer Treatment

By 30 years after the cancer diagnosis, 73% of childhood cancer survivors have at least one chronic health condition, with 42% experiencing a severe, life-threatening or disabling condition or death due to a chronic condition [152]. Endocrinopathies are among the most frequently reported chronic medical conditions in childhood cancer survivors, particularly in those exposed to high doses of alkylating agents and radiotherapy [153]. Survivors of central nervous system (CNS) tumors and Hodgkin lymphoma, as well as alloHCT recipients, are at especially high risk for the development of endocrine disturbances, which may include linear growth disturbance due to growth hormone deficiency, thyroid dysfunction, ACTH deficiency, gonadal dysfunction leading to pubertal arrest and/or impaired fertility, reduced bone mineral density, and metabolic disorders. Acute lymphoblastic leukemia survivors are at increased risk for insulin resistance, type 2 diabetes mellitus, and leptin dysregulation [154–156]. These late complications can impact survivors' physical health and psychosocial development – especially during childhood and adolescence.

In addition to the endocrinopathies, childhood cancer survivors are at high risk for cardiac late effects [157]. Patients treated with anthracyclines and/or chest radiation are at elevated risk of cardiac late effects and require careful, lifelong screening [30]. Anthracycline-induced cardiotoxicity may present as asymptomatic left ventricular dysfunction, cardiomyopathy, or congestive heart failure. Risk appears to increase with higher cumulative anthracycline dose, younger age at treatment, time from exposure, female gender [158], and specific genetic polymorphisms [159].

Neurocognitive deficits have also been noted in childhood cancer survivors of CNS tumors and those treated with cranial radiotherapy and/or antimetabolite chemotherapy, particularly when administered at a very young age [160–162]. Survivors may demonstrate impairment in one or more neurocognitive domains, which may impact childhood and adult learning and ultimately lead to low self-esteem and lack of academic and professional success. The COG recommends frequent neurocognitive assessment in high-risk patients [163] in order to facilitate early implementation of supportive services and advocacy for survivors with disabilities [164].

Second Primary Malignancy in Childhood Cancer Survivors

Childhood cancer survivors have a significantly increased risk of SPM [165]. The most common types of SPMs in this population include nonmelanoma skin cancer, adult carcinomas (e.g., breast, thyroid, colorectal cancer), and sarcomas. Radiation exposure has been linked in a dose-dependent fashion with SPMs of the thyroid, breast, and CNS tumors such as gliomas and meningiomas. Patients treated with chemotherapy, such as alkylating agents and/or topoisomerase II inhibitors, and/or radiotherapy, are also at risk for therapy-related myeloid neoplasms such as AML and myelodysplastic syndrome.

Recommendations for Follow-Up of Childhood Cancer Survivors

In 2003, the COG released the Long-Term Follow-Up Guidelines for Survivors of Childhood, Adolescent, and Young Adult Cancers, an on-line set of evidence-informed, consensus-based recommendations for long-term follow-up of childhood cancer, based on therapeutic exposures [30]. These guidelines are periodically updated and are currently being harmonized with other international groups [166].

Special Population: The Elderly Cancer Survivor

The majority of cancer survivors in the US are older adults; 60% of all cancer survivors are older than age 65 years and 22% are older than age 80. By year 2020 there will be 11 million elderly cancer survivors in the US [167].

Functional Decline

Elderly cancer survivors are at high risk for functional decline [168] that could lead to inability to perform activities of daily living and loss of independence. Functional decline is usually multifactorial: fatigue, poor nutrition, cancer treatment side effects (e.g. neuropathy), anemia, and poor dental and oral health may contribute [169]. Healthcare providers should pay attention to subtle changes in a cancer survivor's functional activity and perform comprehensive geriatric assessment when needed. Timely referral to physical therapy and supportive services to delay functional dependency is important [170].

Cognitive Decline

Elderly cancer survivors are at risk for cognitive decline following cancer treatment [171]. Often cognitive decline remains undiagnosed and thus untreated with significant impact on survivors' quality of life and ability to live independently [172]. Risk factors include a history of chemotherapy with specific agents (cyclophosphamide, methotrexate, 5-fluororuracil, bleomycin, etoposide, cisplatin, and taxanes) [173–175] and higher dose of chemotherapy [174, 176]. Physicians should pay particular attention for any sign or symptom of cognitive decline. Taking a detailed history of precancer cognitive status, depression, anxiety, fatigue, malnutrition, and social support status, is often helpful, as these precancer factors often contribute to worsening cognitive function among elderly cancer survivors.

Conclusions

As described in the preceding sections of this chapter, cancer survivors are susceptible to a wide range of long-term and late effects. Ongoing follow-up will increase in importance as this population continues to grow. Therefore timely diagnosis and treatment of late effects for cancer survivors will require risk-based care [2, 4, 177]. As outlined by the Institute of Medicine, risk-based care necessitates the systematic plan of periodic screening, surveillance, and prevention that includes an assessment of individual health risks based on the previous cancer and its treatment, genetic and familial factors, comorbid conditions, and lifestyle behaviors such as diet and exercise [2].

In light of the detailed cancer history and treatment information required for this type of care, it is imperative that cancer survivors are provided with a summary of their cancer treatment and survivorship care plan (example, Figure 32.1) [178]. This document is typically provided to cancer survivors at the end of their treatment or upon transition back to the primary care provider. As such, it should include information about key aspects of cancer diagnosis and treatment as well as recommendations for ongoing follow-up. Notably, the survivorship care plan does not appear to cause undue worry among survivors [179]. Nonetheless, the survivorship care plan is likely to be most beneficial in the setting of a comprehensive system of care that includes ongoing communication between providers and that in some way designates those survivors at highest risk for late effects [4].

In conclusion, care of the cancer survivor can be challenging and complex. Commitment to this high-risk group entails dedication to their well-being as well as knowledge of the long-term and late effects of cancer and its treatment.

Acknowledgments

This collaborative effort was completed by the members of the MSKCC Early Career Investigator in Survivorship Research Working Group, supported in part by a grant from the National Cancer Institute (K05CA160724; PI: Oeffinger KC), entitled "Survivorship: Mentoring and Bridging Primary Care and Oncology".

References

1 Miller KD, Siegel RL, Lin CC, *et al*. Cancer treatment and survivorship statistics, 2016. *CA Cancer J Clin* 2016;66:271–89.

2 Hewitt M, Greenfield S, Stovall E. *From Cancer Patient to Cancer Survivor: Lost in Transition*. Washington, D.C.: National Academies Press, 2005.

3 Hewitt M, Weiner SL, Simone JV. *Childhood Cancer Survivorship: Improving Care and Quality of Life*. Washington, D.C.: The National Academies Press, 2003.

4 Oeffinger KC, McCabe MS. Models for delivering survivorship care. *J Clin Oncol* 2006;24:5117–24.

5 Hobbie WL, Stuber M, Meeske K, *et al*. Symptoms of posttraumatic stress in young adult survivors of childhood cancer. *J Clin Oncol* 2000;18:4060–6.

6 von Essen L, Enskar K, Kreuger A, Larsson B, Sjoden PO. Self-esteem, depression and anxiety among Swedish children and adolescents on and off cancer treatment. *Acta Paediatr* 2000;89:229–36.

7 Weaver KE, Forsythe LP, Reeve BB, *et al*. Mental and physical health-related quality of life among U.S. cancer survivors: population estimates from the 2010 National Health Interview Survey. *Cancer Epidemiol Biomarkers Prev* 2012;21:2108–17.

8 Berger AM, Gerber LH, Mayer DK. Cancer-related fatigue: implications for breast cancer survivors. *Cancer* 2012;118:2261–9.

9 Ostroff J, Dhingra L. Smoking cessation and cancer survivors. In: Feuerstein M (ed.) *Handbook of Cancer Survivorship*. New York, NY: Springer, 2007.

10 Karam-Hage M, Cinciripini PM, Gritz ER. Tobacco use and cessation for cancer survivors: an overview for clinicians. *CA Cancer J Clin* 2014;64:272–90.

11 Wolin KY, Carson K, Colditz GA. Obesity and cancer. *Oncologist* 2010;15:556–65.

12 Demark-Wahnefried W, Platz EA, Ligibel JA, *et al.* The role of obesity in cancer survival and recurrence. *Cancer Epidemiol Biomarkers Prev* 2012;21:1244–59.

13 Kroenke CH, Chen WY, Rosner B, Holmes MD. Weight, weight gain, and survival after breast cancer diagnosis. *J Clin Oncol* 2005;23:1370–8.

14 Chlebowski RT, Blackburn GL, Thomson CA, *et al.* Dietary fat reduction and breast cancer outcome: interim efficacy results from the Women's Intervention Nutrition Study. *J Natl Cancer Inst* 2006;98:1767–76.

15 Tonorezos ES, Robien K, Eshelman-Kent D, *et al.* Contribution of diet and physical activity to metabolic parameters among survivors of childhood leukemia. *Cancer Causes Control* 2013;24:313–21.

16 Pierce JP, Natarajan L, Caan BJ, *et al.* Influence of a diet very high in vegetables, fruit, and fiber and low in fat on prognosis following treatment for breast cancer: the Women's Healthy Eating and Living (WHEL) randomized trial. *JAMA* 2007;298:289–98.

17 Beasley JM, Newcomb PA, Trentham-Dietz A, *et al.* Post-diagnosis dietary factors and survival after invasive breast cancer. *Breast Cancer Res Treat* 2011;128:229–36.

18 Meyerhardt JA, Niedzwiecki D, Hollis D, *et al.* Association of dietary patterns with cancer recurrence and survival in patients with stage III colon cancer. *JAMA* 2007;298: 754–64.

19 Schmitz KH, Courneya KS, Matthews C, *et al.* American College of Sports Medicine roundtable on exercise guidelines for cancer survivors. *Med Sci Sports Exerc* 2010;42:1409–26.

20 Wolin KY, Schwartz AL, Matthews CE, Courneya KS, Schmitz KH. Implementing the exercise guidelines for cancer survivors. *J Support Oncol* 2012;10:171–7.

21 Speck RM, Courneya KS, Masse LC, Duval S, Schmitz KH. An update of controlled physical activity trials in cancer survivors: a systematic review and meta-analysis. *J Cancer Surviv* 2010;4:87–100.

22 Cramp F, Byron-Daniel J. Exercise for the management of cancer-related fatigue in adults. *Cochrane Database Syst Rev* 2012;11:CD006145.

23 Craft LL, Vaniterson EH, Helenowski IB, Rademaker AW, Courneya KS. Exercise effects on depressive symptoms in cancer survivors: a systematic review and meta-analysis. *Cancer Epidemiol Biomarkers Prev* 2012;21:3–19.

24 Services UDoHaH. Physical Activity Guidelines Advisory Committee, 2008.

25 Howard-Anderson J, Ganz PA, Bower JE, Stanton AL. Quality of life, fertility concerns, and behavioral health outcomes in younger breast cancer survivors: a systematic review. *J Natl Cancer Inst* 2012;104:386–405.

26 Wakefield CE, Butow P, Fleming CA, Daniel G, Cohn RJ. Family information needs at childhood cancer treatment completion. *Pediatr Blood Cancer* 2012;58:621–6.

27 Metzger ML, Meacham LR, Patterson B, *et al.* Female reproductive health after childhood, adolescent, and young adult cancers: guidelines for the assessment and management of female reproductive complications. *J Clin Oncol* 2013;31:1239–47.

28 Kenney LB, Cohen LE, Shnorhavorian M, *et al.* Male reproductive health after childhood, adolescent, and young adult cancers: a report from the Children's Oncology Group. *J Clin Oncol* 2012;30:3408–16.

29 Ruddy KJ, Partridge AH. Fertility (male and female) and menopause. *J Clin Oncol* 2012;30:3705–11.

30 Group CsO. Long-Term Follow-Up Guidelines for Survivors of Childhood, Adolescent, and Young Adult Survivors of Cancer Available from URL:www.survivorshipguidelines.org (accessed 8 September 2017).

31 Lee SJ, Schover LR, Partridge AH, *et al.* American Society of Clinical Oncology recommendations on fertility preservation in cancer patients. *J Clin Oncol* 2006;24:2917–31.

32 McCabe MS, Bhatia S, Oeffinger KC, *et al.* American Society of Clinical Oncology statement: achieving high-quality cancer survivorship care. *J Clin Oncol* 2013;31:631–40.

33 Kwan W, Jackson J, Weir LM, *et al.* Chronic arm morbidity after curative breast cancer treatment: prevalence and impact on quality of life. *J Clin Oncol* 2002;20:4242–8.

34 Erickson VS, Pearson ML, Ganz PA, Adams J, Kahn KL. Arm edema in breast cancer patients. *J Natl Cancer Inst* 2001;93:96–111.

35 Shaitelman SF, Cromwell KD, Rasmussen JC, *et al.* Recent progress in the treatment and prevention of cancer-related lymphedema. *CA Cancer J Clin* 2015;65:55–81.

36 Clarke M, Collins R, Darby S, *et al.* Effects of radiotherapy and of differences in the extent of surgery for early breast cancer on local recurrence and 15-year survival: an overview of the randomised trials. *Lancet* 2005;366:2087–106.

37 Cheang MC, Voduc D, Bajdik C, *et al.* Basal-like breast cancer defined by five biomarkers has superior prognostic value than triple-negative phenotype. *Clin Cancer Res* 2008;14:1368–76.

38 Foulkes WD, Smith IE, Reis-Filho JS. Triple-negative breast cancer. *N Engl J Med* 2010;363:1938–48.

39 Gao X, Fisher SG, Emami B. Risk of second primary cancer in the contralateral breast in women treated for early-stage breast cancer: a population-based study. *Int J Radiat Oncol Biol Phys* 2003;56:1038–45.

40 Early Breast Cancer Trialists' Collaborative G. Effects of chemotherapy and hormonal therapy for early breast cancer on recurrence and 15-year survival: an overview of the randomised trials. *Lancet* 2005;365:1687–717.

41 Runowicz CD, Leach CR, Henry NL, *et al.* American Cancer Society/American Society of Clinical Oncology Breast Cancer Survivorship Care Guideline. *J Clin Oncol* 2016;34:611–35.

42 Runowicz CD, Leach CR, Henry NL, *et al.* American Cancer Society/American Society of Clinical Oncology Breast Cancer Survivorship Care Guideline. *CA Cancer J Clin* 2016;66:43–73.

43 Khatcheressian JL, Hurley P, Bantug E, *et al.* Breast cancer follow-up and management after primary treatment: american society of clinical oncology clinical practice guideline update. *J Clin Oncol* 2013;31:961–5.

44 Miller DC, Sanda MG, Dunn RL, *et al.* Long-term outcomes among localized prostate cancer survivors: health-related

quality-of-life changes after radical prostatectomy, external radiation, and brachytherapy. *J Clin Oncol* 2005;23:2772–80.

45 Evans HS, Moller H, Robinson D, *et al.* The risk of subsequent primary cancers after colorectal cancer in southeast England. *Gut* 2002;50:647–52.

46 Fransson P, Widmark A. Late side effects unchanged 4–8 years after radiotherapy for prostate carcinoma: a comparison with age-matched controls. *Cancer* 1999;85:678–88.

47 Steineck G, Helgesen F, Adolfsson J, *et al.* Quality of life after radical prostatectomy or watchful waiting. *N Engl J Med* 2002;347:790–6.

48 Herr HW, O'Sullivan M. Quality of life of asymptomatic men with nonmetastatic prostate cancer on androgen deprivation therapy. *J Urol* 2000;163:1743–6.

49 Kintzel PE, Chase SL, Schultz LM, O'Rourke TJ. Increased risk of metabolic syndrome, diabetes mellitus, and cardiovascular disease in men receiving androgen deprivation therapy for prostate cancer. *Pharmacotherapy* 2008;28:1511–22.

50 Smith MR, Egerdie B, Toriz NH, *et al.* Denosumab in men receiving androgen-deprivation therapy for prostate cancer. *N Engl J Med* 2009;361:745–55.

51 Smith MR, McGovern FJ, Zietman AL, *et al.* Pamidronate to prevent bone loss during androgen-deprivation therapy for prostate cancer. *N Engl J Med* 2001;345:948–55.

52 Nieder AM, Porter MP, Soloway MS. Radiation therapy for prostate cancer increases subsequent risk of bladder and rectal cancer: a population based cohort study. *J Urol* 2008;180:2005–9; discussion 2009–10.

53 Skolarus TA, Wolf AM, Erb NL, *et al.* American Cancer Society prostate cancer survivorship care guidelines. *CA Cancer J Clin* 2014;64:225–49.

54 Jansen L, Koch L, Brenner H, Arndt V. Quality of life among long-term (>/=5 years) colorectal cancer survivors – systematic review. *Eur J Cancer* 2010;46:2879–88.

55 Kidwell KM, Yothers G, Ganz PA, *et al.* Long-term neurotoxicity effects of oxaliplatin added to fluorouracil and leucovorin as adjuvant therapy for colon cancer: results from National Surgical Adjuvant Breast and Bowel Project trials C-07 and LTS-01. *Cancer* 2012;118:5614–22.

56 Andre T, Boni C, Navarro M, *et al.* Improved overall survival with oxaliplatin, fluorouracil, and leucovorin as adjuvant treatment in stage II or III colon cancer in the MOSAIC trial. *J Clin Oncol* 2009;27:3109–16.

57 Wolf S, Barton D, Kottschade L, Grothey A, Loprinzi C. Chemotherapy-induced peripheral neuropathy: prevention and treatment strategies. Eur J Cancer 2008:1507–15.

58 Liu L, Herrinton LJ, Hornbrook MC, *et al.* Early and late complications among long-term colorectal cancer survivors with ostomy or anastomosis. *Dis Colon Rectum* 2010;53:200–12.

59 Green RJ, Metlay JP, Propert K, *et al.* Surveillance for second primary colorectal cancer after adjuvant chemotherapy: an analysis of Intergroup 0089. *Ann Intern Med* 2002;136:261–9.

60 Mysliwiec P, Cronin K, Schatzkin A. New malignancies following cancer of the colon, rectum, and anus. In: RE Curtis, DM Freedman, E Ron *et al.* (eds) *New Malignancies Among Cancer Survivors: SEER Cancer Registries, 1973–2000.* Bethesda, MD: National Cancer Institute, 2006:111–44.

61 El-Shami K, Oeffinger KC, Erb NL, *et al.* American Cancer Society Colorectal Cancer Survivorship Care Guidelines. *CA Cancer J Clin* 2015;65:428–55.

62 Carpentier MY, Vernon SW, Bartholomew LK, Murphy CC, Bluethmann SM. Receipt of recommended surveillance among colorectal cancer survivors: a systematic review. *J Cancer Surviv* 2013;7:464–83.

63 Desch CE, Benson AB, 3rd, Somerfield MR, *et al.* Colorectal cancer surveillance:2005 update of an American Society of Clinical Oncology practice guideline. *J Clin Oncol* 2005;23:8512–19.

64 Aleman BM, van den Belt-Dusebout AW, De Bruin ML, *et al.* Late cardiotoxicity after treatment for Hodgkin lymphoma. *Blood* 2007;109:1878–86.

65 Blanco JG, Sun CL, Landier W, *et al.* Anthracycline-related cardiomyopathy after childhood cancer: role of polymorphisms in carbonyl reductase genes – a report from the Children's Oncology Group. *J Clin Oncol* 2012;30:1415–21.

66 Hull MC, Morris CG, Pepine CJ, Mendenhall NP. Valvular dysfunction and carotid, subclavian, and coronary artery disease in survivors of hodgkin lymphoma treated with radiation therapy. *JAMA* 2003;290:2831–7.

67 Press OW, Unger JM, Rimsza LM, *et al.* Phase III randomized intergroup trial of CHOP plus rituximab compared with CHOP chemotherapy plus (131)iodine-tositumomab for previously untreated follicular non-Hodgkin lymphoma: SWOG S0016. *J Clin Oncol* 2013;31:314–20.

68 Carson KR, Evens AM, Richey EA, *et al.* Progressive multifocal leukoencephalopathy after rituximab therapy in HIV-negative patients: a report of 57 cases from the Research on Adverse Drug Events and Reports project. *Blood* 2009;113:4834–40.

69 Engert A, Diehl V, Franklin J, *et al.* Escalated-dose BEACOPP in the treatment of patients with advanced-stage Hodgkin's lymphoma:10 years of follow-up of the GHSG HD9 study. *J Clin Oncol* 2009;27:4548–54.

70 Travis LB, Hill DA, Dores GM, *et al.* Breast cancer following radiotherapy and chemotherapy among young women with Hodgkin disease. *JAMA* 2003;290:465–75.

71 Henderson TO, Amsterdam A, Bhatia S, *et al.* Systematic review: surveillance for breast cancer in women treated with chest radiation for childhood, adolescent, or young adult cancer. *Ann Intern Med* 2010;152:444–55; W144–454.

72 Travis LB, Gospodarowicz M, Curtis RE, *et al.* Lung cancer following chemotherapy and radiotherapy for Hodgkin's disease. *J Natl Cancer Inst* 2002;94:182–92.

73 Swerdlow AJ, Higgins CD, Smith P, *et al.* Second cancer risk after chemotherapy for Hodgkin's lymphoma: a collaborative British cohort study. *J Clin Oncol* 2011;29:4096–104.

74 van den Belt-Dusebout AW, Aleman BM, Besseling G, *et al.* Roles of radiation dose and chemotherapy in the etiology of stomach cancer as a second malignancy. *Int J Radiat Oncol Biol Phys* 2009;75:1420–29.

75 Sigurdson AJ, Ronckers CM, Mertens AC, *et al.* Primary thyroid cancer after a first tumour in childhood (the Childhood Cancer Survivor Study): a nested case-control study. *Lancet* 2005;365:2014–23.

76 Bhatti P, Veiga LH, Ronckers CM, *et al.* Risk of second primary thyroid cancer after radiotherapy for a childhood cancer in a

large cohort study: an update from the childhood cancer survivor study. *Radiat Res* 2010;174:741–52.

77 Lichter MD, Karagas MR, Mott LA, *et al.* Therapeutic ionizing radiation and the incidence of basal cell carcinoma and squamous cell carcinoma. *The New Hampshire Skin Cancer Study Group. Arch Dermatol* 2000;136:1007–11.

78 National Comprehensive Cancer Network. Hodgkin lymphoma. Version 2.2016. www.nccn.org. Accessed October 18, 2016.

79 Ligibel JA, Denlinger CS. New NCCN Guidelines® for Survivorship Care. *J Natl Compr Canc Netw* 2013;11:640–4.

80 Heidenreich PA, Schnittger I, Strauss HW, *et al.* Screening for coronary artery disease after mediastinal irradiation for Hodgkin's disease. *J Clin Oncol* 2007;25:43–9.

81 Huddart RA, Norman A, Shahidi M, *et al.* Cardiovascular disease as a long-term complication of treatment for testicular cancer. *J Clin Oncol* 2003;21:1513–23.

82 Meinardi MT, Gietema JA, van der Graaf WT, *et al.* Cardiovascular morbidity in long-term survivors of metastatic testicular cancer. *J Clin Oncol* 2000;18:1725–32.

83 van den Belt-Dusebout AW, Nuver J, de Wit R, *et al.* Long-term risk of cardiovascular disease in 5-year survivors of testicular cancer. *J Clin Oncol* 2006;24:467–75.

84 Brydoy M, Fossa SD, Klepp O, *et al.* Paternity following treatment for testicular cancer. *J Natl Cancer Inst* 2005;97:1580–8.

85 Beck SD, Bey AL, Bihrle R, Foster RS. Ejaculatory status and fertility rates after primary retroperitoneal lymph node dissection. *J Urol* 2010;184:2078–80.

86 Heidenreich A, Albers P, Hartmann M, *et al.* Complications of primary nerve sparing retroperitoneal lymph node dissection for clinical stage I nonseminomatous germ cell tumors of the testis: experience of the German Testicular Cancer Study Group. *J Urol* 2003;169:1710–14.

87 Pettus JA, Carver BS, Masterson T, Stasi J, Sheinfeld J. Preservation of ejaculation in patients undergoing nerve-sparing postchemotherapy retroperitoneal lymph node dissection for metastatic testicular cancer. *Urology* 2009;73:328–31; discussion 331–22.

88 Subramanian VS, Nguyen CT, Stephenson AJ, Klein EA. Complications of open primary and post-chemotherapy retroperitoneal lymph node dissection for testicular cancer. *Urol Oncol* 2010;28:504–9.

89 Bokemeyer C, Berger CC, Hartmann JT, *et al.* Analysis of risk factors for cisplatin-induced ototoxicity in patients with testicular cancer. *Br J Cancer* 1998;77:1355–62.

90 Hansen SW, Helweg-Larsen S, Trojaborg W. Long-term neurotoxicity in patients treated with cisplatin, vinblastine, and bleomycin for metastatic germ cell cancer. *J Clin Oncol* 1989;7:1457–61.

91 Haugnes HS, Bosl GJ, Boer H, *et al.* Long-term and late effects of germ cell testicular cancer treatment and implications for follow-up. *J Clin Oncol* 2012;30:3752–63.

92 Sprauten M, Darrah TH, Peterson DR, *et al.* Impact of long-term serum platinum concentrations on neuro- and ototoxicity in Cisplatin-treated survivors of testicular cancer. *J Clin Oncol* 2012;30:300–7.

93 Travis LB, Fossa SD, Schonfeld SJ, *et al.* Second cancers among 40,576 testicular cancer patients: focus on long-term survivors. *J Natl Cancer Inst* 2005;97:1354–65.

94 van den Belt-Dusebout AW, de Wit R, Gietema JA, *et al.* Treatment-specific risks of second malignancies and cardiovascular disease in 5-year survivors of testicular cancer. *J Clin Oncol* 2007;25:4370–8.

95 National Comprehensive Cancer Network. Testicular cancer. Version 2.2016. www.nccn.org.

96 Cohen EE, LaMonte SJ, Erb NL, *et al.* American Cancer Society Head and Neck Cancer Survivorship Care Guideline. *CA Cancer J Clin* 2016;66:203–39.

97 De Boer MF, McCormick LK, Pruyn JF, Ryckman RM, van den Borne BW. Physical and psychosocial correlates of head and neck cancer: a review of the literature. *Otolaryngol Head Neck Surg* 1999;120:427–36.

98 Chaplin JM, Morton RP. A prospective, longitudinal study of pain in head and neck cancer patients. *Head Neck* 1999;21:531–7.

99 Hutcheson KA, Lewin JS, Barringer DA, *et al.* Late dysphagia after radiotherapy-based treatment of head and neck cancer. *Cancer* 2012;118:5793–9.

100 van Wilgen CP, Dijkstra PU, van der Laan BF, Plukker JT, Roodenburg JL. Shoulder complaints after nerve sparing neck dissections. *Int J Oral Maxillofac Surg* 2004;33:253–7.

101 Shafer RB, Nuttall FQ, Pollak K, Kuisk H. Thyroid function after radiation and surgery for head and neck cancer. *Arch Intern Med* 1975;135:843–6.

102 Rose BS, Jeong JH, Nath SK, Lu SM, Mell LK. Population-based study of competing mortality in head and neck cancer. *J Clin Oncol* 2011;29:3503–9.

103 Smith GL, Smith BD, Buchholz TA, *et al.* Cerebrovascular disease risk in older head and neck cancer patients after radiotherapy. *J Clin Oncol* 2008;26:5119–25.

104 Argiris A, Brockstein BE, Haraf DJ, *et al.* Competing causes of death and second primary tumors in patients with locoregionally advanced head and neck cancer treated with chemoradiotherapy. *Clin Cancer Res* 2004;10:1956–62.

105 Mell LK, Dignam JJ, Salama JK, *et al.* Predictors of competing mortality in advanced head and neck cancer. *J Clin Oncol* 2010;28:15–20.

106 Khuri FR, Kim ES, Lee JJ, *et al.* The impact of smoking status, disease stage, and index tumor site on second primary tumor incidence and tumor recurrence in the head and neck retinoid chemoprevention trial. *Cancer Epidemiol Biomark Prev* 2001;10:823–9.

107 Cooper JS, Pajak TF, Rubin P, *et al.* Second malignancies in patients who have head and neck cancer: Incidence, effect on survival and implications based on the RTOG experience. *Int J Rad Oncol Biol Phys* 1989;17:449–56.

108 Jones AS, Morar P, Phillips DE, *et al.* Second primary tumors in patients with head and neck squamous cell carcinoma. *Cancer* 1995;75:1343–53.

109 Warnakulasuriya KA, Robinson D, Evans H. Multiple primary tumours following head and neck cancer in southern England during 1961–98. *J Oral Pathol Med* 2003;32:443–9.

110 Leon X, Quer M, Diez S, *et al.* Second neoplasm in patients with head and neck cancer. *Head Neck* 1999;21:204–10.

111 Wender R, Fontham ET, Barrera E, Jr., *et al.* American Cancer Society lung cancer screening guidelines. *CA Cancer J Clin* 2013;63:107–17.

112 Lao-Sirieix P, Fitzgerald RC. Screening for oesophageal cancer. *Nat Rev Clin Oncol* 2012;9:278–87.

113 Marchant FE, Lowry LD, Moffitt JJ, Sabbagh R. Current national trends in the posttreatment follow-up of patients with squamous cell carcinoma of the head and neck. *Am J Otolaryngol* 1993;14:88–93.

114 Pfister DG, Ang KK, Brizel DM, *et al.* National Comprehensive Cancer Network Clinical Practice Guidelines in Oncology. Head and neck cancers. *J Natl Compr Canc Netw* 2011;9:596–650.

115 Yang P, Cheville AL, Wampfler JA, *et al.* Quality of life and symptom burden among long-term lung cancer survivors. *J Thorac Oncol* 2012;7:64–70.

116 Vijayvergia N, Shah PC, Denlinger CS. Survivorship in non-small cell lung cancer: challenges faced and steps forward. *J Natl Compr Canc Netw* 2015;13:1151–61.

117 Huang J, Logue AE, Ostroff JS, *et al.* Comprehensive long-term care of patients with lung cancer: development of a novel thoracic survivorship program. *Ann Thorac Surg* 2014;98:955–61.

118 Hewitt M, Rowland JH, Yancik R. Cancer survivors in the United States: age, health, and disability. *J Gerontol A Biol Sci Med Sci* 2003;58:82–91.

119 Sarna L, Padilla G, Holmes C, *et al.* Quality of life of long-term survivors of non–small-cell lung cancer. *J Clin Oncol* 2002;20:2920–9.

120 Sarna L, Evangelista L, Tashkin D, *et al.* Impact of respiratory symptoms and pulmonary function on quality of life of long-term survivors of non-small cell lung cancer. *Chest* 2004;125:439–45.

121 Coups EJ, Park BJ, Feinstein MB, *et al.* Physical activity among lung cancer survivors: changes across the cancer trajectory and associations with quality of life. *Cancer Epidemiol Biomarkers Prev* 2009;18:664–72.

122 Burns DM. Tobacco-related diseases. *Semin Oncol Nurs* 2003;19:244–9.

123 National Comprehensive Cancer Network. Small cell lung cancer. Version 2.2017. www.nccn.org.

124 Ettinger DS, Akerley W, Borghaei H, *et al.* Non-small cell lung cancer, version 2.2013. *J Natl Compr Canc Netw* 2013;11:645–53; quiz 653.

125 Colt HG, Murgu SD, Korst RJ, *et al.* Follow-up and surveillance of the patient with lung cancer after curative-intent therapy: diagnosis and management of lung cancer, 3rd edn: American College of Chest Physicians evidence-based clinical practice guidelines. *Chest* 2013;143:e437S–454S.

126 Majhail NS, Tao L, Bredeson C, *et al.* Prevalence of hematopoietic cell transplant survivors in the United States. *Biol Blood Marrow Transplant* 2013;19:1498–501.

127 Bhatia S. Long-term health impacts of hematopoietic stem cell transplantation inform recommendations for follow-up. *Expert Rev Hematol* 2011;4:437–52; quiz 453–4.

128 Chemaitilly W, Sklar CA. Endocrine complications of hematopoietic stem cell transplantation. *Endocrinol Metab Clin North Am* 2007;36:983–98; ix.

129 Dvorak CC, Gracia CR, Sanders JE, *et al.* NCI, NHLBI/ PBMTC first international conference on late effects after pediatric hematopoietic cell transplantation: endocrine challenges-thyroid dysfunction, growth impairment, bone

130 Sanders JE, Hoffmeister PA, Woolfrey AE, *et al.* Thyroid function following hematopoietic cell transplantation in children: 30 years' experience. *Blood* 2009;113:306–8.

131 Tauchmanova L, Selleri C, Rosa GD, *et al.* High prevalence of endocrine dysfunction in long-term survivors after allogeneic bone marrow transplantation for hematologic diseases. *Cancer* 2002;95:1076–84.

132 McAvoy S, Baker KS, Mulrooney D, *et al.* Corticosteroid dose as a risk factor for avascular necrosis of the bone after hematopoietic cell transplantation. *Biol Blood Marrow Transplant* 2010;16:1231–6.

133 Ebeling PR, Thomas DM, Erbas B, *et al.* Mechanisms of bone loss following allogeneic and autologous hemopoietic stem cell transplantation. *J Bone Miner Res* 1999;14: 342–50.

134 Loren AW, Chow E, Jacobsohn DA, *et al.* Pregnancy after hematopoietic cell transplantation: a report from the late effects working committee of the Center for International Blood and Marrow Transplant Research (CIBMTR). *Biol Blood Marrow Transplant* 2011;17:157–66.

135 Baker KS, Chow E, Steinberger J. Metabolic syndrome and cardiovascular risk in survivors after hematopoietic cell transplantation. *Bone Marrow Transplant* 2012;47: 619–25.

136 Baker KS, Ness KK, Steinberger J, *et al.* Diabetes, hypertension, and cardiovascular events in survivors of hematopoietic cell transplantation: a report from the bone marrow transplantation survivor study. *Blood* 2007;109:1765–72.

137 Armenian SH, Sun CL, Kawashima T, *et al.* Long-term health-related outcomes in survivors of childhood cancer treated with HSCT versus conventional therapy: a report from the Bone Marrow Transplant Survivor Study (BMTSS) and Childhood Cancer Survivor Study (CCSS). *Blood* 2011;118:1413–20.

138 Chow EJ, Simmons JH, Roth CL, *et al.* Increased cardiometabolic traits in pediatric survivors of acute lymphoblastic leukemia treated with total body irradiation. *Biol Blood Marrow Transplant* 2010;16:1674–81.

139 Oudin C, Simeoni MC, Sirvent N, *et al.* Prevalence and risk factors of the metabolic syndrome in adult survivors of childhood leukemia. *Blood* 2011;117:4442–8.

140 Armenian SH, Sun CL, Mills G, *et al.* Predictors of late cardiovascular complications in survivors of hematopoietic cell transplantation. *Biol Blood Marrow Transplant* 2010;16:1138–44.

141 Bhatia S, Francisco L, Carter A, *et al.* Late mortality after allogeneic hematopoietic cell transplantation and functional status of long-term survivors: report from the Bone Marrow Transplant Survivor Study. *Blood* 2007;110:3784–92.

142 Pallua S, Giesinger J, Oberguggenberger A, *et al.* Impact of GvHD on quality of life in long-term survivors of haematopoietic transplantation. *Bone Marrow Transplant* 2010;45:1534–9.

143 Riemens A, te Boome L, Imhof S, Kuball J, Rothova A. Current insights into ocular graft-versus-host disease. *Curr Opin Ophthalmol* 2010;21:485–94.

144 Treister N, Chai X, Kurland B, *et al*. Measurement of oral chronic GVHD: results from the Chronic GVHD Consortium. *Bone Marrow Transplant* 2013;48:1123–8.

145 Meier JK, Wolff D, Pavletic S, *et al*. Oral chronic graft-versus-host disease: report from the International Consensus Conference on clinical practice in cGVHD. *Clin Oral Investig* 2011;15:127–39.

146 Demarosi F, Lodi G, Carrassi A, Soligo D, Sardella A. Oral malignancies following HSCT: graft versus host disease and other risk factors. *Oral Oncol* 2005;41:865–77.

147 Majhail NS, Rizzo JD, Lee SJ, *et al*. Recommended screening and preventive practices for long-term survivors after hematopoietic cell transplantation. *Hematol Oncol Stem Cell Ther* 2012;5:1–30.

148 Socié G, Baker KS, Bhatia S. Subsequent malignant neoplasms after hematopoietic cell transplantation. *Biol Blood Marrow Transplant* 2012;18:S139–S150.

149 Mohty B, Mohty M. Long-term complications and side effects after allogeneic hematopoietic stem cell transplantation: an update. *Blood Cancer J* 2011;1:e16.

150 Landgren O, Gilbert ES, Rizzo JD, *et al*. Risk factors for lymphoproliferative disorders after allogeneic hematopoietic cell transplantation. *Blood* 2009;113:4992–5001.

151 Phillips SM, Padgett LS, Leisenring WM, *et al*. Survivors of childhood cancer in the United States: prevalence and burden of morbidity. *Cancer Epidemiol Biomarkers Prev* 2015;24:653–63.

152 Oeffinger KC, Mertens AC, Sklar CA, *et al*. Chronic health conditions in adult survivors of childhood cancer. *N Engl J Med* 2006;355:1572–82.

153 Chemaitilly W, Sklar CA. Endocrine complications in long-term survivors of childhood cancers. *Endocr Relat Cancer* 2010;17:R141–159.

154 Meacham LR, Sklar CA, Li S, *et al*. Diabetes mellitus in long-term survivors of childhood cancer. Increased risk associated with radiation therapy: a report for the childhood cancer survivor study. *Arch Intern Med* 2009;169:1381–8.

155 Oeffinger KC, Adams-Huet B, Victor RG, *et al*. Insulin resistance and risk factors for cardiovascular disease in young adult survivors of childhood acute lymphoblastic leukemia. *J Clin Oncol* 2009;27:3698–704.

156 Tonorezos ES, Vega GL, Sklar CA, *et al*. Adipokines, body fatness, and insulin resistance among survivors of childhood leukemia. *Pediatr Blood Cancer* 2012;58:31–6.

157 Kremer LC, van Dalen EC, Offringa M, Ottenkamp J, Voute PA. Anthracycline-induced clinical heart failure in a cohort of 607 children: long-term follow-up study. *J Clin Oncol* 2001;19:191–6.

158 Barry E, Alvarez JA, Scully RE, Miller TL, Lipshultz SE. Anthracycline-induced cardiotoxicity: course, pathophysiology, prevention and management. *Expert Opin Pharmacother* 2007;8:1039–58.

159 Blanco JG, Leisenring WM, Gonzalez-Covarrubias VM, *et al*. Genetic polymorphisms in the carbonyl reductase 3 gene CBR3 and the NAD(P)H:quinone oxidoreductase 1 gene NQO1 in patients who developed anthracycline-related congestive heart failure after childhood cancer. *Cancer* 2008;112:2789–95.

160 Mulhern RK, Merchant TE, Gajjar A, Reddick WE, Kun LE. Late neurocognitive sequelae in survivors of brain tumours in childhood. *Lancet Oncol* 2004;5:399–408.

161 Kadan-Lottick NS, Zeltzer LK, Liu Q, *et al*. Neurocognitive functioning in adult survivors of childhood non-central nervous system cancers. *J Natl Cancer Inst* 2010;102:881–93.

162 Conklin HM, Krull KR, Reddick WE, *et al*. Cognitive outcomes following contemporary treatment without cranial irradiation for childhood acute lymphoblastic leukemia. *J Natl Cancer Inst* 2012;104:1386–95.

163 Krull KR, Okcu MF, Potter B, *et al*. Screening for Neurocognitive impairment in pediatric cancer long-term survivors. *J Clin Oncol* 2008;26:4138–43.

164 Nathan PC, Patel SK, Dilley K, *et al*. Guidelines for identification of, advocacy for, and intervention in neurocognitive problems in survivors of childhood cancer: a report from the Children's Oncology Group. *Arch Pediatr Adolesc Med* 2007;161:798–806.

165 Friedman DL, Whitton J, Leisenring W, *et al*. Subsequent neoplasms in 5-year survivors of childhood cancer: the Childhood Cancer Survivor Study. *J Natl Cancer Inst* 2010;102:1083–95.

166 Kremer LC, Mulder RL, Oeffinger KC, *et al*. A worldwide collaboration to harmonize guidelines for the long-term follow-up of childhood and young adult cancer survivors: a report from the International Late Effects of Childhood Cancer Guideline Harmonization Group. *Pediatr Blood Cancer* 2013;60:543–9.

167 Parry C, Kent EE, Mariotto AB, Alfano CM, Rowland JH. Cancer survivors: a booming population. *Cancer Epidemiol Biomarkers Prev* 2011;20:1996–2005.

168 Sweeney C, Schmitz KH, Lazovich D, Virnig BA, Wallace RB, Folsom AR. Functional limitations in elderly female cancer survivors. *J Natl Cancer Inst* 2006;98:521–9.

169 Luciani A, Jacobsen PB, Extermann M, *et al*. Fatigue and functional dependence in older cancer patients. *Am J Clin Oncol* 2008;31:424–30.

170 Morey MC, Snyder DC, Sloane R, *et al*. Effects of home-based diet and exercise on functional outcomes among older, overweight long-term cancer survivors: RENEW: a randomized controlled trial. *JAMA* 2009;301:1883–91.

171 Ahles TA, Saykin AJ, McDonald BC, *et al*. Longitudinal assessment of cognitive changes associated with adjuvant treatment for breast cancer: impact of age and cognitive reserve. *J Clin Oncol* 2010;28:4434–40.

172 Argyriou AA, Assimakopoulos K, Iconomou G, Giannakopoulou F, Kalofonos HP. Either called "chemobrain" or "chemofog," the long-term chemotherapy-induced cognitive decline in cancer survivors is real. *J Pain Symptom Manage* 2010;41:126–39.

173 Schagen SB, Boogerd W, Muller MJ, *et al*. Cognitive complaints and cognitive impairment following BEP chemotherapy in patients with testicular cancer. *Acta Oncol* 2008;47:63–70.

174 Schagen SB, Muller MJ, Boogerd W, Mellenbergh GJ, van Dam FS. Change in cognitive function after chemotherapy: a prospective longitudinal study in breast cancer patients. *J Natl Cancer Inst* 2006;98:1742–5.

175 Vardy J, Tannock I. Cognitive function after chemotherapy in adults with solid tumours. *Crit Rev Oncol Hematol* 2007;63:183–202.

176 Collins B, Mackenzie J, Tasca GA, Scherling C, Smith A. Cognitive effects of chemotherapy in breast cancer patients: a dose-response study. *Psychooncology* 2012;22:1517–27.

177 Ganz PA, Earle CC, Goodwin PJ. Journal of Clinical Oncology update on progress in cancer survivorship care and research. *J Clin Oncol* 2012;30:3655–6.

178 Salz T, Oeffinger KC, McCabe MS, Layne TM, Bach PB. Survivorship care plans in research and practice. *CA Cancer J Clin* 2012;62:101–17.

179 Spain PD, Oeffinger KC, Candela J, *et al*. Response to a treatment summary and care plan among adult survivors of pediatric and young adult cancer. *J Oncol Pract* 2012;8:196–202.

180 Matesich SM, Shapiro CL. Second cancers after breast cancer treatment. *Semin Oncol* 2003;30:740–8.

181 Davies C, Pan H, Godwin J, *et al*. Long-term effects of continuing adjuvant tamoxifen to 10 years versus stopping at 5 years after diagnosis of oestrogen receptor-positive breast cancer: ATLAS, a randomised trial. *Lancet* 2013;381:805–16.

182 Bowles EJ, Wellman R, Feigelson HS, *et al*. Risk of heart failure in breast cancer patients after anthracycline and trastuzumab treatment: a retrospective cohort study. *J Natl Cancer Inst* 2012;104:1293–305.

183 Slamon D, Eiermann W, Robert N, *et al*. Adjuvant trastuzumab in HER2-positive breast cancer. *N Engl J Med* 2011;365:1273–83.

184 Darby SC, Ewertz M, McGale P, *et al*. Risk of ischemic heart disease in women after radiotherapy for breast cancer. *N Engl J Med* 2013;368:987–98.

185 Disipio T, Rye S, Newman B, Hayes S. Incidence of unilateral arm lymphoedema after breast cancer: a systematic review and meta-analysis. *Lancet Oncol* 2013;14:500–15.

186 Kim M, Kim SW, Lee SU, *et al*. A model to estimate the risk of breast cancer-related lymphedema: combinations of treatment-related factors of the number of dissected axillary nodes, adjuvant chemotherapy, and radiation therapy. *Int J Radiat Oncol Biol Phys* 2013;86:498–503.

187 Mincey BA, Duh MS, Thomas SK, *et al*. Risk of cancer treatment-associated bone loss and fractures among women with breast cancer receiving aromatase inhibitors. *Clin Breast Cancer* 2006;7:127–132.

188 Petrek JA, Naughton MJ, Case LD, *et al*. Incidence, time course, and determinants of menstrual bleeding after breast cancer treatment: a prospective study. *J Clin Oncol* 2006;24:1045–51.

189 Panjari M, Bell RJ, Davis SR. Sexual function after breast cancer. *J Sex Med* 2011;8:294–302.

190 Day R, National Surgical Adjuvant Breast and Bowel Project P-1. Quality of life and tamoxifen in a breast cancer prevention trial: a summary of findings from the NSABP P-1 study. *Ann N Y Acad Sci* 2001;949:143–50.

191 Hershman DL, Weimer LH, Wang A, *et al*. Association between patient reported outcomes and quantitative sensory tests for measuring long-term neurotoxicity in breast cancer survivors treated with adjuvant paclitaxel chemotherapy. *Breast Cancer Res Treat* 2011;125:767–74.

192 Sparano JA, Wang M, Martino S, *et al*. Weekly paclitaxel in the adjuvant treatment of breast cancer. *N Engl J Med* 2008;358:1663–71.

Index

The American Cancer Society's Principles of Oncology: Prevention to Survivorship, First Edition. Edited by The American Cancer Society.
© 2018 The American Cancer Society. Published 2018 by John Wiley & Sons, Inc.